An Invitation to Health

An Invitation to Health
The Power of Now

Dianne Hales

17th Edition

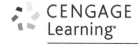

CENGAGE
Learning·

Australia • Brazil • Mexico • Singapore • United Kingdom • United States

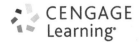

An Invitation to Health: The Power of Now,
17th Edition
Dianne Hales

Product Manager: Krista Mastroianni

Content Developers: Nedah Rose, Trudy Brown

Product Assistant: Victor Luu

Marketing Manager: Ana Albinson

Content Project Manager: Tanya Nigh

Art Director: Michael Cook

Manufacturing Planner: Karen Hunt

Production Service and Compositor: Graphic
    World, Inc.

Photo and Text Researcher: Lumina
    Datamatics Ltd.

Text Designer: Liz Harasymczuk

Cover Designer: Michael Cook

Cover Image: iStockphoto/mel-nik

Library of Congress Control Number: 2015945046

Student Edition:

ISBN: 978-1-305-63800-6

Loose-leaf Edition:

ISBN: 978-1-305-86929-5

Cengage Learning
20 Channel Center Street
Boston, MA 02210
USA

Cengage Learning is a leading provider of customized learning solutions
with employees residing in nearly 40 different countries and sales in more
than 125 countries around the world. Find your local representative at
www.cengage.com.

Cengage Learning products are represented in Canada by Nelson
Education, Ltd.

To learn more about Cengage Learning Solutions, visit **www.cengage.com.**

Purchase any of our products at your local college store or at our preferred
online store **www.cengagebrain.com.**

Printed in the United States of America
Print Number: 02   Print Year: 2017

Brief Contents

Contents

Key Features

YOUR STRATEGIES FOR PREVENTION

Preface

To the Student: Starting Now

College prepares you for the future. But when it comes to health, your future starts *now!*

Every day you make choices and take actions that may or may not have long-term consequences in the future. Yet they do have immediate effects on how you feel now. Here are some examples:

- You stay up late and get less than five hours' sleep. The next day you feel groggy, your reflexes are off, and you find it harder to concentrate.

- You scarf down a double cheeseburger with bacon, a supersized side of fries, and a milkshake. By the time you're done with your meal, harmful fats are coursing through your bloodstream.

- You chug a combo of Red Bull and vodka and keep partying for hours. Even before you finish your first drink, your heart is racing and your blood pressure rising. If you keep drinking, you'll reach dangerous levels of intoxication—probably without realizing how inebriated you are.

- Too tired to head to the gym, you binge-watch streaming videos for hours. Your metabolism slows; your unexercised muscles weaken.

- Just this once, you have sex without a condom. You wake up the next morning worrying about a sexually transmitted infection (STI) or a possible pregnancy.

- You don't have time to get to the student health center for a flu shot. Then your roommate comes down with the flu.

- You text while driving—and don't notice that the traffic light is changing.

There are countless other little things that can have very big consequences on your life today as well as through all the years to come. But they don't have to be negative. Consider these alternatives:

- Get a solid night's sleep after studying, and you'll remember more course material and probably score higher on a test.

- Eat a meal of a low-fat protein, vegetables, and grains, and you'll feel more energetic.

- Limit your alcohol intake, and you'll enjoy the evening and feel better the morning after.

- Go for a 10-minute walk or bike ride, and you'll feel less stressed and weary.

- Practice safe sex always, and you won't have to wonder if you've jeopardized your sexual health.

- Keep up with your vaccinations, and you lower your odds of serious sicknesses.

- Pay attention to the road when you drive, and you can avoid accidents.

In addition to their immediate effects, the impact of health behaviors continues for years and decades to come. Consider these facts:

- More than 40 percent of college students are already overweight or obese.

- One in four college students may have at least one risk factor for cardiovascular disease.

- Nine in ten college students report feeling stressed.

- One in three reports binge drinking at least once in the previous two weeks.

Such risky behaviors take a toll. According to an international study, young Americans are less likely to survive until age 55 than their peers in other developed nations. Those who do live to middle age and beyond are more likely to suffer serious chronic diseases and disabilities.

You do not have to be among them. *An Invitation to Health: The Power of Now* shows you how to start living a healthier, happier, fuller life now and in the years to come.

To the Instructor

You talk to your students about their future because it matters. But in the whirl of undergraduates' busy lives, today matters more. As recent research has documented, payoffs in the present are more powerful motivators for healthful behaviors than future rewards. Individuals exercise more, eat better, quit smoking, and make positive changes when immediate actions yield short-term as well as long-term benefits.

An Invitation to Health: The Power of Now incorporates this underlying philosophy throughout its chapters. As you can see in the Preface for students, we consistently point out the impact that everyday choices have on their health now and in the future. Each chapter highlights specific, practical steps that make a difference in how students feel and function. The "Health Now!" feature gives students step-by-step guidance on how to apply what they're learning in their daily lives. "The Power of Now!" checklist at each chapter's end reinforces key behavioral changes that can enhance and safeguard health.

I also am introducing a new interactive "check-in" feature that engages students as they read by posing questions that relate directly to their lives, experiences, and perspectives. After the definitions of wellness in Chapter 1, for instance, a "check-in" asks "What does wellness mean to you?" In the section on healthy habits, another "check-in" instructs students to rate their own health habits. As they learn about behavioral changes, this feature prompts them to identify a health-related change they want to make and their stage of readiness for change.

As an instructor, you can utilize the "check-in" features in different ways. For instance, you might suggest that students use them to test their comprehension of the material in the chapter. You might assign them to write a brief reflection on one or more "check-ins." Or you might draw on the "check-ins" to spark classroom discussion and increase student engagement.

This textbook is an invitation to you as an instructor. I invite you to share your passion for education and to enter into a partnership with the editorial team at Cengage Learning. We welcome your feedback and suggestions. Please let us hear from you at **www.cengage.com/health.**

I personally look forward to working with you toward our shared goal of preparing a new generation for a healthful future.

What's New in *An Invitation to Health: The Power of Now*

Some things don't change: as always, this *Invitation* presents up-to-date, concise, research-based coverage of all the dimensions of health. It also continues to define health in the broadest sense of the word—not as an entity in itself, but as an integrated process for discovering, using, and protecting all possible resources within the individual, family, community, and environment.

What is new is the theme that threads through every chapter: providing students with practical knowledge and tools they can apply immediately to improve their health and their lives. One of the keys to doing so is behavioral change, which has always been fundamental to *An Invitation to Health*. The one feature that has appeared in every edition—and that remains the most popular—is "Your Strategies for Change."

Every chapter concludes with "The Power of Now!," a checklist that students can use to assess their current status and work toward specific goals, whether by creating better relationships (Chapter 5), getting in better shape (Chapter 8), or taking charge of their alcohol intake (Chapter 13). Chapter 17, Consumer Health, contains updated information on the Affordable Care Act as well as ways to evaluate health information, prepare for a medical exam, get quality traditional and alternative health care, and navigate the health-care system.

Throughout this edition, the focus is on students, with real-life examples, the latest statistics on undergraduate behaviors and attitudes, and coverage of new campus health risks, including alcohol mixed with energy drinks (AmEDs), HPV, piercing and body art, electronic cigarettes and vaping, hookah (water pipe) smoking, the combination of binge drinking and disordered drinking, polysubstance abuse, "bath salts," cyberbullying, and campus stalking.

An interactive feature, "On Campus Now," showcases the latest research on student behavior, including their sleep habits (Chapter 2), stress levels (Chapter 4), weight (Chapter 7), and sexual experiences (Chapter 9). "Health Now!" presents practical, ready-to-use tips related to real-life issues such as recognizing substance abuse (Chapter 12), infection protection (Chapter 16), preventing accidents (Chapter 18), and going green (Chapter 19).

Other popular features that have been retained and updated include "Health on a Budget" and "Consumer Alert." A "Self Survey" for each chapter can be found within MindTap. End-of-chapter resources include "Review Questions," "Critical Thinking Questions," and "Key Terms." At the end of the book is a full Glossary as well as complete chapter references.

Because health is an ever-evolving field, this edition includes many new topics, including the latest reports on dietary guidelines for Americans, students' mental health, merging tobacco products, the impact of stress, campus hookups, same-sex marriage, self-injury, suicide prevention, vitamin supplements, exercise guidelines, STIs, gun violence, attention-deficit/hyperactivity disorder (ADHD), autism spectrum disorder, caffeinated alcoholic beverages, binge drinking, weight management, metabolic syndromes, myalgic encephalomyelitis/chronic fatigue syndrome (ME/CFS), and the latest recommendations for prevention and treatment of infectious illnesses.

All the chapters have been updated with the most current research, including many citations published in 2015, and incorporating the latest available statistics. The majority come from primary sources, including professional books; medical, health, and mental health journals; health education periodicals; scientific meetings, federal agencies, and consensus panels; publications from research laboratories and universities; and personal interviews with specialists in a number of fields. In addition, "What's Online" presents reliable Internet addresses where students can turn for additional information.

As I tell students, *An Invitation to Health: The Power of Now* can serve as an owner's manual to their bodies and minds. By using this book and taking your course, they can acquire a special type of power—the power to make good decisions, to assume responsibility, and to create and follow a healthy lifestyle. This textbook is our invitation to them to live what they learn and make the most of their health—now and in the future.

An Overview of Changes and Updates

Following is a chapter-by-chapter listing of some of the key topics that have been added, expanded, or revised for this edition.

Chapter 1: The Power of Now
College and health; occupational health; dimensions of health; student health norms; self-affirmation theory; health belief model (HBM)

Chapter 2: Your Psychological and Spiritual Well-Being
Positive psychology and positive psychiatry; most effective positive psychology interventions; positive effects of optimism, autonomy, and self-compassion; most effective gratitude interventions; tracking moods; sense of purpose; sleep times; sleep and sex; electronic devices and sleep onset; napping; snoring; Exploding Head Syndrome

Chapter 3: Caring for Your Mind
Mental health on campus; top concerns of undergraduates; students at risk; recognizing the characteristics of depression; ADHD; autism spectrum disorder; self-injury; suicide; psychiatric medications

Chapter 4: Personal Stress Management
Stress in America; occupational stress; discrimination and stress; stress and the heart; stress-management apps; self-compassion; burnout

Chapter 5: Your Social Health
Loneliness; companion pets; cyberstalking and cyberbullying; college students' cell phone use; the brain in love; trends in sexual relationships; hookup culture; same-sex marriage; long-term health consequences of divorce

Chapter 6: Personal Nutrition
Preliminary 2015 Dietary Guidelines for Americans; calorie balance; eating patterns in the United States and worldwide; student use of dietary supplements; food allergies; Mediterranean diet; nutrition labels; artificially sweetened drinks; sugar consumption; fruit and fruit juices; vitamin supplements

Chapter 7: Managing Your Weight
Weight on campus; body mass index (BMI); evaluating weight loss programs; CAM for obesity; emotional eating

Chapter 8: The Joy of Fitness
"Exercise Is Medicine," countering dangers of sedentary living, how much exercise is enough, barefoot running, bariatric surgery, salt supplements

Chapter 9: Sexual Health
Changes in sexual behavior; casual sex on campus; sex among young adults; why students hook up; culture and sexual messages; homophobia; LGBT health disparities; female ejaculation; sexual dysfunction

Chapter 10: Reproductive Choices
Contraceptive information sources for young adults; impact of contraception on women's lives; statistical "snapshot" of current birth control in the United States; reproductive coercion on campus; student access to condoms; long-acting reversible contraceptives (LARCs); female condoms; abortion; pregnancy-related mortality rates

Chapter 11: Lowering Your Risk of Sexually Transmitted Infections
Risks factors for sexually transmitted infections (STIs); update on Human papillomavirus (HPV); meeting sex partners online; bacterial vaginosis (BV); syphilis

Chapter 12: Addictions
Drugs in America; students and drugs; substance-free reinforcement; polysubstance abuse; gambling disorders; caffeine-containing energy drinks (CCEDs); stimulants; marijuana's effects on health; medical marijuana; legalized marijuana; artificial reproductive technology

Chapter 13: Alcohol
Alcohol-free programs on campus; drinking in America; toll of alcohol; drinking on campus; how schools are sobering up; work hours and drinking; discrimination and drinking; alcohol-related cues; alcohol mixed with energy drinks (AmEDs); alcohol poisoning; cirrhosis; consequences of light drinking; trauma and abuse as risk factors for drinking; behavioral therapies; medicines for alcohol recovery

Chapter 14: Tobacco
Smoking in America; smoke- and tobacco-free policies on campus; tobacco bans; smoking and mortality; health consequences of smoking; emerging tobacco products; electronic cigarettes; vaping; hookahs; secondhand smoke; thirdhand smoke

Chapter 15: Major Diseases
Importance of "now" for health; global toll of obesity; American Heart Association's steps to safeguard health; evaluating metabolic risk; role of healthy diet and weight; diabetes; blood pressure; hypertension in the young; high cholesterol; psychological factors; impact of stress; benefit of antidepressants; women and heart disease; reducing heart disease risk; cancer in America; external causes of cancer; internal causes of cancer; cancer staging; risk factors for skin cancer; lowering the risk of breast cancer; treatments for breast cancer

Chapter 16: Infectious Illnesses
New tick-borne pathogen; new guidelines for treating allergic rhinitis; childhood and adult vaccinations; common cold treatments; drug-resistant superbugs; tests and treatments for hepatitis C; myalgic encephalomyelitis/chronic fatigue syndrome; Ebola outbreaks; bacterial *Clostridium difficile (C. difficile)* infections

Chapter 17: Consumer Health
Update on the Affordable Care Act (Obamacare), consumer-driven health care, personal health apps and monitors, privacy of personal health information, trends in plastic surgery, CAM use in America and on college campuses

Chapter 18: Personal Safety
Risk factors for unintentional injury in young adults; factors that impair driving; bicycle fatalities; cell phone use and driving; gun violence; mass shootings; mental illness and violent crime; sexual coercion and violence; hate crimes; victimization based on sexual orientation; sexting; dating violence

Chapter 19: A Healthier Environment
Effects of global warming on health; pollution's health impact; indoor and outdoor air quality; electromagnetic fields; cell phone dangers; energy-efficient lightbulbs

Chapter 20: A Lifetime of Health
Health problems of seniors; impact of feeling younger than actual age; Mediterranean diet and longevity; quality of sleep and aging; disabilities in older Americans; age-related memory loss; Alzheimer's disease; advance health directives; quality of life in final years

Supplemental Resources

Health MindTap for *An Invitation to Health: The Power of Now!* (Instant Access Code: ISBN-13: 978-1-305-86621-8)
MindTap is a personalized teaching experience with relevant assignments that guide students to analyze, apply, and improve thinking, allowing you to measure skills and outcomes with ease.

- Personalized Teaching: Becomes yours with a Learning Path that is built with key student objectives. Control what students see and when they see it. Use it as-is or match to your syllabus exactly—hide, rearrange, add, and create your own content.

- Guide Students: A unique learning path of relevant readings, multimedia and activities that move students up the learning taxonomy from basic knowledge and comprehension to analysis and application.

- Promote Better Outcomes: Empower instructors and motivate students with analytics and reports that provide a snapshot of class progress, time in course, engagement, and completion rates.

Diet & Wellness Plus
Diet & Wellness Plus helps you gain a better understanding of how nutrition relates to your personal health goals. It enables you to track your diet and activity, generate reports, and analyze the nutritional value of the food you eat. It includes more than 55,000 foods in the database, custom food and recipe features, the latest Dietary References, as well as your goal and actual percentages of essential nutrients, vitamins, and minerals. It also helps you to identify a problem behavior and make a positive change. After you complete a Wellness Profile questionnaire, Diet & Wellness Plus rates the level of concern for eight different areas of wellness, helping you determine the areas where you are most at risk. It then helps you put together a plan for positive change by helping you select a goal to work toward, complete with a reward for all your hard work.

Diet & Wellness Plus is also available as an app that can be accessed from the app dock in MindTap and can be used throughout the course to track diet and activity, as well as behavior change.

Instructor Companion Site
This site offers everything you need for your course in one place! This collection of book-specific lecture and class tools is available online via www.cengage.com/login. Access and download PowerPoint presentations, images, the instructor's manual, videos, and more.

Cengage Learning Testing Powered by Cognero

Cengage Learning Testing Powered by Cognero is a flexible online system that allows you to:

- Author, edit, and manage test bank content from multiple Cengage Learning solutions
- Create multiple test versions in an instant
- Deliver tests from your LMS, your classroom, or wherever you want

Global Health Watch (Instant Access Code: ISBN-13: 978-1-111-37733-5; Printed Access Card: ISBN-13: 978-1-111-37731-1)

Updated with today's current headlines, Global Health Watch is a one-stop resource for classroom discussion and research projects. This resource center provides access to thousands of trusted health sources, including academic journals, magazines, newspapers, videos, podcasts, and more. It is updated daily to offer the most current news about topics related to your health course.

Careers in Health, Physical Education, and Sport, 2nd edition (ISBN-13: 978-0-495-38839-5)

This unique booklet takes students through the complicated process of choosing the type of career they want to pursue; explains how to prepare for the transition into the working world; and provides insight into different types of career paths, education requirements, and reasonable salary expectations. A designated chapter discusses some of the legal issues that surround the workplace, including discrimination and harassment. This supplement is complete with personal development activities designed to encourage students to focus on and develop better insight into their futures.

Acknowledgments

One of the joys of writing each edition of *An Invitation to Health* is the opportunity to work with a team I consider the best of the best in textbook publishing. I thank Krista Mastroianni, product manager, for her enthusiasm and support. Nedah Rose, senior content developer, contributed in countless ways to many editions, making each one stronger. I applaud Alexandria Brady for taking over the reins and shepherding this edition through completion. Michael Cook, senior designer, provided the evocative cover and eye-catching design. I am also grateful to Yolanda Cossio, both personally and professionally, for her wisdom and guidance.

I thank Victor Luu, our editorial assistant, for his invaluable aid; Tanya Nigh, senior content project manager, for expertly shepherding this edition from conception to production; Liz Harasymczuk for the vibrant new design; and Evelyn Dayringer of Graphic World Publishing Services for her supervision of the production process. Veerabhagu Nagarajan, our photo researcher, provided images that capture the diversity and energy of today's college students. Ganesh Krishnan coordinated text permissions, and Christine Myaskovsky managed the overall permissions process.

My thanks to Ana Albinson, marketing manager; to Alexandria Brady, who managed the creation of MindTap; and to Kellie Petruzzelli, who guided the ancillaries.

Finally, I would like to thank the reviewers whose input has been so valuable through these many editions.

Ghulam Aasef, *Kaskaskia College*
Andrea Abercrombie, *Clemson University*
Daniel Adame, *Emory University*
Lisa Alastuey, *University of Houston*

Carol Allen, *Lone Community College*
Lana Arabas, *Truman State University*
Judy Baker, *East Carolina University*
Marcia Ball, *James Madison University*
Jeremy Barnes, *Southeast Missouri State University*
Rick Barnes, *East Carolina University*
Lois Beach, *SUNY-Plattsburg*
Liz Belyea, *Cosumnes River College*
Betsy Bergen, *Kansas State University*
Nancy Bessette, *Saddleback College*
Carol Biddington, *California University of Pennsylvania*
David Black, *Purdue University*
Jill M. Black, *Cleveland State University*
Cynthia Pike Blocksom, *Cincinnati Health Department*
Laura Bounds, *Northern Arizona University*
James Brik, *Willamette University*
Mitchell Brodsky, *York College*
Jodi Broodkins-Fisher, *University of Utah*
Elaine D. Bryan, *Georgia Perimeter College*
James G. Bryant, Jr., *Western Carolina University*
Conswella Byrd, *California State University East Bay*
Marsha Campos, *Modesto Junior College*
Richard Capriccioso, *University of Phoenix*
James Lester Carter, *Montana State University*
Jewel Carter-McCummings, *Montclair State University*
Peggy L. Chin, *University of Connecticut*
Olga Comissiong, *Kean University*
Patti Cost, *Weber State University*
Maxine Davis, *Eastern Washington University*
Maria Decker, *Marian Court College*
Laura Demeri, *Clark College*
Lori Dewald, *Shippensburg University of Pennsylvania*
Julie Dietz, *Eastern Illinois University*
Peter DiLorenzo, *Camden County College*
Robert Dollinger, *Florida International University College of Medicine*
Rachelle D. Duncan, *Oklahoma State University*
Sarah Catherine Dunsmore, *Idaho State University*
Gary English, *Ithaca College*
Victoria L. Evans, *Hendrix College*
Melinda K. Everman, *Ohio State University*
Michael Felts, *East Carolina University*
Lynne Fitzgerald, *Morehead State University*
Matthew Flint, *Utah Valley University*
Kathie C. Garbe, *Kennesaw State College*
Gail Gates, *Oklahoma State University*
Dawn Graff-Haight, *Portland State University*
Carolyn Gray, *New Mexico State University*
Mary Gress, *Lorain County Community College*
Janet Grochowski, *University of St. Thomas*
Jack Gutierrez, *Central Community College*
Autumn R. Hamilton, *Minnesota State University*
Christy D. Hawkins, *Thomas Nelson Community College*
Stephen Haynie, *College of William and Mary*
Amy Hedman, *Mankato State University*
Ron Heinrichs, *Central Missouri State University*
Candace H. Hendershot, *University of Findlay*
Michael Hoadley, *University of South Dakota*
Debbie Hogan, *Tri County Community College*
Margaret Hollinger, *Reading Area Community College*
Harold Horne, *University of Illinois at Springfield*
Linda L. Howard, *Idaho State University*
Mary Hunt, *Madonna University*
Kim Hyatt, *Weber State University*
Bill Hyman, *Sam Houston State University*
Dee Jacobsen, *Southeastern Louisiana University*
John Janowiak, *Appalachian State University*
Peggy Jarnigan, *Rollins College*
Jim Johnson, *Northwest Missouri State University*
Chester S. Jones, *University of Arkansas*
Herb Jones, *Ball State University*
Jane Jones, *University of Wisconsin, Stevens Point*
Lorraine J. Jones, *Muncie, Indiana*
Walter Justice, *Southwestern College*
Becky Kennedy-Koch, *The Ohio State University*
Margaret Kenrick, *Los Medanos College*

About the Author

Dianne Hales is one of the most widely published and honored freelance journalists in the country. She is the author of 15 trade books, including *Mona Lisa: A Life Discovered*; *La Bella Lingua*; *Just Like a Woman*; *Think Thin, Be Thin*; and *Caring for the Mind*, with translations into Chinese, Japanese, Italian, French, Spanish, Portuguese, German, Dutch, Swedish, Danish and Korean.

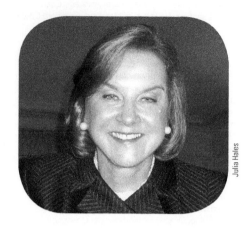

Julia Hales

Hales has received the highest honor the government of Italy can bestow on a foreigner, an honorary knighthood, with the title *Cavaliere dell' Ordine della Stella della Solidarietà Italiana* (Knight of the Order of the Star of Italian Solidarity) in recognition of her book *La Bella Lingua: My Love Affair with Italian, the World's Most Enchanting Language*, as "an invaluable tool for promoting the Italian language."

Hales is a former contributing editor for *Parade*, *Ladies' Home Journal*, *Working Mother*, and *American Health* and has written more than 1,000 articles for publications including *Family Circle*, *Glamour*, *Good Housekeeping*, *Health*, *The New York Times*, *Reader's Digest*, *The Washington Post*, *Woman's Day*, and *The World Book Encyclopedia*.

Hales has received writing awards from the American Psychiatric Association and the American Psychological Association, an EMMA (Exceptional Media Merit Award) for health reporting from the National Women's Political Caucus and Radcliffe College, three EDI (Equality, Dignity, Independence) awards for print journalism from the National Easter Seal Society, the National Mature Media Award, and awards from the Arthritis Foundation, California Psychiatric Society, CHADD (Children and Adults with Attention Deficit/Hyperactivity Disorder), Council for the Advancement of Scientific Education, and New York City Public Library.

An Invitation to Health

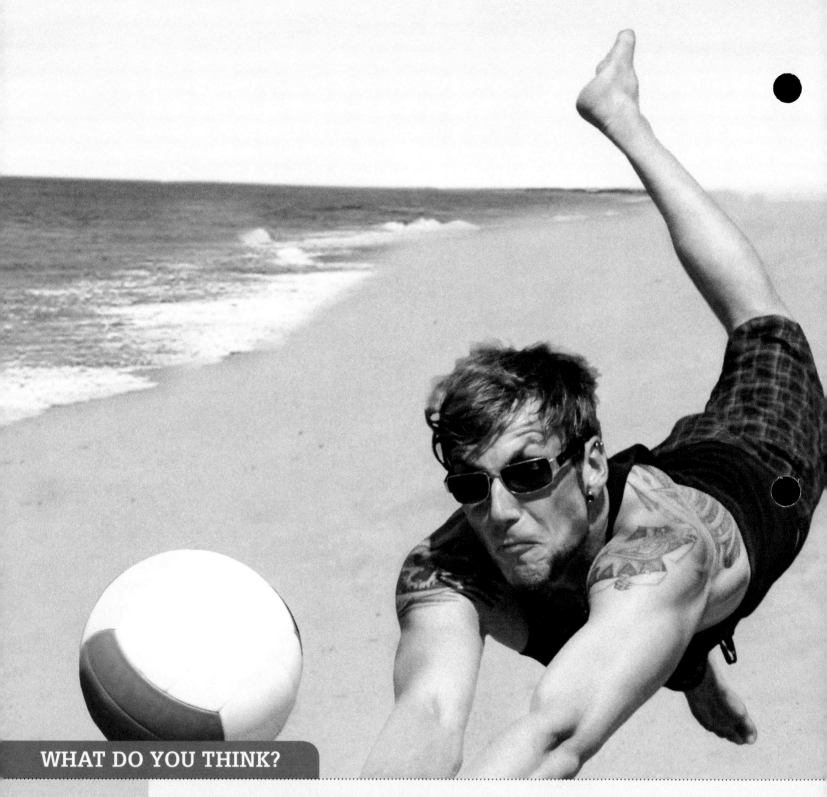

WHAT DO YOU THINK?

- What does "health" mean to you?
- How healthy are today's college students?
- Do race and gender affect health?
- Can people successfully change their health behaviors?

1

The Power of Now

Keisha always thought of health as something you worry about when you get older. Then her twin brother developed a health problem she'd never heard of: prediabetes (discussed in Chapter 15), which increased his risk of diabetes and heart disease. At a health fair on campus, she found out that her blood pressure was higher than normal. She also learned that young adults with high blood pressure could be at greater risk of heart problems in the future.[1]

"Maybe I'm not too young to start thinking about my health," Keisha concluded. Neither are you, whether you're a traditional-age college student or, like an ever-increasing number of undergraduates, years older. **<**

After reading this chapter, you should be able to:

1.1 Define health and wellness and outline the dimensions of health.

1.2 Assess the current health status of Americans, including health goals and health disparities.

1.3 Compare the health trends of students with those of Americans in general.

1.4 Explain the influences on behavior that support or impede healthy change.

1.5 Identify the stages of change.

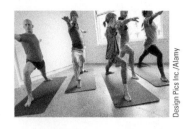

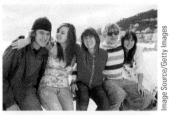

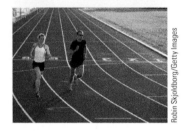

Health is the process of discovering, using, and protecting all the resources within our bodies, minds, spirits, families, communities, and environment.

An Invitation to Health is both *about* and *for* you; it asks you to go beyond thinking about your health to taking charge and making healthy choices for yourself and your future. This book includes material on your mind and your body, your spirit and your social ties, your needs and your wants, your past and your potential. It will help you explore options, discover possibilities, and find new ways to make your life worthwhile.

What you learn from this book and in this course depends on you. You have more control over your life and well-being than anything or anyone else does. Through the decisions you make and the habits you develop, you can influence how well—and perhaps how long—you will live.

The time to start is *now*. Every day you make choices that have short- and long-term consequences for your health. Eat a high-fat meal, and your blood chemistry changes. Spend a few hours slumped in front of the television, and your metabolism slows. Chug a high-caffeine energy drink, and your heart races. Have yet another beer, and your reflexes slow. Text while driving, and you may weave into another lane. Don't bother with a condom, and your risk of sexually transmitted infection (STI) skyrockets.

Sometimes making the best choices demands making healthy changes in your life. This chapter will show you how—and how to live more fully, more happily, and more healthfully. This is an offer that you literally cannot afford to refuse. Your life may depend on it—starting now.

Health and Wellness

By simplest definition, **health** means being sound in body, mind, and spirit. The World Health Organization defines *health* as "not merely the absence of disease or infirmity" but "a state of complete physical, mental, and social well-being.[2] Health is the process of discovering, using, and protecting all the resources within our bodies, minds, spirits, families, communities, and environment.

Health has many dimensions: physical, psychological, spiritual, social, intellectual, and environmental. Some add an "emotional" and a "cultural" dimension. This book integrates these aspects into a *holistic* approach that looks at health and the individual as a whole rather than part by part.

Your own definition of health may include different elements, but chances are you and your classmates agree that it includes at least some of the following:

- A positive, optimistic outlook
- A sense of control over stress and worries; time to relax
- Energy and vitality; freedom from pain or serious illness
- Supportive friends and family and a nurturing intimate relationship with someone you love
- A personally satisfying job or intellectual endeavor
- A clean, healthful environment

✓**check-in** How would you define *health*?

Wellness can be defined as purposeful, enjoyable living or, more specifically, a deliberate lifestyle choice characterized by personal responsibility and optimal enhancement of physical, mental, and spiritual health. In the broadest sense, wellness is

- A decision you make to move toward optimal health
- A way of life you design to achieve your highest potential
- A process of developing awareness that health and happiness are possible in the present
- The integration of body, mind, and spirit
- The belief that everything you do, think, and feel has an impact on your state of health and the health of the world

✓**check-in** What does *wellness* mean to you?

The Dimensions of Health

Scientists are discovering that various dimensions and the interplay among them can affect us at a molecular level. For instance, a lack of education—an indicator of poor intellectual health—has long been linked with poor physical health and relatively early death. However, other factors—such as having meaningful relationships with others (part of social health) and a sense of meaning and purpose in life (an indicator of spiritual health)—can overcome the disadvantages associated with poverty or minimal schooling.

By learning more about the six dimensions of health, you gain insight into the complex interplay of factors that determine your level of wellness.

health A state of complete well-being, including physical, psychological, spiritual, social, intellectual, and environmental dimensions.

wellness A deliberate lifestyle choice characterized by personal responsibility and optimal enhancement of physical, mental, and spiritual health.

The following are the most commonly recognized dimensions of health and wellness, but some models treat emotional, cultural, or financial health as separate categories rather than aspects of psychological, social, or occupational health.

✓ check-in What do you consider the most important *or relevant* dimensions of health?

Physical Health   Webster's 1913 dictionary defined *health* as "the state of being hale, sound, or whole, in body, mind, or soul, especially the state of being free from physical disease or pain." More recent definitions conceive health as "an optimal state of physical, mental, and social well-being, not merely the absence of disease or infirmity."

Health is not a static state but a process that depends on the decisions we make and the behaviors we practice every day. To ensure optimal physical health, we must feed our bodies nutritiously, exercise them regularly, avoid harmful behaviors and substances, watch for early signs of sickness, and protect ourselves from accidents.

Psychological Health   Like physical well-being, psychological health, discussed in the following chapters, is more than the absence of problems or illness. Psychological health refers to both our emotional and mental states—that is, to our feelings and our thoughts. It involves awareness and acceptance of a wide range of feelings in oneself and others, as well as the ability to express emotions, to function independently, and to cope with the challenges of daily stressors.

Spiritual Health   Spiritually healthy individuals identify their own basic purpose in life; learn how to experience love, joy, peace, and fulfillment; and help themselves and others achieve their full potential. As they devote themselves to others' needs more than their own, their spiritual development produces a sense of greater meaning in their lives. (See Chapter 2 for an in-depth discussion of spiritual and emotional well-being.)

Social Health   Social health refers to the ability to interact effectively with other people and the social environment, to develop satisfying interpersonal relationships, and to fulfill social roles. It involves participating in and contributing to your community, living in harmony with fellow human beings, developing positive interdependent relationships, and practicing healthy sexual behaviors. (See Chapter 5.)

Health educators are placing greater emphasis on social health in its broadest sense as they expand the traditional individualistic concept of health to include the complex interrelationships between one person's health and the health of the community and environment. This change in perspective has given rise to a new emphasis on **health promotion**, which educators define as "any planned combination of educational, political, regulatory, and organizational supports for actions and conditions of living conducive to the health of individuals, groups, or communities." Examples on campus include establishing smoke-free policies for all college buildings, residences, and dining areas; prohibiting tobacco advertising and sponsorship of campus social events; promoting safety at parties; and enforcing alcohol laws and policies.

Intellectual Health   Your brain is the only one of your organs capable of self-awareness. Every day you use your mind to gather, process, and act on information; to think through your values; to make decisions, set goals, and figure out how to handle a problem or challenge. Intellectual health refers to your ability to think and learn from life experience, your openness to new ideas, and your capacity to question and evaluate information. Throughout your life, you'll use your critical thinking skills, including your ability to evaluate health information, to safeguard your well-being.

Environmental Health   You live in a physical and social setting that can affect every aspect of your health. Environmental health refers to the impact your world has on your well-being. It involves protecting yourself from dangers in the air, water, and soil, as well as in products you use—and working to preserve the environment itself. (Chapter 19 offers a thorough discussion of environmental health.)

Occupational Health   In the coming decades, you will devote much of your time and energy to your career. Ideally, you will contribute your unique talents and skills to work that is rewarding in many ways—intellectually, emotionally, creatively, financially. Yet every job presents physical, psychological, and mental challenges that can affect your well-being. College provides the opportunity for you to choose and prepare for a career that is consistent with your personal values and beliefs. Now is also the time to build the healthy habits and coping skills that will enable you to balance work and other endeavors throughout your life.

✓ check-in How do you rate yourself on each of these dimensions of health?

health promotion Any planned combination of educational, political, regulatory, and organizational supports for actions and conditions of living conducive to the health of individuals, groups, or communities.

Health in America

Although the United States ranks among the wealthiest nations in the world, it is far from the healthiest. We spend more than any other nation on health care: a whopping $2.9 trillion, about 18 percent of our GDP (gross domestic product).

Life expectancy at birth in the United States has increased to an all-time high of 76.4 years for men and 81.2 years for women, but citizens of other affluent nations, such as Japan and Switzerland, live significantly longer.[3] A major study by the National Research Council and Institute of Medicine concluded that "Americans live shorter lives and experience more injuries and illnesses than people in other high-income countries."[4] Among the diseases taking the greatest toll on Americans' well-being are hypertension, heart disease, diabetes, arthritis, and autoimmune disorders.[5]

Rather than focus solely on life expectancy, experts are calculating healthy life expectancy (HALE), based on years lived without disease or disability. On average, life expectancy at birth for Americans averages about age 79, but the average HALE is considerably shorter: about 68 years.[6]

If you are under age 50, you may think this doesn't apply to you. Think again. The Americans experiencing the greatest health deficits and most years lost to illness, disability, and premature death are not the elderly but young adults. As a young American, your probability of reaching your 50th birthday is lower than in almost every other high-income nation.[7]

In comparison with almost all of 16 high-income "peer" countries—Australia, Austria, Canada, Denmark, Finland, France, Germany, Italy, Japan, Norway, Portugal, Spain, Sweden, Switzerland, the Netherlands, and the United Kingdom—Americans have shorter life expectancies.

Deaths before age 50 account for about two-thirds of the difference in life expectancy for American men and one-third of the difference for American women, compared with their counterparts in other nations.[8]

....
✓ **check-in** How do you think your life
....
expectancy and your healthy life expectancy
....
(HALE) compare?
....

How We Lag Behind

Here are some of the key areas in which the United States lags behind other first-world nations:

- **Birth outcomes.** Although infant mortality rates have improved, they remain higher in the United States than in other nations. American babies also are more likely to have low birth weights. Our children are less likely to live to age 5 than those in other developed countries.

- **Injuries and homicides.** Since the 1950s, American adolescents and young adults have died at higher rates from traffic accidents and violence than their counterparts in other countries.

- **Teen pregnancy and sexually transmitted infections (STIs).** Adolescents in the United States have the highest rates of pregnancy among developed nations and are more likely to acquire an STI.

- **HIV and AIDS.** The United States has the second-highest prevalence of HIV infections among its peer nations and the highest incidence of AIDS.

- **Drug-related mortality.** Americans lose more years of life to alcohol and other drugs than people in peer countries, even when deaths from drunk driving are excluded.

- **Obesity and diabetes.** The United States has the highest obesity rate among high-income countries in every age group. From age 20 onward, Americans have the highest prevalence of diabetes and high glucose levels (discussed in Chapter 15) among peer countries.

- **Heart disease.** Americans who survive to age 50 have more cardiovascular risk factors (discussed in Chapter 15) than their counterparts in Europe. Adults over age 50 are more likely to develop and die from cardiovascular disease than those in other high-income countries.

- **Chronic lung disease.** Lung disease is more prevalent and deadly in the United States than in European countries.

- **Disability.** Adults in the United States report a higher prevalence of arthritis and activity limitations than their counterparts in other affluent nations.

Closing the Gap

Americans could be living both longer and healthier lives, but only a minority have adopted healthy behaviors. Here are the latest findings on our health and habits from the Centers for Disease Control and Prevention (CDC):

- **Fitness:** Fewer than 20 percent of men and women exercise regularly.

- **Weight:** The percentage of obese Americans has risen from 30 percent in 2000 to 34 percent today. Two-thirds of the population are either overweight or obese.

- **Overall health:** Ten percent of all Americans describe their health as fair or poor. This percentage increases to 18 percent of those over age 65.

- **Medical conditions:** Almost one-third (33 percent) of Americans over age 20 have hypertension; 15 percent have high cholesterol; 12 percent have diabetes. About 18 percent of Americans over age 65 have had cancer.

- **Health care:** Almost one-quarter (23 percent) of men and women between ages 18 and 44 did not see a health-care professional in the previous year.

✓**check-in** How would you rate your health habits?

Healthy People 2020

Every decade since 1980, the U.S. Department of Health and Human Services (HHS) has published a comprehensive set of national public health objectives as part of the Healthy People Initiative. The department's vision is to create a society in which all people can live long, healthy lives. Its mission includes identifying nationwide health improvement priorities, increasing public awareness of health issues, and providing measurable objectives and goals.

Drawing on the lessons learned and needs identified in *Healthy People 2010*, HHS has set the following overarching goals for *Healthy People 2020*:

- Eliminate preventable disease, disability, injury, and premature death.

- Achieve health equity, eliminate disparities, and improve the health of all groups.

- Create social and physical environments that promote good health for all.

- Promote healthy development and healthy behaviors across every stage of life.

Here are examples of specific new recommendations that have been added to the national health agenda for 2020:

- **Nutrition and weight status:** Prevent inappropriate weight gain in youths and adults.

- **Tobacco use:** Increase smoking-cessation success by adult smokers.

- **Sexually transmitted infections:** Increase the proportion of adolescents who abstain

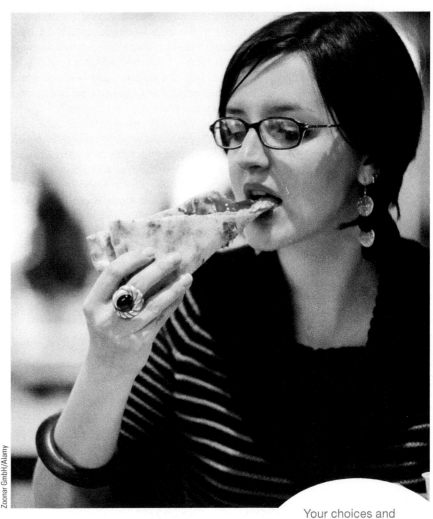

Zoonar GmbH/Alamy

from sexual intercourse or use condoms if sexually active.

- **Substance abuse:** Reduce misuse of prescription drugs.

- **Heart disease and stroke:** Increase overall cardiovascular health in the U.S. population.

- **Injury and violence prevention:** Reduce sports and recreation injuries.

✓**check-in** If you were setting personal health objectives to attain by 2020, what would they be?

Health Disparities

Despite improvements in the overall health of the nation, Americans who are members of racial and ethnic groups—including black or African Americans, American Indians, Alaska Natives, Asian Americans, Hispanics, Latinos, and Pacific Islanders— are more likely than whites to suffer disease and

Your choices and behaviors during your college years can influence how healthy you will be in the future.

disability. "Multiple disadvantages," as researchers refer to the extra challenges minorities face, increase the likelihood of major depression, poor physical health, functional limitations, and premature death.[9] The longevity gap between white and black women is four years; for white and black men it is six years.

Genetic variations, environmental influences, and specific health behaviors contribute to health disparities, but poverty is a key factor. Many minorities have not been able to afford the tests and treatments that could prevent illness or overcome it at the earliest possible stages. According to public health experts, low income may account for one-third of the racial differences in death rates for middle-aged African American adults.

✓**check-in** Are you a member of a racial or ethnic minority? If so, do you think this status affects your health or health care?

If you are a member of a racial or ethnic minority, you need to educate yourself about your health risks, take responsibility for those within your control, and become a savvy, assertive consumer of health-care services. The federal Office of Minority Health and Health Disparities (www.cdc.gov/omhd), which provides general information and the latest research and recommendations, is a good place to start.

YOUR STRATEGIES FOR PREVENTION

If You Are at Risk

Certain health risks may be genetic, but behavior influences their impact. Here are specific steps you can take to protect your health:

- **Ask if you are at risk for any medical conditions or disorders based on your family history or racial or ethnic background.**

- **Find out if there are tests that could determine your risks.** Discuss the advantages and disadvantages of such testing with your doctor.

- **If you or a family member requires treatment for a chronic illness, ask your doctor whether any medications have proved particularly effective for your racial or ethnic background.**

- **If you are African American, you are significantly more likely to develop high blood pressure, diabetes, and kidney disease.** Being overweight or obese adds to the danger. The information in Chapters 6, 7, and 8 can help you lower your risk by keeping in shape, making healthy food choices, and managing your weight.

- **Hispanics and Latinos have disproportionately high rates of respiratory problems, such as asthma, chronic obstructive lung disease, and tuberculosis.** To protect your lungs, stop smoking and avoid secondary smoke. Learn as much as you can about the factors that can trigger or worsen lung diseases.

Why Race Matters If, like many other Americans, you come from a racially mixed background, your health profile may be complex. Here are just some of the differences race makes:

- Black Americans lose substantially more years of potential life to homicide (nine times as many), stroke (three times as many), and diabetes (three times as many) as whites. Also, compared with whites, blacks have more new AIDS cases.

- About one in three Hispanics has prediabetes; only about half of Hispanics with diabetes have it under control.[10]

- American Indian and Alaska Native women are less likely to receive prenatal care, and Asian American women have significantly lower rates of mammography.

- Caucasians are prone to osteoporosis (progressive weakening of bone tissue); cystic fibrosis; skin cancer; and phenylketonuria (PKU), a metabolic disorder that can lead to cognitive impairment

- Native Americans, including those indigenous to Alaska, are more likely to die young than the population as a whole, primarily as a result of accidental injuries, cirrhosis of the liver, homicide, pneumonia, and complications of diabetes.

- The suicide rate among American Indians and Alaska Natives is 50 percent higher than the national rate. The rates of co-occurring mental illness and substance abuse (especially alcohol abuse) are also higher among Native American youth and adults.

Cancer Screening and Management Overall, black Americans are more likely to develop cancer than persons of any other racial or ethnic group. As discussed in Chapter 15, medical scientists have debated whether the reason might be that treatments are less effective in blacks or whether many are not diagnosed early enough or treated rigorously enough:

- Black women have higher rates of colon, pancreatic, and stomach cancer. Black men have higher rates of prostate, colon, and stomach cancer.

- African Americans have the highest death rates for lung cancer of any racial or ethnic group in the United States.

- African American women are more than twice as likely to die of cervical cancer as are white women and are more likely to die of breast cancer than are women of any racial or ethnic group except Native Hawaiians.

- Native Hawaiian women have the highest rates of breast cancer. Women from many racial minorities, including those of Filipino, Pakistani, Mexican, and Puerto Rican descent, are more likely to be diagnosed with late-stage breast cancer than white women.

Cardiovascular Disease   Heart disease and stroke are the leading causes of death for all racial and ethnic groups in the United States, but mortality rates of death from these diseases are higher among African American adults than among white adults. African Americans also have higher rates of high blood pressure (hypertension), develop this problem earlier in life, suffer more severe hypertension, and have higher rates of stroke.

Diabetes   American Indians and Alaska Natives, African Americans, and Hispanics are twice as likely to be diagnosed with diabetes as are non-Hispanic whites.

Infant Mortality   African American, American Indian, and Puerto Rican infants have higher death rates than white infants.

Mental Health   American Indians and Alaska Natives suffer disproportionately from depression and substance abuse. Minorities have less access to mental health services and are less likely to receive needed high-quality mental health services.

Infectious Disease   Asian Americans and Pacific Islanders have much higher rates of hepatitis B than other racial groups. Black teenagers and young adults become infected with hepatitis B three to four times more often than those who are white. Black people also have a higher incidence of hepatitis C infection than white people. Almost 80 percent of reported cases affect racial and ethnic minorities.

HIV and Sexually Transmitted Infections   Although African Americans and Hispanics represent only about one-quarter of the U.S. population, they account for about two-thirds of adult AIDS cases and more than 80 percent of pediatric AIDS cases. Yet only one in three HIV-infected black Americans is receiving treatment.[11]

Sex, Gender, and Health

Medical scientists define *sex* as a classification, generally as male or female, according to the reproductive organs and functions that derive from the chromosomal complement. *Gender* refers to a person's self-representation as male or female

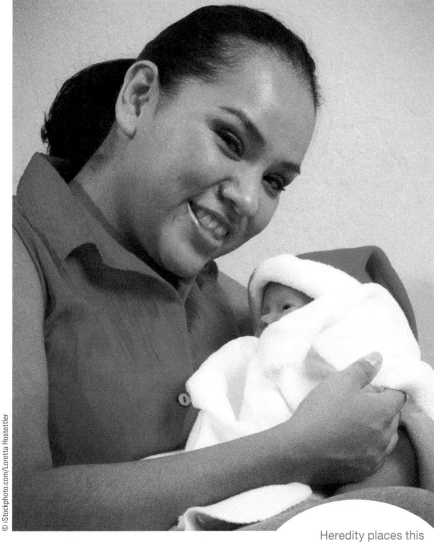

© iStockphoto.com/Loretta Hostettler

Heredity places this Pima Indian infant at higher risk of developing disease, but environmental factors also play a role.

or how social institutions respond to a person, on the basis of the individual's gender presentation. Gender is rooted in biology and shaped by environment and experience.

The experience of being male or female in a particular culture and society can and does have an effect on physical and psychological well-being. In fact, sex and gender may have a greater impact than any other variable on how our bodies function, how long we live, and the symptoms, course, and treatment of the diseases that strike us. (See Figure 1.1.)

Here are some health differences between men and women:

- Although many assume that men are the stronger sex, they die at a higher rate than women. About 115 males are conceived for every 100 females, but more males die before birth.

- Boys are more likely to be born prematurely, to suffer birth-related injuries, and to die before their first birthdays than girls.

He:

- averages 12 breaths a minute
- has lower core body temperature
- has a slower heart rate
- has more oxygen-rich hemoglobin in his blood
- is more sensitive to sound
- produces twice as much saliva
- has a 10 percent larger brain
- is 10 times more likely to have attention deficit disorder
- as a teen, has an attention span of 5 minutes
- is more likely to be physically active
- is more prone to lethal diseases, including heart attacks, cancer, and liver failure
- is five times more likely to become an alcoholic
- has a life expectancy of 76 years

She:

- averages 9 breaths a minute
- has higher core body temperature
- has a faster heart rate
- has higher levels of protective immunoglobulin in her blood
- is more sensitive to light
- takes twice as long to process food
- has more neurons in certain brain regions
- is twice as likely to have an eating disorder
- as a teen, has an attention span of 20 minutes
- is more likely to be overweight
- is more vulnerable to chronic diseases, like arthritis and autoimmune disorders, and age-related conditions like osteoporosis
- is twice as likely to develop depression
- has a life expectancy of 81 years

© Cengage Learning

FIGURE 1.1 Some of the Many Ways Men and Women Are Different

- Men's overall mortality rate is 41 percent higher than women's. They have higher rates of cancer, heart disease, stroke, lung disease, kidney disease, liver disease, and HIV/AIDS. They are four times more likely to take their own lives or to be murdered than women.

- Cardiovascular disease is the leading cause of death for women in the United States, yet only about one-third of clinical trial subjects in cardiovascular research are female, and just 31 percent of studies that include women report outcomes by sex.[12]

- Lung cancer is the leading cause of cancer death among women, with increased rates particularly among young female nonsmokers.[13]

- Women are 70 percent more likely than men to suffer from depression over the course of their lifetimes.[14]

✓**check-in** How do you think your gender affects your health?

Among the reasons that may contribute to the health and longevity gap between the sexes are:

- **Biological factors:** For example, women have two X chromosomes and men only one, and men and women have different levels of sex hormones (particularly testosterone and estrogen).

- **Social factors:** These include work stress, hostility levels, and social networks and supports.

- **Behavioral factors:** Men and women differ in risky behavior, aggression, violence, smoking, and substance abuse.

- **Health habits:** The sexes vary in terms of regular screenings, preventive care, and minimizing symptoms.

Sexual orientation also can affect health. Lesbian, gay, bisexual, and transgender individuals are more likely to encounter health disparities linked to social stigma, discrimination, and denial of their human and civil rights. Such discrimination has been implicated as a cause of high rates of psychiatric disorders, substance abuse, and suicide. The *Healthy People 2020* initiative has made improvements in LGBTQ health one of its new goals.

Health on Campus

As one of an estimated 21 million college students in the United States, you are part of a remarkably diverse group. Today's undergraduates come from every age group and social, racial, ethnic, economic, political, and religious background. Some 12 million are female; 9 million, male. You may have served in the military, started a family, or emigrated from another country. You might be enrolled in a two-year college, a four-year university, or a technical school. Your classrooms might be in a busy city or a small town—or they might exist solely as a virtual campus. Although the majority of undergraduates are "traditional" age (between 18 and 24 years old), more of you than ever before—8 million—are over age 25.[15]

Today's college students are both similar to and different from previous generations in many ways. Among the unique characteristics of current undergraduates are the following:

- They are the first generation of "digital natives," who've grown up in a wired world.

- They are the most diverse in higher-education history. About 15 percent are black; an equal percentage are Hispanic.

- They are both more connected and more isolated than their predecessors, with a "tribe" of friends, family, and acquaintances in constant contact through social media but with weak interpersonal, communications, and problem-solving skills.

- More students are working, working longer hours, taking fewer credits, requiring more time to graduate, and leaving college with large student loan debts.

- They are more coddled and protected by parents, who remain very involved in their daily lives.

- They were born into a nation enduring "unrelenting and profound change at a speed and magnitude never before experienced."

- They face a future in which the pace and scale of change will constantly accelerate.

√**check-in** A recent analysis of community college students identified four types of entering undergraduates: dreamers, drifters, passengers, and planners. What kind are you?

If you're a dreamer, seek guidance to fill in the details of your "big picture" goal for college.

If you're a drifter, focus on developing specific strategies to reach your educational goals.

If you're a passenger, find a mentor or advisor to help you interpret what you learn.

If you're a planner, look for help in applying the information you've gathered to your unique situation.[16]

College and Health

Although the words "college health" often appear together, they are, in fact, two different things

that profoundly influence each other. Healthier students get better grades and are more likely to graduate. A college education boosts health status, income, and community engagement later in life.[17]

Yet the transition from high school to college is considered an at-risk period for health and healthy behaviors. As studies in both the United States and Europe have documented, from their final year of high school to the second year of college, students are likely to do the following:

- Gain weight. In a recent study, undergraduates put on around six pounds—nine pounds for the men; four pounds for the women.[18]

- Cut back on their participation in sports—perhaps because they move away from hometown teams or they lack free time.

- Decrease some sedentary behaviors, such as viewing TV/DVDs and playing computers, but increase others, such as Internet use and studying.

- Eat less fruit and fewer vegetables.

- Consume more alcohol.[19]

Although healthier than their peers who are not attending college, undergraduates have significant health issues that can affect their overall well-being and ability to perform well in an academic environment:

- More than half report common acute illnesses, such as colds and flus, that interfere with their studies.

- A significant proportion report symptoms of depression, anxiety, and other mental disorders.

- For many, poor sleep has an impact on academic performance.

- Undergraduates are more likely to use alcohol and drugs than nonstudents their age.

- College students experience higher rates of interpersonal violence.

- On the positive side, college students are less likely to be overweight or obese, to smoke, to consume high-fat and low-fiber foods, to have high cholesterol levels, and to engage in high-risk sexual behavior than young adults who are not attending college.[20]

College also represents a rite of passage, when undergraduates typically engage in "adult" behaviors, such as drinking, getting involved in intimate relationships, and taking personal responsibility for health behaviors (such as sleep schedules and nutrition) that their parents may have previously supervised. Students cramming for a big

SNAPSHOT: ON CAMPUS NOW

Student Health

Percentage of students who describe their health as good, very good, or excellent:

Men	Women	Average
92.7	90.6	91.2

Top Ten Health Problems

	Percent
1. Allergies	19.7
2. Sinus infection	16.9
3. Back pain	12.6
4. Strep throat	10.6
5. Urinary tract infection	10
6. Asthma	9.1
7. Migraine headache	7.8
8. Broken bone/fracture/sprain	7.7
9. Ear infection	7.0
10. Bronchitis	6.2

Proportion of college students who reported being diagnosed or treated for these health problems in the past year.

Source: American College Health Association. *American College Health Association–National College Health Assessment II: Reference Group Executive Summary, Spring 2014*. Hanover, MD: American College Health Association, 2014.

exam may decide not to sleep and accept the short-term consequences on their health. Others, thinking ahead to future goals, may consciously choose to avoid behaviors, such as unsafe sex or drug use, that may jeopardize their plans.[21]

√ **check-in** Do you feel that today's undergraduates face unique pressures that can take a toll on physical and psychological health?

How Healthy Are Today's Students?

In the American College Health Association's National College Health Assessment (ACHA-NCHA) survey, more than 9 in 10 undergraduates rated their health as good, very good, or excellent (see Snapshot: On Campus Now). Yet the habits of young Americans often aren't healthy:

- Adults in the United States between the ages of 20 and 34 have the highest BMIs (body mass indexes) of any developed country. (See Chapter 7 on weight.)[22]

- In the ACHA survey, half (50.4 percent) of undergraduates got the recommended amounts of physical activity (discussed in Chapter 8).

- Some 67 percent had drunk alcohol at least once in the previous months; 42.7 percent reported having consumed five or more drinks in a single sitting within the past two weeks. (See Chapter 13.)

- Of those engaging in vaginal intercourse, only about half reported having used a condom mostly or always. (See Chapter 11.)

- About 12 percent reported having smoked at least once in the past month. (See Chapter 14.)

- A higher percentage—18.3 percent—had used marijuana in the previous month. (See Chapter 12.)

- Only 11.9 percent of students said they get enough sleep to feel rested in the morning six or more days a week; 10 percent said they never feel rested. (See Chapter 2.)

- College athletes, according to a recent longitudinal study, have lower health-related quality of life than their same-age peers who did not or no longer play college sports.[23]

✓**check-in** How do you think your current health behaviors may affect your future?

Colleges and universities have tried various interventions to improve students' health choices and habits. Do they work? In a meta-analysis of 41 studies, most conducted in the United States, 34 yielded significant improvements in one of several key outcomes, including these:

• Physical activity: more steps per day, more time in vigorous and/or moderate exercise, greater maximum oxygen consumption, and improved muscle strength, endurance, and flexibility

• Nutrition: lower calorie intake, more fruits and vegetables, reduced fat consumption, more macronutrients, and better overall diet quality

• Weight: improved weight, lower body fat, and healthier waist circumference and waist-to-hip ratio[24]

The most effective interventions spanned a semester or less, targeted only nutrition rather than multiple behaviors, and were imbedded within college courses. As the researchers noted, "universities and colleges are an ideal setting for implementation of health promotion programs." Why?

• They reach a large student population during a crucial life transition.

• They offer access to world-class facilities, technology, and highly educated staff in various health disciplines.

• They reach young adults at an age "where health behaviors that impact on health later in life can be provided."[25]

Why "Now" Matters

The choices you make today have an immediate impact on how you feel as well as long-term consequences, including the following:

• Individuals who begin using tobacco or alcohol in their teens and 20s are more likely to continue to do so as they get older.

• Obese children often grow into obese adolescents and obese adults, with ever-increasing risks of diabetes and cardiovascular disease.

• People in their 20s who have even mildly elevated blood pressure face an increased risk of clogged heart arteries by middle age.

• Young adults who acquire an STI may jeopardize both their future fertility and their health.

At any age, health risks are not inevitable. As recent research has shown, young adults with high aerobic fitness (discussed in Chapter 8) have a reduced risk of cardiovascular disease later in life.[20] Your current health habits may affect your mind as well as your body as you age. According to a large-scale new study, the more physically active you are at age 25, the better your thinking, memory, and cognitive skills in middle age.[26]

Simple steps, such as those listed in Health Now! can get you started in the right direction now!

Student Health Norms

Psychologists use the term *norm*, or **social norm**, to refer to a behavior or an attitude that a particular group expects, values, and enforces. Norms influence a wide variety of human activities, including health habits. However, perceptions of social norms are often inaccurate. Only anonymous responses to a scientifically designed questionnaire can reveal what individuals really do—the actual social norms—as compared to what they may say they do to gain social approval.

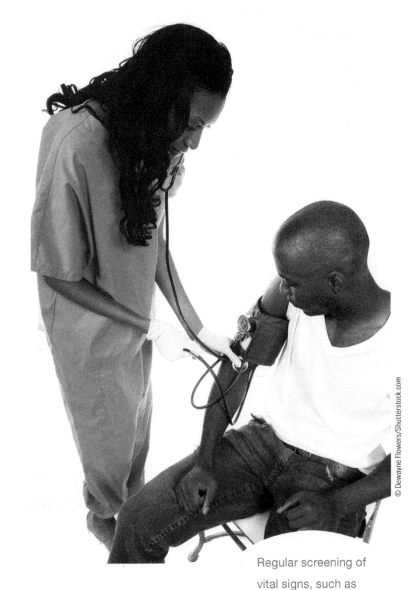

© Dewayne Flowers/Shutterstock.com

Regular screening of vital signs, such as blood pressure, can lead to early detection of a potentially serious health problem.

social norm A behavior or an attitude that a particular group expects, values, and enforces.

HEALTH NOW!

First Steps

- To lower your risk of heart disease, get your blood pressure and cholesterol checked. Don't smoke. Stay at a healthy weight. Exercise regularly.

- To lower your risks of major diseases, get regular check-ups. Make sure you are immunized against infectious illnesses.

- To lower your risks of sub-stance abuse and related illnesses and injuries, don't drink, or limit how much you drink. Avoid illegal drugs.

- To lower your risk of sexually transmitted infections or unwanted pregnancy, abstain from sex. If you engage in sexual activities, protect yourself with contraceptives, condoms, and spermicides.

- To prevent car accidents, stay off the road in hazard-ous circumstances, such as bad weather. Wear a seat belt when you drive and use defensive driving techniques.

Identify your top preventive health priority—lowering your risk of heart disease, for instance, or avoiding accidents. Write down a single action you can take this week that will reduce your health risks. As soon as you take this step, write a brief reflection in your online journal.

prevention Information and support offered to help healthy people identify their health risks, reduce stressors, prevent potential medical problems, and enhance their well-being.

protection Measures that an individual can take when participating in risky behavior to prevent injury or unwanted risks.

Throughout this text, we rely on the most comprehensive survey of college students, the ACHA-NCHA, to provide actual social norms for student behaviors. Its most recent survey included a national sample of 94,197 students from 168 schools.[27]

Undergraduates are particularly likely to mis-judge what their peers are—and aren't—doing. In recent years, colleges have found that publicizing research data on behaviors such as drinking, smok-ing, and drug use helps students get a more accu-rate sense of the real health norms on campus.

The gap between students' misperceptions and accurate health norms can be enormous. For example, undergraduates in the ACHA survey esti-mated that only 8.9 percent of students had never smoked cigarettes. In fact, 71.4 percent never had. Students guessed that only 3.2 percent of their peers never drank alcohol. In reality, 20.1 percent never did.[28] Providing accurate information on drinking norms on campus has proven effective in changing students' perceptions and in reducing alcohol consumption by both men and women.

✓**check-in** Do you think your peers have better or worse health habits than you?

The Promise of Prevention

You may think you are too young to worry about serious health conditions. Yet many chronic prob-lems begin early in life:

- Two percent of college-age women already have osteoporosis, a bone-weakening disease; another 15 percent have osteopenia, low bone densities that put them at risk of osteoporosis.

- Many college students have several risk factors for heart disease, including high blood pres-sure and high cholesterol. Others increase their risk by eating a high-fat diet and not exercising regularly. The time to change is now.

No medical treatment, however successful or sophisticated, can compare with the power of **prevention**. Two out of every three deaths and one in three hospitalizations in the United States could be prevented by changes in six main risk factors: tobacco use, alcohol abuse, accidents, high blood pressure, obesity, and gaps in screen-ing and primary health care.

Prevention remains the best weapon against cancer and heart disease. One of its greatest successes has come from the anti-smoking cam-paign, which in the past 40 years has prevented 8 million premature deaths in the United States, giving these ex-smokers an average of nearly 20 additional years of life.[29]

Protecting Yourself

There is a great deal of overlap between pre-vention and **protection**. Some people might think of immunizations as a way of preventing illness; others see them as a form of protection against dangerous diseases. Unfortunately, many adults are not getting the immunizations they need—and are putting their health in jeopardy as a result.[23] (See Chapter 16 to find out which vaccinations you should receive.)

You can prevent STIs or unwanted pregnancy by abstaining from sex. But if you decide to engage in sexual activities, you can protect your-self with condoms and spermicides.

Similarly, you can prevent many automobile accidents by not driving when road conditions are hazardous. But if you do have to drive, you can protect yourself by wearing a seat belt and using defensive driving techniques.

✓**check-in** What steps are you taking to protect your health?

Understanding Risky Behaviors

Today's students face different—and potentially deadlier—risks than undergraduates did a gener-ation or two ago. The problem is not that students who engage in risky behavior feel invulnerable or do not know the danger. Young people, accord-ing to recent research, actually overestimate the risk of some outcomes. However, they also over-estimate the benefit of immediate pleasure when, for instance, engaging in unsafe sex, and they underestimate the negative consequences, such as an STI.

College-age men are more likely than women to engage in risky behaviors—to use drugs and alcohol, to have unprotected sex, and to drive dangerously. Men also are more likely to be hospitalized for injuries and to commit suicide. Three-fourths of the deaths in the 15- to 24-year age range are men.

Drinking has long been part of college life and, despite efforts across U.S. college campuses to curb alcohol abuse, two out of five students engage in binge drinking—consumption of five or more drinks at a single session for men or four for women. Heavy drinking increases the likeli-hood of other risky behaviors, such as smoking cigarettes, using drugs, and having multiple sexual partners. New trends, such as drinking caffeinated alcoholic beverages (discussed in Chapter 13), smoking tobacco from a hookah or water pipe (Chapter 14), and using dangerous stimulants called "bath salts" (Chapter 12) present new risks.

Invest in Yourself

As the economy has declined, visits to doctors have dropped, and millions of people are not taking prescribed medications. However, trying to save money in the short term by doing without needed health care can cost you a great deal—financially and physically—in the long term. Here are some ways to keep medical costs down without sacrificing your good health:

- **Stay healthy.** Use this book to learn the basics of a healthy lifestyle and then live accordingly. By eating nutritiously, exercising, getting enough sleep, not smoking, and getting regular immunizations, you'll reduce your risk of conditions that require expensive treatments.

- **Build a good relationship with a primary care physician.** Although your choices may be limited, try to schedule appointments with the same doctor. A physician who knows you, your history, and your concerns can give the best advice on staying healthy.

- **Don't go to a specialist without consulting your primary care provider,** who can help you avoid overtesting and duplicate treatments.

- **If you need a prescription, ask if a generic form is available.** Brand names cost more, and most insurers charge higher copayments for them.

- **Take medications as prescribed.** Skipping doses or cutting pills in two may seem like easy ways to save money, but you may end up spending more for additional care because the treatment won't be as effective.

- **Don't go to an emergency department unless absolutely necessary.** Call your doctor for advice or go to the student health service. Emergency departments are overburdened with caring for the very ill and for injured people, and their services are expensive.

✓**check-in** What is the greatest health risk you've ever taken?

Making Healthy Changes

In terms of human health, the 1800s were the century of hygiene, with life-saving advances in sanitation and clean drinking water. The 1900s were the century of medicine, with breakthroughs in diagnosing and treating major illnesses. The 2000s may become the century of behavioral change, when individuals take charge of their health by breaking unhealthy habits and creating healthier new ones. (See Health on a Budget.)

✓**check-in** What health-related change would you like to make?

If you would like to improve your health behavior, you have to realize that change isn't easy. Between 40 and 80 percent of those who try to kick bad health habits lapse back into their unhealthy ways within six weeks.

Fortunately, our understanding of change has itself changed. Thanks to decades of research, we now know what sets the stage for change, the way change progresses, and the keys to lasting change. We also know that personal change

is neither mysterious nor magical but rather a methodical science that anyone can master.

Understanding Health Behavior

Three types of influences shape behavior: predisposing, enabling, and reinforcing factors (Figure 1.2).

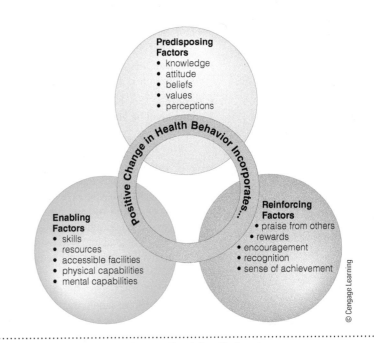

Predisposing Factors
- knowledge
- attitude
- beliefs
- values
- perceptions

Positive Change in Health Behavior Incorporates...

Enabling Factors
- skills
- resources
- accessible facilities
- physical capabilities
- mental capabilities

Reinforcing Factors
- praise from others
- rewards
- encouragement
- recognition
- sense of achievement

© Cengage Learning

FIGURE 1.2 Factors That Shape Positive Behavior

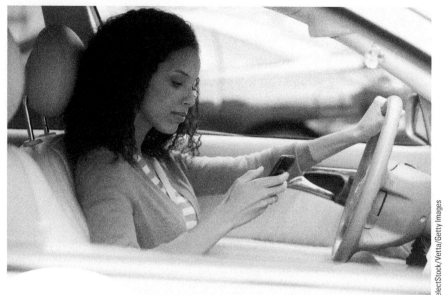
SelectStock/Vetta/Getty Images

Your stated knowledge-based belief may be that unsafe driving can cause accidents. Your actual belief is that it won't happen to you.

predisposing factors The beliefs, values, attitudes, knowledge, and perceptions that influence our behavior.

enabling factors The skills, resources, and physical and mental capabilities that shape our behavior.

reinforcing factors Rewards, encouragement, and recognition that influence our behavior in the short run.

health belief model (HBM) A model of behavioral change that focuses on the individual's attitudes and beliefs.

Predisposing Factors **Predisposing factors** include knowledge, attitudes, beliefs, values, and perceptions. Unfortunately, knowledge isn't enough to cause most people to change their behavior; for example, people fully aware of the grim consequences of smoking often continue to puff away. Nor is attitude—one's likes and dislikes—sufficient; an individual may dislike the smell and taste of cigarettes but continue to smoke anyway.

Beliefs are more powerful than knowledge and attitudes, and researchers report that people are most likely to change health behavior if they hold three beliefs:

- **Susceptibility:** They acknowledge that they are at risk for the negative consequences of their behavior.

- **Severity:** They believe that they may pay a very high price if they don't make a change.

- **Benefits:** They believe that the proposed change will be advantageous to their health.

Enabling Factors **Enabling factors** include skills, resources, accessible facilities, and physical and mental capacities. Before you initiate a change, assess the means available to reach your goal. No matter how motivated you are, you'll become frustrated if you keep encountering obstacles. Breaking down a task or goal into step-by-step strategies is very important in behavioral change.

Reinforcing Factors **Reinforcing factors** may be praise from family members and friends, rewards from teachers or parents, or encouragement and recognition for meeting a goal. Although these help a great deal in the short run, lasting change depends not on external rewards but on an internal commitment and sense of achievement. To make a difference, reinforcement must come from within.

A decision to change a health behavior should stem from a permanent, personal goal not from a desire to please or impress someone else. If you lose weight for the homecoming dance, you're almost sure to regain pounds afterward. But if you shed extra pounds because you want to feel better about yourself or get into shape, you're far more likely to keep off the weight.

✓**check-in** What goal would motivate you to change?

How and Why People Change

Change can simply happen. You get older. You put on or lose weight. You have an accident. Intentional change is different: A person consciously, deliberately sets out either to change a negative behavior, such as chronic procrastination, or to initiate a healthy behavior, such as daily exercise. For decades psychologists have studied how people intentionally change and have developed various models that reveal the anatomy of change.

In the *moral model*, you take responsibility for a problem (such as smoking) and its solution; success depends on adequate motivation, while failure is seen as a sign of character weakness. In the *enlightenment model*, you submit to strict discipline to correct a problem; this is the approach used in Alcoholics Anonymous. The *behavioral model* involves rewarding yourself when you make positive changes. The *medical model* sees the behavior as caused by forces beyond your control (a genetic predisposition to being overweight, for example) and employs an expert to provide advice or treatment. For many people, the most effective approach is the *compensatory model*, which doesn't assign blame but puts responsibility on individuals to acquire whatever skills or power they need to overcome their problems.

Health Belief Model

Psychologists developed the **health belief model (HBM)** about 50 years ago to explain and predict health behaviors by focusing on the attitudes and beliefs of individuals. (Remember that your attitudes and beliefs are predisposing influences on your capacity for change.) According to this model, people will take a health-related action (e.g., use condoms) if they

- feel susceptible to a possible negative consequence, such as a sexually transmitted infection (STI)

- perceive the consequence as serious or dangerous

- think that a particular action (using a condom) will reduce or eliminate the threat (of STIs)

- feel that they can take the necessary action without difficulty or negative consequences

- believe that they can successfully do what's necessary—for example, use condoms comfortably and confidently[30]

Readiness to act on health beliefs, in this model, depends on how vulnerable individuals feel, how severe they perceive the danger to be, the benefits they expect to gain, and the barriers they think they will encounter. Another key factor is self-efficacy, their confidence in their ability to take action.

In a study that tested the relationship between college students' health beliefs and cancer self-examinations, women were more likely to examine their breasts than men were to perform testicular exams. However, students of both sexes were more likely to do self-exams if they felt susceptible to developing cancer, if they felt comfortable and confident doing so, and if they were given a cue to action (such as a recommendation by a health professional).[31]

Self-Determination Theory

This approach, developed several decades ago by psychologists Edward Deci and Richard Ryan, focuses on whether an individual lacks motivation, is externally motivated, or is intrinsically motivated. Someone who is "amotivated" does not value an activity, such as exercise, or does not believe it will lead to a desired outcome, such as more energy or lower weight. Individuals who are externally motivated may engage in an activity like exercise to gain a reward or avoid a negative consequence (such as a loved one's nagging). Some people are motivated by a desired outcome; for instance, they might exercise for the sake of better health or longer life. Behavior becomes self-determined when someone engages in it for its own sake, such as exercising because it's fun.

Numerous studies have evaluated self-determination as it relates to health behavior. In research on exercise, individuals with greater self-determined motivation are less likely to stop exercising; they have stronger intentions to continue exercise, higher physical self-worth, and lower social anxiety related to their physique.

Motivational Interviewing

Health professionals, counselors, and coaches use motivational interviewing, developed by psychologists William Miller and Stephen Rollnick, to inspire individuals, regardless of their enthusiasm for change, to move toward improvements that could make their lives better. The United States Public Health Service, based on its assessment of current research, recommends motivational interviewing as an effective way to increase all tobacco users' willingness to quit.[32] Building a collaborative partnership, the therapist does not persuade directly but uses empathy and respect for the patient's perspective to evoke recognition of the desirability of change.

Self-Affirmation Theory

Affirmations, discussed in Chapter 2, can improve integrity, problem solving, self-worth, and self-regulation. They also are effective in encouraging behavioral change. According to self-affirmation theory, thinking about core personal values, important personal strengths, or valued relationships can provide reassurance and reinforce self-worth. Repeating an affirmation is one of the fastest ways to restructure thought patterns, develop new pathways in the brain, and make individuals less defensive about changing health behaviors.[33]

Recent neuroimaging studies have revealed how self-affirmations may increase the effectiveness of many health interventions. Using functional magnetic resonance imaging (fMRI), scientists were able to visualize changes in the brains of volunteers as they were reciting affirmations in their minds. These internal messages produced more activity in a region of the brain associated with positive responses.[34]

✓ **check-in** Some common self-affirmations are "I am strong" or "I can handle this challenge." What would you say to yourself to encourage a behavioral change?

Transtheoretical Model

Psychologist James Prochaska and his colleagues, by tracking what they considered to be universal

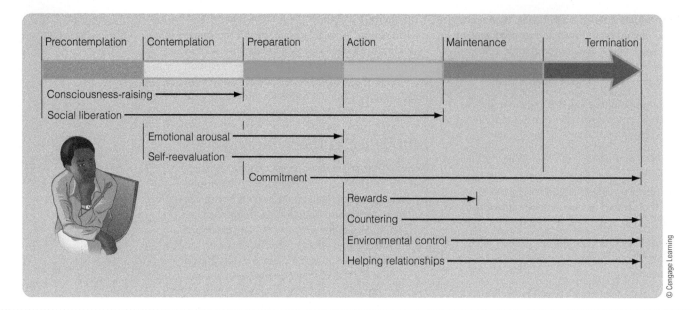

FIGURE 1.3 The Stages of Change and Some Change Processes

These change processes can help you progress through the stages of change. Each may be most useful at particular stages.

stages in the successful recovery of drug addicts and alcoholics, developed a way of thinking about change that cuts across psychological theories. Their **transtheoretical model** focuses on universal aspects of an individual's decision-making process rather than on social or biological influences on behavior.

The transtheoretical model has become the foundation of programs for smoking cessation, exercise, healthy food choices, alcohol cessation, weight control, condom use, drug use cessation, mammography screening, and stress management. Recent studies have demonstrated that it is more effective in encouraging weight loss than physical activity.[35]

The following sections describe these key components of the transtheoretical model:

- **Stages of change**

- **Processes of change**—cognitive and behavioral activities that facilitate change

- **Self-efficacy**—the confidence people have in their ability to cope with challenge

The Stages of Change According to the transtheoretical model of change, individuals progress through a sequence of stages as they make a change (Figure 1.3). No one stage is more important than another, and people often move back and forth between them. Most people "spiral" from stage to stage, slipping from maintenance to contemplation or from action to precontemplation before moving forward again.

People usually cycle and recycle through the stages several times. Smokers, for instance, report making three or four serious efforts to quit before they succeed.

The six stages of change are

1. **Precontemplation:** You are at this stage if you, as yet, have no intention of making a change. You are vaguely uncomfortable, but this is where your grasp of what is going on ends. You may never think about exercise, for instance, until you notice that it's harder to zip your jeans or that you get winded walking up stairs. Still, you don't quite register the need to do anything about it.

   During precontemplation, change remains hypothetical, distant, and vague. Yet you may speak of something bugging you and wish that things were somehow different.

2. **Contemplation:** In this stage, you still prefer not to have to change, but you start to realize that you can't avoid reality. Maybe none of your jeans fit anymore, or you feel sluggish and listless. In this stage, you may alternate between wanting to take action and resisting it.

√**check-in** Are you contemplating change? You may be if you find yourself thinking

- "I hate it that I keep . . ."
- "I should . . ."
- "Maybe I'll do it someday—not tomorrow, but someday."

transtheoretical model A model of behavioral change that focuses on the individual's decision making; it states that an individual progresses through a sequence of six stages as he or she makes a change in behavior.

3. **Preparation:** At some point, you stop waffling, make a clear decision, and feel a burst of energy. This decision heralds the preparation stage. You gather information, make phone calls, do research online, and look into exercise classes at the gym. You begin to think and act with change specifically in mind. If you were to eavesdrop on what you're saying to yourself, you would hear statements such as, "I am going to do this."

4. **Action:** You are actively modifying your behavior according to your plan. Your resolve is strong, and you know you're on your way to a better you. You may be getting up 15 minutes earlier to make time for a healthy breakfast or to walk to class rather than take the shuttle. In a relatively short time, you acquire a sense of comfort and ease with the change in your life.

5. **Maintenance:** This stabilizing stage, which follows the flurry of specific steps taken in the action stage, is absolutely necessary to retain what you've worked for and to make change permanent. In this stage, you strengthen, enhance, and extend the changes you've initiated. By securing the progress you've made, even if you hit a plateau or slip backward, you can regain your footing and keep moving forward.

6. **Termination:** At this stage, your "change" has become status quo. While it may take two to five years, the behavior has become so deeply ingrained that you can't imagine abandoning it.

Research on college students has shown that attitudes and feelings are related to stages of change. Smokers who believe that continuing to smoke would have only a minor or no impact on their health remain in the precontemplation stage; those with respiratory symptoms move on to contemplation and preparation.

✓**check-in** Do you want to change a health behavior? If so, what stage of change are you in?

The Processes of Change   Anything you do to modify your thinking, feeling, or behavior can be called a *change process*. The nine processes of change included in the transtheoretical model are shown in Figure 1.3, in their corresponding stages:

• **Consciousness-raising:** This most widely used change process involves increasing knowledge about yourself or the nature of your problem. As you learn more, you gain understanding and feedback about your behavior.

Example: Reading Chapter 6 on making healthy food choices.

• **Social liberation:** In this process, you take advantage of alternatives in the external environment that can help you begin or continue your efforts to change.

Example: Spending as much time as possible in nonsmoking areas.

• **Emotional arousal:** This process, also known as dramatic relief, works on a deeper level than consciousness-raising and is equally important in the early stages of change. Emotional arousal means experiencing and expressing feelings about a problem behavior and its potential solutions.

Example: Resolving never to drink and drive after the death of a friend in a car accident.

• **Self-reevaluation:** This process requires a thoughtful reappraisal of your problem, including an assessment of the person you might be once you have changed the behavior.

Example: Recognizing that you have a gambling problem and imagining yourself as a nongambler.

• **Commitment:** In this process, you acknowledge—first privately and then publicly—that you are responsible for your behavior and the only one who can change it.

Example: Joining a self-help or support group.

• **Rewards:** In this process, you reinforce positive behavioral changes with self-praise or small gifts.

Example: Getting a massage after a month of consistent exercise.

• **Countering:** Countering, or counterconditioning, involves substituting healthy behaviors for unhealthy ones.

Example: Chewing gum rather than smoking.

• **Environmental control:** This is an action-oriented process in which you restructure your environment so you are less likely to engage in a problem behavior.

Example: Getting rid of your stash of sweets.

• **Helping relationships:** In this process, you recruit individuals—family, friends, therapist, coach—to provide support, caring, understanding, and acceptance.

Example: Finding an exercise buddy.

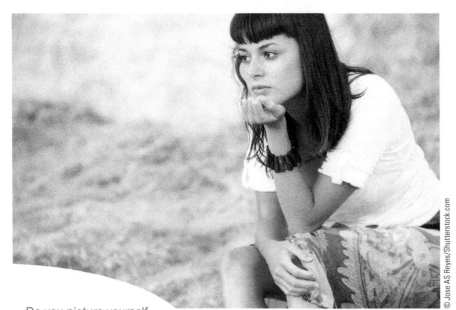

and will succeed in making a change. In his research on self-efficacy, psychologist Albert Bandura of Stanford University found that the individuals most likely to reach a goal are those who believe they can. The stronger their faith in themselves, the more energy and persistence they put into making a change. The opposite is also true, especially for health behaviors: Among people who begin an exercise program, those with lower self-efficacy are more likely to drop out.

√**check-in** How "internal" or "external" do you rate your locus of control?

If you believe that your actions will make a difference in your health, your locus of control is internal. If you believe that external forces or factors play a greater role, your locus of control is external. Hundreds of studies have compared people who have these different perceptions of control:

- "Internals," who believe that their actions largely determine what happens to them, act more independently, enjoy better health, are more optimistic about their future, and have lower mortality rates.[36]

- "Externals," who perceive that chance or outside forces determine their fate, find it harder to cope with stress and feel increasingly helpless over time. When it comes to weight, for instance, they see themselves as destined to be fat.

Do you picture yourself as master of your own destiny? You are more likely to achieve your health goals if you do.

self-efficacy Belief in one's ability to accomplish a goal or change a behavior.

locus of control An individual's belief about the sources of power and influence over his or her life.

Self-Efficacy and Locus of Control   Do you see yourself as master of your fate, asserting control over your destiny? Or do so many things happen in your life that you just hang on and hope for the best? The answers to these questions reveal two important characteristics that affect your health: your sense of **self-efficacy** (the belief in your ability to change and to reach a goal) and your **locus of control** (the sense of being in control of your life).

Your confidence in your ability to cope with challenge can determine whether you can

WHAT DID YOU DECIDE?

- What does "health" mean to you?
- How healthy are today's college students?
- Do race and gender affect health?
- Can people successfully change their health behaviors?

THE POWER OF NOW!

Making Healthy Changes

Ultimately, you have more control over your health than anyone else. Use this course as an opportunity to zero in on at least one less-than-healthful behavior and improve it. Here are some suggestions for small steps that can have a big payoff. Check those that you commit to making today, this week, this month, or this term. Indicate "t," "w," "m," or "term," and repeat this self-evaluation throughout the course.

_____ Use seat belts. In the past decade, seat belts have saved more than 40,000 lives and prevented millions of injuries.

_____ Eat an extra fruit or vegetable every day. Adding more fruits and vegetables to your diet can improve your digestion and lower your risk of several cancers.

_____ Get enough sleep. A good night's rest provides the energy you need to make it through the following day.

_____ Take regular stress breaks. A few quiet minutes spent stretching, looking out the window, or simply letting yourself unwind are good for body and soul.

_____ Lose a pound. If you're overweight, you may not think a pound will make a difference, but it's a step in the right direction.

_____ If you're a woman, examine your breasts regularly. Get in the habit of performing a breast self-examination every month after your period (when breasts are least swollen or tender).

_____ If you're a man, examine your testicles regularly. These simple self-exams can help you spot signs of cancer early, when it is most likely to be cured.

_____ Get physical. Just a little exercise will do some good. A regular workout schedule will be good for your heart, lungs, muscles, bones—even your mood.

_____ Drink more water. You need eight glasses a day to replenish lost fluids, prevent constipation, and keep your digestive system working efficiently.

_____ Do a good deed. Caring for others is a wonderful way to care for your own soul and connect with others.

What's Online

CENGAGE brain .com   Visit www.cengagebrain.com to access course materials for this text, including the Behavior Change Planner, interactive quizzes, tutorials, and more.

self survey

Are You in Control of Your Health?

To test whether you are the master of your fate, asserting control over your destiny, or just hanging on, hoping for the best, take the test below. Depending on which statement you agree with, check either a or b for each of the following.

1. (a) Many of the unhappy things in people's lives are partly due to bad luck. _____

   (b) People's misfortunes result from mistakes they make. _____

2. (a) One of the major reasons why we have wars is that people don't take enough interest in politics. _____

   (b) There will always be wars, no matter how hard people try to prevent them. _____

3. (a) In the long run, people get the respect they deserve in this world. _____

   (b) Unfortunately, an individual's worth often passes unrecognized no matter how hard he tries. _____

4. (a) The idea that teachers are unfair to students is nonsense. _____

   (b) Most students don't realize the extent to which their grades are influenced by accidental happenings. _____

5. (a) Without the right breaks, one cannot be an effective leader. _____

   (b) Capable people who fail to become leaders have not taken advantage of their opportunities. _____

6. (a) No matter how hard you try, some people just don't like you. _____

   (b) People who can't get others to like them don't understand how to get along with others. _____

7. (a) I have often found that what is going to happen will happen. _____

   (b) Trusting to fate has never turned out as well for me as making a decision to take a definite course of action. _____

8. (a) In the case of the well-prepared student, there is rarely, if ever, such a thing as an unfair test. ____

   (b) Many times exam questions tend to be so unrelated to course work that studying is really useless. ____

9. (a) Becoming a success is a matter of hard work; luck has little or nothing to do with it. ____

   (b) Getting a good job depends mainly on being in the right place at the right time. ____

10. (a) The average citizen can have influence in government decisions. ____

    (b) This world is run by the few people in power, and there is not much the little guy can do about it. ____

11. (a) When I make plans, I am almost certain that I can make them work. ____

    (b) It is not always wise to plan too far ahead because many things turn out to be a matter of luck anyway. ____

12. (a) In my case, getting what I want has little or nothing to do with luck. ____

    (b) Many times we might just as well decide what to do by flipping a coin. ____

13. (a) What happens to me is my own doing. ____

    (b) Sometimes I feel that I don't have enough control over the direction my life is taking. ____

Scoring

Give yourself one point for each of the following answers:
1a, 2b, 3b, 4b, 5a, 6a, 7a, 8b, 9b, 10b, 11b, 12b, 13b
You do not get any points for other choices.
Add up the totals. Scores can range from 0 to 13. A high score indicates an external locus of control, the belief that forces outside yourself control your destiny. A low score indicates an internal locus of control, a belief in your ability to take charge of your life.

Source: Based on J. B. Rotter, "Generalized Expectancies for Internal versus External Control of Reinforcement," *Psychological Monographs*, Vol. 80, Whole No. 609 (1966).

If you turned out to be external on this self-assessment quiz, don't accept your current score as a given for life. If you want to shift your perspective, you can. People are not internal or external in every situation. At home you may go along with your parents' or roommates' preferences and let them call the shots. In class you might feel confident and participate without hesitation.

Take inventory of the situations in which you feel most and least in control. Are you bold on the basketball court but hesitant on a date? Do you feel confident that you can resolve a dispute with your friends but throw up your hands when a landlord refuses to refund your security deposit? Look for ways to exert more influence in situations in which you once yielded to external influences. See what a difference you can make.

MAKING THIS CHAPTER WORK FOR YOU

Review Questions

(LO 1.1) 1. _____ is defined as a state of complete physical, mental, and social well-being.
   a. Volatility
   b. Welfare
   c. Health
   d. Spirituality

(LO 1.1) 2. _____ refers to the ability to learn from life experience and the capacity to question and evaluate information.
   a. Psychological health
   b. Intellectual health
   c. Social health
   d. Spiritual health

(LO 1.2) 3. Which of the following statements is true of the health differences between men and women?
   a. The overall mortality rate of women is higher than that of men.
   b. Girls are more likely to be born prematurely than boys.
   c. Women die at a younger age than men.
   d. Women are more likely to suffer from depression than men.

(LO 1.2) 4. Which of the following statements is true about the health and habits of Americans, according to the latest findings from the Centers for Disease Control and Prevention?
a. More than 50 percent of men and women exercise regularly.
b. Two-thirds of the population are either over-weight or obese.
c. Five percent of all Americans over age 20 have hypertension.
d. Almost one-quarter of men and women between ages 18 and 44 saw a health-care professional in the previous year.

(LO 1.3) 5. Which of the following statements is true about the impact of unhealthy choices on young Americans?
a. Obese children often grow into obese adults, with risks of diabetes and cardiovascular disease.
b. A mild rise in blood pressure during young adulthood does not increase the risk of clogged heart arteries by middle age.
c. Young adults who begin using tobacco or alcohol in their teens and 20s are less likely to continue to do so as they get older.
d. Aerobic fitness has little impact on the cardiovascular health of individuals in later years.

(LO 1.3) 6. Which of the following statements is true about risky behaviors among college students?
a. Three-fourths of the deaths in the 15- to 24-year age range are men.
b. College-age women are more likely than men to engage in binge drinking.
c. Suicide rates are higher among women than men.
d. Men are more likely to avoid risky behaviors than women.

(LO 1.4) 7. Which of the following factors that influence health behavior include knowledge, attitudes, beliefs, values, and perceptions?
a. Enabling factors
b. Risk factors
c. Reinforcing factors
d. Predisposing factors

(LO 1.4) 8. In the transtheoretical model, which of the following processes of change involves acknowledging—first privately and then publicly—that you are responsible for your behavior and are the only one who can change it?
a. Consciousness-raising
b. Self-reevaluation
c. Commitment
d. Social liberation

Answers to these questions can be found on page 623.

Critical Thinking

1. Where are you on the wellness–illness continuum? What variables might affect your place on the scale? What do you consider your optimum state of health to be?
2. Talk to classmates from different racial or ethnic backgrounds than yours about their culture's health attitudes. Ask them what is considered healthy behavior in their cultures. For example, is having a good appetite a sign of health? What kinds of self-care practices did their parents and grandparents use to treat colds, fevers, rashes, and other health problems? What are their attitudes about the health-care system?
3. Jocelyn has been experiencing a great deal of fatigue and frequent headaches for the past couple of months. She doesn't have health insurance and doesn't want to spend money on a doctor visit. So she did some research on the Internet about ways to relieve her symptoms and was considering taking a couple of herbal supplements that were touted as potential treatments. If she asked you for your advice, what would you tell her? Do you think that self-care is appropriate in this situation?

Key Terms

The terms listed are used on the page indicated. Definitions of the terms are in the glossary at the end of the book.

enabling factors 14
health 2
health belief model (HBM) 14
health promotion 3
locus of control 18
predisposing factors 14
prevention 12

protection 12
reinforcing factors 14
self-efficacy 18
social norm 11
transtheoretical model 16
wellness 2

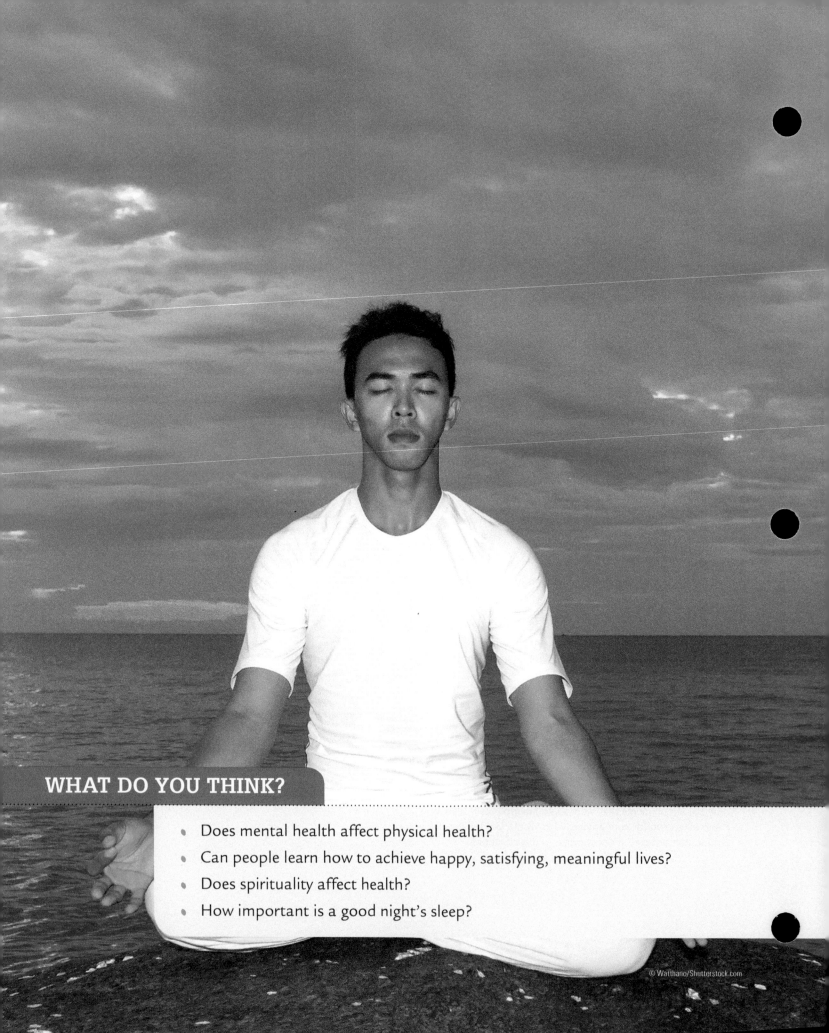

WHAT DO YOU THINK?

- Does mental health affect physical health?
- Can people learn how to achieve happy, satisfying, meaningful lives?
- Does spirituality affect health?
- How important is a good night's sleep?

© Watthano/Shutterstock.com

2

Your Psychological and Spiritual Well-Being

Josh never considered himself a spiritual person until he enrolled in a class on the science of personal well-being. For a homework assignment, he had to pursue different paths to happiness. As part of his experiment, he went to a Mardi Gras celebration and partied all night to see if having fun made him happier. To test whether doing good makes a person happy, Josh volunteered to help build a house for a homeless family. "I can't remember the name of a single person I met at the party," he says. "But I'll never forget the look on the family's faces when we handed them the keys to their new home."

For his final project, Josh, who did not have a religious upbringing, focused on developing a richer spiritual life. "The spirituality didn't end with the term," he says. "I continue to meditate, do yoga, and read religious texts because I believe a more spiritual life will help me in the long run with happiness and health." <

After reading this chapter, you should be able to:

2.1 Identify the characteristics of emotionally healthy individuals.

2.2 Summarize the components of positive psychology that can lead to a happy and purposeful life.

2.3 Describe the roles of autonomy and self-assertion in boosting self control.

2.4 Discuss the impact of spirituality on individuals.

2.5 Review the relationship of sleep and health.

The quest for a more fulfilling and meaningful life is attracting more people of all ages. The reason? As the burgeoning field of positive psychology has resoundingly proved, people who achieve emotional and spiritual health are more creative and productive, earn more money, attract more friends, enjoy better marriages, develop fewer illnesses, and live longer.

This chapter reports the latest findings on making the most of psychological strengths, enhancing happiness, and developing the spiritual dimension of your health and your life.

Emotional and Mental Health

"A sound mind in a sound body" was, according to the ancient Roman poet Juvenal, something all should strive for. This timeless advice still holds. Almost 2,000 years later, we understand on a much more scientific level that physical and mental health are interconnected in complex and vital ways. One does not guarantee the other, but recent research has found that individuals whose lifestyle includes the following four fundamental behaviors are less likely to become depressed, be overwhelmed by stress, or suffer poor mental health:

- Regular exercise
- A healthful diet
- Moderate alcohol use
- No tobacco

✓**check-in** Do you practice these four key behaviors?

Unlike physical health, psychological well-being cannot be measured, tested, X-rayed, or dissected. Yet psychologically healthy men and women generally share certain characteristics:

- They value themselves and strive toward happiness and fulfillment.
- They establish and maintain close relationships with others.
- They accept the limitations as well as the possibilities that life has to offer.
- They feel a sense of meaning and purpose that makes the gestures of living worth the effort required.

✓**check-in** How many of these characteristics do you have?

Psychological health encompasses both our emotional and mental states—that is, our feelings and our thoughts. **Emotional health** generally refers to feelings and moods, both of which are discussed later in this chapter. Characteristics of emotionally healthy persons include the following:

- Determination and effort to be healthy
- Flexibility and adaptability to a variety of circumstances
- Development of a sense of meaning and affirmation of life
- An understanding that the self is not the center of the universe
- Compassion for others
- The ability to be unselfish in serving or relating to others
- Increased depth and satisfaction in intimate relationships
- A sense of control over the mind and body that enables the person to make health-enhancing choices and decisions

Mental health describes our ability to perceive reality as it is, to respond to its challenges, and to develop rational strategies for living. A mentally healthy person doesn't try to avoid conflicts and distress but can cope with life's transitions, traumas, and losses in a way that allows for emotional stability and growth. The characteristics of mental health include:

- The ability to function and carry out responsibilities
- The ability to form relationships
- Realistic perceptions of the motivations of others
- Rational, logical thought processes
- The ability to adapt to change and to cope with adversity

✓**check-in** How would you assess yourself on each of these characteristics?

Culture also helps to define psychological health. In one culture, men and women may express feelings with great intensity, shouting in joy or wailing in grief, while in another culture, such behavior might be considered abnormal or unhealthy. In our diverse society, many cultural influences affect Americans' sense of who they are, where they came from, and what they believe. Cultural rituals help bring people together, strengthen their bonds, reinforce the values and beliefs they share, and provide a sense of belonging, meaning, and purpose.

emotional health The ability to express and acknowledge one's feelings and moods and exhibit adaptability and compassion for others.

mental health The ability to perceive reality as it is, respond to its challenges, and develop rational strategies for living.

culture The set of shared attitudes, values, goals, and practices of a group that are internalized by an individual within the group.

To find out where you are on the psychological well-being scale, take the Self Survey: Well-Being Scale.

The Lessons of Positive Mental Health

Positive psychology (the scientific study of ordinary human strengths and virtues) and positive psychiatry (which promotes positive psychosocial development in those with or at high risk of mental or physical illness) focus on the aspects of human experience that lead to happiness and fulfillment—in other words, on what makes life worthwhile.[1] This perspective has expanded the definition of psychological well-being.

According to psychologist Martin Seligman, Ph.D., who popularized the positive psychology movement, everyone, regardless of genes or fate, can achieve a happy, gratifying, meaningful life. The goal is not simply to feel good momentarily or to avoid bad experiences but to build positive strengths and virtues that enable us to find meaning and purpose in life. The core philosophy is to add a "build what's strong" approach to the "fix what's wrong" focus of traditional psychotherapy.[2]

Among the positive psychology interventions that have proven effective in enhancing emotional, cognitive, and physical well-being, easing depression, lessening disease and disability, and even increasing longevity are

- Counting one's blessings
- Savoring experiences
- Practicing kindness
- Pursuing meaning
- Setting personal goals
- Expressing gratitude
- Building compassion for one's self and others
- Identifying and using one's strengths (which may include traits such as kindness or perseverance)
- Visualizing and writing about one's best possible self at a time in the future[3]

Neuroscientists, using sophisticated imaging techniques, have been able to identify specific areas in the brain associated with positive emotions, such as love, hope, and enthusiasm. As

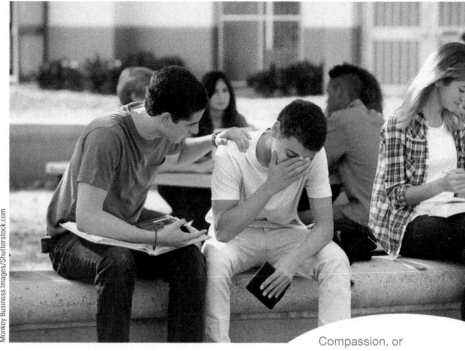

Monkey Business Images/Shutterstock.com

people change, the processing of emotions in the brain appears to change, with older adults responding more to positive information and filtering out irrelevant negative stimuli.[4]

✓**check-in** Practice positive psychology.

- The next time you think, "I've never tried that before," also say to yourself, "This is an opportunity to learn something new."
- When something seems too complicated, remind yourself to tackle it from another angle.
- If you get discouraged and feel that you're never going to get better at some new skill, tell yourself to give it another try. (See Health Now! for more suggestions.)

Know Yourself

Why do some students consistently invest in taking the best possible care of themselves while others repeatedly put their well-being at risk? The answers may lie within their personalities. Two personality traits in particular—conscientiousness (striving for competence and achievement, self-discipline, orderliness, reliability, deliberativeness) and extraversion (being active, talkative, assertive, social, stimulation-seeking)—correlate with very different health behaviors.

College students who rate high in conscientiousness tend to wear seat belts, get enough sleep, drive safely, use safer sex practices, exercise, not smoke, drink less, and eat fruits and vegetables.

Compassion, or caring for others, is a characteristic of an emotionally healthy person.

Accentuate the Positive

Try some of these strategies from positive psychology and comment on your experience in your online journal.

Do

- **Smile.** Putting on a happy face makes for a happy spirit.

- **Focus.** By being fully present in the moment, you'll experience it more intensely.

- **Share your joy.** Talking about and celebrating good experiences extends positive feelings over and above the positive event.

- **Travel through time.** Vividly remembering or anticipating positive events—a technique psychologists call "positive mental time travel"—boosts levels of happiness and life satisfaction.

Don't

- **Don't hide your feelings.** Suppressing positive feelings—because of shyness or a sense of modesty, for instance—diminishes them and may have physiological consequences on your health.

- **Don't get distracted.** Unrelated worries and thoughts detract from the here-and-now of a positive experience.

- **Don't find fault.** Paying attention to negative aspects of otherwise positive experiences sabotages levels of happiness, optimism, self-esteem, and life satisfaction.

- **Don't go there.** "Negative mental time travel"—reflecting on what went wrong or what may go wrong—can lower self-esteem and foster depressive symptoms.

self-compassion A healthy form of self-acceptance in the face of perceived inadequacy or failure.

The reason may be that they carefully weigh the risks and benefits of their behavior. They also can delay immediate gratification for the sake of long-term benefits, such as preventing cardiovascular disease or sexually transmitted infections.

Although they're more likely to participate in vigorous exercise, students who score high in extraversion are more likely to put their health at risk. They often drink more alcohol, binge-drink, smoke, engage in risky sexual behaviors, and don't get enough sleep. The reasons may involve brain chemistry. Individuals with low levels of neurochemical arousal may pursue highly stimulating (though risky) behaviors to feel more alert and excited.

✓**check-in** Is personality destiny? Not at all. If you see yourself as low in conscientiousness or high in extraversion, you can take deliberate steps that will safeguard your health. For instance, you might fulfill your need for stimulation and excitement with less risky alternatives, such as extreme sports competitions, rock-climbing, or volunteering with student-led emergency response services.

Develop Self-Compassion

Self-compassion is a healthy form of self-acceptance and a way of conceptualizing our favorable and unfavorable attitudes about ourselves and others. Some psychologists describe it as being kind to yourself in the face of suffering and practicing a "reciprocal golden rule," in which you treat yourself with the kindness usually reserved for others. This includes accepting your flaws; letting go of regrets, illusions, and disappointments; and taking responsibility for actions that may have harmed others without feeling a need to punish yourself.

Individuals high in self-compassion tend to

- Be understanding toward themselves when they make mistake

- Recognize that all humans are imperfect

- Not ruminate about their errors in judgment or behavior

- When feeling inadequate engage in soothing and positive self-talk

- Recognize that failure is an unavoidable part of the human experience so, they feel a greater sense of connection to others, even in the face of disappointment

- Not exaggerate the significance of painful thoughts (though they're mindful of them)

- Manage frustration by quelling self-pity and melodrama

In contrast, individuals low in self-compassion are extremely critical of themselves, believe they are unique in their imperfection, and obsessively fixate on their mistakes. After a traumatic life event, self-compassion may help individuals recognize the need to care for themselves, reach out for social support, engage in less self-blame and self-criticism, and look back on the time as an emotionally difficult event rather than an experience that defines or changes them.[5] Therapists have developed specific cognitive treatments that can increase the attributes of compassion for self and others and alleviate feelings of anxiety and depression.

✓**check-in** How do you practice self-compassion?

Boost Emotional Intelligence

A person's "IQ"—or intelligence quotient—was once considered the leading predictor of achievement. However, psychologists have determined that another "way of knowing," dubbed **emotional intelligence**, makes an even greater difference in personal and professional success.

"EQ" (for emotional quotient) is the ability to monitor and use emotions to guide thinking and actions. Neuroscientists have mapped the brain regions involved in emotional intelligence, which overlap significantly with those involved in general intelligence. Among the emotional competencies that most benefit students are focusing on clear, manageable goals and identifying and understanding emotions rather than relying on "gut" feelings.

✓**check-in** How emotionally intelligent do you think you are?

People with high EQ are more likely to enjoy good mental and physical health and are more productive at work and happier at home. They're also less prone to stress, depression, and anxiety, and they bounce back more quickly from serious illnesses.

Meet Your Needs

Newborns are unable to survive on their own. They depend on others for the satisfaction of their physical needs for food, shelter, warmth, and protection, as well as their less tangible emotional needs. In growing to maturity, children take on more responsibility and become more independent.

No one, however, becomes totally self-sufficient. As adults, we easily recognize our basic physical needs, but we often fail to acknowledge our emotional needs. Yet they, too, must be met if we are to be as fulfilled as possible.

The humanist theorist Abraham Maslow believed that human needs are the motivating factors in personality development. First, we must satisfy basic physiological needs, such as those for food, shelter, and sleep. Only then can we pursue fulfillment of our higher needs—for safety and security, love and affection, and self-esteem. Few individuals reach the state of **self-actualization**, in which one functions at the highest possible level and derives the greatest possible satisfaction from life (Figure 2.1).

✓**check-in** Where do you see yourself on Maslow's pyramid of needs?

Boost Self-Esteem

Each of us wants and needs to feel significant as a human being, with unique talents, abilities, and roles in life. A sense of **self-esteem**, of belief or pride in ourselves, gives us confidence to dare to attempt to achieve at school or work and to reach out to others to form friendships and close relationships. Self-esteem is the little voice that whispers, "You're worth it. You can do it. You're okay."

Self-esteem is based not on external factors like wealth or beauty but on what you believe about yourself. It's not something you're born with; self-esteem develops over time. It's also not something anyone else can give to you, although those around you can either help boost or diminish your self-esteem.

The seeds of self-esteem are planted in childhood when parents provide the assurance and appreciation youngsters need to push themselves toward new accomplishments: crawling, walking, forming words and sentences, learning control over their bladder and bowels.

Adults, too, must consider themselves worthy of love, friendship, and success if they are to be loved, to make friends, and to achieve their goals. Low self-esteem is more common in people who have been abused as children and in those with psychiatric disorders, including depression, anxiety, alcoholism, and drug dependence.

One of the most useful techniques for bolstering self-esteem and achieving your goals is developing the habit of positive thinking and talking.

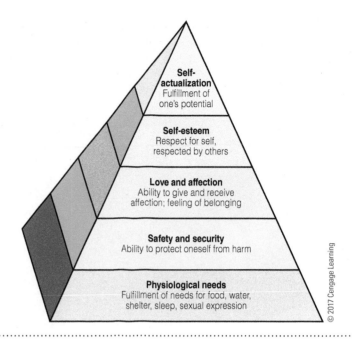

FIGURE 2.1 The Maslow Pyramid

To attain the highest level of psychological health, you must first satisfy your needs for safety and security, love and affection, and self-esteem.

While negative observations—such as constant criticisms or reminders of the most minor faults—can undermine self-image, positive affirmations—compliments, kudos, encouragements—have proved effective in enhancing self-esteem and psychological well-being. Individuals who fight off negative thoughts fare better psychologically than those who collapse when a setback occurs or who rely on others to make them feel better.

✓**check-in** How positive are the messages you send to yourself?

Pursue Happiness

"Imagine a drug that causes you to live eight or nine years longer, to make $15,000 more a year, to be less likely to get divorced," says Martin Seligman, the "father" of positive psychology. "Happiness seems to be that drug." As a meta-analysis of long-term studies has shown, happiness even reduces the risk of dying—both in healthy people and in those with diagnosed diseases. But even if just about everyone might benefit from smiling more and scowling less, can almost anyone learn to live on the brighter side of life?

Skeptics who dismiss "happichondria" as the latest feel-good fad are dubious. However, happiness researchers, backed by thousands of scientific studies, cite mounting evidence suggesting

emotional intelligence The ability to monitor and use emotions to guide thinking and actions.

self-actualization A state of wellness and fulfillment that can be achieved once certain human needs are satisfied; living to one's full potential.

self-esteem Confidence and satisfaction in oneself.

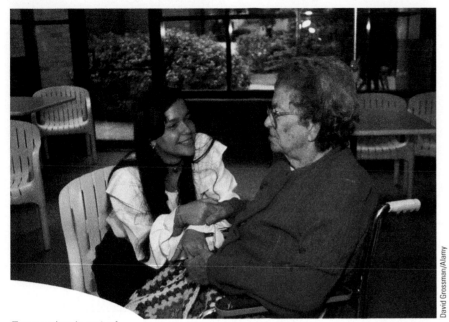

Even a simple act of kindness, such as visiting an elderly relative, can produce a profound sense of happiness and satisfaction.

David Grossman/Alamy

diagnosed with epilepsy face a lifetime of uncertainty about the occurrence of seizures.

What Does and Doesn't Make Us Happy

Many people assume that they can't be happy unless they get into a certain school, earn a certain grade, win a certain job, make a certain income, find a perfect mate, or look a certain way. But according to psychologist Sonja Lyubomirsky, author of *The Myths of Happiness*, such notions are false. "People find a way to be happy in spite of unwanted life circumstances," she notes, "and many people who are blessed by wealth and good fortune aren't any happier than those who lack these fortunes."[9]

Unfortunately, most of us look for happiness in the wrong places. We assume that external things—a bigger house, a better job, a winning lottery ticket—will gladden our lives. While they do bring temporary delight, the thrill invariably fades.

The joy we feel when we get something we desire—whether it's a new car or a sports trophy—doesn't last because of "hedonic habituation," the capacity to become accustomed to life changes and take them for granted. The bliss of acquiring a new cell phone or flat-screen TV generally fades in 6 to 12 weeks; the bliss of making a new friend, which is more dynamic and engaging, lasts longer. Children, despite all the challenges they bring, yield more joy than many possessions, according to studies of parents.[10]

Positive activities also boost positive emotions like happiness. One of the most effective is performing small acts of kindness. While there is no set formula for their variety and frequency, Lyubomirsky advises a minimum of once a week, which provides as much a boost as a thrice-weekly activity. She also recommends variety—taking out the trash when it's your roommate's turn one time, for instance, and buying a hot chocolate for a homeless person the next—because simple repetitions lose their ability to boost happiness.

In surveys of college students, the happiest generally shared one distinctive characteristic: a rich and fulfilling social life. Almost all were involved in a romantic relationship as well as in rewarding friendships. The happiest students spent the least time alone, and their friends rated them as highest on good relationships.

Even people we don't know may make us happy. By analyzing 20 years of data on the social ties of almost 5,000 participants in the Framingham Heart Study, researchers found that happy people spread happiness to others. Spouses, neighbors, relatives, and friends benefit most, but so did more distant contacts. The more happy people you surround yourself with, the happier you—and your social network—are likely to be in the future.

that happiness is, to a significant degree, a learned behavior. (See Health on a Budget, page 29.)

Among 5,000 students in 280 countries who completed a massive online open course (MOOC) on happiness, positive feelings kept going up as the course progressed. The students registered progressively less sadness, anger, and increasing fear and more amusement, enthusiasm, and affection.[6]

The Roots of Happiness

Psychological research has identified three major factors that contribute to a sense of well-being:

- Your happiness set point—a genetic component that contributes about 50 percent to individual differences in contentment

- Life circumstances such as income or marital status, which account for about 10 percent

- Thoughts, behaviors, beliefs, and goal-based activities, which may account for up to 40 percent of individual variations[7]

Education may protect against mental disorders, but it doesn't guarantee happiness. Asked if they were "feeling good and functioning well," people with varying levels of education had similar odds of high levels of emotional well-being.[8]

Intelligence, gender, and race do not matter much for happiness. Health has a greater impact on happiness than does income, but pain and anxiety take an even greater toll. People seem to be less able to adapt to the unpredictability of certain health conditions than they are to others. The well-being of individuals who can no longer walk after an accident, for example, typically returns to its pre-accident levels, while many

Happiness for Free!

Money can't buy happiness. As long as you have enough money to cover the basics, you don't need more wealth or more possessions for greater joy. Even people who win a fortune in a lottery return to their baseline of happiness within months. So rather than spend money on lottery tickets, try these ways to put a smile on your face:

- **Make time for yourself.** It's impossible to meet the needs of others without recognizing and fulfilling your own.

- **Up your appreciation quotient.** Regularly take stock of all the things for which you are grateful. To deepen the impact, write a letter of gratitude to someone who's helped you along the way.

- **String beads.** Think of every positive experience during the day as a bead on a necklace. This simple exercise focuses you on positive experiences, such as a cheery greeting from a cashier or a funny e-mail from a friend, and encourages you to act more kindly toward others.

- **Create a virtual DVD.** Visualize several of your happiest memories in as much detail as possible. Smell the air. Feel the sun. Hear the sea. Play this video in your mind when your spirits slump.

- **Fortify optimism.** Whenever possible, see the glass as half-full. Keep track of what's going right in your life. Imagine and write down your vision for your best possible future and track your progress toward it.

- **Immerse yourself.** Find activities that delight and engage you so much that you lose track of time. Experiment with creative outlets. Look for ways to build these passions into your life.

- **Seize the moment.** Rather than wait to celebrate big birthday-cake moments, savor a bite of cupcake every day. Delight in a child's cuddle, a glorious sunset, a lively conversation. Cry at the movies. Cheer at football games. This life is your gift to yourself. Open it!

This may also be true online—at least to a certain extent. According to a recent study of college students, their feelings of well-being increase along with the number of their Facebook friends—perhaps because seeing friends' photos reminds them of their social connections and enhances their feelings of self-worth. (See Chapter 5 for more on social media.)

✓**check-in** What are the greatest sources of happiness in your life?

Become Optimistic

Mental health professionals define **optimism** as the "extent to which individuals expect favorable outcomes to occur." Studies have established "significant relationships" between optimism and cardiovascular health, stroke risk, immune function, cancer prognoses, physical symptoms, pain, and mortality rates.[11]

For various reasons—because they believe in themselves, because they trust in a higher power, because they feel lucky—optimists expect positive experiences from life. When bad things happen, they tend to see setbacks or losses as specific, temporary incidents. In their eyes, a disappointment is "one of those things" that happens every once in a while rather than the latest in a long string of disasters.

In terms of health, optimists not only expect good outcomes—for instance, that a surgery will be successful—but take steps to increase this likelihood. Pessimists, expecting the worst, are more likely to deny or avoid a problem, sometimes through drinking or other destructive behaviors.

Individuals aren't born optimistic or pessimistic. Researchers have documented changes over time in the ways that individuals view the world and what they expect to experience in the future.[12] Cognitive-behavioral techniques (discussed in chapter 3) have proven effective in helping pessimists become more optimistic. In research on college students, learning to decrease automatic negative thoughts and increase more constructive ones reduced episodes of moderate depression.

✓**check-in** Do you usually anticipate the best or the worst possible outcome?

Manage Your Moods

Feelings come and go within minutes. A **mood** is a more sustained emotional state that colors our view of the world for hours or days. According to surveys by psychologist Randy Larsen of the University of Michigan, bad moods descend upon us an average of 3 out of every 10 days. "A few people—about 2 percent—are happy just about every day," he says. "About 5 percent report bad moods four out of every five days."[13]

There are gender differences in mood management: Men typically try to distract themselves (a partially successful strategy) or use alcohol or drugs (an ineffective tactic). Women are more

optimism The tendency to seek out, remember, and expect pleasurable experiences.

mood A sustained emotional state that colors one's view of the world for hours or days.

likely to talk to someone (which can help) or to ruminate on why they feel bad (which doesn't help). Learning effective mood-boosting, mood-regulating strategies can help both men and women pull themselves up and out of an emotional slump.

The most effective way to banish a sad or bad mood is by changing what caused it in the first place—if you can figure out what made you upset and why. "Most bad moods are caused by loss or failure in work or intimate relationships," says Larsen. "The questions to ask are: What can I do to fix the failure? What can I do to remedy the loss? Is there anything under my control that I can change? If there is, take action and solve it."

Rewrite the report. Ask to take a makeup exam. Apologize to the friend whose feelings you hurt. Tell your parents you feel bad about the argument you had.

If there's nothing you can do, accept what happened and focus on doing things differently next time. "In our studies, resolving to try harder actually was as effective in improving mood as taking action in the present," says Larsen.

You also can try to think about what happened in a different way and put a positive spin on it. This technique, known as *cognitive reappraisal,* or *reframing,* helps you look at a setback in a new light: What lessons did it teach you? What would you have done differently? Could there be a silver lining or hidden benefit?

··
√**check-in** Track your moods

Fear   Enthusiasm   Anger   Affection   Sadness   Amusement

··
Every day, rate how much each emoji
··
matches how you have been feeling on a
··
scale of 1 to 10. At the end of the week,
··
average your daily ratings into a collec-
··
tive score. Track how your feelings change
··
throughout the term.
··

Feeling in Control

Although no one has absolute control over destiny, we can do a great deal to control how we think, feel, and behave. By assessing our life situations realistically, we can make plans and preparations that allow us to make the most of our circumstances. By doing so, we gain a sense of mastery.

In nationwide surveys, Americans who feel in control of their lives report greater psychological well-being than those who do not, as well as extraordinarily positive feelings of happiness.

One way to boost self-control is with a short bout of moderately intense exercise. In an analysis of two dozen studies, a workout, such as a half-hour run or bike ride, improved "executive" brain functions, such as self-control, in people under age 35.[14]

Develop Autonomy

One goal that many people strive for is **autonomy**, or independence. Both family and society influence our ability to grow toward independence. Autonomous individuals are true to themselves. As they weigh the pros and cons of any decision, whether it's using or refusing drugs or choosing a major or career, they base their judgment on their own values, not those of others. Their ability to draw on internal resources and cope with challenges has a positive impact on both their psychological well-being and their physical health, including recovery from illness.

Those who've achieved autonomy may seek the opinions of others, but they do not allow their decisions to be dictated by external influences. For autonomous individuals, their locus of control—that is, where they view control as originating—is *internal* (from within themselves) rather than *external* (from others). (See Chapter 1.)

Autonomy also contributes to a sense of personal mastery, the tendency to feel that life circumstances are under one's control. A sense of mastery reflects general expectations about an individual's coping resources rather than confidence in performing specific behaviors. Closely rated to self-efficacy and an internal locus of control, mastery is associated with better cardiometabolic health and reduced risk for disease or death.[15]

Assert Yourself

Being assertive means recognizing your feelings and making your needs and desires clear to others. Unlike aggression, a far less healthy means of expression, assertiveness usually works. You can change a situation you don't like by communicating your feelings and thoughts in nonprovocative words, by focusing on specifics, and by making sure you're talking with the person who is directly responsible.

Becoming assertive isn't always easy. Many people have learned to cope by being passive and not communicating their feelings or opinions. Sooner or later they become so irritated, frustrated, or overwhelmed that they explode in an outburst—which they think of as being assertive. However, such behavior is so distasteful to them that they'd rather be passive. But assertiveness doesn't mean screaming or telling someone off. You can communicate your wishes calmly and clearly. Assertiveness is a behavior that respects your rights and the rights of other people even when you disagree.

Even at its mildest, assertiveness can make you feel better about yourself and your life. The reason: When you speak up or take action, you're in the driver's seat. And that's always much less stressful than taking a backseat and trying to hang on for dear life.

✓**check-in** When was the last time you asserted yourself? When was the last time you wished you had?

Spiritual Health

Whatever your faith, whether or not you belong to any formal religion, you are more than a body of a certain height and weight occupying space on the planet. You have a mind that equips you to learn and question. And you have a spirit that animates everything you say and do. **Spiritual health** refers to this breath of life and to our ability to identify our basic purpose in life and experience the fulfillment of achieving our full potential. Spiritual readings or practices can increase calmness, inner strength, and meaning; improve self-awareness; and enhance your sense of well-being. Religious support has also been shown to help lower depression and increase life satisfaction beyond the benefits of social support from friends and family.

Spirituality is a belief in what some call a higher power, in someone or something that transcends the boundaries of self. It gives rise to a strong sense of purpose, values, morals, and ethics. Throughout life you make choices and decide to behave in one way rather than another because your spirituality serves as both a compass and a guide.

The terms *religiosity* and *religiousness* refer to various spiritual practices. That definition

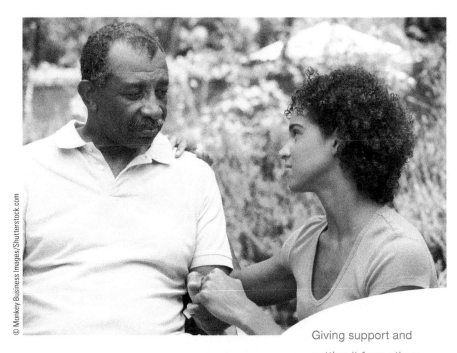

© Monkey Business Images/Shutterstock.com

Giving support and getting it from others are fundamental to good psychological health and emotional well-being.

may seem vague, but one thing is clear. According to thousands of studies on the relationship between religious beliefs and practices and health, religious individuals are less depressed, less anxious, and better able to cope with crises such as illness or divorce than are nonreligious ones. The more that a believer incorporates spiritual practices—such as prayer, meditation, or attending services—into daily life, the greater his or her sense of satisfaction with life.

In a ten-year study of young adults (average age 29), those who considered religion or spirituality "highly important" were 76 percent less likely to experience an episode of major depression—regardless of their religious denomination or whether they attended religious services. Other research has found that religiosity affects patterns of alcohol use[16] and vulnerability to eating disorders.[17]

✓**check-in** How would you describe your spiritual self?

Spirituality and Physical Health

A growing body of scientific evidence indicates that faith and spirituality can enhance health—and perhaps even extend life. Individuals who pray and report greater spiritual well-being consistently describe themselves as enjoying greater psychological and overall well-being.

Among the positive traits that correlate with a lower risk for heart disease, stroke, brain deterioration, or premature death is a strong sense of purpose, defined as "a sense of meaning and

spiritual health The ability to identify one's basic purpose in life and to achieve one's full potential.

spirituality A belief in someone or something that transcends the boundaries of self.

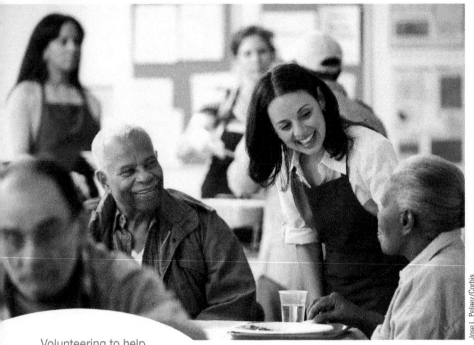
Jose L. Peláez/Corbis

Volunteering to help others, like these students serving meals to homeless people, can contribute to your sense of life satisfaction.

spiritual intelligence The capacity to sense, understand, and tap into ourselves, others, and the world around us.

values The criteria by which one makes choices about one's thoughts, actions, goals, and ideals.

reframing, acceptance, and humor. This implies that students who are already religious use their spirituality to bolster resources to focus on the problem at hand. Those who did not score high in spirituality but turned to religion in a crisis were more likely to do so as a way of avoiding or denying the problem, along with such maladaptive strategies as trying to distract themselves from it.[20]

Deepen Your Spiritual Intelligence

Mental health professionals have recognized the power of **spiritual intelligence**, which some define as "the capacity to sense, understand, and tap into the highest parts of ourselves, others, and the world around us." Spiritual intelligence, unlike spirituality, does not center on the worship of a God above, but on the discovery of a wisdom within.

All of us are born with the potential to develop spiritual intelligence, but most of us aren't even aware of it—and do little or nothing to nurture it. Part of the reason is that we confuse spiritual intelligence with religion, dogma, or old-fashioned morality.

"You don't have to go to church to be spiritually intelligent; you don't even have to believe in God," says Reverend Paul Edwards, a retired Episcopalian priest and therapist in Fullerton, California. "It is a scientific fact that when you are feeling secure, at peace, loved, and happy, you see, hear, and act differently than when you're feeling insecure, unhappy, and unloved. Spiritual intelligence allows you to use the wisdom you have when you're in a state of inner peace. And you get there by changing the way you think, basically by listening less to what's in your head and more to what's in your heart."

Clarify Your Values

Your **values** are the criteria by which you evaluate things, people, events, and yourself; they represent what's most important to you. In a world of almost dizzying complexity, values can provide guidelines for making decisions that are right for you. If understood and applied, they help give life meaning and structure.

When you confront a situation in which you must choose different paths or behaviors, follow these steps:

direction in one's life, which gives the feeling that life is worth living."[18] In older adults, a strong purpose in life lowers the risk of brain damage, dementia, and stroke.[19]

Church attendance may account for an additional two to three years of life (by comparison, exercise may add three to five extra years), according to researchers' calculations. According to data on nearly 95,000 participants in the landmark Women's Health Initiative, attending a weekly church service, regardless of an individual's faith, lowers the risk of death by 20 percent, compared with those who don't attend at all. Attending less frequently also reduces the risk, but by a smaller percentage. How does going to church add years to a life? Researchers speculate that the reason may be the sense of community or support or that people feel less depressed when they join in religious services.

Prayer and other religious experiences, including meditation, may actually change the brain—for the better. Using neuroimaging techniques, scientists have documented alterations in various parts of the brain that are associated with stress and anxiety. This effect may slow down the aging process, reduce psychological symptoms, and increase feelings of security, compassion, and love.

In a recent study, undergraduates with higher levels of spirituality coped with challenges by "turning to religion" along with other practical problem-solving strategies, such as positive

1. Carefully consider the consequences of each choice.

2. Choose freely from among all the options.

3. Publicly affirm your values by sharing them with others.

4. Act out your values.

Values clarification is not a once-in-a-lifetime task but an ongoing process of sorting out what matters most to you. Values are more than ideals we'd like to attain; they should be reflected in the way we live day by day.

✓**check-in** Do you put your values into action? If you believe in protecting the environment, for instance, do you shut off lights or walk rather than drive in order to conserve energy? Do you recycle newspapers, bottles, and cans?

Enrich Your Spiritual Life

Whatever role religion plays in your life, you have the capacity for deep, meaningful spiritual experiences that can add great meaning to everyday existence. You don't need to enroll in theology classes or commit to a certain religious preference. The following simple steps can start you on an inner journey to a new level of understanding:

- **Sit quietly.** The process of cultivating spiritual intelligence begins in solitude and silence. "There is an inner wisdom," says Dr. Dean Ornish, the pioneering cardiologist who incorporates spiritual health into his mind–body therapies, "but it speaks very, very softly." To tune into its whisper, turn down the volume in your busy, noisy, complicated life and force yourself to do nothing at all. This may sound easy; it's anything but.

- **Start small.** Create islands of silence in your day. Don't reach for the radio dial as soon as you get in the car. Leave your ear buds on as you walk across campus but turn off the music. Shut the door to your room, take a few huge deep breaths, and let them out very, very slowly. Don't worry if you're too busy to carve out half an hour for quiet contemplation. Even 10 minutes every day can make a difference.

- **Step outside.** For many people, nature sets their spirit free. Being outdoors, walking by the ocean, or looking at the hills puts the little hassles of daily living into perspective. As you wait for the bus or for a traffic light to change, let your gaze linger on silvery ice glazing a branch or an azalea bush in wild bloom. Follow the flight of a bird; watch clouds float overhead. Gaze into the night sky and think of the stars as holes in the darkness, letting the light of heaven shine through.

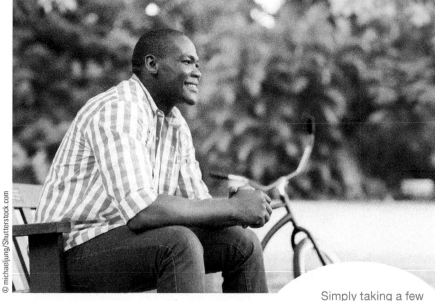

© michaeljung/Shutterstock.com

Simply taking a few moments to stop and enjoy the day can help quiet your mind and soothe your spirit.

- **Use activity to tune into your spirit.** Spirituality exists in every cell of the body, not just in the brain. As a student, you devote much of your day to mental labor. To tap into your spirit, try a less cerebral activity, such as singing, chanting, dancing, or drumming. Alternative ways of quieting your mind and tuning into your spirit include gardening, walking, arranging flowers, listening to music that touches your soul, or immersing yourself in a simple process like preparing a meal.

- **Ask questions of yourself.** Some people use their contemplative time to focus on a line of scripture or poetry. Others ask open-ended questions, such as What am I feeling? What are my choices? Where am I heading?

- **Trust your spirit.** While most of us rely on gut feelings to alert us to danger, our inner spirits usually nudge us not away from but toward some action that will somehow lead to a greater good—even if we can't see it at the time. You may suddenly feel the urge to call or e-mail a friend you've lost touch with—only to discover that he just lost a loved one and was grateful for the comfort of your caring.

- **Develop a spiritual practice:**

  - **If you are religious:** Deepen your spiritual commitment through prayer, more frequent church attendance, or participation in a prayer group.

  - **If you are not religious:** Keep an open mind about the value of religion or spirituality. Consider visiting a church or synagogue. Read the writings of inspired people of deep faith, such as Rabbi Harold Kushner and Rev. Martin Luther King, Jr.

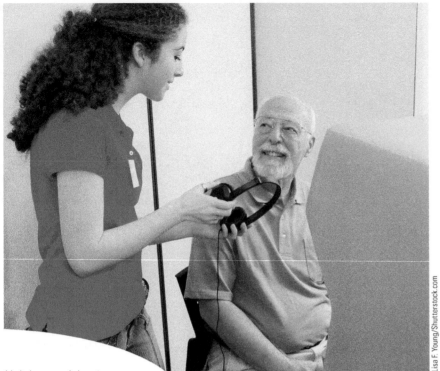

Helping or giving to others enhances self-esteem, relieves stress, and protects psychological well-being.

Lisa F. Young/Shutterstock.com

- **If you are not ready to consider religion:** Try nonreligious meditation or relaxation training. Research has shown that focusing the mind on a single sound or image can slow heart rate, respiration, and brain waves; relax muscles; and lower stress-related hormones—responses similar to those induced by prayer.

✓**check-in** Live your legacy. Write a one-page essay detailing your legacy as if you were a biographer recounting a long, fruitful life. Consider traits, accomplishments, and behaviors that you hope to be remembered for. Then consider what you do on an average day and how these activities align with the legacy you'd like to leave behind.

Consider the Power of Prayer

Prayer, a spiritual practice of millions, is the most commonly used form of complementary and alternative medicine. However, only in recent years has science launched rigorous investigations of the healing power of prayer.

Petitionary prayer—praying directly to a higher power—affects both the quality and quantity of life, says Dr. Harold Koenig, director of Duke University's Center for Spirituality, Theology and Health. "It boosts morale; lowers agitation, loneliness, and life dissatisfaction; and enhances ability to cope in men, women, the elderly, the young, the healthy, and the sick."

People who pray regularly have significantly lower blood pressure and stronger immune systems than those who are less religious. They're also hospitalized less often, less prone to alcoholism, and less likely to smoke heavily.[21]

Prayer may foster a state of peace and calm that could lead to beneficial changes in the cardiovascular and immune systems. Sophisticated brain imaging techniques have shown that prayer and meditation cause changes in blood flow in particular regions of the brain that may lead to lower blood pressure, slower heart rate, decreased anxiety, and an enhanced sense of well-being. However, praying for others, regardless of the type of prayer or religion, has not been shown to improve either symptoms or recovery of patients undergoing various medical procedures.

Will science ever be able to prove the power of prayer? No one is certain. "While I personally believe that God heals people in supernatural ways, I don't think science can shape a study to prove it," says Koenig. "But we now know enough, based on solid scientific research, to recommend prayer, much like exercise and diet, as one of the best and most cost-effective ways of protecting and enhancing health."

✓**check-in** Do you pray? Is there a specific reason why or why not?

Cultivate Gratitude

A grateful spirit brightens mood, boosts energy, and infuses daily living with a sense of glad abundance. Although giving thanks is an ancient virtue, only recently have researchers focused on the "trait" of gratitude—appreciation not just for a special gift but for everything that makes life a bit better. Feelings of gratitude are associated with better mood, improved sleep, less fatigue, less inflammation, and lower risk of heart failure.[22] Here are some of its psychological effects:

- More frequent and intense positive emotions
- More positive views of the social environment
- More productive coping strategies
- Greater appreciation of life and possessions

College students who keep gratitude journals report higher levels of happiness, feel better about their lives as a whole, are more likely to

3. Publicly affirm your values by sharing them with others.

4. Act out your values.

Values clarification is not a once-in-a-lifetime task but an ongoing process of sorting out what matters most to you. Values are more than ideals we'd like to attain; they should be reflected in the way we live day by day.

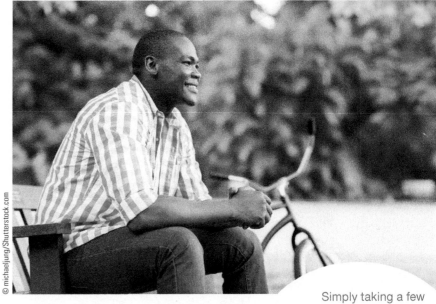
© michaeljung/Shutterstock.com

✓ **check-in** Do you put your values into action? If you believe in protecting the environment, for instance, do you shut off lights or walk rather than drive in order to conserve energy? Do you recycle newspapers, bottles, and cans?

Enrich Your Spiritual Life

Whatever role religion plays in your life, you have the capacity for deep, meaningful spiritual experiences that can add great meaning to everyday existence. You don't need to enroll in theology classes or commit to a certain religious preference. The following simple steps can start you on an inner journey to a new level of understanding:

• **Sit quietly.** The process of cultivating spiritual intelligence begins in solitude and silence. "There is an inner wisdom," says Dr. Dean Ornish, the pioneering cardiologist who incorporates spiritual health into his mind–body therapies, "but it speaks very, very softly." To tune into its whisper, turn down the volume in your busy, noisy, complicated life and force yourself to do nothing at all. This may sound easy; it's anything but.

• **Start small.** Create islands of silence in your day. Don't reach for the radio dial as soon as you get in the car. Leave your ear buds on as you walk across campus but turn off the music. Shut the door to your room, take a few huge deep breaths, and let them out very, very slowly. Don't worry if you're too busy to carve out half an hour for quiet contemplation. Even 10 minutes every day can make a difference.

• **Step outside.** For many people, nature sets their spirit free. Being outdoors, walking by the ocean, or looking at the hills puts the little hassles of daily living into perspective. As you wait for the bus or for a traffic light to change, let your gaze linger on silvery ice glazing a branch or an azalea bush in wild bloom. Follow the flight of a bird; watch clouds float overhead. Gaze into the night sky and think of the stars as holes in the darkness, letting the light of heaven shine through.

• **Use activity to tune into your spirit.** Spirituality exists in every cell of the body, not just in the brain. As a student, you devote much of your day to mental labor. To tap into your spirit, try a less cerebral activity, such as singing, chanting, dancing, or drumming. Alternative ways of quieting your mind and tuning into your spirit include gardening, walking, arranging flowers, listening to music that touches your soul, or immersing yourself in a simple process like preparing a meal.

• **Ask questions of yourself.** Some people use their contemplative time to focus on a line of scripture or poetry. Others ask open-ended questions, such as What am I feeling? What are my choices? Where am I heading?

• **Trust your spirit.** While most of us rely on gut feelings to alert us to danger, our inner spirits usually nudge us not away from but toward some action that will somehow lead to a greater good—even if we can't see it at the time. You may suddenly feel the urge to call or e-mail a friend you've lost touch with—only to discover that he just lost a loved one and was grateful for the comfort of your caring.

• **Develop a spiritual practice:**

  • **If you are religious:** Deepen your spiritual commitment through prayer, more frequent church attendance, or participation in a prayer group.

  • **If you are not religious:** Keep an open mind about the value of religion or spirituality. Consider visiting a church or synagogue. Read the writings of inspired people of deep faith, such as Rabbi Harold Kushner and Rev. Martin Luther King, Jr.

Simply taking a few moments to stop and enjoy the day can help quiet your mind and soothe your spirit.

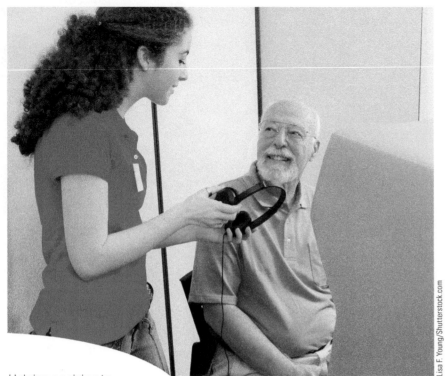

Helping or giving to others enhances self-esteem, relieves stress, and protects psychological well-being.

• **If you are not ready to consider religion:** Try nonreligious meditation or relaxation training. Research has shown that focusing the mind on a single sound or image can slow heart rate, respiration, and brain waves; relax muscles; and lower stress-related hormones—responses similar to those induced by prayer.

√**check-in** Live your legacy. Write a one-page essay detailing your legacy as if you were a biographer recounting a long, fruitful life. Consider traits, accomplishments, and behaviors that you hope to be remembered for. Then consider what you do on an average day and how these activities align with the legacy you'd like to leave behind.

Consider the Power of Prayer

Prayer, a spiritual practice of millions, is the most commonly used form of complementary and alternative medicine. However, only in recent years has science launched rigorous investigations of the healing power of prayer.

Petitionary prayer—praying directly to a higher power—affects both the quality and quantity of life, says Dr. Harold Koenig, director of Duke University's Center for Spirituality, Theology and Health. "It boosts morale; lowers agitation, loneliness, and life dissatisfaction; and enhances ability to cope in men, women, the elderly, the young, the healthy, and the sick."

People who pray regularly have significantly lower blood pressure and stronger immune systems than those who are less religious. They're also hospitalized less often, less prone to alcoholism, and less likely to smoke heavily.[21]

Prayer may foster a state of peace and calm that could lead to beneficial changes in the cardiovascular and immune systems. Sophisticated brain imaging techniques have shown that prayer and meditation cause changes in blood flow in particular regions of the brain that may lead to lower blood pressure, slower heart rate, decreased anxiety, and an enhanced sense of well-being. However, praying for others, regardless of the type of prayer or religion, has not been shown to improve either symptoms or recovery of patients undergoing various medical procedures.

Will science ever be able to prove the power of prayer? No one is certain. "While I personally believe that God heals people in supernatural ways, I don't think science can shape a study to prove it," says Koenig. "But we now know enough, based on solid scientific research, to recommend prayer, much like exercise and diet, as one of the best and most cost-effective ways of protecting and enhancing health."

√**check-in** Do you pray? Is there a specific reason why or why not?

Cultivate Gratitude

A grateful spirit brightens mood, boosts energy, and infuses daily living with a sense of glad abundance. Although giving thanks is an ancient virtue, only recently have researchers focused on the "trait" of gratitude—appreciation not just for a special gift but for everything that makes life a bit better. Feelings of gratitude are associated with better mood, improved sleep, less fatigue, less inflammation, and lower risk of heart failure.[22] Here are some of its psychological effects:

• More frequent and intense positive emotions

• More positive views of the social environment

• More productive coping strategies

• Greater appreciation of life and possessions

College students who keep gratitude journals report higher levels of happiness, feel better about their lives as a whole, are more likely to have made progress toward important personal goals, exercise more regularly, and report fewer negative health symptoms.

Among the most effective "gratitude interventions"—proven techniques for increasing appreciation—is keeping a diary and recording three things you are grateful for every day. In clinical studies, this approach has proven as effective as the rigorously developed and tested techniques used in psychotherapy. In experiments with students, expressions and displays of gratitude not only increased the helpers' sense of self-worth by making them feel valued but also spurred them to do more to help others.

....
√**check-in** Three Good Things
....
Every night, write down three good things
....
that happened during the day. They can
....
be big or small but should be specific (e.g.
....
"having a great dinner with close friends"
....
rather than "having great friends"). This
....
exercise takes practice, but as you train
....
yourself to notice and remember the little
....
things that make a difference, you'll feel
....
their impact more.[23]
....

Forgive

Being angry, harboring resentments, or reliving hurts over and over again is bad for your health in general and your heart in particular. The word *forgive* comes from the Greek for "letting go," and that's what happens when you forgive: You let go of all the anger and pain that have been demanding your time and draining your energy.

People may feel more in control, more powerful, when they're filled with anger, but forgiving instills a much greater sense of power. Forgiving a friend or family member may be more difficult than forgiving a stranger because the hurt occurs in a context in which people deliberately make themselves vulnerable. Forgiving yourself may be even harder.

When you forgive, you reclaim your power to choose. It doesn't matter whether someone deserves to be forgiven; you deserve to be free. However, forgiveness isn't easy. It's not a one-time thing but a process that takes a lot of time and work and involves both the conscious mind and the unconscious mind.

Forgiveness-based interventions for individuals, couples, and groups and for specific conditions such as bereavement and alcohol abuse have resulted in greater self-esteem and hopefulness, positive emotions toward others, less depression and anxiety, and improved resistance

How to Forgive

- **Compose an apology letter.** Address it to yourself and write it from someone who's hurt you. This simple task enables you to get a new perspective on a painful experience.

- **Leap forward in time.** In a visualization exercise, imagine that you are very old, meet a person who hurt you long ago, and sit down together on a park bench on a beautiful spring day. You both talk until everything that needs to be said finally is said. This allows you to benefit from the perspective time brings without having to wait years to achieve it.

- **Talk with "safe" people.** Vent your anger or disappointment with a trusted friend or a counselor, without the danger of saying or doing anything you'll regret later. And if you can laugh about what happened with a friend, the laughter helps dissolve the rage.

- **Forgive the person, not the deed.** In themselves, abuse, rape, murder, and betrayal are beyond forgiveness. But you can forgive people who couldn't manage to handle their own suffering, misery, confusion, and desperation.

to drug use. In college students, such interventions have helped relieve symptoms of depression and reduce suicidal thoughts and behavior.

....
√**check-in** Is there someone in your life
....
you haven't forgiven—yet?
....

Sleepless on Campus

You stay up late cramming for a final. You drive through the night to visit a friend at another campus. You get up for an early class during the week but stay in bed until noon on weekends. And you wonder: "Why am I so tired?" The answer: You're not getting enough sleep. You're hardly alone. According to the Centers for Disease Control and Prevention (CDC),

- Only one-third of Americans say they get enough sleep.

- An estimated 50 to 70 million American adults suffer from sleep and wakefulness disorders.

- Women are more likely than men to report not getting enough sleep.

- African Americans reported getting less sleep compared with all other ethnic groups.

SNAPSHOT: ON CAMPUS NOW

📷 Sleepy Students

Over the past seven days, students getting enough sleep to feel rested in the morning:

	Percent (%)		
	Male	Female	Average
0 days	8.0	10.2	9.5
1–2 days	26.2	30.9	29.3
3–5 days	51.1	48.5	49.3
6+ days	14.7	10.4	11.9

Students often feeling tired, dragged out, or sleepy during the day:

	Percent (%)		
	Male	Female	Average
0 days	12.2	6.0	8.2
1–2 days	35.0	28.3	30.6
3–5 days	40.7	46.3	44.3
6+ days	12.1	19.3	16.9

Impact of sleepiness on daytime activities:

	Percent (%)		
	Male	Female	Average
No problem	14.0	7.8	9.9
A little problem	49.8	48.4	48.8
More than a little problem	22.4	25.6	24.5
A big problem	9.8	13.0	11.9
A very big problem	3.9	5.3	4.9

Source: American College Health Association. *American College Health Association–National College Health Assessment II: Reference Group Executive Summary, Spring 2014.* Hanover, MD: American College Health Association, 2014.

> ✓**check-in** Are you getting enough sleep? The National Sleep Foundation recommends seven to nine hours for men and women ages 18 to 25. How do you compare?

Student Night Life

College students are notorious for their erratic sleep schedules and late bedtimes. In various studies, 25 to 50 percent of undergraduates have reported significant daytime sleepiness, which may affect academic performance as well as daily tasks such as driving. In the National College Health Assessment, about one in five college students said that sleep difficulties have affected their academic performance, ranking behind stress and anxiety.[24] (See Snapshot: On Campus Now.)

Alcohol compounds many students' sleep problems. Poor-quality sleepers report drinking more alcohol than good sleepers and are twice as likely to use alcohol to induce sleep as are better sleepers. Students who drink more alcohol go to bed later, sleep less, and show greater differences between weekday and weekend sleep timing and duration. In general, students who do not adhere to a regular bedtime and rising schedule are more likely to be poor sleepers.

Female students generally have poorer sleep patterns than males and suffer more consequences as a result. Women report more sleep disturbances than men and are at greater risk for poor academic performance and more physical, social, and emotional problems. Men sleep better at the beginning of the academic year, but their sleep quality decreases. Women's sleep quality worsens only slightly over the school year. Students reporting poor quality sleep feel more tense, irritable, anxious, depressed, angry, and confused than others.

On average, college students go to bed 1 to 2 hours later and sleep 1 to 1.6 hours less than students of a generation ago. In comparisons of exhaustion levels reported by workers in various occupations, college students consistently score high. Figure 2.2 shows a campus campaign to encourage students to get more sleep.

Fortunately, college students can learn to sleep better. In an experiment with introductory psychology students—mostly freshmen—those who learned basic sleep skills significantly improved their overall sleep quality compared with students who did not receive such training.

✓**check-in** Do you feel rested every day?

Sleep's Impact on Health

The following are some of the key ways in which your nighttime sleep affects your daytime well-being:

- **Learning and memory.** When you sleep, your brain helps "consolidate" new information, so you are more likely to retain it in your memory.

- **Metabolism and weight.** The less you sleep, the more weight you may gain.[25] Chronic sleep deprivation may cause weight gain by altering metabolism (for example, changing the way individuals process and store carbohydrates) and by stimulating excess stress hormones. Loss of sleep also reduces levels of the hormones that regulate appetite, which may be why, in one study, young normal-weight men ate larger portions of high-calorie junk foods than they did after a normal night of sleep.[26]

- **Safety.** People who don't get adequate nighttime sleep are more likely to fall asleep during the daytime. Daytime sleepiness can cause falls, medical errors, air traffic mishaps, and road accidents.

- **Mood/quality of life.** Too little sleep—whether just for a night or two or for longer periods—can cause psychological symptoms, such as irritability, impatience, inability to concentrate, lack of motivation, moodiness, and lowered long-term life satisfaction.

- **Immunity.** Sleep deprivation alters immune function, including the activity of the body's killer cells. If you get less than seven hours of sleep a night, you're three times more likely to catch a cold. And if you sleep poorly, you're five times more susceptible.

- **Mental disorders.** Disturbed sleep can be an early sign of mental illness; sleep loss may trigger or may be an early sign of a manic episode (see the discussion of bipolar disorder on page 58).[27] Too much (10 or more hours a night) or too little (5 or fewer hours) sleep, according to recent research, can increase the risk of depression.

- **Major diseases and death.** Serious sleep disorders such as insomnia and sleep apnea have been linked to hypertension, increased

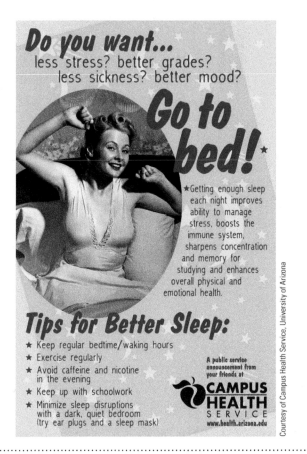

FIGURE 2.2 "Go to Bed" campaign poster

stress hormone levels, irregular heartbeats, and increased inflammation (which, as discussed in Chapter 15, may play a role in heart attacks). Inadequate sleep also has been linked to higher overall death rates.

- **Sexuality.** In a study of college women, those who slept longer were more likely to engage in sexual activity the following day. On average the women slept 7 hours, 22 minutes, with each hour of sleep increasing the women's sexual desire and likelihood of sexual activity.[28]

What Happens When We Sleep?

A normal night of sleep consists of several distinct stages of sleep, divided into two major types: an active state, characterized by rapid eye movement (REM) and called REM sleep (or dream sleep), and a quiet state, referred to as non-REM or NREM sleep, that consists of four stages:

- In **Stage 1**, a twilight zone between full wakefulness and sleep, the brain produces small, irregular, rapid electrical waves. The muscles of the body relax, and breathing is smooth and even.

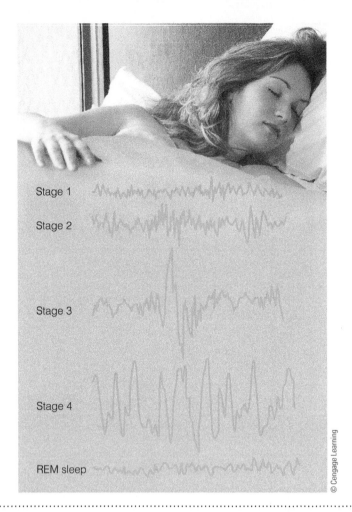

Stage 1

Stage 2

Stage 3

Stage 4

REM sleep

© Cengage Learning

FIGURE 2.3 Stages of Sleep

Differences in brain wave patterns characterize the various stages of sleep.

- In **Stage 2**, brain waves are larger and punctuated with occasional sudden bursts of electrical activity. The eyes are no longer responsive to light. Bodily functions slow still more.

- **Stages 3 and 4** constitute the most profound state of unconsciousness. The brain produces slower, larger waves, and this is sometimes referred to as "delta" or slow-wave sleep (Figure 2.3).

After about an hour in the four stages of non-REM sleep, sleepers enter the time of vivid dreaming called REM sleep, when brain waves resemble those of waking more than those of quiet sleep. The large muscles of the torso, arms, and legs are paralyzed and cannot move—possibly to prevent sleepers from acting out their dreams. The fingers and toes may twitch; breathing is quick and shallow; blood flow through the brain speeds up; men may have partial or full erections.

How Much Sleep Do You Need?

Over the last century, we have cut our average nightly sleep time by 20 percent. More than half of us try to get by with less than seven hours of shut-eye a night. College students are no exception, with an average sleep time slightly less than seven hours, with little difference between men and women.

No formula can say how long a good night's sleep should be. Normal sleep times range from five to ten hours; the average is seven and a half. About one or two people in a hundred can get by with just five hours; another small minority needs twice that amount. Each of us seems to have an innate sleep *appetite* that is as much a part of our genetic programming as hair color and skin tone.

√ **check-in** Do you use an electronic device before bedtime? If so, it may be disrupting your sleep. In a study of 10,000 young men and women, the use of any electronic device—computer, smartphone, tablet, video game console, television, MP3 player—during the day, particularly in the hour before bedtime, increased time before falling sleep. Time before falling asleep increased with more than two hours of screen time late in the day.[29]

To figure out your sleep needs, keep your wake-up time the same every morning and vary your bedtime. Are you groggy after six hours of shut-eye? Does an extra hour give you more stamina? What about an extra two hours? Since too much sleep can make you feel sluggish, don't assume that more is always better. Listen to your body's signals, and adjust your sleep schedule to suit them.

Are you better off pulling an all-nighter before a big test or closing the books and getting a good night's sleep? According to researchers, that depends on the nature of the exam. If it's a test of facts—Civil War battles, for instance—cramming all night works. However, if you will have to write analytical essays in which you compare, contrast, and make connections, you need to sleep to make the most of your reasoning abilities.

To Nap or Not to Nap?

Is napping good or bad for you? That depends. In a recent study, a late-afternoon nap proved to undo the negative impact on hormones and immunity of a lost night of sleep.[30] However, napping can disrupt the sleep-wake cycle, which can lead to negative health consequences such as depression, metabolic abnormalities, and hormonal disruptions. Longer naps are associated with poorer overall sleep quality than shorter ones and can cause "sleep inertia," a lethargy that can last for several hours. In a study of college students, quantity and quality sleep as well as GPA and class attendance suffered in those who did the following:

- Napped more than three times a week
- Napped for more than two hours
- Napped between 6:00 and 9:00 p.m.[31]

✓**check-in** Do you nap at least once a week? Four in ten college students say they do.[32]

Sleep Disorders

Three of four Americans struggle to get a good night's sleep at least a few nights a week. According to the National Commission on Sleep Disorders Research, 40 million adults suffer from a specific sleep disorder, such as chronic insomnia or sleep apnea; an additional 20 to 30 million have occasional sleep difficulties. The estimated economic cost of sleeplessness may be higher than $300 million a year.

✓**check-in** Are you a poor sleeper? In a recent study, about six in ten colleges students were characterized as poor sleepers. The causes include irregular sleep-wake schedules, late-to-bed times, a noisy/bright/disruptive sleep environment, and early morning classes.[33]

Insomnia Individuals with insomnia—a lack of sleep so severe that it interferes with functioning during the day—may toss and turn for an hour or more when they get into bed, wake frequently in the night, wake up too early, or not be able to sleep long enough to feel alert and energetic the next day. Most often insomnia is transient, typically occurring before or after a major life event (such as a job interview) and lasting for three or four nights. During periods of prolonged stress (such as a marriage breakup), short-term insomnia may continue for several weeks. Chronic or long-term insomnia, which can begin at any age, may persist for long periods. About three-fourths of insomniacs struggle to sleep more for at least a year; almost half, for three years.

For about a third of those with chronic insomnia, the underlying problem is a mental disorder, most often depression or an anxiety disorder. Many substances, including alcohol, medications,

and drugs of abuse, often disrupt sleep. About 15 percent of those seeking help for chronic insomnia suffer from "learned" or "behavioral" insomnia. While a life crisis may trigger their initial sleep problems, each night they try harder and harder to get to sleep, but they cannot—although they often doze off while reading or watching a movie.

Sleeping pills may be used for a specific, time-limited problem—always with a physician's supervision. (See Consumer Alert, p. 39.) In the long term, behavioral approaches, including the following, have proved more effective:

- **Relaxation therapy,** which may involve progressive muscle relaxation, diaphragmatic breathing, hypnosis, or meditation
- **Cognitive therapy,** which challenges misconceptions about sleep and helps shift a poor sleeper's mind away from anxiety-inducing thoughts
- **Stimulus control therapy,** in which individuals who do not fall asleep quickly must get up and leave their beds until they are very sleepy

⊙ CONSUMER ALERT

Sleeping Pill Precautions

Chances are you've taken some form of sleep medication. After aspirin, they are the most widely used drugs in the United States. If sleeping pills seem the best option at a certain time in your life, use them with caution.

Facts to Know

- **Sleeping pills** are not a long-term solution to a sleep problem, but they can be helpful if travel, injury, or illness interfere with your nightly rest.
- **Prescription and over-the-counter sleep aids** can interact with other medications or a medical condition, so always check with your doctor before taking them.
- **If taken too often** or for more than several nights, some sleeping pills may cause rebound insomnia—sleeplessness that returns in full force when you stop taking the medication.

Steps to Take

- **Read carefully.** Take time to read through the informational materials and

warnings on pill containers. Make sure you understand the potential risks and the behaviors to avoid.

- **If you are a woman, take half the standard dose.** The FDA has found that women metabolize sleeping medications much more slowly than men so their effects linger longer.
- **Avoid alcohol.** Never mix alcohol and sleeping pills. Alcohol increases the sedative effects of the pills. Even a small amount of alcohol combined with sleeping pills can make you feel dizzy, confused, or faint.
- **Quit carefully.** When you're ready to stop taking sleeping pills, follow your doctor's instructions or the directions on the label. Some medications must be stopped gradually.
- **Watch for side effects.** If you feel sleepy or dizzy during the day, talk to your doctor about changing the dosage or discontinuing the pills.

- **Sleep restriction therapy,** in which sleep times are sharply curtailed in order to improve the quality of sleep

Breathing Disorders (Snoring and Sleep Apnea)

Although most people snore in certain positions or when they have stuffed-up noses, snoring can be a sign of a serious problem and increases the likelihood of health problems and of accidents. Caused by the vibration in tissues in the mouth and throat as a sleeper tries to suck air into the lungs, snoring can be so loud that it disrupts a bed partner or others in the same house. In young people, the cause is most likely to be enlarged tonsils or adenoids. In adults, extreme snoring may be a symptom of sleep apnea, which may itself be harmful to health. Heavy snorers and people with sleep apnea may be more likely to develop memory and thinking problems at younger ages than their better-rested peers.[34]

Translated from the Greek words meaning "no" and "breath," apnea is exactly that: the absence of breathing for a brief period. People with sleep apnea may briefly stop breathing dozens or even hundreds of times during the night. As they struggle for breath, they may gasp for air, snore extremely loudly, or thrash about.

Although apnea, which can lead to high blood pressure, stroke, and cardiovascular disease, may affect as many as 10 million Americans, most are unaware of the problem. More physical activity and fewer hours sitting can lead to improvements. Effective treatments include weight loss (if obesity is contributing to the problem), a nasal mask that provides continuous positive airway pressure (CPAP) to ensure a steady flow of air into the lungs, and, in severe cases, surgery to enlarge the upper airway. Treatment can reduce snoring, improve quality of sleep, and boost performance at work or school.

Movement Disorders

Restless legs syndrome, which may affect 12 million Americans, is a movement disorder characterized by symptoms that patients describe as pulling, burning, tingling, creepy-crawly, grabbing, buzzing, jitteriness, or gnawing. Many people with these symptoms have difficulty falling or staying asleep but do not realize that the cause is a medical disorder that can be treated with regular physical activity. Medications also are available.

Circadian Rhythm Sleep Disorders

Problems involving the timing of sleep are called circadian rhythm disorders because they affect the basic circadian ("about a day") rhythm that influences many biological processes. The most common causes are jet lag and shift work. Jet lag generally improves on its own within two to seven days, depending on the length of the trip and the individual's response. Avoiding caffeine and alcohol and immediately switching to the new time zone's schedule can help in overcoming jet lag.

A "shift work" circadian rhythm disorder consists of any inability to sleep when one wants or to stay alert when needed because of frequently changing work shifts. Behavioral strategies and good sleep habits can help. In addition, phototherapy—exposure to bright light for periods ranging from 30 minutes to two hours—has shown promise as an experimental treatment to help shift workers adjust to their changing schedules.

√**check-in** Have you experienced Exploding Head Syndrome? An estimated 18 percent of college students have heard loud sounds (a bomb going off or gunshots) or sensed an explosion in their heads as they were falling asleep or waking up. Most had recurrent episodes. Although not physically painful, Exploding Head Syndrome produces intense fear and apprehension, which causes significant distress or impairment for some students.[35]

Sleeping Pills

The use of prescription sleeping pills has more than doubled in the last decade, and increasing numbers of teenagers and young adults use these medications either occasionally or regularly. An even greater number buy nonprescription or over-the-counter (OTC) sleep inducers. Others rely on herbal remedies, antihistamines, and other medications to get to sleep.

In the long run, good sleep habits, regular exercise, and a tranquil sleep environment are the cornerstones of high-quality sleep. But if circumstances, travel, injury, or illness have disrupted your sleep, you may consider sleep medications. Here is what you need to know about them. (See Consumer Alert.)

- **Over-the-counter medications.** Various over-the-counter sleeping pills, sold in any pharmacy or supermarket, contain antihistamines, which induce drowsiness by working against the central nervous system chemical histamine. They may help for an occasional sleepless night, but the more often you take them, the less effective they become.

- **Dietary supplements.** The most widely publicized dietary supplement is the hormone melatonin, which may help control your body's internal clock. The melatonin supplements most often found in health food stores and pharmacies are synthetic versions of the natural hormone. Although these supplements may help some people fall asleep or stay asleep and may sometimes help prevent jet lag, there are many unanswered questions about melatonin. Reported side effects include drowsiness, headaches, stomach discomfort, confusion, decreased body temperature, seizures, and drug interactions. The optimal dose isn't certain, and the long-term effects are unknown. Other supplements—such as valerian, chamomile, and kava—have yet to be fully studied for safety or effectiveness in relieving insomnia.

- **Prescription medications.** The newest sleep drugs—nonbenzodiazepine hypnotic medications such as Lunesta (eszopiclone), Ambien/Ambien CR (zolpidem), and Sonata (zaleplon)—quiet the nervous system, which helps induce sleep. They're metabolized quickly, which helps reduce the risk of side effects the next day. These medications, which can interact with other medications, are mainly intended for short-term or intermittent use.

WHAT DID YOU DECIDE?

- Does mental health affect physical health?
- Can individuals learn how to achieve happy, satisfying, meaningful lives?
- Does spirituality affect health?
- How important is a good night's sleep?

THE POWER OF NOW!
Building a Fulfilling Life

Just like physical health, psychological well-being involves more than an absence of problems. By developing your inner strengths and resources, you become the author of your life, capable of confronting challenges and learning from them. As positive psychologists have discovered, you have greater control over how happy, optimistic, upbeat, and lovable you are than anyone or anything else. But only by consciously taking charge of your life can you find happiness and fulfillment.

Here are some suggestions to enhance your emotional health now and in the future. Check the ones that you already practice and then work on adding others.

____ Recognize and express your feelings. Pent-up emotions tend to fester inside, building into anger or depression.

____ Don't brood. Rather than merely mulling over a problem, try to find solutions that are positive and useful.

____ Take one step at a time. As long as you're taking some action to solve a problem, you can take pride in your ability to cope.

____ Spend more time doing those activities you know you do best. For example, if you are a good cook, prepare a meal for someone.

____ Separate what you do, especially any mistakes you make, from who you are. Instead of saying, "I'm so stupid," tell yourself, "That wasn't the smartest move I ever made, but I'll learn from it."

____ Use affirmations, positive statements that help reinforce the most positive aspects of your personality and experience. Every day, you might say, "I am a loving, caring person," or "I am honest and open in expressing my feelings." Write some affirmations of your own on index cards and flip through them occasionally.

____ List the things you would like to have or experience. Construct the statements as if you were already enjoying the situations you list, beginning each sentence with "I am." For example, "I am feeling great about doing well in my classes."

What's Online

CENGAGE
brain
.com

Visit www.cengagebrain.com to access course materials for this text, including the Behavior Change Planner, interactive quizzes, tutorials, and more.

self survey

Well-Being Scale

Part I

The following questions contain statements and their opposites. Notice that the statements extend from one extreme to the other. Where would you place yourself on this scale? Place a circle on the number that is most true for you at this time. Do not put your circles between numbers.

Life Purpose and Satisfaction

#	Statement	Low end	Scale	High end
1.	During most of the day, my energy level is	very low	1 2 3 4 5 6 7	very high
2.	As a whole, my life seems	dull	1 2 3 4 5 6 7	vibrant
3.	My daily activities are	not a source of satisfaction	1 2 3 4 5 6 7	a source of satisfaction
4.	I have come to expect that every day will be	exactly the same	1 2 3 4 5 6 7	new and different
5.	When I think deeply about life	I do not feel there is any purpose to it	1 2 3 4 5 6 7	I feel there is a purpose to it
6.	I feel that my life so far has	not been productive	1 2 3 4 5 6 7	been productive
7.	I feel that the work[1] I am doing	is of no value	1 2 3 4 5 6 7	is of great value
8.	I wish I were different than who I am.	agree strongly	1 2 3 4 5 6 7	disagree strongly
9.	At this time, I have	no clearly defined goals for my life	1 2 3 4 5 6 7	clearly defined goals for my life
10.	When sad things happen to me or other people	I cannot feel positive about life	1 2 3 4 5 6 7	I continue to feel positive about life
11.	When I think about what I have done with my life, I feel	worthless	1 2 3 4 5 6 7	worthwhile
12.	My present life	does not satisfy me	1 2 3 4 5 6 7	satisfies me
13.	I feel joy in my heart	never	1 2 3 4 5 6 7	all the time
14.	I feel trapped by the circumstances of my life.	agree strongly	1 2 3 4 5 6 7	disagree strongly
15.	When I think about my past	I feel many regrets	1 2 3 4 5 6 7	I feel no regrets
16.	Deep inside myself	I do not feel loved	1 2 3 4 5 6 7	I feel loved
17.	When I think about the problems that I have	I do not feel hopeful about solving them	1 2 3 4 5 6 7	I feel very hopeful about solving them

Part II

Self-Confidence during Stress (Answer according to how you feel during stressful times.)

#	Statement	Low end	Scale	High end
1.	When there is a great deal of pressure being placed on me	I get tense	1 2 3 4 5 6 7	I remain calm
2.	I react to problems and difficulties	with a great deal of frustration	1 2 3 4 5 6 7	with no frustration
3.	In a difficult situation, I am confident that I will receive the help that I need.	disagree strongly	1 2 3 4 5 6 7	agree strongly
4.	I experience anxiety	all the time	1 2 3 4 5 6 7	never

[1]The definition of work is not limited to income-producing jobs. It includes childcare, housework, studies, and volunteer services.

42   CHAPTER 2 • Your Psychological and Spiritual Well-Being

5.	When I have made a mistake	I feel extreme dislike for myself	1 2 3 4 5 6 7	I continue to like myself
6.	I find myself worrying that something bad is going to happen to me or those I love	all the time	1 2 3 4 5 6 7	never
7.	In a stressful situation	I cannot concentrate easily	1 2 3 4 5 6 7	I can concentrate easily
8.	I am fearful	all the time	1 2 3 4 5 6 7	never
9.	When I need to stand up for myself	I cannot do it	1 2 3 4 5 6 7	I can do it easily
10.	I feel less than adequate in most situations.	agree strongly	1 2 3 4 5 6 7	disagree strongly
11.	During times of stress, I feel isolated and alone.	agree strongly	1 2 3 4 5 6 7	disagree strongly
12.	In really difficult situations	I feel unable to respond in positive ways	1 2 3 4 5 6 7	I feel able to respond in positive ways
13.	When I need to relax	I experience no peace—only thoughts and worries	1 2 3 4 5 6 7	I experience a peacefulness—free of thoughts and worries
14.	When I am frightened	I panic	1 2 3 4 5 6 7	I remain calm
15.	I worry about the future	all the time	1 2 3 4 5 6 7	never

Scoring

The number you circled is your score for that question. Add your scores in each of the two sections and divide each sum by the number of questions in the section.

- Life Purpose and Satisfaction: _____ ÷ 17 = ____.__
- Self-Confidence during Stress: _____ ÷ 15 = ____.__
- Combined Well-Being: (add scores for both) _____ ÷ 32 = ____.__

Each score should range between 1.00 and 7.00 and may include decimals (for example, 5.15).

Interpretation

VERY LOW: 1.00 TO 2.49
MEDIUM LOW: 2.50 TO 3.99
MEDIUM HIGH: 4.00 TO 5.49
VERY HIGH: 5.50 TO 7.00

These scores reflect the strength with which you feel these positive emotions. Do they make sense to you? Review each scale and each question in each scale. Your score on each item gives you information about the emotions and areas in your life where your psychological resources are strong, as well as the areas where strength needs to be developed.

If you notice a large difference between the LPS and SCDS scores, use this information to recognize which central attitudes and aspects of your life most need strengthening. If your scores on both scales are very low, talk with a counselor or a friend about how you are feeling about yourself and your life.

MAKING THIS CHAPTER WORK FOR YOU

Review Questions

(LO 2.1)   1. _____ describes our ability to perceive reality as it is, to respond to its challenges, and to develop rational strategies for living.
   a. Emotional health
   b. Spiritual health
   c. Physical health
   d. Mental health

(LO 2.1)   2. Which of the following statements is true of the psychological health of a person?
   a. It encompasses the physical and spiritual health of a person.
   b. It encompasses the emotional and mental health of a person.
   c. It can be measured and tested.
   d. It considers "IQ," or intelligence, quotient as the leading predictor of achievement.

(LO 2.2)   3. Treating yourself with kindness usually reserved for others is a feature of _____.
   a. self-compassion
   b. self-schema
   c. self-actualization
   d. self-esteem

(LO 2.2)   4. Which of the following approaches to practicing positive psychology requires a person to expect positive experiences from life?
   a. Boosting his or her intelligence quotient
   b. Relying on others to make them feel better
   c. Becoming optimistic
   d. Concentrating on constant criticisms

(LO 2.3)   5. People who are autonomous _____.
   a. allow their decisions to be dictated by external influences
   b. have absolute control over their destiny
   c. are true to themselves
   d. have difficulty coping with challenges

(LO 2.3)   6. Having a sense of mastery over your own destiny includes _____.
   a. not communicating your feelings and opinions
   b. being frustrated when things don't go your way
   c. insisting on your own rights
   d. making your needs and desires clear to others

(LO 2.4)   7. Which of the following statements is true of the relationship between spirituality and physical health?
   a. Spirituality can enhance physical health.
   b. Spiritual beliefs and practices lead to depression and anxiety.
   c. Spiritual individuals are more likely to attempt suicide than others.
   d. Spirituality does not center on the worship of a God above but on the discovery of a wisdom within.

(LO 2.4)   8. What is the first step in the process of values clarification?
   a. Publicly affirm your values by sharing them with others.
   b. Act out your values.
   c. Choose freely from among all available options.
   d. Carefully consider the consequences of each choice.

(LO 2.5)   9. According to the Centers for Disease Control and Prevention, which of the following statements is true of sleep-related problems among Americans?
   a. Normal sleep times range from 10 to 20 hours.
   b. Women are more likely than men to report not getting enough sleep.
   c. Poor-quality sleepers report drinking less alcohol than good sleepers.
   d. Asian Americans report getting less sleep compared with all other ethnic groups.

(LO 2.5)   10. The most widely publicized dietary supplement for relieving insomnia contains _____.
   a. chamomile
   b. antihistamines
   c. antipyretic
   d. melatonin

Answers to these questions can be found on page 623.

Critical Thinking

1. Would you say that you view life positively or negatively? Would your friends and family agree with your assessment? Ask two of your closest friends for feedback about what they perceive are your typical responses to a problematic situation. Are these indicative of positive attitudes? If not, what could you do to become more psychologically positive?

2. Were you raised in a religious family? If yes, have you continued the same religious practices from your childhood? Why or why not? If no, have you been to places of worship to explore religious practices? Why or why not?

3. What is your personal experience with lack of sleep? Have you suffered effects described in the text? Has cramming all night ever worked for you? Why or why not?

Additional Online Resources

www.ppc.sas.upenn.edu
This positive psychology website at the University of Pennsylvania has questionnaires on authentic happiness and gratitude.

www.apa.org
The APA is the scientific and professional organization for psychology in the United States. Its website provides up-to-date information on psychological issues.

www.spiritualityhealth.com
Developed by the Publishing Group of Trinity Church, Wall Street in New York City, this website offers self-tests, guidance on spiritual practices, resources for people on spiritual journeys, and subscriptions to a bimonthly print magazine.

www.beliefnet.com
An eclectic, informative guide to different forms of religion and spirituality.

Key Terms

The terms listed are used on the pages indicated. Definitions of the terms are in the glossary at the end of the book.

autonomy 30	self-actualization 27
culture 24	self-compassion 26
emotional health 24	self-esteem 27
emotional intelligence 27	spiritual health 31
mental health 24	spiritual intelligence 32
mood 29	spirituality 31
optimism 29	values 32

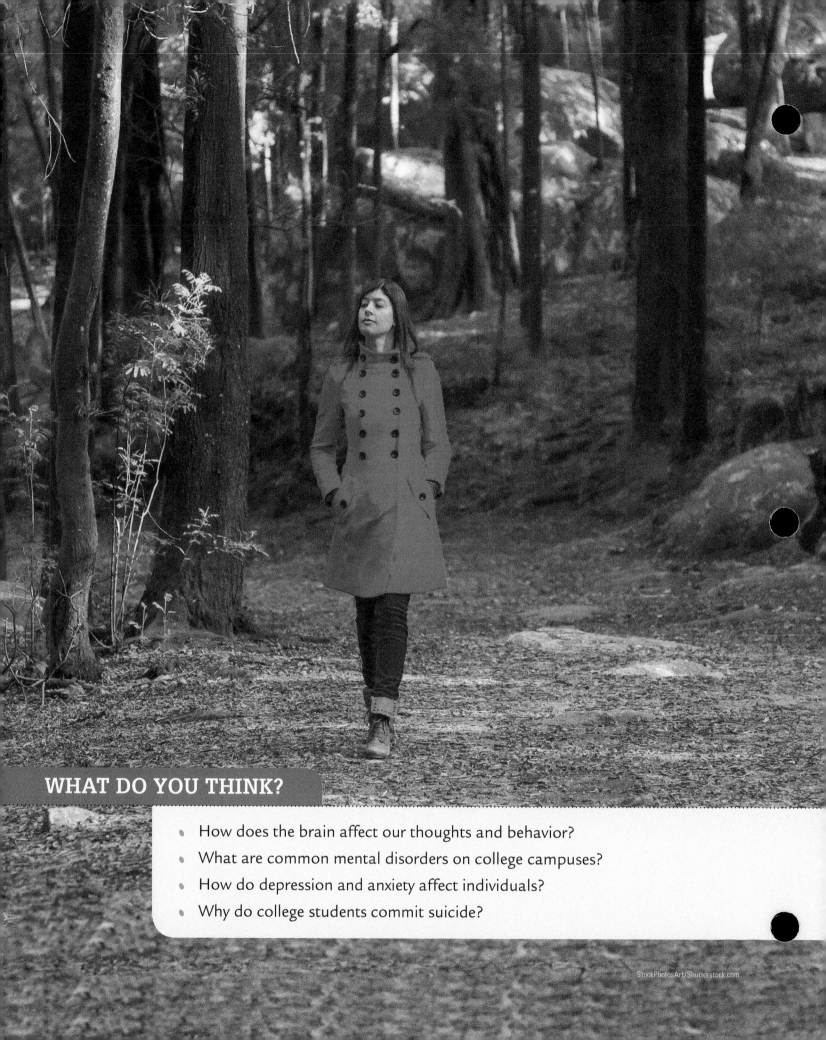

WHAT DO YOU THINK?

- How does the brain affect our thoughts and behavior?
- What are common mental disorders on college campuses?
- How do depression and anxiety affect individuals?
- Why do college students commit suicide?

3

Caring for Your Mind

For years, Travis put on his "happy face" around his friends and family. Popular and athletic in high school, he never let anyone know how desperately unhappy he actually felt. "Whatever I was doing during the day, nothing was on my mind more than wanting to die," he recalls. On a perfectly ordinary day in his senior year, Travis tried to kill himself with an overdose of pills. Rushed to a hospital, Travis recovered, resumed his studies, and

entered college. By the middle of his freshman year, he was struggling once more with feelings of hopelessness. This time he realized what was happening and sought help from a therapist. "I thought college was supposed to be the happiest time of your life," he said. "What went wrong?"

This is a question many young people might ask. Although youth can seem a golden time, when body and mind glow with potential, the process of becoming an adult is a challenging one in every culture and country. Psychological health can make the difference between facing this challenge with optimism

and confidence or feeling overwhelmed by expectations and responsibilities.

This isn't always easy. At some point in life almost half of Americans develop an emotional disorder. Many, including bipolar illness (manic depression) and schizophrenia, often develop in early adulthood. The saddest fact is not that so many people of every age feel so bad, but that so few realize they can get better. Only a third of those with a mental disorder receive any treatment at all. Yet 80 to 90 percent of those treated for psychological problems recover, most within a few months.

After reading this chapter, you should be able to:

3.1 Review the structures and communication pathways of the human brain.

3.2 Distinguish between mental health and mental disorders.

3.3 Describe the key factors related to depressive disorders, their symptoms, and treatments.

3.4 Summarize four categories of anxiety disorders.

3.5 Identify the risk factors, symptoms, and therapeutic approaches for other mental disorders discussed in this chapter.

3.6 Outline the patterns of committing or attempting suicide among Americans.

3.7 List treatment options available for mental disorders.

By learning about psychological disorders covered in this chapter, you may be able to recognize early warning signals in yourself or your loved ones so you can deal with potential difficulties or seek professional help for more serious problems. <

The Brain: The Last Frontier

The brain has intrigued scientists for centuries, but only recently have its explorers made dramatic progress in unraveling its mysteries. Leaders in **neuropsychiatry**—the field that brings together the study of the brain and the mind—remind us that 95 percent of what is known about brain anatomy, chemistry, and physiology has been learned in the last 25 years. These discoveries have reshaped our understanding of the organ that is central to our identity and well-being and have fostered great hope for more effective therapies for the more than 1,000 disorders—psychiatric and neurologic—that affect the brain and nervous system.

Inside the Brain

The human brain, the most complex organ in the body, controls the central nervous system (CNS) and regulates virtually all our activities, including involuntary, or "lower," actions like heart rate, respiration, and digestion, and conscious, or "higher," mental activity like thought, reason, and abstraction. More than one hundred billion **neurons**, or nerve cells, within the brain are capable of electrical and chemical communication with tens of thousands of other nerve cells. (The basic anatomy of the brain is shown in Figure 3.1.)

The neurons are the basic working units of the brain. Like snowflakes, no two are exactly the same. Each consists of a cell body containing the **nucleus**; a long fiber called the **axon**,

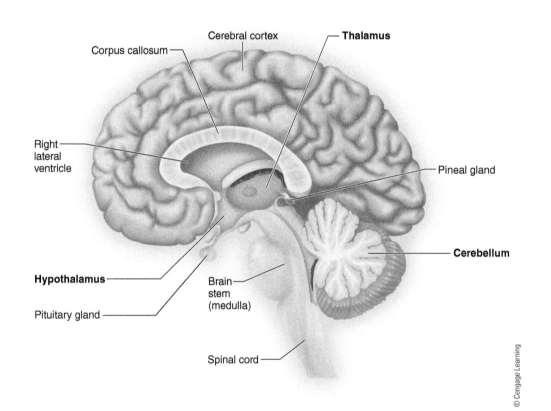

neuropsychiatry The study of the brain and mind.

neurons Nerve cells; the basic working units of the brain, which transmit information from the senses to the brain and from the brain to specific body parts; each neuron consists of a cell body, an axon terminal, and dendrites.

nucleus The central part of a cell, contained in the cell body of a neuron.

axon The long fiber that conducts impulses from the neuron's nucleus to its dendrites.

© Cengage Learning

FIGURE 3.1 The Brain

The three major parts of the brain are the cerebrum, cerebellum, and brainstem (medulla). The cerebrum is divided into two hemispheres—the left, which regulates the right side of the body, and the right, which regulates the left side of the body. The cerebellum plays the major role in coordinating movement, balance, and posture. The brainstem contains centers that control breathing, blood pressure, heart rate, and other physiological functions.

which can range from less than an inch to several feet in length; an **axon terminal**, or ending; and multiple branching fibers called **dendrites** (Figure 3.2). The **glia** serve as the scaffolding for the brain, separate the brain from the bloodstream, assist in the growth of neurons, speed up the transmission of nerve impulses, and engulf and digest damaged neurons.

Until quite recently scientists believed no new neurons or synapses formed in the brain after birth. This theory has been soundly disproved. The brain and spinal cord contain stem cells, which turn into thousands of new neurons a day. The process of creating new brain cells and synapses occurs most rapidly in childhood but continues throughout life, even into old age. Whenever you learn and change, you establish new neural networks.

Anatomically, the brain consists of three parts: the forebrain, midbrain, and hindbrain. The forebrain includes the several lobes of the cerebral cortex that control higher functions, while the mid- and hindbrain are more involved with unconscious, autonomic functions. The normal adult human brain typically weighs about three pounds.

Communication within the Brain

Neurons "talk" with each other by means of electrical and chemical processes (see Figure 3.2). An electric charge, or impulse, travels along an axon to the terminal, where packets of chemicals called **neurotransmitters** are stored. When released, these messengers flow out of the axon terminal and cross a **synapse**, a specialized site at which the axon terminal of one neuron comes extremely close to a dendrite from another neuron.

On the surface of the dendrite are **receptors**, protein molecules designed to bind with neurotransmitters. It takes only about a ten-thousandth of a second for a neurotransmitter and a receptor to come together. Neurotransmitters that do not connect with receptors may remain in the synapse until they are reabsorbed by the cell that produced them—a process called **reuptake**—or broken down by enzymes.

A malfunction in the release of a neurotransmitter, in its reuptake or elimination, or in the receptors or secondary messengers may result in abnormalities in thinking, feeling, or behavior. Some of the most promising and exciting

axon terminal The ending of an axon, from which impulses are transmitted to a dendrite of another neuron.

dendrites Branching fibers of a neuron that receive impulses from axon terminals of other neurons and conduct these impulses toward the nucleus.

glia Support cells for neurons in the brain and spinal cord that separate the brain from the bloodstream, assist in the growth of neurons, speed transmission of nerve impulses, and eliminate damaged neurons.

neurotransmitters Chemicals released by neurons that stimulate or inhibit the action of other neurons.

synapse A specialized site at which electrical impulses are transmitted from the axon terminal of one neuron to a dendrite of another.

receptors Molecules on the surface of neurons on which neurotransmitters bind after their release from other neurons.

reuptake Reabsorption by the originating cell of neurotransmitters that have not connected with receptors and have been left in synapses.

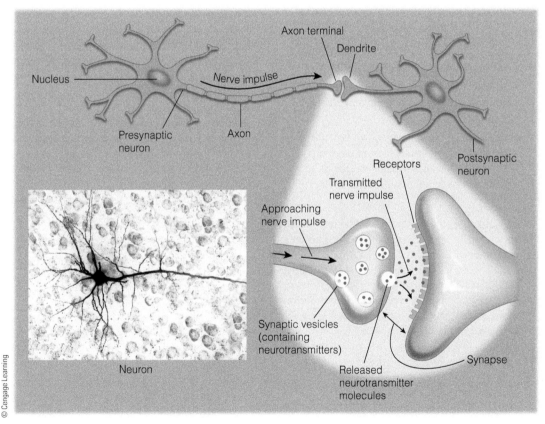

© Cengage Learning

FIGURE 3.2 Brain Messaging: Anatomy of a Neuron
This figure shows how nerve impulses are transmitted from one neuron to another within the brain.

research in neuropsychiatry is focusing on correcting such malfunctions.

The neurotransmitter serotonin and its receptors have been shown to affect mood, sleep, behavior, appetite, memory, learning, sexuality, and aggression and to play a role in several mental disorders. The discovery of a possible link between low levels of serotonin and some cases of major depression has led to the development of more precisely targeted antidepressant medications that boost serotonin to normal levels. (See "Psychiatric Drugs" later in the chapter.)

Sex Differences in the Brain

From birth, male and female brains differ in a variety of ways.

- Overall, a woman's brain, like her body, is 10 to 15 percent smaller than a man's, yet the regions dedicated to higher cognitive functions such as language are more densely packed with neurons—and women use more of them.

- When a male puts his mind to work, neurons turn on in highly specific areas. When females set their minds on similar tasks, cells light up all over the brain.

- A man's eyes are more sensitive to bright light and retain their ability to see well at long distances longer in life.

- A woman hears a much broader range of sounds, and her hearing remains sharper longer.

- According to neuroimaging studies, the genders respond differently to emotions, especially sadness, which activates, or turns on, neurons in an area eight times larger in women than men.

Neither gender's brain is "better." Intelligence *per se* appears equal in both. The greatest gender differences appear at both the top and bottom of the intelligence scales. Nevertheless, more than half the time, regardless of the type of test, most women and men perform more or less equally—even though they may well take different routes to arrive at the same answers.

✓**check-in** Are women or men more intelligent?
The essayist Samuel Johnson may have given the best response: "Which man? Which woman?"

The Teenage and 20-Something Brain

If you are under the age of 25, your brain is a work in progress. As neuroimaging techniques such as PET scans (positron-emission tomography) and fMRIs (functional magnetic resonance imaging) have revealed, the brain continues to develop throughout the first quarter-century of life.

The number of synapses surges in the "tween" years before adolescence, followed by a "pruning" of nonessential connections. In a sense, each individual determines which synapses stay and which are deleted.

If you started to play the piano as a child and continue as an adolescent, for instance, you retain the synapses involved in this skill. If you don't practice regularly, your brain will prune the unused synapses, and your piano-playing ability will diminish. Inadequate pruning of synapses may contribute to mental disorders such as schizophrenia, which usually first occur in late adolescence.

Brain areas responsible for tasks such as organizing, controlling impulses, planning, and strategizing do not fully develop until the mid-20s. Brain chemicals such as dopamine that help distinguish between what is worthy of attention and what is mere distraction also do not reach optimal levels until then.

The brains of teens and young adults function differently than those of older individuals. In dealing with daily life, they rely more on the amygdala, a small almond-shaped region in the medial and temporal lobes that processes emotions and memories. This is one reason why any setback—a poor grade or a friend's snub—can feel like a major crisis. As individuals age, the frontal cortex, which governs reason and forethought, plays a greater role and helps put challenges into perspective.

A young, "maturing" brain does not necessarily lead to poor judgments and risky behaviors. However, be aware that your brain may not always grasp the long-term consequences of your actions, set realistic priorities, or restrain potentially harmful impulses. In addition,

- Learn to center yourself.
- Seek the counsel of others.
- Tame your temper so you don't fly off the handle.
- Be cautious about drugs and alcohol, which are especially toxic to the developing brain and increase the risk of acts you may later regret.

✓**check-in** Are you under age 25?

Understanding Mental Health

Mentally healthy individuals value themselves, perceive reality as it is, accept their limitations and possibilities, carry out their responsibilities, establish and maintain close relationships, pursue work that suits their talent and training, and feel a sense of fulfillment that makes the efforts of daily living worthwhile (Figure 3.3).

The state of mental health around the world is far from ideal. Psychiatric illness and substance abuse affect 450 million people worldwide and cause more premature deaths than any other factor.[1]

The most common psychiatric conditions are depression, alcohol dependence and abuse, bipolar disorder, schizophrenia, Alzheimer's and other forms of dementia, panic disorder, and drug dependence and abuse.

Across the globe, depression is the leading cause of years of health lost to disease in both men and women. The worldwide rate of depression among women is 50 percent higher than in men, and women and girls have higher rates of anxiety disorders, migraine, and Alzheimer's disease. Men's rates of alcohol and substance abuse are nearly seven times higher than women's.[2]

Preventive steps can help maintain and enhance your psychological health, just as similar actions boost physical health. (See "Self-Help Strategies" on page 67.)

Despite public education campaigns, the level of prejudice and discrimination against people with a serious mental illness has changed little over the last ten years. More people now attribute problems like depression and substance abuse to neurobiological causes—and are more likely to favor providing treatment.

What Is a Mental Disorder?

While laypeople may speak of "nervous breakdowns" or "insanity," these are not scientific terms. The U.S. government's official definition states that a serious mental illness is "a diagnosable mental, behavioral, or emotional disorder that interferes with one or more major activities in life, like dressing, eating, or working."

About one in four adults in the United States suffers from mental illness at some point in life.[3] Psychiatrists define a **mental disorder** as a clinically significant behavioral or psychological syndrome or pattern that is associated with present distress (a painful symptom) or disability (impairment in one or more important areas of functioning) or with a significantly increased risk of suffering death, pain, disability, or an important loss of freedom.[4]

Diagnosis is based on a pattern of symptoms, or diagnostic criteria, spelled out in the American Psychiatric Association's *Diagnostic and Statistical Manual,* 5th edition (DSM-5).

Mental disorders can affect every aspect of life, including its length. Individuals with a serious mental illness tend to die at younger ages than peers without disorders from both medical conditions and "unnatural causes" such as suicide and accidents. Conditions such as chronic depression, anxiety, or schizophrenia typically rob people of nearly a decade of life and account for about one in nine deaths worldwide, or approximately 8 million deaths each year. Individuals with mental disorders may be at greater risk because of poor diets, lack of exercise, smoking, lack of social support, or problems getting needed medical care or complying with treatments.[5]

Mental disorders, also undermine physical well-being. Major depression is associated with lower bone density in young men and in adolescent girls. Anxiety can lead to intensified asthmatic reactions, skin conditions, and digestive disorders. Stress as discussed in Chapter 4, can play a role in hypertension, heart attacks, sudden cardiac death, and immune disorders in the young as well as in older individuals.

✓**check-in** Do you feel that your mental health affects your physical well-being—and vice versa?

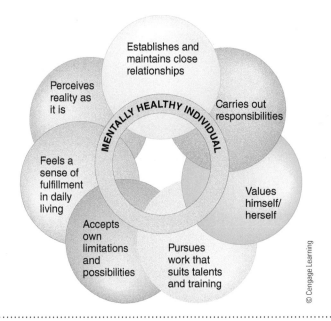

FIGURE 3.3 The Mentally Healthy Individual
Mental well-being is a combination of many factors.

mental disorder A behavioral or psychological syndrome associated with distress or disability or with a significantly increased risk of suffering death, pain, disability, or loss of freedom.

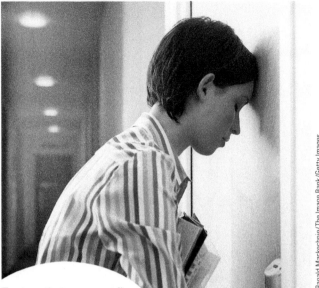

Factors that can contribute to feelings of distress among college students include stressful events, poor academic performance, loneliness, and relationship problems.

Personality and Health Various personality types and behaviors have also been linked to certain illnesses. Aggressive, impatient, Type A people may be more prone to heart disease, high blood pressure, high cholesterol levels, and increased stomach acid secretion than more relaxed Type B people.

Some have proposed that individuals with a Type C personality—hard-working, highly responsible, quiet, courteous—may suppress negative emotions (especially anger), avoid conflicts, never retaliate, and rarely pursue their own desires. However, there have not been conclusive findings that these behavioral and emotional characteristics increase the risk of cancer.

The Type D (for distressed) personality, characterized by tendencies both to experience

negative emotions and to inhibit these emotions while avoiding contact with others, has emerged as an independent risk factor for heart disease, a poor prognosis if cardiovascular problems develop, and increased mortality.[6]

Mental Health on Campus

Students have always faced challenges when they begin post-secondary education. Many are leaving home for the first time and taking on new responsibilities in unfamiliar settings. During the transition to college life, freshmen often report homesickness, problems concentrating, sleep difficulties, and mood swings.[7] Even older students with more life experiences must cope with academic pressures, financial concerns, personal relationships, and post-graduation plans.[8] (See Table 3.1 on common concerns of college students.)

According to the American College Health Association (ACHA) National College Health Assessment, the most common mental disorders among students are anxiety, depression, panic attacks, and attention deficit/hyperactivity disorder.[9]

Concern about mental health on college and university campuses has grown in recent years as campus shootings have killed and injured dozens. There also have been increases in the numbers of students seeking psychological services and in the severity of problems they report, such as drug use, alcohol abuse, sexual assaults, self-injury, and suicide.

Here is a statistical snapshot of mental health among today's undergraduates:

- About 10 percent have been diagnosed with or treated for depression over the past 12 months.[10]

- Incoming students rated their emotional health at the lowest point in the last two decades.[11]

- Some schools report that the number of students diagnosed with depression or anxiety has more than doubled in recent years.[12]

- Students seeking care report more severe and persistent problems—for example, poor mental health for 15 or more days in the last month.[13]

- Students who live off campus are more likely to be depressed or anxious, perhaps because of the added stress of dealing with rent, household expenses, and housekeeping tasks.[14]

- Transfer students score higher in anxiety than other undergraduates, while depression, anxiety, and stress ratings typically increase as students progress through college and are higher in upperclassmen than underclassmen.[15]

- Students who are veterans or currently serving in the military do not have higher rates

TABLE 3.1 Top Concerns of College Students

- Academic performance
- Pressure to succeed
- Post-graduation plans
- Financial concerns
- Quality of sleep
- Relationship with friends
- Relationship with family
- Overall health
- Body image
- Self-esteem

Source: Beiter, R., et al. "The prevalence and correlates of depression, anxiety, and stress in a sample of college students." *Journal of Affective Disorders* 173 (2015): pp. 90–96.

Wavebreakmedia/Shutterstock.com

of mental disorders, regardless of whether they have been deployed on hazardous duty. Thanks to what some have dubbed "the healthy warrior effect," the challenges of military service may impart qualities or skills that help in coping with college pressures.[16]

✓ **check-in** Do you feel that more undergraduates today are experiencing mental health issues than in the past?

Students at Risk According to the ACHA survey, about one in four undergraduates has been diagnosed or treated for a mental disorder. (See Snapshot: On Campus Now.) Here are some of the factors that increase vulnerability:

- **History of a mental disorder.** Many undergraduates arrive on campus with a history of psychological problems. Medications for common disorders such as depression and attention-deficit/hyperactivity disorder have made it possible for young people who might otherwise not have been able to function in a college setting to pursue higher education.

- **Ongoing psychiatric issues.** Some undergraduates are dealing with ongoing issues such as bulimia, self-cutting, and childhood sexual abuse.

- **Breakup.** Many students become distressed following a romantic breakup or loss. In the survey, about one in eight individuals reported a breakup in the previous year. Their odds of having a psychiatric disorder are significantly higher than those who hadn't been through a breakup.

- **Financial pressures.** Student loans amount to a staggering $1 trillion, with the average graduate owing $23,300. Student loan debt may not only induce stress and worry but also increase stress in other ways, such as forcing students to delay marriage or parenthood or to forgo home ownership or other life goals.[17]

- **Discrimination.** Racial discrimination may be experienced more intensely than other forms of discrimination and may have a more ominous impact on mental and physical well-being. As research in psychology, sociology, and epidemiology has confirmed, the harmful effects of racial discrimination on African Americans include distress, depression, anxiety, and psychiatric symptoms.[18] Among African American students, a sense of hopelessness can contribute to or intensify symptoms of depression and anxiety.[19]

- **Increased risk of other disorders.** Undergraduate women with symptoms of depression, for instance, are less likely to use protective behavioral strategies (described in Chapter 13) when they drink, which can lead to drinking more often and more heavily.[20]

- **Minority status.** The few studies that have looked into ethnic differences in psychological health have yielded conflicting or inconclusive results: Some found no differences; others suggested higher rates of depression among Indian, Korean, and South Asian students. Various racial, ethnic, and sexual minority groups report less of a sense of belonging and a lack of mentoring and peer support.

✓ **check-in** Has a psychological or emotional problem ever affected your ability to study or your academic performance?

The Toll on Students Psychological and emotional problems can affect every aspect of a student's life, including physical health, overall satisfaction, and relationships. Students who struggle with symptoms of anxiety or depression, which can interfere with concentration, study habits, classroom participation, and testing, commonly report struggling with academics.

In the ACHA's national assessment, 21.8 percent of students reported that anxiety had impaired their ability to learn and earn higher grades; 13.5 percent said that depression had affected their academic performance.[21] Some estimate that 5 percent of undergraduates may not complete their degrees because of psychological problems.

The impact of mental health problems extends beyond an individual student to roommates, friends, classmates, family, and instructors. Suicides or suicide attempts affect all members of the campus community, who may experience profound sadness and grief. (See the discussion of suicide later in this chapter.)

Seeking Help Although serious mental disorders may begin or worsen during young adulthood, 18- to 24-year-olds are less likely to seek and receive mental health care than any other age group.[22] In a survey of students at 26 colleges, fewer than one in four with symptoms of depression or suicidal thoughts in the previous 12 months received treatment during that time.

Among the barriers that keep students from seeking help are these:

- Financial concerns

- Belief that they could handle the problem without treatment and didn't need help

- Lack of time

- Belief that treatment would not be helpful

HEALTH NOW!

Count Your Blessings

As discussed in Chapter 2, gratitude has proven as effective in brightening mood and boosting energy as the standard, well-studied techniques used in psychotherapy. Below are some simple steps to cultivating and expressing gratitude.

- Every day write down ten new things for which you are grateful. You can start with this list and keep adding to it: your bed, your cell phone and every person whose efforts led to its development, every road you take, loyalty, your toothbrush, your toes, the sky, ice cream, etc.

- Record the ways you express gratitude. How do you feel when doing so?

- Create a daily practice of appreciation. This may be as simple as saying a few words of thanks before each meal (if only to yourself) or writing down your feelings of gratitude.

- Make a list of ten people— teachers, coaches, neighbors, relatives—to whom you owe a debt of gratitude. Write a one-to two-page letter to each of them, stating your appreciation of what he or she has contributed to you and your well-being. You do not have to send the letters. What is important is that you focus deeply on the contribution of each person and allow feelings of gratitude to come as they may.

🔲 Student Mental Health

Within the past 12 months, students diagnosed or treated by a professional for the following:

	Percent (%)		
	Male	Female	Average
Anorexia	0.5	1.5	1.1
Anxiety	8.0	17.5	14.3
Attention-deficit/hyperactivity disorder	5.8	4.9	5.3
Bipolar disorder	1.3	1.5	1.4
Bulimia	0.5	1.3	1.0
Depression	7.6	14.2	12
Obsessive-compulsive disorder	1.6	2.6	2.3
Panic attacks	3.1	8.5	6.7
Phobia	0.4	0.1	0.3
Schizophrenia	0.5	0.1	0.3
Substance abuse or addiction	1.2	0.8	1.0
Other addiction	0.7	0.3	0.5
Other mental health condition	1.8	2.6	2.4
Students reporting none of the above	83.4	73.9	77.1
Students reporting only one of the above	7.7	9.1	8.6
Students reporting both depression and anxiety	4.8	10.4	8.6
Students reporting any two or more of the above, excluding the combination of depression and anxiety	4.2	7.4	6.4

Source: American College Health Association. *American College Health Association–National College Health Assessment II: Reference Group Executive Summary, Spring 2014.* Hanover, MD: American College Health Association, 2014.

- Belief that others would have a negative opinion of them if they sought help
- Unawareness of where to get treatment[23]

As in the general population, minority college students, including black, Latino, and Asian undergraduates, are less likely to seek and get needed mental health care. Concerns about stigma keep many, particularly racial/ethnic minorities, from seeking mental health care.[24] Among African American students, women in their junior and senior year are more likely to utilize mental health care services than male students or underclassmen.[25] Asian Americans between ages 15 and 24, who feel the stress of high expectations as the "model minority," have significantly higher suicidal rates than other racial/ethnic groups of the same age range, yet they typically do not seek mental health services because of cultural stigma attached to mental health problems.[26] The young adults most likely to receive needed mental health care tend to be whites or American Indians living at home.[27]

√**check-in** In a national survey of undergraduates, about eight in ten of those with high ratings for depression or suicidal thoughts sought help from nonclinical sources, primarily family and friends.[28] Where would you turn for help with a mental health concern?

Depressive Disorders

Depression, the world's most common mental ailment, affects more than 13 million adults in the United States every year and costs billions of dollars for treatment and lost productivity and lives.

Those most likely to have major depression are

- Women
- Racial and ethnic minorities
- Those without a high school education
- Divorced or never-married individuals
- Those without jobs
- Those without health insurance

Depression in Students

An estimated 15 to 40 percent of college-age men and women (18- to 24-year-olds) may develop depression, but the number may be rising. Screening all students at college health centers has identified a large percentage of minority students with depression. (See the Self Survey, "Recognizing Depression.")

Key contributors to depression in college students are the following:

- **Stress.** As they adjust to campus life, undergraduates face the ongoing stress of forging a new identity and finding a place for themselves in various social hierarchies. This triggers the release of the so-called stress hormones (discussed in Chapter 4), which can change brain activity. A lack of social support can increase stress and depressive symptoms in first-year students.[30] Drugs and alcohol, widely used on campus, also affect the brain in ways that make managing stress even harder.

- **Too little sleep.** Computers, the Internet, around-the-clock television, and the college tradition of pulling all-nighters can contribute to sabotaging rest and increasing vulnerability to depression.

- **Academic and athletic pressures.** Depression has been linked to poorer academic performance and increased likelihood of dropping out before graduation. Students engaged in intercollegiate sports, according to a recent study, are twice as likely to be depressed as former athletes. The reasons may include overtraining, injury, pressure to perform, lack of free time, and the stress of juggling athletics and schoolwork.[31] Concussions may increase the risk of depression as well as academic problems in some college athletes.[32]

Gender and Depression

Female Depression   Depression is twice as common in women as men. However, this gender gap decreases or disappears in studies of men and women in similar socioeconomic situations, such as college students, civil servants, and the Amish community.

Black women are much less likely to report suffering from depression than white women are. About 10 percent of black women report struggling with the mental health disorder at some point in their lives, compared with 21 percent of white women. The reason may be that they have developed resources and coping strategies to deal with stressful circumstances, such as supportive social ties, religious participation, group identity, and a strong sense of mastery and self-esteem.[33]

Women may not necessarily be more likely to develop depression, this research suggests, but may have an underlying predisposition that puts them at greater risk under various social stressors.

Brain chemistry and sex hormones may play a role in the following ways:

- Women produce less of certain metabolites of serotonin, a messenger chemical that helps regulate mood.

- Women's brains register sadness much more intensely than men's.

- Women, more sensitive to changes in light and temperature, are at least four times more

week before onset of menstruation, an estimated 1.8 to 5.8 percent of women experience the characteristic symptoms of PDD:[35]

- Marked mood swings, tearfulness, sadness, or sensitivity to rejection
- Marked irritability, anger, or conflicts with others
- Marked depressed moods, hopelessness, or self-deprecating thoughts
- Marked anxiety, tension, or feelings of being on edge

Other symptoms may include the following:

- Decreased interest in usual activities
- Difficulty concentrating
- Lethargy or lack of energy
- Change in appetite, overeating, or food cravings
- Sleeping much more or less than usual
- Sense of being overwhelmed
- Physical symptoms such as breast tenderness or pain, joint or muscle pain, bloating, and/or weight gain

√**check-in** If you are a woman, have you ever experienced any symptoms of premenstrual dysphoric disorder?

Symptoms start to improve within a few days after menstruation begins and end or become minimal in the following week.[36]

Pregnancy, contrary to what many people assume, does not "protect" a woman from depression, and women who discontinue treatment when they become pregnant are at risk of a relapse. Women and their psychiatrists must carefully weigh the risks and benefits of psychiatric medications during pregnancy.

Male Depression More than 6 million men in the United States—1 in every 14—suffer from this insidious disorder, many without recognizing what's wrong. Experts describe male depression as an "under" disease: underdiscussed, underrecognized, underdiagnosed, and undertreated.

Depression "looks" different in men than in women in the following ways:

- Irritability or tremendous fatigue rather than sadness
- A sense of being dead inside, of worthlessness, hopelessness, helplessness, of losing their life force
- Physical symptoms such as headaches, pain, and insomnia
- Attempts to "self-medicate" with alcohol or drugs

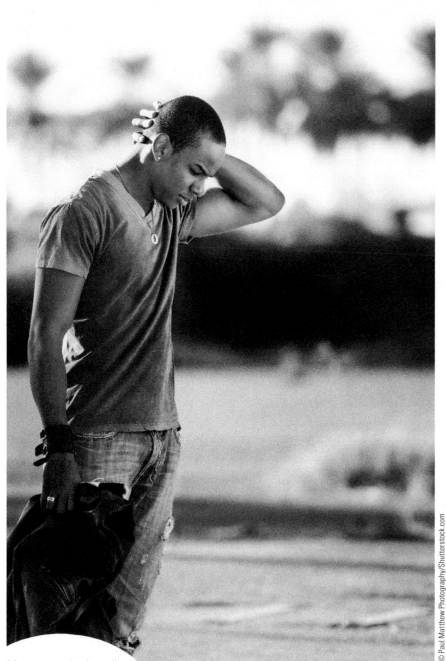

Many men don't realize that a sense of hopelessness, worthlessness, helplessness, or feeling dead inside can be a symptom of depression.

likely than men to develop seasonal affective disorder (SAD) and to become depressed in the dark winter months.

- Some women also seem more sensitive to their own hormones or to the changes in them that occur at puberty, during the menstrual cycle, after childbirth, or during perimenopause and menopause.[34]

The DSM-5 classifies premenstrual dysphoric disorder (PDD), which is not the same as premenstrual syndrome (PMS), discussed in Chapter 8, as a depressive disorder. In the final

Genes may make some men more vulnerable than others, but chronic stress of any sort plays a major role in male depression, possibly by raising levels of the stress hormone cortisol and lowering testosterone. Men also are more likely than women to become depressed following divorce, job loss, or a career setback.

Whatever its roots, male depression alters brain chemistry in potentially deadly ways. Four times as many men as women kill themselves; depressed men are two to four times more likely to take their own lives than are depressed women.

Major Depressive Disorder

The simplest definition of a **major depressive disorder** is sadness that does not end. The incidence of major depression has soared over the past two decades, especially among young adults, to an estimated lifetime prevalence of about 16 percent.[37] An estimated 5 percent of college students suffer a major depressive disorder.[38]

Major depression can destroy a person's joy for living. Food, friends, sex, or any form of pleasure no longer appeals. It is impossible to concentrate on work and responsibilities. Unable to escape a sense of utter hopelessness, depressed individuals may fight back tears throughout the day and toss and turn through long, empty nights. Thoughts of death or suicide may push into their minds.

The characteristic symptoms of major depression include the following:

- **Feeling depressed,** sad, empty, discouraged, or tearful most of the day, nearly every day
- **Losing of interest** or pleasure in once-enjoyable activities
- **Eating more or less** than usual and either gaining or losing a significant amount of weight
- **Having trouble sleeping** or sleeping much more than usual
- **Feeling slowed down** or restless and unable to sit still
- **Lacking energy** or fatigue nearly every day
- **Feeling helpless,** hopeless, worthless, inadequate, or inappropriately guilty
- **Having difficulty thinking or concentrating;** indecisiveness
- **Having persistent thoughts of death** or suicide[39]

As many as half of major depressive episodes are not recognized because the symptoms are "masked." Rather than feeling sad or

YOUR STRATEGIES FOR PREVENTION
How to Help Someone Who Is Depressed

- **Express your concern, but don't nag.** You might say, "I'm concerned about you. You are struggling right now. We need to find some help."

- **Don't be distracted by behaviors like drinking or gambling, which can disguise depression in men.**

- **Encourage the individual to remain in treatment** until symptoms begin to lift (which takes several weeks).

- **Provide emotional support.** Listen carefully. Offer hope and reassurance that with time and treatment, things will get better.

- **Do not ignore remarks about suicide.** Report them to the person's doctor or, in an emergency, call 911.

depressed, individuals may experience low energy, insomnia, difficulty concentrating, and physical symptoms.

Treating Depression

The most recent guidelines for treating depression, developed by the American Psychiatric Association, call for an individualized approach tailored to each patient's symptoms. Specific treatments might include medication, healthy behaviors, exercise (proven to reduce depressive symptoms, especially in older adults and those with chronic medical problems), and psychotherapy.

The rate of depression treatment, particularly with **antidepressants**, has increased in the past decade. Medication has become the most common approach, while fewer patients receive psychotherapy than in the past, possibly because of limited insurance coverage. A combination of psychotherapy and medication is considered the most effective approach for most patients. (See Consumer Alert.)

Psychotherapy helps individuals pinpoint the life problems that contribute to their depression, identify negative or distorted thinking patterns, explore behaviors that contribute to depression, and regain a sense of control and pleasure in life. Two specific psychotherapies—cognitive-behavioral therapy and interpersonal therapy (described later in this chapter)—have proved as helpful as antidepressant drugs, although they take longer than medication to achieve results.

Even without treatment, depression generally lifts after six to nine months. However, in more than 80 percent of people, it recurs, with each episode lasting longer and becoming more severe and difficult to treat.

major depressive disorder
Sadness that does not end; ongoing feelings of utter helplessness.

antidepressants Drugs used primarily to treat symptoms of depression.

The Pros and Cons of Antidepressants

Millions of individuals have benefited from the category of antidepressant drugs called selective serotonin reuptake inhibitors (SSRIs). However, like all drugs, they can cause side effects that range from temporary physical symptoms, such as stomach upset and headaches, to more persistent problems, such as sexual dysfunction. The most serious—and controversial—risk is suicide. Some studies have shown an association between SSRIs and an increased risk of suicide, especially during the first months of treatment,[40] but more recent reports have not confirmed this link in adults.[41]

Facts to Know

- The FDA has issued a "black box" warning about the risk of suicidal thoughts, hostility, and aggression in both children and young adults.
- This risk of suicide while taking an antidepressant is about 1 in 3,000; the risk of a serious attempt is 1 in 1,000.

Steps to Take

- If you are younger than age 20, be aware of the increased suicide risk with the use

of SSRIs. Talk these over carefully with a psychiatrist. Discuss alternative treatments, such as psychotherapy.

- For individuals older than age 20, the benefits of antidepressants have proved to outweigh their risks in most cases. Adults treated with SSRIs are 40 percent less likely to commit suicide than depressed individuals who do not receive this therapy.
- In patients initially treated with antidepressants, two approaches based on mindfulness (discussed in Chapter 4)—mindfulness-based cognitive therapy and mindfulness meditation—have proven as effective as continuing drug therapy in preventing a return of depression symptoms.
- Whatever your age, arrange for careful monitoring and follow-up with a psychiatrist when you start taking an antidepressant. Familiarize yourself with possible side effects, and seek help immediately if you begin to think about taking your own life.

Bipolar Disorder

bipolar disorder Severe depression alternating with periods of manic activity and elation.

anxiety disorders A group of psychological disorders involving episodes of apprehension, tension, or uneasiness, stemming from the anticipation of danger and sometimes accompanied by physical symptoms, which cause significant distress and impairment to an individual.

phobias Anxiety disorders marked by an inordinate fear of an object, a class of objects, or a situation, resulting in extreme avoidance behaviors.

Bipolar disorder, known as manic depression in the past, consists of mood swings that may take individuals from manic states of feeling euphoric and energetic to depressive states of utter despair. In episodes of full mania, they may become so impulsive and out of touch with reality that they endanger their careers, relationships, health, or even survival. Psychiatrists view bipolar symptoms on a spectrum that includes depression and states of acute irritability and distress.

During a manic episode, individuals may make grandiose plans, feel little need for sleep, talk more than usual, and get involved in activities with a high potential for painful consequences (such as buying sprees or sexual indiscretions). During a hypomanic episode, people may feel an elevated, expansive, or irritable mood and abnormally and persistently increased activity or energy along with symptoms similar to those of mania.

Often those with bipolar disorder plunge from these exhilarating states into major depressive episodes, in which they may feel sad, hopeless, and helpless and develop other characteristic symptoms of depression.[42]

Bipolar and related disorders affect approximately 4 percent of the population.[43] Men tend to develop bipolar disorder earlier in life (between ages 16 and 25), but women have higher rates overall. About 50 percent of patients with bipolar illness have a family history of the disorder.

The characteristic symptoms of bipolar disorder include these:

- **Mood swings**—from happy to miserable, optimistic to despairing, and so on
- **Changes in thinking**—thoughts speeding through one's mind, unrealistic self-confidence, difficulty concentrating, delusions, hallucinations
- **Changes in behavior**—sudden immersion in plans and projects, talking very rapidly and much more than usual, excessive spending, impaired judgment, impulsive sexual involvement
- **Changes in physical condition**—less need for sleep, increased energy, fewer health complaints than usual

Professional therapy is essential in treating bipolar disorders. Bipolar disorder decreases the life expectancy of patients diagnosed at age 15 by 11 years or more.[44] An estimated 25 to 50 percent of bipolar patients attempt suicide at least once. About 1 percent take their own lives every year. Mood-stabilizing medications are the keystone of treatment, although psychotherapy plays a critical role in helping individuals understand their illness and rebuild their lives. Most individuals continue taking medication indefinitely after remission of their symptoms because the risk of recurrence is high.

Anxiety Disorders

Anxiety disorders, which affect an estimated 10 to 15 percent of psychiatric patients, are more common than depression (diagnosed in 7 to 10 percent of patients).[45] They may involve inordinate fears of certain objects or situations (**phobias**); episodes of sudden, inexplicable terror (**panic attacks**); chronic distress (generalized anxiety disorder [GAD]); or persistent, disturbing thoughts. These disorders can increase the risk of developing depression. Although postpartum depression has been widely recognized, new studies show that anxiety is far more common, with about one in five new mothers reporting acute anxiety in the days after giving birth. However, these symptoms tended to drop rapidly by six months after delivery.[46]

Over a lifetime, as many as one in four Americans may experience an anxiety disorder. More than 40 percent are never correctly diagnosed and treated. Yet most individuals who do get treatment, even for severe and disabling problems, improve dramatically.

√ **check-in** Are you feeling any of the following characteristics of anxiety?

__ Apprehensive

__ Panicky

__ Trembly

__ Shaky

__ Dry mouth

__ Difficulty breathing

__ Pounding heart

__ Sweaty palms

__ Worried about performance or lack of control[47]

Specific Phobia

Phobias—the most prevalent type of anxiety disorder—are out-of-the-ordinary, irrational, intense, persistent fears of certain objects or situations. About 2 million Americans develop such acute terror that they go to extremes to avoid whatever it is that they fear, even though they realize that these feelings are excessive or unreasonable.

The most common phobias involve

- Animals, particularly dogs, snakes, insects, and mice

- The sight of blood

- Closed spaces (*claustrophobia*)

- Heights (*acrophobia*)

- Air travel

- Being in open or public places or situations from which one perceives it would be difficult or embarrassing to escape (*agoraphobia*)

Although various medications have been tried, the best approach is behavioral therapy, which consists of gradual, systematic exposure to the feared object (a process called *systematic desensitization*). Numerous studies have proved that exposure—especially in vivo exposure, in which individuals are exposed to the actual source of their fear rather than simply imagining it—is

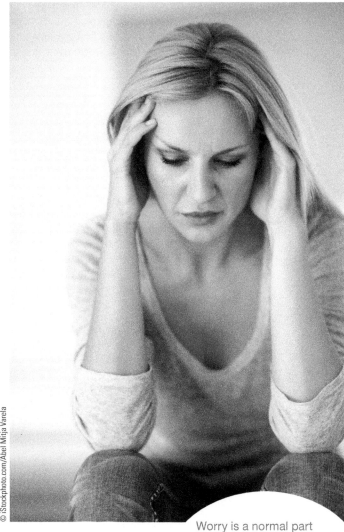

© iStockphoto.com/Abel Mitja Varela

highly effective. Medical hypnosis—the use of induction of an altered state of consciousness—also can help.

√ **check-in** Does any particular object or situation make you fearful or anxious?

Panic Attacks and Panic Disorder

Individuals who have had panic attacks describe them as the most frightening experiences of their lives. Without reason or warning, their hearts race wildly. They may become light-headed or dizzy. Because they can't catch their breath, they may start breathing rapidly and hyperventilate. Parts of their bodies, such as their fingers or toes, may tingle or feel numb. Worst of all is the terrible sense that something horrible is about to happen: that they will die, lose their minds, or have a heart attack.

Worry is a normal part of daily life, but individuals with generalized anxiety disorder worry constantly about everything that might go wrong.

panic attacks Short episodes characterized by physical sensations of light-headedness, dizziness, hyperventilation, and numbness of extremities, accompanied by an inexplicable terror, usually of a physical disaster such as death.

Most attacks reach peak intensity within 10 minutes. Afterward, individuals live in dread of another one. In the course of a lifetime, your risk of having a single panic attack is 7 percent.

√**check-in** Have you ever had a panic attack?

Panic disorder develops when attacks recur or apprehension about them becomes so intense that individuals cannot function normally. Full-blown panic disorder occurs in about 2 percent of all adults in the course of a lifetime and usually develops before age 30. Women are more than twice as likely as men to experience panic attacks, although no one knows why. Parents, siblings, and children of individuals with panic disorders also are more likely to develop them than are others.

The two primary treatments for panic disorder are

- Cognitive-behavioral therapy (CBT), which teaches specific strategies for coping with symptoms like rapid breathing

- Medication

Treatment helps as many as 90 percent of those with panic disorder either improve significantly or recover completely, usually within six to eight weeks.

Generalized Anxiety Disorder

About 10 million adults in the United States suffer from a **generalized anxiety disorder (GAD)**, excessive or unrealistic apprehension that causes physical symptoms, such as restlessness, fatigue, and muscle tension, and lasts for six months or longer. It usually starts when people are in their 20s. Unlike fear, which helps us recognize and avoid real danger, GAD is an irrational or un-warranted response to harmless objects or situations of exaggerated danger.

The most common symptoms are

- Increased heart rate
- Sweating
- Increased blood pressure
- Muscle aches
- Intestinal pains
- Irritability
- Sleep problems
- Difficulty concentrating

Undergraduates with generalized anxiety may find it especially difficult to deal with physical discomfort, uncertainty, negative emotions, ambiguity, and frustration.[48]

Chronically anxious individuals worry—not just some of the time, and not just about the stresses and strains of ordinary life—but constantly, about almost everything: their health, families, finances, marriages, potential dangers. Treatment for GAD may consist of a combination of psychotherapy, behavioral therapy, and antianxiety drugs.

Other Common Disorders

Obsessive-Compulsive Disorder

An estimated 1.9 to 3.3 percent of Americans have an **obsessive-compulsive disorder (OCD)**.[49] Some of these individuals suffer only from an *obsession*, a recurring idea, thought, or image that they realize, at least initially, is senseless.

The most common obsessions are these:

- Repetitive thoughts that usually involve harm and danger

- Contamination (for example, becoming infected by shaking hands)

- Doubt (for example, wondering whether one has performed some act, such as having hurt someone in a traffic accident)

Most people with OCD also suffer from a *compulsion*, a repetitive behavior performed according to certain rules or in a stereotyped fashion. The most common compulsions include the following:

- Handwashing
- Cleaning
- Repeating words silently
- Counting
- Checking (for example, making sure dozens of times that a door is locked)

Individuals with OCD realize that their thoughts or behaviors are bizarre, but they cannot resist or control them. Eventually, the obsessions or compulsions consume a great deal of time and significantly interfere with normal routines, job functioning, or usual social activities or relationships with others. A young woman who must follow a very rigid dressing routine may always be late for class, for example; a student who must count each letter of the alphabet as he types may not be able to complete a term paper.

Treatment may consist of cognitive therapy to correct irrational assumptions, behavioral

panic disorder An anxiety disorder in which the apprehension or experience of recurring panic attacks is so intense that normal functioning is impaired.

generalized anxiety disorder (GAD) An anxiety disorder characterized as chronic distress.

obsessive-compulsive disorder (OCD) An anxiety disorder characterized by obsessions and/or compulsions that impair one's ability to function and form relationships.

techniques such as progressively limiting the amount of time someone obsessed with cleanliness can spend washing and scrubbing, and medication. Deep brain stimulation, which is used to treat Parkinson's, has helped patients with severe OCD.[50]

Other related disorders include excoriation (skin-picking), hoarding (persistent difficulty discarding or parting with possessions), body dysmorphic disorder (preoccupation with perceived physical defects or flaws), and trichotillomania (hair-pulling).[51]

Attention-Deficit/Hyperactivity Disorder

Attention-deficit/hyperactivity disorder (ADHD) is the most common mental disorder in childhood. In a recent meta-analysis of 86 studies, 5.9 percent to 7.1 percent of children and adolescents meet the diagnostic criteria for ADHD—as do 5 percent of adults.[52]

The characteristic symptoms of ADHD are

- Inattention—wandering off task, difficulty sustaining focus, being disorganized, lacking persistence

- Hyperactivity—excessive movements, such as fidgeting or tapping

- Impulsivity—hasty actions done without forethought and with high potential for harm[53]

For many youngsters, ADHD persists into adolescence and adulthood. About one in three young adults (29 percent) diagnosed with childhood ADHD still had the disorder at an average age of 27. About twice as many (57 percent) had at least one other mental health issue, such as alcohol abuse, depression, or chronic anxiety.

Adults with ADHD also are at increased risk. If they do not take medication for their disorder, they are nearly 50 percent more likely to be in a serious car crash.[54] Researchers also have documented a greater risk of premature death in individuals with ADHD.

ADHD on Campus An estimated 2 to 8 percent of young adult college students report clinically significant ADHD symptoms.[55]

In the ACHA survey, 7.8 percent of students reported that they had been diagnosed with ADHD: The normal challenges of college—navigating the complexities of scheduling, planning courses, and honing study skills—may be especially daunting for these students, who may find it hard to concentrate, read, make decisions, complete complex projects, and meet deadlines. Undergraduates with ADHD report greater anxiety[56] and are at higher risk of becoming smokers, abusing alcohol and drugs, and having automobile accidents.

Relationships with peers also can become more challenging. Young people with ADHD may become frustrated easily, have a short fuse, and erupt into angry outbursts. Some become more argumentative, negative, and defiant than most other teens.

In a Canadian study, undergraduates diagnosed with ADHD maintained average GPAs but reported significant psychological distress and difficulty functioning in everyday life.[57] Male students with ADHD typically begin dating at a later age, have fewer romantic relationships, and experience more rejection than undergraduate men without ADHD. Young women diagnosed with ADHD as children generally engage in fewer romantic relationships than others. In a recent study, female undergraduates with ADHD reported more difficulties regulating their emotions, more stress, more conflict, and lower satisfaction in their romantic relationships than other female students.[58]

Sleep problems, including sleeping much more or less than normal, are common. The likelihood of developing other emotional problems, including depression and anxiety disorders, is higher. As many as 20 percent of those diagnosed with depression, anxiety, or substance abuse also have ADHD.

The risk of substance use disorders for individuals with ADHD is twice that of the general population. According to several reports, between 15 and 25 percent of adults with substance use disorders have ADHD.

Treating ADHD The medications used for this disorder include stimulants (such as Ritalin), which improve behavior and cognition for about 70 percent of adolescents with ADHD. Extended-release preparations (including a skin patch) are longer acting, so individuals do not have to take these medications as often as in the past.

As discussed in Chapter 12, an estimated 17 percent of college students misuse stimulant medications.[59] Some may be self-medicating themselves for attention problems. In one survey, 10 percent of those who had never been diagnosed with ADHD had high levels of ADHD symptoms. However, it's not clear whether they suffer from true ADHD. Emergency department visits involving abuse of ADHD drugs have doubled in the past decade.

An alternative nonstimulant treatment is Strattera (atomoxetine), which treats ADHD and coexisting problems such as depression and anxiety but does not seem to have any known

attention-deficit/hyperactivity disorder (ADHD) A spectrum of difficulties in controlling motion and sustaining attention, including hyperactivity, impulsivity, and distractibility.

potential for abuse. Adverse effects include drowsiness, loss of appetite, nausea, vomiting, and headaches. Its long-term effects are not known.

√**check-in** If you have an attention disorder, how do you cope with it?

Many students with ADHD benefit from strategies such as sitting in the front row to avoid distraction, recording lectures if they have difficulty listening and taking notes at the same time, being allowed extended time for tests, and taking oral rather than written exams. Some students have tried to feign ADHD to qualify for such special treatment or to obtain prescriptions for stimulants. However, a thorough examination by an experienced therapist can usually determine whether a student actually suffers from ADHD.

Autism Spectrum Disorder

Autism, a complex neurodevelopmental disability that causes social and communication impairments, is a "spectrum" disorder that affects individuals to varying degrees. Found in all racial, ethnic, and socioeconomic groups, this disorder can affect every aspect of an individual's life. As many as 70 percent of autistic individuals may also have another mental disorder requiring treatment.

According to recent estimates from the CDC, about 1 in 68 children has **autism spectrum disorder**.[60] Boys are four to five times more likely to be diagnosed with autism spectrum disorder (ASD) than girls, perhaps because of genetic vulnerability.[61]

Among the possible factors that may increase the risk of autism spectrum disorder are genetic factors,[62] maternal illness or trauma during pregnancy, abnormalities in brain circuitry,[63] low birth weight, and parental age.[64] In a study of more than 2 million children born in Sweden, researchers found that those born to fathers aged 45 and older were more prone to autism spectrum disorder as well as problems such as ADHD, poor grades in school, low IQ scores, and substance abuse.[65]

There is no scientific evidence that any part of a vaccine or combination of vaccines causes autism, nor is there proof that any material used to produce the vaccine, such as thimerosal, a mercury-containing preservative, plays a role in causing autism. Although past research fraudulently linked vaccines to autism, further investigations have refuted those findings[66] and found no link, even in youngsters with siblings with autism.

Autism spectrum disorder symptoms, which include repetitive patterns of thoughts and behavior and deficits in communication and social interactions, usually start before age 2 and can create delays or problems in many different skills that develop from infancy to adulthood. The earlier interventions begin, the more effective they have proved to be.[67]

Treatments for managing autism spectrum disorders include the following:

- Behavioral therapy to reinforce wanted behaviors and reduce unwanted behaviors
- Speech-language therapy to improve ability to communicate
- Social skills training to enhance interactions with others
- Physical therapy to build motor control and improve posture and balance
- School-based educational programs

There are no medications specifically for the treatment of autism, but various medicines can help manage associated symptoms.

Autism Spectrum Disorder on Campus
Increasing numbers of adolescents and young adults diagnosed with ASD—an estimated two percent of all undergraduates with disabilities—are entering colleges and universities. Although many have the cognitive ability to succeed academically, a high percentage of ASD-diagnosed undergraduates do not complete their postsecondary programs. One reason may be social exclusion, often based on misconceptions about autism.[68] Specific interventions, such as online training, have been shown to increase undergraduates' understanding and acceptance of their peers with autism.[69]

√**check-in** How would you rate your knowledge of autism spectrum disorder and your attitude toward individuals with this disorder?

Adults with autism have significantly increased rates of all major psychiatric disorders, including depression, anxiety, bipolar disorder, obsessive–compulsive disorder, schizophrenia, and suicide attempts, as well as physical illnesses such as immune conditions, digestive and sleep disorders, seizures, obesity, hypertension, and diabetes.[70]

Schizophrenia

Schizophrenia, one of the most debilitating mental disorders, profoundly impairs an individual's

autism spectrum disorder A neurodevelopmental disorder that causes social and communication impairments.

schizophrenia A general term for a group of mental disorders with characteristic psychotic symptoms, such as delusions, hallucinations, and disordered thought patterns during the active phase of the illness, and a duration of at least six months.

sense of reality. As the National Institute of Mental Health (NIMH) puts it, schizophrenia, which is characterized by abnormalities in brain structure and chemistry, destroys "the inner unity of the mind" and weakens "the will and drive that constitute our essential character." This disorder, which is diagnosed in about 1 percent of people worldwide, affects every aspect of psychological functioning, including the ways in which people think, feel, view themselves, and relate to others.[71]

The symptoms of schizophrenia include the following:

- Hallucinations

- Delusions

- Disorganized thinking

- Talking in rambling or incoherent ways

- Making odd or purposeless movements or not moving at all

- Repeating others' words or mimicking their gestures

- Showing few, if any, feelings; responding with inappropriate emotions

- Lacking will or motivation to complete a task or accomplish something

- Functioning at a much lower level than in the past at work, in interpersonal relations, or in taking care of themselves

Schizophrenia, which affects .3 to .7 percent of the world's population, is one of the leading causes of disability among young adults. Schizophrenia usually develops in the early to mid-20s in men and the late 20s in women.[72] Although symptoms do not occur until then, they almost certainly result from failure in brain development that occurs very early in life, probably before birth. Schizophrenia has a strong genetic basis and is not the result of upbringing, social conditions, or traumatic experiences.

For the vast majority of individuals with schizophrenia, antipsychotic drugs are the foundation of treatment. Newer agents are more effective in making most people with schizophrenia feel more comfortable and in control of themselves, helping organize chaotic thinking, and reducing or eliminating delusions or hallucinations, allowing fuller participation in normal activities. Aerobic exercise also has proven beneficial.[73]

Nonsuicidal Self-Injury

Deliberately harming oneself may take any form of damage to the body: cutting, burning, stabbing, hitting, excessive rubbing. The intent is not to take one's life but to obtain relief from painful feelings or thoughts, to resolve an interpersonal difficulty, or to induce positive feelings, such as relief. A diagnosis of nonsuicidal self-injury is based on intentional self-damage occurring on five or more days within the past year.[74]

Self-injury most often starts in the early teens and can continue for many years. Admission to hospitals for self-inflicted injuries peaks between the ages of 20 and 29 and then declines. In the ACHA survey, 5.5 percent of college students—3.8 percent of men and 6.3 percent of women—reported intentionally cutting, burning, bruising, or otherwise injuring themselves.[75]

Approximately 17 percent of college students have engaged in nonsuicidal self-injury at some point in their lives; 14 percent have done so in the previous 12 months. A significant proportion begin self-injury during college, particularly during freshman year.

Students at risk for nonsuicidal self-injury may experience elevated internal distress, become involved in dysfunctional relationships, and attempt to cope with difficulties in unhealthy ways, including disordered eating and self-injury. Younger first-year students may be at greater risk because they feel less connected to campus life and lack strong social support. Undergraduates who identify as a sexual or racial/ethnic minority also are at increased risk of both self-injury and suicidal behavior, perhaps because of a sense of isolation and stigma. In a recent study, a third of those who reported self-injury also attempted suicide during the previous year.[76]

Among the factors associated with self-injury in college students are

- Bisexual or questioning sexual orientation

- History of abuse or neglect

- Psychological and emotional distress

- Symptoms of depression or anxiety

- Childhood separation

- Interpersonal difficulties

- Eating disorders

- Cigarette smoking

- Substance abuse[77]

Suicide

Suicide is the third leading cause of death among 10- to 24-year-olds in the United States.[79] The most common methods are guns, hanging and poisoning. Suicide, often the tragic

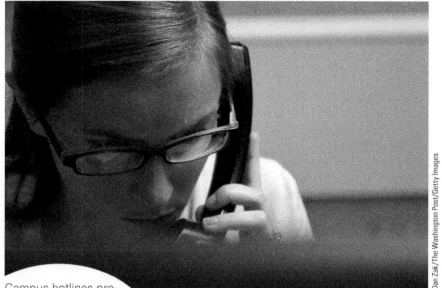

Campus hotlines provide peer support to students who may be feeling overwhelmed but don't know where to turn for help.

Long considered a threat to younger and older Americans, suicide has increased significantly among middle-aged men and women. Although the reasons are unknown, researchers speculate that baby boomers, who also had high suicide rates in adolescence, may be particularly vulnerable to self-inflicted harm. They also tend to choose the most lethal suicide methods, such as guns and hanging.[78] At all ages, men *commit* suicide three to four times more frequently than women, but women *attempt* suicide much more often than men (see Table 3.2).

Suicide on Campus

More than 1,100 college students take their own lives every year; many more—an estimated 1.2 percent of undergraduates—attempt to do so.

An estimated 18 percent of undergraduates have seriously considered suicide at some point in their lives; 40 to 50 percent of these students report multiple episodes of suicidal thoughts. Some 8 to 15 percent of college students act on their suicidal thoughts and plan or attempt suicide.[80] College students who are serving or have served in the military do not have higher rates of depression and are not more likely to plan or attempt suicide than other undergraduates. [81]

Suicide rarely stems from a single cause. Researchers have identified several common ones for college students, including the following:

consequence of emotional and psychological problems, affects millions of lives every year:

- An estimated 8.5 million American adults (3.8 percent) report having had serious thoughts of suicide in the past year.

- 1.1 million (.5 percent) attempt suicide.

- Some 38,000 Americans—among them many young people who seem to have "everything to live for"—commit suicide.

- An average of 105 suicides occur in the United States every day.

- An estimated 811,000 people attempt to take their own lives per year.

- There may be 4.5 million suicide "survivors" in the United States.

- The suicide rate for African American and Caucasian men peaks between ages 20 and 40 and rises again after age 65 among white men and after age 75 among blacks.

- In general, whites are at highest risk for suicide, followed by American Indians, African Americans, Hispanic Americans, and Asian Americans.

- Depression.

- Depressive symptoms.

- Family history of mental illness.

- Personality traits such as hopelessness, helplessness, impulsivity, and aggression.

- Alcohol use and binge drinking. (Among college students, binge drinkers are significantly more likely to contemplate suicide, to have attempted suicide in the past, and to believe they would make a future suicide attempt than non-binge drinkers.)

- Interpersonal difficulties with a romantic partner, family, or friends, which may reflect what researchers call "thwarted belongingness" or a lack of connection with peers, loved ones, and the school community.[82]

- Ineffective problem solving and coping skills.

- Recent sexual or physical victimization; being in an emotionally or physically abusive relationship.

- Family problems.

- Exposure to trauma or stress.

TABLE 3.2 Suicide Risk

	Who Attempts Suicide?	Who Commits Suicide?
Sex	Female	Male
Age	Under 35	Under 20 or over 60
Means	Less deadly, such as a wrist slashing	More deadly, such as a gun
Circumstances	High chance of rescue	Low chance of rescue

© Cengage Learning

- Feelings of loneliness or social isolation.
- Harassment because of sexual orientation.

The stress of acculturation (the psychosocial adjustments that occur when an ethnic minority interacts with the ethnic majority may also play a role. Blacks who take their own lives tend to be younger, less likely to have been depressed, and less likely to have financial problems, chronic illness, or substance abuse problems.

Although many schools offer counseling and crisis services, students often don't know where to turn when they feel hopeless or are thinking about suicide. In a study of undergraduates with suicidal thoughts, 44 percent did not seek treatment for reasons that included ambivalence, stigma, and financial concerns.

Colleges are sponsoring more screening and educational programs on suicide.[83] In preliminary studies of online risk assessments, this approach increased the willingness of students at risk to talk to a friend or family member and to consider and engage in mental health treatment.[84]

Factors That Lead to Suicide

The most important risk factors for suicide appear to be impulsivity, high levels of arousal and aggression, and past suicidal behavior (see Table 3.3).

Suicidal Behavior Disorder According to the American Psychiatric Association's DSM-5, a suicide attempt, defined as a self-initiated sequence of behaviors intended to lead to death, within the previous 24 months is the characteristic symptom of suicidal behavior disorder. Individuals who have tried to take their own lives are at higher risk for further attempts and for death in the two years following a failed attempt. About 25 to 30 percent of persons who try to kill themselves attempt to do so again.[85]

Mental Disorders More than 95 percent of those who commit suicide have a mental disorder. Two in particular—depression and alcoholism—account for two-thirds of all suicides. Suicide also is a risk for those with other disorders, including schizophrenia, posttraumatic stress disorder, personality disorders; and untreated depression; the lifetime suicide rate for people with major depression is 15 percent. Panic attacks increase the risk in depressed individuals.[86]

Substance Abuse Many of those who commit suicide drink beforehand, and their

TABLE 3.3 Risk Factors for Suicide

Biopsychosocial Risk Factors

- Mental disorders, particularly depressive disorders, schizophrenia, and anxiety disorders
- Alcohol and other substance use disorders
- Hopelessness
- Impulsive and/or aggressive tendencies
- History of trauma or abuse
- Some major physical illness
- Previous suicide attempt
- Family history of suicide

Environmental Risk Factors

- Job or financial loss
- Relational or social loss
- Easy access to lethal means
- Local clusters of suicide that have a contagious influence

Sociocultural Risk Factors

- Lack of social support and sense of isolation
- Stigma associated with help-seeking behavior
- Barriers to accessing health care, especially mental health and substance abuse treatment
- Certain cultural and religious beliefs (for instance, the belief that suicide is a noble resolution of a personal dilemma)
- Exposure to suicide, including through the media, and the influence of others who have died by suicide

Source: Suicide Prevention Resource Center: http://www.sprc.org/

use of alcohol may lower their inhibitions and intensify despondent feelings. Alcoholics who attempt suicide often have other risk factors, including major depression, poor social support, serious medical illness, and unemployment.

Hopelessness When hope dies, individuals view every experience in negative terms and come to expect the worst possible outcomes for their problems. Given this way of thinking, suicide often seems a reasonable response to a life seen as not worth living.

Combat Stress According to the Department of Veterans Affairs, an estimated 22 military veterans kill themselves every day—one every 65 minutes. Most (64 percent) are age 50 or older. Conditions that may increase a veteran's risk of suicide include depression, PTSD, traumatic brain injury, and lack of social support. The Veterans Administration has set up a Suicide Prevention Hotline number: 1-800-274-TALK.

Family History One of every four people who attempt suicide has a family member who

YOUR STRATEGIES FOR PREVENTION

Steps to Prevent Suicide

If you worry that someone you know may be contemplating suicide, express your concern. Here are some specific guidelines:

- **Ask concerned questions.** Listen attentively. Show that you take the person's feelings seriously and truly care.

- **Don't offer trite reassurances.** Don't list reasons to go on living, try to analyze the person's motives, or try to shock or challenge him or her.

- **Suggest solutions or alternatives to problems.** Make plans. Encourage positive action, such as getting away for a while to gain a better perspective on a problem.

- **Don't be afraid to ask whether your friend has considered suicide.** The opportunity to talk about thoughts of suicide may be an enormous relief and—contrary to a long-standing myth—will not fix the idea of suicide more firmly in a person's mind.

- **Don't think that people who talk about killing themselves never carry out their threat.** Most individuals who commit suicide give definite indications of their intent to die.

- **Watch out for behavioral clues.** If your friend begins to behave unpredictably or suddenly emerges from a severe depression into a calm, settled state of mind, these could signal increased danger of suicide. Don't leave your friend alone. Call a suicide hotline, or get in touch with a mental health professional.

- **If a friend expresses suicidal thoughts on Facebook, report the post to its "Report Suicidal Content" link.** The person who posted the suicidal content will receive an e-mail or call from the National Suicide Prevention Lifeline (1-800-273-TALK).

If you are thinking about suicide . . .

- **Talk to a mental health professional.** If you have a therapist, call immediately. If not, call a suicide hotline.

- **Find someone you can trust and talk honestly about what you're feeling.** If you suffer from depression or another mental disorder, educate trusted friends or relatives about your condition so they are prepared if called upon to help.

- **Write down your more uplifting thoughts.** Even if you are despondent, you can help yourself by taking the time to retrieve some more positive thoughts or memories. A simple record of your hopes for the future and the people you value in your life can remind you of why your own life is worth continuing.

- **Avoid drugs and alcohol.** Most suicides are the results of sudden, uncontrolled impulses, and drugs and alcohol can make it harder to resist these destructive urges.

- **Go to the hospital.** Hospitalization can sometimes be the best way to protect your health and safety.

also tried to commit suicide. While a family history of suicide is not in itself considered a predictor of suicide, two mental disorders that can lead to suicide—depression and bipolar disorder (manic depression)—do run in families.

Physical Illness People who commit suicide are likely to be ill or to believe that they are. About 5 percent actually have a serious physical disorder, such as AIDS or cancer. While suicide may seem to be a decision rationally arrived at in persons with serious or fatal illness, depression, not uncommon in such instances, can warp judgment. When the depression is treated, the person may no longer have suicidal intentions.

Brain Chemistry Investigators have found abnormalities in the brain chemistry of individuals who complete suicide, especially low levels of a metabolite of the neurotransmitter serotonin. Individuals with a deficiency in this substance may have as much as a ten times greater risk of committing suicide than those with higher levels.

Access to Guns For individuals with predisposing factors, access to a means of committing suicide, particularly guns, can add to the risk. Unlike other methods of suicide, guns almost always work. Although only 5 percent of suicide attempts involve firearms, more than 90 percent of these attempts are fatal. States with stricter gun-control laws have much lower rates of suicide than states with more lenient laws.

Other Factors Individuals who kill themselves have often gone through more major life crises—job changes, births, financial reversals, divorce, retirement—in the previous six months, compared with others. Long-standing, intense conflict with family members or other important people may add to the danger. In some cases, suicide may be an act of revenge that offers a sense of control—however temporary or illusory. By rejecting life, a person also rejects a partner or parent who abandoned or betrayed them.

✓**check-in** Do you know anyone who attempted or committed suicide?

Overcoming Problems of the Mind

At any given time, about 25 percent of men, women, and children meet the criteria for a mental disorder, yet 75 percent of those in need of

HEALTH ON A BUDGET

The Exercise Prescription

Imagine a drug so powerful it can alter brain chemistry, so versatile it can help prevent or treat many common mental disorders, so safe that moderate doses cause few, if any, side effects, and so inexpensive that anyone can afford it. This wonder drug, proved in years of research, is exercise.

Chapter 8 provides detailed information on improving your fitness. To make a difference in the way you look and feel, follow these simple guidelines:

- **Work in short bouts.** Three 10-minute intervals of exercise can be just as effective as exercising for 30 minutes straight.

- **Mix it up.** Combine moderate and vigorous intensity exercises to meet the guidelines. For instance, you can walk briskly two days a week and jog at a faster pace on the other days.

- **Set aside exercise times.** Schedule exercise in advance so you can plan your day around it.

- **Find exercise buddies.** Recruit roommates, friends, family, coworkers. You'll have more fun on your way to getting fit.

---

psychological help never receive the treatment they need. As discussed earlier in this chapter, college students are especially likely to delay getting help for a psychological problem.

The median delay for all disorders is nearly 10 years. Those with social phobia and separation anxiety disorders may not get help for more than 20 years. The earlier in life that a disorder begins, the longer individuals tend to delay treatment.

Without treatment, mental disorders take a toll on every aspect of life, including academics, relationships, careers, and risk-taking. Symptoms or episodes of a disorder typically become more frequent or severe. Individuals with one mental disorder are at high risk of having a second one; this is called *comorbidity*.

Self-Help Strategies

Self-care can contribute enormously to both physical and psychological health.

Eating Right Both body and mind require good nutrition to run efficiently. Poor eating habits—skipping meals, wolfing them down, munching on junk foods—can make people psychologically uneasy and unable to concentrate on tasks at hand, relax, or enjoy being with others. A healthful, balanced diet is essential to a feeling of well-being.

People who are depressed need to be especially watchful because they may lose their appetite, eat less, lose weight, and be at risk for nutritional deficiencies. Although various nutritional "cures" for depression have been touted over the years, none has been scientifically validated.

Excessive caffeine (discussed in Chapters 6 and 12) can cause many symptoms associated with anxiety or panic. Anyone troubled by an anxiety disorder should avoid caffeinated beverages.

Many people increase the amount of alcohol they drink when under stress. Depressed individuals may try to drown their sorrows; those who are anxious may drink to calm their "nerves." However, drinking only makes these problems worse. As discussed in Chapter 13, alcohol, a central nervous system depressant, can intensify a depressed mood or exacerbate anxiety.

Exercise In addition to its head-to-toe physical benefits, discussed in Chapter 8, exercise may be, as one therapist puts it, the single most effective way to lift a person's spirits and to restore feelings of potency about all aspects of life (see Health on a Budget). People who exercise regularly report a more cheerful mood, higher self-esteem, and less stress. Their sleep and appetite also tend to improve. In clinical studies, exercise has proved effective as a treatment for depression and anxiety disorders. But remember: Although exercise can help prevent and ease problems for many people, it's no substitute for professional treatment of serious psychiatric disorders.

Books and Websites A wealth of informational and motivational material is available online and in books. Research has shown that such "low-intensity interventions," which do not require the expense and time of a professional therapist, can help individuals with mild or moderate depression or anxiety. In a recent study in Great Britain, individuals with more severe mental disorders also benefited, perhaps because the information and activities helped them better manage their symptoms.[87]

Virtual Support Increasingly, mental health professionals are utilizing "e-health" or "m-health" (the delivery of health care by electronic means via the Internet using phones, watches, and other devices). Such technology makes psychological support available 24 hours a day, 7 days a week—a boon for many patients.[88] Online sites such as PatientsLikeMe offer patients tools to track mental health symptoms and enhance peer learning and social support.[89]

Peer Support   Support groups have long been a staple of treatment for individuals who have a chronic illness; are wrestling with a substance use disorder; have experienced common traumatic experiences, such as child abuse; or are dealing with similar challenges, such as widowhood. Often these groups do not have a professional leader or formal structure. Their primary goal is to provide support and encouragement, overcome a sense of isolation, and share information.

Peer support has long been available on many university campuses. More recently, some schools have begun offering online peer support forums for students with problems such as symptoms of depression. They have proven helpful in increasing problem-solving skills, decreasing alienation and isolation, and lowering stress.[90]

With an estimated half million veterans, active-duty personnel, reservists, and National Guardsmen attending college, more peer support groups for fellow service members or veterans are appearing on campus. Compared with their civilian counterparts, they focus on issues such as the challenge of adjusting from military service to student life, tobacco- and alcohol-related risky behaviors, psychological symptoms, and suicide risk.

✓ **check-in Do** you need help?
Consider therapy if you
__ Feel an overwhelming and prolonged sense of helplessness and sadness, which does not lift despite your efforts and help from family and friends
__ Find it difficult to carry out everyday activities such as homework, and your academic performance is suffering
__ Worry excessively, expect the worst, or are constantly on edge
__ Are finding it hard to resist or are engaging in behaviors that are harmful to you or others, such as drinking too much alcohol, abusing drugs, or becoming aggressive or violent
__ Have persistent thoughts or fantasies of harming yourself or others

psychiatrists Licensed medical doctors with additional training in psychotherapy, psychopharmacology, and treatment of mental disorders.

psychologists Mental health care professionals who have completed a doctoral or graduate program in psychology and are trained in psychotherapeutic techniques, but who are not medically trained and do not prescribe medications.

Where to Turn for Help

About 10 percent of students seek care from a mental health counseling center on campus. Your health education instructor can tell you about general and mental health counseling available on campus, school-based support groups, community-based programs, and special emergency services. On campus, you can also turn to the student health services or the office of the dean of student services or student affairs.

Within the community, you may be able to get help through the city or county health department and neighborhood health centers. Local hospitals often have special clinics and services, and there are usually local branches of national service organizations, such as United Way or Alcoholics Anonymous, other 12 Step programs, and various support groups. You can call the psychiatric or psychological association in your city or state for the names of licensed professionals. (Check the telephone directory for listings.) Your primary physician may also be able to help.

Search the Internet for special programs, found either by the nature of the service, by the name of the neighborhood or city, or by the name of the sponsoring group. In addition to suicide-prevention programs, look for crisis intervention, violence prevention, and child-abuse prevention programs; drug-treatment information; shelters for battered women; senior citizen centers; and self-help and counseling services. Many services have special hotlines for coping with emergencies. Others provide information as well as support over the phone, or by e-mail or texts.

Types of Therapists   Only professionally trained individuals who have met state licensing requirements are certified as psychiatrists, psychologists, or social workers. Before selecting any of these mental health professionals, be sure to check the person's background and credentials.

Psychiatrists are licensed medical doctors (M.D.) who complete medical school; a year-long internship; and a three-year residency that provides training in various forms of psychotherapy, psychopharmacology, and both outpatient and inpatient treatment of mental disorders. They can prescribe medications and make medical decisions. *Board-certified* psychiatrists have passed oral and written examinations following completion of residency training.

Psychologists complete a graduate program (including clinical training and internships) in human psychology but do not study medicine and cannot prescribe medication. They must be licensed in most states in order to practice independently.

Certified social workers or licensed clinical social workers (LCSWs) usually complete a two-year graduate program and have specialized training in helping people with mental problems in addition to conventional social work.

Psychiatric nurses have nursing degrees and have passed a state examination. They usually have special training and experience in mental health care, although no specialty licensing or certification is required.

Marriage and family therapists, licensed in some but not all states, usually have a graduate degree, often in psychology, and at least two years of supervised clinical training in dealing with relationship problems.

Other therapists include pastoral counselors, members of the clergy who offer psychological counseling; hypnotherapists, who use hypnosis for problems such as smoking and obesity; stress-management counselors, who teach relaxation methods; and alcohol and drug counselors, who help individuals with substance use problems. Anyone can use these terms themselves professionally, and there are no licensing requirements.

Choosing a Therapist Ask your physician or another health professional. Call your local or state psychological association. Consult your university or college department of psychology or health center. Contact your area community mental health center. Inquire at your church or synagogue.

- A good rapport with your psychotherapist is critical. Choose someone with whom you feel comfortable and at ease.
- Ask the following questions:
  - Are you licensed?
  - How long have you been practicing?
  - I have been feeling (anxious, tense, depressed, etc.), and I'm having problems (with school, relationships, eating, sleeping, etc.). What experience do you have helping people with these types of problems?
  - What are your areas of expertise—phobias? ADHD? depression?
  - What kinds of treatments do you use? Have they proved effective for dealing with my kind of problem or issue?
  - What are your fees? (Fees are usually based on a 45-minute to 50-minute session.) Do you have a sliding-scale fee policy?
  - How much therapy would you recommend?
  - What types of insurance do you accept?

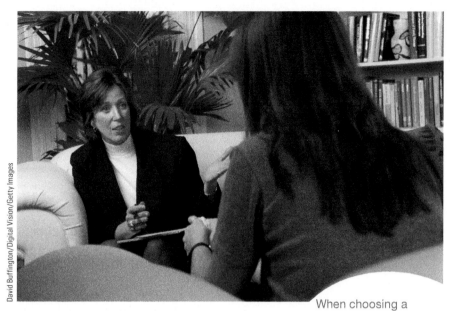

David Buffington/Digital Vision/Getty Images

As you begin therapy, establish clear goals with your therapist. Some goals require more time to reach than others. You and your therapist should decide at what point you might expect to begin to see progress.

✓**check-in** Where would you turn if you wanted help with a psychological issue?

Types of Therapy

The term **psychotherapy** refers to any type of counseling based on the exchange of words in the context of the unique relationship that develops between a mental health professional and a person seeking help. The process of talking and listening can lead to new insight, relief from distressing psychological symptoms, changes in unhealthy or maladaptive behaviors, and more effective ways of dealing with the world. "Spirituality oriented" psychotherapy pays particular attention to the roles that religion and spiritual and religious beliefs play in an individual's psychological life.

Psychotherapy does not just benefit the mind but actually changes the brain. In studies comparing psychotherapy and psychiatric medications as treatments for depression, both proved about equally effective. But a particular group of patients—those who had lost a parent at an early age or had experienced childhood trauma, including physical or sexual abuse—gained greater benefits with talk therapy.

Most mental health professionals today are trained in a variety of psychotherapeutic techniques and tailor their approach to the problem,

When choosing a therapist, always consider professional qualifications, such as education, as well as personal qualities, such as compassion.

certified social workers or licensed clinical social workers (LCSWs) Persons who have completed a two-year graduate program in counseling people with mental problems.

psychiatric nurses Nurses with special training and experience in mental health care.

marriage and family therapists Psychiatrists, psychologists, or social workers who specialize in marriage and family counseling.

psychotherapy Treatment designed to produce a response by psychological rather than physical means, such as suggestion, persuasion, reassurance, and support.

personality, and needs of each person seeking their help. Because skilled therapists may combine different techniques in the course of therapy, the lines between the various approaches often blur.

Brief Psychotherapies Short-term treatments (which may consist of psychodynamic, behavioral, cognitive, interpersonal, or other approaches) typically focus on a central issue and typically conclude in less than 6 months or 24 sessions. The individuals most likely to benefit are those who are interested in solving immediate problems rather than changing their characters, who can think in psychological terms, whose issues are not highly complex or severe, and who are motivated to change.

Psychodynamic Psychotherapy For the most part, today's mental health professionals base their assessment of individuals on a **psychodynamic** understanding that takes into account the role of early experiences and unconscious influences in *actively* shaping behavior. (This is the *dynamic* in psychodynamic.) Psychodynamic treatments work toward the goal of providing greater insight into problems and bringing about behavioral change. Therapy may be brief, intermittent, or longer term, continuing for several years.[91]

Cognitive-Behavioral Therapy (CBT) Cognitive-behavioral therapy (CBT) focuses on inappropriate or inaccurate thoughts or beliefs to help individuals break out of a distorted, mal-adaptive way of thinking.[92] The techniques of **cognitive therapy** include identification of an individual's beliefs and attitudes, recognition of negative thought patterns, and education in alternative ways of thinking. Individuals with major depression or anxiety disorders are most likely to benefit, usually in 15 to 25 sessions. In a recent study, telephone CBT proved as effective as face-to-face therapy.[93]

Behavioral Therapy The goal of **behavioral therapy** is to substitute healthier ways of behaving for maladaptive patterns used in the past. Some therapists believe that changing behavior also changes how people think and feel. As they put it, "Change the behavior, and the feelings will follow." Behavioral therapies work best for disorders characterized by specific, abnormal patterns of acting—such as alcohol and drug abuse, anxiety disorders, and phobias—and for individuals who want to change habits.

CBT has proven effective for treating depression, often in combination with medication; anxiety; trauma-related disorders; bipolar disorder as an addition to medication; and eating disorders.

Family-Focused Therapy (FFT) This approach is based on the assumption that a patient's relationship with family members is vital to successful management of his or her illness. Therapists trained in FFT involve family members in therapy and identify difficulties and conflicts that may be worsening the patient's condition. FFT also focuses on the stresses on family members caring for a relative with a mental disorder and helps prevent burnout.

Interpersonal Therapy (IPT) Originally developed for research into the treatment of major depression, **interpersonal therapy (IPT)** does not deal with the psychological origins of symptoms but rather concentrates on current problems of getting along with others. The emphasis is on the here and now and on interpersonal—rather than intrapsychic—issues. Individuals with major depression, chronic difficulties developing relationships, and chronic mild depression are most likely to benefit. IPT usually consists of 12 to 16 sessions.

Other Treatment Options

Psychiatric Drugs Thanks to the development of more precise and effective **psychiatric drugs**, success rates for treating many common and disabling disorders—depression, panic disorder, schizophrenia, and others—have soared. Often used in conjunction with psychotherapy, these medications have revolutionized mental health care.

At some point in their lives, about half of all Americans will take a psychiatric drug. The reason may be depression, anxiety, a sleep difficulty, an eating disorder, alcohol or drug dependence, impaired memory, or another disorder that disrupts the intricate chemistry of the brain.

√**check-in** Have you ever taken a psychiatric drug?

Psychiatric medications, among the most commonly prescribed drugs in the United States, account for almost 12 percent of drug prescriptions in the United States. Sedatives and hypnotics are the most widely prescribed, followed by antidepressants. Adverse reactions to psychiatric medications, including antidepressants, lead to about 90,000 visits to emergency departments every year.[94] Serotonin-boosting medications (SSRIs), the drugs of choice in treating depression, also are effective in treating obsessive-compulsive

psychodynamic Interpreting behaviors in terms of early experiences and unconscious influences.

cognitive therapy A technique used to identify an individual's beliefs and attitudes, recognize negative thought patterns, and educate in alternative ways of thinking.

behavioral therapy A technique that emphasizes application of the principles of learning to substitute desirable responses and behavior patterns for undesirable ones.

interpersonal therapy (IPT) A technique used to develop communication skills and relationships.

psychiatric drugs Medications that regulate a person's mental, emotional, and physical functions to facilitate normal functioning.

disorder, panic disorder, social phobia, posttraumatic stress disorder, premenstrual dysphoric disorder, and generalized anxiety disorder. In patients who don't respond, psychiatrists may add another drug to boost the efficacy of the treatment.

Alternative Mind–Mood Products Some "natural" products, such as herbs and enzymes, claim to have psychological effects. However, they have not undergone rigorous scientific testing. The most well known is St. John's wort, which has been used to treat anxiety and depression in Europe for many years. In 10 carefully controlled studies in the United States, the herb did not prove more effective than a placebo. Side effects include dizziness, abdominal pain and bloating, constipation, nausea, fatigue, and dry mouth. St. John's wort should not be taken in combination with other prescription antidepressants. An added precaution: It can lower the efficacy of oral contraceptives and increase the risk of unwanted pregnancy.

Daily meditation (discussed in Chapter 4) might help relieve anxiety and depression, according to an analysis of 47 studies that examined the effects of meditation on various conditions. The researchers concluded that meditation produced "moderate" benefits in depressed or anxious individuals.

- How does the brain affect our thoughts and behavior?
- What are common mental disorders on college campuses?
- How do depression and anxiety affect individuals?
- Why do college students commit suicide?

THE POWER OF NOW!
Taking Care of Your Mental Health

Like physical health, psychological well-being is not a fixed state of being but a process. The way you live every day affects how you feel about yourself and the world. Here are some basic guidelines that you can rely on to make the most of the process of living. Check those that you commit to making part of your mental and psychological self-care:

____ Accept yourself. As a human being, you are, by definition, imperfect. Come to terms with the fact that you are a worthwhile person despite your mistakes.

____ Respect yourself. Recognize your abilities and talents. Acknowledge your competence and achievements and take pride in them.

____ Trust yourself. Learn to listen to the voice within you and let your intuition be your guide.

____ Love yourself. Be happy to spend time by yourself. Learn to appreciate your own company and to be glad you're you.

____ Stretch yourself. Be willing to change and grow, to try something new and dare to be vulnerable.

____ Look at challenges as opportunities for personal growth. "Every problem brings the possibility of a widening of consciousness," psychologist Carl Jung once noted. Put his words to the test.

____ When your internal critic—the negative inner voice we all have—starts putting you down, force yourself to think of a situation that you handled well.

____ Set a limit on self-pity. Tell yourself, "I'm going to feel sorry for myself this morning, but this afternoon, I've got to get on with my life."

____ Recognize and express your feelings. Pent-up emotions tend to fester inside, building into anger or depression.

____ Don't brood. Rather than merely mull over a problem, try to find solutions that are positive and useful.

____ Take one step at a time. As long as you're taking some action to solve a problem, you can take pride in your ability to cope.

____ Spend more time doing activities you know you do well. For example, if you are a good cook, prepare a meal for someone.

____ Use affirmations. These positive statements help reinforce the most positive aspects of your personality and experience. Every day, you might say, "I am a loving, caring person" or "I am honest and open in expressing my feelings." Write some affirmations of your own on index cards or in the Notes app on your phone and flip through them occasionally.

____ List the things you would like to have or experience. Construct the statements as if you were already enjoying the situations you list, beginning each sentence with "I am." For example, "I am feeling great about doing well in my classes."

What's Online

CENGAGE Visit www.cengagebrain.com to access course materials for this text, including the Behavior Change Planner, interactive quizzes, tutorials. and more.

Recognizing Depression

Depression comes in different forms, just like other illnesses such as heart disease. Not everyone with a depressive disorder experiences every symptom. The number and severity of symptoms may vary among individuals and also over time.

Read through the following list, and check all the descriptions that apply.

- ❏ I am often restless and irritable.

- ❏ I am having irregular sleep patterns—either too much or not enough.

- ❏ I don't enjoy hobbies, my friends, family, or leisure activities anymore.

- ❏ I am having trouble managing my diabetes, hypertension, or other chronic illness.

- ❏ I have nagging aches and pains that do not get better no matter what I do.

- ❏ Specifically, I often experience

  - ❏ Digestive problems

  - ❏ Headache or backache

  - ❏ Vague aches and pains like joint or muscle pains

  - ❏ Chest pains

  - ❏ Dizziness

- ❏ I have trouble concentrating or making simple decisions.

- ❏ Others have commented on my mood or attitude lately.

- ❏ My weight has changed a considerable amount.

- ❏ I have had several of the symptoms I checked above for more than two weeks.

- ❏ I feel that my functioning in my everyday life (work, family, friends) is suffering because of these problems.

- ❏ I have a family history of depression.

- ❏ I have thought about suicide.[1]

Checking several items on this list does not mean that you have a depressive disorder because many conditions can cause similar symptoms. However, you should take this list with you to discuss with your health-care provider or mental health therapist. Even though it can be difficult to talk about certain things, your health-care provider is knowledgeable, trained, and committed to helping you.

If you can't think of what to say, try these conversation starters:

"I just don't feel like myself lately."

"My friend (parent, roommate, spouse) thinks I might be depressed."

"I haven't been sleeping well lately."

"Everything seems harder than before."

"Nothing's fun anymore."

If you are diagnosed with depression, remember that it is a common and highly treatable illness with medical causes. Your habits or personality did not cause your depression, and you do not have to face it alone.

[1]University of Michigan Depression Center, 800-475-MICH, http://www.depression center.org/

MAKING THIS CHAPTER WORK FOR YOU

Review Questions

(LO 3.1)   1. Neurons _____.
   a. transmit information within the brain and throughout the body by means of electrical impulses and chemical messengers
   b. are specialized support cells that travel through the spinal cord, carrying signals related to movement
   c. are protein molecules designed to bind with neurotransmitters
   d. cross a synapse before reuptake

(LO 3.1)   2. One of the ways that male and female brain differ is _____.
   a. women's brains are larger relative to overall body size than men's
   b. men's hearing is sharper than women's
   c. women's eyes are more sensitive to bright light than men's
   d. when men actively think about something, neurons turn on in highly specific areas of the brain

(LO 3.2)   3. Among other serious impacts, mental disorders tend to _____.
   a. shorten the lives of those who have a disorder
   b. increase the risk of obesity
   c. increase the risk of type 2 diabetes
   d. increase the likelihood of contracting an STI

(LO 3.2)   4. Factors that increase vulnerability to a mental disorder among undergraduates include which of the following?
   a. Trouble with roommates
   b. Long-term relationship
   c. Financial pressures
   d. Belonging to a fraternity or sorority

(LO 3.3)   5. Which of the following observations is true of gender differences in depression?
   a. Women are more likely than men to become depressed following a divorce, job loss, or career setback.
   b. Women are more sensitive to changes in light and temperature than men.
   c. Men's brains register sadness much more intensely than women's.
   d. Depressed women are more likely to take their own lives than are depressed men.

(LO 3.5)   6. Which of the following is a characteristic symptom of bipolar disorder?
   a. Lack of energy
   b. Persistent thoughts of death
   c. Mood swings
   d. Eating more or less than usual

(LO 3.4)   7. Which of the following anxiety disorders is treated with a process called systematic desensitization?
   a. Panic attack
   b. Phobia
   c. Generalized anxiety disorder
   d. Obsessive-compulsive disorder

(LO 3.4)   8. Panic attacks _____.
   a. occur more frequently among men than women
   b. always require hospitalization
   c. occur more frequently among parents, siblings, and children or individuals with panic disorder
   d. are resistant to treatment by therapy and medication

(LO 3.5)   9. Which of the following strategies will benefit students with attention-deficit/hyperactivity disorder (ADHD)?
   a. Stand in the last row rather than sitting in the front row.
   b. Draw images rather than writing notes.
   c. Take written exams rather than oral exams.
   d. Record lectures rather than taking notes.

(LO 3.5)   10. According to the National Institute of Mental Health, _____ is characterized by abnormalities in brain structure and chemistry, destroys "the inner unity of the mind," and weakens "the will and drive that constitute our essential character."
   a. phobia
   b. schizophrenia
   c. attention-deficit/hyperactivity disorder
   d. depression

(LO 3.6)   11. Which of the following observations is true of suicide?
   a. Individuals with a high level of serotonin may have a greater risk of committing suicide than those with lower levels.
   b. White Americans are at the lowest risk for suicide.
   c. Women attempt suicide much more often than men.
   d. Suicide often stems from a single cause.

(LO 3.6)   12. Which of the following mental disorders is most common among those who commit suicide?
   a. Depression
   b. Attention-deficit/hyperactivity disorder
   c. Phobia
   d. Obsessive-compulsive disorder

(LO 3.7) 13. _____ takes into account the role of early experiences and unconscious influences in *actively* shaping behavior.
a. Family-focused therapy
b. Cognitive-behavioral therapy
c. Interpersonal therapy
d. Psychodynamic psychotherapy

(LO 3.7) 14. Which of the following therapies focuses on modifying inappropriate or inaccurate thoughts or beliefs to help individuals break out of a distorted, maladaptive way of thinking?
a. Family-focused therapy
b. Cognitive-behavioral therapy
c. Interpersonal therapy
d. Psychodynamic psychotherapy

Answers to these questions can be found on page 623.

Critical Thinking Questions

1. Jake, who took antidepressants to recover from depression in high school, began feeling the same troubling symptoms. A physician at the student health center prescribed the same medication that had helped him in the past, but this time Jake noticed the warning about an increased risk of suicide. He has had thoughts of killing himself, and he worries whether or not to start the medication. When he did some online research, he learned that the risk of suicide is greater if depression is untreated than it is with medication. How would you counsel Jake? How would you weigh the risks and benefits of taking an antidepressant? Do you know someone who might benefit from taking antidepressants but is afraid to take them because of the possible risk of suicide? What might you say to this person based on what you have read in this chapter?

2. Research has indicated that many homeless men and women are in need of outpatient psychiatric care, often because they suffer from chronic mental illnesses or alcoholism. Yet government funding for the mentally ill is inadequate, and homelessness itself can make it difficult, if not impossible, for people to gain access to the care they need. How do you feel when you pass homeless individuals who seem disoriented or out of touch with reality? Who should take responsibility for their welfare? Should they be forced to undergo treatment at psychiatric institutions?

Additional Online Resources

www.save.org
This site offers research, facts, survivor support, and more.

www.nimh.nih.gov
The National Institute of Mental Health is a federally sponsored organization that provides useful information on a variety of mental health topics including current mental health research.

www.apa.org
The APA is the scientific and professional organization for psychology in the United States. Its website provides up-to-date information on psychological issues and disorders.

www.mentalhealthamerica.net
This site features fact sheets on a variety of mental health topics, including depression screening, college initiative, substance abuse prevention, and information for families. Also available are current mental health articles, an e-mail newsletter, and a bookstore.

www.afsp.org
This site provides facts and statistics about suicide and depression, as well as information about current research and educational projects. It also provides support information for survivors.

http://activeminds.org
This site provides fact sheets on mental illness and information about starting an Active Minds chapter and planning events at your campus to create awareness about mental health.

Key Terms

The terms listed are used on the page indicated. Definitions of the terms are in the glossary at the end of the book.

antidepressants 57

anxiety disorders 58

attention-deficit/hyperactivity disorder (ADHD) 61

autism spectrum disorder 62

axon 48

axon terminal 49

behavioral therapy 70

bipolar disorder 58

certified social workers or licensed clinical social workers (LCSWs) 69

cognitive therapy 70

dendrites 49

generalized anxiety disorder (GAD) 60

glia 49

interpersonal therapy (IPT) 70

major depressive disorder 57

marriage and family therapists 69

mental disorder 51

neurons 48

neuropsychiatry 48

neurotransmitters 49

nucleus 48

obsessive-compulsive disorder (OCD) 60

panic attacks 59

panic disorder 60

phobias 58

psychiatric drugs 70

psychiatric nurses 69

psychiatrists 68

psychodynamic 70

psychologists 68

psychotherapy 69

receptors 49

reuptake 49

schizophrenia 62

synapse 49

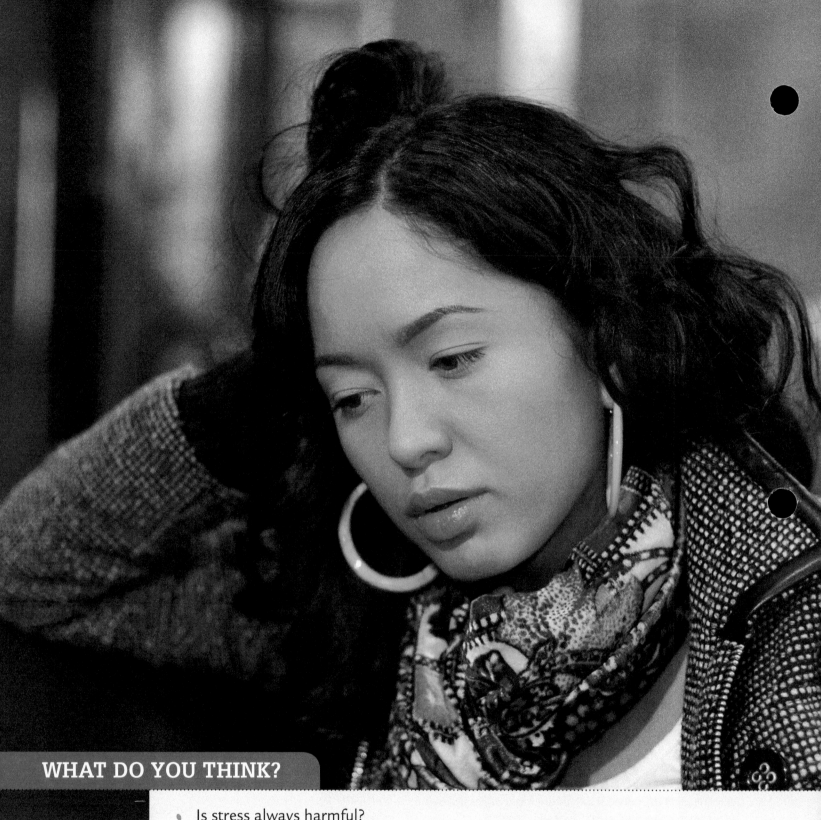

WHAT DO YOU THINK?

- Is stress always harmful?
- What stressors do college students typically encounter?
- How does the body respond to stress?
- What are some effective ways of managing stress?

© cloki/Shutterstock.com

4

Personal Stress Management

Getting laid off felt like a punch in the stomach. Chayla had heard rumors that all part-time positions would be eliminated. But her boss always said she was the best assistant they had ever hired. And now she was without a job—with tuition, rent, and insurance bills all due in a month. And so in between writing papers and preparing for finals, Chayla would have to look for another job. Just thinking about all she had to do made her head throb. <

After reading this chapter, you should be able to:

4.1 Outline the types of stress and the effects of stress on people.

4.2 Identify stressors commonly reported by different groups across America.

4.3 Examine some common causes of stress that individuals face.

4.4 Summarize the incidence, symptoms, and treatment of the stress disorders associated with traumatic life events.

4.5 Outline the ways in which the body responds to stress.

4.6 Describe how stress can affect a person's heart, immune system, gastrointestinal system, and susceptibility to cancer.

4.7 Explain psychological responses to stress.

4.8 Discuss practical techniques of stress management.

4.9 Summarize how time management can help prevent stress.

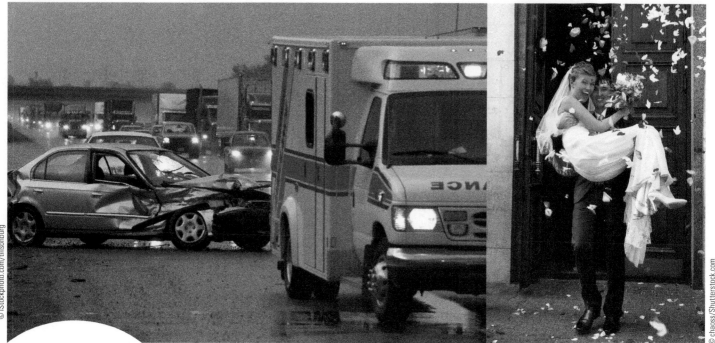

An automobile accident is an acute negative stressor. A wedding is an example of a positive stressor that triggers both joy and anxiety.

Like Chayla, you live with stress every day, whether you're studying for exams, meeting people, facing new experiences, or figuring out how to live on a budget. You're not alone. College students rank stress as the number-one barrier to academic achievement, according to the American College Health Association (ACHA) national survey. Almost a third of undergraduates report clinical levels of distress.[1]

During a typical semester, about half of undergraduates report high levels of stress; some describe their stress levels as nothing less than "tremendous." Freshmen, female, minority, and first-generation students register the most stress, but no one is immune. However old you are, wherever you come from, whatever your goals, stress is and always will be part of your life.

Yet stress in itself isn't necessarily bad. What matters most is not a stressful situation but an individual's response to it. This chapter will help you learn to anticipate stressful events, to manage day-to-day hassles, to prevent stress overload, and to find alternatives to running endlessly on a treadmill of alarm, panic, and exhaustion.

stress The nonspecific response of the body to any demands made upon it; may be characterized by muscle tension and acute anxiety, or may be a positive force for action.

stressor A specific or nonspecific agent or situation that causes the stress response in a body.

eustress Positive stress, which stimulates a person to function properly.

distress A negative stress that may result in illness.

What Is Stress?

The word **stress** comes from the Latin *stringere*, which means "to draw tight." Many people use the word loosely to refer to an external force that

causes someone to become tense or upset, to the internal state of arousal, and to the physical response of the body when it must adapt, cope, or adjust to a challenge.

Hans Selye, a pioneer in studying physiological responses to challenge, defined *stress* as "the non-specific response of the body to any demand made upon it." Through years of research, he noted that laboratory animals and people responded in the same way to a **stressor** (anything that triggers a state of arousal), regardless of whether it was positive or negative.

You experience stress when you confront what you perceive as a potential challenge or a threat that you don't think you can handle. This thought stimulates feelings, such as fear and anxiety, which lead to unconscious physiological responses as well as to conscious, deliberate behaviors.

Eustress and Distress

Not all stressors are negative. Some of life's happiest moments—births, reunions, weddings—are enormously stressful. We weep with the stress of frustration or loss; we weep, too, with the stress of love and joy.

Selye coined the term **eustress** for positive stress in our lives (*eu* is a Greek prefix meaning "good"). Eustress challenges us to grow, adapt, and find creative solutions in our lives.

Distress refers to the negative effects of stress that can deplete or even destroy life energy.

Ideally, the level of stress in our lives should be just high enough to motivate us to satisfy our needs and not so high that it interferes with our ability to reach our fullest potential.

Stress and the Dimensions of Health

From a **holistic** perspective, which looks at health and an individual as a whole rather than part by part, stress can have an impact on every dimension of well-being.

Physical Stress, whether physical or psychological, triggers molecular changes within your body that affect your heart, muscles, immune system, bones, blood vessels, skin, lungs, gastrointestinal (digestive) tract, and reproductive organs.

Psychological Chronic stress affects both thoughts and feelings, impairing your ability to learn and to remember and contributing to anxiety and depression. However, positive emotions and attitudes, such as compassion and gratitude, can buffer the ill effects of stress and enhance satisfaction and genuine happiness.

Spiritual Stress can sidetrack our quest to identify our basic purpose in life and to experience the fulfillment of achieving our full potential. But your spirit, when nurtured, can help you both resist and recover from stress.

Social Your relationships with your family, friends, coworkers, and loved ones affect and are affected by the stress in your life. Social support has proven effective in easing stress, loneliness, and depression in college students.[2]

Intellectual Even mild stressors can interfere with your brain's functioning by impairing sleep, dampening creativity, disrupting concentration and memory, and undermining your ability to make good choices and decisions.

Occupational Most undergraduates—about 70 percent—are employed, with 20 percent working full-time year-round. They are more likely to feel overwhelmed and report greater anxiety and stress than students without jobs.[3] In the workforce, employees with dead-end jobs with little or no control or status are especially vulnerable to stress-related problems such as hypertension. The workplace itself can contribute to stress if it's noisy, crowded, poorly lit and ventilated, or tolerant of insensitive jokes and comments. Yet as pressured as a job may be, losing one can be even more stressful. In various studies, unemployment has emerged as a major stressor that causes significant anxiety, depression, and health complaints.

Environmental External forces such as pollution, noise, natural disasters, exposure to toxic chemicals, and threats to your safety can cause or intensify the stress in your life. These days, you also have to cope with a byproduct of our 24/7, nonstop digital world: technostress, created by an unending barrage of texts, tweets, e-mails, notifications, pins, pokes and other digital distractions.

√**check-in** How does stress affect the various dimensions of your health?

holistic A perspective that looks at health and an individual as a whole rather than part by part.

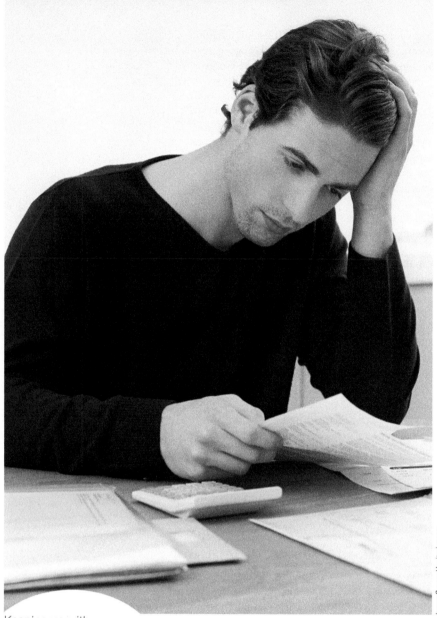

Keeping up with paperwork and figuring out how to stay on a budget can add to a student's stress level.

Types of Stressors

Stressors come in all varieties: big, small, brief, long, intense, mild, trivial, terrible. Here are some of the most common stressors:

- **Acute time-limited stressors** include anxiety-provoking situations such as having to give a talk in public or work out a math problem, such as calculating a tip or dividing a bill, under pressure. Even small daily hassles like misplacing your keys or cell phone can add to your stress.

- **Brief naturalistic stressors** are more serious challenges such as taking the SAT or meeting a deadline for a big project

- **Life change events** include planned and predictable occurrences, such as graduation or marriage, as well as unexpected ones,

such as the loss of a home in a fire or flood. Stress experts Thomas Holmes and Richard Rahe first documented an association between stressful life events and the onset of a disease. Their Schedule of Recent Experiences (SRE) evaluates individual levels of stress and potential for coping on the basis of life change units, determined by the degree of readjustment necessary to adapt successfully to an event. The death of a partner or parent ranks high on the list, but even positive events, such as a vacation trip, involve some degree of stress. Life changes do not in themselves cause diseases, however. Their actual impact depends on your response and coping skills.

- **Chronic stressors** are ongoing demands caused by life-changing circumstances, such as permanent disability following an accident or caregiving for a parent with dementia, that do not have any clear end point.

- **Distant stressors** are traumatic experiences that occurred long ago, such as child abuse or combat, yet continue to have an emotional and psychological impact.

✓**check-in** Which types of stressors have you encountered?

Stress in America

Every year the American Psychological Association (APA) asks men and women across the country to rank their stress level on a scale of 1 (little or no stress) to 10 (a great deal of stress). In the APA's most recent *Stress in America* survey, the average stress level was 4.9, lower than previous years but higher than the 3.7 Americans see as a healthy stress rating.[4]

✓**check-in** What's your stress level? Rank your current state of stress on a scale from 1 (low) to 10 (extreme). How does it compare with the national average of 4.9? What do you think is a healthy stress level?

Here are some key findings from the APA report:

- Younger respondents report higher stress levels. Compared to older Americans, a higher percentage of millennials (18- to 35-year-olds) and Gen Xers (36- to 49-year-olds) say that their overall stress has increased in the last year. (See Figure 4.1.)

Image Source/Jupiterimages

- About eight in ten younger Americans report experiencing at least one stress-related symptom in the last month.

- About four in ten of those surveyed say they are not doing enough or aren't sure if they're doing enough to manage their stress. One in five never engages in any activity to help relieve or manage stress.

- The most common source of stress—reported by about two-thirds of respondents—is money, followed by work, the economy, family responsibilities, and health concerns.

- The most common symptoms of stress in the past month were feeling irritable/angry; being nervous/anxious; lacking interest/motivation; feeling fatigued; feeling overwhelmed; and being depressed/sad. Women are more likely than men to report these symptoms in the past month.

- Many stressed Americans blame their anxiety for unhealthy behaviors, such as lying in bed awake at night or eating too much or choosing unhealthy foods. About three in ten blame stress for getting in the way of exercising.

- Millennials rely on more sedentary stress management techniques than other generations, including listening to music, watching television or videos for more than two hours a day, and going online and surfing the Internet.[5]

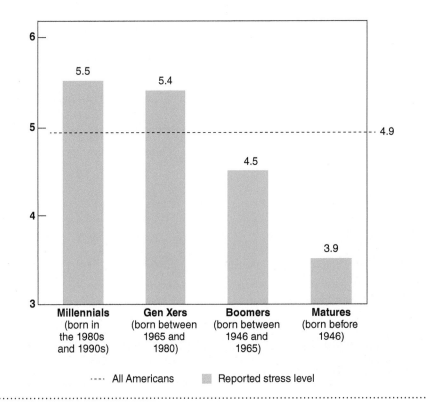

FIGURE 4.1 Stress levels are highest among younger Americans.

Source: *Stress in America*

Stress on Campus

Being a student—full-time or part-time, in your late teens, early 20s, or later in life—can be extremely stressful. You may feel pressure to perform well to qualify for a good job or graduate school. To meet steep tuition payments, you may have to juggle part-time work and coursework. You may feel stressed about choosing a major, getting along with a difficult roommate, passing a particularly hard course, or living up to your parents' and teachers' expectations. If you're an older student, you may have children, jobs, housework, and homework to balance. Your days may seem so busy and your life so full that you worry about coming apart at the seams.

In the American College Health Association's national survey, about 9 in 10 students rated the overall level of stress they experienced in the previous 12 months as "average," "more than average," or "tremendous."[6] More than 86 percent—77 percent of men and 91.6 percent of women—reported feeling overwhelmed by all they had to do at some point in the past 12 months.[7] (See Snapshot: On Campus Now.) Common stressors reported by students around the world include test pressures; financial problems; frustrations, such as delays in reaching goals; problems in friendships and dating relationships; and daily hassles.[8]

🔘 Stressed-Out Students

Within the past 12 months, students' ratings of the overall level of stress experienced:

	Percent (%)		
	Male	**Female**	**Average**
No stress	3.0	0.6	1.5
Less than average stress	12.1	4.4	7.1
Average stress	39.0	35.7	36.7
More than average stress	37.7	46.9	43.7
Tremendous stress	8.2	12.5	11.0

This table summarizes the levels of stress reported by college students in the previous 12 months. How does your stress level compare?

Source: American College Health Association. *American College Health Association–National College Health Assessment II: Reference Group Executive Summary, Spring 2014.* Hanover, MD: American College Health Association, 2014.

Stress and Student Health

Students say they react to stress in various ways:

- Physiologically—by sweating, stuttering, trembling, or developing physical symptoms

- Emotionally—by becoming anxious, fearful, angry, guilty, or depressed

- Behaviorally—by crying, eating, smoking, or being irritable or abusive

- Cognitively—by thinking about and analyzing stressful situations and strategies that might be useful in dealing with them

Students under stress may engage in behaviors that can harm their health, including smoking, excessive drinking, and substance abuse.

The undergraduates who report higher stress levels differ from their classmates in various ways. They are

- Less likely to exercise regularly

- Less likely to consume fruits and vegetables

- More likely to consume junk food and soft drinks

- Shown to report more symptoms of depression and anxiety[9]

In addition to its impact on health, stress can affect students physically, emotionally, academically, and socially. Among its documented effects are the following:

- Difficulty paying attention and concentrating

- Poor or inadequate sleep

- Lack of exercise

- Increased consumption of junk food

- Greater risk of anxiety and depression

- Lessened life satisfaction

To get a sense of your personal stress level, complete Self Survey: Student Stress Scale, modified to include college-specific stressors such as a failing grade or a change in major. If you score high, think about the reasons your life may be in turmoil. Of course, some events, such as your parents' divorce or a meningitis outbreak, are beyond your control. Even so, you can respond with coping techniques that will protect your long-term well-being.

✓**check-in** What is your greatest source of stress?

Gender Differences If you're a woman, you're more likely than your male classmates to be stressed about finances, social relationships, and daily hassles. In the ACHA survey, more female than male students reported feeling hopeless, overwhelmed, or exhausted (but not from physical activity). Women also scored higher than men in feeling stressed about having too many things to do at once, being separated from people they care about, financial burdens, and important decisions about their education.

Neither gender necessarily handles stress better. College men are more likely to "disengage" by using alcohol. College women report more emotion-focused strategies, such as expressing feelings, seeking emotional support, and positive reframing. They're also more prone to acting impulsively and not dealing with a problem directly, sometimes by spending more time online.[10]

Students under Age 25 Those of you between the ages of 18 and 25 are in the life stage termed "emerging adulthood." During this potentially risky transition period, young men and women of every racial and ethnic group are more likely to engage in behaviors that can increase stress and imperil health, such as eating more junk food, smoking, not exercising, and taking risks.

As neuroimaging research has revealed, the brain continues to develop throughout the first quarter-century of life, and this affects cognitive and problem-solving skills. In dealing with daily stressors, for instance, a teenage or 20-something brain relies more on the amygdala, a small almond-shaped region in the medial and temporal lobes that processes emotions and memories. This is one reason any stressor—a poor grade or a friend's snub, for instance—feels as intensely upsetting as a major crisis. As individuals age, the frontal cortex, which governs reason and forethought, plays a greater role and helps put challenges into perspective.

✓**check-in** If you are under 25:
- Be aware that your brain may not always grasp the long-term consequences of your actions.
- Set realistic priorities.
- Restrain potentially harmful impulses.
- Learn to center yourself with the breathing and relaxation techniques described on pages 94–95.

Students over Age 25 The number of older undergraduates is skyrocketing, with an estimated increase of 21 percent by 2016. Many of these students, often parents with full- or part-time jobs, find themselves playing multiple roles and facing multiple stressors, including pressure to perform well to qualify for a better job or graduate school. Veterans may be processing their experiences in distant and dangerous lands. Finances are a huge source of stress, and many worry about the costs of housing and child care and fear incurring additional debt.

Family typically emerges as the greatest source of both stress and support for women returning to school. On the one hand, women feel stressed about not earning money, missing special occasions like their children's track meets or dance recitals, and keeping up with endless household chores. On the other, they feel that short-term sacrifices will pay off in greater long-term security for their families. Single mothers face the most acute stressors, such as not being able to complete an assignment on time because they have to care for a sick child.

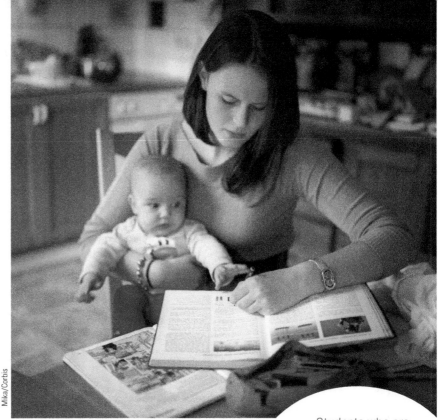

Mika/Corbis

Students who are parents must deal with the stress of juggling multiple tasks and responsibilities— often at the same time.

Minority Students *Minority stress* refers to negative experiences in the campus environment that students perceive to be linked to the social, physical, or cultural attributes characteristic of their racial or ethnic group. Among its forms are the following:

- **University social climate stress,** which arises from perceptions of the campus environment as unwelcoming to members of the student's group.

- **Intergroup stress,** based on perceptions of negative relations among students from different racial and ethnic groups, primarily white students.

- **Discrimination stress,** which reflects concerns related to personal experiences of prejudice and discrimination. As research in psychology, sociology, and epidemiology has confirmed, discrimination can cause chronic stress and take a significant toll on emotional well-being. Racial discrimination, which may be experienced more intensely than other forms of bias, has been linked to increased distress, depression, anxiety, and psychiatric symptoms in African Americans.[11]

- **Within-group stress,** which stems from perceived pressure to conform to the norms of the student's group regarding language, behaviors, and ways of thinking.

- **Achievement stress,** which reflects students' concerns about the relative inadequacy of their academic preparation and ability.

- **For instance,** Asian Americans between ages 15 and 24, who feel the stress of high expectations as the "model minority," have significantly higher suicidal rates than other racial/ethnic groups in the same age range.[12]

- **Acculturative stress,** the tension and anxiety that accompany efforts to adapt to the orientation and values of a dominant culture. Nearly half of Latinos who immigrated to the United States report discrimination on a daily basis, with young Latinos, including those born in the United States, reporting high levels of discrimination-related stress, anxiety, and depression.[13]

Minority stress can have an influence on many physical and mental health conditions, including hypertension, depression, substance dependence, and anxiety disorders. In studies of minority freshmen, Asian, Filipino, African American, and Native American students all felt more sensitive and vulnerable to the college social climate, to interpersonal tensions between themselves and nonminority students and faculty, to experiences of actual or perceived racism, and to discrimination.

✓**check-in** Have you experienced any form of minority stress?

Minority students, despite scoring above the national average on the SAT, may not feel accepted as legitimate undergraduates and may sense that others view them as unworthy beneficiaries of affirmative action initiatives. While many minority students say that overt racism is rare and relatively easy to deal with, subtle racial expressions—sometimes termed **microaggressions**—may undermine their academic confidence and their ability to bond with the university. Researchers have identified three common types:

- **Microassaults.** These are conscious and intentional actions or slurs, such as using racial epithets, displaying swastikas, or deliberately responding to a white customer before a person of color in a restaurant or store.

- **Microinsults.** These verbal and nonverbal communications subtly convey rudeness and insensitivity and demean a person's racial heritage or identity. An example is a student implying that a classmate won admission to a university on the basis of race rather than merit.

- **Microinvalidations.** These communications subtly exclude, negate, or nullify the thoughts, feelings, or experiential reality of a person of color—for instance, asking Asian Americans where they were born, which conveys the message that they are perpetual foreigners in their own land.

✓**check-in** Have you ever encountered microaggressions on your campus?

Entering Freshmen The first year of college is the most stressful for all undergraduates, even when they begin with positive expectations and attitudes.[14] However, it is even more challenging for first-generation college students—those whose parents never experienced at least one full year of college. They are less likely to share details of campus life and course work with family and friends, who may not be able to relate to and understand college-related stressors. This lack of social support itself adds to their stress levels because they have no experience, even vicarious, to draw from as they negotiate the transition to university life. Often first-generation students see themselves taking on the challenging roles of being trailblazers and role models in addition to the usual academic and personal demands.

Students whose parents and perhaps grandparents attended college may have several advantages, including more knowledge of college life, greater social support, more preparation for college in high school, a greater focus on college activities, and more financial resources. However, some report increased stress because of the high expectations of their college-educated parents.

✓**check-in** Did your parents attend college?

microaggressions Subtle racial expressions.

microassaults Conscious and intentional actions and slurs.

microinsults Verbal and nonverbal communications that subtly convey rudeness and insensitivity.

microinvalidations Communications that subtly exclude, negate, or nullify the thoughts, feelings, or experiential reality of a person of color.

YOUR STRATEGIES FOR PREVENTION

How to Handle Test Stress

- **Plan ahead.** A month before finals, map out a study schedule for each course. Set aside a small amount of time every day or every other day to review the course materials.

- **Be positive.** Picture yourself taking your final exam. Imagine yourself walking into the exam room feeling confident, opening up the test booklet, and seeing questions for which you know the answers.

- **Take regular breaks.** Get up from your desk, breathe deeply, stretch, and visualize a pleasant scene. You'll feel more refreshed than you would if you chugged another cup of coffee.

- **Practice.** Some teachers are willing to give practice finals to prepare students for test situations, or you and your friends can test each other.

- **Talk to other students.** Chances are that many of them share your fears about test taking and may have discovered some helpful techniques of their own. Sometimes talking to your adviser or a counselor can also help.

- **Be satisfied with doing your best.** You can't expect to ace every test; all you can and should expect is your best effort. Once you've completed the exam, allow yourself the sweet pleasure of relief that it's over.

HEALTH ON A BUDGET

How to Handle Economic Stress

Whether or not you have a job—or have lost one—the recent economic downturn has probably affected you or those close to you. But as always, what matters most isn't how stressful circumstances may be but how you react to them:

- **Pause but don't panic.** Pay attention to what's happening around you but refrain from getting caught up in doom-and-gloom hype, which can lead to high levels of anxiety and bad decision making.

- **Avoid the tendency to overreact or to become passive.** Remain calm and stay focused.

- **Identify your financial stressors and make a plan.** Although this can be anxiety provoking in the short term, putting things down on paper can reduce stress.

Write down specific ways you can reduce expenses or manage your finances more efficiently.

- **If you are having trouble paying bills or staying on top of debt, reach out for help by calling your bank or credit card company.** Credit counseling services and financial planners can help you take control over your money situation.

- **Recognize how you deal with stress related to money.** In tough economic times, some people turn to unhealthy activities like smoking, drinking, gambling, or emotional eating. If these behaviors are causing you trouble, seek help from a campus counselor before the problem gets worse.

Source: Based on materials from the American Psychological Association.

Test Stress How many tests have you taken in your life? Hundreds? Thousands? After so much experience, you'd think that tests would be no big deal. And they're not—unless you have developed a thought pattern that sets you up to stress out. For some students, test anxiety provokes a marked elevation in blood pressure, a potential threat to their cardiovascular health. Even if you react this intensely, you can take steps to ease your stressful feelings.

Students feel stressed by tests because they are afraid of a negative outcome, whether it's failing or just not getting an excellent grade. Sometimes they become so preoccupied with the possibility of failing that they can't concentrate on studying. Bright students may freeze up during tests and be unable to comprehend multiple-choice questions or write essay answers, even if they know the material.

Locus of control, discussed in Chapter 1, is crucial. If you see external forces as determining how well you do on tests, you give away your power, and your sense of helplessness creates disabling symptoms of anxiety. The students most susceptible to exam stress are those who believe they'll do poorly and who see tests as extremely threatening.

Unfortunately, negative thoughts often become a self-fulfilling prophecy. As they study, these students keep wondering, "What good will studying do? I never do well on tests." As their fear increases, they try harder. Fueled by caffeine, munching on sugary snacks, they become edgy and find it harder to concentrate. By the time of the test, they're nervous wrecks, scarcely able to sit still and focus on the exam.

You can overcome test stress by knowing—even mastering—the subject and by controlling the way you think about and talk to yourself about tests. Rather than waste energy worrying about the test, shift your attention to studying and the pleasure of learning. Rather than remind yourself of tests you blew in the past, train yourself to ace tests in the future.

Relaxation training also helps. Students who learn relaxation techniques—such as controlled breathing, meditation, progressive relaxation, and guided imagery (visualization)—before finals tend to have higher levels of immune cells during the exam period and feel in better control during their tests.

....
✓**check-in** How would you rate your test anxiety?
....

Other Stressors

At every stage of life, you will encounter challenges and stressors. Among the most common are those related to money, anger, work, and illness. (See Health on a Budget.)

The Anger Epidemic

Experts single out three primary culprits for the anger epidemic: time, technology, and tension. Americans are working longer hours than anyone else in the world. The cell phones and pagers that were supposed to make our lives easier have put us on call 24/7/365. People are tense and low on patience, and the less patience they have, the less they monitor their behavior. In the ACHA survey, 37.4 percent of undergraduates reported having felt overwhelming anger at some point in the previous 12 months.[15]

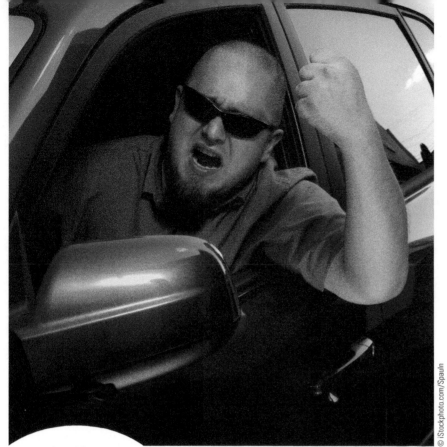

Aggressive drivers who lose control of their anger may contribute to half of all motor vehicle accidents.

For years therapists encouraged people to "vent" their anger. However, research now shows that letting anger out only makes it worse. Over time, temper tantrums sabotage physical health as well as psychological equanimity. By churning out stress hormones, chronic anger revs the body into a state of combat readiness, multiplying the risk for stroke and heart attack—even in healthy individuals. In recent years, violent, aggressive driving—which some dub *road rage*—has exploded. Driver aggression contributes to half of all motor vehicle accidents (see Chapter 18).

To deal with anger, you have to figure out what's really making you mad. Usually the jammed soda machine is the final straw that unleashes bottled-up fury over a more difficult issue, such as a recent breakup or a domineering parent or boss. Also monitor yourself for early signs of exhaustion and overload. While stress alone doesn't cause a blowup, it makes you more vulnerable to overreacting.

✓**check-in** Do you have trouble controlling your temper?

Economic Stress

With the recent economic slump, millions of Americans have confronted a serious new stressor: unemployment. Workers who are laid off must deal with multiple losses: the loss of a job; the possible loss of

the financial ability to support themselves; the loss of self-respect, security, and a daily routine; and—for some people—the loss of identity. More undergraduates are feeling financial stress. Many worry about their ability to pay for their education, particularly if they have a parent who is unemployed and can no longer help with tuition and other costs.[16]

Although money cannot buy happiness, it does buffer the ill effects of stress. According to a recent study, psychological distress, particularly when combined with poverty, can shorten life expectancy. Even when wealthier people have high levels of stress, money seems to serve as a buffer against lasting distress.[17]

✓**check-in** Do you think you would be less stressed if you had more money?

Job Stress

More today than ever before, many people find that they are working more and enjoying it less. Many, including working parents, spend 55 to 60 hours a week on the job. More people are caught up in an exhausting cycle of overwork, which causes stress, which makes work harder, which leads to more stress.

High job strain—defined as high psychological demands combined with low control or decision-making ability over one's job—may increase blood pressure, particularly among men. People who become obsessed by their work and careers can turn into workaholics, so caught up in racing toward the top that they forget what they're racing toward and why. In some cases, they throw themselves into their work to mask or avoid painful feelings or difficulties in their own lives.

As pressured as a job may be, not having one is even more stressful. In various studies, unemployment has emerged as a major stressor that causes significantly more anxiety, depression, health complaints, and a shortened lifespan.[18] For the employed, an insecure position can cause as much stress as not having a job at all.[19]

✓**check-in** If you work, what aspects of your job do you find most stressful?

Burnout

You don't need a job to experience **burnout**, a state of physical, emotional, and mental exhaustion brought on by constant or repeated emotional pressure. Many people, especially those caring for others at work or at home, get to a point where there's an imbalance between their own feelings and dealing with difficult, distressful issues on a day-to-day basis. If they don't recognize what's

burnout A state of physical, emotional, and mental exhaustion resulting from constant or repeated emotional pressure.

going on and make some changes, their health and the quality of their work suffer.

The risk of burnout may depend on your perception of anxiety, a low-intensity fear triggered by apprehension about ongoing or future challenges. Individuals who perceive anxiety as motivational may be energized and channel this energy into productive effort so they outperform under stress, while those who experience anxiety as debilitating or unpleasant may if perform to their full potential in stressful circumstances.[20]

The early signs of burnout overlap with the symptoms of stress: exhaustion; sleep problems or nightmares; increased anxiety or nervousness; muscular tension (headaches, backaches, and the like); increased use of alcohol or medication; digestive problems (such as nausea, vomiting, or diarrhea); loss of interest in sex; frequent body aches or pain; quarrels with family or friends; negative feelings about everything; problems concentrating; job mistakes and accidents; and feelings of depression, hopelessness, or helplessness.

Illness and Disability

Just as the mind can have profound effects on the body, the body can have an enormous impact on our emotions. Whenever we come down with the flu or pull a muscle, we feel under par. When we face a more serious or persistent problem—a chronic disease like diabetes, for instance, or a lifelong hearing impairment—the emotional stress of constantly coping with it is even greater.

A common source of stress for college students is learning disabilities, which may affect 1 of every 10 Americans. Most people with learning disabilities have average or above-average intelligence, but they rarely live up to their ability in school. Some have only one area of difficulty, such as reading or math. Others have problems with attention, writing, communicating, reasoning, coordination, and social skills.

√**check-in** Have you ever experienced stress because of an illness or a disability?

Traumatic Life Events

Bad things happen. Cars crash. Close friends and relatives die. Floods, tornadoes, and earthquakes wreak havoc on communities. Armed students shoot senselessly at classmates and professors. Bombs explode in peaceful public places.

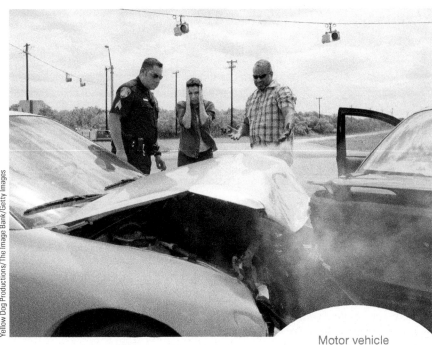

Yellow Dog Productions/The Image Bank/Getty Images

Motor vehicle accidents are the most frequently reported traumatic experiences.

According to epidemiological studies, about 60 percent of men and 50 percent of women experience at least one potentially traumatic event—natural or human-caused, large-scale or small—during the course of their lives.[21] Nine in 10 college women report having directly experienced at least one traumatic event, usually involving a threat to their own lives or to others. The most frequently reported trauma was motor vehicle accident.

√**check-in** Have you ever experienced a traumatic event?

As profoundly disturbing as such experiences can be, recent research has shown that after a trauma, the vast majority of people, including children, cope well, continue to meet the demands of their daily lives, and recover fully.

Acute Stress Disorder

In acute stress disorder, disabling symptoms occur within three days to a month after exposure to a traumatic event, such as threatened or actual personal or sexual assault, mugging, violence, physical or sexual abuse, kidnapping, being taken hostage, terrorist attack, natural disaster, airplane crash, or severe industrial or automobile accident.

Symptoms of acute stress disorder may include

• Recurrent, involuntary, and intrusive distressing memories of the trauma

• Recurrent distressing dreams related to the trauma

YOUR STRATEGIES FOR CHANGE

How to Cope with Distress after a Trauma

Senseless acts of violence or terrorism can trigger a variety of emotions, including shock, sorrow, fear, anger, and grief. You may have problems sleeping, concentrating, or going about simple chores. Because the world seems more dangerous, it may take a while for you to regain your sense of equilibrium. The following recommendations from the American Psychological Association can help.

- **Talk about it.** Ask for support from people who will listen to your concerns. It often helps to speak with others who have shared your experience so you do not feel so different or alone.

- **Strive for balance.** Remind yourself of people and events that are meaningful and comforting, even encouraging.

- **Take a break.** While you may want to keep informed, limit your exposure to news on television, the Internet, newspapers, or magazines. Schedule breaks to focus on something you enjoy.

- **Take care of yourself.** Engage in healthy behaviors, such as exercise, that will enhance your ability to cope. Avoid alcohol and drugs because they can suppress your feelings rather than help you to manage your distress.

- **Help others or do something productive.** Try volunteering at your school or within your community. Helping someone else often helps you feel better too.

- Dissociative reactions, such as flashbacks, in which an individual feels that the traumatic event is recurring

- Persistent inability to experience happiness, satisfaction, or other positive emotions

- Altered sense of the reality of one's surroundings or oneself, such as time slowing down

- Inability to remember an important aspect of the traumatic event

- Efforts to avoid distressing memories, thoughts, or feelings related to the trauma

- Efforts to avoid reminders, such as certain people, places, activities, objects, or situations, that arouse distressing feelings or thoughts

- Sleep disturbances, including difficulty falling or staying asleep and restless sleep

- Irritable behavior and angry outbursts

- Hypervigilance

- Problems with concentration

- Intensified startle response[22]

posttraumatic stress disorder (PTSD) The repeated reliving of a trauma through nightmares or recollection.

Acute stress disorder causes significant distress and interferes with a person's ability to work, study, relate to others, and maintain usual routine and social activities. People with acute stress disorder initially need protection, consolation, assurance of safety, and assistance with decisions and plans. Self-compassion, discussed in Chapter 2, can help survivors of traumatic events reach out for social support, engage in less self-blame and self-criticism, and view the memory as an emotionally difficult event rather than an experience that defines or changes them.[23]

Posttraumatic Stress Disorder (PTSD)

In the past, **posttraumatic stress disorder (PTSD)** was viewed as a psychological response to out-of-the-ordinary stressors, such as captivity or combat. However, other experiences can also forever change the way people view themselves and their world. Individuals with PTSD directly experience or witness a trauma, learn of an actual or threatened act of violence toward a family member or friend, or experience repeated or extreme exposure to the traumatic events (as happens with soldiers in combat and first responders).

An estimated 9 percent of all college students suffer from PTSD. According to a recent study of almost 500 undergraduates, those with PTSD drink more alcohol than other students, potentially worsening their symptoms and leading to even heavier drinking.[23]

In the general population, an estimated 8 to 10 percent of women and 4 to 5 percent of men develop PTSD in their lifetime.[24] Women are most vulnerable between the ages of 44 and 51, while men are more prone to PTSD from ages 41 to 45.[25] Childhood traumas occur equally in both sexes. Adult men encounter more traumas— accidents, violence, combat, terrorism, disasters, injuries—than adult women. Women experience more sexual assaults and abuse.

Symptoms of PTSD, which usually begin within the first three months after a trauma, include the following:

- Recurrent, involuntary, and intrusive distressing memories of the traumatic event

- Recurrent distressing dreams related to the trauma

- Persistent avoidance of external reminders and distressing memories of the trauma

- Persistent feelings of guilt, shame, anger, horror, fear, or other negative emotions

- Hypervigilance and other changes in arousal and alertness.[26]

Some individuals reexperience their terror and helplessness again and again in their dreams or intrusive thoughts. Some engage in aggressive, reckless, or self-destructive behavior. Others enter a state of emotional numbness and no longer can respond to people and experiences the way they once did, especially when it comes to showing tenderness or affection.

Individuals with PTSD may require different types of help at different stages. During the first days after a trauma, protection, reassurance of safety, help making decisions and plans, and the support of those closest to them can be most significant in easing their distress.[27] Some approaches, such as immediate "debriefing" to release emotions or treatment with anxiety-reducing medications, may not help and may even hinder long-term recovery. Behavioral, cognitive, and psychodynamic therapy, sometimes along with psychiatric medication, can help individuals suffering with PTSD. Mind–body practices, such as exercise, mindfulness, meditation, and deep breathing (described later in this chapter), also have proven effective.

Without recognition and treatment, PTSD can last for decades, with symptoms intensifying during periods of stress. When identified and treated, more than half of affected persons achieve complete recovery. The odds of recovery are greatest when symptoms develop soon after the trauma, when the individual had previously been in good psychological condition, when there are strong social supports, and when there are no other mental or medical disorders. In time, individuals with PTSD can learn to increase their control over anguishing memories and feelings and come to accept what happened, however horrible, as a tragic reality of the past that does not have to shape their future.

Mental health professionals have found that no single approach to treatment works for all trauma victims. Some approaches, such as immediate "debriefing" to release emotions or treatment with anxiety-reducing medications, may not help and may even hinder long-term recovery. Behavioral, cognitive, and psychodynamic therapy, sometimes along with psychiatric medication (described in Chapter 3), also can help individuals suffering with PTSD. Mind–body practices, such as exercise, mindfulness, meditation, and deep breathing, have proven effective in treating PTSD.[28]

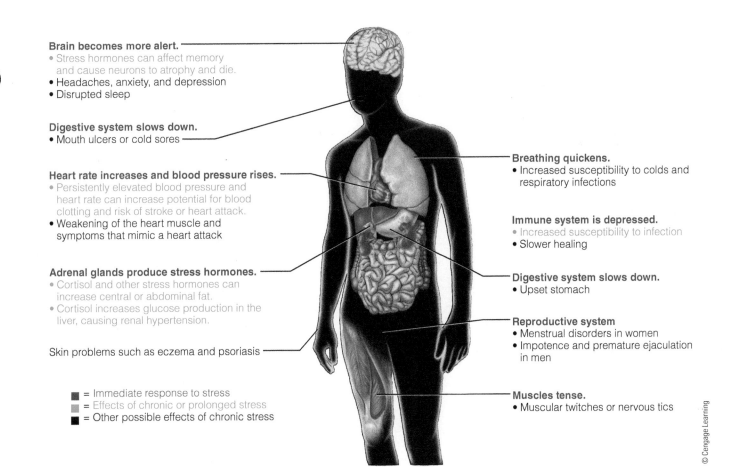

Brain becomes more alert.
- Stress hormones can affect memory and cause neurons to atrophy and die.
- Headaches, anxiety, and depression
- Disrupted sleep

Digestive system slows down.
- Mouth ulcers or cold sores

Heart rate increases and blood pressure rises.
- Persistently elevated blood pressure and heart rate can increase potential for blood clotting and risk of stroke or heart attack.
- Weakening of the heart muscle and symptoms that mimic a heart attack

Adrenal glands produce stress hormones.
- Cortisol and other stress hormones can increase central or abdominal fat.
- Cortisol increases glucose production in the liver, causing renal hypertension.

Skin problems such as eczema and psoriasis

■ = Immediate response to stress
■ = Effects of chronic or prolonged stress
■ = Other possible effects of chronic stress

Breathing quickens.
- Increased susceptibility to colds and respiratory infections

Immune system is depressed.
- Increased susceptibility to infection
- Slower healing

Digestive system slows down.
- Upset stomach

Reproductive system
- Menstrual disorders in women
- Impotence and premature ejaculation in men

Muscles tense.
- Muscular twitches or nervous tics

© Cengage Learning

FIGURE 4.2 The Effects of Stress on the Body

The Stress Response

The **stress response** refers to a cascade of internal changes that mobilize the body's resources for action (see Figure 4.2):

- When you confront a stressor, the adrenal glands, two crescent-shaped glands that sit atop the kidneys, respond by producing stress hormones, including catecholamines, cortisol (hydrocortisone), and epinephrine (adrenaline), that speed up heart rate and raise blood pressure and prepare the body to deal with the threat. This "fight-or-flight" response prepares you for quick action.

- Your heart works harder to pump more blood to your legs and arms.

- Your muscles tense.

- Your breathing quickens.

- Your brain becomes extra alert.

- Because it's nonessential in a crisis, your digestive system practically shuts down.

stress response The cascade of internal changes that mobilize the body's resources for action.

tend and befriend A behavioral response to stress characterized by increased feelings of trust.

homeostasis The body's natural state of balance or stability.

Just as your body instinctively mobilizes to deal with potential danger, once the threat passes, it restores a state of homeostasis, or balance. Breathing and heart rate slow. Blood pressure and body temperature drop. Muscles relax. Routine processes such as digestion, energy storage, tissue repair, and growth return to normal. Your body regenerates and restores itself.

Oxytocin, produced by the pituitary gland, plays a special role at this stage. The so-called cuddle chemical fine-tunes the brain's social network, increases empathy, and fosters willingness to help and support others. As an additional benefit, it protects the cardiovascular system by stimulating natural anti-inflammatory agents that help the heart regenerate and grow stronger. Oxytocin may also contribute to a behavioral response to stress dubbed **tend and befriend** by increasing feelings of trust.[29] Although the classic "fight-or-flight" response to threats is better known, researchers have noted that women in particular may respond to stress by reaching out to others—both to care for those in need and to be cared for in turn.

General Adaptation Syndrome (GAS)

In his GAS model of the stress response, Hans Selye postulated that our bodies continually strive to maintain a stable and consistent physiological state, called **homeostasis** (see Figure 4.3). When a stressor disrupts this state, it triggers a nonspecific physiological response, consisting of three distinct stages:

1. **Alarm.** As it becomes aware of a stressor, the body mobilizes various systems for action. Levels of certain hormones (discussed in Chapter 3) rise; blood pressure and flow to the muscles increase; the digestive and immune systems slow down.

2. **Resistance.** If the stress continues, the body draws on its internal resources to try to sustain homeostasis, but this requires greater and greater effort. If, for example, a loved one is seriously hurt in an accident, you initially respond intensely and feel great anxiety. During the subsequent stressful period of recovery, you struggle to carry on as normally as possible, but this requires considerable effort.

3. **Exhaustion.** If stress continues long enough, normal functioning becomes impossible. Even a small amount of additional stress at this point can lead to a breakdown. In animal experiments, Selye found that persistent stress caused illnesses similar to those seen in humans, such as heart attacks, stroke, kidney disease, and rheumatoid arthritis.

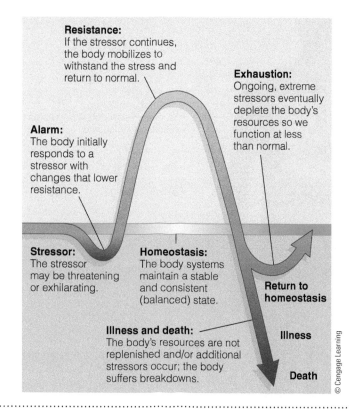

Resistance: If the stressor continues, the body mobilizes to withstand the stress and return to normal.

Exhaustion: Ongoing, extreme stressors eventually deplete the body's resources so we function at less than normal.

Alarm: The body initially responds to a stressor with changes that lower resistance.

Stressor: The stressor may be threatening or exhilarating.

Homeostasis: The body systems maintain a stable and consistent (balanced) state.

Return to homeostasis

Illness and death: The body's resources are not replenished and/or additional stressors occur; the body suffers breakdowns.

Illness

Death

© Cengage Learning

FIGURE 4.3 General Adaptation Syndrome (GAS)
The three stages of Selye's GAS are alarm, resistance, and exhaustion.

Some critics of Selye's theory argue that it is overly abstract and comprehensive and does not take into account variation among individuals and differences between minor and major stresses. However, GAS remains fundamental to understanding the physiology of stress.

Cognitive Transactional Model

Psychologist Richard Lazarus based his cognitive transactional model on the interrelationship between stress, which has a powerful impact on well-being, and health, which affects a person's ability to cope with stress. In his view, stress is "neither an environmental stimulus, a characteristic of the person, nor a response but a relationship between demands and the power to deal with them without unreasonable or destructive costs."[30]

When individuals confront a challenge, they make immediate judgments about whether it poses a threat and whether they will be able to respond to it. Lazarus identified four stages in this process:

- During the *primary appraisal*, you judge the severity of a threat, based on previous experience, self-knowledge, and available information about the challenge. If you do not perceive it as dangerous, no stress develops.

- If you perceive the situation as threatening, you proceed to the *secondary appraisal* and assess whether you have the power and resources to act.

- In the *coping* stage, you do whatever you can to deal with the challenge.

- In the fourth stage, *reappraisal*, you evaluate whether the original stressor has been eliminated or whether you need to try again or use a different approach.

Yerkes-Dodson Law

With too little stress, you might not be motivated enough to get out of bed in the morning and work toward your goals. With too much, you can't function at your best. But when your stress level is neither too high nor too low but just right, you are energized, effective, and efficient.

Psychology explains this phenomenon in terms of the Yerkes-Dodson Law (named for the psychologists who first described it in 1908). In laboratory experiments, these researchers found that mild electrical shocks motivated rats to complete a maze, but when the shocks became too strong, the rats scurried around in random directions to escape. Their conclusion: Increasing stress can boost performance—but only up to a certain point.

√**check-in** How do you rate your current stress level: Too little? Too much? About right?

The Impact of Stress

In recent years, stress has been implicated as a culprit in a range of medical problems. While stress alone doesn't cause disease, it triggers molecular changes throughout the body that make us more susceptible to many illnesses.

Stress and the Heart

The links between stress, behavior, and the heart are complex. Scientists continue to explore the impact of acute and chronic stress, gender, race, and socioeconomic status. One way in which stress increases the risk of heart attack and other cardiovascular problems is by pushing people toward bad habits. Men and women with high stress levels smoke and drink more and exercise less—and have higher rates of heart attacks, strokes, and bypass surgeries.

Stress may be as great a threat for cardiovascular disease as smoking, hypertension, and other major risk factors (discussed in Chapter 15)—depending on how individuals respond to a stressor. According to a recent large-scale longitudinal study, men with low stress resilience in adolescence faced a greater danger of cardiovascular illness in middle age—perhaps because of unhealthy habits they acquired at an early age or because of inadequate coping skills.[31]

Chronic stress, whether because of finances, a demanding job, racial discrimination, or marital problems, can contribute to hypertension (discussed in depth in Chapter 15). Ruminating—mulling over stressful events or upsetting thoughts—may be the mechanism that elevates blood pressure even hours or days after a stressful occurrence. The relaxation technique that has proven most effective in reducing blood pressure is meditation (discussed later in this chapter).

Stress and Immunity

The immune system is the network of organs, tissues, and white blood cells that defend against disease. Impaired immunity makes the body more susceptible to many diseases, including infections (from the common cold to tuberculosis) and disorders of the immune system itself. Acute time-limited stressors, the type that produce a fight-or-flight response, prompt the immune system to ready itself for the possibility of infections resulting from bites, punctures, or other wounds.

However, long-term, or chronic, stress creates excessive wear and tear, and the system breaks down. Chronic stressors, so profound and persistent that they seem endless and beyond a person's control, suppress immune responses the most. The longer the stress, the more the immune system shifts from potentially adaptive changes to potentially harmful ones, first in cellular immunity and then in broader immune function. Traumatic stress, such as losing a loved one through death or divorce, can impair immunity for as long as a year.

Stress and the Gastrointestinal System

The "brain–gut axis," as gastroenterologists have called it, links the brain with the organs involved in digesting food as it enters your mouth, moves down the esophagus to the stomach, passes through the small and large intestines, and finally exits through your rectum and anus. During this journey, stress can

- Decrease saliva so your mouth becomes dry (a frequent occurrence when under the stress of speaking in public)

- Cause contractions in the esophagus that interfere with swallowing

- Increase the amount of hydrochloric acid in the stomach

- Constrict blood vessels in the digestive tract

- Alter the rhythmic movements of the small and large intestines necessary for the transport of food (leading to diarrhea if too fast or constipation if too slow)

- Contribute to or exacerbate GERD (gastro-esophageal reflux disease)

- Lead to blockage of the bile and pancreatic ducts

- Increase the risk of pancreatitis (inflammation of the pancreas), ulcerative colitis, and irritable bowel syndrome.[32]

For many years stress alone was blamed for causing stomach ulcers, but scientists have discovered that a bacterium, *Helicobacter pylori*, infects the digestive system and sets the stage for ulcers. However, stress may increase susceptibility by reducing the protective gastric mucus that lines the stomach so ulcers develop more readily. With other chronic digestive diseases, such as irritable bowel syndrome, stress can be both a contributor and a consequence, causing or worsening symptoms that in turn intensify stress.

Stress directly affects what researchers call our "drive to eat." Under any type of stress, individuals eat more, binge more, and choose "palatable nonnutritious foods" (better known as junk foods) like candy and cookies rather than healthier options. Foods high in sugar and fat may target pleasure centers in the brain and provide temporary comfort and relief. However, sweet treats can send blood sugar levels on a roller-coaster ride—up one moment and down the next.

Even if they don't consume more calories, some people, perhaps especially sensitive to cortisol, put on "belly," or visceral, fat (deposited deep within the central abdominal area of the body) when stressed. This type of fat poses a greater health threat than subcutaneous (under-the-skin) fat because it enters the bloodstream more readily, raises levels of harmful cholesterol, and heightens the risk of diseases such as diabetes, high blood pressure, and stroke. (See Chapter 7.)

Stress and Cancer

Cutting-edge research has not only transformed cancer treatments but has also deepened understanding of the role of psychosocial factors, including stress, in vulnerability to and recovery from cancer.[33] Among the latest findings from psycho-oncology, the field that combines medical and psychological approaches to cancer, are the following:

- Stress-related abnormalities in cortisol, inflammation, and the sympathetic nervous system can affect cancer growth.

- Stressful life experiences and depression are associated with poorer survival and greater mortality from various types of cancer, including breast, lung, and head and neck tumors.

- Psychosocial support and improved coping skills help even terminally ill patients to live better at the end of life—and in some cases to live longer as well.[34]

Other Stress Symptoms

The first signs of stress include muscle tightness, tension headaches, backaches, upset stomach, and sleep disruptions (caused by stress-altered brain-wave activity). Some people feel fatigued, their hearts may race or beat faster than usual at rest, and they may feel tense all the time, easily frustrated, and often irritable. Others feel sad; lose their energy, appetite, or sex drive; and develop psychological problems, including depression, anxiety, and panic attacks.

Stress also is closely linked to skin conditions. If you break out the week before an exam, you know firsthand that skin can be extremely sensitive to stress. Skin conditions worsened by stress include acne, psoriasis, herpes, hives, and eczema. With acne, increased touching of the face, perhaps while cramming for a test, may be partly responsible. Other factors, such as temperature, humidity, and cosmetics and toiletries, may also play a role.

Psychological Responses to Stress

Sometimes we respond to stress or challenge with self-destructive behaviors, such as drinking or using drugs. These responses can lead to psychological problems, such as anxiety or depression, and physical problems, including psychosomatic illnesses.

Defense Mechanisms

Defense mechanisms, such as those described in Table 4.1, are another response to stress. These psychological devices are mental processes that help us cope with personal problems. Such responses also are not the answer to stress—and learning to recognize them in yourself will enable you to deal with your stress in a healthier way.

Cognitive Restructuring

Every day about 60,000 thoughts pass through our brains as we plan, evaluate, judge, interpret, and remember. Some of these thoughts are as precise as a mathematical equation, but others are misleading or inappropriate. These inaccurate or self-defeating thoughts are the target of cognitive-behavioral therapy (CBT), a highly effective psychological treatment described in Chapter 3.

Cognitive restructuring, one of the techniques of CBT, can reduce stress by helping people examine unhappy, negative thoughts that are making them anxious, challenging these thoughts, and in many cases rewriting the negative thinking that lies behind them. Because thoughts create feelings and drive behavior, this approach enables people to approach stressful situations in a positive frame of mind. Here are the basic steps:

- The first step is becoming aware of automatic thoughts that enter your brain, such as "I will never understand this material," "I'm going to flunk this test," or "No one wants to talk with me."

- Challenge these negative assumptions with counterarguments such as "I felt the same way in chemistry class, and eventually I figured it out," "If I focus on the questions I do know, I'll be okay," or "I can try smiling and striking up a conversation."

- Develop specific action techniques to blunt negative thoughts and lessen stress. For instance, you could master some of the relaxation and test-taking techniques described in this chapter.

Managing Stress

College is a perfect time to learn and practice the art of stress reduction. You can start applying the techniques and concepts outlined in this chapter immediately. You may want to begin by doing some relaxation or awareness exercises. They can give you the peace of mind you need to focus more effectively on larger issues, goals, and decisions.

You needn't see stress as a problem to solve on your own. Reach out to others. As you build friendships and intimate relationships, you may find that some irritating problems are easier to

defense mechanisms Psychological processes that alleviate anxiety and eliminate mental conflict; include denial, displacement, projection, rationalization, reaction formation, and repression.

TABLE 4.1 Common Defense Mechanisms Used to Alleviate Anxiety and Eliminate Conflict

Defense Mechanism	Example
Denial: the refusal to accept a painful reality	You don't accept as true the news that a loved one is seriously ill.
Displacement: the redirection of feelings from their true object to a more acceptable or safer substitute	Instead of lashing out at a coach or teacher, you snap at your best friend.
Projection: the attribution of unacceptable feelings or impulses to someone else	When you want to end a relationship, you project your unhappiness onto your partner.
Rationalization: the substitution of "good," acceptable reasons for the real motivations of our behavior	You report a classmate who has been mean for cheating on an exam and explain that cheating is unfair to other students.
Reaction formation: adopting attitudes and behaviors that are the opposite of what we feel	You lavishly compliment an acquaintance whom you really despise.
Repression: the way we keep threatening impulses, fantasies, memories, feelings, or wishes from becoming conscious	You don't "hear" the alarm after the late night, or you "forget" to take out the trash.

© Cengage Learning

HEALTH NOW!

Write It Out!

One of the most effective ways of coping with stress and other psychological challenges is by using a journal to monitor and express your feelings. Try the following stress-reducing exercises and record your responses and reflections in your online journal:

- **Assess your stress.** Take a strain inventory of your body every day to determine where things aren't feeling quite right. Ask yourself, "What's keeping me from feeling terrific today?" Focusing on problem spots such as stomach knots or neck tightness increases your sense of control over stress.

- **Reconstruct stressful situations.** Think about a recent episode of distress; then write down three ways it could have gone better and three ways it could have gone worse. This should help you see that the situation wasn't as disastrous as it might have been and help you find ways to cope better in the future.

- **Practice self-compassion.** As discussed in Chapter 2, treating yourself kindly in the face of stressful circumstances helps turn wisdom and awareness inward and provides a sense of perspective and connectedness.

- **Soothe yourself.** List some of the nice things you can do to soothe yourself, and include at least three of them in your daily routine. Make notes on how you feel after such experiences and which ones seem to have the most lasting impact.

progressive relaxation A method of reducing muscle tension by contracting, then relaxing, certain areas of the body.

put into perspective. Don't be afraid to laugh at yourself and to look for the comic or absurd aspects of a situation.

Although many students experience high levels of stress, relatively few seek counseling. Yet various approaches, including online stress management interventions, have proven effective in reducing perceived stress and symptoms of anxiety, depression, and stress.[35] Apps for smartphones, watches, and other mobile devices are offering novel ways to monitor stressful situations and modify reactions to them.[36]

√ **check-in** Do you—or would you—use a stress-management app?

Journaling

One of the simplest yet most effective ways to work through stress is by putting your feelings into words that only you will read. The more honest and open you are as you write, the better. (See Health Now!)

College students who wrote in their journals about traumatic events felt much better afterward than those who wrote about superficial topics. Focus on intense emotional experiences and "autopsy" them to try to understand why they affected you the way they did. Rereading and thinking about your notes may reveal the underlying reasons for your response.

√ **check-in** Have you ever tried journaling?

Exercise

Regular physical activity can relieve stress, boost energy, lift mood, and keep stress under control. Young adults who adopt and continue regular aerobic exercise show less intense cardiovascular responses to stress, which may protect them against coronary heart disease as they age. Strength training may have similar benefits. (See Chapter 8.)

There is a correlation between physical activity and stress in college students. Students who report higher levels of leisure-time exercise, along with a good social network and time management skills, generally enjoy better mental health, even when they report as much stress as less active undergraduates.

√ **check-in** Try an experiment with yourself: Keep track of the days when you work out in some way and those you don't. Rate your stress level every day, and see if exercise makes a difference for you.

Routes to Relaxation

Relaxation is the physical and mental state opposite that of stress. Rather than gear up for fight or flight, during relaxation our bodies and minds grow calmer and work more smoothly. We're less likely to become frazzled, and we're more capable of staying in control. A growing number of studies have confirmed the benefits of relaxation techniques. Although they differ in many ways, the various approaches may alter brain chemistry in fundamental ways, such as increasing the levels of pleasure-inducing chemicals in the brain.

When you practice **progressive relaxation**, you intentionally increase and then decrease tension in the muscles. While sitting or lying down in a quiet, comfortable setting, you tense and release various muscles, beginning with those of the hand, for instance, and then proceeding to the arms, shoulders, neck, face, scalp, chest, stomach, buttocks, genitals, and so on, down each leg to the toes. Relaxing the muscles can quiet the mind and restore internal balance.

Visualization, **or guided imagery**, involves creating mental pictures that calm you down and focus your mind. Some people use this technique to promote healing when they are ill. Visualization skills require practice and, in some cases, instruction by qualified health professionals.

Biofeedback is a method of obtaining feedback, or information, about some physiological activity occurring in the body. An electronic monitoring device attached to the body detects a change in an internal function and communicates it to the person through a tone, light, or meter. By paying attention to this feedback, most people can gain some control over functions previously thought to be beyond conscious control, such as body temperature, heart rate, muscle tension, and brain waves.

The goal of biofeedback for stress reduction is a state of tranquility, usually associated with the brain's production of alpha waves (which are slower and more regular than normal waking waves).

Meditation and Mindfulness

Meditation has been practiced in many forms over the ages, from the yogic techniques of the Far East to the Quaker silence of more modern times. Brain scans have shown that meditation activates the sections of the brain in charge of the autonomic nervous system, which governs bodily functions, such as digestion and blood pressure, that we cannot consciously control. Research with a group of Tibetan monks and lay practitioners with extensive experience in meditation has demonstrated that meditation produces changes in various regions of the brain and can actually cause people to be more compassionate. The effects continue even after sessions of meditation.

Although many studies have documented the benefits of meditation for overall health, it may be particularly helpful for people dealing with stress-related medical conditions such as high blood pressure and heart problems, as well as for preventing stress-induced changes in the immune system. (See Figure 4.4.)

Meditation helps a person reach a state of relaxation, with the goal of achieving inner peace and harmony. There is no one right way to meditate, and many people have discovered how to meditate on their own, without even knowing what it is they are doing.

Increasing numbers of college students are turning to meditation as a way of coping with stress. Most forms of meditation have common elements: sitting quietly for 15 to 20 minutes once or twice a day, concentrating on a word or an image, and breathing slowly and rhythmically. If you wish to try meditation, it often helps to have someone guide you through your first sessions. Or try tape recording your own voice (with or without favorite music in the background) and playing it back to yourself, freeing yourself to concentrate on the goal of turning the attention within.

Regular practice of transcendental meditation has reduced sleepiness in college students and improved their alertness and brain functioning. Undergraduates who began meditating during the first week of the term report being less tired and more resistant to the stress of finals than others.

Mindfulness is a modern form of an ancient Asian technique that involves maintaining awareness in the present moment. Some define it as "an awareness that emerges by paying attention deliberately in the present to an experience as it happens moment by moment."[37]

In mindful meditation, you tune in to each part of your body, scanning from head to toe, noting every sensation, however slight. You allow whatever you experience—an itch, an ache, a feeling of warmth—to enter your awareness. Then you open yourself to focus on all the thoughts, sensations, sounds, and feelings that enter your awareness. Mindfulness keeps you in the here and now, thinking about *what is* rather than about *what if* or *if only*. For college students, mindfulness has proven to improve confidence in the ability to handle the complex challenges of adulthood.[38]

Mindfulness-Based Stress Reduction, a group program that focuses on progressive acquisition of mindful awareness, has been used for patients with a wide variety of health problems as well as in healthy people coping with daily stress. Its

The Benefits of Meditation

- Reduces activation of the sympathetic nervous system—which, in turn, dilates the blood vessels and reduces stress hormones, such as adrenaline, noradrenaline, and cortisol.
- Reduces high blood pressure and need for hypertension medications
- Reduces atherosclerosis
- Reduces constriction of blood vessels
- Reduces thickening of coronary arteries
- Reduces mortality rates
- Slows aging
- Reduces hospitalization rates
- Decreases medical care utilization and hospitalization
- Increases creativity
- Improves memory
- Increases intelligence
- Decreases anxiety
- Reduces alcohol abuse
- Increases productivity

© Cengage Learning

FIGURE 4.4 Millions of college students use meditation as a way of coping with stress. Have you tried it?

proven psychological benefits include greater self-compassion and decreased absentmindedness, difficulty regulating emotions, fear of emotion, worry, and anger. Researchers have documented benefits for individuals suffering from chronic pain (including fibromyalgia), cancer, anxiety disorders, depression, and the stresses of the transition from high school to college.[39]

Yoga

An estimated 14.9 million Americans practice yoga, which has been defined as a union of mind, body, and spirit. In addition to easing conditions such as lower-back pain, migraine, asthma, and hypertension, yoga has proven to reduce anxiety and cortisol levels in those with moderate levels of stress. Compared with other forms of exercise, yoga has a greater positive impact on mood and anxiety, possibly because it increases antidepressant neurotransmitters (messenger chemicals) in the brain.

Yoga (also discussed in Chapter 8) has proven effective in alleviating stress-related symptoms.[40] Research on college students found yoga to be as effective as aerobic exercise in boosting feelings of well-being.[41]

Yoga may lower harmful compounds associated with stress that increase inflammation. "Expert" yoga practitioners, with a year or two of yoga practice, generally have lower levels of markers of chronic inflammation than novices. Yoga may be beneficial because it increases flexibility and allows relaxation, which can lower stress.

visualization, or guided imagery An approach to stress control, self-healing, or motivating life changes by means of seeing oneself in the state of calmness, wellness, or change.

biofeedback A technique of becoming aware, with the aid of external monitoring devices, of internal physiological activities in order to develop the capability of altering them.

meditation A group of approaches that use quiet sitting, breathing techniques, and/or chanting to relax, improve concentration, and become attuned to one's inner self.

mindfulness A method of stress reduction that involves experiencing the physical and mental sensations of the present moment.

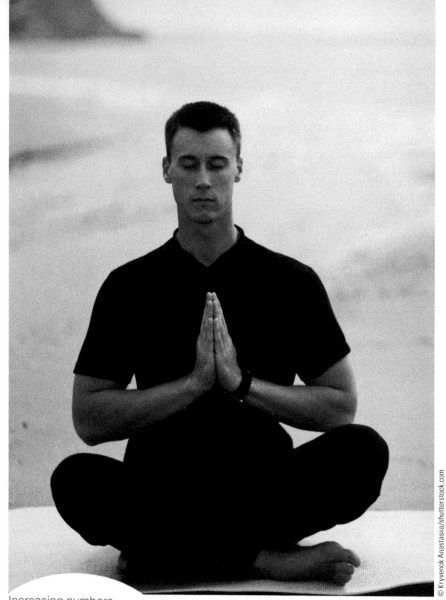

Increasing numbers of college students are turning to meditation as a way of coping with stress.

painful, the individuals often look back at them as bringing positive changes into their lives.

Researchers have studied various factors that enable individuals to thrive in the face of adversity. These include the following:

- **An optimistic attitude.** Rather than react to a stressor simply as a threat, resilient men and women view it as a challenge—one they believe they can and will overcome. Researchers have documented that individuals facing various stressors, including serious illness and bereavement, are more likely to report experiencing growth if they have high levels of hope and optimism.

- **Self-efficacy.** A sense of being in control of one's life can boost health, even in times of great stress.

- **Stress inoculation.** People who deal well with adversity often have had previous experiences with stress that toughened them in various ways, such as teaching them skills that enhanced their ability to cope and boosting their confidence in their ability to weather a rough patch.

- **Secure personal relationships.** Individuals who know they can count on the support of their loved ones are more likely to be resilient.

- **Spirituality or religiosity.** Religious coping may be particularly related to growth and resilience. In particular, two types seem most beneficial: spiritually-based religious coping (receiving emotional reassurance and guidance from God) and good-deeds coping (living a better, more spiritual life that includes altruistic acts).

Resilience

Adversity—whether in the form of a traumatic event or chronic stress—has different effects on individuals. Some people never recover and continue on a downward slide that may ultimately prove fatal. Others return, though at different rates, to their prior level of functioning. Life challenges, according to recent research, may increase mental toughness, build resilience, and help people cope with adversity.

Resilience can take many forms. A father whose child is kidnapped and killed may become a nationwide advocate for victims' rights. A student whose roommate dies in a car crash after a party may campaign for tougher laws against drunk driving. A couple whose premature baby spends weeks in a neonatal intensive care unit may find that their marriage has grown closer and stronger. Even though their experiences were

Resilience sometimes means developing new skills simply because, in order to get through the stressful experience, people had to learn something they hadn't known how to do before—for instance, wrangling with insurance companies or other bureaucracies. By mastering such skills, they become more fit to deal with an unpredictable world and develop new flexibility in facing the unknown.

Individuals who engage in proactive coping, a concept based on the principles of positive psychology discussed in Chapter 2, perceive stressful situations as challenges instead of threats. Teaching such skills to incoming freshmen, recent research shows, builds their resilience and helps them deal better with the transition to college.[35]

Along with new coping abilities comes the psychological sense of mastery. "I survived this," an individual may say, "so I'll be able to deal with other hard things in the future." Such

© Kryvenok Anastasiia/shutterstock.com

confidence keeps people actively engaged in the effort to cope and is itself a predictor of eventual success. Stress also can make individuals more aware of the fulfilling aspects of life, and they may become more interested in spiritual pursuits. Certain kinds of stressful experiences also have social consequences. If a person experiencing a traumatic event finds that the significant others in his or her life can be counted on, the result can be a strengthening of their relationship.

√ **check-in** Have you experienced life challenges that helped build your resilience?

Stress Prevention: Taking Control of Your Time

Although you may struggle to cram all that you need and want to do into your allotted 24 hours each day, you can take control of how you use the time you have. Becoming conscious of time and how you use it is crucial to reducing stressors and preventing stress overload.

Every day you make dozens of decisions, and the choices you make about how to use your time directly affect your stress level. If you have a big test on Monday and a term paper due Tuesday, you may plan to study all weekend. Then, when you're invited to a party Saturday night, you go. Although you set the alarm for 7:00 a.m. on Sunday, you don't pull yourself out of bed until noon. By the time you start studying, it's 4:00 p.m., and anxiety is building inside you.

√ **check-in** Do you feel that you are losing control of your time?

Are You Running Out of Time?

How can you tell if you've lost control of your time? The following are telltale symptoms of poor time management:

• Rushing

• Chronic inability to make choices or decisions

• Fatigue or listlessness

• Constantly missed deadlines

• Not enough time for rest or personal relationships

YOUR STRATEGIES FOR CHANGE

How to Become More Resilient

The following pointers may be helpful to consider in developing your own strategy for building resilience.

• **Make connections.** Accepting help and support from those who care about you and will listen to you strengthens resilience. Assisting others in their time of need can also benefit the helper.

• **Avoid seeing crises as insurmountable problems.** You can't change the fact that highly stressful events happen, but you can change how you interpret and respond to these events. Try looking beyond the present to how future circumstances may be a little better.

• **Accept that change is a part of living.** Certain goals may no longer be attainable as a result of adverse situations. Accepting circumstances that cannot be changed can help you focus on circumstances that you can alter.

• **Move toward your goals.** Think about possible solutions to the problems you are facing and decide what realistic goals you want to achieve. Do something regularly—even if it seems like a small accomplishment—that enables you to move forward. Ask yourself, "What's one thing I know I can accomplish today that helps me move in the direction I want to go?"

• **Take decisive actions.** Act on adverse situations as much as you can. Take decisive actions rather than detaching from problems and stresses and wishing they would just go away. Being active instead of passive helps people more effectively manage adversity.

• **Find positive ways to reduce stress and negative feelings.** Positive distractions such as exercising, going to a movie, or reading a book can help renew you so you can refocus on meeting challenges in your life. Avoid numbing your unpleasant feelings with alcohol or drugs.

• **Look for opportunities for self-discovery.** Many people who have experienced tragedies and hardship have reported better relationships, greater sense of strength even while feeling vulnerable, increased sense of self-worth, a more developed spirituality, and heightened appreciation for life.

• **Nurture a positive view of yourself.** Developing confidence in your ability to solve problems and trusting your instincts helps build resilience.

• **Keep things in perspective.** Even when facing very painful events, try to consider the stressful situation in a broader context and keep a long-term perspective. Avoid blowing the event out of proportion.

• **Maintain a hopeful outlook.** An optimistic outlook enables you to expect that good things will happen in your life. Try visualizing what you want rather than worrying about what you fear. Take care of yourself. Pay attention to your own needs and feelings. Engage in activities that you enjoy and find relaxing and that contribute to good health, including regular exercise and healthy eating.

Source: Adapted from materials available at the American Psychological Association's Help Center. http://www.apapracticecentral.org/outreach/building-resilience.aspx

• A sense of being overwhelmed by demands and details and having to do what you don't want to do most of the time

One of the hard lessons of being on your own is that your choices and your actions have consequences. Stress is just one of them. But by thinking ahead, being realistic about your workload, and sticking to your plans, you can gain better control over your time and your stress levels.

Time Management

Time management involves skills that anyone can learn, but they require commitment and practice to make a difference in your life. It may help to know the techniques that other students have found most useful:

- **Schedule your time.** Use a calendar or planner. Beginning the first week of class, mark down deadlines for each assignment, paper, project, and test scheduled that semester. Develop a daily schedule, listing very specifically what you will do the next day, along with the times. Block out times for working out, eating dinner, calling home, and talking with friends, as well as for studying.

- **Develop a game plan.** Allow at least two nights to study for any major exam. Set aside more time for researching and writing papers. Make sure to allow time to revise and print out a paper—and to deal with emergencies like a computer breakdown. Set daily and weekly goals for every class. When working on a big project, don't neglect your other courses. Whenever possible, try to work ahead in all your classes.

- **Identify time robbers.** For several days, keep a log of what you do and how much time you spend doing it. You may discover that disorganization is eating away at your time or that you have a problem getting started. (See the following section, "Overcoming Procrastination.")

- **Make the most of classes.** Read the assignments before class rather than wait until just before you have a test. By reading ahead of time, you'll make it easier to understand the lectures. Go to class yourself. Your own notes will be more helpful than a friend's or those from a note-taking service. Read your lecture notes at the end of each day or at least at the end of each week.

- **Develop an efficient study style.** Some experts recommend studying for 50 minutes and then breaking for 10 minutes. Small incentives, such as allowing yourself to call or visit a friend during those 10 minutes, can provide the motivation to keep you at the books longer. When you're reading, don't just highlight passages. Instead, write notes or questions to yourself in the margins, which will help you retain more information. Even

if you're racing to start a paper, take a few extra minutes to prepare a workable outline. This will help you better structure your paper when you start writing.

- **Focus on the task at hand.** Rather than worry about how you did on yesterday's test or how you'll ever finish next week's project, focus intently on whatever you're doing at any given moment. If your mind starts to wander, use any distraction—the sound of the phone ringing or a noise from the hall—as a reminder to stay in the moment.

- **Turn elephants into hors d'oeuvres.** Cut a huge task into smaller chunks so it seems less enormous. For instance, break down your term paper into a series of steps, such as selecting a topic, identifying sources of research information, taking notes, developing an outline, and so on.

- **Keep your workspace in order.** Even if the rest of your room is a shambles, try to keep your desk clear. Piles of papers are distracting, and you can end up wasting lots of time searching piles for notes you misplaced or an article you have to read by morning. Try to spend the last 10 minutes of the day getting your desk in order so you get a fresh start on the next day.

Overcoming Procrastination

Putting off until tomorrow what should be done today creates a great deal of stress for many students. In various studies, 30 to 60 percent of undergraduates have reported postponing academic tasks, such as studying for exams, writing papers, and reading weekly assignments, so often that their performance and grades have suffered. Occasional delay becomes a more serious problem when it triggers internal discomfort, such as anxiety, irritation, regret, despair, and self-blame, as well as external consequences, such as poor performance and lost opportunities.

✓**check-in** Do you have a procrastination problem?

The three most common types of procrastination are

- Putting off unpleasant things
- Putting off difficult tasks
- Putting off tough decisions

Procrastinators are most likely to delay by wishing they didn't have to do what they must or by telling themselves they "just can't get started," which means they never do.

To get out of the procrastination trap, keep track of the tasks you're most likely to put off and try to figure out why you don't want to tackle them. Think of alternative ways to get tasks done. If you put off library readings, for instance, is the problem getting to the library or the reading itself? If it's the trip to the library, arrange to walk over with a friend whose company you enjoy.

Do what you like least first. Once you have that out of the way, you can concentrate on the tasks you enjoy. Build time into your schedule for interruptions, unforeseen problems, and unexpected events so you aren't constantly racing around. Establish ground rules for meeting your own needs (including getting enough sleep and making time for friends) before saying yes to any activity. Learn to live according to a three-word motto: Just do it!

- Is stress always harmful?
- What stressors do college students typically encounter?
- How does the body respond to stress?
- What are some effective ways of managing stress?

THE POWER OF NOW!
Strengthening Your Stress Muscles

If you decide to run a charity 5-kilometer race, you don't start training by heading for the gym or track and immediately going the full distance. You build up your muscles and your aerobic capacity by starting with a lap or two and gradually increasing your distance and pace. Similarly, with stress management, you need to acquire and enhance fundamental skills that lay the foundation for developing all kinds of new, more complex habits and skills. Check the strategies you might use to manage stress better in your daily life:

____ Think back to times in the past week or so when you managed stress well. Write down the practical skills you used. Go further into the past and think about other times you handled stress successfully. Also add these to your list of strengths.

____ Review the times in the past when you did not handle stress well. Write down why you think you handled stress badly in certain situations. Identify specific steps or skills that would have enabled you to handle the situations better.

____ In assessing your strengths and weaknesses in handling stress, separate what you did, especially any mistakes you made, from who you are. Instead of saying, "I'm so stupid," tell yourself, "That wasn't the smartest move I ever made, but I learned from it."

____ Pause but don't panic when confronting a stressor. Pay attention to what's happening around you and analyze the situation thoughtfully but refrain from getting caught up in gloom-and-doom thinking, which can lead to high levels of anxiety and poor decision making.

____ Avoid the tendency to overreact or to become passive. Remain calm and stay focused.

____ If you find yourself turning more to escape routes such as drinking, gambling, or emotional eating, seek help from a campus counselor before the problem gets worse.

What's Online

CENGAGE brain.com   Visit www.cengagebrain.com to access course materials for this text, including the Behavior Change Planner, interactive quizzes, tutorials, and more.

Student Stress Scale

The Student Stress Scale, an adaptation of Holmes and Rahe's Life Events Scale for college-age adults, provides a rough indication of stress levels and possible health consequences.

In the Student Stress Scale, each event, such as beginning or ending school, is given a score that represents the amount of readjustment a person has to make as a result of the change. In some studies, using similar scales, people with serious illnesses have been found to have high scores.

To determine your stress score, add up the number of points corresponding to the events you have experienced in the past 12 months.

1.	Death of a close family member	100
2.	Death of a close friend	73
3.	Divorce of parents	65
4.	Jail term	63
5.	Major personal injury or illness	63
6.	Marriage	58
7.	Getting fired from a job	50
8.	Failing an important course	47
9.	Change in the health of a family member	45
10.	Pregnancy	45
11.	Sex problems	44
12.	Serious argument with a close friend	40
13.	Change in financial status	39
14.	Change of academic major	39
15.	Trouble with parents	39
16.	New girlfriend or boyfriend	37
17.	Increase in workload at school	37
18.	Outstanding personal achievement	36
19.	First quarter/semester in college	36
20.	Change in living conditions	31
21.	Serious argument with an instructor	30
22.	Getting lower grades than expected	29
23.	Change in sleeping habits	29
24.	Change in social activities	29
25.	Change in eating habits	28
26.	Chronic car trouble	26
27.	Change in number of family get-togethers	26
28.	Too many missed classes	25
29.	Changing colleges	24
30.	Dropping more than one class	23
31.	Minor traffic violations	20

Total Stress Score _____

Here's how to interpret your score: If your score is 300 or higher, you're at high risk for developing a health problem. If your score is between 150 and 300, you have a 50–50 chance of experiencing a serious health change within two years. If your score is below 150, you have a one in three chance of a serious health change.

Source: Mullen, Kathleen, and Gerald Costello. *Health Awareness Through Discovery*. Minneapolis: Burgess Publishing Company, 1981.

MAKING THIS CHAPTER WORK FOR YOU

Review Questions

(LO 4.1) 1. Stress is defined as _____.
   a. a negative emotional state related to fatigue and similar to depression
   b. the physiological and psychological response to any event or situation that either upsets or excites us
   c. the end result of the general adaptation syndrome
   d. a motivational strategy for making life changes

(LO 4.1) 2. Another term for looking at an individual's health as a whole rather than part by part is _____.
   a. comprehensive
   b. holistic
   c. unrealistic
   d. transcendental

(LO 4.2) 3. Stress levels in college students _____.
- a. may be high due to stressors such as academic pressures, financial concerns, learning disabilities, and relationship problems
- b. are usually low because students feel empowered living independently of their parents
- c. are typically highest in seniors because their self-esteem diminishes during the college years
- d. are lower in minority students because they are used to stressors such as a hostile social climate and actual or perceived discrimination

(LO 4.2) 4. The most common source of stress, as reported by about two-thirds of the people who responded to a recent American Psychological Association survey, is _____.
- a. relationship problems
- b. parenting problems
- c. money
- d. job

(LO 4.3) 5. Burnout is _____.
- a. the aftermath of extreme anger triggered by stress
- b. a feeling of complete defeat
- c. the feeling that comes after a long evening of partying
- d. a state of exhaustion brought on by constant or repeated emotional pressure

(LO 4.3) 6. "Venting" anger _____.
- a. is considered by therapists to be a healthy way of relieving anger
- b. can lead to a calm state that helps you concentrate
- c. can sabotage health over time by churning out stress hormones
- d. is acceptable if done in private

(LO 4.4) 7. Traumatic events that may trigger acute stress disorder include which of the following?
- a. Loss of a friend in an accident
- b. Breakup of a relationship
- c. Personal or physical assault
- d. Failing a course

(LO 4.4) 8. Which of the following is true of posttraumatic stress disorder (PTSD)?
- a. Individuals with PTSD require standard forms of help at all stages.
- b. Without recognition and treatment, PTSD can last decades, with symptoms intensifying during periods of stress.
- c. The odds of recovering from PTSD are worst when symptoms develop soon after the trauma.
- d. Immediate "debriefing" to release emotions or treatment with anxiety-reducing medications is the best approach to treat PTSD.

(LO 4.4) 9. A person suffering from posttraumatic stress disorder may experience which of the following symptoms?
- a. procrastination
- b. constant thirst
- c. drowsiness
- d. terror-filled dreams

(LO 4.5) 10. According to the general adaptation syndrome theory, how does the body typically respond to an acute stressor?
- a. The heart rate slows, blood pressure declines, and eye movement increases.
- b. The body enters a physical state called eustress and then moves into the physical state referred to as distress.
- c. If the stressor is viewed as a positive event, there are no physical changes.
- d. The body demonstrates three stages of change: alarm, resistance, and exhaustion.

(LO 4.5) 11. Which of the following is produced by the pituitary gland as a response to stress and is also called the "cuddle chemical"?
- a. Melanin
- b. Cortisol
- c. Epinephrine
- d. Oxytocin

(LO 4.6) 12. Which of the following statements is true of stress and the gastrointestinal system?
- a. Stress can constrict blood vessels in the digestive tract.
- b. Stress can increase saliva in the mouth.
- c. Stress can decrease the amount of hydrochloric acid in the stomach.
- d. Stress can dilate the esophagus.

(LO 4.6) 13. _____ produce a fight-or-flight response and prompt the immune system to ready itself for the possibility of infections resulting from bites, punctures, or other wounds.
- a. Distant stressors
- b. Acute time-limited stressors
- c. Chronic stressors
- d. Brief naturalistic stressors

(LO 4.7) 14. Which of the following illustrates the defense mechanism of displacement?
- a. You have a beer in the evening after a tough day.
- b. You act as if nothing has happened after you have been laid off from your job.
- c. You start an argument with your sister after being laid off from your job.
- d. You argue with your boss after he lays you off from your job.

(LO 4.7) 15. Which of the following is a factor that enables individuals to thrive in the face of adversity?
  a. Self-inoculation
  b. Self-schema
  c. Self-actualization
  d. Self-efficacy

(LO 4.7) 16. Which of the following relaxation techniques involves an electronic monitoring device attached to the body that detects a change in an internal function and communicates it back to the person through a tone, light, or meter?
  a. Biofeedback
  b. Visualization
  c. Progressive relaxation
  d. Guided imagery

(LO 4.8) 17. A relaxed, peaceful state of being can be achieved with which of the following activities?
  a. An aerobic exercise class
  b. Playing a computer game
  c. Meditating for 15 minutes
  d. Attending a rap concert

(LO 4.9) 18. Which of the following techniques will help a student with time management?
  a. Chunking smaller tasks together into larger tasks
  b. Focusing on past activities
  c. Providing small incentives at regular intervals
  d. Seeking a note-taking service

(LO 4.9) 19. The best way an individual can deal with procrastination is by _____.
  a. wishing he or she didn't have to do the required task
  b. figuring out why he or she doesn't want to tackle the required task
  c. focusing on just one way to get the required task done
  d. doing the task he or she likes least last

Answers to these questions can be found on page 623.

Critical Thinking

1. Identify three stressful situations in your life and determine whether they are examples of eustress or distress. Describe both the positive and negative aspects of each situation.
2. Can you think of any ways in which your behavior or attitudes might create stress for others? What changes could you make to avoid doing so?
3. What advice might you give an incoming freshman at your school about managing stress in college? What techniques have been most helpful for you in dealing with stress? Suppose that this student is from a different ethnic group than you. What additional suggestions would you have for this student?

Additional Online Resources

www.teachhealth.com
This comprehensive website is written specifically for college students by Steven Burns, M.D. It features the following topics: signs of how to recognize stress, two stress surveys for adults and college students, information on the pathophysiology of stress, the genetics of stress and stress tolerance, and information on how to best manage and treat stress.

www.mindtools.com/smpage.html
This site covers a variety of topics on stress management, including recognizing stress, exercise, time management, coping mechanisms, and more. The site also features a free comprehensive personal self-assessment with questions pertaining to work and home stressors, physical and behavioral signs and symptoms, as well as personal coping skills and resources.

Key Terms

The terms listed are used on the page indicated. Definitions of the terms are in the glossary at the end of the book.

biofeedback 95

burnout 86

defense mechanisms 93

distress 78

eustress 78

holistic 79

homeostasis 90

meditation 95

microaggressions 84

microassaults 84

microinsults 84

microinvalidations 84

mindfulness 95

posttraumatic stress disorder (PTSD) 88

progressive relaxation 94

stress 78

stressor 78

stress response 90

tend and befriend 90

visualization, or guided imagery 95

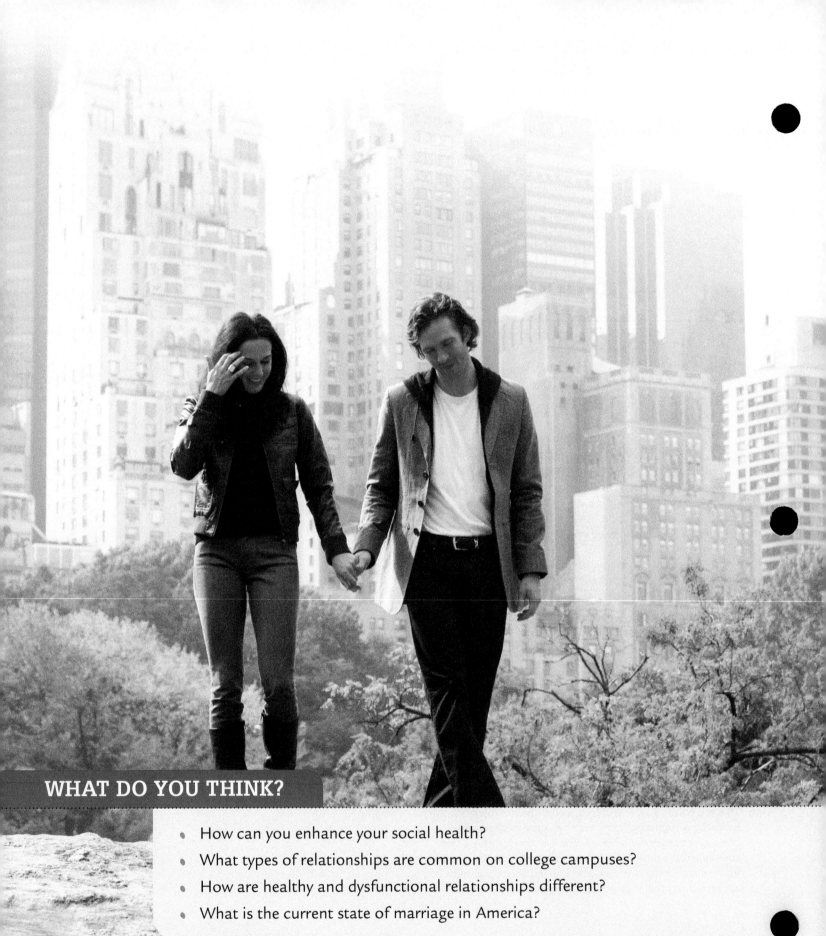

WHAT DO YOU THINK?

- How can you enhance your social health?
- What types of relationships are common on college campuses?
- How are healthy and dysfunctional relationships different?
- What is the current state of marriage in America?

Radius Images/Getty Images

5

Your Social Health

Andrea got her first cell phone on her eighth birthday. She opened an e-mail account when she was 11, joined Facebook at 13, started tweeting and posting YouTube videos at 16, and signed onto LinkedIn after getting her first summer job at 17. No matter where she goes, Andrea posts photos on Pinterest, Flickr, and Instagram. With 800-plus Facebook friends, 400 Instagram followers, and 300 Twitter followers, Andrea says she can't imagine feeling lonely—as long as she doesn't misplace her cell phone and its battery doesn't die. <

After reading this chapter, you should be able to:

5.1 Explain the meaning of the term *social health*, using examples.

5.2 Outline various ways of communicating.

5.3 Examine how relationships contribute to the social health of individuals.

5.4 Evaluate the impact of modern technology on communicating.

5.5 Identify current trends in dating among young people.

5.6 Explain the significance of love to an individual's well-being.

5.7 Summarize the impact of dysfunctional relationships.

5.8 Describe the trends, factors, and forms of long-term partnering in America.

5.9 Summarize the changes that have taken place in the American household over time.

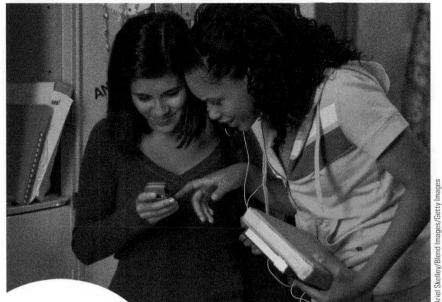

No one yet knows the impact that digital communication may have on relationships. Do you think texting might someday take the place of talking?

The Social Dimension of Health

Social health refers to the ability

- To interact effectively with other people and with the social environment
- To develop satisfying interpersonal relationships
- To fulfill social roles

Social health doesn't necessarily mean joining organizations or mingling in large groups, but it does involve participating in your community, living in harmony with others, communicating clearly, and practicing healthy sexual behaviors (discussed in Chapter 9).

✓ **check-in** How would you assess your social health? Excellent? Good? Not as good as you'd like?

Is Andrea the poster child for social health in the twenty-first century? Or is her virtual socializing somehow undermining her overall well-being? Scientists who study relationships are just beginning to explore the impact of our digital world. Will 140-character tweets and emoticons replace conversation? Could online social networking make face-to-face friendships obsolete?

No one knows the answers to these questions yet, but as much as technology may change our lives, one thing remains constant: We always have craved and always will crave human connection. As individuals and as part of society, we need to care about others and to know that others care about us, to feel for others and have others feel for us, to share what we know and to learn from what others know.

Your relationships with your family, friends, coworkers, and loved ones may amaze, irritate, exhilarate, frustrate, and delight you. They also may affect your health. As noted in Chapter 1, your ability to communicate, to develop satisfying relationships, and to live in harmony with others is an important dimension of health and wellness.

This chapter discusses the social needs we all share, the ways some of us respond` to those needs, healthy and unhealthy relationships, and the possibilities that exist for coming together from our solitude to warm ourselves in each other's glow.

As huge epidemiological studies have demonstrated beyond any doubt, supportive relationships buffer us from stress, distress, and disease. People with close ties to others have stronger cardiovascular and immune systems, resist colds better, and are less vulnerable to serious illness and premature death.

Specific qualities in a relationship, particularly *social support*, affect physical health. This term refers to the ways in which we provide information or assistance, show affection, comfort, and confide in others. As mounting evidence shows, people of all ages function best in socially supportive environments.

This is particularly true of college students, who report more stress and more physical symptoms when they feel a lack of family support. More than any other component of social support, a sense of belonging may have the greatest impact on college students' health. Because college is a transition time, forming new attachments may be especially important—and beneficial to overall health.

Your social support network might consist of people you see almost every day; more casual acquaintances; and friends, followers, and bloggers you get to know online. (Social networking is covered later in this chapter.) Simply staying in touch and sharing each other's lives bolster feelings of self-worth, security, and belonging.

√**check-in** Who is in your social support network?

According to the concept of **social contagion**, friends, friends of friends, acquaintances, and others in our social circle influence our behavior and our health—both positively and negatively. Among the 15,000 people followed over three generations in the Framingham heart study, various health-related factors, such as weight gain, drinking, and smoking, changed not just individually over time but among clusters of people. The conclusion: Just as people are connected, so is their health. The reasons may include peer pressure or "mirror neurons" in the brain that automatically mimic what we see in the people around us.

According to social scientists, each of us is linked within three degrees (to a friend, a friend of a friend, and that friend's friend) to more than 1,000 people. Think of this social web as an opportunity. By your good health behaviors you can, in theory, influence 1,000 individuals to become healthier, fitter, and happier. And if you choose your friends wisely, they will do the same for you.

√**check-in** Has your social network influenced any of your health behaviors? How do you think you may have influenced others?

Communicating

Healthy, mutually beneficial relationships add joy to our years and maybe even years to our life. Unhealthy or dysfunctional ones can be so toxic that they undermine health as well as happiness. By mastering skills to communicate more clearly and by being responsible and responsive in your interactions with others, you can cultivate what psychologist Daniel Goleman called "social intelligence" and create relationships worth cherishing.

Learning to Listen

Communication stems from a desire to know and a decision to tell. The first step is learning how to listen. Then you mostly choose what information about yourself to disclose and what to keep private. In opening up to others, you increase your own self-knowledge and understanding.

A great deal of daily communication focuses on facts: on the who, what, where, when, and how. Information is easy to convey and

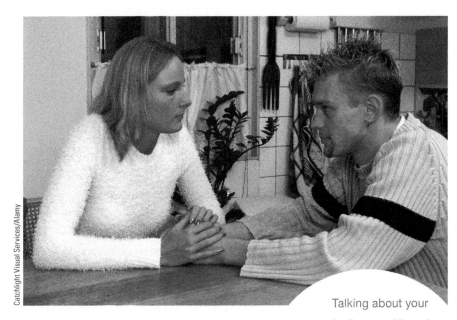

Catchlight Visual Services/Alamy

Talking about your feelings and listening intently move a relationship to a deeper and more meaningful level.

comprehend. Emotions are not. Some people have great difficulty saying "I appreciate you" or "I care about you," even though they are genuinely appreciative and caring. Others find it hard to know what to say in response and how to accept such expressions of affection.

Some people feel that relationships shouldn't require any effort, that there's no need to talk of responsibility between people who care about each other. Yet responsibility is implicit in our dealings with anyone or anything we value—and what can be more valuable than those with whom we share our lives? Friendships and other intimate relationships always demand an emotional investment, but the rewards they yield are great.

√**check-in** Do you put effort into maintaining and strengthening your close relationships?

Being Agreeable but Assertive

There's an old saying that "nice guys finish last," but that's not the case. Psychologists translate "niceness" into a personality trait called "agreeableness," which includes being helpful, unselfish, generally trusting, considerate, cooperative, sympathetic, warm, and concerned for others. Among the benefits that agreeable people enjoy are strong relationships, less conflict, happy marriages, better job performance, healthier eating habits and behaviors, less stress, and fewer medical complaints.

Agreeable people aren't so "nice" that other people can easily influence or take advantage of them. In situations that call for it, they make their

social contagion The process by which friends, friends of friends, acquaintances, and others in our social circle influence our behavior and our health—both positively and negatively.

YOUR STRATEGIES FOR CHANGE

How to Assert Yourself

- **Use "I" statements to explain your feelings.** This allows you to take ownership of your opinions and feelings without putting down others for how they feel and think.

- **Listen to and acknowledge what the other person says.** After you speak, find out if the other person understands your position. Ask how he or she feels about what you've said.

- **Be direct and specific.** Describe the problem as you see it, using neutral language rather than assigning blame. Also suggest a specific solution, but make it clear that you'd like the lines of communication and negotiation to remain open.

- **Don't think you have to be obnoxious in order to be assertive.** It's most effective to state your needs and preferences without any sarcasm or hostility.

needs and desires clear by being assertive—but not aggressive.

Assertiveness doesn't mean screaming or telling someone off. You can communicate your wishes calmly and clearly. Assertiveness involves respecting your rights and the rights of other people even when you disagree. (See "Your Strategies for Change: How to Assert Yourself.")

You can change a situation you don't like by communicating your feelings and thoughts in nonprovocative words, by focusing on specifics, and by making sure you're talking with the person who is directly responsible.

✓**check-in** Do you feel comfortable asserting yourself?

How Men and Women Communicate

Gender differences in communication start early. By age 1, boys make less eye contact than girls and pay more attention to moving objects like cars than to human faces. Both mothers and fathers talk less about feelings (except anger) to sons than daughters, and boys' vocabularies include fewer "feeling" words. On the playground, if not at home, boys learn to choke back tears and show no fear. Their faces—once as openly emotional as girls'—become less expressive as they move through the elementary years.

As adults, men use fewer words and talk, at least in public, as a means of putting themselves in a one-up situation—unlike women, who talk to draw others closer. Even with friends, men mainly swap information as they talk shop, sports, cars, and computers.

In studies of language, linguists have identified the following gender differences, which may be based on sex or gender roles:

Men:

- Speak more often and for longer periods in public.

- Interrupt more, breaking in on another's monologue if they aren't getting the information they need.

- Look into a woman's eyes more often when talking than they would if talking with another man.

- When writing, use more numbers, more prepositions, and articles such as *an* and *the*.

- Write briefer, more utilitarian e-mails.

- In blogs or chat rooms, are more likely to make strong assertions, disagree with others, and use profanity and sarcasm.

Women:

- Speak more in private, usually to build better connections with others.

- Are generally better listeners, facilitating conversation by nodding, asking questions, and signaling interest by saying "uh-huh" or "yes."

- Are more likely to wait for a speaker to finish rather than interrupt.

- Look into another woman's eyes more often than they would if talking with a man.

- When writing, use more words overall; more words related to emotion (positive and negative); more idea words; more hearing, feeling, and sensing words; more causal words (such as *because*); and more modal words (*would, should, could*).

- Write e-mails in much the same way they talk, using words to build a connection with people.

- In blogs or chat rooms, are more prone to posing questions, making suggestions, and including polite expressions. Communication researchers studying the differences between "he-mails" and "she-mails" have also found that people who are not generally verbally expressive—mainly but not exclusively men—often convey more feelings in e-mails than they do in face-to-face conversations.

✓**check-in** What do you feel you can learn from the communication style of the "other" sex?

Nonverbal Communication

More than 90 percent of communication may be nonverbal. While we speak with our vocal cords, we communicate with our facial expressions, tone of voice, hands, shoulders, legs, torsos, posture. Body language is the building block upon which more advanced verbal forms of communication rest.

Culture has a great deal of influence over body language. In some cultures, for example, establishing eye contact is considered hostile or challenging; in others, it conveys friendliness. A person's sense of personal space—the distance he or she feels most comfortable keeping from others—also varies in different societies.

√**check-in** What does your body language say about you?

Forming Relationships

We first learn how to relate as children. Our relationships with parents and siblings change dramatically as we grow toward independence. Relationships between friends also change as they move or develop different interests; between lovers, as they come to know more about each other; between spouses, as they pass through life together; and between parents and children, as youngsters develop and mature. But throughout life, close relationships, tested and strengthened by time, allow us to explore the depths of our souls and the heights of our emotions. (See the Self Survey "What's Your Intimacy Quotient?")

Even a relationship with a pet can be beneficial. "Companion animals" have proven beneficial in lessening the symptoms of several mental disorders, easing the sting of rejection, and boosting a sense of well-being. They also can enhance feelings of self-worth and serve as catalysts for forming new relationships with other pet owners and neighbors.[1]

Friendship

Friendship has been described as "the most holy bond of society." Every culture has prized the ties of respect, tolerance, and loyalty that friendship builds and nurtures. An anonymous writer put it well:

A friend is one who knows you as you are,
Understands where you've been,
Accepts who you've become,
And still gently invites you to grow.

Friends can be a basic source of happiness, a connection to a larger world, a source of solace in times of trouble. Although we have different friends throughout life, often the friendships of adolescence and young adulthood are the closest ones we ever form. They ease the normal break from parents and the transition from childhood to independence.

On average, we devote 40 percent of our limited social time to the five most important people we know, who represent just 3 percent of our social world. Having more than five best friends is impossible when we interact face-to-face because of time constraints. But thanks to social networking online, it's possible to accumulate hundreds, or even thousands, of virtual friends.

Even so, most of us can maintain no more than 150 meaningful relationships online and off—a total called "Dunbar's number," in recognition of the researcher who came up with it. At one time, when almost all humans on Earth lived in small, rural, interconnected communities, everyone in a village may have known the same 150 people.

In our modern mobile society, we move time and again, leaving behind old friends. Emotional closeness, Dunbar found, declines by around 15 percent a year in the absence of face-to-face contact. Facebook, at the least, provides us an opportunity to maintain friendships that would otherwise rapidly wither away. Online status reports and, more effectively, everyday images of faraway friends can provide some of the same benefits as in-person friendship, including enhanced self-esteem and happiness.

√**check-in** How many truly close friends do you have? How many "friendly" relationships do you have, both online and offline?

Loneliness

More so than many other countries, ours is a nation of loners. Recent trends—longer work hours, busy family schedules, frequent moves, high divorce rates—have created even more lonely people. Only about one-quarter of Americans say they're never lonely. In the most recent American College Health Association (ACHA) survey, 59.2 percent of undergraduates reported feeling very lonely at some time in the past 12 months.[2] (See Snapshot: On Campus Now on page 110.)

√**check-in** Have you felt very lonely at some time in the past 12 months?

Loneliness, defined as "feelings of distress and dysphoria resulting from a discrepancy between a person's desired and achieved social relations," has been identified as a risk factor for depression

SNAPSHOT: ON CAMPUS NOW

All the Lonely Students

Students who say they felt very lonely:

	Percent (%)		
	Male	Female	Average
No, never	28.9	18.7	22.3
No, not in the past 12 months	19.7	18.0	18.6
Yes, in the past 2 weeks	20.1	26.1	24.1
Yes, in the past 30 days	11.0	14.6	13.3
Yes, in the past 12 months	20.2	22.6	21.7
Anytime within the past 12 months	51.3	63.3	59.2

Source: American College Health Association. *American College Health Association–National College Health Assessment II: Reference Group Executive Summary, Spring 2014.* Hanover, MD: American College Health Association, 2014.

and poor psychological health. However, it may also threaten physical well-being. In a review of studies involving more than 3 million people, both feeling lonely and social isolation—having few or no social contacts or activities—increased the risk of an earlier death for both men and women, particularly those under the age of 65.[3]

Loneliest of all are adolescents and elderly people; those who are divorced, separated, or widowed; and adults who live alone or solely with children. Loneliness is most likely to cause emotional distress when it is chronic rather than episodic. Chronic loneliness may impair the immune system and increase pain, depression, and fatigue.[4]

To combat loneliness, people may join groups, fling themselves into projects and activities, or surround themselves with superficial acquaintances. Others avoid the effort of trying to connect, sometimes limiting most of their personal interactions to their computers and mobile devices.

The true keys to overcoming loneliness are developing resources to fulfill our own potential and learning to reach out to others. In this way, loneliness can become a means to personal growth and discovery.

Shyness and Social Anxiety Disorder

Many people are uncomfortable meeting strangers or speaking or performing in public. In some surveys, as many as 40 percent of people describe themselves as shy or socially anxious.

social anxiety disorder A fear and avoidance of social situations.

Some shy people—an estimated 10 to 15 percent of children—are born with a predisposition to shyness. Others become shy because they don't learn proper social responses or because they experience rejection or shame.

Some people are "fearfully" shy; that is, they withdraw and avoid contact with others and experience a high degree of anxiety and fear in social situations. Others are "self-consciously" shy. They enjoy the company of others but become highly self-aware and anxious in social situations.

In studies of college students, men have reported somewhat more shyness than women. Students may develop symptoms of shyness or social anxiety when they go to a party or are called on in class. Some experience symptoms when they try to perform any sort of action in the presence of others, even such everyday activities as eating in public, using a public restroom, or going to the grocery store.

About 7 percent of the population could be diagnosed with a **social anxiety disorder** (social phobia), in which individuals typically fear and avoid various social situations. Childhood shyness, emotional abuse, neglect, and chronic illness increase the likelihood of this problem.[5] Asian cultures typically show the lowest rates; Russian and American, the highest.

Adolescents and young adults with severe social anxiety are at increased risk of major depression. The key difference between these problems and normal shyness and self-consciousness is the degree of distress and impairment that individuals experience.

√**check-in** Do you think of yourself as shy?

If you're shy, you can overcome much of your social apprehensiveness on your own, in much the same way as you might set out to stop smoking or lose weight. For example, you can improve your social skills by pushing yourself to introduce yourself to a stranger at a party or to chat about the weather or the food selections with the person next to you in a cafeteria line. Gradually, you'll acquire a sense of social timing and a verbal ease that will take the worry out of close encounters with others. Those with more disabling social anxiety may do best with psychotherapy and medication, which have been shown to be highly effective.

Building a Healthy Community

"No man is an island," the English poet John Donne wrote in 1624. In today's global society, this phrase rings just as true. In addition to our families, friendships, and social networks, we are part of communities—our campus, our neighborhood, our town or city. (Chapter 19 discusses the community we are all citizens of: planet Earth.)

Contributing to your community can take many forms, from volunteering at a Habitat for Humanity building project to singing in a church choir. By giving to others, you get a great deal in return. As researchers have documented, **altruism**—helping or giving to others—enhances self-esteem, relieves physical and mental stress, and protects psychological well-being.

√**check-in** What do you do to contribute to your community?

Doing Good

Helping or giving to others enhances self-esteem, relieves physical and mental stress, and protects psychological well-being. Hans Selye, the father of stress research, described cooperation with others for the self's sake as altruistic egotism, whereby we satisfy our own needs while helping others satisfy theirs. This concept is essentially an updated version of the golden rule: Do unto others as you would have them do unto you. The important difference is that you earn your neighbor's love and help by offering him or her love and help.

Volunteerism helps those who give as well as those who receive. People involved in community organizations, for instance, consistently report a surge of well-being called *helper's high*, which they describe as a unique sense of calmness, warmth, and enhanced self-worth. College students who provided community service as part of a semester-long course reported changes in attitude (including a decreased tendency to blame

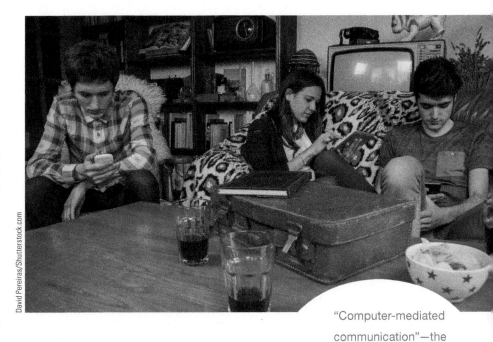

David Pereiras/Shutterstock.com

people for their misfortunes), self-esteem (primarily a belief that they can make a difference), and behavior (such as a greater commitment to do more volunteer work). Volunteering also may lower risk factors for cardiovascular disease.[6]

√**check-in** Do you volunteer?

The options for giving of yourself are limitless: Volunteer to serve a meal at a homeless shelter. Collect donations for a charity auction. Teach in a literacy program. Perform the simplest act of charity: Pray for others.

"Computer-mediated communication"—the conveying of written text via the Internet— is changing the ways we relate to others.

Living in a Wired World

Modern technology is changing our social DNA. Today you can use a smartphone to call, text, or video chat with almost anyone almost anywhere. You also may blog, tweet, follow Facebook or other networking services, upload photos, and give the world (or selected citizens) front-row seats to your life.

Some experts say that with social networking, humans are only doing what comes naturally—but now with twenty-first-century tools. Our brains seem wired to connect. As neuroimaging studies have shown, the amygdala, a brain region involved in processing emotional reactions, is bigger in individuals with large, complex social networks.

altruism Acts of helping or giving to others without thought of self-benefit.

These networks are getting bigger than ever—thanks to "computer-mediated communication"—the conveying of written text via the Internet—whether by Facebook, Twitter, or ever-evolving new networks, sites, and apps.

According to recent research, individuals who socialize online show the same psychological sense of community as those who interact in person, although Facebook users report greater social support than Twitter users.[7]

✓**check-in** Do you feel a sense of community with your online social network?

Social Networking on Campus

College-age young adults may be the most wired age group. More than nine in ten college students maintain a social networking profile, with Facebook the most popular choice. College students ages 18 to 24 spend an average of 32.2 hours a month online; those ages 25 to 34 spend 35.8 hours.[8]

Social networks are especially appealing to college students, who often have to completely reorganize their social connections, particularly if they leave home and move to a campus where they know few, if any, people. Many incoming students use online social networks to maintain relationships with the friends and family members they left behind and to learn more about the new acquaintances they are making.

✓**check-in** How much time do you spend online every day?

Facebook

The world's most popular website was created by a college student for college students in 2004. More than 800 million users around the globe have since joined and spend an average of 19 minutes a day on the site. Men and women between ages 18 and 25 make up about one-third of Facebook users. However, these days your parents and their friends are as likely as your peers to have Facebook pages.

In one survey of more than 1,500 college students, respondents reported checking Facebook five or more times on a typical day and spending more than 100 minutes on the site. Students spend more time observing content than actually posting, and they check up on others more frequently than they send private messages. Such "lurking," according to studies, is one of the most popular Facebook activities among college students. They also engage in electronic interactions with friends by means of posting, commenting, or replying to messages and in self-presentation through photos, wall posts, "likes," or friend lists.[9]

The most common motivations undergraduates give for their Facebook use are

- Nurturing or maintaining existing relationships
- Seeking new relationships
- Enhancing their reputation (being cool)
- Avoiding loneliness
- Keeping tabs on other people
- Feeling better about themselves

Students feeling stressed or down report a psychological boost in self-esteem after viewing their Facebook profiles, perhaps because when they do so, they are reminded of the personal traits and relationships that they value most.[10] Simply having a certain number of Facebook friends boosts feelings of happiness, researchers have found. Even more meaningful is getting support from online acquaintances—but only if it comes in response to an honest presentation of oneself.

In general, women tend to use social networking sites to compare themselves with others and search for information. Men are more likely to look at other people's profiles to find friends. The sexes even differ in their profile photos: Women usually add portraits, while men prefer full-body shots.

College students of both sexes try to present themselves as positively as possible—but some of the most intense Facebook users attribute others' seeming success and happiness to their personalities. As researchers in a recent study of undergraduates at a state university in Utah found, students, particularly those who included more people they did not know among their Facebook friends, were most likely to agree that others on Facebook "are happier and having better lives than I am."

In another study, freshmen who had a stronger emotional connection to, and spent more time on, Facebook reported having fewer friends on campus and experiencing more emotional and academic difficulties in adjusting to college life. However, students seemed to learn to use Facebook effectively with their peers, with the result that upperclassmen on Facebook showed greater positive social adjustment and more attachment to their schools.

✓**check-in** What are your reasons for being on Facebook—or not?

Self-Disclosure and Privacy in a Digital Age

A key element of relationships—whether friendships or romantic relationships—is **self-disclosure**—that is, how much we reveal about ourselves to another person. What you share about yourself is a critical building block that

self-disclosure Sharing personal information and experiences with another that he or she would not otherwise discover; self-disclosure involves risk and vulnerability.

affects the nature and quality of the bonds you establish with others.

Social networking has transformed the issues of privacy and disclosure. Rather than confide in a trusted friend, individuals may go online and reveal highly personal information to a stranger—or, if a comment or video makes its way onto a public site, to many strangers.

Previously personal moments now play out in public—sometimes by choice (as in an engagement announced via a change in status on Facebook), sometimes by chance (as when someone uploads a video of drunk beer-pong players).

In surveys of teenagers and young adults with online profiles, one-third to one-half had posted photos or videos depicting what researchers call "negative health risk behaviors," such as drinking and using drugs. Many viewed the images (of drinking more than drug use) in positive ways. Parents, friends of parents, siblings, coworkers, and employers often have a very different perspective.

Digital Sexual Disclosures

"Sexting"—sending sexually explicit text messages or digital photos—is fairly common among teens. The reasons for its popularity include peer pressure, the search for romance, and trust that the recipient will respond positively. Despite warnings about potential misuse of such messages, adolescents tend not to consider the potential for negative fallout down the road.

Sexual disclosure in texts or online continues in college. In an analysis of sexual references on the Facebook profiles of college freshmen, researchers found that those displaying sexual information were more likely to be considering sexual activity than those who refrained from posting sexual content.[11] (See Consumer Alert.)

Sexual posts can have unanticipated consequences. In one study, women's sexy pictures or comments increased the sexual expectations of male students. "The sexier the pictures, the wilder you know they are," commented one young man. "Sexual pictures equal sexual activity being around the corner," said another.

Yet at the same time, sexual or suggestive material lessens the guys' interest in a serious relationship with the young women. "I don't want to show my friends a girl I like on Facebook and have them see sexual pictures and her all drunk," a student remarked. Sexual references generate powerful "subconscious impressions," the researchers concluded—and could put female students at risk for unwanted sexual advances.

❗ CONSUMER ALERT

Online Flirting and Dating

Virtual flirtations can be fun, but they also entail some risks, particularly if you decide to go offline and meet in person. Here are some guidelines.

Facts to Know

- Remember that you have no way of verifying whether a correspondent is telling the truth about anything—sex, age, occupation, marital status. If your online partner seems insincere or strange in any way, stop corresponding.

- Be careful of what you type. Anything you put on the Internet can end up almost anywhere, including with potential employers. To avoid embarrassment, don't say anything you wouldn't want to see in newspaper print.

Steps to Take

- Don't give out your address, telephone number, or any other identifying information. The people you meet online are strangers, and you should keep your guard up.

- Don't "date" on an office or university computer. You could end up supplying your professors, classmates, or coworkers with unintentional entertainment. Also, many organizations and institutions consider e-mail messages company property.

- Don't rely on the Internet as your only method of meeting people. Continue to get out in the real world and meet potential dates the old-fashioned way: live and in person.

- If you do decide to meet someone you met online, make your first face-to-face encounter a double or group date and make it somewhere public, like a café or museum. Don't plan a full-day outing. Coffee or a drink in a crowded place makes the best transition from e-mail.

- Don't let your expectations run wild. Finding Mr. or Ms. Right is no easier in cyberspace than anywhere else, so be realistic about where your relationship might lead.

✓**check-in** How do you react to sexual tests or online posts?

Problematic Cell Phone and Internet Use

College students primarily use cell phones for leisure rather than school or work. Researchers have classified those who are on their phones 10 or more hours a day as "high users," while those who spend three hours or less on their cell phones qualify as low users. In terms of personality characteristics, the low users showed a higher preference for challenge and were least susceptible to boredom. The high users reported greater distress and more susceptibility to boredom.[12]

Too much connectivity can be hazardous to your health. In a recent study of about 500 male and female undergraduates "high-frequency cell phone users" reported higher levels of anxiety, less satisfaction with life, and lower grades than peers who use their cell phones less.[13] On average, the students reported spending 279 minutes—almost 5 hours—a day using their

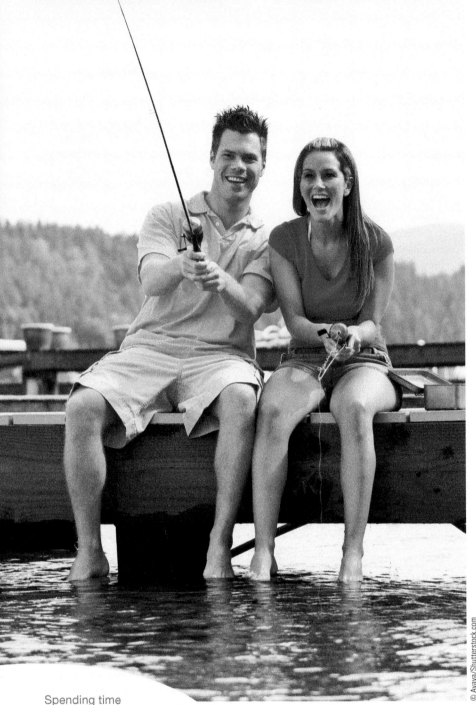

Spending time together gives couples a chance to have fun and share their likes, dislikes, and interests.

© Avava/Shutterstock.com

✓**check-in** How much time do you spend on your cell phone every day?

College students often consider social networking and other online activities a "guilty pleasure," but only online video viewing is associated with less time spent on schoolwork.[15]

A minority of Internet users—from 1 to 10 percent in various studies—report symptoms associated with addictive behavior. Like other addictions (discussed in Chapter 12), "problematic" Internet use may lead to preoccupation, withdrawal, difficulty with control, disregard for harmful consequences, loss of other interests, desire for escape, hiding the behavior, and harmful effects on relationships or work- or school-related performance. Adverse physical effects include carpal tunnel syndrome, dry eyes, headaches, and altered sleep patterns.

Estimates of problematic Internet use among college students range from 1 to 6 percent. In the ACHA survey, 13.2 percent of students—more than the percentage citing relationship difficulties or depression—ranked Internet use/computer games as having a negative impact on their academic performance.[16]

Undergraduates reporting problematic Internet use are equally likely to be male or female but more likely to be younger, single, and of Asian or Pacific Islander descent. The higher their Internet use, the lower their GPAs and levels of physical activity. They also are more stressed and depressed and engage in more online compulsive behaviors, including shopping and pornography viewing.[17]

✓**check-in** Has your Internet use ever caused problems for you?

For some the Internet has become an outlet for anger. Various "rant" websites allow anonymous users to adopt a screen name and engage in back-and-forth online screaming. This behavior may seem harmless, but as research shows, individuals who engage in virtual venting may initially feel more relaxed but overall tend to experience more anger in general and express it in maladaptive ways.[18]

Cyberbullying consists of deliberate, repeated, and hostile actions that use information and communication technologies, including online web pages, and text messages, with the intent of harming others by means of intimidation, control, manipulation, false accusations, or humiliation. Cyberbullies may know their victims or strike randomly.

Its prevalence on college campuses ranges from 8 to 21 percent.[19] Involvement in cyberbullying increases the odds of depression for

cell phones and sending 77 text messages a day. As cell phone use increased, so did anxiety—and, as another study demonstrated, fitness levels declined.[14]

Cell phone use itself may not make people anxious, the researchers noted, but the more time you spend with your phone, the less time you have to engage in other stress reducers, such as getting exercise, being alone and having time to think, talking with a friend face to face, and engaging in other activities you truly enjoy.

affects the nature and quality of the bonds you establish with others.

Social networking has transformed the issues of privacy and disclosure. Rather than confide in a trusted friend, individuals may go online and reveal highly personal information to a stranger—or, if a comment or video makes its way onto a public site, to many strangers.

Previously personal moments now play out in public—sometimes by choice (as in an engagement announced via a change in status on Facebook), sometimes by chance (as when someone uploads a video of drunk beer-pong players).

In surveys of teenagers and young adults with online profiles, one-third to one-half had posted photos or videos depicting what researchers call "negative health risk behaviors," such as drinking and using drugs. Many viewed the images (of drinking more than drug use) in positive ways. Parents, friends of parents, siblings, coworkers, and employers often have a very different perspective.

Digital Sexual Disclosures

"Sexting"—sending sexually explicit text messages or digital photos—is fairly common among teens. The reasons for its popularity include peer pressure, the search for romance, and trust that the recipient will respond positively. Despite warnings about potential misuse of such messages, adolescents tend not to consider the potential for negative fallout down the road.

Sexual disclosure in texts or online continues in college. In an analysis of sexual references on the Facebook profiles of college freshmen, researchers found that those displaying sexual information were more likely to be considering sexual activity than those who refrained from posting sexual content.[11] (See Consumer Alert.)

Sexual posts can have unanticipated consequences. In one study, women's sexy pictures or comments increased the sexual expectations of male students. "The sexier the pictures, the wilder you know they are," commented one young man. "Sexual pictures equal sexual activity being around the corner," said another.

Yet at the same time, sexual or suggestive material lessens the guys' interest in a serious relationship with the young women. "I don't want to show my friends a girl I like on Facebook and have them see sexual pictures and her all drunk," a student remarked. Sexual references generate powerful "subconscious impressions," the researchers concluded—and could put female students at risk for unwanted sexual advances.

✓**check-in** How do you react to sexual tests or online posts?

Problematic Cell Phone and Internet Use

College students primarily use cell phones for leisure rather than school or work. Researchers have classified those who are on their phones 10 or more hours a day as "high users," while those who spend three hours or less on their cell phones qualify as low users. In terms of personality characteristics, the low users showed a higher preference for challenge and were least susceptible to boredom. The high users reported greater distress and more susceptibility to boredom.[12]

Too much connectivity can be hazardous to your health. In a recent study of about 500 male and female undergraduates "high-frequency cell phone users" reported higher levels of anxiety, less satisfaction with life, and lower grades than peers who use their cell phones less.[13] On average, the students reported spending 279 minutes—almost 5 hours—a day using their

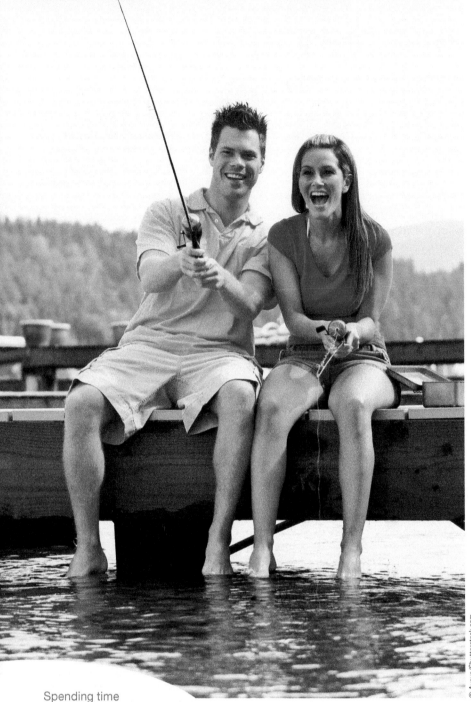

Spending time together gives couples a chance to have fun and share their likes, dislikes, and interests.

© Avava/Shutterstock.com

✓**check-in** How much time do you spend on your cell phone every day?

College students often consider social networking and other online activities a "guilty pleasure," but only online video viewing is associated with less time spent on schoolwork.[15]

A minority of Internet users—from 1 to 10 percent in various studies—report symptoms associated with addictive behavior. Like other addictions (discussed in Chapter 12), "problematic" Internet use may lead to preoccupation, withdrawal, difficulty with control, disregard for harmful consequences, loss of other interests, desire for escape, hiding the behavior, and harmful effects on relationships or work- or school-related performance. Adverse physical effects include carpal tunnel syndrome, dry eyes, headaches, and altered sleep patterns.

Estimates of problematic Internet use among college students range from 1 to 6 percent. In the ACHA survey, 13.2 percent of students—more than the percentage citing relationship difficulties or depression—ranked Internet use/computer games as having a negative impact on their academic performance.[16]

Undergraduates reporting problematic Internet use are equally likely to be male or female but more likely to be younger, single, and of Asian or Pacific Islander descent. The higher their Internet use, the lower their GPAs and levels of physical activity. They also are more stressed and depressed and engage in more online compulsive behaviors, including shopping and pornography viewing.[17]

✓**check-in** Has your Internet use ever caused problems for you?

For some the Internet has become an outlet for anger. Various "rant" websites allow anonymous users to adopt a screen name and engage in back-and-forth online screaming. This behavior may seem harmless, but as research shows, individuals who engage in virtual venting may initially feel more relaxed but overall tend to experience more anger in general and express it in maladaptive ways.[18]

Cyberbullying consists of deliberate, repeated, and hostile actions that use information and communication technologies, including online web pages, and text messages, with the intent of harming others by means of intimidation, control, manipulation, false accusations, or humiliation. Cyberbullies may know their victims or strike randomly.

Its prevalence on college campuses ranges from 8 to 21 percent.[19] Involvement in cyberbullying increases the odds of depression for

cell phones and sending 77 text messages a day. As cell phone use increased, so did anxiety—and, as another study demonstrated, fitness levels declined.[14]

Cell phone use itself may not make people anxious, the researchers noted, but the more time you spend with your phone, the less time you have to engage in other stress reducers, such as getting exercise, being alone and having time to think, talking with a friend face to face, and engaging in other activities you truly enjoy.

both bully and victim, particularly if it includes unwanted sexual advances.[20]

Cyberstalking, a form of cyberbullying, uses online sites, e-mail messages, and social media to harass victims and try to damage their reputation or turn others against them. Cyberstalking may include false accusations, threats, identity theft, damage to data or equipment, or the solicitation of minors for sex. Both cyberbullying and cyberstalking can be criminal offenses punishable by imprisonment.

Cyberstalking occurs most often in the context of ex-partner relationships. Most of its perpetrators are male and its victims female. Its negative psychological impact on a victim's well-being is comparable to real-life stalking.[21]

√**check-in** Have you ever experienced cyberbullying or cyberstalking?

Another negative impact of Facebook, according to researchers, may be distortion of students' perceptions of drinking norms (see Chapter 1 for a discussion of social norms). In one study of college students on Facebook, about one-third reported posting pictures of themselves with alcohol-related content. Other researchers have found alcohol-related content on more than three-quarters of students' Facebook pages. Undergraduates who view alcohol-related content on Facebook estimate college drinking norms to be higher than those who did not.[22] (See Chapter 13 for more on actual and perceived alcohol use on campus.)

Dating on Campus

Dating isn't what it used to be. Many young people socialize in groups until a couple pairs off into a romantic relationship. Rather than the conventional dinner and a movie, college students may just get together to hang out. Is one person interested in something more? Is the other? Often it can take a while for couples to figure out if they are in fact dating.

Sexual relations also have changed. As discussed in Chapter 9, sexual initiation is occurring earlier—at about age 16 for both genders. More women—about 15 percent of those ages 20 to 24—report having had sex with another woman. The percentage of men having sex with men has not changed over recent decades. Men report more lifetime sex partners than women, but the difference has narrowed over time.[23]

Hooking Up

An estimated 56 to 86 percent of college students report engaging in some form of casual sex (also discussed in Chapter 9). A **hookup** might involve a range of physically intimate behaviors—from kissing to intercourse—characterized by a lack of any expectation of emotional intimacy or a romantic relationship. Some students have defined it more informally as "making out with no future" or "a one-time experience without any kind of responsibility to each other."[24]

Although popular media have described a pervasive "hookup culture" on campuses, researchers have challenged its prevalence. In one study, recent undergraduates did not report more sexual partners since age 19, more frequent sex, or more partners during the past year than those enrolled from 1988 to 1996. However, they were more likely to report sex with a casual date/pickup and less likely to report sex with a spouse or regular partner.[25] Other studies have documented a pattern in college hookups, which tend to peak between spring semester of the first year of college and fall semester of the second year, followed by a gradual decline over subsequent terms.[26]

√**check-in** How common are hookups on your campus?

A college hookup usually involves two people who have met earlier in the evening, often at a bar, fraternity house, club, or party, and agree to engage in some sexual behavior for which there is little or no expectation of future commitment. There is often minimal communication, and the hookup ends when one partner leaves, falls asleep, or passes out.

According to recent studies, students most likely to engage in hookups tend to

- Be white
- Be attractive
- Be outgoing
- Be nonreligious
- Have higher-income and/or divorced parents
- Have a history of middle and high school hookups
- Have greater-than-typical alcohol use
- Be in a situation, such as spring break, that encourages hookups
- More frequently view pornography[27]

Individuals who have never hooked up prefer not being the center of attention, have no fear of intimacy, and do not take a "game-playing"

cyberbullying Deliberate, repeated, and hostile actions that use information and communication technologies, including online web pages and text messages, with the intent of harming others by means of intimidation, control, manipulation, false accusations, or humiliation.

cyberstalking A form of cyberbullying that uses online sites, Twitter, e-mail messages, and social media to harass victims and try to damage their reputation or turn others against them.

hookup Refers to a range of physically intimate behaviors—from kissing to intercourse—with no expectation of emotional intimacy or a romantic relationship.

approach to romance. Those who engage in "coital hookups" (involving oral, vaginal, or anal intercourse) tend to avoid attachment, be impulsive or rebellious, and have a "game-playing" relationship style and a lower concern for personal safety than those who stop short of sexual intercourse.[28]

In a study of 210 students at a two-year liberal arts college in the southeastern United States, the majority (60 percent) reported having had at least one hookup experience. Men and women were equally likely to hook up, while significantly more whites than African Americans or Asians and more sophomores than freshmen reported doing so. Virtually all the students (99 percent) said they were aware of the danger of STIs in a casual sex encounter; 9 in 10 also were aware of the risks of negative emotional and mental health consequences.[29]

....
√ **check-in** What is your opinion of hooking up?
....

Why Students Hook Up Students may engage in or endorse casual, commitment-free sexual encounters for various reasons, including a belief that hooking up is harmless because it requires no emotional commitment, that hooking up is fun, that hooking up will enhance their status in a peer group, that hooking up allows them to assert control over their sexuality, and that hooking up is a reflection of sexual freedom.

Five factors increase the likelihood of a hookup:

• Alcohol use

• Attractiveness of a potential hookup partner

• Past hookup experience

• An outgoing personality

• Membership in certain social networks/clubs

Social norms are another influence. Even students who say they've never engaged in any type of casual sex believe that almost everyone else is hooking up. Students who had hooked up in high school are likely to continue this behavior in college. Those who describe themselves as religious or who attend religious services report fewer hookups and less likelihood of intercourse during a hookup.

Consequences of Hooking Up Although hookups imply no conditions and no expectations, they can and do have unanticipated consequences, including unwanted pregnancy, sexually transmitted infections, sexual violence, embarrassment, regret, and loss of self-respect.[30]

Some earlier studies suggested that hookups were more likely to lead to psychological distress for women, who expressed greater guilt and regret and less enjoyment of sex, than for men. However, a more recent, much larger analysis of almost 4,000 students ages 18 to 25 at 30 campuses came up with more complex results.[31] As discussed in Chapter 9, emotional and psychological responses to a hookup vary, depending on the nature and duration of the hookup as well individual characteristics.[32]

In a recent study of 483 first-year college women, half reported engaging in oral or vaginal hookup sex (compared with 62 percent who had sex with romantic partners). Hooking up was significantly correlated with depression, for several reasons that the researchers identified:

• Unfavorable attitudes toward sex outside a committed relationship

• Risk of acquiring a bad reputation

• Failure for the hookup to lead to a romantic relationship

• Unsatisfying sex

• Pressure to go further sexually than desired

Approximately one-quarter of the women reported at least one instance of sexual violence, including physical force, threats of harm, or incapacitation with drugs or alcohol. Hookups also increased the incidence of STIs.[33]

Asked to identify positive aspects of hooking up, students selected "it is fun to be spontaneous," "a hookup might turn into a relationship," and "you don't have to deal with the hassle of maintaining a relationship." Yet the majority expressed interest in finding a romantic relationship.

Two-thirds of those who had ever had a hookup experienced regrets, including these:

• Drinking too much and losing control

• Choosing a partner who did not meet their usual standards

• Disappointment because a hookup failed to lead to an ongoing relationship

• For men, embarrassment over their sexual performance, particularly premature ejaculation

• For women, disappointment over a lack of orgasm

• Guilt about cheating on a partner or hooking up with someone who was in a relationship

• Hurting or losing a friendship

The motivations for a hookup may affect a participant's emotional and psychological responses. In a sample of 528 undergraduates followed for an academic year, men and women who hooked up for "autonomous," or deliberate, independently motivated reasons (such as sexual desire, pleasure, physical attraction, experimenting, exploring, novelty, excitement) did not experience depression, anxiety, lower self-esteem, or other negative impacts on their well-being. However, men and women who hooked up for "nonautonomous" reasons (low self-esteem, peer pressure, need for self-affirmation, social status, material rewards, intoxication with alcohol or drugs) were more likely to experience depression, anxiety, lower self-esteem, and lower overall well-being.[34]

Friends with Benefits

Like hookups, relationships between "friends with benefits" include varied sexual behaviors but occur between two individuals who have a friendship extending beyond a one-time sexual encounter. About 45 to 50 percent of college students report having engaged in a friends-with-benefits relationship in the preceding 12 months. A significant number also were involved in other sexual relationships, often with other friends.

The more committed that two partners felt to both the friendship and the sexual aspects of the relationship, the less likely they were to use condoms. Men were more likely to desire no change in such a relationship, while women preferred either to go back to being "just friends" or to move into a committed romantic relationship.

✓**check-in** Do you think sexual "benefits" affect a friendship?

Loving and Being Loved

You may not think of love as a basic need like food and rest, but it is essential for both physical and psychological well-being. Mounting evidence suggests that people who lack love and commitment are at high risk for a host of illnesses, including infections, heart disease, and cancer.

Intimate Relationships

The term **intimacy**—the open, trusting sharing of close, confidential thoughts and feelings—comes from the Latin word for *within*. Intimacy doesn't happen at first sight, or in a day or a week or a number of weeks. Intimacy requires time and nurturing; it is a process of revealing

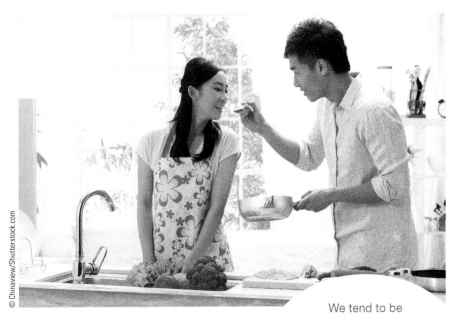

© Chinaview/Shutterstock.com

rather than hiding, of wanting to know another and to be known by that other. Although intimacy doesn't require sex, an intimate relationship often includes a sexual relationship, heterosexual or homosexual.

In an intimate relationship, empathy becomes even more important. You can develop your capacity for empathy by pulling back periodically, particularly in moments of stress or conflict, and asking yourself: "What is my partner or spouse feeling right now? What does he or she need?"

✓**check-in** Are you in a committed intimate relationship?

Committed intimate relationships may be beneficial for college students' physical and mental health, just as marriage is for spouses. In a study of more than 1,600 undergraduates between ages 18 and 25, those in committed relationships experienced fewer mental health problems, were less likely to be overweight/obese, and engaged in fewer risky behaviors (such as binge drinking).

The reasons may be that these students have less time for risky behavior, that being in a relationship fosters a less impulsive lifestyle, or that partners who use drugs or drink heavily may be unable to keep a romantic partner. Simply having fewer sexual partners lowers general stress as well as the risk of sexual infections or assaults. The study found no difference in physical health between those in and not in intimate relationships, possibly because most students are young and healthy to begin with.

In another survey of undergraduates between ages 18 and 23, in the long term men received greater emotional benefits than women from the

> We tend to be attracted to people who are similar to ourselves in age, race, ethnicity, socioeconomic class, and education.

intimacy A state of closeness between two people, characterized by the desire and ability to share one's innermost thoughts and feelings with each other either verbally or nonverbally.

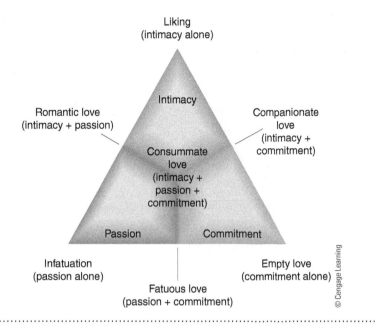

FIGURE 5.1 Sternberg's Love Triangle

The three components of love are intimacy, passion, and commitment. The various kinds of love are composed of different combinations of the three components.

positive aspects of romance and were more likely than women to be emotionally harmed by the stress of a rocky patch.

What Attracts Two People to Each Other?

Scientists have tried to analyze the combination of factors that attracts two people to each other. In several studies of college students, four predictors ranked as the most important reasons for attraction:

- Warmth and kindness
- Desirable personality
- Something specific about the person
- Reciprocal liking

Economic factors, including money or lack thereof, didn't make the list. In a recent study, physical attractiveness had similar modest to strong effects on both sexes, while earning prospects mattered little to men and women.[35]

Infatuation

It is tempting to think of love as scenes from a movie script: blazing sunsets and misty nights, fiery glances and passionate embraces, consuming desire and happy-ever-after endings. However, movies last only two hours; ideally, love lasts a lifetime. Infatuation falls somewhere in between.

Certainly, falling in love is an intense, dizzying experience. A person not only enters our life but also takes possession. We are intrigued, flattered, captivated, delighted—but is this love or a love of loving?

At the time you're experiencing it, there is no difference between infatuation and lasting love. You feel the same giddy, wonderful way. However, if it's infatuation, it won't last. Infatuation refers only to falling in love. People genuinely in love with each other do more than fall: They start building a relationship together.

Being head over heels in love can have such an impact on the brain that it reduces pain. Stanford University researchers studied 15 undergraduates in the infatuation stage of love and inflicted pain with a handheld thermal probe. Those looking at a photograph of their beloved not only reported less pain but showed the same brain changes as those induced by drugs like cocaine.

Infatuation also can be a disguise for something quite different: a strong sex drive, a fear of loneliness, loneliness itself, or a hunger for approval. Sometimes lovers in love with love may become infatuated with someone who doesn't even exist: the projection of their unmet needs for unconditional love.

The Science of Romantic Love

We like to think of this powerful force, a source of both danger and delight, as something that defies analysis. However, scientists have provided new perspectives on its true nature.

A Psychological View According to psychologist Robert Sternberg, love can be viewed as a triangle with three faces: passion, intimacy, and commitment (Figure 5.1). Each person brings his or her own triangle to a relationship. If they match well, their relationship is likely to be satisfying.

Sternberg also identified six types of love:

- **Liking:** The intimacy friends share
- **Infatuation:** The passion that stems from physical and emotional attraction
- **Romantic love:** A combination of intimacy and passion
- **Companionate love:** A deep emotional bond in a relationship that may have had romantic components
- **Fatuous love:** A combination of passion and commitment in two people who lack a deep emotional intimacy
- **Consummate love:** A combination of passion, intimacy, and commitment over time

An Anthropological View When you first fall in love, you may be sure that no one else has ever known the same dizzying, wonderful feelings. Yet, while every romance may be unique, romantic love is anything but. Anthropologists have found evidence of romantic love between individuals in most of the cultures they have studied.

As anthropologist Helen Fisher, author of *Anatomy of Love: The Natural History of Monogamy, Adultery and Divorce*, explains, romantic love pulled men and women of prehistoric times into the sort of partnerships that were essential to child rearing. But after about four years—just "long enough to rear one child through infancy," says Fisher—romantic love seemed to wane, and primitive couples tended to break up and find new partners.

A Biochemical View The heart is the organ we associate with love, but the brain may be where the action really is. In a recent study of "speed-dating," mutual attraction activated key areas in the brain involved in making choices.[36]

According to research on neurotransmitters (the messenger chemicals within the brain), love sets off a chemical chain reaction that causes our skin to flush, our palms to sweat, and our lungs to breathe more deeply and rapidly.

Neuroimaging studies reveal that viewing images of a romantic partner activates the areas of the brain that produce the so-called "love chemicals"—dopamine, norepinephrine, and phenylethylamine (PEA)—involved in various rewarding experiences, including beauty and love.[37]

Infatuation may indeed be a natural high, but like other highs, this rush doesn't last—possibly because the body develops tolerance for love-induced chemicals, just as it does with amphetamines. However, as the initial lover's high fades, other brain chemicals may come into play: the endorphins, morphine-like chemicals that can help produce feelings of well-being, security, and tranquility. These feel-good molecules may increase in partners who develop a deep attachment.

....
√**check-in** Do these theories help you
understand love better?
....

Mature Love

Social scientists have distinguished between *passionate love* (characterized by intense feelings of elation, sexual desire, and ecstasy) and *companionate love* (characterized by friendly affection and deep attachment). Often relationships begin with passionate love and evolve into a more companionate love. Sometimes the opposite happens

and two people who know each other well discover that their friendship has "caught fire," and the sparks have flamed an unexpected passion.

Mature love is a complex combination of sexual excitement, tenderness, commitment, and—most of all—an overriding passion that sets it apart from all other love relationships in one's life. This passion isn't simply a matter of orgasm but also entails a crossing of the psychological boundaries between oneself and one's lover. You feel as if you're becoming one with your partner while simultaneously retaining a sense of yourself.

Dysfunctional Relationships

Mental health professionals define a **dysfunctional** relationship as one that doesn't promote healthy communication, honesty, and intimacy and here either person is made to feel worthless or incompetent. Feelings of insecurity and anxiety about a dysfunctional relationship may boost stress hormones and impair the immune system, according to recent research.[38] Individuals with addictive behaviors or dependence on drugs or alcohol (see Chapters 12 and 13), and the children or partners of such people, are especially likely to find themselves in a dysfunctional relationship.

Often partners have magical, unrealistic expectations (e.g., they expect that a relationship with the right person will make their life okay), and one person uses the other almost as if he or she were a mood-altering drug. The partners may compulsively try to get the other to act the way they want. Both persons may distrust or may deceive each other. Often they isolate themselves from others, thus trapping themselves in a recurring cycle of pain.

Physical symptoms, such as headaches, digestive troubles, tics, and inability to sleep well, can be signs of a destructive relationship. Yet, although one person may repeatedly attack, abandon, betray, badger, bully, criticize, deceive, dominate, or demean the other, the responsibility for changing the unhealthy dynamic belongs to both.

Intimate Partner Violence

Dysfunction can lead to violence, discussed in Chapter 18. Nearly half of all couples experience some form of physical aggression. Couples who are cohabiting (see page 123) experience more aggression than married partners and those who are dating but living separately. In teenage couples, dating violence has been linked with higher

dysfunctional Characterized by negative and destructive patterns of behavior between partners or between parents and children.

TABLE 5.1 Abusive Relationships on Campus

Within the past 12 months, college students reported experiencing:

	Men	Women	Average
An emotionally abusive intimate relationship	6.3	10.5	9.1
A physically abusive intimate relationship	1.7	2	2
A sexually abusive intimate relationship	1	2.1	1.7

Source: American College Health Association. *American College Health Association–National College Health Assessment II: Reference Group Executive Summary, Spring 2014.* Hanover, MD: American College Health Association, 2014

levels of jealousy, verbal conflict, and cheating and can lead to depression in young adults.[39] In the most recent ACHA survey, about 2 percent of students had been in a physically abusive relationship in the preceding 12 months; 9.1 percent reported being in an emotionally abusive intimate relationship.[40] (See Table 5.1.)

Women attending urban commuter colleges may be at particular risk if they have partners who seek to control or limit their college experience or who feel threatened by what they may achieve by attending college.[41]

Minority stress (discussed in Chapter 4) may contribute to violence among lesbian, gay, bisexual, and transgender (LGBT) partners, who are much less likely than other couples to disclose what happened. In one recent study, only about a third (compared to roughly three-quarters of heterosexuals) revealed a violent episode to any person, most often a friend. The reasons for nondisclosure include a feeling that it was "not a big

deal," a desire for privacy, and concern about others' reactions.[42]

✓**check-in** What do victims of intimate partner violence say are the most helpful responses of friends they confide in?

Empathic support; listening and talking; practical support. The least helpful: giving advice.[43]

Emotional Abuse

Abuse consists of any behavior that uses fear, humiliation, or verbal or physical assaults to control and subjugate another human being. Rather than being physical, emotional abuse takes many forms:

• Berating

• Belittling or demeaning

• Constant criticism

• Name calling

• Blaming

• Threatening

• Accusing

• Judging

• Trivializing, minimizing, or denying what a person says or feels

Even if done for the sake of "teaching" or "helping," emotional abuse wears away at self-confidence, sense of self-worth, and trust and belief in oneself. Because it is more than skin deep, emotional abuse can leave deeper, longer-lasting scars.

HEALTH ON A BUDGET

Money Can't Buy Love

The things that matter most in a healthy relationship don't come with a price tag. Here are some guidelines for what you should invest in to have a healthy, happy relationship:

• **Recognize that both people in the relationship have the right to be accepted as they are,** to be treated with respect, to feel safe, to ask for what they want, to say no without feeling guilty, to express themselves, to give and receive affection, and to make some mistakes and be forgiven.

• **Remember that no one in a relationship has the right to force the other to do anything,** to tell the other where or when to speak up or go out, to humiliate the other in public or private, to isolate the other from friends and family, to read personal material without permission, to pressure the other to give up goals or interests, or to abuse the other person verbally or physically.

• **Be willing to open up.** The more you share, the deeper the bond between you and your friend will become.

• **Be sensitive to your friend's or partner's feelings.** Keep in mind that, like you, he or she has unique needs, desires, and dreams.

• **Express appreciation.** Be generous with your compliments. Let your friends and family know you recognize their kindnesses.

• **Know that people will disappoint you from time to time.** We are only human. Accept your loved ones as they are. Admitting their faults need not reduce your respect for them.

• **Talk about your relationship.** If you have any gripes or frustrations, air them.

No one wants to get into an abusive relationship, but often people who were emotionally abused in childhood find themselves in similar circumstances as adults. Dealing with an emotional abuser, regardless of how painful, may feel familiar or even comfortable. Individuals who think very little of themselves also may pick partners who treat them as badly as they believe they deserve.

Abusers also may have grown up with emotional abuse and view it as a way of coping with feelings of fear, hurt, powerlessness, or anger. They may seek partners who see themselves as helpless and who make them feel more powerful.

Among the signs of emotional abuse are

- **Attempting to control various aspects of your life,** such as what you say or wear
- **Frequently humiliating you** or making you feel bad about yourself
- **Making you feel as if you are to blame** for what your partner does
- **Wanting to know where you are** and whom you're with at all times
- **Becoming jealous or angry** when you spend time with friends
- **Threatening to harm you** if you break up
- **Trying to coerce you** into unwanted sexual activity with statements such as "If you loved me, you would . . ."

If you can never get what you need or if you're afraid, you need to get out of the relationship. Take whatever steps necessary to ensure your safety. Find a trusted friend who can help. Don't isolate yourself from family and friends. This is a time when you need their support and often the support of a counselor, minister, or doctor as well. (See "Your Strategies for Change: How to Cope with an Unhealthy Relationship.")

Codependency

The definition of **codependency** has expanded to include any maladaptive behaviors learned by family members in order to survive great emotional pain and stress, such as an addiction, chronic mental or physical illness, and abuse. Some therapists refer to codependency as a "relationship addiction" because codependent people often form or maintain relationships that are one-sided, emotionally destructive, or abusive. First identified in studies of the relationships in families of alcoholics, codependent behavior can occur in any dysfunctional family.

YOUR STRATEGIES FOR CHANGE
How to Cope with an Unhealthy Relationship

- **Start a dialogue.** Focus on communication, not confrontation. Start with a positive statement, for instance, saying what you really value in the relationship. Volunteer what you might do to make it better and state what you need from the other person.

- **Distance yourself.** Take a vacation from a toxic friendship. Skip the family reunion or Thanksgiving dinner. When forced into proximity, be polite. If you refuse to engage—not arguing, not getting angry, not trying to make things better—toxic people give up trying to get under your skin.

- **Consult a professional.** A therapist or minister can help people recognize and change toxic behavior patterns. Changes you make in how you act and react may trigger changes in others.

- **Save yourself.** If you can never get what you need in a relationship, you may need to let it go. Nothing is worth compromising your mental or physical health.

Signs of Codependency   Among the characteristics of codependency are

- An exaggerated sense of responsibility for the actions of others
- An attraction to people who need rescuing
- Always trying to do more than one's share
- Doing anything to cling to a relationship and avoid feeling abandoned
- An extreme need for approval and recognition
- A sense of guilt about asserting needs and desires
- A compelling need to control others
- Lack of trust in self and/or others
- Fear of being alone
- Difficulty identifying feelings
- Rigidity/difficulty adjusting to change
- Chronic anger
- Lying/dishonesty
- Poor communications
- Difficulty making decisions

Because the roots of codependency run so deep, people don't just "outgrow" this problem or magically find themselves in a healthy relationship. Treatment to resolve childhood hurts and deal with emotional issues may take the form of individual or group therapy, education, or programs such as Co-Dependents Anonymous (www.coda.org). The goal is to help individuals get in touch with long-buried feelings and build healthier family and relationship dynamics.

codependency An emotional and psychological behavioral pattern in which the spouses, partners, parents, children, and friends of individuals with addictive behaviors allow or enable their loved ones to continue their self-destructive habits.

Assessing a Relationship

If you're currently involved with someone, read through the following list of positive indicators of a healthy relationship and check all that apply.

___ You feel at ease with your partner.

___ You feel good about your partner when you're together and when you're not.

___ Your partner is open with you about his or her life—past, present, and future.

___ You can say no to each other without feeling guilty.

___ You feel cared for, appreciated, and accepted as you are.

___ Your partner really listens to what you have to say.

The more items you've checked, the more reasons you have to keep seeing each other. Read through the list of negative indicators below and check those that apply. In this case, every check is a red flag warning of dangers ahead.

___ You don't feel comfortable together.

___ You feel angry or let down when you're together or apart.

___ Your partner is very secretive about his or her life.

___ You feel your partner isn't attentive to you.

___ You don't feel cared for and appreciated.

Reflect on the pluses and minuses of your relationship in your online journal.

enabling Unwittingly contributing to a person's addictive or abusive behavior. Components of enabling include shielding or covering up for an abuser/addict, controlling him or her, taking over responsibilities, rationalizing addictive behavior, and cooperating with him or her.

Enabling Experts on the subject of addiction first identified traits of codependency in spouses of alcoholics, who followed a predictable pattern of behavior: While intensely trying to control the drinkers, the codependent mates would act in ways that allowed the drinkers to keep drinking. For example, if an alcoholic found it hard to get up in the morning, his wife would wake him up, pull him out of bed and into the shower, and drop him off at work. If he was late, she made excuses to his boss. The husband was the one with the substance-abuse problem, but without realizing it, his wife was **enabling** him to continue drinking. In fact, he might not have been able to keep up his habit without her unintentional cooperation.

Codependency progresses just as an addiction does, and codependents excuse their own behavior with many of the same defense mechanisms used by addicts, such as rationalization ("I cut class so I could catch up on my reading, not to keep an eye on my partner") and denial ("He likes to gamble, but he never loses more than he can afford"). In time, codependents lose sight of everything but their loved one. They feel that if they can only "fix" this person, everything will be fine.

When Love Ends

As the old song says, breaking up is indeed hard to do. Sometimes two people grow apart gradually, and both of them realize that they must go their separate ways. More often, one person falls out of love first. It hurts to be rejected; it also hurts to inflict pain on someone who once meant a great deal to you.

In surveys, college students say it's more difficult to initiate a breakup than to be rejected. Those who decide to end a relationship report greater feelings of guilt, uncertainty, discomfort, and awkwardness than their girlfriends or boyfriends. However, students with high levels of jealousy are likely to feel a desire for vengeance that can lead to aggressive behavior.

Research suggests that people do not end their relationships because of the disappearance of love. Rather, a sense of dissatisfaction or unhappiness develops, which may then cause love to stop growing. The fact that love does not dissipate completely may be why breakups are so painful.

While the pain does ease over time, it can help both parties if they end their relationship in a way that shows kindness and respect. Your basic guideline should be to think of how you would like to be treated if someone were breaking up with you:

- Would it hurt more to find out from someone else?

- Would it be more painful if the person you cared for lied to you or deceived you, rather than admitting the truth?

Saying "I don't feel the way I once did about you; I don't want to continue our relationship" is hard, but it's also honest and direct.

✓ **check-in** Have you ever broken up with someone? Has someone ever broken up with you?

Partnering across the Lifespan

Even though men and women today may have more sexual partners than in the past, most still yearn for an intense, supportive, exclusive relationship, based on mutual commitment and enduring over time. In our society, most such relationships take the form of heterosexual marriages, but partners of the same sex or heterosexual partners who never marry also may sustain long-lasting, deeply committed relationships.

These couples are much like married people: They make a home, handle daily chores, cope with problems, celebrate special occasions, plan for the future—all the while knowing that they are not alone, that they are part of a pair that adds up to far more than just the sum of two individual souls.

The New Transition to Adulthood

Growing up is not what it used to be. Social scientists have identified "emerging adulthood" as a unique developmental period that spans the late teens and the 20s, marked by volatility and identity formation. Traditionally the milestones of this life stage were completing school, leaving home, becoming financially independent, marrying, and having a child.

Today more than 95 percent of Americans consider the most important markers of adulthood to be completing school, establishing an independent household, and being employed full time. Only about half consider it necessary to marry or have children to be regarded as an adult. Unlike their parents and grandparents, young people view these markers as life choices rather than requirements.

✓ **check-in** Do you think of graduation, living on your own, or getting a full-time job as a marker of maturity or a life choice?

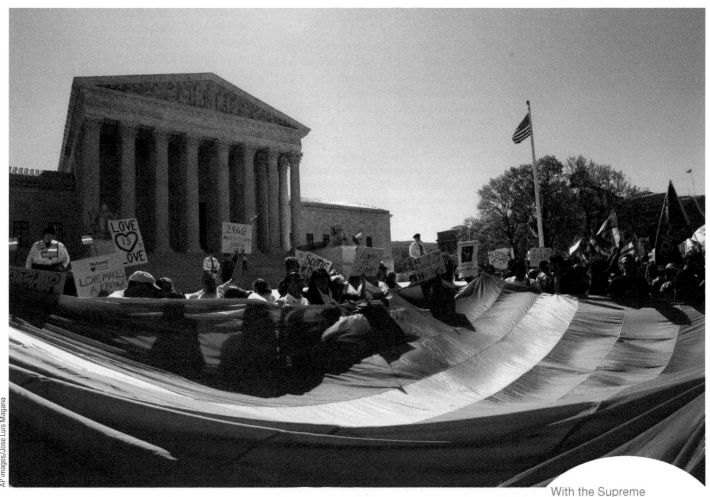

AP images/Jose Luis Magana

The changing time table for adulthood has affected the timing and nature of intimate relationships, or, as sociologists describe them, "partnerships." Although just as eager for intimacy—emotional and sexual—younger adults are following a different pattern than past generations. Among a smorgasbord of romantic options, they may do the following:

- Enter into casual, short-term relationships

- Commit to a long-term monogamous relationship

- Live with a partner with or without the intent of getting married

- View marriage as the final step in a relationship that may take place after sexual involvement, shared living, and even childbearing and parenting

Nearly half of young people live with their parents. This percentage drops below 1 in 7 by the late 20s and below 1 in 10 by the early 30s. Women are typically younger than men when they leave home because they complete college earlier, form cohabiting unions earlier, and marry about two years earlier.

In 1970, two-thirds of 20-somethings were married. Now just about one-quarter are. Emerging adults who want to get married in their 20s generally express greater religiosity and more conservative sexual attitudes, are less sexually active, and engage in fewer risky health behaviors (smoking, drinking, drug use, etc.).

Cohabitation

Although couples have always shared homes in informal relationships without any official ties, "living together," or **cohabitation**, has become more common. The majority of young adults have lived with a partner by their mid-20s, but they do not view it as a permanent alternative to marriage. Although cohabitation has been increasing steadily for decades, the number of couples living together has spiked in recent years.

One reason may be economic. Partners may not have enough money to live alone but don't plan to get married until they have more money—which is harder to get in a bad economy. Social acceptance may also contribute. A few generations ago, "shacking up" seemed shocking. Today fewer than half of Americans think living together is a bad idea.

With the Supreme Court's historic ruling on marriage equality, same-sex partners won the legal right to marry anywhere in the United States.

cohabitation Two people living together as a couple, without official ties such as marriage.

About one-quarter of unmarried women ages 25 to 39 are currently living with a partner; an additional one-quarter lived with a partner in the past. Couples live together before more than half of all marriages, a practice that was practically unknown 50 years ago. In addition, the proportion of cohabiting women between the ages of 20 and 50 has tripled in the past 50 years.

Cohabitation can be a prelude to marriage, an alternative to living alone, or an alternative to marriage. Couples choose to cohabit for different reasons. In one study, spending more time together and convenience were the most common motivations. Personal traits, such as physical attractiveness, personality, and grooming, matter less when choosing a partner to live with than they do when selecting a prospective spouse.[44] Couples who move in together to "test" their relationship report more problems—including more negative communication, physical aggression, and symptoms of depression and anxiety—than others.

The timing of a decision to move in together also matters. Couples who cohabited before getting engaged later reported less marital satisfaction, dedication, and confidence as well as more negative communication and greater potential for divorce than those who lived together after engagement or after getting married.

Asians and non-Hispanic white couples are the least likely to cohabit. A higher percentage of Native American, black, and Hispanic couples are unmarried. "Cohabiters" tend to have lower income and education levels. They also are younger—on average, some 12 years younger than married men and women.

Committed couples, both heterosexual and homosexual, can register as domestic partners in certain areas. This may enable them to qualify for benefits such as health insurance. Recent court rulings have placed domestic partners on the same legal footing as married couples in dealings with businesses.

Long-Term Relationships

Both heterosexual ("straight") and same-sex couples progress through various stages as their relationships develop:

- Blending, a time of intense passion and romantic love
- Nesting (starting a home together)
- Building trust and dependability
- Merging assets
- Establishing a strong sense of partnership

Gay and lesbian relationships are comparable to straight relationships in other ways. However, because there are no social norms for same-sex unions, researchers describe these relationships as more egalitarian. Each partner tends to be more self-reliant, and homosexual men and women tend to be more willing to communicate and experiment in terms of sexual behaviors. But many same-sex couples have to deal with everyday ups-and-downs in a social context of isolation from family, workplace prejudice, and other social barriers.

Compared to straight couples, gay and lesbian couples use more affection and humor when they bring up a disagreement and remain more positive after a disagreement. They also display less belligerence, domineering, and fear with each other than straight couples do. When they argue, they are better able to soothe each other, so they show fewer signs of physiological arousal, such as an elevated heart rate or sweaty palms, than heterosexual couples.

Regardless of sexual orientation, couples influence—or try to influence—a partner's health behaviors. In straight couples, women are most likely to play this role. In gay and lesbian couples, partners mutually influence one another's health choices and habits.

Marriage

A generation ago, nearly 70 percent of Americans were married; now only about half are. The proportion of married people, especially among younger age groups, has been declining for decades. Here are the most recent statistics on Americans' unions:

- The median age for first marriage, which has gone up about a year every decade since the 1960s, has risen to 28.2 years for men and 26.1 years for women.
- Men in every age bracket through age 34 are more likely to be single than are women.
- Black men and women are less likely to be married than whites, with Hispanics between the two.
- Most young adults view marriage positively, and 95 percent expect to marry in the future—except for young African Americans, who have significantly lower expectations of being wed than their white counterparts.

If you aren't already married, simply getting a college degree increases your odds of entering into matrimony in the future. College-educated women are most likely to be currently married, in part because they are more likely to stay married or remarry after divorce or widowhood. Less well-educated Americans are less likely to marry; in addition, if they do, their unions are more likely to end in divorce.

Preparing for Marriage

Most people say they marry for one far-from-simple reason: love. However, with more than half of all marriages ending in divorce, there's little doubt that modern marriages aren't made in heaven.

There are scientific ways of predicting marital happiness. Some premarital assessment inventories identify strengths and weaknesses in many aspects of a relationship: realistic expectations, personality issues, communication, conflict resolution, financial management, leisure activities, sex, children, family and friends, egalitarian roles, and religious orientation. Couples who become aware of potential conflicts by means of such inventories may be able to resolve them through professional counseling. In some cases, they may want to reconsider or postpone their wedding.

Other common predictors of marital discord, unhappiness, and separation are

- A high level of arousal during a discussion
- Defensive behaviors such as making excuses and denying responsibility for disagreements
- A wife's expressions of contempt
- A husband's stonewalling (showing no response when a wife expresses her concerns)

By looking for such behaviors, researchers have been able to predict with better than 90 percent accuracy whether a couple will separate within the first few years of marriage.

The Benefits of Marriage

Despite its problems, marriage endures because it is a fulfilling way for two people to live. As researchers have proved, saying "I do" can do wonders for health. Compared to those who are divorced, widowed, never-married, or living with a partner, married people

- Are healthier
- Live longer
- Have lower rates of coronary disease and cancer
- Are less likely to suffer back pain, headaches, and other common illnesses
- Recover faster and have a better chance of surviving a serious illness
- Have lower rates of most mental disorders than single or divorced individuals

For years researchers thought that marriage was especially beneficial to men. Married men have lower rates of alcohol and drug abuse, depression, and risk-taking behavior than divorced men. They also earn more money—possibly because they have more incentive to do so. However, more recent research indicates that a happy marriage boosts mental health and well-being in both spouses.

Among the theories of why marriage benefits health are

- **Selection:** People in better physical and psychological health may be more likely to get married in the first place and to remain married.
- **Social support:** Marriage may provide people with emotional satisfaction that buffers them against daily life stressors. In a recent study, people who felt that their spouses are always helpful in times of difficulty were less likely to show early signs of heart disease.[45]
- **Behavioral regulation:** Marriage partners may monitor each other's behaviors, discourage risky behaviors like smoking, and encourage healthier ones such as driving safely.

Marriage Equality

Same-sex marriage, also called gay or single-sex or gender-neutral marriage, refers to a governmentally, socially, or religiously recognized marriage in which two people of the same sex live together as a family.

In a landmark decision in June 2015, the U.S. Supreme Court ruled that the Constitution guarantees a right to marriage for all Americans, regardless of their sexual orientation or gender. Marriage is a "keystone of our social order," the majority of justices ruled, noting that all citizens are entitled to "equal dignity in the eyes of the law."

Same-sex marriage triggered intense controversy for decades. Some people opposed gay unions on religious and moral grounds, while others argued that marriage is a right based on procreation and designed to protect the children of a man and a woman. Advocates of single-sex marriage campaigned for years to win the same civil rights and legal protections as heterosexual couples.

Same-sex marriages have accounted for about 2 to 7 percent of all marriages contracted in a single year in the United States. The median age at marriage tends to be higher for persons in gay marriages, followed by those in lesbian marriages, and then in heterosexual marriages.

Same-sex couples live together and marry for similar reasons as heterosexual couples: At least a half million same-sex couples live together in the United States, and their numbers are expected to grow. More than nine in ten lesbians and eight in ten gay youth expect to have monogamous partners by age 30. Because access to legal marriage was long denied, marriage may take on special significance for gay couples, although their reasons for marrying are similar to those of

same-sex marriage Governmentally, socially, or religiously recognized marriage in which two people of the same sex live together as a family.

heterosexuals: to indicate long-term commitment, provide emotional support, establish a family, and share life together.[46] Just as for heterosexual couples, marriage brings not only economic and psychosocial benefits but also improved health.[47]

In terms of physical well-being, researchers found no difference between heterosexual and homosexual spouses. Being in a legally recognized relationship reduces nervousness, hopelessness, and depression in same-sex partners.[48]

Children adopted into lesbian and gay families appear to be as well adjusted as those adopted by heterosexual couples, according to recent research. Earlier studies have shown that children born to homosexual parents follow normal patterns of general development and are virtually indistinguishable from other youngsters.

Issues Couples Confront

No two people can live together in perfect harmony all the time. Some of the issues that crop up in any long-term relationship include expectations, money, sex, and careers.

Money Money may make the business world go around, but it has the opposite effect on relationships: It knocks them off their tracks, brings them to a halt, twists them upside down. However, even though almost all couples quarrel about money, they rarely fight over how much they have. What matters more—whether they make $10,000 or $100,000 a year—is what money means to both partners.

√**check-in** Have you ever had to deal with money issues in an intimate relationship?

To avoid fighting over money, understand that having different money values or expectations doesn't make one of you right and the other wrong:

- Recognize the value of unpaid work. A partner who's finishing school or taking care of the children is making an important contribution to the family and its future.

- Go over your finances together so that you have a firm basis in reality for what you can and can't afford.

- Talk about the financial goals you hope to attain five years from now.

- Set aside money for each of you to spend without asking or answering to the other. Even a small amount can make each partner feel more independent.

Sex Like every other aspect of a relationship, sex evolves and changes over the course of marriage. The red-hot sexual chemistry of the early stages of intimacy invariably cools down. Even

so, the happiest couples have sex more often than unhappily married pairs do.

What matters most isn't quantity alone, but the quality of sexual activity and intimacy. Here are some common questions that arise in a marriage:

- Are both partners satisfied with their sexual relationship?

- Does one partner always initiate sex?

- Do the partners talk about their preferences and pleasures?

- Do the partners acknowledge and adapt to the changes in sexuality that time brings?

- Do they feel sufficiently at ease with each other to discuss anxieties about sex?

The answers to these questions can determine how sexually gratifying a marriage is for both spouses.

Extramarital Affairs How faithful are American mates? The answer depends on the questions researchers ask and who they ask. In face-to-face interviews, University of Chicago researchers found that 25 percent of men and 15 percent of women had had affairs and that 94 percent of the married subjects had been monogamous in the past year. Another survey of Americans found that one out of six Americans had had an extramarital relationship.

High or low, numbers are little comfort when affairs do occur. A husband or wife who learns about a spouse's affair typically feels a devastating sense of betrayal as well as deep feelings of shame, fear of abandonment, depression, and anger. Two crucial questions determine whether a marriage can survive: Do the spouses still feel a serious commitment to each other? Do they love each other and want to remain together?

Two-Career Couples More than 75 percent of women with children work—a dramatic increase from the 1960s, when only 30 percent of mothers worked outside the home. Two careers can bring pressure to a relationship: Both individuals may come home tired and irritable; both may have to spend a great deal of time on their jobs; both may have to travel or work on weekends. Two-career couples must be able to discuss their problems openly to resolve these pressures.

√**check-in** Couples pursuing individual careers sometimes face difficult choices. What if you or your partner is offered a promising job in another city? Would you quit your job, pack up, and move?

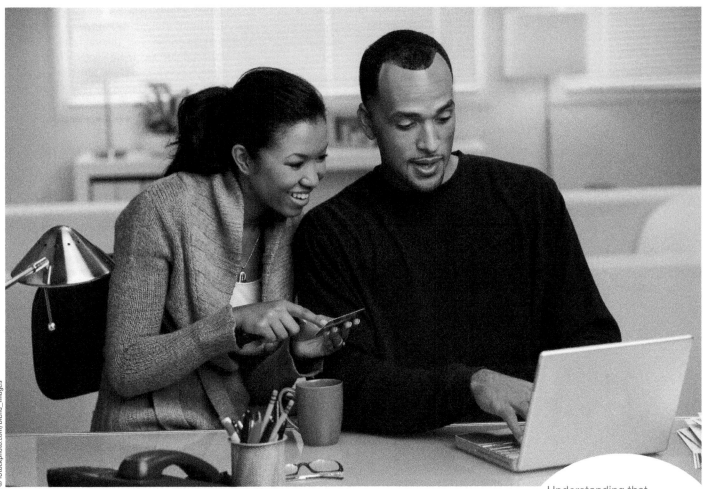
© iStockphoto.com/Blend_Images

Some couples resolve such dilemmas by working in different cities and spending weekends together. Others try to alternate career and home priorities. However imperfect these arrangements may be, they work for some couples.

Conflict in Marriage While all couples may wish to live happily and peacefully ever after, sooner or later, they disagree. In a five-year study of newly married couples, 36 percent sought some form of help for their relationship, most often from books on relationships and marital therapy.[49] Years of research have shown that while conflict is inevitable, the key difference between happy and unhappy couples is the way they handle disagreements.

Happier couples interject positive interactions, like a joke or a smile, into their arguments. As long as the ratio of positive to negative interactions remains at least five to one, the relationship remains intact. By comparison, unhappy couples unfurl a barrage of negative words, gestures, criticisms, and hostility at their mates, with hardly any positive interactions.

Saving Marriages Fewer than two-thirds of couples—64 percent of husbands and 60 percent of wives—say their marriages are very happy (down from 70 percent of men and 66 percent of women a generation ago).

According to recent research, happy marriages allow both partners to self-actualize (discussed in Chapter 2) and develop to their fullest potential. Some refer to this mutual benefit as "co-actualization." Others refer to the process of using a relationship to accumulate knowledge and experiences as "self-expansion." The more self-expansion that people experience from their partner, the more committed and satisfied they are in the relationship.

Among the other suggestions therapists offer couples are these:

- **Focus on friendship.** If a marriage is not built on a strong friendship, it may be difficult to stay connected over time.

- **Remember what you loved and admired in your partner in the first place.** Focusing on these qualities can foster a much more positive attitude toward him or her.

Understanding that your partner may have a different perspective on saving and spending money can help avoid arguments.

- **Show respect.** Your spouse deserves the same courtesy and civility that your colleagues do. Without respect, love cannot survive.

- **Compliment what your partner does right.** Noticing the positive can change how both of you feel about each other.

- **Forgive one another.** When your partner hurts your feelings but then reaches out, don't reject his or her attempts to make things better.

Each year, hundreds of thousands of couples go into counseling in an effort to make their unions happier. Marriage education consists of workshops that teach couples practical skills so they get along better. Some studies indicate that graduates of these programs have a lower divorce rate than unhappy couples who do not enroll in them.

Couples therapy, also called marriage counseling or marriage therapy, uses a variety of psychological techniques to help couples understand and overcome their conflicts. These include the following:

- **Behavioral marital therapy,** which teaches partners to communicate better and to improve their conflict resolution skills.

- **Emotionally focused therapy,** which helps couples identify and break free of destructive emotional cycles.

- **Insight-oriented marital therapy,** which combines behavioral therapy with techniques for understanding negative behaviors, such as power struggles, within the relationship.

Divorce

According to the most recent estimates, 40 to 50 percent of first marriages end in divorce, affecting about 2.5 million adults a year.

The leveling of divorce among persons born since 1980, especially college-educated women, may reflect a delay in getting married, increasing selectivity when choosing partners, or a preference for cohabitation rather than marriage.[50]

In addition to age, other factors lower the risk of divorce, including

- Having some college education

- Earning an income higher than $50,000

- Marrying at age 25 or older

- Not having a baby during the first seven months after the wedding

- Coming from an intact family

- Having some religious affiliation

families Groups of people united by marriage, blood, or adoption—each residing in the same household; maintaining a common culture; and interacting with one another on the basis of their roles within the group.

Children whose parents divorced are less likely to marry and to stay married. Race also influences marriage and divorce rates. African American couples are more likely to break up than white couples, and black divorcées are less likely to marry again. Researchers have found that African Americans place an equally high value on marriage. However, there is a smaller "marriageable pool" of black men for a variety of reasons, including a higher mortality rate. An analysis of marital stability in interracial marriages found higher divorce rates for Latino/white intermarriages but not for black/white intermarriages.

Many marriages dissolve simply because one partner's commitment to maintaining the relationship declines. Even couples who are initially very happy can go on to divorce if they begin to engage in more negative communication and emotion and provide less mutual support.

Divorce can have long-term consequences for mental and physical health, including these:

- Long-term decreases in life satisfaction

- Heightened risk for a range of illnesses

- Poor prognosis for those already ill

- Increased risk of early death[52]

- Higher chance of heart attack[53]

✓**check-in** How would you assess your "risk" of divorce?

Family Ties

A century ago, most households contained children under age 18. In 1960, slightly fewer than half did. Only about one-third of households now include children. Attitudes also have changed. While many traditionally viewed having children as the primary purpose for getting married, nearly 70 percent of Americans now cite another reason.

In 1960 the average woman had 3.5 children (statistically speaking) over the course of her life. Today's woman has an average of about 2 children, which is lower than the "replacement level" of 2.1 children per woman—that is, the level at which the population would be replaced by births alone. In most European and several Asian countries, fertility has dropped even lower.

✓**check-in** Do you have children? Do you want to have children someday?

Diversity within Families

Families have become as diverse as the American population and reflect different traditions, beliefs, and values:

- Within African American families, for instance, traditional gender roles are often reversed, with women serving as head of the household, a kinship bond uniting several households, and a strong religious commitment or orientation.

- In Chinese American families, both spouses may work and see themselves as bread-winners, but the wife may not have an equal role in decision making.

- In Hispanic families, wives and mothers are acknowledged and respected as healers and dispensers of wisdom. At the same time, they are expected to defer to their husbands, who see themselves as the strong, protective, dominant head of the family.

As time passes and families from different cultures become more integrated into American life, traditional gender roles and decision-making patterns often change, particularly among the youngest family members.

American families are diverse in other ways. *Multigenerational families*, with children, parents, and grandparents, make up 3.7 percent of households. They occur most often in areas where new immigrants live with relatives, where housing shortages or high costs force families to double up their living arrangements, or where high rates of out-of-wedlock childbearing force unwed mothers to live with their children in their parents' home.

Three of every 10 households consist of **blended families**, formed when one or both of the partners bring children from a previous union. In the future, social scientists predict, American families will become even more diverse, or pluralistic. But as norms or expectations about the configurations of families have changed, values or ideas about the intents and purposes of families have not. American families of every type still support each other and strive toward values such as commitment and caring.

The traditional family with a breadwinner and a homemaker has been replaced by what some call "the juggler family." Two working parents or an unmarried working parent head 70 percent of American families with children. As a result, American parents have fewer hours to spend with their children. Women, balancing multiple roles as parents, spouses, caregivers, and employees, often give their own personal needs the lowest priority.

√**check-in** How would you describe the family you grew up in?

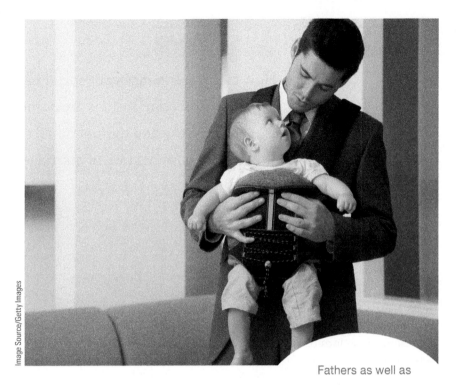

Image Source/Getty Images

Fathers as well as mothers often find themselves juggling the needs of their children and the demands of their jobs.

Unmarried Parents

The proportion of babies born to unmarried parents has grown from about 4 percent in 1940 to about 40 percent today. About 7 in 10 African American babies and half of Hispanic babies are born out of wedlock. African American mothers have the lowest rates of marriage and cohabitation and the highest breakup rates. Mexican immigrant mothers have the highest rates of marriage and cohabitation and the lowest breakup rates.

Many unmarried parents are in a romantic relationship when their baby is born, with about half cohabiting and the others living apart. The majority are not able to establish stable unions. One-third of fathers virtually disappear from their children's lives within five years.

An increasing number of college students have children. Here are recent statistics:

- The percentage of undergraduates who are unmarried parents has nearly doubled over the past 20 years, from 7 percent to just over 13 percent.

- Overall, 8 percent of male undergraduates and 17 percent of female undergraduates are unmarried parents.

- More than one-third of African American college women and 15 percent of African American college men are unmarried parents, as are 20 percent of Native American undergraduates, 16 percent of all Latino undergraduates, and 10 percent of whites.

blended families Families formed when one or both of the partners bring children from a previous union to the new marriage.

- How can you enhance your social health?
- What types of relationships are common on college campuses?
- How are healthy and dysfunctional relationships different?
- What is the current state of marriage in America?

THE POWER OF NOW!
Creating Better Relationships

We are born social. From our first days of life, we reach out to others, struggle to express ourselves, strive to forge connections. The fabric of our lives becomes richer as family and friends weave through it the threads of their experiences. No solitary pleasure can match the gifts that we gain by reaching out and connecting with others.

As with other significant endeavors, good relationships require work—through hard times, despite conflicts, over months and years and decades. As you strive to improve the ties that bind you to others, keep in mind the characteristics of a good relationship. Check the ones that are most important to you.

____ Trust. Partners are able to confide in each other openly, knowing their confidences will be respected.

____ Togetherness. In a healthy relationship, two people create a sense of both intimacy and autonomy. They enjoy each other's company but also pursue solitary interests.

____ Expressiveness. Partners in healthy relationships say what they feel, need, and desire.

____ Staying power. People in committed relationships keep their bond strong through tough times by proving that they will be there for each other.

____ Security. Because a good relationship is strong enough to absorb conflict and anger, partners know they can express their feelings honestly. They also are willing to risk vulnerability for the sake of becoming closer.

____ Laughter. Humor keeps things in perspective—always crucial in any sort of ongoing relationship or enterprise.

____ Support. Partners in good relationships continually offer each other encouragement, comfort, and acceptance.

____ Physical affection. Sexual desire may fluctuate or diminish over the years, but partners in loving, long-term relationships usually retain some physical connection.

____ Personal growth. In the best relationships, partners are committed to bringing out the best in each other and have the other's best interests at heart.

____ Respect. Caring partners are aware of each other's boundaries, need for personal space, and vulnerabilities. They do not take each other or their relationship for granted.

What's Online

CENGAGE brain .com Visit www.cengagebrain.com to access course materials for this text, including the Behavior Change Planner, interactive quizzes, and more.

Diversity within Families

Families have become as diverse as the American population and reflect different traditions, beliefs, and values:

- Within African American families, for instance, traditional gender roles are often reversed, with women serving as head of the household, a kinship bond uniting several households, and a strong religious commitment or orientation.

- In Chinese American families, both spouses may work and see themselves as breadwinners, but the wife may not have an equal role in decision making.

- In Hispanic families, wives and mothers are acknowledged and respected as healers and dispensers of wisdom. At the same time, they are expected to defer to their husbands, who see themselves as the strong, protective, dominant head of the family.

As time passes and families from different cultures become more integrated into American life, traditional gender roles and decision-making patterns often change, particularly among the youngest family members.

American families are diverse in other ways. *Multigenerational families*, with children, parents, and grandparents, make up 3.7 percent of households. They occur most often in areas where new immigrants live with relatives, where housing shortages or high costs force families to double up their living arrangements, or where high rates of out-of-wedlock childbearing force unwed mothers to live with their children in their parents' home.

Three of every 10 households consist of **blended families**, formed when one or both of the partners bring children from a previous union. In the future, social scientists predict, American families will become even more diverse, or pluralistic. But as norms or expectations about the configurations of families have changed, values or ideas about the intents and purposes of families have not. American families of every type still support each other and strive toward values such as commitment and caring.

The traditional family with a breadwinner and a homemaker has been replaced by what some call "the juggler family." Two working parents or an unmarried working parent head 70 percent of American families with children. As a result, American parents have fewer hours to spend with their children. Women, balancing multiple roles as parents, spouses, caregivers, and employees, often give their own personal needs the lowest priority.

√**check-in** How would you describe the family you grew up in?

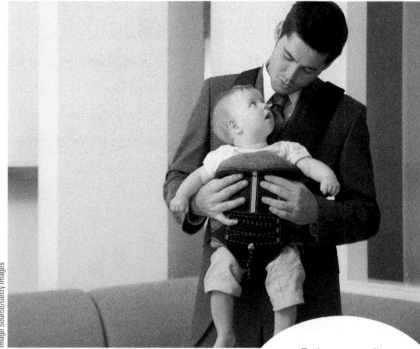

Image Source/Getty Images

Fathers as well as mothers often find themselves juggling the needs of their children and the demands of their jobs.

Unmarried Parents

The proportion of babies born to unmarried parents has grown from about 4 percent in 1940 to about 40 percent today. About 7 in 10 African American babies and half of Hispanic babies are born out of wedlock. African American mothers have the lowest rates of marriage and cohabitation and the highest breakup rates. Mexican immigrant mothers have the highest rates of marriage and cohabitation and the lowest breakup rates.

Many unmarried parents are in a romantic relationship when their baby is born, with about half cohabiting and the others living apart. The majority are not able to establish stable unions. One-third of fathers virtually disappear from their children's lives within five years.

An increasing number of college students have children. Here are recent statistics:

- The percentage of undergraduates who are unmarried parents has nearly doubled over the past 20 years, from 7 percent to just over 13 percent.

- Overall, 8 percent of male undergraduates and 17 percent of female undergraduates are unmarried parents.

- More than one-third of African American college women and 15 percent of African American college men are unmarried parents, as are 20 percent of Native American undergraduates, 16 percent of all Latino undergraduates, and 10 percent of whites.

blended families Families formed when one or both of the partners bring children from a previous union to the new marriage.

Family Ties   **129**

- How can you enhance your social health?
- What types of relationships are common on college campuses?
- How are healthy and dysfunctional relationships different?
- What is the current state of marriage in America?

THE POWER OF NOW!
Creating Better Relationships

We are born social. From our first days of life, we reach out to others, struggle to express ourselves, strive to forge connections. The fabric of our lives becomes richer as family and friends weave through it the threads of their experiences. No solitary pleasure can match the gifts that we gain by reaching out and connecting with others.

As with other significant endeavors, good relationships require work—through hard times, despite conflicts, over months and years and decades. As you strive to improve the ties that bind you to others, keep in mind the characteristics of a good relationship. Check the ones that are most important to you.

____ Trust. Partners are able to confide in each other openly, knowing their confidences will be respected.

____ Togetherness. In a healthy relationship, two people create a sense of both intimacy and autonomy. They enjoy each other's company but also pursue solitary interests.

____ Expressiveness. Partners in healthy relationships say what they feel, need, and desire.

____ Staying power. People in committed relationships keep their bond strong through tough times by proving that they will be there for each other.

____ Security. Because a good relationship is strong enough to absorb conflict and anger, partners know they can express their feelings honestly. They also are willing to risk vulnerability for the sake of becoming closer.

____ Laughter. Humor keeps things in perspective—always crucial in any sort of ongoing relationship or enterprise.

____ Support. Partners in good relationships continually offer each other encouragement, comfort, and acceptance.

____ Physical affection. Sexual desire may fluctuate or diminish over the years, but partners in loving, long-term relationships usually retain some physical connection.

____ Personal growth. In the best relationships, partners are committed to bringing out the best in each other and have the other's best interests at heart.

____ Respect. Caring partners are aware of each other's boundaries, need for personal space, and vulnerabilities. They do not take each other or their relationship for granted.

What's Online

CENGAGE brain .com   Visit www.cengagebrain.com to access course materials for this text, including the Behavior Change Planner, interactive quizzes, and more.

Diversity within Families

Families have become as diverse as the American population and reflect different traditions, beliefs, and values:

- Within African American families, for instance, traditional gender roles are often reversed, with women serving as head of the household, a kinship bond uniting several households, and a strong religious commitment or orientation.

- In Chinese American families, both spouses may work and see themselves as bread-winners, but the wife may not have an equal role in decision making.

- In Hispanic families, wives and mothers are acknowledged and respected as healers and dispensers of wisdom. At the same time, they are expected to defer to their husbands, who see themselves as the strong, protective, dominant head of the family.

As time passes and families from different cultures become more integrated into American life, traditional gender roles and decision-making patterns often change, particularly among the youngest family members.

American families are diverse in other ways. *Multigenerational families*, with children, parents, and grandparents, make up 3.7 percent of households. They occur most often in areas where new immigrants live with relatives, where housing shortages or high costs force families to double up their living arrangements, or where high rates of out-of-wedlock childbearing force unwed mothers to live with their children in their parents' home.

Three of every 10 households consist of **blended families**, formed when one or both of the partners bring children from a previous union. In the future, social scientists predict, American families will become even more diverse, or pluralistic. But as norms or expectations about the configurations of families have changed, values or ideas about the intents and purposes of families have not. American families of every type still support each other and strive toward values such as commitment and caring.

The traditional family with a breadwinner and a homemaker has been replaced by what some call "the juggler family." Two working parents or an unmarried working parent head 70 percent of American families with children. As a result, American parents have fewer hours to spend with their children. Women, balancing multiple roles as parents, spouses, caregivers, and employees, often give their own personal needs the lowest priority.

....
✓**check-in** How would you describe the family you grew up in?
....

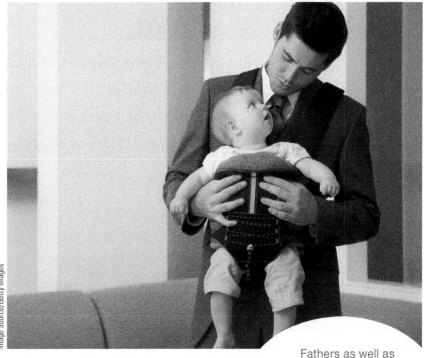

Fathers as well as mothers often find themselves juggling the needs of their children and the demands of their jobs.

Unmarried Parents

The proportion of babies born to unmarried parents has grown from about 4 percent in 1940 to about 40 percent today. About 7 in 10 African American babies and half of Hispanic babies are born out of wedlock. African American mothers have the lowest rates of marriage and cohabitation and the highest breakup rates. Mexican immigrant mothers have the highest rates of marriage and cohabitation and the lowest breakup rates.

Many unmarried parents are in a romantic relationship when their baby is born, with about half cohabiting and the others living apart. The majority are not able to establish stable unions. One-third of fathers virtually disappear from their children's lives within five years.

An increasing number of college students have children. Here are recent statistics:

- The percentage of undergraduates who are unmarried parents has nearly doubled over the past 20 years, from 7 percent to just over 13 percent.

- Overall, 8 percent of male undergraduates and 17 percent of female undergraduates are unmarried parents.

- More than one-third of African American college women and 15 percent of African American college men are unmarried parents, as are 20 percent of Native American undergraduates, 16 percent of all Latino undergraduates, and 10 percent of whites.

blended families Families formed when one or both of the partners bring children from a previous union to the new marriage.

Family Ties   **129**

- How can you enhance your social health?
- What types of relationships are common on college campuses?
- How are healthy and dysfunctional relationships different?
- What is the current state of marriage in America?

THE POWER OF NOW!
Creating Better Relationships

We are born social. From our first days of life, we reach out to others, struggle to express ourselves, strive to forge connections. The fabric of our lives becomes richer as family and friends weave through it the threads of their experiences. No solitary pleasure can match the gifts that we gain by reaching out and connecting with others.

As with other significant endeavors, good relationships require work—through hard times, despite conflicts, over months and years and decades. As you strive to improve the ties that bind you to others, keep in mind the characteristics of a good relationship. Check the ones that are most important to you.

____ Trust. Partners are able to confide in each other openly, knowing their confidences will be respected.

____ Togetherness. In a healthy relationship, two people create a sense of both intimacy and autonomy. They enjoy each other's company but also pursue solitary interests.

____ Expressiveness. Partners in healthy relationships say what they feel, need, and desire.

____ Staying power. People in committed relationships keep their bond strong through tough times by proving that they will be there for each other.

____ Security. Because a good relationship is strong enough to absorb conflict and anger, partners know they can express their feelings honestly. They also are willing to risk vulnerability for the sake of becoming closer.

____ Laughter. Humor keeps things in perspective—always crucial in any sort of ongoing relationship or enterprise.

____ Support. Partners in good relationships continually offer each other encouragement, comfort, and acceptance.

____ Physical affection. Sexual desire may fluctuate or diminish over the years, but partners in loving, long-term relationships usually retain some physical connection.

____ Personal growth. In the best relationships, partners are committed to bringing out the best in each other and have the other's best interests at heart.

____ Respect. Caring partners are aware of each other's boundaries, need for personal space, and vulnerabilities. They do not take each other or their relationship for granted.

What's Online

CENGAGE
brain.com

Visit www.cengagebrain.com to access course materials for this text, including the Behavior Change Planner, interactive quizzes, and more.

What's Your Intimacy Quotient?

Creating and maintaining close relationships require essential skills, including those listed below. Read through the following brief descriptions, and answer the questions at the end of each with a "yes" or "no."

Scoring:

Count up the number of "yes's" to calculate your score from "0" to "10." A higher score indicates that you have mastered some of the key skills for establishing significant relationships. But focus on the "no's" as well as the "yes's" so you can identify the skills that require greater attention. You might want to focus on a specific skill to strengthen during this term. However, it's important to keep working to deepen and enrich your relationships throughout life.

1. **Self-love.**

   Self-love means being at ease with your positive qualities and forgiving yourself for your faults and failings. Don't confuse this with narcissism, or excessive admiration of one's self. *Self-intimacy*, getting to know and feel comfortable with yourself, is the cornerstone of intimacy with others. If you do not understand and accept yourself, how can you expect to understand and accept others and how can you expect others to think that you will be any more interested in or accepting of them? When you know and like yourself, you can reach out to connect with others. And you can extend to them the same care and appreciation you extend to yourself.

   Do you spend time often keeping in touch with yourself by journaling or another structured activity? _____

2. **Receptivity.**

   If you are text messaging or checking e-mail while talking to your partner, friend, or child, you're not really tuning in to what they have to say. In fact, the message you're sending them is, "Don't bother me. I've got something better to do." You signal genuine receptivity by smiling, making eye contact, and turning away from other distractions. Be open and attentive to another's requests for attention.

   Do you spend some time every day simply sitting and reconnecting with your partner? Do you spend some time every day simply sitting and reconnecting with yourself? _____

3. **Listening.**

   The greatest gift you can give another person is your full attention. Ask questions. Look into your partner's eyes. Nod your head. Don't interrupt or judge. See things from your partner's perspective. (See the "Listen Up" lab for more suggestions.)

   Do you spend time every day listening to your partner? _____

   Do you spend time every day listening to yourself? _____

4. **Expressing yourself.**

   Relationships begin with signals: yes's, no's, and maybe's. It's your responsibility to make the signals and messages you send as clear as possible. Don't expect your partner to read your mind. Avoid the "if you loved me, you'd know" trap. Make sure your words and actions match your feelings. Pay attention to your body language. Use "I" statements, such as "I feel sad because I missed you." Avoid fuzzy expressions like "sort of," "kind of," and "maybe."

   Do you spend time every day communicating your thoughts, needs, and wishes to yourself and your partner?

   _____

5. **Support and acceptance.**

   When you love someone, support him or her. When you become truly intimate, the nature of the support becomes more complex and less conventional. Being willing to say difficult things without aggression, to tell the truth in the least accusatory and most tender way, is an art worth achieving. Only by being willing to reveal your own weaknesses do you create an island of safety where intimacy flourishes. Only by being willing to reveal the truth about yourself can you request the truth from your partner and achieve the utmost intimacy. Only by knowing and acknowledging the intentions behind each act you make can you create a safe place in which your and your partner's faults and foibles are acknowledged without attack or scolding. Do not seek perfection, in the sense of banishing every false step or idiosyncrasy, in your partner or in yourself.

   Do you consciously create this special support and acceptance every day? _____

6. **Affection.**

   Infinite possibilities exist for expressing affection. Some are obvious, like a handwritten note. The more subtle ones may go unnoticed but stem from serious contemplation of your partner's nature and needs. When you know and care for someone deeply, you sense when to approach and when to retreat, when to speak and when to be silent. You also communicate, in ways beyond mere words, that you are and always will be there for your partner.

   Love is a noun. Love is a verb. Do you seek, create, and act on opportunities to "verb" your love every day? _____

7. **Touch.**

As humans, we're wired to respond to loving touches. Watch doting parents with their babies or toddlers. They can't keep their hands off them: they hug, hold, kiss, cuddle, and enfold them in their arms. Physical displays of affection show that you feel a sense of warmth and security with your partner.

Do you spend time often kissing or caressing your partner or simply lying in each other's arms? _____

8. **Trust.**

Love—or at least infatuation—can strike in a heart-pounding, head-spinning moment, but trust builds as slowly as a coral reef. With each promise kept, each secret safeguarded, and each inch of soul exposed, something soft and squishy between two people grows stronger and firmer. In an intimate relationship, trust creates a safe harbor where you can be who you are without being attacked, rejected, or abandoned—and without attacking, rejecting, or abandoning.

Do you honor the trust between you and your partner every day by following a basic rule: no secrets, no lies, no deceptions, no excuses, no illusions? _____

9. **Respect.**

Your partner in an intimate relationship may like the same music, pursue the same interests, and even share the same favorite ice cream flavor. However, your partner is not you but a unique individual with his or her own desires, needs, and—face it—quirks. Respect means acknowledging, understanding, and accepting what makes your partner different from you and you different from your partner.

Do you show respect for your partner every day? _____

Source: Dianne Hales and Kenneth W. Christian, Labs for An Invitation to Personal Change, Belmont, CA: Wadsworth, 2009.

MAKING THIS CHAPTER WORK FOR YOU

Review Questions

(LO 5.1)   1. Which of the following statements is true of social health?
   a. It involves complete sexual abstinence.
   b. It involves periodic withdrawal from large groups.
   c. It primarily involves joining large social organizations.
   d. It involves developing interpersonal relationships.

(LO 5.1)   2. The process by which friends, friends of friends, acquaintances, and others in our social circle influence our behavior and our health, both positively and negatively, is termed _____.
   a. social connection
   b. social contagion
   c. social adjustment
   d. cyberbullying

(LO 5.2)   3. Which of the following traits is essential to communicating clearly?
   a. Being assertive
   b. Being loud
   c. Being aggressive
   d. Being humble

(LO 5.2)   4. Which of the following statements is true regarding the gender differences in communication?
   a. Men are generally better listeners.
   b. Women speak more in private, usually to build better connections with others.
   c. Men facilitate conversation better by nodding, asking questions, and signaling interest.
   d. Women interrupt more if they aren't getting the information they need.

(LO 5.3)   5. "Dunbar's number" limits the online and offline meaningful relationships maintained by most people to _____.
   a. 1,500
   b. 500
   c. 150
   d. 50

(LO 5.3)   6. Which of the following is true of "helper's high"?
   a. It is a social anxiety disorder.
   b. It is a form of infatuation.
   c. It leads to loneliness.
   d. It is a surge of well-being.

(LO 5.4)   7. Sexting involves _____.
   a. sending sexual text messages or photos by cell phone
   b. seeking help for sexual abuse from online support programs
   c. the online dissemination of information on sexually transmitted diseases
   d. abstaining from sex for a period of time

(LO 5.4)   8. Which of the following uses online sites, forums, and social media to harass victims and tries to damage their reputation or turn others against them?
   a. Cyber-terrorism
   b. Cybersquatting
   c. Facebook "lurking"
   d. Cyberstalking

(LO 5.5)   9. Which of the following statements is true of people who engage in hookups?
   a. They look forward to the attachment.
   b. They avoid being the center of attention.
   c. They believe it is a reflection of sexual freedom.
   d. They have a higher concern for personal safety.

(LO 5.5)   10. A friends-with-benefits relationship is a relationship _____.
   a. that involves casual sex for pay
   b. between friends that includes sexual intimacy
   c. that involves a one-time-only sexual encounter between friends
   d. between friends who take monetary favors from each other

(LO 5.6) 11. _____ is a state of closeness between two people, characterized by the desire and ability to share one's innermost thoughts and feelings with each other either verbally or nonverbally.
   a. Intimacy
   b. Infatuation
   c. Fatuous love
   d. Hooking up

(LO 5.6) 12. According to Robert Sternberg's psychological view, which of the following types of love is a deep emotional bond in a relationship that may have had romantic components?
   a. Consummate love
   b. Romantic love
   c. Companionate love
   d. Fatuous love

(LO 5.7) 13. A relationship that doesn't promote healthy communication, honesty, and intimacy and in which either person is made to feel worthless or incompetent is termed _____.
   a. fatuous love
   b. dysfunctional
   c. friends-without-benefits
   d. cyberbullying

(LO 5.7) 14. Which of the following terms refers to unwittingly contributing to a person's addictive or abusive behavior?
   a. Blending
   b. Cohabiting
   c. Enabling
   d. Coercing

(LO 5.8) 15. Which of the following is the first stage of a relationship?
   a. Establishing a strong sense of partnership
   b. Building trust and dependability
   c. Nesting
   d. Blending

(LO 5.8) 16. Which of the following statements is true of marriages and divorces among Americans?
   a. Children whose parents are divorced are more likely to marry.
   b. Married people have lower rates of coronary disease and cancer.
   c. Well-educated Americans are less likely to marry, and if they do, their unions are more likely to end in divorce.
   d. Having a baby during the first seven months after the wedding lowers the risk of divorce.

(LO 5.9) 17. Which of the following statements is true of American families?
   a. The average household has more children under age 18 now than a century ago.
   b. In white American families, wives and mothers are acknowledged and respected as healers and dispensers of wisdom.
   c. The primary purpose cited by the current American population for getting married is having children.
   d. In African American families, traditional gender roles are often reversed.

(LO 5.9) 18. Blended families are families _____.
   a. in which one or both of the partners bring children from a previous union
   b. in which children, parents, and grandparents live in the same house
   c. with two working parents or an unmarried working parent
   d. with same-sex parents

Answers to these questions can be found on page 623.

Critical Thinking Questions

1. Do you consider yourself a shy person? Why? Describe situations in which you may find yourself socially anxious. Discuss strategies to overcome anxieties in these situations.

2. What do you think of social networking? Which online social network do you use? Give reasons for your choice. On a typical day, how much time do you spend on it? Describe the activities you engage in. How has it impacted your health? How much have you disclosed about yourself on the site? What kind of information do you think should not be shared on social networks?

3. Describe the relationship between your parents. How has their relationship impacted you while you were growing up? What attracts you to another person? What is your opinion on long-term relationships? When would you consider marriage and having children? Explain.

Additional Online Resources

http://goaskalice.columbia.edu
Sponsored by the health education and wellness program of the Columbia University Health Service, this site features educators' answers to questions on a wide variety of topics, including those related to relationships and marriage and family.

www.apa.org/helpcenter
The American Psychological Association provides a wealth of articles and information on sustaining healthy relationships.

www1.extension.umn.edu/family/cyfc
This site offers research, programs, publications, and information on all types of parenting, relationships, and family issues.

Key Terms

The terms listed are used on the pages indicated. Definitions of the terms are in the glossary at the end of the book.

altruism 111	families 128
blended families 129	hookup 115
codependency 121	intimacy 117
cohabitation 123	same-sex marriage 125
cyberbullying 115	self-disclosure 112
cyberstalking 115	social contagion 107
dysfunctional 119	social anxiety disorder 110
enabling 122	

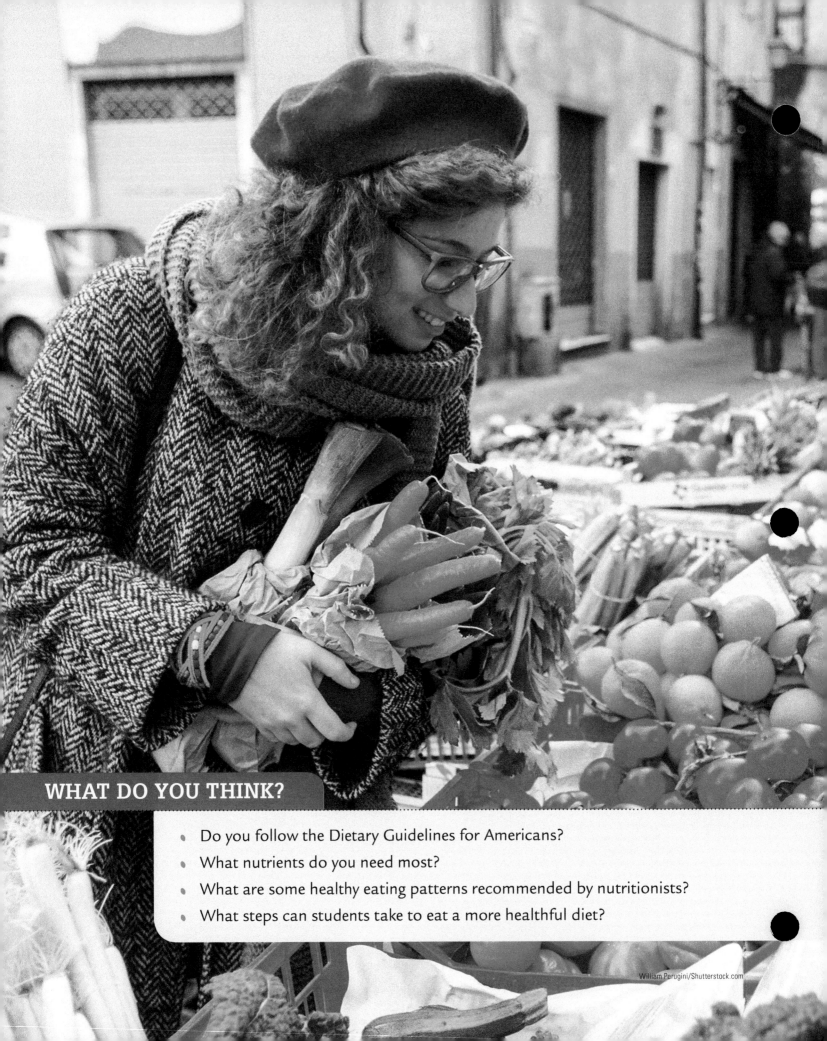

WHAT DO YOU THINK?

- Do you follow the Dietary Guidelines for Americans?
- What nutrients do you need most?
- What are some healthy eating patterns recommended by nutritionists?
- What steps can students take to eat a more healthful diet?

William Perugini/Shutterstock.com

6

Personal Nutrition

Matt, a second-year student at a community college in the Northwest, doesn't spend much time thinking about nutrition and health. He has a more pressing concern: getting enough food to eat. Even though he works 20 hours a week, with tuition and student fees rising, he struggles to pay for basic necessities, including food.

Matt's not unusual. A growing percentage of undergraduates—from 39 to 69 percent at different schools—report that at some point in the previous academic year, they could not afford enough to eat. About one in three have to choose between paying tuition and purchasing food.[1] Many report hunger, dizziness, difficulty concentrating, and other health problems.

"Food insecurity" (discussed on pages 161–162), researchers note, can potentially affect students' "cognitive, academic, and psychosocial development."[2] Other undergraduates face a different danger: diets that are high in calories but low in

nutrients and that put them at risk of obesity (discussed in Chapter 7) and a host of medical problems.

About half of American adults—some 117 million people—have one or more preventable chronic diseases. Poor eating patterns, overconsumption of **calories,** and lack of physical activity directly contribute to these disorders.[3]

Globally people are eating more healthy foods like fruits and vegetables but even more unhealthy ones such as sugar-sweetened drinks and processed meat. In higher-income nations, people do somewhat better, increasing their intake of healthy foods and slightly decreasing consumption of unhealthy ones.[4] <

After reading this chapter, you should be able to:

6.1 Analyze how the key recommendations of the *Dietary Guidelines for Americans* might affect food choices.

6.2 Review the roles played by macronutrients and micronutrients in fulfilling the requirements of the human body.

6.3 Assess the impact of eating habits on the health of many Americans.

6.4 Specify the steps you can take to ensure a balanced intake of nutrients.

6.5 Discuss the causes, effects, and prevention of foodborne infections.

6.6 Outline steps to follow in order to safeguard yourself from nutrition quackery.

At every stage of life, **nutrition**—the connection between our bodies and the foods we eat—matters. Healthful eating can provide energy for our daily tasks, can protect us from many chronic illnesses, and may even extend longevity. A high-quality diet also enhances day-to-day vitality, energy, and well-being.

This chapter can help you make healthier food choices, regardless of your financial or time constraints. It translates the latest scientific research and government dietary guidelines into specific advice designed both to promote health and to prevent chronic disease. By learning more about nutrients, food groups, eating patterns, nutrition labels, and safety practices, you can nourish your body with foods that not only taste good but also are good for you.

✓**check-in** How would you rate your knowledge of nutrition: Excellent? Good? Average? Poor? Ask yourself this same question at the end of this course

Dietary Guidelines for Americans

At least every five years, as mandated by federal law, the Department of Agriculture assembles a panel of registered dietitian nutritionists, health professionals, and representatives of the food industry to review the latest research on nutrition and health and develop *Dietary Guidelines for Americans*. These recommendations serve as "the cornerstone of all federal nutrition policy, education, outreach, and food assistance programs." Their primary purpose is to provide "science-based advice for healthy people ages 2 years and older to assist them in their efforts to make food and physical activity choices that promote health and prevent the risk of disease."[5]

The principal recommendations of the 2010 *Dietary Guidelines for Americans* encompassed two overarching concepts:

- **The key to achieving and sustaining a healthy weight is to maintain calorie balance.** People with healthy weights consume only enough calories from foods and beverages to meet their needs and expend excess calories through physical activity. (See page 140.)

- **Americans should focus on consuming nutrient-dense foods and beverages.** Rather than getting calories from solid fats, added sugars, and refined grains, we should limit such foods and increase our intake of foods that pack more nutritional power, such as vegetables, fruits, whole grains, nonfat or low-fat milk and milk products, seafood, lean meats, poultry, eggs, beans, peas, nuts, and seeds.

The 2010 *Dietary Guidelines* emphasized that excessive amounts of certain foods and food components—sodium, solid fats (major sources of saturated and *trans*-fatty acids), added sugars, refined grains, cholesterol, and alcohol—may increase the risks to health by adding excess and often "empty" calories to a daily diet. Even in normal-weight individuals, these foods could increase the risk of some of the most common chronic diseases in the United States.

The 2015 *Dietary Guidelines* generally reinforce the messages of the previous guidelines, with some modifications:

- Limit sodium, saturated fats, and trans fat. One good way to do so is cutting down on "mixed" dishes—foods like burgers, tacos, and pizza—that contribute about 44 percent of sodium and 38 percent of saturated fat to the American diet.

- Cut way back on sweet treats and sugary soda, prime sources of added sugars, salt, and saturated fat.

- Eat plenty of fruits and vegetables, good sources of the vitamins and minerals lacking in many Americans' diets.

- Don't worry about the cholesterol in foods such as eggs and shellfish. As the panel notes, diet influences about 20 percent of a person's blood cholesterol levels; the rest is governed by genetics. However, as many as one in four people may be genetically predisposed to create unhealthy levels of cholesterol in their bodies, and they must continue limiting dietary cholesterol.

- Limit coffee to three to five cups a day. This amount of caffeine is not linked to any long-term health risks and, in fact, has been associated with a reduced risk of type 2 diabetes and heart disease.

- Follow a "lifestyle" diet, such as the DASH diet, Mediterranean diet, or the USDA eating patterns (discussed later in this chapter). Although they vary somewhat, all recommend consuming fruits and vegetables, whole grains, and low- or no-fat dairy foods, limited red and processed meat, more poultry and seafood, and healthy sources of fat such as nuts and olive oil and avoiding foods made with lots of sugar and refined flour.[6]

calories The amount of energy required to raise the temperature of 1 gram of water by 1 degree Celsius. In everyday usage related to the energy content of foods and the energy expended in activities, a calorie is actually the equivalent of a thousand such calories, or a kilocalorie.

nutrition The science devoted to the study of dietary needs for food and the effects of food on organisms.

The Building Blocks of Good Nutrition

The digestive system (Figure 6.1) breaks down food into **macronutrients**, the nutrients required by the human body in the greatest amounts. We also need vitamins and minerals, the so-called **micronutrients**, but in only very small amounts. (See pages 146–155.)

Calories

Calories are the measure of the amount of energy that can be derived from food. How many calories you need depends on your gender, age, body-frame size, weight, percentage of body fat, and your **basal metabolic rate (BMR)**—the number of calories needed to sustain your body at rest. Your activity level also affects your calorie requirements (See Table 6.1). Regardless of

macronutrients Nutrients required by the human body in the greatest amounts, including water, carbohydrates, proteins, and fats.

micronutrients Vitamins and minerals needed by the body in very small amounts.

basal metabolic rate (BMR) The number of calories required to sustain the body at rest.

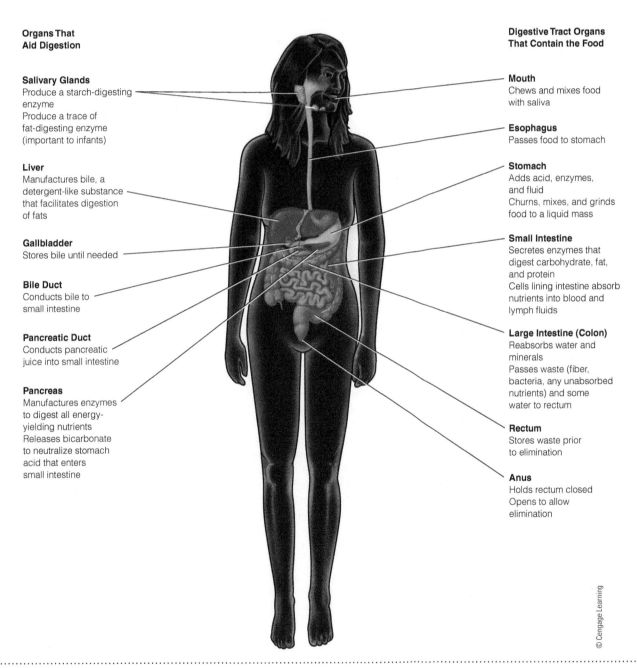

Organs That Aid Digestion

Salivary Glands
Produce a starch-digesting enzyme
Produce a trace of fat-digesting enzyme (important to infants)

Liver
Manufactures bile, a detergent-like substance that facilitates digestion of fats

Gallbladder
Stores bile until needed

Bile Duct
Conducts bile to small intestine

Pancreatic Duct
Conducts pancreatic juice into small intestine

Pancreas
Manufactures enzymes to digest all energy-yielding nutrients
Releases bicarbonate to neutralize stomach acid that enters small intestine

Digestive Tract Organs That Contain the Food

Mouth
Chews and mixes food with saliva

Esophagus
Passes food to stomach

Stomach
Adds acid, enzymes, and fluid
Churns, mixes, and grinds food to a liquid mass

Small Intestine
Secretes enzymes that digest carbohydrate, fat, and protein
Cells lining intestine absorb nutrients into blood and lymph fluids

Large Intestine (Colon)
Reabsorbs water and minerals
Passes waste (fiber, bacteria, any unabsorbed nutrients) and some water to rectum

Rectum
Stores waste prior to elimination

Anus
Holds rectum closed
Opens to allow elimination

© Cengage Learning

FIGURE 6.1 The Digestive System
The organs of the digestive system break down food into nutrients that the body can use.

TABLE 6.1 Estimated Calorie Needs per Day by Age, Gender, and Physical Activity Level

Estimated amounts of calories needed to maintain calorie balance for various gender and age groups at three different levels of physical activity. The estimates are rounded to the nearest 200 calories. An individual's calorie needs may be higher or lower than these average estimates.

Gender	Age (years)	Physical Activity Level		
		Sedentary	Moderately Active	Active
Female	19–30	1,800–2,000	2,000–2,200	2,400
	31–50	1,800	2,000	2,200
	51+	1,600	1,800	2,000–2,200
Male	19–30	2,400–2,600	2,600–2,800	3,000
	31–50	2,200–2,400	2,400–2,600	2,800–3,000
	51+	2,000–2,200	2,200–2,400	2,400–2,800

© Cengage Learning

Calorie balance The relationship between calories consumed from foods and beverages and calories expended in normal body functions and through physical activity. If the calories consumed equal calories expended, you will have calorie balance.

essential nutrients Nutrients that the body cannot manufacture for itself and must obtain from food.

proteins Organic compounds composed of amino acids; one of the essential nutrients.

amino acids Organic compounds containing nitrogen, carbon, hydrogen, and oxygen; the essential building blocks of proteins.

complete protein Proteins that contain all the amino acids needed by the body for growth and maintenance.

incomplete protein Proteins that lack one or more of the amino acids essential for protein synthesis.

complementary proteins Incomplete proteins that, when combined, provide all the amino acids essential for protein synthesis.

whether you consume fat, protein, or carbohydrates, if you take in more calories than required to maintain your size and don't work them off in some sort of physical activity, your body will convert the excess to fat (see Chapter 7). On average, daily calorie needs are as follows:

- Most women, some older adults, children ages 2 to 6: 1,600
- Average adult: 2,000
- Most men, active women, teenage girls, older children: 2,200
- Active men, teenage boys: 2,800

Calorie balance refers to the relationship between calories consumed from foods and beverages and calories expended in normal body functions and through physical activity. You cannot control the calories your body burns to maintain temperature and other basic processes. However, you can control what you eat and drink and how many calories you use in physical activity. To maintain a healthy weight, you must expend as much energy (calories) as you take in.

Among the best ways to balance this energy equation are

- Limiting portion sizes (discussed later in this chapter).
- Substituting nutrient-dense foods (such as raw vegetables or low-fat soups) for nutrient-poor foods (such as candy and cake).
- Limiting added sugars, solid fats, and alcoholic beverages.
- Increasing physical activity. As discussed in Chapter 7, adults may need up to 60 minutes

of moderate to vigorous physical activity—the equivalent of 150 to 200 calories, depending on body size—daily to prevent unhealthy weight gain. Men and women who have lost weight may need 60 to 90 minutes to keep off excess pounds.

√**check-in** How do you balance the calories you consume with the calories you use?

Essential Nutrients

Every day your body needs certain **essential nutrients** that provide energy, build and repair body tissues, and regulate body functions. The six classes of essential nutrients are water, protein, carbohydrates, fats, vitamins, and minerals (Figure 6.2, page 141).

Water Water, essential for health and survival, makes up 85 percent of blood, 70 percent of muscles, and about 75 percent of the brain and performs many essential functions, including the following:

- Carrying nutrients
- Maintaining temperature
- Lubricating joints
- Helping with digestion
- Ridding the body of waste through urine
- Contributing to the production of sweat, which evaporates from the skin to cool the body

Research has correlated high fluid intake with a lower risk of kidney stones, colon cancer, and bladder cancer. (See Chapter 19 for a discussion of bottled water.)

You lose about 64 to 80 ounces of water a day—the equivalent of 8 to 10 8-ounce glasses—through perspiration, urination, bowel movements, and normal exhalation. You lose water more rapidly if you exercise, live in a dry climate or at a high altitude, drink a lot of caffeine or alcohol (which increases urination), skip a meal, or become ill. To ensure adequate water intake, nutritionists advise drinking enough so that your urine is not dark in color. Healthy individuals can get adequate hydration from beverages other than plain water, including juice.

√**check-in** How much water to you drink every day?

Protein Every living cell in the body contains protein. Critical for growth and repair, **proteins** form the basic framework for our muscles, bones, blood, hair, and fingernails.

Twenty different **amino acids** join together to make all types of protein. Our bodies cannot make nine of these amino acids. These are known as *essential* amino acids that we must get from our diets. Dietary protein sources are categorized according to how many of the essential amino acids they provide:

- A **complete protein**, or high-quality protein, source provides all the essential amino acids. Animal-based foods such as meat, poultry, fish, milk, eggs, and cheese are considered complete protein sources.

- An **incomplete protein** source is low in one or more of the essential amino acids.

- **Complementary proteins** are two or more incomplete protein sources that together provide adequate amounts of all the essential amino acids. Two good examples are rice and dry beans, which together can provide adequate amounts of all the essential amino acids the body needs.

You need to eat protein every day because your body doesn't store it the way it stores fats or carbohydrates. The average person needs 50 to 65 grams of protein daily. This is the amount in 4 ounces of meat plus 1 cup of cottage cheese.

Protein Sources Protein is found in the following foods:

- Meats, poultry, and fish
- Legumes (dry beans and peas)
- Tofu
- Eggs
- Nuts and seeds
- Milk and milk products
- Grains, some vegetables, and some fruits (only small amounts relative to other sources)

Most people eat more protein than they need without harmful effects. However, protein contributes to calorie intake, so if you eat too much, your overall calorie intake could be greater than your calorie needs, and you could gain weight. Animal proteins also are sources of saturated fat, which has been linked to elevated low-density lipoprotein (LDL) cholesterol, a risk factor for cardiovascular disease.

Red meat in particular may increase the risk of death from cancer and heart disease—and the more of it that men and women eat, the greater the risk. Processed meats, such as bologna and hot dogs, also contain high amounts of sodium, unhealthy saturated fats, and nitrates, preservatives that have been linked to cancer.

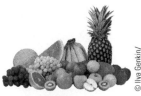
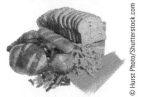

1. CARBOHYDRATES are substances in food that each consist of a single sugar molecule, or of multiple sugar molecules in various forms. They provide the body with energy.

Simple sugars are the most basic type of carbohydrates. Examples include glucose (blood sugar), sucrose (table sugar), and lactose (milk sugar). **Starches** are complex carbohydrates consisting primarily of long, interlocking chains of glucose units. **Dietary fiber** consists of complex carbohydrates found principally in plant cell walls. Dietary fiber cannot be broken down by human digestive enzymes.

....

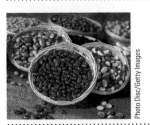

2. PROTEINS are substances in food that are composed of amino acids. Amino acids are specific chemical substances from which proteins are made. Of the 20 amino acids, 9 are "essential," or a required part of our diet.

....

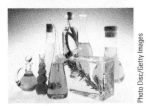

3. FATS are substances in food that are soluble in fat, not water.

Saturated fats are found primarily in animal products, such as meat, butter, and cheese, and in palm and coconut oils. Diets high in saturated fat may elevate blood cholesterol levels. **Unsaturated fats** are found primarily in plant products, such as vegetable oil, nuts, and seeds, as well as in fish. Unsaturated fats tend to lower blood cholesterol levels. **Essential fatty acids** are two specific types of unsaturated fats that are required in the diet. *Trans* **fats** are a type of unsaturated fat present in hydrogenated oil, margarine, shortening, pastries, and some cooking oils that increase the risk of heart disease. **Cholesterol** is a fat-soluble, colorless liquid primarily found in animals. It can be manufactured by the liver.

....

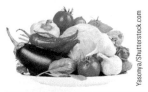

4. VITAMINS are chemical substances found in food that perform specific functions in the body. Humans require 13 different vitamins in their diet.

....

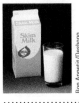

5. MINERALS are chemical substances that make up the "ash" that remains when food is completely burned. Humans require 15 different minerals in their diet.

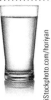

6. WATER is essential for life. Most adults need about 11–15 cups of water each day from food and fluids.

....

FIGURE 6.2 Six Categories of Nutrients
© Cengage Learning

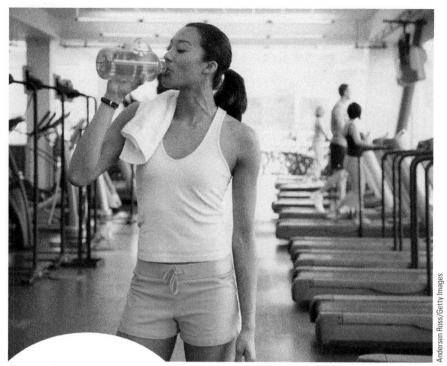

Be sure to get an adequate supply of water whenever and wherever you exercise.

Andersen Ross/Getty Images

....
√**check-in** How much meat do you eat in a week?
....

The *Dietary Guidelines* recommend a balanced variety of protein sources to get more nutrients and health benefits. Certain nuts—peanuts, walnuts, almonds, and pistachios—reduce risk factors for cardiovascular disease but, because they are high in calories, should be eaten only in small amounts.

....
√**check-in** Go nuts! In a recent study of more than 200,000 people, those who ate more nuts, including peanuts and peanut butter, had lower rates of premature death from heart disease and other causes. The recommended daily amount: about two tablespoons of shelled peanuts.[7]
....

The 2010 *Dietary Guidelines* included a quantitative recommendation for seafood: 8 or more ounces a week or about 20 percent of total protein intake. Currently Americans consume about 3.5 ounces of seafood every week. Because it is rich in omega-3 fatty acids, seafood has been linked with fewer cardiac deaths among individuals with or without cardiovascular disease.

These benefits outweigh the risks associated with methyl mercury, a heavy metal found in varying levels in different types of seafood. The types of seafood that are generally lower in mercury include salmon, anchovies, herring, sardines, Pacific oysters, trout, and Atlantic and Pacific mackerel (but not king mackerel, which is high in mercury).

....
√**check-in** How much seafood do you eat each week?
....

Because some vegetarians avoid eating all (or most) animal foods, they must rely on plant-based sources of protein to meet their protein needs. With some planning, a vegetarian diet can easily meet the recommended protein needs (see pages 159–160).

Carbohydrates **Carbohydrates** are organic compounds that provide our brains and bodies with *glucose*, their basic fuel. The major sources of carbohydrates are plants—including grains, vegetables, fruits, and beans—and milk. There are two types: *simple carbohydrates* (sugars) and *complex carbohydrates* (starches and fiber). All carbohydrates provide 4 calories per gram. Both adults and children should consume at least 130 grams of carbohydrates each day, the minimum needed to produce enough glucose for the brain to function.

Simple carbohydrates include *natural sugars*, such as the lactose in milk and the fructose in fruit, and *added sugars* that are found in candy, soft drinks, fruit drinks, pastries, and other sweets.

On average, Americans consume more than 20 teaspoons of sweet calories a day. Some come from the teaspoons of sucrose (simple sugar) you add to coffee or tea. Those whose diets are higher in added sugars typically have lower intakes of other essential nutrients. Even relatively low amounts of added sugar may increase the risk of cardiovascular disease and mortality.[8]

....
√**check-in** How much sugar do you consciously add to your diet every day?
....

A common hidden source of simple carbohydrates is high-fructose corn syrup, a sweetener and preservative made by changing the sugar glucose in cornstarch to fructose. Because it extends the shelf life of processed foods and is cheaper than sugar, high-fructose corn syrup has become a popular ingredient in many sodas, fruit-flavored drinks, and other processed foods. Although not intrinsically less healthy than sugar, high-fructose corn syrup might stimulate the pancreas to produce more insulin. It also makes beverages very sweet, which may increase consumption and contribute to obesity and other health problems.

carbohydrates Organic compounds, such as starches, sugars, and glycogen, that are composed of carbon, hydrogen, and oxygen and are sources of bodily energy.

simple carbohydrates Sugars; like all other carbohydrates, they provide the body with glucose.

Sugar consumption, especially added sugar, has been implicated as a major cause of several chronic diseases, including obesity, heart disease, diabetes, and dental cavities. Americans have cut back on added sugars over the past 14 years, but health authorities are calling for greater reductions to as low as 5 percent of total calories. However, some nutritionists contend that the amount of added sugars even in nutrient-rich, recommended foods such as yogurt and whole grains may make this goal difficult to achieve.[9]

The major sources of added sugars are

- Soda, energy drinks, and sports drinks
- Grain-based desserts
- Sugar-sweetened fruit drinks
- Dairy-based desserts
- Candy

✓**check-in** Do you think foods high in added sugars should be taxed or restricted to reduce their consumption?

Complex carbohydrates include grains, cereals, vegetables, beans, and nuts. Americans get most of their complex carbohydrates from refined grains, which have been stripped of fiber and many nutrients, in breads and desserts.

Far more nutritious are whole grains, which can help lower the risk of diabetes and heart disease and are associated with lower mortality rates.[10] They consist of all components of the grain, including

- The *bran*—the fiber-rich outer layer
- The middle layer, called the *endosperm*
- The *germ*—the nutrient-packed inner layer

Fewer than 5 percent of Americans consume the minimum recommended amount of whole grains—about 3 ounce-equivalents a day—which can reduce the risk of diabetes and cardiovascular disease.

✓**check-in** Are half of the grains you consume every day whole grains? (They should be.)

To get more grains in your diet try the following:

- **Check labels of rolls and bread** and choose those with at least 2 to 3 grams of fiber per slice.
- **Add brown rice or barley** to soups.
- **Choose whole-grain,** ready-to-eat cereals.
- **Have a whole-grain cereal for breakfast.** According to a recent study, people who eat breakfast cereal generally eat less total fat, saturated fat, and sugar than those who do not, and they have better intakes of protein and important micronutrients, such as iron, vitamins, and calcium, throughout the day.

Fiber Dietary fiber is the nondigestible form of complex carbohydrates that occurs naturally in plant foods, such as leaves, stems, skins, seeds, and hulls. **Functional fiber** consists of isolated, nondigestible carbohydrates that may be added to foods and that provide beneficial effects in humans. Total fiber is the sum of both.

The various forms of fiber enhance health in different ways:

- They slow the emptying of the stomach, which creates a feeling of fullness and aids in weight control.
- They interfere with absorption of dietary fat and cholesterol, which reduces the risk of heart disease and stroke in both middle-aged and elderly individuals.
- They help prevent constipation and diabetes. However, a high-fiber diet does not lower the risk of diverticulosis (a painful inflammation of the bowel).
- They may contribute to a longer lifespan. In a study of almost 400,000 people ages 50 to 71, those who ate a diet rich in whole grains, fruits, and vegetables were significantly less likely to die of cardiovascular disease, infectious illnesses, and respiratory disorders over a nine-year period. A high-fiber diet also was associated with fewer cancer deaths in men, but not in women.

The Institute of Medicine has set recommendations for daily intake levels of total fiber (dietary plus functional fiber):

- 38 grams of total fiber for men.
- 25 grams for women.
- For men and women over 50 years of age, who consume less food, the recommendations are, respectively, 30 and 21 grams.

✓**check-in** Are you getting enough fiber in your daily diet?

Good fiber sources include wheat and corn bran (the outer layer); leafy greens; the skins of fruits and root vegetables; oats, beans, and barley; and the pulp, skin, and seeds of many vegetables and fruits, such as apples and strawberries (see Table 6.2). Because sudden increases in fiber can cause symptoms like bloating and gas, experts recommend gradually adding more fiber

complex carbohydrates Starches, including cereals, fruits, and vegetables.

dietary fiber The nondigestible form of carbohydrates found in plant foods, such as leaves, stems, skins, seeds, and hulls.

functional fiber Isolated, nondigestible carbohydrates that have beneficial effects in humans.

TABLE 6.2 High-Fiber Foods

Grains

Whole-grain products provide about 1 to 2 grams (or more) of fiber per serving:

- 1 slice whole-wheat, pumpernickel, rye bread
- 1 oz ready-to-eat cereal (100% bran cereals contain 10 grams or more)
- ½ cup cooked barley, bulgur, grits, oatmeal, brown rice, quinoa

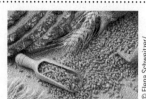

Vegetables Grains

Most vegetables contain about 2 to 3 grams of fiber per serving:

- 1 cup raw bean sprouts
- ½ cup cooked broccoli, brussels sprouts, cabbage, carrots, cauliflower, collards, corn, eggplant, green beans, green peas, kale, mushrooms, okra, parsnips, potatoes, pumpkin, spinach, sweet potatoes, swiss chard, winter squash
- ½ cup chopped raw carrots, peppers

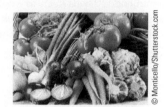

Fruits

Fresh, frozen, and dried fruits have about 2 grams of fiber per serving:

- 1 medium apple, banana, kiwi, nectarine, orange, pear
- ½ cup applesauce, blackberries, blueberries, raspberries, strawberries

Fruit juices contain very little fiber.

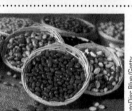

Legumes

Many legumes provide about 6 to 8 grams of fiber per serving:

- ½ cup cooked baked beans, black beans, black-eyed peas, kidney beans, navy beans, pinto beans

Some legumes provide about 5 grams of fiber per serving:

- ½ cup cooked garbanzo beans, great northern beans, lentils, lima beans, split peas

to your diet, with an additional serving or two of vegetables, fruit, or whole-wheat bread.

✓**check-in** Do you avoid gluten?
You should if you're among the estimated three million adults and children (about 1 percent of the population) with celiac disease. In this autoimmune disorder, immune cells attack the lining of the small intestine, through which nutrients are absorbed. For genetically susceptible people, gluten, a protein in wheat, barley, rye, and other grains, can trigger symptoms such as abdominal pain, bloating, diarrhea, headache, and fatigue. If you don't have celiac disease or a sensitivity to gluten, doctors caution that a gluten-free diet can do more harm than good because it may not provide necessary vitamins, minerals, and fiber.

Glycemic Index and Glycemic Load The glycemic index is a ranking of carbohydrates, gram for gram, based on their immediate effect on blood glucose (sugar) levels. Carbohydrates that break down quickly during digestion and trigger a fast, high glucose response have the highest glycemic index rating. Those that break down slowly, releasing glucose gradually into the bloodstream, have low glycemic index ratings. Potatoes, which raise blood sugar higher and faster than apples, for instance, earn a higher glycemic index rating than apples. Glycemic index does not account for the amount of food you typically eat in a serving.

Glycemic load is a measure of how much a typical serving size of a particular food raises blood glucose. For example, the glycemic index of table sugar is high, but you use so little to sweeten your coffee or tea that its glycemic load is low.

Low-Carb Foods The popularity of diets that restrict carbohydrate intake, discussed in Chapter 7, prompted an explosion in products

touted as "low-carb." You can get low-carb versions of everything from beer to bread. However, the Food and Drug Administration (FDA), which regulates health claims on food labels in the United States, hasn't defined what "low-carb" means. Words like "low-carb," "carb-wise," or "carb-free" are marketing terms created by manufacturers to sell their products.

Although many people may buy low-carb foods because they believe that they're healthier, that isn't necessarily the case. A low-carb nutrition bar, for instance, may be high in saturated fat and calories. Some low-carb food products cause digestive symptoms because food companies often replace the carbohydrates in a cookie or cracker with substances such as the sweetener sorbitol, which can cause diarrhea or stomach cramps.

Dieters often buy low-carb products in order to lose weight. According to proponents of low-carb diets, if carbohydrates raise blood sugar and insulin levels and cause weight gain, a decrease in carbs should result in lower blood sugar and insulin levels—and weight loss. With limited carbohydrates in the diet, the body would break down fat to provide needed energy.

Some people do lose weight when they switch to low-carb foods, but the reasons are probably that they consume fewer calories, lose water weight, and have decreased appetite because of a buildup of ketones (a by-product of fat metabolism) in the blood. As discussed in Chapter 7, a low-carb diet can lead to fairly rapid weight loss but is no easier to maintain over the long run than any other diet.

Refined Grains The refining of whole grains removes vitamins, minerals, and fiber. Although most refined grains are enriched with iron, thiamin, riboflavin, niacin, and folic acid before being used as food ingredients, not all of the vitamins and minerals and none of the dietary fiber are routinely added back. Many refined grain products, such as cookies and cake, also are high in solid fats and added sugars.

On average, Americans consume the equivalent of 6.3 ounces of refined grains per day. The recommended amount is no more than 3 ounce-equivalents. The *Dietary Guidelines* urge replacing refined grains with whole grains so that at least half of all the grains you consume are whole.

Fats Fats carry the fat-soluble vitamins A, D, E, and K; aid in their absorption in the intestine; protect organs from injury; regulate body temperature; and play an important role in growth and development. They provide 9 calories per gram—more than twice the amount in carbohydrates or proteins.

Both high- and low-fat diets can be unhealthy. When people eat very low levels of fat and very high levels of carbohydrates, their levels of high-density lipoprotein, the so-called *good cholesterol*, decline. On the other hand, high-fat diets can lead to obesity and its related health dangers.

Solid fats make up an average of 19 percent of the total calories in the average daily diet, but contribute few essential nutrients and no dietary fiber. Reducing solid fats, most commonly consumed in grain-based desserts, pizza, regular cheese, processed meat products, and fried potatoes, can reduce extra calories, saturated fats, *trans*-fatty acids, and cholesterol.

Forms of Fat *Saturated fats* and *unsaturated fats* are distinguished by the type of fatty acids in their chemical structures. All dietary fats are a mix of saturated and unsaturated fats but are predominantly one or the other. **Saturated fats** have long been considered a major threat to cardiovascular health, although recent research has raised some questions about their impact.[11]

However, there is ample evidence that lowering saturated fats to the recommended 10 percent of all calories—or lower—can significantly reduce the risk of cardiovascular disease. The American Heart Association recommends that people restrict saturated fats to as little as 5 percent of daily calories—roughly 2 tablespoons of butter or 2 ounces of Cheddar cheese if you are consuming 2,000 calories a day.

To reduce your saturated fat intake:

- **Cut back on the major sources of saturated fats in your diet:** regular (full-fat) cheese, pizza, grain-based desserts (cakes, cookies, pies, sweet rolls, pastries, doughnuts, etc.), dairy-based desserts (ice cream, frozen yogurt, milkshakes, pudding, etc.), sausages, franks, bacon, and ribs.

- **Switch to nonfat or low-fat milk and dairy products.**

- When preparing or ordering fish, **choose grilled, baked, broiled, or poached fish,** not fried. Fried fish at fast-food restaurants is often low in omega-3 fatty acids and high in *trans* and saturated fats.

- **Trim all visible fat from meat**.

- **Use oils that are rich in monounsaturated fatty acids,** such as canola, olive, and safflower oils, or polyunsaturated fatty acids, such as soybean, corn, and cottonseed oils.

saturated fats A chemical term indicating that a fat molecule contains as many hydrogen atoms as its carbon skeleton can hold. These fats are normally solid at room temperature.

Unsaturated fats can be divided into mono-unsaturated or polyunsaturated, again depending on their chemical structure. Unsaturated fats, like oils, are likely to be liquid at room temperature, and saturated fats, like butter, are likely to be solid. In general, vegetable and fish oils are unsaturated, and animal fats are saturated.

Olive, soybean, canola, cottonseed, corn, and other vegetable oils are unsaturated fats. Olive oil is considered a good fat and one of the best vegetable oils for salads and cooking. Used for thousands of years, this staple of the Mediterranean diet (discussed later in this chapter) has been correlated with a lower incidence of heart disease, including strokes and heart attacks.

Omega-3 and omega-6 are polyunsaturated fatty acids with slightly different chemical compositions. Regular consumption of omega-3 fatty acids, found in fatty fish such as salmon and sardines, flaxseed, and walnuts, helps prevent blood clots, protect against irregular heartbeats, and lower blood pressure, especially among people with high blood pressure or atherosclerosis. Omega-6 fatty acids are found in vegetable oils, nuts, seeds, meat, poultry, and eggs.

Some fish, such as mackerel, shark, tilefish, tuna, and swordfish, contain potentially harmful levels of mercury. To balance the benefits and risks of eating fish, the American Heart Association recommends two servings of fish a week, although even a single fish meal a month may be beneficial.

Fish oil supplements are not recommended.[12] As numerous clinical trials have shown, they do not provide any significant protection against macular degeneration or other age-related eye diseases.[13] A recent analysis of all available data from decades of testing further concluded that fish oil supplements show "no clear, considerable benefit" in enhancing health in individuals with or without cardiovascular disease.[14]

Cholesterol The body makes more cholesterol than it uses, and people do not need additional amounts. The main sources of cholesterol, which is found only in animal foods, include eggs, chicken, and beef.

Trans-Fatty Acids These substances, found naturally in some foods and formed during food processing, are not essential in the diet. An increased intake of *trans*-fatty acids has been linked with higher levels of LDL (low-density lipoprotein) and heart-harming cholesterol and greater danger of cardiovascular disease.

In response to consumer and health professionals' demand for less saturated fat in the food supply, many manufacturers switched to partially hydrogenated oils. The process of hydrogenation creates unsaturated fatty acids called ***trans fat***. They are found in some margarine products and most foods made with partially hydrogenated oils, such as baked goods and fried foods.

Even though *trans* fats are unsaturated, they have an even more harmful effect on cholesterol than saturated fats because they increase harmful LDL and, in large amounts, decrease helpful HDL (blood fats are discussed in Chapter 15). There is no safe level for *trans* fats, which occur naturally in meats as well as in foods prepared with partially hydrogenated vegetable oils.

Some food manufacturers have reduced or eliminated *trans* fats in snacks and other products. Cities and communities across the country have banned *trans* fats in restaurants. Some campuses also have stopped using *trans* fats in their dining halls and food outlets. The Centers for Disease Control and Prevention (CDC) reports that blood levels of *trans*-fatty acids have dropped by 58 percent since 2000.

To cut down on both saturated and *trans* fats

- Choose oils such as soybean, canola, corn, olive, safflower, and sunflower, which are naturally free of *trans* fats and lower in saturated fats.

- Look for reduced-fat, low-fat, fat-free, and *trans*-fat-free versions of baked goods, snacks, and other processed foods. Some choices—such as butter versus margarine—are more difficult to make (see Figure 6.3).

Oils As discussed previously, fats with a high percentage of monounsaturated and polyunsaturated fatty acids are usually liquid at room temperature and so are referred to as oils. The *Dietary Guidelines* recommend replacing some solid fats with oils in order to lower cholesterol and promote heart health. However, because oils are high in calories, you should use them in small amounts. Some easy ways to replace solid with liquid fats are to use vegetable oils instead of butter for cooking and to use a soft margarine rather than stick margarine or butter. (See Figure 6.3, page 147.)

Vitamins   Americans generally get adequate amounts of most micronutrients. However, intakes of several nutrients are low enough to be of concern:

- **For adults:** Vitamins A, C, and E, calcium, magnesium, potassium, and fiber.

- **For children:** Vitamin E, calcium, magnesium, potassium, and fiber.

unsaturated fats A chemical term indicating that a fat molecule contains fewer hydrogen atoms than its carbon skeleton can hold. These fats are normally liquid at room temperature.

omega-3 and omega-6 Polyunsaturated fatty acids with recognized health benefits. Omega-3 fatty acids are found in fatty fish such as salmon and sardines, flaxseed, and walnuts. Omega-6 fatty acids are found in vegetable oils, nuts, seeds, meat, poultry, and eggs.

***trans* fat** Fat formed when liquid vegetable oils are processed to make table spreads or cooking fats; also found in dairy and beef products; considered to be especially dangerous dietary fats.

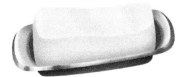
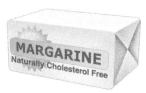
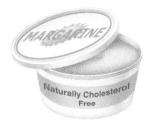
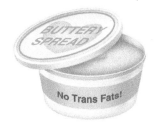

| Butter | Margarine (stick) | Margarine (tub) | Buttery spread |

Nutrition Facts

Serving Size 1 Tbsp (14g)
Servings per container about 32

Amount per serving	
Calories 100 Calories from Fat 100	
	%Daily Value*
Total Fat 11g	17%
Saturated Fat 7g	37%
Trans Fat 0g	
Cholesterol 30mg	10%
Sodium 95mg	4%
Total Carbohydrate 0g	0%
Protein 0g	

Vitamin A 8%

Not a significant source of dietary fiber, sugars, vitamin C, calcium, and iron.

*Percent Daily Values are based on a 2,000 calorie diet.

INGREDIENTS: Cream, salt.

Nutrition Facts

Serving Size 1 Tbsp (14g)
Servings per container about 32

Amount per serving	
Calories 100 Calories from Fat 100	
	%Daily Value*
Total Fat 11g	17%
Saturated Fat 2g	11%
Trans Fat 2.5g	
Polyunsaturated Fat 3.5g	
Monounsaturated Fat 2.5g	
Cholesterol 0mg	0%
Sodium 105mg	4%
Total Carbohydrate 0g	0%
Protein 0g	

Vitamin A 10%

Not a significant source of dietary fiber, sugars, vitamin C, calcium, and iron.

*Percent Daily Values are based on a 2,000 calorie diet.

INGREDIENTS: Liquid soybean oil, partially hydrogenated soybean oil, water, buttermilk, salt, soy lecithin, sodium benzoate (as a preservative), vegetable mono and diglycerides, artificial flavor, vitamin A palmitate, colored with beta carotene (provitamin A).

Nutrition Facts

Serving size 1 Tbsp (14g)
Servings per container about 32

Amount per serving	
Calories 100 Calories from Fat 100	
	%Daily Value*
Total Fat 11g	17%
Saturated Fat 2.5g	13%
Trans Fat 2g	
Polyunsaturated Fat 4g	
Monounsaturated Fat 2.5g	
Cholesterol 0mg	0%
Sodium 80mg	3%
Total Carbohydrate 0g	0%
Protein 0g	

Vitamin A 10%

Not a significant source of dietary fiber, sugars, vitamin C, calcium, and iron.

*Percent Daily Values are based on a 2,000 calorie diet.

INGREDIENTS: Liquid soybean oil, partially hydrogenated soybean oil, buttermilk, water, butter (cream, salt), salt, soy lecithin, vegetable mono and diglycerides, sodium benzoate added as a preservative, artificial flavor, vitamin A palmitate, colored with beta carotene.

Nutrition Facts

Serving size 1 Tbsp (14g)
Servings per container about 24

Amount per serving	
Calories 100 Calories from Fat 100	
	%Daily Value*
Total Fat 11g	17%
Saturated Fat 3.5g	18%
Trans Fat 0g	
Polyunsaturated Fat 3.5g	
Monounsaturated Fat 3.5g	
Cholesterol 0mg	0%
Sodium 120mg	5%
Total Carbohydrate 0g	0%
Protein 0g	

Vitamin A 0%

Not a significant source of dietary fiber, sugars, vitamin C, calcium, and iron.

*Percent Daily Values are based on a 2,000 calorie diet.

INGREDIENTS: Expeller pressed natural oil blend (soybean palm fruit, canola and olive), filtered water, pure salt, natural flavor, soy protein, soy lecithin, lactic acid (non-dairy, derived from sugar beets), and beta-carotene color (from natural source).

© Cengage Learning

FIGURE 6.3 Butter or Margarine?

Most of the fat in butter is saturated fat. Most of the fat in margarine is unsaturated, but the *trans* fats are twice as damaging as saturated fat. If the list of ingredients includes partially hydrogenated oils, you know the food contains *trans* fat. The closer "partially hydrogenated oil" is to the beginning of the ingredients list, the more *trans* fat the product contains. There are a handful of margarine alternatives that do not contain *trans* fats.

Among the groups at highest risk of nutritional deficiencies are these:

- **Teenage girls**
- **Women of child-bearing age:** Iron and folic acid
- **People over age 50:** Vitamin B$_{12}$
- **The elderly, people with dark skin, and those who do not get adequate exposure to sunshine**: Vitamin D

✓**check-in** Are you getting enough of the key nutrients?

Vitamins, which help put proteins, fats, and carbohydrates to use, are essential to regulating growth, maintaining tissue, and releasing energy from foods. Together with the enzymes in the body, they help produce the right chemical reactions at the right times. Table 6.3 on pages 148–150 provides more detailed information on vitamins, including their primary functions, consequences of deficiency and overdose, and primary food sources.

The body produces some vitamins, such as vitamin D, which is manufactured in the skin after exposure to sunlight. Other vitamins must be ingested.

vitamins Organic substances that the body needs in very small amounts and that carry out a variety of functions in metabolism and nutrition.

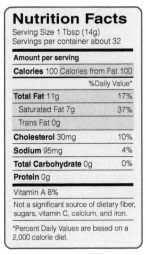

The Building Blocks of Good Nutrition   147

TABLE 6.3 Key Information about Vitamins

The water-soluble vitamins

	Primary functions	Consequences of deficiency	Consequences of overdose	Primary food sources
Thiamin (vitamin B$_1$) AI^a women: 1.1 mg men: 1.2 mg	• Helps body release energy from carbohydrates ingested • Facilitates growth and maintenance of nerve and muscle tissues • Promotes normal appetite	• Fatigue, weakness • Nerve disorders, mental confusion, apathy • Impaired growth • Swelling • Heart irregularity and failure	• High intakes of thiamin are rapidly excreted by the kidneys. Oral doses of 500 mg/day or less are considered safe.	• Grains and grain products (cereals, rice, pasta, bread) • Pork • Nuts
Riboflavin (vitamin B$_2$) AI women: 1.1 mg men: 1.3 mg	• Helps body capture and use energy released from carbohydrates, proteins, and fats • Aids in cell division • Promotes growth and tissue repair • Promotes normal vision	• Reddened lips, cracks at both corners of the mouth • Fatigue	• None known. High doses are rapidly excreted by the kidneys.	• Milk, yogurt, cheese • Grains and grain products (cereals, rice, pasta, bread) • Liver, fish, beef • Eggs
Niacin (vitamin B$_3$) RDA women: 14 mg men: 16 mg UL: 35 mg (from supplements and fortified foods)	• Helps body capture and use energy released from carbohydrates, proteins, and fats • Assists in the manufacture of body fats • Helps maintain normal nervous system functions	• Skin disorders • Nervous and mental disorders • Diarrhea, indigestion • Fatigue	• Flushing, headache, cramps, rapid heartbeat, nausea, diarrhea, decreased liver function with doses above 0.5 g per day	• Meats (all types), fish • Grains and grain products (cereals, rice, pasta, bread) • Nuts
Vitamin B$_6$ (pyridoxine) AI women: 1.3 mg men: 1.3 mg UL: 100 mg	• Needed for reactions that build proteins and protein tissues • Assists in the conversion of tryptophan to niacin • Needed for normal red blood cell formation • Promotes normal functioning of the nervous system	• Irritability, depression • Convulsions, twitching • Muscular weakness • Dermatitis near the eyes • Anemia • Kidney stones	• Bone pain, loss of feeling in fingers and toes, muscular weakness, numbness, loss of balance (mimicking multiple sclerosis)	• Meats (all types) • Breakfast cereals • Bananas, avocados • Potatoes, Brussels sprouts, sweet peppers
Folate (folacin, folic acid) RDA women: 400 mcg men: 400 mcg UL: 1000 mcg (from supplements and fortified foods)	• Needed for reactions that utilize amino acids (the building blocks of protein) for protein tissue formation • Promotes the normal formation of red blood cells	• Megaloblastic anemia • Diarrhea • Red, sore tongue • Increased rise of neural tube defects and other malformations, preterm delivery • Elevated blood levels of homocysteine	• May mask signs of vitamin B$_{12}$ deficiency (pernicious anemia)	• Fortified, refined grain products (cereals, bread, pasta) • Dark green vegetables (spinach, collards, romaine) • Dried beans

AI (Adequate Intakes) and RDAs (Recommended Dietary Allowances) are for 19–30-year-olds; UL (Upper Limits) are for 19–70-year-olds.

TABLE 6.3 Key Information about Vitamins *(continued)*

Vitamin B₁₂ (cyanocobalamin) AI women: 2.4 mcg men: 2.4 mcg	• Helps maintain nerve tissues • Aids in reactions that build up protein and bone tissues • Needed for normal red blood cell development	• Neurological disorders (nervousness, tingling sensations and numbness in fingers and toes, brain degeneration) • Pernicious anemia characterized by large, oval-shaped red blood cells • Fatigue • Sore, beefy red, smooth tongue	• None known. Excess vitamin B₁₂ is rapidly excreted by the kidneys or is not absorbed into the bloodstream. • Vitamin B₁₂ injections may cause a temporary feeling of heightened energy.	• Fish, seafood • Meat • Milk and cheese • Ready-to-eat cereals
Biotin AI women: 30 mcg men: 30 mcg	• Needed for the body's manufacture of fats, proteins, and glycogen	• Seizures • Vision problems • Muscular weakness • Hearing loss	• None known. Excesses are rapidly excreted.	• Grain and cereal products • Meats, dried beans, cooked eggs • Vegetables
Pantothenic acid (pantothenate) AI women: 5 mg men: 5 mg	• Needed for the release of energy from fat and carbohydrates	• Fatigue, sleep disturbances, impaired coordination, vomiting, nausea	• None known. Excesses are rapidly excreted.	• Many foods, including meats, grains, vegetables, fruits, and milk
Vitamin C (ascorbic acid) RDA women: 75 mg men: 90 mg UL: 2000 mg	• Needed for the manufacture of collagen • Helps the body fight infections, repair wounds • Acts as an antioxidant • Enhances iron absorption	• Bleeding and bruising easily due to weakened blood vessels, cartilage, and other tissues containing collagen • Slow recovery from infections and poor wound healing • Fatigue, depression	• High intakes of 1 g or more per day can cause nausea, cramps, and diarrhea and may increase the risk of kidney stones.	• Fruits: guava, oranges, lemons, limes, strawberries, cantaloupe, grapefruit, kiwi fruit • Vegetables: broccoli, green and red peppers, collards, tomato, potatoes • Ready-to-eat cereals
Choline AI women: 425 mg men: 550 mg UL: 3.5g	• Serves as a structural and signaling component of cell membranes • Required for the normal development of memory and attention processes during early life • Required for the transport and metabolism of fat and cholesterol	• Fatty liver • Infertility • Hypertension	• Low blood pressure • Sweating, diarrhea • Fishy body odor • Liver damage	• Meat (all types) • Eggs • Dried beans • Milk
The fat-soluble vitamins				
Vitamin A₁.Retinol RDA women: 700 mcg men: 900 mcg UL: 3000 mcg	• Needed for the formation and maintenance of mucous membranes, skin, bone • Needed for vision in dim light	• Increased incidence and severity of infectious diseases • Impaired vision, blindness • Inability to see in dim light	• Vitamin A toxicity (hypervitaminosis A) with acute doses of 500,000 IU, or long-term intake of 50,000 IU per day. • Nausea, irritability, blurred vision, weakness, headache • Increased pressure in the skull, hip fracture • Liver damage • Hair loss, dry skin • Birth defects	• Vitamin A is found in animal products only. • Liver, clams, low-fat milk, eggs • Ready-to-eat cereals

TABLE 6.3 Key Information about Vitamins *(continued)*

	Primary functions	Consequences of deficiency	Consequences of overdose	Primary food sources
Beta-carotene (a vitamin A precursor or "provitamin") No RDA; suggested intake: 6 mg	• Acts as an antioxidant; prevents damage to cell membranes and the contents of cells by repairing damage caused by free radicals	• Deficiency disease related only to lack of vitamin A	• High intakes from supplements may increase lung damage in smokers. • With high intakes and supplemental doses (over 12 mg/day for months), skin may turn yellow-orange.	• Deep orange, and dark green vegetables. • Carrots, sweet potatoes, pumpkin, spinach, collards, cantaloupe, apricots, vegetable juice
Vitamin E (alpha-to-copherol) RDA women: 15 mg men: 15 mg UL: 1000 mg	• Acts as an antioxidant, prevents damage to cell membranes in blood cells, lungs, and other tissues by repairing damage caused by free radicals • Participates in the regulation of gene expression	• Muscle loss, nerve damage • Anemia • Weakness	• Intakes of up to 800 IU per day are unrelated to toxic side effects; over 800 IU per day may increase bleeding (blood-clotting time). • Avoid supplement use if aspirin, anticoagulants, or fish oil supplements are taken regularly.	• Nuts and seeds • Vegetable oils • Salad dressings, mayonnaise • Whole grains, wheat germ • Leafy, green vegetables, asparagus
Vitamin D **(vitamin D$_2$ = ergocalciferol, vitamin D$_3$ = cholecalciferol)** RDA women: 15 mcg (600 IU) men: 15 mcg (600 IU) UL: 100 mcg (4000 IU)	• Needed for the absorption of calcium and phosphorus, and for their utilization in bone formation, nerve and muscle activity. • Inhibits inflammation • Involved in insulin secretion and blood glucose level maintenance	• Weak, deformed bones (children) • Loss of calcium from bones (adults), osteoporosis • Increased risk of chronic inflammation • Increased risk of death from all causes	• Mental retardation in young children • Abnormal bone growth and formation • Nausea, diarrhea, irritability, weight loss • Deposition of calcium in organs such as the kidneys, liver, and heart • Toxicity possible with long-term use of 10,000 IU daily	• Vitamin D-fortified milk, cereals, and other foods • Fish and shellfish
Vitamin K **(phylloquinone, menaquinone)** AI women: 90 mcg men: 120 mcg	• Is an essential component of mechanisms that cause blood to clot when bleeding occurs • Aids in the incorporation of calcium into bones	• Bleeding, bruises • Decreased calcium in bones • Deficiency is rare. May be induced by the long-term use (months or more) of antibiotics.	• Toxicity is only a problem when synthetic forms of vitamin K are taken in excessive amounts. That may cause liver disease.	• Leafy, green vegetables • Grain products

Vitamins A, D, E, and K are fat soluble; they are absorbed through the intestinal membranes and stored in the body. The B vitamins and vitamin C are water soluble; they are absorbed directly into the blood and then used up or washed out of the body in urine and sweat. They must be replaced daily.

antioxidants Substances that prevent the damaging effects of oxidation in cells.

Antioxidants prevent the harmful effects caused by oxidation within the body. They include vitamins C and E and beta-carotene (a form of vitamin A), as well as compounds like carotenoids and flavonoids. All share a common target: renegade oxygen cells called free radicals released by normal metabolism as well as by pollution, smoking, radiation, and stress.

Diets high in antioxidant-rich fruits and vegetables have been linked with lower rates of esophageal, lung, colon, and stomach cancer. Nevertheless, scientific studies have not proved conclusively that any specific antioxidant, particularly in supplement form, can prevent cancer.

Folic Acid **Folic acid**, or folate, a B vitamin, reduces the risk of neural tube defects in children. Women planning to become pregnant are advised to take a daily supplement of folic acid starting one month before conception. Another potential benefit, based on a study of more than 85,710 new mothers, may be lower risk of the most severe form of autism.[15] However, folic acid supplementation does not substantially decrease—or increase—the incidence of cancer overall or of specific types, such as cancer of the breast, lung, prostate, or large intestine.[16]

Vitamin D This vitamin, essential for bone health, cognitive function, pain control, and many other processes within the body, comes in two forms:

- Vitamin D_2, from plants (that have been exposed to sunlight) and foods fortified with vitamin D, such as milk, cheese, bread, and juice.

- Vitamin D_3, formed in the skin after exposure to the sun's ultraviolet rays and ingested from animal sources, including some fish.

The benefits of vitamin D include

- Better absorption of calcium.

- Formation and maintenance of strong bones.

- Lower risk of heart disease. Calcium deposits that stiffen the arteries are more likely to develop in people with low levels of vitamin D.

- Enhanced immunity. Adequate amounts of vitamin D may help the body fight off the flu, tuberculosis, and infections of the upper respiratory tract.

Low levels of vitamin D have been linked to heart disease, falls and broken bones, breast cancer, prostate cancer, depression, memory loss, Parkinson's disease, and stroke. In a recent analysis of data on more than a million people, adults with lower levels of vitamin D had a significantly increased risk of dying from heart disease, cancer, or other causes.[17] However, it is not clear if low vitamin D causes disease or simply reflects behaviors that contribute to poor health, such as a sedentary lifestyle, smoking, and a diet high in processed and otherwise unhealthy foods.

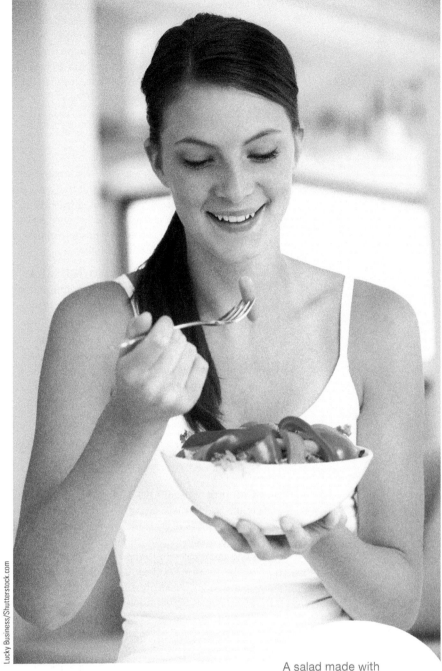

Lucky Business/Shutterstock.com

A salad made with fresh vegetables, rich in antioxidants, can be a nutritious meal choice.

Nearly half of American adults have taken vitamin D supplements. Studies of their effectiveness have yielded mixed results. In one, middle-aged and older adults taking vitamin D_3 had lower overall mortality rates.[18] Others have found "suggestive" but not "highly convincing" evidence that vitamin D can protect against fractures[19] and little or no reduction in the risk of heart attack, stroke, cancer, or bone fractures in the general population.[20] In a meta-analysis of recent research, vitamin D supplements were not effective in lowering blood pressure.[21]

folic acid A form of folate used in vitamin supplements and fortified foods.

Unless used in people with confirmed vitamin D deficiency, vitamin D supplements might actually cause harm.[22] Many experts suggest holding off on vitamin D supplements but improving vitamin D levels with a balanced diet and 30 minutes of sunlight twice a week. Foods fortified with vitamin D may also be beneficial.[23]

✓ **check-in** Have you ever taken a vitamin D supplement?

Minerals Carbon, oxygen, hydrogen, and nitrogen make up 96 percent of our body weight. The other 4 percent consists of **minerals** that help build bones and teeth, aid in muscle function, and help our nervous systems transmit messages. Every day we need the following:

- About one-tenth of a gram (100 milligrams) or more of the major minerals: sodium, potassium chloride, calcium, phosphorus, magnesium, and sulfur

- About one-hundredth of a gram (10 milligrams) or less of each of the trace minerals: iron (although young women need more, particularly if they are physically active), zinc, selenium, molybdenum, iodine, copper, manganese, fluoride, and chromium

Table 6.4 provides more information about minerals.

Calcium Calcium, the most abundant mineral in the body, builds strong bone tissue throughout life and plays a vital role in blood clotting and muscle and nerve functioning. Nursing women need more calcium to meet the additional needs of their babies' bodies. Calcium may also help control high blood pressure, prevent colon cancer in adults, and promote weight loss. Adequate calcium and vitamin D intake during childhood, adolescence, and young adulthood is crucial to prevent osteoporosis, a bone-weakening disease that strikes one of every four women over the age of 60.

The safest way to ensure adequate calcium and vitamin D is by adding foods rich in these nutrients to your diet. Here are the recommended daily intake amounts:

- For women ages 19 to 50 and men ages 19 to 70: 1000 mg

- For women older than 50 and men over 70: 1200 mg

minerals Naturally occurring inorganic substances, small amounts of some being essential in metabolism and nutrition.

Amounts greater than 2000 mg can cause constipation and kidney stones and may put individuals at risk for calcification within their blood vessels and other serious health threats.

In both men and women, bone mass peaks between the ages of 25 and 35. Over the next 10 to 15 years, bone mass remains fairly stable. At about age 40, bone loss equivalent to 0.3 to 0.5 percent per year begins in both men and women. Women may experience greater bone loss, at a rate of 3 to 5 percent, at the time of menopause. This decline continues for approximately 5 to 7 years and is the primary factor leading to postmenopausal osteoporosis.

The higher an individual's peak bone mass, the longer it takes for age- and menopause-related bone loss to increase the risk of fractures. Osteoporosis is less common in groups with higher peak bone mass—men versus women, blacks versus whites. More than 60 percent of middle-aged and older women regularly take calcium supplements, but they may pose potential dangers.

The U.S. Preventive Services Task Force (USPSTF) has recommended against low-dose calcium and vitamin D supplements, citing a possible increased risk of kidney stones and a lack of evidence that they actually prevent fractures. Other studies have linked calcium supplements with other risks, including higher death rates from all causes and from cardiovascular disease.

✓ **check-in** Are you taking steps to strengthen your bones?

Sodium Sodium helps maintain proper fluid balance, regulates blood pressure, transmits muscle impulses, and relaxes muscles. However, excess sodium contributes to high blood pressure, a leading cause of heart disease, kidney disorders, and stroke, and can directly harm the blood vessels, heart, kidneys, and brain.[24] African Americans, who have higher rates of high blood pressure and diseases related to hypertension, such as stroke and kidney failure, tend to be more sensitive to salt.

Nine in 10 Americans consume more sodium (primarily in the form of salt) than they need. The average intake for Americans over age 2 is about 3266 mg per day—much higher than the 1500 mg that the Institute of Medicine has set as the "adequate intake" for individuals ages 9 to 50 and its "tolerable upper limit" of 2300 mg for adolescents over age 14 and all adults. African Americans; individuals with hypertension, diabetes, or chronic kidney disease; and those older than age 51 should cut back to 1500 mg a day.

Salt added at the table and in cooking provides only a small proportion of the sodium Americans

TABLE 6.4 Key Information about Minerals

	Primary functions	Consequences of deficiency	Consequences of overdose	Primary food sources
Calcium AI[a] women: 1000 mg men: 1000 mg UL: 2500 mg	• Component of bones and teeth • Needed for muscle and nerve activity, blood clotting	• Poorly mineralized, weak bones (osteoporosis) • Rickets in children • Osteomalacia (rickets in adults) • Stunted growth in children • Convulsions, muscle spasms	• Drowsiness • Calcium deposits in kidneys, liver, and other tissues • Suppression of bone remodeling • Decreased zinc absorption	• Milk and milk products (cheese, yogurt) • Calcium-fortified foods (some juices, breakfast cereals, soy milk)
Phosphorus RDA women: 700 mg men: 700 mg UL: 4000 mg	• Component of bones and teeth • Component of certain enzymes and other substances involved in energy formation • Needed to maintain the right acid–base balance of body fluids	• Loss of appetite • Nausea, vomiting • Weakness • Confusion • Loss of calcium from bones	• Muscle spasms • Increased risk of cardiovascular disease and osteoporosis	• Milk and milk products (cheese, yogurt) • Meats • Seeds, nuts • Phosphates added to foods
Magnesium RDA women: 310 mg men: 400 mg UL: 350 mg (from supplements only)	• Component of bones and teeth • Needed for nerve activity • Activates hundreds of enzymes involved in energy and protein formation and other body processes	• Stunted growth in children • Weakness • Muscle spasms • Personality changes	• Diarrhea • Dehydration • Impaired nerve activity due to disrupted utilization of calcium	• Plant foods (dried beans, nuts, potatoes, green vegetables) • Ready-to-eat cereals
Iron RDA women: 18 mg men: 8 mg UL: 45 mg	• Transports oxygen as a component of hemoglobin in red blood cells • Component of myoglobin (a muscle protein) • Needed for certain reactions involving energy formation	• Iron deficiency • Iron-deficiency anemia • Weakness, fatigue • Pale appearance • Reduced attention span and resistance to infection • Hair loss • Mental retardation, developmental delay in children • Ice craving • Decreased resistance to infection	• Hemochromatosis ("iron poisoning") • Vomiting, abdominal pain, diarrhea • Blue coloration of skin • Iron deposition in liver and heart • Decreased zinc absorption • Oxidation-related damage to tissues and organs	• Liver, beef, pork • Dried beans • Iron-fortified cereals • Prunes, apricots, raisins • Spinach • Bread
Zinc RDA women: 8 mg men: 11 mg UL: 40 mg	• Required for the activation of many enzymes involved in the reproduction of proteins • Component of insulin, many enzymes	• Growth failure • Delayed sexual maturation • Slow wound healing • Loss of taste and appetite • In pregnancy, low-birth-weight infants and preterm delivery	• Over 25 mg/day is associated with nausea, vomiting, weakness, fatigue, susceptibility to infection, copper deficiency, and metallic taste in mouth. • Increased blood lipids	• Meats (all kinds) • Dried beans • Grains • Nuts • Ready-to-eat cereals
Fluoride AI women: 3 mg men: 4 mg UL: 10 mg	• Component of bones and teeth (enamel) • Helps rebuild enamel that is beginning to decay	• Tooth decay and other dental diseases	• Fluorosis • Brittle bones • Mottled teeth • Nerve abnormalities	• Fluoridated water and foods and beverages made with it • White grape juice • Raisins • Wine

TABLE 6.4 Key Information about Minerals *(continued)*

	Primary functions	Consequences of deficiency	Consequences of overdose	Primary food sources
Iodine RDA women: 150 mcg men: 150 mcg UL: 1100 mcg	• Required for the synthesis of thyroid hormones that help regulate energy production, growth, and development	• Goiter, thyroid disease • Cretinism (mental retardation, hearing loss, growth failure)	• Over 1 mg/day may produce pimples, goiter, decreased thyroid function, and thyroid disease.	• Iodized salt • Milk and milk products • Seaweed, seafoods • Bread from commercial bakeries
Selenium RDA women: 55 mcg men: 55 mcg UL: 400 mcg	• Acts as an antioxidant in conjunction with vitamin E (protects cells from damage due to exposure to oxygen) • Needed for thyroid hormone production	• Anemia • Muscle pain and tenderness • Keshan disease (heart failure), Kashin-Beck disease (joint disease)	• "Selenosis," which includes symptoms of hair and fingernail loss, weakness, liver damage, irritability, and "garlic" or "metallic" breath.	• Fish • Eggs
Copper RDA women: 900 mcg men: 900 mcg UL: 10,000 mcg	• Component of enzymes involved in the body's utilization of iron and oxygen • Functions in growth, immunity, cholesterol and glucose utilization, brain development	• Anemia • Seizures • Nerve and bone abnormalities in children • Growth retardation	• Wilson's disease (excessive accumulation of copper in the liver and kidneys) • Vomiting, diarrhea • Tremors • Liver disease	• Potatoes • Grains • Dried beans • Nuts and seeds • Seafood • Ready-to-eat cereals
Manganese AI women: 2.3 mg men: 1.8 mg	• Needed for the formation of body fat and bone	• Weight loss • Rash • Nausea and vomiting	• Infertility in men • Disruptions in the nervous system, learning impairment • Muscle spasms	• Whole grains • Coffee, tea • Dried beans • Nuts
Chromium AI women: 35 mcg men: 25 mcg	• Required for the normal utilization of glucose and fat	• Elevated blood glucose and triglyceride levels • Weight loss	• Kidney and skin damage	• Whole grains • Wheat germ • Liver, meat • Beer, wine • Oysters
Molybdenum RDA women: 45 mcg men: 45 mcg UL: 2000 mcg	• Component of enzymes involved in the transfer of oxygen from one molecule to another	• Rapid heartbeat and breathing • Nausea, vomiting • Coma	• Loss of copper from the body • Joint pain • Growth failure • Anemia • Gout	• Dried beans • Grains • Dark green vegetables • Liver • Milk and milk products
Sodium AI women: 1500 mg men: 1500 mg UL: 2300 mg	• Needed to maintain the right acid–base balance in body fluids • Helps maintain an appropriate amount of water in blood and body tissues • Needed for muscle and nerve activity	• Weakness • Apathy • Poor appetite • Muscle cramps • Headache • Swelling	• High blood pressure in susceptible people • Kidney disease • Heart problems	• Foods processed with salt • Cured foods (corned beef, ham, bacon, pickles, sauerkraut) • Table and sea salt • Bread • Milk, cheese • Salad dressing

TABLE 6.4 Key Information about Minerals *(continued)*

Potassium AI women: 4700 mg men: 4700 mg UL: Not determined	• Same as for sodium	• Weakness • Irritability, mental confusion • Irregular heartbeat • Paralysis	• Irregular heartbeat, heart attack	• Plant foods (potatoes, squash, lima beans, tomatoes, plantains, bananas, oranges, avocados) • Meats • Milk and milk products • Coffee
Chloride AI women: 2300 mg men: 2300 mg UL: 3600 mg	• Component of hydrochloric acid secreted by the stomach (used in digestion) • Needed to maintain the right acid–base balance of body fluids • Helps maintain an appropriate water balance in the body	• Muscle cramps • Apathy • Poor appetite • Long-term mental retardation in infants	• Vomiting	• Same as for sodium (most of the chloride in our diets comes from salt)

consume. The most common sources are commercially packaged and restaurant foods.[25]

Here is what you can do to lower your sodium intake:

• **Look for labels that say "low sodium."** They contain 140 mg or less of sodium per serving.

• **Learn to use spices and herbs** rather than salt to enhance the flavor of food.

• **Go easy on condiments** such as soy sauce, pickles, olives, ketchup, and mustard, which can add a lot of salt to your food.

• **Always check the amount of sodium in processed foods,** such as frozen dinners, packaged mixes, cereals, salad dressings, and sauces. The amount in different types and brands can vary widely.

✓**check-in** Are you consuming too much sodium?

Vegetables and Fruits The *Dietary Guidelines* recommend eating more vegetables and fruits because they

• Provide many nutrients that many Americans lack.

• Lower the risk of many chronic illnesses, including type 2 diabetes, cardiovascular disease (including heart attack and stroke), and certain cancers.

• Help individuals reach and maintain a healthy weight.

• Lessen the risk of dying. In a recent study, individuals who ate seven or more portions of fresh fruits and vegetables a day had a 42 percent lower risk of death at any age than those who ate less than one portion a day. Even those who ate just one portion had lower death rates.[26]

Fewer than one-third of American adults eat the recommended amounts of fruits and vegetables. College-age young adults between ages 18 and 24 eat the fewest vegetables. Nearly four-fifths of this group don't put vegetables on their plates—or scrape them to the side if they do. About one in four teenagers eats fruit less than once a day.

American adults average about one cup of fruit a day—half the recommended amount. Two-thirds comes from whole fruit; one-third, from juice.

To increase your fruit and vegetable intake try these tips:

• **Toss fruit into a green salad** for extra flavor, variety, color, and crunch.

• **Start the day with a daily double:** a glass of juice and a banana or other fruit on cereal.

• **Buy precut vegetables** for snacking or dipping (instead of chips).

• **Fill half your dinner plate with vegetables.**

• **Make or order sandwiches** with extra tomatoes or other vegetable toppings.

(See Snapshot: On Campus Now.)

✓**check-in** Which is better for you: fruit or fruit juice? As long as you drink 100-percent juice, you can choose either—or, better yet, both. According to a nutritional analysis, a combination of whole fruit and 100-percent juice boosts potassium and vitamin C

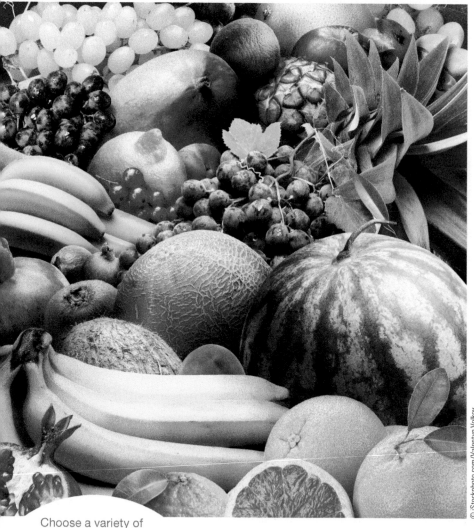

Choose a variety of fruits and vegetables to get the full range of nutrients.

access to a variety of fruits and is a cost-effective way to help people meet fruit recommendations.[27]

Milk and Milk Products Dairy products provide many nutrients, including calcium, vitamin D, and potassium, and may improve bone health, lower blood pressure, and reduce the risk of cardiovascular disease and type 2 diabetes. The *Dietary Guidelines* recommend 3 cups a day or the equivalent for adults—ideally from nonfat or low-fat dairy products. Soy beverages fortified with calcium and vitamins A and D are considered part of the dairy product food group.

Alcohol As discussed in Chapter 12, about half of Americans regularly drink alcohol. Depending on the amount consumed, age, and other factors, alcohol can have harmful or beneficial effects. However, there is no nutritional need for alcohol. The *Dietary Guidelines* note that no one should begin drinking or drink more frequently on the basis of potential health benefits because moderate alcohol consumption, though associated with a lower risk of cardiovascular disease, also is linked with increased risks of breast cancer, violence, drowning, and injuries from falls and motor vehicle crashes.

Phytochemicals **Phytochemicals**, compounds that exist naturally in plants, serve many functions, including helping a plant protect itself from bacteria and disease, giving tomatoes their red color, and putting "fire" into hot peppers. In the body, they act as antioxidants, mimic hormones, and reduce the risk of various illnesses, including cancer and heart disease (see Table 6.5 for good sources). Good sources include broccoli, tomatoes, and soybeans.

without significantly increasing total calories. Not only does 100-percent fruit juice deliver essential nutrients and phytonutrients, but it also provides year-round

© iStockphoto.com/Valentyn Volkov

SNAPSHOT: ON CAMPUS NOW

Are You Eating Your Veggies?

College students who report:	Male	Female	Average
Eating no servings of fruits and vegetables a day	7.4	4.9	5.8
Eating one to two servings	60.1	56.1	57.5
Eating three to four servings	26.9	32.0	30.2
Eating five or more servings	5.6	7.0	6.5

✓ **check-in** For a three-day period (including one weekend day), keep track of your veggie intake. Put a star by those you like most. If you aren't getting at least five servings a day, add at least one of your favorites every day. Record your observations in your online journal.

Source: American College Health Association. *American College Health Association–National College Health Assessment II: Reference Group Executive Summary, Spring 2014.* Hanover, MD: American College Health Association, 2014.

Phytochemicals give tomatoes their red color and hot peppers their "fire." In the body, they act as antioxidants, mimic hormones, and reduce the risk of various illnesses, including cancer and heart disease (see Table 6.5). Broccoli may contain as many as 10,000 different phytochemicals, each capable of influencing some action or organ in the body. Tomatoes provide lycopene, a powerful antioxidant that seems to offer protection against cancers of the esophagus, lungs, prostate, and stomach. Soybeans, a rich source of an array of phytochemicals, appear to slow the growth of breast and prostate cancer.

Dietary Supplements   About half of adults in the United States use dietary supplements, most often multivitamins to improve or maintain overall health.[28] However, many supplements, including vitamins C and E, have failed to deliver on their promised benefits in rigorous, randomized controlled trials. Folic acid and other B vitamins, once believed to prevent heart disease and strokes, may increase cancer risk in high doses. Here are the most recent findings:

- Treatment with beta-carotene, vitamin A, and vitamin E may increase mortality, whereas vitamin D supplementation may reduce mortality.

- Vitamin B supplementation may protect against stroke but has no effect on cardiovascular disease or cancer.

- Omega-3 fatty acids have shown no protective effects on cardiovascular disease.[29]

Years of research have found no clear evidence of a beneficial effect of supplements on all-cause mortality, cardiovascular disease, or cancer.

In a study at five American universities, about two-thirds of students took dietary supplements

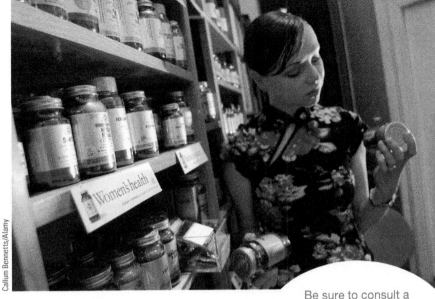

Callum Bennetts/Alamy

at least once a week, while 12 percent consumed five or more supplements a week. The most commonly used were these:

- Multivitamins (42 percent)
- Vitamin C (18 percent)
- Protein/amino acids (17 percent)
- Calcium (13 percent)

Students take supplements primarily to promote general health, provide more energy, increase muscle strength, or enhance performance. Yet, researchers note, college students typically are not deficient in crucial nutrients, and there is little or no evidence that the supplements provide the desired benefits.[30]

√**check-in** Do you take dietary supplements? If so, why do you use them?

Be sure to consult a health professional and read labels carefully before you start taking a dietary supplement.

phytochemicals Chemicals such as indoles, coumarins, and capsaicin, which exist naturally in plants and have disease-fighting properties.

TABLE 6.5 Color-Coding Your Vegetables and Fruits

Color	Phytochemical Antioxidant	Vegetable and Fruit Sources
Red	Lycopene (*lie-co-peen*)	Tomatoes, red raspberries, watermelon, strawberries, red peppers
Yellow-green	Lutein zeaxanthin (*lou-te-in, ze-ah-zan-thun*)	Leafy greens, avocado, honeydew melon, kiwi fruit
Red-purple	Anthocyanins (*antho-sigh-ah-nins*)	Grapes, berries, wine, red apples, plums, prunes
Orange	Beta-carotene	Carrots, mangos, papayas, apricots, pumpkins, yams
Orange-yellow	Flavonoids (*fla-von-oids*)	Oranges, tangerines, lemons, plums, peaches, cantaloupe
Green	Glucosinolates (*glu-co-sin-oh-lates*)	Broccoli, brussels sprouts, kale, cabbage
White-green	Allyl sulfides (*al-lill sulf-ides*)	Onions, leeks, garlic

© Cengage Learning

YOUR STRATEGIES FOR CHANGE

Creating a Healthy Eating Pattern

- **Limit calorie intake to the amount needed** to attain or maintain a healthy weight.

- **Consume foods from all food groups** in nutrient-dense forms and in recommended amounts.

- **Reduce intake of solid fats**.

- **Replace solid fats with oils**.

- **Reduce intake of added sugars**.

- **Reduce intake of refined grains** and replace some refined grains with whole grains.

- **Reduce intake of sodium**.

- If consumed, **limit alcohol intake to moderate levels**.

- **Increase intake of vegetables and fruits**.

- **Increase intake of whole grains**.

- **Increase intake of milk and milk products** and replace whole milk and full-fat milk products with nonfat or low-fat choices to reduce solid fat intake.

- **Increase seafood intake** by replacing some meat or poultry with seafood.

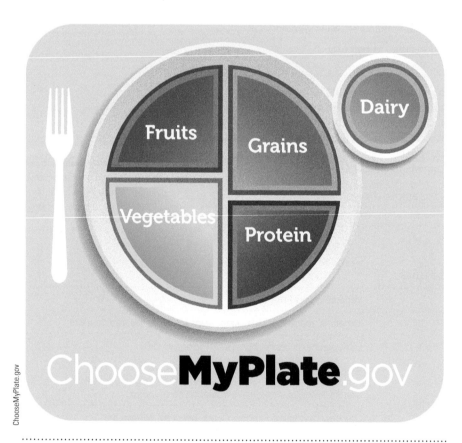

FIGURE 6.4 The MyPlate System

The most recent food pattern from the USDA reminds Americans to balance calories, increase foods such as fruits and vegetables, and drink fat-free or low-fat milk.

Healthy Eating Patterns

There is no one "right" way to eat. A healthy eating pattern is not a rigid prescription but an array of options that can accommodate cultural, ethnic, traditional, and personal preferences as well as food costs and availability.

Although healthy eating patterns vary around the world, most

- Are abundant in vegetables and fruits

- Emphasize whole grains

- Suggest moderate amounts

- Emphasize a variety of foods high in protein (seafood, beans and peas, nuts, seeds, soy products, meat, poultry, eggs)

- Include only limited amounts of food high in added sugars

- May include more oils than solid fats

- Are generally low in full-fat dairy products, although some include substantial amounts of low-fat milk and milk products

Compared to typical American diets, these patterns tend to have a high unsaturated to saturated fat ratio and a high dietary fiber and potassium content. Some are also relatively low in sodium compared to current American intake.

✓**check-in** How does your diet compare with this healthy eating pattern?

Among the research-based healthy eating patterns are the U.S. Department of Agriculture's (USDA's) MyPlate and Food Patterns, the Dietary Approaches to Stop Hypertension (DASH) plan, the Mediterranean diet, and vegetarian diets.

MyPlate

In 2011 the USDA introduced a new food pattern icon: MyPlate. Rather than providing specific directives, it serves as a visual reminder for healthy eating (see Figure 6.4), based on the key themes of the most recent *Dietary Guidelines*:

Balancing Calories

- Enjoy your food but eat less.

- Avoid oversized portions.

Foods to Increase

- Make half your plate fruits and vegetables.
- Make at least half your grains whole grains.
- Switch to nonfat or low-fat (1%) milk.

Foods to Reduce

- Compare sodium in foods like soup, bread, and frozen meals and choose those with lower numbers.
- Drink water instead of sugary drinks.

The USDA Food Patterns

These approaches identify daily amounts of foods to eat from five major food groups and subgroups: vegetables, fruits and juices, grains, milk and milk products, and protein foods. They also include an allowance for oils and limits on the maximum number of calories that should be consumed from solid fats and added sugars. Amounts and limits are given at different calorie levels, ranging from 1,000 to 3,200. All the USDA Food Patterns emphasize selection of a variety of foods in nutrient-dense forms—that is, with little or no solid fats and added sugars—from each food group.

The USDA Food Patterns include a vegan pattern, which consists of only plant foods and substitutes calcium-fortified beverages and foods for dairy products, and a lacto-ovo-vegetarian pattern, which includes milk, milk products, and eggs.

The DASH Eating Plan

DASH emphasizes vegetables, fruits, and low-fat milk and milk products; includes whole grains, poultry, seafood, and nuts; and is lower in sodium, red and processed meats, sweets, and sugar-containing beverages than typical intakes in the United States (See Table 6.6). In research studies, DASH approaches have proven to lower blood pressure, improve blood lipids, and reduce the risk of cardiovascular disease.

The Mediterranean Diet

Because many cultures and agricultural patterns exist in the countries that border the Mediterranean Sea, the "Mediterranean diet" is not one set way of eating but an eating pattern that emphasizes vegetables, fruits and nuts, olive oil, and grains (often whole grains), with only small amounts of meats and full-fat milk and milk products.

Scientists have identified antioxidants in red wine and olive oil that may account for the beneficial effects on the heart of the Mediterranean diet, which features lots of fruits and vegetables,

TABLE 6.6 The DASH Eating Plan

USDA/DASH recommendations for a 2,000-calorie daily diet include

- Fruit Group—2–2.5 cups (4–5 servings) of fresh, frozen, canned, or dried fruit, with only limited juice
- Vegetable Group—2–2.5 cups (4–5 servings)
- Dark greens, such as broccoli and leafy greens—3 cups per week
- Orange vegetables, such as carrots and sweet potatoes—2 cups per week
- Legumes, such as pinto or kidney beans, split peas, or lentils—3 cups per week
- Starchy vegetables—3 cups per week
- Other vegetables—6.5 cups per week

- Grain Group—6–8 ounce-equivalents of cereal, bread, crackers, rice, or pasta, with at least 50% whole grain

- Meat and Beans Group—5.5–6 ounce-equivalents of baked, broiled, or grilled lean meat, poultry, or fish, eggs, nuts, seeds, beans, peas, or tofu

- Milk Group—2–3 cups low-fat/fat-free milk, yogurt, or cheese, or lactose-free, calcium-fortified products

- Oils—2–6 teaspoons

- Discretionary—267 calories; for example, solid fats (saturated fat such as butter, margarine, shortening, or lard) or added sugar

www.usda.gov

legumes, nuts, and grains (see Figure 6.5). Among its health benefits are

- Reduced risk of asthma and progressive lung disease, as well as cardiovascular disease
- Lower body mass index (BMI), body fat, and waist-to-hip ratios
- Lower risk of metabolic syndrome and cardiovascular disease[31] (discussed in Chapter 10)
- Less narrowing of the arteries in the legs[32]
- Lower risk of stroke[33]

Strict adherence to the Mediterranean diet has proven so beneficial that many physicians recommend its use for the general population, regardless of gender, age, family history of heart disease, diabetes, smoking status, hypertension, or fitness.[34]

Vegetarian Diets

Among the followers of vegetarian diets are

- Lacto-ovo-pesco-vegetarians, who eat dairy products, eggs, and fish but not red meat.
- Lacto-vegetarians, who eat dairy products as well as grains, fruits, and vegetables.
- Ovo-lacto-vegetarians, who also eat eggs.
- Vegans, or pure vegetarians, who eat only plant foods. They may take vitamin B_{12} supplements because that vitamin is normally found only in animal products.

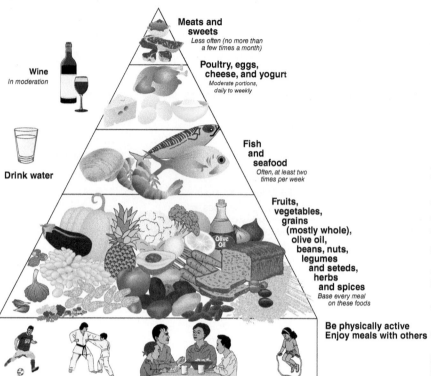

Mediterranean Diet Pyramid
A contemporary approach to delicious, healthy eating

Meats and sweets
Less often (no more than a few times a month)

Wine
In moderation

Poultry, eggs, cheese, and yogurt
Moderate portions, daily to weekly

Drink water

Fish and seafood
Often, at least two times per week

Fruits, vegetables, grains (mostly whole), olive oil, beans, nuts, legumes and seeds, herbs and spices
Base every meal on these foods

Be physically active
Enjoy meals with others

FIGURE 6.5 The Traditional Healthy Mediterranean Diet Pyramid

The key to getting sufficient protein from a vegetarian diet is understanding the concept of complementary proteins. Recall that meat, poultry, fish, eggs, and dairy products are complete proteins that provide the nine essential amino acids—substances that the human body cannot produce itself. Incomplete proteins, such as legumes or nuts, may have relatively low levels of one or two essential amino acids but fairly high levels of others.

By combining complementary protein sources, vegetarians can make sure their bodies make the most of the nonanimal proteins they eat. Many cultures rely heavily on complementary foods for protein. In Middle Eastern cooking, sesame seeds and chickpeas are a popular combination; in Latin American dishes, beans and rice, or beans and tortillas; in Chinese cuisine, soy and rice.

Vegetarians can best meet their nutrient needs by paying special attention to protein, iron, vitamin B_{12}, calcium, and vitamin D. Instead of a 6-ounce serving of meat, they can substitute one egg, 1.5 ounces of nuts, or 2/3 cup of legumes. Those who avoid milk because of its lactose content may obtain all the nutrients of milk by using lactose-reduced milk or eating other calcium-rich foods, such as broccoli, calcium-fortified orange juice, and fortified soy milk.

Vegetarian diets have proven health benefits, including the following:

- Lower cholesterol levels
- Healthier weight
- Decreased risk of heart disease
- Lower incidences of breast, colon, and prostate cancer; high blood pressure; and osteoporosis

Even people who are not strict vegetarians but who eat more plant foods (whole grains, beans, vegetables, fruits, nuts) than animal products lower their risk of dying from heart disease or a stroke.[35]

√**check-in** Are you a vegetarian? If so, which type? How do you ensure an adequate amount of protein in your diet?

Ethnic Cuisines

Whatever your cultural heritage, you have probably sampled Chinese, Mexican, Indian, Italian, and Japanese foods. If you belong to any of these ethnic groups, you may eat these cuisines regularly. Each type of ethnic cooking has its own nutritional benefits and potential drawbacks.

The cuisine served in Mexico features rice, corn, and beans, which are low in fat and high in nutrients. However, the dishes Americans think of as Mexican are far less healthful. Burritos, especially when topped with cheese and sour cream, are very high in fat. Although guacamole has a high fat content, it contains mostly monounsaturated fatty acids, a better form of fat.

African American cuisine traces some of its roots to food preferences from western Africa (for example, peanuts, okra, and black-eyed peas), as well as to traditional American foods, such as fish, game, greens, and sweet potatoes. It uses many nutritious vegetables, such as collard greens and sweet potatoes, as well as legumes. However, some dishes include high-fat food products such as peanuts and pecans or involve frying, sometimes in saturated fat.

The mainland Chinese diet, which is plant-based, high in carbohydrates, and low in fats and animal protein, is considered one of the most healthful in the world. However, Chinese restaurants in the United States serve more meat and sauces than are generally eaten in China. According to laboratory tests of typical take-out dishes from Chinese restaurants, many have more fats and cholesterol than hamburger or egg dishes from fast-food outlets.

Traditional French cuisine, which includes rich, high-fat sauces and dishes, has never been considered healthful. Yet, nutritionists have been stumped to explain the so-called French paradox. Despite a diet high in saturated fats, the French have had one of the lowest rates of coronary artery disease in the world. The French diet increasingly resembles the American diet, but French portions tend to be one-third to one-half the size of American portions.

Many Indian dishes highlight healthful ingredients such as vegetables and legumes (beans and peas). However, many also use *ghee* (a form of butter), which is rich in harmful saturated fats. The best advice in an Indian restaurant is to ask how each dish is prepared. Good choices include *daal* or *dal* (lentils), *karbi* or *karni* (chickpea soup), and *chapati* (tortilla-like bread).

The traditional Japanese diet is very low in fat, which may account for the low incidence of heart disease in Japan. Dietary staples include soybean products, fish, vegetables, noodles, and rice. A variety of fruits and vegetables are also included in many dishes. However, Japanese cuisine is high in salted, smoked, and pickled foods. Watch out for deep-fried dishes such as tempura and salty soups and sauces.

Table 6.7 summarizes some of the ethnic food choices by food group.

The Way We Eat

Your ethnic background and family makeup influenced the way you ate as a child. In college, you probably will find yourself eating in different—and not necessarily better—ways. Because the United States is so diverse, you also will have the opportunity to sample the cuisines of many cultures. However, in this country and others, many do not have enough to eat.

Campus Cuisine: How College Students Eat

Often on their own for the first time, college students typically change their usual eating patterns. When they are making meal choices, the top two influences on students are price and convenience, with nutrition coming in third.

As mentioned at the beginning of this chapter, a growing problem on many campuses is "food insecurity," defined as limited or uncertain availability of healthful foods and limited or uncertain ability to acquire healthful foods. In a survey of 354 students at an Oregon university, 59 percent reported difficulty getting enough healthy food—four

TABLE 6.7 Ethnic Food Choices

	Grains	Vegetables	Fruits	Meats and Legumes	Milk
Asian	Rice, noodles, millet	Amaranth, baby corn, bamboo shoots, chayote, bok choy, mung bean sprouts, sugar peas, straw mushrooms, water chestnuts, kelp	Carambola, guava, kumquat, lychee, persimmon, melons, mandarin orange	Soybeans and soy products such as soy milk and tofu, squid, duck eggs, pork, poultry, fish and other seafood, peanuts, cashews	Usually excluded
Mediterranean	Pita pocket bread, pastas, rice, couscous, polenta, bulgur, focaccia, Italian bread	Eggplant, tomatoes, peppers, cucumbers, grape leaves	Olives, grapes, figs	Fish and other seafood, gyros, lamb, chicken, beef, pork, sausage, lentils, fava beans	Ricotta, provolone, parmesan, feta, mozzarella, and goat cheeses; yogurt
Mexican	Tortillas (corn or flour), taco shells, rice	Chayote, corn, jicama, tomato salsa, cactus, cassava, tomatoes, yams, chilies	Guava, mango, papaya, avocado, plantain, bananas, oranges	Refried beans, fish, chicken, chorizo, beef, eggs	Cheese, custard

Becky Luigart-Stayner/Encyclopedia/Corbis

Photodisc/Getty Images

Mitch Hrdlicka/PhotoDisc/Getty Images

YOUR STRATEGIES FOR CHANGE

Make Smart Choices

Do

- **Choose a healthy snack:** an apple, peanut butter on whole-wheat crackers, or a small handful of nuts, sunflower seeds, and dried fruit instead of a bag of chips.

- **Add a salad to your lunch or dinner** (with low-fat dressing!).

- **At one meal (or more) a day, drink water or skim milk.**

Don't

- **Supersize your fries.**

- **Eat when you are feeling lonely or sad.**

- **Choose a candy bar at the vending machine:** choose trail mix instead.

times higher than the nearly 15 percent of U.S. households that report a lack of food and fear of Employed students including those working full time, were almost twice as likely to report food insecurity.

Many factors may be contributing to the increase in food insecurity, including rising costs for tuition, room, and board; parents' more limited resources; greater competition for work-study jobs; and lack of food stamps or other safety-net services. However, eating healthfully doesn't have to cost more. (See Health on a Budget.)

Even when cost is not an issue, college students don't necessarily get all the nutrients they need. The proportion of 18- to 24-year-olds who eat the recommended amounts of fruits and vegetables is generally lower than in the population as a whole. College men eat fewer fruits and vegetables than women do; Caucasian and Asian students eat more than African American undergraduates. Both African American and Hispanic students consume less than multiracial or other racial/ethnic groups.

Time pressures often affect students' food choices. More than half say they tend to eat on the run, and they consume more soft drinks, fast food, total fat, and saturated fat. A significant number of undergraduates feel they don't have time to sit down and share a meal with friends or family. Yet students who take time for a social meal make better food choices, including eating more fruits and vegetables.

Some colleges are doing their part to improve student nutrition. Many post nutritional information in dining halls; some have expanded their offerings to include more salads, fewer fried foods, and more ethnic dishes. A few have started to offer free bag lunches to students who might otherwise go hungry.

✓**check-in** Are nutritious food choices easily available at your school?

HEALTH ON A BUDGET

Frugal Food Choices

Many people feeling a budget squeeze opt for the cheapest foods they can find, even if they're high in fat and calories and low in nutrients. Such short-term choices can lead to long-term health problems. Here are some ways to eat healthfully for less:

- **Drink tap water.** It's cheaper than bottled and just as safe. Don't waste money on fortified drinks, which offer no proven additional nutritional value. Sugar-sweetened drinks add extra calories as well as extra costs.

- **Consider the cost of convenience.** Prepackaged grab-and-go items such as individual packets of baby carrots or crackers and cheese may be handy but cost more. Buy larger bags or boxes and create your own easy-carry single servings with small reusable containers.

- **Avoid fad fruits.** Pomegranates and other exotic fruits are indeed rich in antioxidants but so are much cheaper oranges and seasonal berries.

- **Freeze.** If you have access to a freezer, take advantage of grocery store sales and stock up on frozen fruits and vegetables, which—thanks to advances in preservation and freezing methods—provide plenty of nutrients.

- **Bulk up.** Join with your roommates or friends and check for low prices on large quantities at the local co-op as well as national mega-stores.

- **Eat seasonally.** Take advantage of the low prices on watermelon in summer or apples in autumn.

- **Look for an Asian grocery store,** if you're a vegan and eat a lot of ramen dishes. Ramen usually costs much less at such stores, but be sure to ask for vegetarian ramen.

- **Sign up for "loyalty" cards** that qualify you for discount or special offers at local grocery stores.

- **Compare unit prices** listed on shelves to get the best price.

Fast Food: Eating on the Run

Young adults (ages 20 to 29) consume approximately 40 percent of their daily calories away from home and eat at fast-food restaurants an average of two to three times a week. Those who frequently eat at burger-and-fries restaurants have a higher intake of sugar-sweetened beverages, total calories, and total fat and saturated fats; a lower intake of healthful foods and key ingredients; and a greater risk of being overweight or obese.

Many fast foods are high in calories, sugar, salt, and fat and low in beneficial nutrients:

- A Burger King Whopper with cheese contains 760 calories and 47 grams of fat, 16 grams from saturated fat.

- A McDonald's Sausage McMuffin with egg has 450 calories and 27 grams of fat, 10 grams from saturated fat.

Although fast-food chains have increased the total number of menu offerings, the average calorie count has not changed much. The average lunch or dinner entrée has 453 calories; the average side dish has 263 calories. (See Table 6.8 on page 164 for more information about choices at fast-food eateries.)

Even a single junk food meal can damage arteries. A recent study compared the effects on blood vessels of a Mediterranean-style meal of salmon, almonds, and vegetables cooked in olive oil and a meal of a sausage, cheese, and egg sandwich with hash browns. Within hours, the junk food meal constricted blood flow through the arteries; the Mediterranean-style meal did not. (See Health Now! for specific strategies to use at fast-food restaurants.)

✓**check-in** How many fast-food meals do you eat in a week?

His Plate, Her Plate: Gender and Nutrition

Men and women do not need to eat different foods, but their nutritional needs are different: Because most men are bigger and taller than most women, they consume more calories. On average, a moderately active 125-pound woman needs 2,000 calories a day; a 175-pound man with a similar exercise pattern needs 2,800 calories.

Here are some gender-specific strategies for better nutrition:

- **Men should cut back on fat and meat.**

- **Women should increase their iron intake** by eating meat (iron from animal sources

is absorbed better than that from vegetable sources) or a combination of meat and vegetable iron sources together (for example, a meat and bean burrito). According to the USDA, most women consume only 60 percent of the recommended 18 milligrams of iron per day. (The recommendation for men is 8 milligrams.)

- **Women should consume more calcium-rich foods,** including low-fat and nonfat dairy products, leafy greens, and tofu.

- **Women who could become pregnant should take a multivitamin** with 400 micrograms of folic acid, which helps prevent neural tube defects such as spina bifida.

You Are What You Drink

Water—tap or bottled, sparkling or still, chilled or room temperature—is the medical experts' beverage of choice. But don't think that "fortified" or "enriched" water is better. There is no evidence that nutrients added to water confer any health benefits. Consumers who assume that they're getting vitamins in their drinks may think they don't need to eat healthful foods and could end up shortchanging themselves of vital nutrients.

Soft Drinks According to a national survey, two-thirds of adults drink sugar-sweetened beverages, averaging 28 ounces per drink and almost 300 calories daily (15 percent of recommended total calories). Soda consumption has decreased among young adults, although one in five still qualify as heavy users.

About 37 percent of the added sugar in Americans' diets comes from sugar-sweetened beverages. One 12-ounce can of regular soda contains 9 teaspoons of sugar (about 140 calories)—enough to put individuals into a higher-risk category for heart disease if they drink soda daily.[36]

✓**check-in** Did you know that drinking a can of soda a day could increase your risk of dying of heart disease by one-third?

Among the health dangers associated with sweetened drinks are

- Increased calorie intake, higher body weight, lower consumption of calcium and other nutrients, and greater risk of diabetes

- Possible greater risk of heart disease

HEALTH NOW!

More Healthful Fast-Food Choices

Fast-food restaurants may be the cheapest option, but unfortunately, they are not usually the most healthful one. Eating just one fast-food meal can pack enough calories, sodium, and fat for an entire day:

- Just two or more high-fat fast-food meals a week have been linked to increased risk of diabetes.

- Seemingly healthful choices, such as a "Mac Snack Wrap," can be low in calories (330) but extremely high in fat (19 grams).

Steps to Take

- **Drink water instead of soda.** One 32-ounce Big Gulp with regular cola packs about 425 calories.

- **Eat your food naked.** Avoid calorie- and fat-packed spreads, cheese, sour cream, and so on. If you sample the salad bar, steer clear of mayonnaise, bacon bits, oily vegetable salads, and rich dressings.

- **Choose small portions.** Since an average fast-food meal can run as high as 1,000 calories or more, don't supersize anything. A single serving often provides enough for two meals. Take half home or divide with a friend.

- **Hold the salt.** Fast-food restaurant food tends to be very high in sodium, so don't add any more.

- **Savor each bite.** If you order fries, eat each one slowly and pay attention to its smell, texture, and taste. Ask yourself, "Do I really need to eat a whole container, or am I satisfied after a handful?"

Try these tips the next time you go to a fast-food restaurant, and describe your experience in your online journal. See Table 6.8 on page 164 for some specific choices.

TABLE 6.8 A Fast-Food Nutrition Survival Guide

Less Healthful Choices	More Healthful Choices
Burger Chains	
Double-patty hamburger with cheese, mayo, special sauce, and bacon	Regular, single-patty hamburger without mayo or cheese
Fried chicken sandwich	Grilled chicken sandwich
Fried fish sandwich	Veggie burger
Salad with toppings such as bacon, cheese, and ranch dressing	Garden salad with grilled chicken and low-fat dressing
Breakfast burrito with steak	Egg on a muffin
French fries	Plain baked potato or a side salad
Milkshake	Yogurt parfait
Chicken "nuggets" or tenders	Grilled chicken strips
Adding cheese, extra mayo, and special sauces	Limiting cheese, mayo, and special sauces
Fried Chicken Chains	
Fried chicken, original or extra-crispy	Skinless chicken breast without breading
Teriyaki wings or popcorn chicken	Honey BBQ chicken sandwich
Caesar salad	Garden salad
Chicken and biscuit "bowl"	Mashed potatoes
Adding extra gravy and sauces	Limiting gravy and sauces
Taco Chains	
Crispy shell chicken taco	Grilled chicken soft taco
Refried beans	Black beans
Steak chalupa	Shrimp ensalada
Crunch wraps or gordita-type burritos	Grilled "fresco"-style steak burrito
Nachos with refried beans	Veggie and bean burrito
Adding sour cream or cheese	Limiting sour cream or cheese
Sub, Sandwich, and Deli Choices	
Foot-long sub	Six-inch sub
High-fat meat such as ham, tuna salad, bacon, meatballs, or steak	Lean meat (roast beef, chicken breast, lean ham) or veggies
The "normal" amount of higher-fat (cheddar, American) cheese	One or two slices of lower-fat cheese (Swiss or mozzarella)
Adding mayo and special sauces	Low-fat dressing or mustard instead of mayo
An "as is" sub with all the toppings	Extra veggie toppings
White bread or "wraps," which are often higher in fat than normal bread	Choosing whole-grain bread or taking the top slice off your sub and eating it open-faced
Asian Food Choices	
Fried egg rolls, spare ribs, tempura	Egg drop, miso, wonton, or hot and sour soup
Battered or deep-fried dishes (sweet-and-sour pork, General Tso's chicken)	Stir-fried, steamed, roasted, or broiled entrées (shrimp chow mein, chop suey)
	Steamed or baked tofu
Deep-fried tofu	Sauces such as ponzu, rice-wine vinegar, wasabi, ginger, and low-sodium soy sauce
Coconut milk, sweet-and-sour sauce, regular soy sauce	
Fried rice	Steamed brown rice
Salads with fried or crispy noodles	Edamame, cucumber salad, stir-fried veggies
Italian and Pizza Restaurant Choices	
Thick-crust pizza with extra cheese and meat toppings	Thin-crust pizza with half the cheese and extra veggies
Garlic bread	Plain rolls or breadsticks
Antipasto with meat	Antipasto with vegetables
Pasta with cream or butter-based sauce	Pasta with tomato sauce and veggies
Entrée with side of pasta	Entrée with side of veggies
Fried ("frito") dishes	Grilled ("griglia") dishes

© Cengage Learning

- Increased likelihood of metabolic syndrome, even with just a single daily soft drink, either diet or regular

- Damage to tooth enamel from sweetened iced tea and many carbonated beverages

- Thinning of hip bones in women who drink regular and diet cola

✓**check-in** Do you love sugary soda? Swapping just one soda a day for water or unsweetened coffee or tea could lower your risk of diabetes by up to 25 percent.[37]

Rather than satisfying a sweet tooth, soft drinks seem to do the opposite and either increase hunger or decrease feelings of satiety or fullness. Even diet drinks made with artificial sweeteners may "condition" people to eat more sweets and increase the risk of diabetes.[38] Diet-soda drinkers who are overweight or obese consume more solid food and calories than those who drink sugary beverages.[39]

Energy Drinks   Energy drinks have become the fastest-growing part of the beverage market in the United States:

- Americans consume more than 6 billion of these caffeinated beverages a year.

- The most frequent users include younger adults, males, Hispanics, blacks, nonmarried individuals, adults with higher family incomes, those living in the South or West, and those who engage in some leisure-time physical activity.

- About 6 percent of young men in the United States report consuming an energy drink every day.

- About eight in ten students at two-year and four-year colleges, online universities, and technical schools, report using energy drinks in the previous year. Although many students use caffeine-fueled concoctions for a physical or mental edge, there is little scientific evidence to indicate that they provide any benefit.

✓**check-in** Do you consume energy drinks? If so, how often?

Some energy drinks contain 15 times the amount of caffeine in a 12-ounce serving of cola. Red Bull, for instance, contains nearly 80 mg of caffeine per can, about the same amount of caffeine as a cup of brewed coffee and twice the caffeine of a cup of tea. Other brands contain several times this amount.

Energy drink formulations vary widely. Some contain fruit juices, teas, and dietary supplements such as ginseng, glucuronolactone, and taurine, a substance that plays an important role in muscle contraction (especially in the heart) and the nervous system. We know very little about the effects of such ingredients, which may work synergistically with caffeine to boost its stimulant power. Frequent or heavy use can trigger physical and psychological complications, including the following:

- Disrupted sleep

- Exaggerated stress response

- Heart palpitations

- Increased risk of high blood pressure

- Panic attacks

- Irritability

- Tremors

- Anxiety

- Depression

- Substance abuse

- Digestive problems

- Cardiac arrhythmia

Toxic levels of caffeine can cause sudden death or life-threatening conditions, such as acute kidney damage, hepatitis, seizures, strokes, coronary artery spasms, and heart attack. Emergency department visits related to energy drinks have more than doubled in recent years.

Doctors recommend that all adults limit their caffeine intake to 500 mg a day, with a lesser amount for those who have heart problems, high blood pressure, or trouble sleeping or who are taking medications. The recommended maximum for adolescents is 100 mg of caffeine a day. (See Table 6.9 for amounts of caffeine in cans and cups.)

The practice of mixing energy drinks with alcohol (discussed in Chapter 13) is especially dangerous, leading to a state some call "wide-awake drunkenness," in which drinkers cannot fully assess their true level of impairment and are more likely to engage in risky behaviors, such as driving while intoxicated. Students consuming alcohol mixed with energy drinks are twice as likely to report being hurt or injured as those who don't.

✓**check-in** How much caffeine do you consume every day?

TABLE 6.9 Caffeine Content of Beverages and Other Products

Energy drinks	Caffeine content (mg)	Other	Caffeine content (mg)
Amp, 8 oz	72	5-Hour Energy	207
BAWLS Guarana, 8 oz	50	Black tea (brewed),[a] 8 oz	55
No Fear, 8 oz	87	Coffee-flavored ice cream,[a] 8 oz	58
Red Bull, 8.4 oz	80	Coffee (brewed),[a] 8 oz	85
Rockstar, 8 oz	80	Coffee (brewed),[a] 16 oz	170
Sodas		Espresso shot,[a] 1 oz	64
Coca-Cola, 12-oz can	35	Excedrin Extra Strength, 2 pills	130
Coca-Cola Zero, 12-oz can	34	Hershey's Kiss, 1	1
Diet Coke, 12-oz can	47	Hershey's milk chocolate bar	12
Diet Pepsi, 12-oz can	36	Hot chocolate,[a] 8 oz	9
Dr Pepper, 12-oz can	42	NoDoz Maximum Strength, 1 pill	200
Mountain Dew, 12-oz can	54	StayAlert gum, 1 piece	100
Pepsi, 12-oz can	38	Vivarin, 1 pill	200
Pepsi MAX, 12-oz can	69		
Vault, 12-oz can	71		

[a]Average values; individual brands may vary.
Source: Center for Military Psychiatry and Neuroscience at the Walter Reed Army Institute of Research.

Taking Charge of What You Eat

You can't control what you don't know. Because of the Nutrition Labeling and Education Act, food manufacturers must provide information about fat, calories, and ingredients in large type on packaged food labels, and they must show how a food item fits into a daily diet of 2,000 calories. The law also restricts nutritional claims for terms such as *healthy*, *low-fat*, and *high-fiber*.

A growing number of cities and states are mandating calorie-posting by fast-food restaurants. Some national health reform proposals would require restaurant chains to post the number of calories, grams of saturated fat, and milligrams of sodium next to menu items, although menu labeling has not proven to affect dietary choices. Often the problem is not a lack of information, health officials note, but a lack of self-control. You can find detailed nutritional information for restaurants of all price levels at www.healthydiningfinder.com.

In evaluating food labels and product claims, keep in mind that while individual foods vary in their nutritional value, what matters is your total diet. If you eat too much of any one food—regardless of what its label states—you may not be getting the variety and balance of nutrients that you need.

Portions and Servings

Consumers often are confused by what a *serving* actually is, especially since many American restaurants have supersized the amount of food they put on their customers' plates. The average bagel has doubled in size in the past 10 to 15 years. A standard fast-food serving of french fries is larger in the United States than in the United Kingdom.

A food-label *serving* is a specific amount of food that contains the quantity of nutrients described on the Nutrition Facts label. A *portion* is the amount of a specific food that an individual eats at one time. Portions can be bigger or smaller than the servings on food labels. According to nutritionists, "marketplace portions"—the actual amounts served to customers—are two to eight times larger than the standard serving sizes defined by the USDA. In fast-food chains, today's portions are two to five times larger than the original sizes. As studies have shown, people presented with larger portions eat 30 to 50 percent more than they otherwise would.

If you are trying to balance your diet or control your weight, it's important to keep track of the size of your portions so that you do not exceed recommended servings. For instance, a 3-ounce serving of meat is about the size of a pack of playing cards—see Figure 6.6. If you eat a larger amount, count it as more than one serving.

Nutrition Labels

The Nutrition Facts label, required on food packages for 20 years, focuses on those nutrients most clearly associated with disease risk and health. The most recent changes proposed by the FDA (see Figure 6.7) include these:

- Information about the amount of "added sugars" or empty calories in a food product.

- Updated serving size requirements to reflect the amounts people actually eat, not what they "should" be eating.

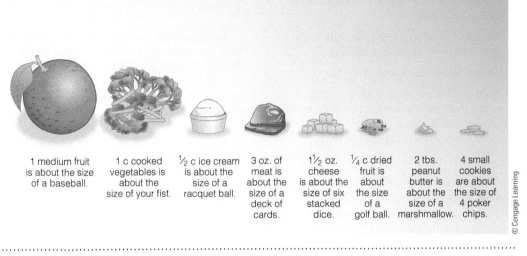

1 medium fruit is about the size of a baseball.

1 c cooked vegetables is about the size of your fist.

½ c ice cream is about the size of a racquet ball.

3 oz. of meat is about the size of a deck of cards.

1½ oz. cheese is about the size of six stacked dice.

¼ c dried fruit is about the size of a golf ball.

2 tbs. peanut butter is about the size of a marshmallow.

4 small cookies are about the size of 4 poker chips.

© Cengage Learning

FIGURE 6.6 Portion Sizes

Quick and easy estimates of portion sizes.

Nutrition Facts

8 servings per container

Serving size	2/3 cup (55g)

Amount per 2/3 cup

Calories 230

% DV*	
12%	**Total Fat** 8g
5%	Saturated Fat 1g
	Trans Fat 0g
0%	**Cholesterol** 0mg
7%	**Sodium** 160mg
12%	**Total Carbs** 37g
14%	Dietary Fiber 4g
	Sugars 1g
	Added Sugars 0g
	Protein 3g
10%	**Vitamin D** 2mcg
20%	**Calcium** 260mg
45%	**Iron** 8mg
5%	**Potassium** 235mg

* Footnote on Daily Values (DV) and calories reference to be inserted here.

© Cengage Learning

FIGURE 6.7 Understanding Nutrition Labels

- Calorie and nutrition information for both "per serving" and "per package" calorie for larger packages that could be consumed in one sitting or multiple sittings.

- Inclusion of potassium and vitamin D, nutrients that some in the U.S. population need more of. Vitamins A and C are no longer required on the label.

- Revised Daily Values (the total amount of a nutrient that the average adult should aim to get or not exceed on a daily basis) for a variety of nutrients such as sodium, dietary fiber, and vitamin D to help consumers understand the nutrition information in the context of a total daily diet.

Nutrition labels can influence purchasing decisions—if consumers are motivated.[40] About a third of Americans say they specifically buy foods labeled "low" or "reduced salt or sodium," but about a fifth of shoppers find it difficult to figure out how much salt is in the foods they eat.[41]

✓**check-in** Do you read nutrition labels on the foods you buy?

What Is Organic?

Foods certified as **organic** by the USDA must meet strict criteria, including the following:

- Processing or preservation only with substances approved by the USDA for organic foods

organic Term designating food produced with, or production based on the use of, fertilizers originating from plants or animals, without the use of pesticides or chemically formulated fertilizers.

- Processing without genetic modification or ionizing radiation
- No use of most synthetic chemicals, such as pesticides, herbicides, or fertilizers
- Fertilization without sewage sludge
- Food-producing animals grown without medication such as antibiotics or hormones, provided with living conditions similar to their natural habitat, and fed organic feed

The primary consumers of organic food are women ages 30 to 45 who have children at home and who are environmentally conscious. College students who are informed about organic products are more likely to choose them. In a recent study, more than half of undergraduates said they would support and purchase organic products on campus.

Are organic foods better for you? There has been limited research on whether organic foods are nutritionally superior to conventional foods. Some studies have shown higher levels of specific nutrients, such as flavonoids, in organic produce, but no one knows if this translates into specific health benefits. However, you can avoid exposure to pesticides and other chemicals by opting for organic foods.

Choosing Healthful Snacks

Snacking has become more widespread on campuses, as in other places. College students snack primarily "to satisfy hunger"; the second most common reason is "no time for meals." Other reasons for munching between meals: "for energy," "to be sociable," and "to relieve stress." One-third snack at 9:00 p.m. or later.

In response to consumer demands for smart snack choices, food manufacturers are offering "better-for-you" options that are lower in salt and sugar or free of *trans* fat and artificial colors. Some new snack items promoted as healthful options, such as sugar-free chocolate or organic potato chips, offer little nutritional value. Meat-based snacks, increasingly popular among young men, also can be high in fat and sodium. Read labels carefully and be sure to check total calories and fat.

A best-for-you option is fruit such as bananas, apples, or berries—rich in vitamins, low in calories, and packed with fiber. Other nutritious snacks include nuts, trail mix, granola bars, yogurt, sunflower seeds, soy nuts, and dried fruit (such as cranberries). If you enjoy fruit juice, buy 100 percent fruit juice without added sugar. Limit yourself to one serving of these calorie-rich beverages a day.

✓ **check-in** What are your favorite snacks?

If you rely on snacks to keep you energized throughout the day, take time to plan in advance so you have choices other than the nearest vending machine. Try to prepare snacks from different food groups: low-fat or nonfat milk and a few graham crackers, for instance, or celery sticks with peanut butter and raisins. Save part of one meal—half of your breakfast bagel or lunch sandwich—to eat a few hours later. If you're trying to add fiber to your diet, eat high-fiber snacks, such as prunes, popcorn, or sunflower seeds.

Food Safety

Foodborne infections cause an estimated 76 million illnesses, 325,000 hospitalizations, and 5,000 deaths in the United States every year. Three organisms—*Salmonella*, *Listeria*, and *Toxoplasma*—are responsible for more than 75 percent of these deaths. Although most foodborne infections cause mild illness, severe infections and serious complications—including death—do occur. College students are one of the most at-risk population groups due to risky food safety behaviors.

Scares about tainted food have led to massive recalls of such popular foods as peanut butter, jalapenos, lettuce, spinach, and tomatoes. As a result, consumer advocates, as well as manufacturers and trade associations, are calling for stricter regulations.

✓ **check-in** What can you do to improve your food safety?

- Pay attention when you hear that a food or product is under suspicion.
- Make note of the brands, the production dates, and the manufacturer(s) involved.
- Check the labels of the foods in your pantry and refrigerator, and throw out any that may be contaminated.

Fight BAC!

"BAC" stands for food bacteria, an invisible threat to your health. To improve food safety awareness and practices, government and private agencies have developed the Fight BAC!

campaign, which identifies four key culprits in foodborne illness:

- Improper cooling
- Improper hand washing
- Inadequate cooking
- Failure to avoid cross-contamination (see Figure 6.8.)

Avoiding *E. Coli* Infection

Eating unwashed produce, such as spinach or lettuce, or undercooked beef, especially hamburger, can increase your risk of infection with *Escherichia coli* (*E. coli*) bacteria. These bacteria, which live in the intestinal tract of healthy people and animals, are usually harmless. However, infection with the strain *E. coli* O157:H7 produces symptoms that can range from mild to life threatening. This strain has made its way into hamburger in fast-food chains and into packaged spinach. *E. coli* can cause severe bloody diarrhea, kidney failure, and even death. Symptoms usually develop within 2 to 10 days and can include severe stomach cramps, vomiting, mild fever, and bloody diarrhea. Most people recover within 7 to 10 days. Others—especially older adults, children under the age of 5, and those with weakened immune systems—may develop complications that lead to kidney failure.

Food Poisoning

Salmonella is a bacterium that contaminates many foods, particularly undercooked chicken, eggs, and sometimes processed meat. Eating contaminated food can result in salmonella poisoning, which causes diarrhea and vomiting. The CDC estimates 40,000 reported cases of salmonella poisoning a year; the actual number of cases could be anywhere from 400,000 to 4 million. The FDA has warned consumers about the dangers of unpasteurized orange juice because of the risk of salmonella contamination.

Another bacterium, *Campylobacter jejuni*, may cause even more stomach infections than salmonella. Found in water, milk, and some foods, campylobacter poisoning causes severe diarrhea and has been implicated in the growth of stomach ulcers.

Bacteria can also cause illness by producing toxins in food. *Staphylococcus aureus* is the most common culprit. When cooked foods are cross-contaminated with the bacteria from raw foods and not stored properly, staph infections

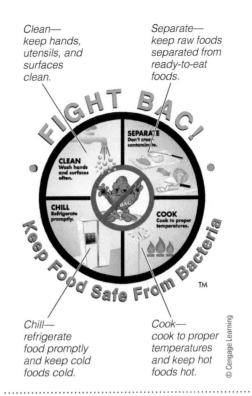

Clean—
keep hands, utensils, and surfaces clean.

Separate—
keep raw foods separated from ready-to-eat foods.

Chill—
refrigerate food promptly and keep cold foods cold.

Cook—
cook to proper temperatures and keep hot foods hot.

© Cengage Learning

FIGURE 6.8 Fight BAC!

can result, causing nausea and abdominal pain anywhere from 30 minutes to 8 hours after ingestion.

An uncommon but sometimes fatal form of food poisoning is botulism, caused by the *Clostridium botulinum* organism. Improper home-canning procedures are the most common cause of this potentially fatal problem.

Even many healthful foods can pose dangers. The FDA has urged consumers to avoid eating raw sprouts because of the risk of getting sick. Sprouts, particularly alfalfa and clover, can be contaminated by *Salmonella* or *E. coli* bacteria. The FDA advises people to either cook sprouts before eating them or request that they be left off sandwiches and other food ordered in restaurants. Home-grown sprouts can also present a risk if they come from contaminated seeds.

There have been several outbreaks of listeriosis, caused by the bacterium *Listeria*, commonly found in deli meats, hot dogs, soft cheeses, raw meat, and unpasteurized milk. Although rare, listeriosis can be life-threatening. At greatest risk are pregnant women, infants, and those with weakened immune systems. You can reduce your risk by cooking meats and leftovers thoroughly and by washing everything that may come into contact with raw meat.

YOUR STRATEGIES FOR PREVENTION

How to Protect Yourself from Food Poisoning

- **Always wash your hands with liquid or clean bar soap before handling food.** Rub your hands vigorously together for 10 to 15 seconds; the soap combined with the scrubbing action dislodges and removes germs.

- **When preparing fresh fruits and vegetables, discard outer leaves, wash under running water, and, when possible, scrub with a clean brush or hands.** Do not wash meat or poultry.

- **To avoid the spread of bacteria to other foods, utensils, or surfaces, do not allow liquids to touch or drip onto other items.** Wipe up all spills immediately.

- **Clean out your refrigerator regularly.** Throw out any leftovers stored for three or four days.

- **To kill bacteria and viruses, sterilize wet kitchen sponges by putting them in a microwave for two minutes.** Make sure they are completely wet to guard against the risk of fire.

Pesticides

Plants and animals naturally produce compounds that act as pesticides to aid in their survival. The vast majority of the pesticides we consume are therefore natural, not added by farmers or food processors. *Commercial pesticides* save billions of dollars of valuable crops from pests, but they also may endanger human health and life. Fearful of potential risks in pesticides, many consumers are purchasing organic foods.

Food Allergies

The National Institute of Allergy and Infectious Diseases defines a food allergy as "an adverse health effect arising from a specific immune response that occurs reproducibly on exposure to a given food." As many as 50 to 90 percent of presumed food allergies are not allergic reactions.

Food allergies are most common in childhood, affecting an estimated 6 to 8 percent of youngsters. Most outgrow allergies to cow's milk, soy, egg, and wheat, but allergies to nuts, fish, and shellfish tend to be lifelong. Early exposure of infants to common allergens may prevent the development of certain allergies later in life.[42] The symptoms that different foods provoke vary. One person might sneeze if exposed to an irritating food; another might vomit or develop diarrhea; others might suffer headaches, dizziness, hives,

or a rapid heartbeat. Symptoms may not develop for up to 72 hours, making it hard to pinpoint which food was responsible.

✓**check-in** Do you have any food allergies? Have they been diagnosed by a physician?

If you suspect that you have a food allergy, see a physician with specialized training in allergy diagnosis. Medical opinion about the merits of many treatments for food allergies is divided. Once you've identified the culprit, the wisest and sometimes simplest course is to avoid it.

Nutritional Quackery

The Academy of Nutrition and Dietetics (AND) describes nutritional quackery as a growing problem for unsuspecting consumers. Because so much nutritional nonsense is garbed in scientific-sounding terms, it can be hard to recognize bad advice when you get it. One basic rule: If the promises of a nutritional claim sound too good to be true, they probably are (see Figure 6.9).

If you seek the advice of a nutrition consultant, know the following:

- Carefully check his or her credentials and professional associations. Because licensing isn't required in all states, almost anyone can use the label "nutritionist," regardless of qualifications.

- Be wary of diplomas from obscure schools and organizations that allow anyone who pays dues to join. (One physician obtained a membership for his dog!)

- A registered dietitian (RD), who has a bachelor's degree and specialized training (including an internship) and who passed a certification examination, is usually a member of the AND, which sets the standard for quality in diets. A nutrition expert with an MD or PhD generally belongs to the AND, the American Institute of Nutrition, or the American Society for Clinical Nutrition, all of which have stringent membership requirements.

Facts to Know

- Nutritional supplements sold in health stores or through health and body-building magazines may contain ingredients that have not been tested and proven safe.

- Be wary of anyone who recommends megadoses of vitamins or nutritional supplements, which can be dangerous. High doses of vitamin A, which some people take to clear up acne, can be toxic.

- A quick way to spot a bad nutrition self-help book is to look in the index for a diet to prevent or treat rheumatoid arthritis (none exists). If you find one, don't buy the book.

Steps to Take

- Before you try any new nutritional approach, check with your doctor or a registered dietitian.

- Don't believe ads or advisers basing their nutritional recommendations on hair analysis, which is not accurate in detecting nutritional deficiencies.

- Question personal testimonies about the powers of some magical pill or powder, and be wary of "scientific articles" in journals that aren't reviewed by health professionals.

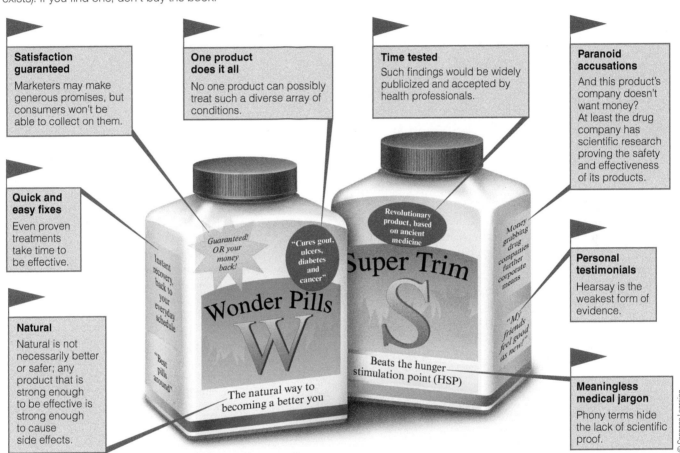

Satisfaction guaranteed
Marketers may make generous promises, but consumers won't be able to collect on them.

One product does it all
No one product can possibly treat such a diverse array of conditions.

Time tested
Such findings would be widely publicized and accepted by health professionals.

Paranoid accusations
And this product's company doesn't want money? At least the drug company has scientific research proving the safety and effectiveness of its products.

Quick and easy fixes
Even proven treatments take time to be effective.

Natural
Natural is not necessarily better or safer; any product that is strong enough to be effective is strong enough to cause side effects.

Personal testimonials
Hearsay is the weakest form of evidence.

Meaningless medical jargon
Phony terms hide the lack of scientific proof.

Guaranteed! OR your money back!

"Cures gout, ulcers, diabetes and cancer"

Instant recovery, back to your everyday schedule

"Best pills around"

Wonder Pills
The natural way to becoming a better you

Revolutionary product, based on ancient medicine

Super Trim
Beats the hunger stimulation point (HSP)

Money grabbing drug companies further corporate means

"My friends feel good as new!"

© Cengage Learning

FIGURE 6.9 Spot the Hype!

- Do you follow the Dietary Guidelines for Americans?
- What nutrients do you need most?
- What are some healthy eating patterns recommended by nutritionists?
- What steps can students take to eat a more healthful diet?

THE POWER OF NOW!
Making Healthful Food Choices

As nutritional knowledge expands and evolves, it's easy to be confused by changing advice on which foods to avoid and which to eat. But even though research may challenge or change thinking on a specific food, some basic principles always apply. Start an online food diary in your journal. For one week, record which of the following healthful eating habits that you follow on most days. Identify at least one other behavior that you would like to adopt. Identify any barriers that are keeping you from implementing this change. Then consciously put it into practice for a week. Write a brief summary of how you did.

_____ Eat breakfast. Easy-to-prepare breakfasts include cold cereal with fruit and low-fat milk, whole-wheat toast with peanut butter, yogurt with fruit, or whole-grain waffles.

_____ Don't eat too much of one thing. Your body needs protein, carbohydrates, fat, and many different vitamins and minerals, such as vitamins C and A, iron, and calcium, from a variety of foods.

_____ Eat more grains, fruits, and vegetables. These foods give you carbohydrates for energy, plus vitamins, minerals, and fiber. Try breads such as whole-wheat, bagels, and pita. Spaghetti and oatmeal are also in the grain group.

_____ Don't ban any food. Fit in a higher-fat food, like pepperoni pizza, at dinner by choosing lower-fat foods at other meals. And don't forget about moderation. If two pieces of pizza fill you up, don't eat a third.

_____ Make every calorie count. Load up on nutrients, not on big portions. Choosing foods that are nutrient dense will help protect against disease and keep you healthy.

_____ Eat five servings of fruits and vegetables per day. For breakfast, have 100% fruit juice or add raisins, berries, or sliced fruit to cereal, pancakes, or waffles. For lunch, have vegetable soup or salad with your meal or pile vegetables on your sandwich. For dinner, choose vegetables that are green, orange (such as carrots or squash), and red (such as tomatoes or bell peppers).

_____ Include three servings of whole-grain foods every day. To identify whole-grain products, check the ingredient list. The first ingredient should be a whole grain, such as "whole-grain oats," "whole-grain wheat," or "whole wheat."

_____ Consume a calcium-rich food at each meal. Good options include low-fat and nonfat milk, cheese, or yogurt; tofu; broccoli; dried beans; spinach; and fortified soy milk.

_____ Eat less meat. Rather than make meat the heart of a meal, think of it as a flavoring ingredient.

_____ Avoid high-fat fast foods. Hot dogs, fried foods, packaged snack foods, and pastries are most likely to be laden with fat.

_____ Check the numbers. When buying prepared foods, choose items that contain no more than 3 grams of fat per 100 calories.

_____ Think small. A dinner-size serving of meat should be about the size of a deck of cards; half a cup is the size of a woman's fist; a pancake is the diameter of a CD.

_____ Read labels carefully. Remember that "cholesterol-free" doesn't necessarily mean fat-free. Avoid products that contain saturated coconut oil, palm oil, lard, or hydrogenated fats.

_____ Switch to low-fat and nonfat dairy products. Rather than buy whole-fat dairy products, choose skim milk, fat-free sour cream, and low- or nonfat yogurt.

_____ The brighter the better. When selecting fruits and vegetables, choose the most intense color. A bright orange carrot has more beta-carotene than a pale one. Dark green lettuce leaves have more vitamins than lighter ones. Orange sweet potatoes pack more vitamin A than yellow ones.

What's Online

CENGAGE brain.com Visit www.cengagebrain.com to access course materials for this text, including the Behavior Change Planner, interactive quizzes, and more.

self survey

How Healthful Is Your Diet?

STEP 1

Keep a food diary for a week, writing down everything you eat and drink for meals and snacks. Include the approximate amount eaten (for example, 1/2 cup, 1 large, 12-oz can, and so on).

	Mon	Tues	Wed	Thurs	Fri	Sat	Sun
Grains							
Vegetables							
Fruits							
Milk, yogurt, cheese							
Meat, poultry, dry beans, eggs, nuts							
Fats, oil, sweets							

STEP 2: Are You Getting Enough Vegetables, Fruits, and Grains?

How often do you eat	Seldom/Never	1–2 times a week	3–5 times a week	Almost daily
At least three servings of vegetables a day?				
Starchy vegetables like potatoes, corn, or peas?				
Foods made with dry beans, lentils, or peas?				
Dark green or deep yellow vegetables (broccoli, spinach, collards, carrots, sweet potatoes, squash)?				
At least two servings of fruit a day?				
Citrus fruits and 100% fruit juices (oranges, grapefruit, tangerines)?				
Whole fruit with skin or seeds (berries, apples, pears)?				
At least six servings of breads, cereals, pasta, or rice a day?				

The best answer for each is "almost daily." Use your food diary to see which foods you should be eating more often.

STEP 3: Are You Getting Too Much Fat?

How often do you eat	Seldom/Never	1–2 times a week	3–5 times a week	Almost daily
Fried, deep-fat fried, or breaded food?				
Fatty meats, such as sausages, luncheon meat, fatty steaks or roasts?				
Whole milk, high-fat cheeses, ice cream?				
Pies, pastries, rich cakes?				
Rich cream sauces and gravies?				
Oily salad dressings or mayonnaise?				
Butter or margarine on vegetables, rolls, bread, or toast?				

Ideally, you should be eating these foods no more than one or two times a week. If your food diary indicates that you're eating them more frequently, your fat intake may well be too high.

STEP 4: Are You Getting Too Much Sodium?

How often do you eat	Seldom/Never	1–2 times a week	3–5 times a week	Almost daily
Cured or processed meats, such as ham, sausage, frankfurters, or luncheon meats?				
Canned vegetables or frozen vegetables with sauce?				
Frozen TV dinners, entrées, or canned or dehydrated soups?				
Salted nuts, popcorn, pretzels, corn chips, or potato chips?				
Seasoning mixes or sauces containing salt?				
Processed cheese?				
Salt added to table foods before you taste them?				

Ideally, you should be eating these high-sodium items no more than one or two times a week. If your food diary indicates that you're eating them more frequently, your sodium intake may well be too high.

MAKING THIS CHAPTER WORK FOR YOU

Review Questions

(LO 6.1)   1. According to the *Dietary Guidelines*, when taken in excess, which of the following food components poses a health risk?
   a. Iron
   b. Zinc
   c. Sodium
   d. Potassium

(LO 6.2)   2. _____ refers to the relationship between calories consumed from foods and beverages and calories expended in normal body functions and through physical activity.
   a. Calorimetry
   b. Bioenergetics
   c. Basal metabolic rate
   d. Calorie balance

(LO 6.2)   3. The classes of essential nutrients include which of the following?
   a. amino acids, antioxidants, fiber, and cholesterol
   b. proteins, calcium, calories, and folic acid
   c. carbohydrates, minerals, fat, and water
   d. iron, whole grains, fruits, and vegetables

(LO 6.2)   4. _____ form the basic framework for our muscles, bones, blood, hair, and fingernails.
   a. Minerals
   b. Fats
   c. Proteins
   d. Carbohydrates

(LO 6.3)   5. _____ are organic compounds that provide our brains and bodies with glucose, their basic fuel.
   a. Carbohydrates
   b. Proteins
   c. Fats
   d. Minerals

(LO 6.3)   6. Antioxidants _____.
   a. are nutrients important in the production of hemoglobin
   b. are substances added to foods to make them more flavorful or physically appealing
   c. are suspected triggers of food allergies
   d. are substances that prevent the harmful effects of free radicals

(LO 6.3)   7. Some vegetarians may _____.
   a. include fish in their diets
   b. avoid vitamin B$_{12}$ supplements if they eat only plant foods
   c. eat only legumes or nuts because these provide complete proteins
   d. have high cholesterol levels because of the saturated fats in fruits and vegetables

(LO 6.3)   8. Which of the following gender-specific strategies paves the way for better nutrition?
   a. Men increasing their iron intake by eating meat
   b. Pregnant women consuming more protein-containing foods
   c. Women consuming more calcium-rich foods
   d. Men eating more fat-free packaged foods

9. Which of the following health dangers is associated with sweetened drinks?
   a. Damage to tooth enamel
   b. Exaggerated stress response
   c. Irritability
   d. Tremors

(LO 6.4) 10. Because Sam plays poker, it's been easy for him to remember that a recommended serving of 3 ounces of meat means a piece of meat about the size of _____.
   a. one deck of cards
   b. eight poker chips
   c. two decks of cards
   d. a roll of quarters

(LO 6.4) 11. According to the FDA, which of the following inclusions is required on a Nutrition Facts label?
   a. Updated portion size requirements to reflect the amounts people should be eating, not what they actually eat
   b. Information about the amount of added sugars or empty calories in a food product
   c. Inclusion of sodium and vitamin E, nutrients that some in the U.S. population lack
   d. Calorie and nutrition information for "per serving" rather than "per package" for larger packages

(LO 6.4) 12. Which of the following criteria must be met by foods that are certified as organic?
   a. Not using preservation techniques
   b. Processing with genetic modification
   c. Processing with ionizing radiation
   d. Not using pesticides or herbicides

(LO 6.5) 13. _____ is a bacterium that contaminates many foods, particularly undercooked chicken, eggs, and sometimes processed meat.
   a. *Staphylococcus aureus*
   b. *Clostridium botulinum*
   c. *Salmonella*
   d. *Campylobacter*

(LO 6.6) 14. A registered dietitian is usually a member of the _____.
   a. American Society for Nutrition
   b. American Society for Clinical Nutrition
   c. Academy of Nutrition and Dietetics
   d. American Institute of Nutrition

Answers to these questions can be found on page 623.

Critical Thinking Questions

1. Discuss the six classes of essential nutrients required by the body. What is the role of vitamins in fulfilling the nutritional requirements of the human body?
2. What is the key to achieving and maintaining a healthy weight? What are the ways to effectively balance the calories consumed?
3. What are organic foods? Do you think organic foods are a better choice? How do you choose healthy snacks?

Additional Online Resources

http://fnic.nal.usda.gov
This comprehensive government website features reports and scientific studies on a variety of nutrition information, including the USDA *Dietary Guidelines 2010*, MyPlate, dietary supplements, dietary assessment, food composition searchable databases, educational brochures, historical food guides, and a topics "A–Z" section.

www.choosemyplate.gov
This interactive site features the MyPlate Plan, which provides suggestions for applying the most recent *Dietary Guidelines*.

Key Terms

The terms listed are used on the pages indicated. Definitions of the terms are in the Glossary at the end of the book.

amino acids   141
antioxidants   150
basal metabolic rate (BMR)   139
calories   138
calorie balance   140
carbohydrates   142
complementary proteins   140
complete protein   140
complex carbohydrates   143
dietary fiber   143
essential nutrients   140
folic acid   151
functional fiber   143

incomplete protein   140
macronutrients   139
micronutrients   139
minerals   152
nutrition   138
omega-3 and omega-6   146
organic   167
phytochemicals   157
proteins   140
saturated fats   145
simple carbohydrates   142
trans fat   146
unsaturated fats   146
vitamins   147

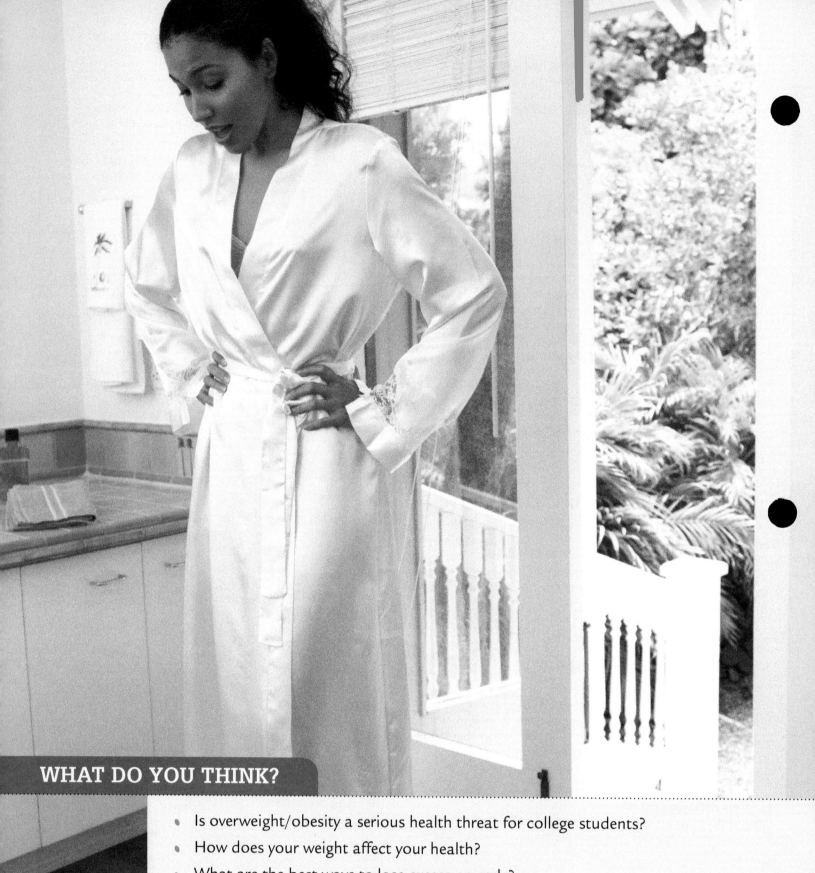

WHAT DO YOU THINK?

- Is overweight/obesity a serious health threat for college students?
- How does your weight affect your health?
- What are the best ways to lose excess pounds?
- What are the most common eating disorders on college campuses?

7

Managing Your Weight

Sarah's mother called it "baby fat." "You'll outgrow it soon enough," she said. Yet Sarah's cheeks grew chubbier and her waist wider every year. "Wait for your growth spurt," her mother reassured her. But Sarah remained one of the shortest girls in her class—and, she was convinced, the roundest.

Sarah went on her first diet in high school. For three days she ate nothing but carrot sticks, cottage cheese, and apples. Then she scarfed down two double cheeseburgers with fries and a chocolate shake. Her other attempts at dieting didn't last much longer. By graduation Sarah was grateful to hide under the flowing black robe as she walked on stage to get her diploma. <

After reading this chapter, you should be able to:

7.1 Summarize differences in weight among different populations in America.

7.2 Compare ways of defining a "healthy" weight.

7.3 Explain the factors that have contributed to the obesity epidemic.

7.4 Discuss the impact of excess weight on health.

7.5 Give an example of a healthy approach to gaining weight.

7.6 Assess ways of attaining and maintaining a healthy weight.

7.7 List the treatment options for extreme obesity.

7.8 Discuss the factors that lead to unhealthy eating on campus.

7.9 Recognize common forms of disordered eating and of eating disorders.

When Sarah heard about the "freshman 15," the extra pounds many students acquire during their first year at college, she groaned at the prospect of putting on more weight. In her Personal Health class, Sarah set one primary goal: not to gain another pound. Rather than going on—and inevitably falling off—one diet after another, she developed a weight management plan that included healthful food choices and regular exercise. Armed with the information and tools provided in this chapter, Sarah, for the first time in her life, took charge of her weight.

You can do the same.

This chapter explains what obesity is and why excess pounds are dangerous, describes current approaches to weight loss, discusses diets that work (and some that don't), offers practical guidelines for exercise and behavioral approaches to losing weight, and examines unhealthy eating patterns and eating disorders. If you're already at a healthy weight, this chapter can ensure that you remain so in the future. If, like two-thirds of Americans, you are overweight, you will find help in these pages. Remember: You *can* choose to lose. And you can start now.

✓**check-in** Do you know your current weight?

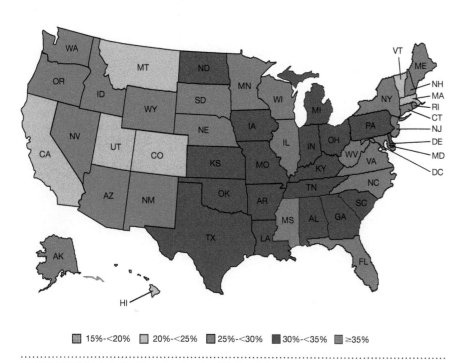

FIGURE 7.1 Adult Obesity in the United States.
The proportion of obese adults varies by state and region.

■ 15%-<20% ■ 20%-<25% ■ 25%-<30% ■ 30%-<35% ■ ≥35%

Weight in America

Over the past 30 years, the proportion of Americans considered overweight (with a body mass index [BMI] of 25 or higher) or obese (with a BMI of 30 or higher) has steadily increased. (BMI is discussed later in this chapter, on page 180.) However, health experts have reported an encouraging change: a significant decline in obesity among children aged 2 to 5 years, which has dropped from 14 percent a decade ago to about 8 percent.[1]

Obesity levels among other age groups seem to be leveling off.[2] Although this trend was initially attributed to hard economic times, health experts now see it as a result of better eating habits that Americans began to adopt about 10 years ago. According to a recent report, long-term efforts to educate Americans about healthy eating habits and food choices are paying off, and people are consuming fewer calories.[3]

However, excess weight continues to be a problem for many Americans (see Figure 7.1):

- More than 2 in 3 adults are overweight or obese.

- More than 1 in 3 adults—some 78 million individuals—are obese.

- More than 1 in 20 adults have extreme obesity.

- More than 1 in 6 children and adolescents ages 6 to 19 are obese.[4]

The prevalence of obesity among women has remained relatively stable, at about 35 percent, since 2000, but the prevalence among men has increased from 27.5 percent to 35.5 percent. Americans of all races carry excess pounds, but there are racial differences.

- Asian Americans have the lowest obesity rates (11.6 percent).

- Obesity is significantly higher in American Indians and Alaska Natives (39.9 percent) and Native Hawaiians and Pacific Islanders (43.5 percent) than in other races.

- Among white people, 66.7 percent are overweight or obese, including 34.3 percent who are obese and 5.7 percent who are extremely obese.

- About 17 percent of children over age 5 and adolescents in the United States are obese, with higher rates among boys (18.6 percent) than girls (15 percent).

✓**check-in** Are you between ages 18 and 35? If so, you are likely to put on weight more quickly than your parents.[5]

Weight on Campus

Whether or not they are enrolled in college, young adults gain an average of 30 pounds between ages 18 and 35. In the last decade, the prevalence of overweight and obesity increased from 62.2 to 67.1 percent among young men and from 51.7 to 55.8 percent among young women ages 20 to 39. Here are some specifics about weight issues on campus:

- About six in ten undergraduates are overweight; about a third are obese.[6]

- Students at two-year colleges may be twice as likely to be obese as those at four-year institutions.[7]

- Bisexual and lesbian female undergraduates are more likely to be obese than heterosexual women and may be at greater risk for unhealthy dietary, exercise, and weight control behaviors.[8]

- In addition to health-related risks, overweight and obesity in college are associated with significantly lower overall academic achievement and more depressive symptoms. Obese male undergraduates have significantly higher rates of lifetime trichotillomania (hair-pulling),

while overweight and obese females report higher rates of panic disorder.[9]

Many factors contribute to weight gain in college. "Millennials," the young adults born between 1980 and 2000, report experiencing high levels of stress and engaging in unhealthy behaviors in response: They get little if any regular exercise; skip breakfast; eat more fast food; drink more sugary sodas, energy drinks, and alcohol; and get less sleep than older Americans. As a result, they're more likely to develop one or more risk factors for cardiovascular disease.[10]

As discussed in Chapter 6, students in a hurry often opt for fast food and consume more fatty foods and sugared drinks, which increase their risks of obesity and other health problems. Students' snack choices tend is become less healthy with each passing week of the semester, with the most "junk food" consumed during finals. However, it is possible to hold the line on calories—and costs. (See Health on a Budget.)

✓**check-in** Do you eat differently in college than you did before? How?

Here are some of the ways weights change in college (also see Snapshot: On Campus Now):

- Only about 5 percent of students gain the legendary "freshman 15" although most put on some weight, an average of about 11 pounds. The students who gain the most

SNAPSHOT: ON CAMPUS NOW

📷 The Weight of Student Bodies

BMI	Percent (%)		
	Male	Female	Average
<18.5, underweight	3.2	5.2	4.5
18.5–24.9, healthy weight	56.3	63.4	60.9
25–29.9, overweight	28.3	19.4	22.5
30–34.9, class I obesity	8.2	7.0	7.5
35–39.9, class II obesity	2.8	2.8	2.8
≥40, class III obesity	1.3	2.1	1.8

✓**check-in** Using the chart on page 181, determine your BMI. Which of the above categories do you fit in? Have you ever been overweight or obese? Are you now? Do you want to lose weight? Why or why not? Record your feelings on your weight today and in the past in your online journal.

Source: American College Health Association. *American College Health Association–National College Health Assessment II: Reference Group Executive Summary, Spring 2014.* Hanover, MD: American College Health Association, 2014.

Hold the Line!

You can leave college a whole lot smarter but no heavier than when you entered—without spending extra money. Here are some suggestions:

- **Plan meals.** Most campus cafeterias post the week's menus in advance. Plan which items you will eat before you see or smell high-fat dishes.

- **Don't linger.** If you use the cafeteria as a social gathering place, you may end up eating with two or three different groups of people. Set a time limit to eat—then leave.

- **Develop alternative behavior.** People who eat when they are stressed or bored need to have substitute activities

ready when they need them. Make a list of things you can do—shower, phone a friend, take a hike—when stress strikes.

- **Eat at "home."** If the dormitory has a small kitchen, cook some healthful dishes and invite friends to join you.

- **Take advantage of physical activity programs.** Many college students become less active during their years in college. Aim to maintain or increase the amount of exercise you did in high school. Join a biking club, take a salsa class, learn yoga, or try tennis or racquetball.

---

weight tend to be less physically active than their peers.

- Percentage of body fat, absolute body fat, and BMI also tend to increase in the first semester at school.

- A certain percentage of incoming students—27 to 34 percent in different studies—lose weight their first year.

- In male students, increased alcohol consumption and peer pressure to drink account for extra pounds.

- In college women, the strongest correlation of weight gain was with an increased workload, which may lead to more stress-related eating, greater snacking, or less exercise.

- An estimated 10 to 13 percent of college students—report using prescription stimulants to lose weight. (See Chapter 12 for more on prescription drug misuse.)

✓**check-in** Have you gained or lost weight since starting college?

What Is a Healthy Weight?

Rather than rely on a range of ideal weights for various heights, as they did in the past, medical experts use various methods to assess body composition and weight. Experts debate which

measure of body composition—BMI, waist circumference, or waist-to-hip ratio—is the best indicator of central or visceral obesity, which increases the risk of heart disease, metabolic syndrome, diabetes, and other illnesses.

Average weight, BMI, and waist circumference have increased in both men and women in the United States in the last quarter century.[11]

Body Mass Index (BMI)

Body mass index (BMI), a ratio between weight and height, is a mathematical formula that correlates with body fat. You can determine your BMI from Figure 7.2. Here is how to interpret the reading:

- A healthy BMI ranges from 18.5 to 24.9.

- A BMI of 25 or greater defines **overweight** and marks the point at which excess weight increases the risk of disease. If your BMI is between 25 (23.4 for Asians) and 29.9, your weight is undermining the quality of your life. You suffer more aches and pains. You find it harder to perform everyday tasks. You run a greater risk of serious health problems.

- A BMI of 30 or greater defines **obesity** and marks the point at which excess weight increases the risk of death. If your BMI is between 30 and 34.9 (class 1 obesity), you face all the preceding dangers plus one more: dying.

- A BMI between 35 and 39.9 (class 2 obesity) means increased risk of premature death.

- A BMI of 40 or higher indicates class 3 or severe obesity, a truly life-threatening condition.

✓**check-in** Do you know your BMI?

body mass index (BMI)
A mathematical formula that correlates with body fat; the ratio of weight to height squared.

overweight A condition of having a BMI between 25.0 and 29.9.

obesity The excessive accumulation of fat in the body; class 1 obesity is defined by a BMI between 30.0 and 34.9; class 2 obesity is a BMI between 35.0 and 39.9; class 3, or severe obesity, is a BMI of 40 or higher.

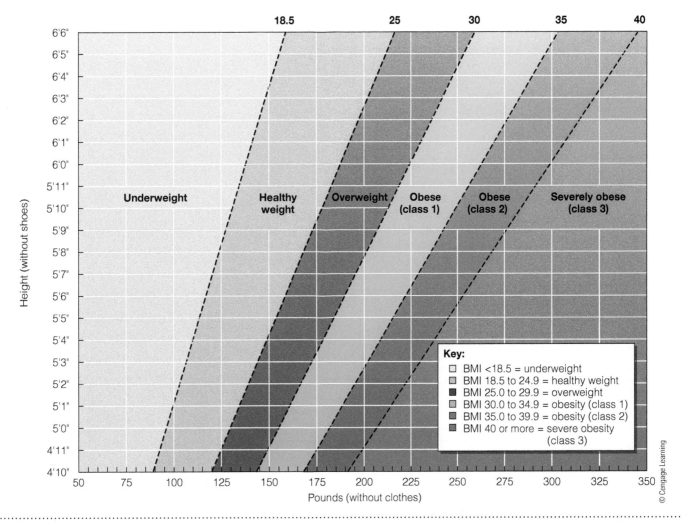

FIGURE 7.2 BMI Values Used to Assess Weight for Adults

Doctors use BMI to determine whether a person is at risk for weight-related diseases such as diabetes. Young adults who maintain a stable BMI into middle age may prevent the progression of cardiovascular risk factors such as high blood pressure, even if they are already overweight.[12] However, some argue that fat distribution, not overall fatness, is a critical of the health risks of obesity.

BMI has other limitations as an assessment tool:

- Muscular individuals, including athletes and body builders, may be miscategorized as overweight or obese because they have greater lean muscle mass.

- BMI does not reliably reflect body fat, an independent predictor of health risk.

- BMI is not useful for growing children, women who are pregnant or nursing, or elderly people.

- BMI, which was developed in Western nations, may not accurately indicate the risk of obesity-related diseases in Asian men and women.

Waist Circumference

A widening waist, or "apple" shape, is a warning signal. In an analysis of 11 studies of more than 600,000 people worldwide, those with larger waist circumferences were at increased risk of developing conditions such as heart disease, lung problems, and cancer and dying younger.[13]

✓**check-in** What is your waist measurement? Place a tape measure around your bare abdomen just above your hip bone. Be sure that the tape is snug but does not compress your skin. Relax, exhale, and measure.

When is a waist too wide? Various studies have produced different results, but the general guideline is that a waist measuring more than 35 inches in a woman or more than 40 inches in a man signals greater health risks. The larger the waist, the greater the risk of premature death.

Waist circumferences indicate "central" obesity, which is characterized by fat deposited deep within the central abdominal area of the body. Such "visceral" fat is more dangerous than "subcutaneous" fat just below the skin because it moves more readily into the bloodstream and directly raises levels of harmful cholesterol.

Waist-to-Hip Ratio (WHR)

Men of all ages are more prone to develop the "apple" shape characteristic of central obesity; women in their reproductive years are more likely to accumulate fat around the hips and thighs and acquire a pear shape (Figure 7.3). An indicator of shape-related health risks is your **waist-to-hip ratio (WHR)**. In addition to measuring your waist, measure your hips at the widest part. Divide your waist measurement by your hip measurement.

....
✓**check-in** What is your WHR?
....

For women, a ratio of 0.80 or less is considered safe; for men, the recommended ratio is 0.90 or less. For both men and women, a 1.0 or higher is considered "at risk" or in the danger zone for undesirable health consequences, such as heart disease and other ailments associated with being overweight.

Measuring Body Fat

waist-to-hip ratio (WHR)
The proportion of one's waist circumference to one's hip circumference.

Ideal body fat percentages for men range from 7 to 25 percent and for women from 16 to 35 percent. Methods of assessing body composition include a variety of approaches.

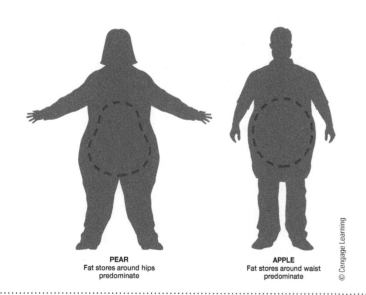

PEAR
Fat stores around hips predominate

APPLE
Fat stores around waist predominate

© Cengage Learning

....
FIGURE 7.3 Pear-Shaped versus Apple-Shaped Bodies

Skinfold Measurement   *Skinfold measurement* is determined using a caliper to measure the amount of skinfold. The usual sites include the chest, abdomen, and thigh for men and the tricep, hip, and thigh for women. Various equations determine body fat percentage, including calculations that take into account age, gender, race, and other factors. This relatively simple and low-cost method requires considerable technical skill for an accurate reading.

Home Body Fat Analyzers   Handheld devices and stand-on monitors sold online and in specialty stores promise to make measuring your body fat percentage as easy as finding your weight. None has been extensively tested.

Laboratory Methods

- **Bioelectrical Impedance Analysis (BIA).** This noninvasive method is based on the principle that electrical current applied to the body meets greater resistance with different types of tissue. Lean tissue, which contains large amounts of water and electrolytes, is a good electrical conductor; fat, which does not, is a poor conductor. In theory, the easier the electrical conduction, the greater an individual's lean body mass.

- **Hydrostatic (underwater) weighing.** According to the Archimedes Principle, a body immersed in a fluid is buoyed by a force equal to the weight of the displaced fluid. Since muscle has a higher density than water and fat has a lower density, fat people tend to displace less water than lean people.

- **Dual-energy X-ray absorptiometry (DXA).** X-rays are used to quantify the skeletal and soft tissue components of body mass. The test requires just 10 to 20 minutes, and radiation dosage is low (800 to 2,000 times lower than a typical chest X-ray). Some researchers believe that DXA will supplant hydrostatic testing as the standard for body composition assessment.

- **The Bod Pod®.** This large, egg-shaped fiberglass chamber uses an approach based on air displacement plethysmography—that is, the calculation of the relationship between pressure and volume—to derive body volume.

....
✓**check-in** Do you know your body fat
....
percentage?
....

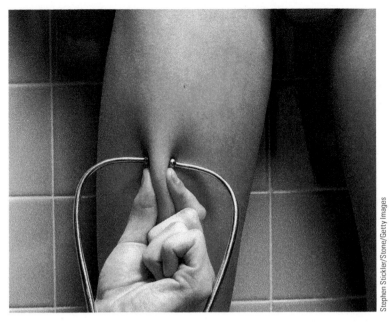

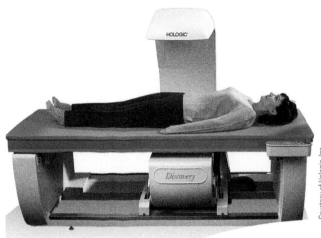

Skinfold measure accuracy depends on the technician's skill; laboratory methods such as DXA don't have that subjective component.

Understanding Weight Problems

Ultimately, all weight problems result from a prolonged energy imbalance—of consuming too many calories and burning too few in daily activities. How many calories you need depends on your gender, age, body-frame size, weight, percentage of body fat, and *basal metabolic rate* (BMR)—the number of calories needed to sustain your body at rest.

Your activity level also affects your calorie requirements. Regardless of whether you consume fat, protein, or carbohydrates, if you take in more calories than required to maintain your size and don't work them off in some sort of physical activity, your body will convert the excess to fat.

How Did So Many Get So Fat?

A variety of factors, ranging from behavior to environment to genetics, played a role in the increase in overweight and obesity in the United States. They include the following:

- **Bigger portions:** As Table 7.1 shows, the size of many popular restaurant and packaged foods has increased two to five times during the past 20 years. According to studies of appetite and satiety, people presented with larger portions eat up to 30 percent more than they otherwise would.

- **Consuming more calories than we burn:** American adults have been eating steadily

fewer calories for almost a decade, despite the continued increase in obesity rates, according to the Centers for Disease Control and Prevention (CDC). Among adults, average daily intake has fallen by about 75 calories. However, Americans may still not be getting enough exercise to burn the calories they do consume.

- **Fast food:** Young adults who eat frequently at fast-food restaurants gain more weight and develop metabolic abnormalities that increase their risk of diabetes in early middle age. (See the discussion of fast food in Chapter 6.)

TABLE 7.1 Supersized Portions

Food/Beverage	Original Size (year introduced)	Today (largest available)
Soda (Coca-Cola)	6.5 oz (1916)	34 oz
French fries (Burger King)	2.6 oz (1954)	6.9 oz
Hamburger (McDonald's; beef only)	1.6 oz (1965)	8 oz
Nestlé Crunch	1.6 oz (1938)	5 oz
Budweiser (bottle)	7 oz (1976)	40 oz

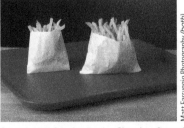
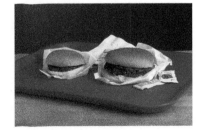

Source: "Are Growing Portion Sizes Leading to Expanding Waistlines?" Academy of Nutrition and Dietetics, www.eatright.org.

- **Physical inactivity:** The heaviest individuals tend to move the least. Obese men and women log fewer hours of vigorous exercise than leaner individuals.[13]

- **Passive entertainment:** Television viewing, a culprit in an estimated 30 percent of new cases of obesity, may increase weight in several ways:

  ○ It takes up time that otherwise might be spent in physical activities.

  ○ It increases food intake since people tend to eat more while watching TV.

  ○ Compared with sewing, reading, driving, or other relatively sedentary pursuits, it lowers metabolic rate so viewers burn fewer calories.

✓**check-in** How much television do you watch every day? Every week?

- **Emotional eating:** College students who are prone to boredom and have difficulty coping with negative emotions are likely to eat when they have nothing else to do or are feeling upset.[14]

- **Genetics:** Scientists have identified a particular variation in a gene associated with fat mass and obesity, called *FTO*, that increases the risk of excess weight by 20 to 30 percent. However, physical activity can counteract its effect.

- **Social networks:** Friends may have a significant effect on the risk of obesity. Young adults who are overweight or obese tend to befriend and date people who also have weight problems. Researchers are not sure if overweight people seek out other overweight people or whether normal-weight individuals become heavier as a result of their relationships with heavier partners.

- **Marriage:** Although marriage confers many health benefits, it also puts on pounds—particularly among the happily married. The reason may be that, having found a mate, spouses no longer try to stay slim to attract a partner.

Health Dangers of Excess Weight

If you have put on weight, you may be most concerned about looking fat or not fitting into your clothes. But the younger individuals are when they gain weight, the more health risks they may face over their lifetimes, including these:

- A 70 percent chance of becoming overweight or obese throughout life.

- Greater likelihood of high total cholesterol levels and other cardiovascular disease risk factors such as elevated blood pressure.

- Higher prevalence of type 2 diabetes.

- Increased risk of premature death. Obesity, smoking, and high blood sugar levels significantly increase the risk of dying before age 55.

- Physiological changes that are the equivalent to 20 years of aging, including increased risk of cardiovascular disease, diabetes, cancer, rheumatoid arthritis, sleep apnea, gout, and liver disease (Figure 7.4), as well as difficulties in walking, balance, and rising from a chair.

The Impact on the Body

Major diseases linked to obesity include

- **Type 2 diabetes:** More than 80 percent of people with type 2 diabetes are overweight. Although the reasons are not known, being overweight may make cells less efficient at using sugar from the blood. This then puts stress on the cells that produce insulin (a hormone that carries sugar from the blood to cells) and makes them gradually fail. Those with BMIs of 35 or more are approximately 20 times more likely to develop diabetes. Excess weight also increases the risk of premature death among people with type 2 diabetes.[15]

  ○ You can lower your risk for developing type 2 diabetes by losing weight and increasing the amount of physical activity you do.

  ○ If you have type 2 diabetes, losing weight and becoming more active can help you control your blood sugar levels and may allow you to reduce the amount of diabetes medication you take.

- **Heart disease and stroke:** People who are overweight are more likely to suffer from high blood pressure, high levels of triglycerides (blood fats) and harmful low-density lipoprotein (LDL) cholesterol, and low levels of beneficial high-density lipoprotein (HDL) cholesterol. Even relatively small amounts of excess fat—as little as 5 pounds—can add to the dangers in those already at risk for hypertension. People with more body fat

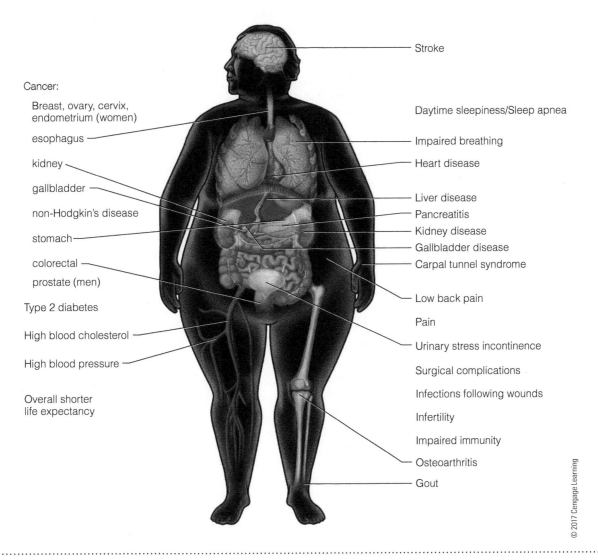

Cancer:

Breast, ovary, cervix, endometrium (women)

esophagus

kidney

gallbladder

non-Hodgkin's disease

stomach

colorectal

prostate (men)

Type 2 diabetes

High blood cholesterol

High blood pressure

Overall shorter life expectancy

Stroke

Daytime sleepiness/Sleep apnea

Impaired breathing

Heart disease

Liver disease

Pancreatitis

Kidney disease

Gallbladder disease

Carpal tunnel syndrome

Low back pain

Pain

Urinary stress incontinence

Surgical complications

Infections following wounds

Infertility

Impaired immunity

Osteoarthritis

Gout

© 2017 Cengage Learning

FIGURE 7.4 Health Dangers of Excess Weight

have higher blood levels of substances that cause inflammation, which may raise heart disease risk. Obese men face a much greater risk of dying from a heart attack, regardless of whether they have other risk factors.

○ Losing 5 to 15 percent of your weight can lower your chances for developing heart disease or having a stroke.

- **Cancer:** Obesity contributes to more than 100,000 cases of cancer—among them cancers of the endometrium, esophagus, pancreas, gallbladder, kidney, breast, ovaries, and colon—in the United States every year. Excess weight may account for 14 percent of all cancer deaths in men and 20 percent of those in women.

○ Obesity quadruples the risk of prostate cancer in black men.[16] Women who were overweight as children or teens may have a greater risk of colon cancer as adults.[17]

○ Losing weight, researchers estimate, could prevent as many as one in every six cancer deaths.

- **Other health problems:** Overweight men and women are also more likely to develop

○ Knee injuries that require surgery to repair.

○ Spinal disc degeneration, a common cause of low back pain.

○ Alterations in various measures of immune function.

○ Greater risk of gall stones, kidney stones, and kidney disease.

○ Less responsiveness to flu vaccination.

○ Cognitive problems and dementia.

○ Worsened symptoms of fibromyalgia, a musculoskeletal disorder.

° Poor sleep, which could add to the risk of medical problems. (See Chapter 2 for a discussion of sleep.)

° Health professionals describe the "plague of obesity" as an epidemic that claims 2.8 million lives around the world every year.[18]

• **Premature death:** Obese American adults die an average of almost four years earlier than those with normal weight, and middle-aged obese adults face the highest risk of early death. According to recent research, obesity is associated with at least a 20 percent increased risk of death from all causes or from heart disease. Overall, obese adults died 3.7 years earlier from all causes and 1.7 years earlier from heart disease, compared with normal-weight adults.[19]

✓**check-in** What do you see as the greatest health risk of excess weight and obesity?

The Emotional Toll

In our calorie-conscious and thinness-obsessed society, obesity also affects quality of life, including sense of vitality and physical pain.

Many see excess weight as a psychological burden, a sign of failure, laziness, or inadequate willpower. Overweight men and women often blame themselves for becoming heavy and feel guilty and depressed as a result. In fact, the psychological problems once considered the cause of obesity may be its consequence.

Obesity also has social consequences. Heavy women are less likely to marry, earn less, and have lower rates of college graduation.

✓**check-in** Do you think that there is a bias against obese people?

If You're Too Thin: How to Gain Weight

Being underweight is not an uncommon problem, particularly among adolescent and young adult men as well as among those who diet excessively or suffer from eating disorders (discussed later in this chapter).

If you lose weight suddenly and don't know the reason, talk to a doctor. Rapid weight loss can be an early symptom of a health problem. Compared to normal-weight folks, those who are excessively thin have nearly twice the risk of death, according to a recent analysis of more than 50 prior studies.[20]

If you're trying to put on pounds, you need to do the opposite of dieters: Consume more calories than you burn. But as with losing weight, you should try to gain weight in healthy ways. Here are some suggestions:

• **Eat more of a variety of foods** rather than more high-fat, high-calorie foods. Get no more than 30 percent of your daily calories from fat. A higher percentage poses a threat to your heart and your health.

• **If your appetite is small, eat more frequently.** Try for five or six smaller meals rather than a big lunch and dinner.

• **Choose some calorie-rich foods,** such as dried fruits rather than fresh ones. Add nuts and cheese to salads and main dishes.

• **Drink juice** rather than regular or diet soda.

• **Try adding a commercial liquid meal** replacement as a snack.

• **Exercise regularly** to build up both appetite and muscle.

A Practical Guide to a Healthy Weight

More than half of college women and about one-third of college men intend to lose weight. However, individuals vary in their readiness to change their diets, increase their physical activity, and seek professional counseling. Take the Self Survey that accompanies this chapter to determine your readiness to lose weight.

There are only two effective strategies for losing weight: eating less and exercising more. Unfortunately, most people search for easier alternatives that almost invariably turn into dietary dead ends or unexpected dangers. Among young people, the most successful strategies for attaining and maintaining a healthy weight include these:

• Drinking less soda

• Eating less junk food

• Drinking more water

• Increasing physical activity

• Weighing themselves regularly

- Adding more protein to their diets
- Watching less television
- Adding more fiber to their diets[21]

✓ **check-in** Have you tried any of these strategies to lose weight?

Why We Overeat

The answer lies not just in the belly but in the brain. Both **hunger**, the physiological drive to consume food, and **appetite**, the psychological desire to eat, influence and control our desire for food. Scientists have discovered appetite receptors within the brain that specifically respond to hunger messages carried by hormones produced in the digestive tract.

A hormone called leptin, produced by fat cells, sends signals that regulate appetite to the brain. When leptin levels are normal, people eat just enough to maintain weight. When leptin is low, the brain responds as if fat stores had been depleted and slows down metabolism. This may be one reason why it is so difficult to lose weight by dieting alone. However, vigorous exercise can lower the hormone ghrelin, which is a natural appetite stimulant.

We usually stop eating when we feel satisfied; this is called **satiety**, a feeling of fullness and relief from hunger. The neurotransmitter serotonin has been shown to produce feelings of satiety. In addition, several peptides, released from the digestive tract as we ingest food, may signal the brain to stop or restrict eating. However, it takes 20 minutes for the brain to register fullness.

Many people eat without regard for their bodies' signals. This "non-hunger" or "emotional" eating is almost always overeating, since it's eating for reasons other than sustenance. The psychological aspects of overeating are discussed later in the chapter.

Weight Loss Diets

Every year, sometimes every season, seems to bring a breakthrough diet that promises to take off pounds, reshape your body, and recharge your life. You can "shred" 4 inches in six weeks, fast your way to a lower weight and longer life, or follow the dictates of Doctors Oz, Phil, or Ornish. Or you can try diets with roots in the Paleolithic Age, South Beach, Beverly Hills, or Park Avenue.

✓ **check-in** Have you ever been on a diet? Which type?

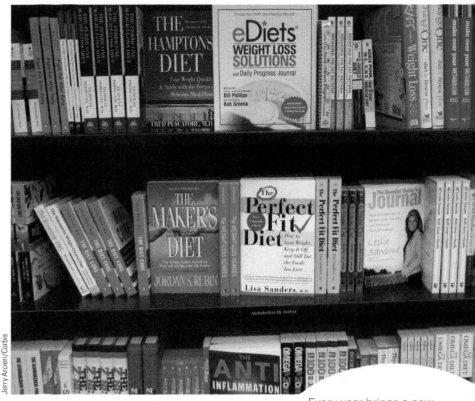

Jerry Arcieri/Corbis

Every year brings a new crop of diet books that promise to help readers lose weight, but reading alone is no substitute for eating less and exercising more.

Some popular diets are high in protein; others are low in complex carbohydrates. Some allow no fat; others ban sugar or gluten. Which ones work? As long as you are burning more calories than you consume, they all do. But not all diets are practical, inexpensive, easy to stay on, or good for your overall nutrition and health. (You can find an authoritative analysis of the latest diets at www.webmd.com/diet/evaluate-latest-diets.)

High-Protein Diets Many popular diets emphasize more protein and fewer carbohydrates. The Institute of Medicine considers a range of 10 to 35 percent of calories from protein as acceptable for adults, and some diets advise even higher levels. Protein is more satiating than carbohydrates and fat, so dieters complain less of hunger. However, severe restriction of carbohydrates can induce ketosis, which is caused by an incomplete breakdown of fats that can lead to nausea, fatigue, and light-headedness and can worsen kidney disease and other medical problems.

Recent studies have shown that high-protein diets are effective in controlling appetite, reducing body fat, maintaining lean body mass, and improving blood pressure and other health biomarkers. Ongoing studies are weighing their long-term impact on weight and well-being.[22]

Low-Carbohydrate, Low-Fat Diets Some popular diets are based on the premise that the

hunger The physiological drive to consume food.

appetite A desire for food, stimulated by anticipated hunger, physiological changes within the brain and body, the availability of food, and other environmental and psychological factors.

satiety The sensation of feeling full after eating.

correct proportions of various nutrients, particularly carbohydrates, fats, and proteins, lead to hormonal balance, weight loss, and greater vitality. They also promise additional health benefits, including lower blood pressure and cholesterol.

While dieters may eat just as much or even more food, they ingest fewer calories and much less fat. This can be so unsatisfying that many people cannot stay on these diets for a sustained period.

The Bottom Line Researchers have identified the key components of a successful diet:

- Daily caloric intake of about 500 calories less than usual (or a recommended 1,200 calories for women and 1,500 for men)

- Relatively high in protein

- Moderately low in calories

- Low glycemic index (discussed on page 144 in Chapter 6)

- A minimum of 30 minutes of daily, moderate-intensity physical exercise

Not all diets are safe or effective. To spot a dubious approach to weight loss, see the Consumer Alert feature.

⚠ CONSUMER ALERT

Dubious Diets

Facts to Know

The National Council Against Health Fraud cautions dieters to watch for these warnings of dangerous or fraudulent programs:

- Promises of very rapid weight loss

- Claims that the diet can eliminate "cellulite" (a term used to describe dimply fatty tissue on the arms and legs)

- "Counselors" who are really salespersons pushing a product or program

- No mention of any risks associated with the diet

- Unproven gimmicks, such as body wraps, starch blockers, hormones, diuretics, or "unique" pills or potions

- No maintenance program

Steps to Take

If you hear about a new diet that promises to melt away fat, don't try it until you get answers to the following questions:

- Does it include a wide variety of nutritious foods?

- Does it provide at least 1,200 calories a day?

- Is it designed to reduce your weight by ½ to 2 pounds per week?

- Does it emphasize moderate portions?

- Does it use foods that are easy to find and prepare?

- Can you follow it wherever you eat—at home, work, restaurants, or parties?

- Is its cost reasonable?

If the answer to any of these questions is no, don't try the diet; then ask yourself one more question: Is losing weight worth losing your well-being?

As randomized controlled trials have conclusively shown, what matters most is total calorie intake—not whether calories come from protein, carbohydrates, or fat. Sticking to diets with strict proportions of fat, carbohydrates, and protein may not be more effective than simply cutting back on total calories.

Although people lose weight on any diet that helps them eat less, most dieters lose only about 5 percent of their initial weight and gain some of that back. However, even a modest weight loss can lower cardiovascular risk factors, such as elevated blood pressure, total cholesterol, and blood glucose.

✓ **check-in** Have you ever lost weight on a diet? Did you keep it off?

Do Weight Loss Programs Work?

✓ **check-in** You've seen the ads. You've heard the promises. Would you turn to a commercial weight-loss program to help you shed excess pounds? Before you answer, read the following section.

Americans spend $2.5 billion a year on programs and products to help them lose weight and keep it off. Yet there has been little scientific evidence to show whether or not these plans lead to successful long-term weight loss. A recent study analyzed published studies on some of the most popular programs. Here are the findings:

- **Counseling plus calorie control** (Weight Watchers and Jenny Craig). These are the only two programs backed by scientific evidence showing that their clients maintained weight loss for at least a year. Nutrisystem clients also lost weight but were followed for only three months.

- **Very-low-calorie and low-calorie meal replacement programs** (Medifast, Optifast, Health Management Resources). Consumers using these products initially reported greater weight loss than those given counseling alone, but attrition was high and the difference was not statistically significant by nine months. The very-low-calorie methods increased the risk of gallstones.

- **Self-directed** (Atkins, Slimfast). Individuals following the Atkins diet reported greater weight loss than those in education-counseling programs at 6 and 12 months. Adherence was not reported; the most common complication was constipation. Slimfast users lost more weight than a control group but had results similar to those who received counseling alone.

- **Internet based programs** (The Biggest Loser Club, eDiets, Lose it!). Results varied, with Biggest Loser Club members showing greater weight loss than a control group at three months but no difference between eDiets and LoseIt! participants and controls.

Since so little solid research is available, the researchers' conclusion was inconclusive: "We still don't know whether a lot of these programs work."[23]

Physical Activity and Exercise

Unplanned daily activity, such as fidgeting or pacing, can make a difference in preventing weight gain. Scientists use the acronym **NEAT (nonexercise activity thermogenesis)** to describe such "nonvolitional" movement, which may be an effective way of burning calories. In research on self-confessed couch potatoes, the thinner ones sat an average of two hours less and moved and stood more often than the heavier individuals.

Although physical activity and exercise can prevent weight gain and improve health, usually they do not lead to significant weight loss. However, when combined with diet, exercise ensures that you lose fat rather than muscle, helps keep off excess pounds, and promotes greater fitness. Moderate exercise, such as 30 to 60 minutes of daily physical activity, reduces the risk of heart disease and other health threats. More exercise— a minimum of 200 to 300 minutes weekly of moderately intense activity—is necessary to maintain weight loss.

Among its other benefits (discussed in Chapter 8), exercise contributes to a healthy weight by

- Increasing energy expenditure
- Building up muscle tissue
- Burning off fat stores
- Stimulating the immune system
- Possibly reprogramming metabolism so that more calories are burned during and after a workout

An exercise program designed for both health benefits and weight loss should include both aerobic activity and resistance training. People who start and stick with an exercise program during or after a weight loss program are consistently

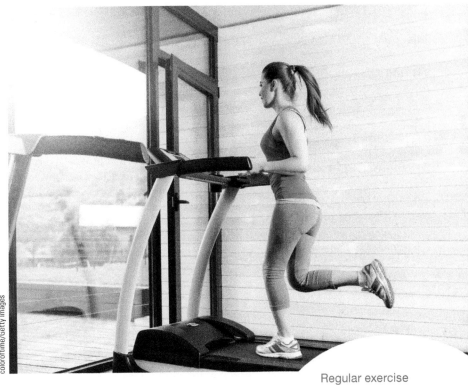

coloroftime/Getty Images

more successful in keeping off most of the pounds they've shed.

Complementary and Alternative Medicine (CAM) for Obesity

As Americans struggle to manage their weight, many are turning to complementary and alternative medicine (CAM), defined as "varied medical and health-care systems, practices, and products that are not considered to be part of any Western health-care system" (see Chapter 17). A recent scientific study reviewed the available scientific evidence on the most widely used approaches. Here are its findings:[24]

- **Herbal supplements.** Medicinal plant extracts, some traditionally used to prevent or treat disease, are being touted—often with misleading labels—as "natural" fat fighters. They include green tea from the leaves of *C. sinensis*, dehydrated fruit rind (*Garcinia cambogia*) used as a cooking ingredient in southern India, and the milkweed *H. gordonii*. Although widely advertised, the researchers concluded that "the evidence in support of their effectiveness is either non-existent or points to a negligible effect."

- **Acupuncture.** In randomized trials, acupuncture was more effective than lifestyle

Regular exercise provides many health benefits while also helping to control weight.

NEAT (nonexercise activity thermogenesis) Nonvolitional movement that can be an effective way of burning calories.

HEALTH NOW!

Thinking Thinner

Do you ease onto your scale, hoping for a certain number to appear—maybe what you weighed when you graduated from high school? If so, you may be setting yourself up for disappointment. Rather than focus on just one number, consider other ways to think about weight:

- **"If-only weight":** A weight you would choose if you could weigh whatever you wanted—just like the height or eye color you'd have chosen if you could.

- **"Happy weight":** A weight that is not the one you'd choose as your ideal but that you'd be happy with.

- **"Acceptable weight":** A weight that would not make you particularly happy but that you could be satisfied with.

- **"Disappointed weight":** A weight that would not be acceptable.

- **"Never-again weight":** The all-time high you never want to hit again.

In your online journal, jot down your if-only weight, happy weight, acceptable weight, disappointed weight, and never-again weight. Then write down your actual weight, as of today. How many pounds is your real weight from your acceptable weight?

Assuming that you can lose a pound a week, how many weeks would it take to get to that weight? How do you envision yourself feeling and behaving once you reach your acceptable weight? Do you have any plans once you reach your acceptable weight, such as buying clothes or taking a weekend trip? How will your life be different?

---

modification and placebo in reducing BMI and weight. However, scientists have criticized the design and validity of the studies.

- **Noninvasive body contouring.** Various methods using ultrasound, laser, and radio frequency may produce modest reductions in fat deposits at specific sites, such as the waist or upper arm, in normal-weight individuals but offer little, if any benefits, to the obese.[25]

- **Mindfulness.** Weight loss programs that incorporate mindfulness (discussed in Chapter 4) along with diet and exercise have proven effective in helping participants shed pounds, but the impact of mindfulness alone is not clear.[26]

✓**check-in:** Out of Sight, Out of Mouth

Want to eat less? Keep food out of sight. Leaving food in plain sight increases the likelihood of consuming it—and gaining weight. Seeing food can trigger thoughts about eating and increase stress about resisting the temptation to do so.[27]

Common Diet Traps

A multi-million-dollar industry thrives on marketing various diet aids, most of dubious value. Here is what you should know about some of the most widespread:

- **Over-the-counter diet pills:** An estimated 15 percent of adults—21 percent of women and 10 percent of men—have used weight loss supplements. The weight loss prescription drug Orlistat (Xenical) is available as an over-the-counter weight loss pill called Alli. The drug, which blocks about one-quarter of the fat consumed, works best with a low-fat diet. If dieters eat a meal made up of more than 15 fat grams, they can suffer nasty side effects, including flatulence, an urgent need to defecate, oily stools, and diarrhea.

- **Diet foods:** Diet products, including diet sodas and low-fat foods, are a very big business. Many people rely on meal replacements, usually shakes or snack bars, to lose or keep off weight. If used appropriately—as actual replacements rather than supplements to regular meals and snacks—they can be a useful strategy for weight loss. Yet people who use these products often gain weight because they think that they can afford to add high-calorie treats to their diets.

- **Artificial sweeteners and fake fats:** Nutritionists caution to use these products in moderation and not as substitutes for basic foods, such as grains, fruits, and vegetables. Foods made with fat substitutes may have fewer grams of fat, but they don't necessarily have significantly fewer calories. Many people who consume reduced-fat, fat-free, or sugar-free sodas, cookies, chips, and other snacks often cut back on more nutritious foods, such as fruits and vegetables. They also tend to eat more of the low- or no-fat foods so that their daily calorie intake either stays the same or actually increases.

Maintaining Weight Loss

Surveys of people who lost significant amounts of weight and kept it off for several years show that most did so on their own—without medication, meal substitutes, or membership in an organized weight loss group. "Weight loss maintainers" are more active, have fewer TVs in their homes, and don't keep high-fat foods in their pantries. (See Strategies for Prevention on page 192.)

Rather than focus on why dieters fail, the creators of the National Weight Control Registry study the habits and lifestyles of those who've maintained a weight loss of at least 30 pounds for at least a year. The nearly 6,000 people in the registry have maintained their weight loss for almost six years.

No one diet or commercial weight loss program helped all these formerly overweight individuals. Many, through years of trial and error, eventually came up with a permanent exercise and eating program that worked for them. Despite the immense variety, their customized approaches share certain characteristics:

- **Personal responsibility for change:** Weight loss winners develop an internal locus of control. Rather than blame others for their weight problem or rely on a doctor or trainer to fix it, they believe that the keys to a healthy weight lie within themselves.

- **Exercise:** Registry members report an hour of moderate physical activity almost every day. Their favorite exercise? Three in four say walking, followed by cycling, weight lifting, aerobics, running, and stair climbing. On average, they burn about 2,545 calories per week through physical activity.

- **Monitoring:** About 44 percent of registry members count calories, and almost all keep track of their food intake in some way, written or not.

- **Vigilance:** Rather than avoid the scale or tell themselves their jeans shrank in the wash, successful losers keep tabs on their weight and size. About one-third check the scale every week. If the scale notches upward or their waistbands start to pinch, they take action.

- **Frequent eating:** In a 10-year study that followed girls from ages 9 and 10 to ages 19 and 20, those who ate frequent meals and snacks put on fewer pounds and gained fewer inches around their waists than those who ate only a couple of times each day. A study of middle-aged women found a similar pattern. Normal-weight women and those who managed to maintain a significant weight loss ate more frequently (an average of three meals and two snacks a day) than those who ate less often.

✓ **check-in** What steps do you take to maintain a healthy weight?

Treating Severe Obesity

The biggest Americans are getting bigger, as the following statistics indicate:

- The prevalence of severe, or "morbid," obesity is increasing faster than obesity itself.

- The number of extremely obese adults—those at least 100 pounds overweight with BMIs over 40—has quadrupled in the past two decades from 1 in 200 to about 1 in every 50 men and women.

- The number with BMIs greater than 50 has jumped from 1 in 2,000 in the 1980s to 1 in 400.

Extreme obesity poses extreme risks to health and survival and undermines quality of life. The options for treating this dangerous condition include medication and surgery.

Prescription Drug Therapy

Xenical (Orlistat, also available in a lower dose as the over-the-counter drug Alli) blocks fat absorption by the gut, and it also inhibits absorption of water and vitamins in some patients and may cause cramping and diarrhea. It produces a weight loss of 2 to 3 percent of initial weight beyond the weight lost by dieting over the course of a year.

The FDA has approved two additional medications: Belviq (lorcaserin hydrochloride) and Qsymia (phentermine and topiramate extended-release). Both are meant for individuals with a BMI higher than 30 or a BMI higher than 27 with at least one weight-related health problem, such as

© iStockphoto.com/esolla

hypertension or diabetes. Each should be taken only under a physician's care.

Potential adverse reactions to Belviq include cognitive changes, neuromuscular symptoms, and digestive problems such as nausea, vomiting, and diarrhea. Qsymia may cause altered mood and thought processes, suicidal thoughts and behaviors, dizziness, drowsiness, and birth defects if taken during the first trimester of pregnancy.

Obesity Surgery

Obesity, or bariatric, surgery is becoming the most popular weight loss approach for the estimated

Vigilance helps keep weight off. If the number on the scale creeps upward, take action immediately.

YOUR STRATEGIES FOR PREVENTION

Keeping the Pounds Off

Once you've reached your weight goal, try the following suggestions for long-term success:

- **Set a danger zone.** Once you've reached your desired weight, don't let your weight climb more than 3 or 4 pounds higher. Take into account normal fluctuations but watch out for an upward trend. Once you hit your upper weight limit, take action immediately rather than wait until you gain 10 pounds.

- **Be patient.** Think of weight loss as a road trip. If you're going across town, you expect to get there in 20 minutes. If your destination is 400 miles away, you know it'll take longer. Give yourself the time you need to lose weight safely and steadily.

- **Try, try again.** Dieters don't usually keep weight off on their first attempt. The people who eventually succeed don't give up. Through trial and error, they find a plan that works for them.

15 million men and women who qualify as "morbidly obese" (100 or more pounds overweight) because of their increased health risks. This year as many as 200,000 Americans will undergo obesity surgery—four times the number who did so in 2000. Eight in 10 are women. A growing number are teenagers. Bariatric surgery seems to offer the same benefits for obese teens as for older patients, but its long-term health consequences are unknown.[28]

The individuals most likely to benefit from obesity surgery generally

- Have a body mass index over 40
- Have a BMI over 35 and a serious obesity-related problem, such as type 2 diabetes or severe sleep apnea (when breathing stops for brief periods during sleep)
- Have made repeated unsuccessful attempts to lose weight
- Do not have any significant or untreated psychological problems
- Are well informed about the risks of the surgery
- Recognize the need for lifestyle changes and daily vitamin and mineral supplements

According to the Agency for Healthcare Research and Quality, three in four bariatric surgery patients lose 50 to 75 percent of their excess weight within two years and keep it off. Among its other potential benefits are the following:

- Improvement in or elimination of diabetes in some people.

- Alleviation of high cholesterol, hypertension, and sleep apnea.
- Reduction of odds of dying by nearly half.
- Reduction of cardiovascular disorder, such as heart attack or stroke, and heart-related deaths.[29]
- Lower risk of gestational (pregnancy) diabetes[30]

The types of procedures are

- **Gastric bypass:** Surgeons create an egg-sized pouch with staples and reroute food around part of the upper intestine to block absorption of calories and nutrients. About 75 percent of bypass patients lose 50 to 75 percent of their excess weight within two years. For the "super obese," a more extensive procedure that bypasses most of the small intestine can lead to a loss of 80 percent of excess weight. However, the latter procedure carries the highest risks of complications, including serious vitamin and mineral deficiencies.

- **Banding:** In this newer, less risky procedure, surgeons slip an inflatable silicon band around the stomach; it can be tightened or loosened at a doctor's office without the need for further surgery. Patients lose about 40 to 55 percent of excess weight but may be more likely to regain lost pounds. The band also may slip or erode.

- **Duodenal switch:** Duodenal switch or biliopancreatic diversion, a more extensive operation that removes a portion of the stomach and bypasses a large portion of the small intestine, may lead to greater long-term weight loss but carries a risk of more complications.[31]

Bariatric operations—particularly in the hands of poorly trained or inexperienced surgeons—pose serious risks, including potentially fatal leaks, infection, bleeding, hernias, and pneumonia. According to federal estimates, 4 in 10 patients suffer complications within six months. The mortality rate averages about 2 deaths in 1,000 operations. Even with excellent medical results, extreme weight loss creates drapes of excess skin that sag over the belly, buttocks, thighs, breasts, or upper arms.[32]

Long-term dangers—both physical and psychological—are unknown, particularly for adolescents. Following gastric bypass surgery, obese teenagers lose weight and no longer suffer from diabetes. The benefits extend beyond the physical, with many reporting better psychological health and social ease.

Unhealthy Eating on Campus

Unhealthy eating behavior takes many forms, ranging from not eating enough to eating too much too quickly. Its roots are complex. In addition to media and external pressures, family history can play a role. Researchers have linked specific genes to some cases of anorexia nervosa and binge eating, but most believe that a variety of factors, including stress and culture, combine to cause disordered eating.

College students—particularly women, including varsity athletes—are at risk for unhealthy eating behaviors. Researchers estimate that only about one-third of college women maintain healthy eating patterns. Some college women have full-blown eating disorders; others develop "partial syndromes" and experience symptoms that are not severe or numerous enough for a diagnosis of anorexia nervosa or bulimia nervosa. Distress about body image increases the risk of all forms of disordered eating.

✓**check-in** Do you think unhealthy eating is common on your campus?

Body Image

Women have long been bombarded by idealized images in the media of female bodies that bear little resemblance to the way most women look. Increasingly, more advertisements and men's magazines are featuring idealized male bodies that bear little resemblance to the bodies most men inhabit. As the gap between reality and ideal grows, both genders struggle with issues related to body image, although men and women report different concerns:

• Women express greater worry about thinness and more dissatisfaction with their lower rather than their upper bodies.

• College women are more likely to overestimate their weight, while men tend to underestimate their actual weight.

• The greater the discrepancy between a woman's current view of her body shape and the ideal she considers most attractive to men, the more likely she is to worry about how others will view her and to doubt her ability to make a desirable impression.

• "Social physique anxiety" occurs often in women who feel they do not measure up to

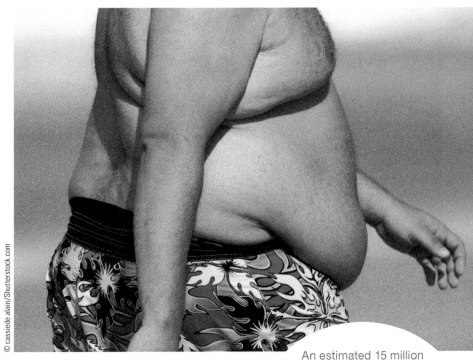

© cassiede alain/Shutterstock.com

An estimated 15 million men and women are "morbidly obese" (100 or more pounds overweight).

what they or others consider most desirable in terms of weight or appearance. Those reporting the greatest distress because of body image are at highest risk for eating disorders (discussed later in this chapter).

• Women compare their appearance to that of celebrities and models as well as peers more frequently than men and worry more that others will think negatively about their looks. Yet appearance matters just as much to men, who are as likely as women to engage in efforts to improve their bodies.

• Men often want either to lose or gain weight or to add muscle and bulk.

• College men in the United States overwhelmingly associate greater muscularity with feeling sexier, more confident, and more attractive to women. Pursuit of this idealized body type can lead to a dangerous obsession called muscle dysmorphia or reverse anorexia. Men with this disorder are at higher risk for depression and anxiety, abuse of substances such as anabolic steroids, and suicide.

College students of different ethnic and racial backgrounds express as much concern about their body shape and weight as whites—and sometimes more. In a study of university students, African American and Caucasian men were similar in their ideals for body size and in their perceptions of their own shapes. Both

African American and white women perceive themselves as smaller than they actually are and desire an even smaller body size. However, African American women are more accepting of larger size.

✓ **check-in** Do you think more realistic media images would affect how you feel about your body?

"Fat Talk"

✓ **check-in** Have you heard or made comments like these?

"I'm so fat."

"I can't fit into my jeans anymore."

"My butt looks enormous."

"I haven't been to the gym in weeks."

All the above statements are examples of what researchers call "fat talk," informal conversations about body image, weight, and shape.[33] Such discussions are especially common on college campuses. Regardless of their weight, undergraduates perceive body talk, including negative comments about size and fitness, as normal.

In studies of college students, most female undergraduates engage in fat talk. Typically, one woman complains about her size or weight, while her peers insist that she is not too fat or too big and argue that they are heavier or have flabbier arms or bigger hips. Women rarely express satisfaction with their appearance or body parts, perhaps because they fear such comments will sound arrogant or unsympathetic to women who are dissatisfied with their bodies.

Female undergraduates who tend to compare themselves to others and those concerned about their own body images are most likely to engage in fat talk. Regardless of whether women are expressing unhappiness with their own bodies, comparing themselves to others, or denying that another woman is or looks fat, the conversation itself increases stress.

College men also talk about their bodies—about a quarter doing so frequently—but in different ways. Men talk most frequently about their abdomens, chests, and overall muscularity, followed by body fat. These discussions are most likely to occur at the gym or while playing sports, although men sometimes talked about their bodies while eating, hanging out with friends, talking about women, or engaging in an activity, such as swimming, where they were removing their clothing.

Men's comments about their bodies—unlike women's—were as likely to be positive as negative. This may be because it seems more acceptable in our culture for men to praise the appearance of their bodies without sounding arrogant. Men also are more likely than women to validate a friend's bodily concerns—for instance, to agree that another man needs to lose weight or has gotten out of shape.

Critical self-talk was associated with more eating disordered comments and behaviors. Simply hearing their peers engage in muscle or fat talk resulted in lower body satisfaction and self-esteem than listening to comments about other subjects.

Disordered Eating

In a survey at a large, public, rural university in the mid-Atlantic states, 17 percent of the women were struggling with disordered eating. Younger women (ages 18 to 21) were more likely than older students to have an eating disorder. In this study, eating disorders equally affected women of different races (white, Asian, African American, Native American, and Hispanic), religions, athletic involvement, and living arrangements (on or off campus; with roommates, boyfriends, or family).

Although the students viewed eating disorders as both mental and physical problems and felt that individual therapy would be most helpful, all said that they would first turn to a friend for help. Women in sororities are at slightly increased risk of an eating disorder compared with those in dormitories. Loneliness also has emerged as a risk factor for eating disorders in college women.

Brief interventions, such as four-hour Healthy Weight programs, have proven effective in preventing the onset of various forms of disordered eating.

Extreme Dieting

Extreme dieters go beyond cutting back on calories or increasing physical activity. They become preoccupied with what they eat and weigh. Although their weight never falls below 85 percent of normal, their weight loss is severe enough to cause uncomfortable physical consequences, such as weakness and sensitivity to cold. Technically, these dieters do not have anorexia nervosa

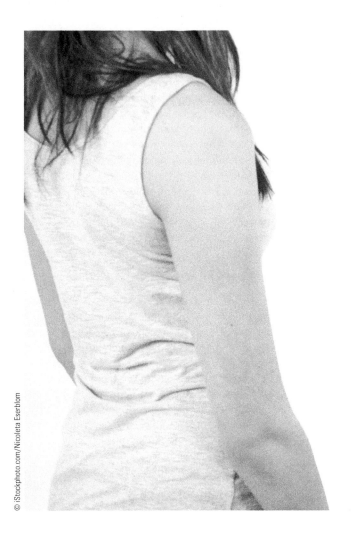

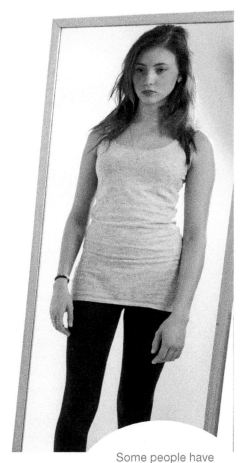

Some people have a distorted view of their weight. How do you decide what your ideal body size is?

(discussed later in this chapter), but they are at increased risk for it.

Extreme dieters may think they know a great deal about nutrition, yet many of their beliefs about food and weight are misconceptions or myths. For instance, they may eat only protein because they believe complex carbohydrates, including fruits and whole-grain breads, are fattening.

Sometimes nutritional education alone can help change these eating patterns. However, many avid dieters who deny that they have a problem with food may need counseling (which they usually agree to only at their family's insistence) to correct dangerous eating behavior and prevent further complications.

√ **check-in** Have you ever tried an extreme diet?

Compulsive Overeating

People who eat compulsively cannot stop putting food in their mouths. They eat fast, and they eat a lot. They eat even when they're full. They may eat around the clock rather than at set mealtimes, often in private because they are embarrassed about how much they consume.

Some mental health professionals describe compulsive eating as a food addiction that is much more likely to develop in women. According to Overeaters Anonymous (OA), an international 12 Step program, many women who eat compulsively view food as a source of comfort against feelings of inner emptiness, low self-esteem, and fear of abandonment.

The following behaviors may signal a potential problem with compulsive overeating:

- **Turning to food** when depressed or lonely, when feeling rejected, or as a reward
- **A history of failed diets** and anxiety when dieting
- **Thinking about food** throughout the day
- **Eating quickly** and without pleasure
- **Continuing to eat** even when no longer hungry

- **Frequently talking about food** or refusing to talk about food
- **Fear of not being able to stop** eating after starting

Recovery from compulsive eating can be challenging because people with this problem cannot give up entirely the substance they abuse. Like everyone else, they must eat. However, they can learn new eating habits and ways of dealing with underlying emotional problems. Most OA members join to lose weight but later feel that the most important effect was their improved emotional, mental, and physical health. As one woman puts it, "I came for vanity but stayed for sanity."

✓**check-in** Have you ever felt a compulsion to eat even when you weren't hungry?

Binge Eating

Binge eating—the rapid consumption of an abnormally large amount of food in a relatively short time—often occurs in compulsive eaters. The 25 million Americans with a binge-eating disorder typically eat a larger-than-ordinary amount of food during a relatively brief period, feel a lack of control over eating, and binge at least once a week for at least a three-month period. During most of these episodes, binge eaters experience at least three of the following:

- **Eating much more rapidly** than usual
- **Eating until they feel uncomfortably full**
- **Eating large amounts of food** when not feeling physically hungry
- **Eating large amounts of food** throughout the day with no planned mealtimes
- **Eating alone** because they are embarrassed by how much they eat and by their eating habits[30]

Binge eaters may spend up to several hours eating and consume 2,000 or more calories in a single binge—more than many people eat in a day. After such binges, they usually do not do anything to control weight but simply get fatter. As their weight climbs, they become depressed, anxious, or troubled by other psychological symptoms to a much greater extent than others of comparable weight.

Binge eating is probably the most common eating disorder. An estimated 8 to 19 percent of obese patients in weight loss programs are binge eaters.

✓**check-in** Have you ever gone on an eating binge?

If you occasionally go on eating binges, use the behavioral technique called *habit reversal* and replace your bingeing with a competing behavior. For example, every time you're tempted to binge, immediately do something—text-message a friend, play solitaire, check your e-mail—that keeps food out of your mouth.

If you binge once a week or more for at least a three-month period, you may have **binge-eating disorder**, a recently recognized psychiatric disorder that can require professional help.[34] Short-term talk treatment, such as cognitive-behavioral therapy, either individually or in a group setting, has proven most effective for binge eating.

Eating Disorders

Eating disorders affect an estimated 5 to 10 million women and 1 million men. Despite evidence that 5 to 10 percent of those with eating disorders are male, many college students believe mainly young white women develop eating disorders. More people—and more types of people—are developing full-blown or "partial syndrome" eating disorders, including young children, boys and men, people of color, and individuals with lower socioeconomic backgrounds.

The most common eating disorders are binge-eating disorder, anorexia nervosa, and bulimia nervosa. Among the factors that increase the risk are

- Genetic predisposition
- Preoccupation with a thin body
- Social pressure
- Perfectionism and excessive cautiousness, which can reflect an obsessive-compulsive personality
- Lite transitions, such as puberty and the transition from adolescence to adulthood[35]

Female college students who spend a lot of time on Facebook tend to be more likely to be concerned about their body image and could be at increased risk for eating disorders, a recent study suggests. More so than other students, they placed greater importance on receiving comments and "likes," frequently untagged photos of themselves, and compared their photos to pictures of friends.[36]

Athletes in sports involving pressure either to maintain ideal body weight or to achieve a weight that might enhance their performance—such as gymnastics, distance running, diving, figure skating, wrestling, and cycling—are more likely to develop eating disorders. Male and female performers, dancers, and models are also at risk.

binge eating The rapid consumption of an abnormally large amount of food in a relatively short time.

binge-eating disorder A psychiatric disorder characterized by binge-eating once a week or more for at least a three-month period.

eating disorders Unusual, often dangerous patterns of food consumption, including anorexia nervosa and bulimia nervosa.

In the few studies of eating disorders in minority college students that have been completed, African American female undergraduates had a slightly lower prevalence of eating disorders than did whites. Asian Americans reported fewer symptoms of eating disorders but more body dissatisfaction, concerns about shape, and more intense efforts to lose weight.

The American Psychiatric Association has developed practice guidelines for the treatment of patients with eating disorders, which include medical, psychological, and behavioral approaches. One of the most scientifically supported is cognitive-behavioral therapy (discussed in Chapter 3).

Anorexia Nervosa Although *anorexia* means "loss of appetite," most individuals with **anorexia nervosa** are, in fact, hungry all the time. For them, food is an enemy—a threat to their sense of self, identity, and autonomy. In the distorted mirror of their mind's eye, they see themselves as fat or flabby even at a normal or below-normal body weight. Some simply feel fat; others think that they are thin in some places and too fat in others, such as the abdomen, buttocks, or thighs.

Anorexia, which affects about 0.4 percent of girls and young women per year, is ten times more common in females than males.[37] Its key characteristics include the following:

- Restriction of food intake, leading to a significantly low body weight for their age, health, and gender

- Intense fear of gaining weight or of becoming fat

- Disturbance in the way individuals experience their body weight or shape[38]

The incidence of anorexia nervosa has increased in the past three decades in most developed countries. The peak ages for its onset are 14.5 to 18 years. Cases are increasing among males, minorities, women of all ages, and possibly preteens.

There are two recognizable forms of anorexia:

- In the *restricting type*, individuals lose weight by avoiding any fatty foods and by dieting, fasting, and exercising. Some start smoking as a way of controlling their weight. Some college women may numb their pain by drinking alcohol, a problem the media have dubbed "drunkorexia."

- In the *binge-eating/purging* type, individuals engage in binge eating, purging (through self-induced vomiting, laxatives, diuretics, or enemas), or both. Obsessed with an intense fear of fatness, they may weigh themselves several times a day, measure various parts of their body, check mirrors to see if they look fat, and try on different items of clothing to see if they feel tight.

What Causes Anorexia Nervosa? Many complex factors interact and contribute to this disorder, including biological, psychological, and social ones. Anorexia is more common among close relatives, particularly sisters, than it is in the general population. The relatives of anorexics also have a higher-than-expected frequency of depressive disorders.

Anorexia is associated with changes within the brain, including abnormalities in the stress hormone cortisol and the neurotransmitters dopamine, serotonin, and norepinephrine—all of which influence appetite and satiety. Brain chemistry returns to normal after treatment and recovery.

Anorexia also may be a response to a personal loss or a sign of a driven, perfectionist personality. Often young anorexics have above-average grades and an unwarranted fear of failure. Girls who develop anorexia often have little insight into or awareness of their feelings, needs, and wants.

In one study that followed 21 college women with eating disorders for six years, 11 got better during their postcollege years, while 10 continued to struggle with disordered eating. The major difference between the two groups revolved around issues of autonomy and relation. Those who could better negotiate the tension between being independent and relating to others had higher self-esteem, a more positive self-concept, and a healthier relationship with food.

About one-third of those with anorexia initially were mildly overweight and cut back on food just to lose a few pounds. Others had normal weights but began to diet to look more attractive or, in the case of male and female athletes and dancers, to gain a performance advantage.

Sometimes illness, stress, or surgery triggers weight loss. Often the initial response to their weight loss—from parents, coaches, or friends—is positive. However, starvation seems to take on a life of its own, and anorexics cannot return to a healthy eating pattern. In time, they may place so much value on thinness that they cannot recognize the dangers to their health.

Health Dangers and Treatment The medical consequences of anorexia nervosa are serious (Figure 7.5).

- Menstrual periods stop in women; testosterone levels decline in men.

anorexia nervosa A psychological disorder in which refusal to eat and/or an extreme loss of appetite leads to malnutrition, severe weight loss, and possibly death.

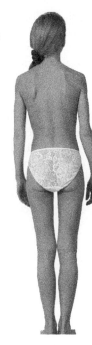

Loss of fat and muscle mass, including heart muscle

Increased sensitivity to cold

Irregular heartbeats

Bloating, constipation, abdominal pain

Amenorrhea (absence of menstruation)

Growth of fine, baby-like hair over body

Abnormal taste sensations

Osteoporosis

Depression

Sudden death

B Bodine/Custom Medical Stock Photo

FIGURE 7.5 Medical Complications of Anorexia Nervosa

- Adolescents with this disorder do not undergo normal sexual maturation, such as breast development, and may not reach their anticipated height.

- Even individuals who look and feel reasonably healthy may have subtle or hidden abnormalities, including heart irregularities and arrhythmias that can increase their risk of sudden death.

- Women who do not menstruate for six months or more may develop osteoporosis and suffer irreversible weakening and thinning of their bones as a result.

Even when they realize that they are jeopardizing their health, people with anorexia tend to fear that treatment will make them worse—that is, fatter. They need repeated reassurance that they will not become overweight and that they can and will find healthier ways of coping with life.

According to current practice guidelines, treatment of anorexia nervosa includes medical therapy (such as "refeeding" to overcome malnutrition) and behavioral, cognitive, psychodynamic, and family therapy. Antidepressant medication sometimes can help, particularly when there is a personal or family history of depression. Most people who get help do return to normal weight, but it can take a long time for

bulimia nervosa Episodic binge eating, often followed by forced vomiting or laxative abuse, and accompanied by a persistent preoccupation with body shape and weight.

their eating behaviors to become normal and for them to deal with troubling body image issues. Nutritional therapy is critical for a return to regular menstrual periods and an improvement in bone density.

Bulimia Nervosa Individuals with **bulimia nervosa** go on repeated eating binges and rapidly consume large amounts of food, usually sweets, stopping only because of severe abdominal pain or sleep, or because they are interrupted. Those with purging bulimia induce vomiting or take large doses of laxatives to relieve guilt and control their weight. In non-purging bulimia, individuals use other means, such as fasting or excessive exercise, to compensate for binges.

The characteristics of bulimia nervosa include these:

- Repeated binge eating

- A feeling of lack of control over eating behavior

- Regular reliance on self-induced vomiting, laxatives, or diuretics

- Strict dieting or fasting, or vigorous exercise, to prevent weight gain

- A minimum average of one bingeing episode a week for at least three months

- A preoccupation with body shape and weight.[39-40]

An estimated 1 to 2 percent of adolescent and young American women develop bulimia. Some experiment with bingeing and purging for a few months and then stop when they change their social or living situation. Others develop longer-term bulimia. Among males, this disorder is about one-tenth as common. The average age for developing bulimia is 18.

What Causes Bulimia Nervosa? Bulimia usually begins after a rigid diet that lasted from several weeks to a year or more. Strict dieting may affect brain chemistry in such a way as to disrupt the normal mechanisms for appetite and satiety. Semi-starvation eventually sets off a binge; bingeing leads to purging. Once dieters realize that vomiting reduces the anxiety triggered by gorging, they no longer fear overeating. When this happens, bingeing may become more frequent and severe until, in time, it becomes an all-purpose way of coping with stress. However, the driving force in this disorder may not be the overeating but the vomiting or laxative use. If individuals felt they couldn't get rid of food, they might not overeat.

Obesity in adolescence may increase the likelihood of bulimia in adulthood. Extremely obese individuals may lose weight by vomiting and not want to stop because they fear regaining it. Sometimes bulimia develops after recovery from anorexia. Purging becomes an alternative way of staying thin. People with bulimia may spend thousands of dollars—a third of their food budget—on foods for binge episodes and for laxatives and diet pills.

As with anorexia, bulimia is associated with changes in brain chemistry, particularly low levels of the peptide cholescystokinin, which produces feelings of satiety. The cycle of bingeing and purging seems to wreak havoc on the biological controls that keep weight at a certain level. Neuroimaging scans show differences in areas of the brain responsible for regulating behavior in individuals with bulimia.

Family conflicts, life stresses such as going away to school, and struggles with the transition to independent adulthood also may play a role. Bulimia also may be a symptom of depression. About 20 to 30 percent of those with this problem are chronically depressed; others have a history of depressive episodes.

Bulimic individuals also are more likely to experience other problems, including anxiety disorders, substance abuse, and impulse disorders, such as shoplifting (kleptomania) and cutting themselves. A significant percentage of bulimics—from a quarter to a half, by some estimates—may have been victims of incest, sexual molestation, or rape, but this correlation is controversial.

Health Dangers and Treatment Bulimia may continue for many years, with binges alternating with periods of normal eating. Physiological

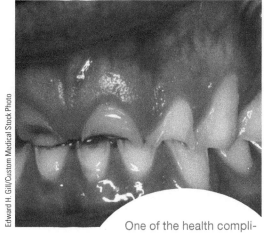

Edward H. Gill/Custom Medical Stock Photo

One of the health complications of purging is erosion and decay of dental enamel from the acid in vomit.

consequences are cumulative. Often dentists are the first to detect bulimia because they notice damage to teeth and gums, including erosion of the enamel from the stomach acids in vomit. Repeated vomiting can lead to other complications as it robs the body of essential nutrients and fluids, causes dehydration and electrolyte imbalances, and impairs the ability of the heart and other muscles to function. Bulimia can trigger cardiac arrhythmias and, occasionally, sudden death.

Cognitive-behavioral therapy has proved more effective than other approaches in improving bulimia symptoms.

- Is overweight/obesity a serious health threat for college students?
- How does your weight affect your health?
- What are the best ways to lose excess pounds?
- What are the most common eating disorders on college campuses?

THE POWER OF NOW!
Taking Control of Your Weight

No diet—high-protein, low-fat, or high-carbohydrate—can produce permanent weight loss. Successful weight management, the Academy of Nutrition and Dietetics has concluded, "requires a lifelong commitment to healthful lifestyle behaviors emphasizing sustainable and enjoyable eating practices and daily physical activity." Studies have shown that successful dieters are highly motivated, monitor their food intake, increase their activity, set realistic goals, and receive social support from others. Another key to long-term success is tailoring any weight loss program to an individual's gender, lifestyle, and cultural, racial, and ethnic values.

Are you following these practical guidelines?

____ Be realistic. Trying to shrink to an impossibly low weight dooms you to defeat. Start off slowly and make steady progress. If your weight creeps up five pounds, go back to the basics of your program.

____ Recognize that there are no quick fixes. Ultimately, quick-loss diets are very damaging physically and psychologically because when you stop dieting and put the pounds back on, you feel like a failure.

____ Note your progress. Make a graph, with your initial weight as the base, to indicate your progress. View plateaus or occasional gains as temporary setbacks rather than disasters.

____ Adopt the 90 percent rule. If you practice good eating habits 90 percent of the time, a few indiscretions won't make a difference. In effect, you should allow for occasional cheating, so that you don't have to feel guilty about it.

____ Look for joy and meaning beyond your food life. Make your personal goals and your relationships your priorities, and treat food as the fuel that allows you to bring your best to both.

____ Try again and again. Remember, dieters usually don't keep weight off on their first attempt. The people who eventually succeed try various methods until they find the plan that works for them.

What's Online

 Visit www.cengagebrain.com to access course materials for this text, including the Behavior Change Planner, interactive quizzes, and more.

Are You Ready to Lose Weight?

As discussed in Chapter 1, people change the way they behave stage by stage and step by step. The same is true for changing behaviors related to weight. If you need to lose excess pounds, knowing your stage of readiness for change is a crucial first step. Here is a guide to identifying where you are right now.

If you are still in the *precontemplation* stage, you don't think of yourself as having a weight problem, even though others may. If you can't fit into some of your clothes, you blame the dry cleaners. Or you look around and think, "I'm no bigger than anyone else in this class." Unconsciously, you may feel helpless to do anything about your weight. So you deny or dismiss its importance.

In the *contemplation* stage, you would prefer not to have to change, but you can't avoid reality. Your coach or doctor may comment on your weight. You wince at the vacation photos of you in a swimsuit. You look in the mirror, try to suck in your stomach, and say, "I've got to do something about my weight."

In the *preparation* stage, you're gearing up by taking small but necessary steps. You may buy athletic shoes or check out several diet books from the library. Maybe you experiment with some minor changes, such as having fruit instead of cookies for an afternoon snack. Internally, you are getting accustomed to the idea of change.

In the *action* stage of change, you are deliberately working to lose weight. You no longer snack all evening long. You stick to a specific diet and track calories, carbs, or points. You hop on a treadmill or stationary bike for 30 minutes a day. Your resolve is strong, and you know you're on your way to a thinner, healthier you.

In the *maintenance* stage, you strengthen, enhance, and extend the changes you've made. Whether or not you have lost all the weight you want, you've made significant progress. As you continue to watch what you eat and to be physically active, you lock in healthy new habits.

Where are you right now? Read each of the following statements and decide which best applies to you.

1.	I never think about my weight.	Precontemplation Stage
2.	I'm trying to zip up a pair of jeans and wondering when was the last time they fit.	Contemplation Stage
3.	I'm downloading a food diary to keep track of what I eat.	Preparation Stage
4.	I have been following a diet for three weeks and have started working out.	Action Stage
5.	I have been sticking to a diet and engaging in regular physical activity for at least six months.	Maintenance Stage

MAKING THIS CHAPTER WORK FOR YOU

Review Questions

(LO 7.1) 1. Which of the following statements is true about the obesity levels in Americans?
   a. There has been a significant decline in obesity among children aged 2 to 5 years.
   b. The prevalence of obesity among men has drastically decreased over the years.
   c. The prevalence of obesity among women has drastically increased over the years.
   d. The levels of obesity in adolescents are higher among girls than among boys.

(LO 7.1) 2. _____ people have the lowest obesity rates.
   a. American Indian
   b. Asian American
   c. Pacific Islander
   d. Native Hawaiian

(LO 7.2) 3. Which of the following statements is true of body mass index (BMI)?
   a. A BMI between 35 to 39.9 means increased risk of premature death.
   b. A healthy BMI ranges from 11.5 to 21.
   c. A BMI of 30 or greater defines overweight.
   d. A BMI that ranges from 20 to 25 defines obesity.

(LO 7.2) 4. Which of the following statements is true about the waist-to-hip ratio?
   a. Women in their reproductive years are more likely to accumulate fat around the hips and thighs.
   b. A ratio of 2.5 or less is considered safe for women.
   c. A ratio of 3.5 or less is considered safe for men.
   d. Men of all ages are less prone to accumulate fat around the belly.

(LO 7.3) 5. _____ refers to the number of calories needed to sustain the human body at rest.
   a. Active metabolic rate
   b. Anaerobic metabolic rate
   c. Aerobic metabolic rate
   d. Basal metabolic rate

(LO 7.3) 6. Which of the following factors has resulted in an increase in overweight and obese people in the United States?
   a. Physical inactivity
   b. Excessive dieting
   c. Active work culture
   d. Excessive protein intake

(LO 7.4) 7. People who are overweight are at increased risk of suffering from _____.
   a. jaundice
   b. tuberculosis
   c. type 1 diabetes
   d. cancer

(LO 7.4) 8. Which of the following statements is true about the social consequences of obesity?
   a. Heavy women are less likely to marry.
   b. Heavy women are more likely to be well settled and earn more.
   c. Heavy women are more likely to be highly qualified.
   d. Heavy women are unlikely to blame themselves for becoming heavy.

(LO 7.5) 9. Which of the following suggestions should be adopted in order to gain weight in healthy ways?
   a. Drink regular or diet soda rather than juice.
   b. Opt for a big lunch or dinner rather than five or six smaller meals.
   c. Eat more of a variety of foods rather than more high-fat, high-calorie foods.
   d. Choose fresh fruits rather than dried ones.

(LO 7.5) 10. Which of the following statements is true about individuals who are underweight?
   a. They have an increased risk of being diagnosed with type 1 diabetes.
   b. They are less likely to engage in physical activity or exercise.
   c. They are more likely than overweight individuals to adopt a sedentary lifestyle.
   d. They have nearly twice the risk of death of normal-weight individuals.

(LO 7.6) 11. A successful strategy for attaining and maintaining a healthy weight is to _____.
   a. drink more soda
   b. check your weight regularly
   c. adopt a sedentary lifestyle
   d. add more sodium to your diet

(LO 7.6) 12. Which of the following statements is true about weight-loss diets?
   a. Diets with strict proportions of fat, carbohydrates, and proteins are always more effective than diets that cut back on total calories.
   b. Many popular diets emphasize more carbohydrates and fewer proteins.
   c. A healthy diet comprises 1,600 calories for women and 2,000 calories for men.
   d. Most dieters lose only about 5 percent of their initial weight and gain some of that back.

(LO 7.7) 13. Which of the following prescription drugs leads to birth defects if taken during the first trimester of pregnancy?
  a. Xenical
  b. Qsymia
  c. Belviq
  d. Lorcaserin

(LO 7.7) 14. Individuals most likely to benefit from obesity surgery _____.
  a. are unaware of the risks of surgery
  b. have failed to recognize the need for lifestyle changes
  c. have a body mass index over 40
  d. do not have any significant symptoms of sleep apnea

(LO 7.8) 15. Which of the following is a common concern of men about their body image?
  a. Men often want either to lose or gain weight or to add muscle and bulk.
  b. College men are most likely to overestimate their weight.
  c. Men express greater worry about thinness.
  d. Men express more dissatisfaction with their lower rather than their upper bodies.

(LO 7.8) 16. Which of the following is a common concern of women about their body image?
  a. Women express more dissatisfaction with their upper bodies rather than their lower bodies.
  b. College women are more likely to underestimate their weight.
  c. Women express greater worry about thinness.
  d. Women are at a higher risk of suffering from muscle dysmorphia.

(LO 7.9) 17. Which of the following behaviors may signal a potential problem with compulsive overeating?
  a. Relishing every bite and deriving pleasure from food
  b. Frequently talking about food or refusing to talk about food
  c. Eating only proteins as they believe carbohydrates are fattening
  d. Being diagnosed with anorexia nervosa

(LO 7.9) 18. For individuals with _____, food is a threat to their sense of self, identity, and autonomy.
  a. compulsive-eating disorder
  b. binge-eating disorder
  c. bulimia nervosa
  d. anorexia nervosa

Answers to these questions can be found on page 623.

Critical Thinking Questions

1. Is eating less and exercising more an effective strategy for losing weight? Discuss the different types of weight loss diets.
2. Discuss the treatment procedures for individuals with severe obesity. How are individuals most likely to benefit from obesity, or bariatric, surgeries?

Additional Online Resources

www.obesity.org
The Obesity Society is the leading organization for advocacy and education on the nation's obesity epidemic. This comprehensive website features statistics on overweight and obesity in the United States, research articles, consumer protection links, prevention topics, library resources, fact sheets on a variety of weight management topics, and more.

http://win.niddk.nih.gov
This government-sponsored website features a variety of publications in English and Spanish on nutrition, physical activity, and weight control for the general public and for health-care professionals. In addition, there are links for research, a newsletter, statistical data, and a bibliographic collection of journal articles on various aspects of weight management and obesity.

www.something-fishy.org
This very comprehensive and popular site features the latest news on eating disorders, as well as links regarding signs to watch for, "Recovery: Reach Out," treatment finders, doctors and patients, cultural issues, and a support chat.

Key Terms

The terms listed are used on the pages indicated. Definitions of the terms are in the glossary at the end of the book.

anorexia nervosa 197	hunger 187
appetite 187	NEAT (nonexercise activity thermogenesis) 189
binge eating 196	
binge-eating disorder 196	obesity 180
body mass index (BMI) 180	overweight 180
bulimia nervosa 198	satiety 187
eating disorders 196	waist-to-hip ratio (WHR) 182

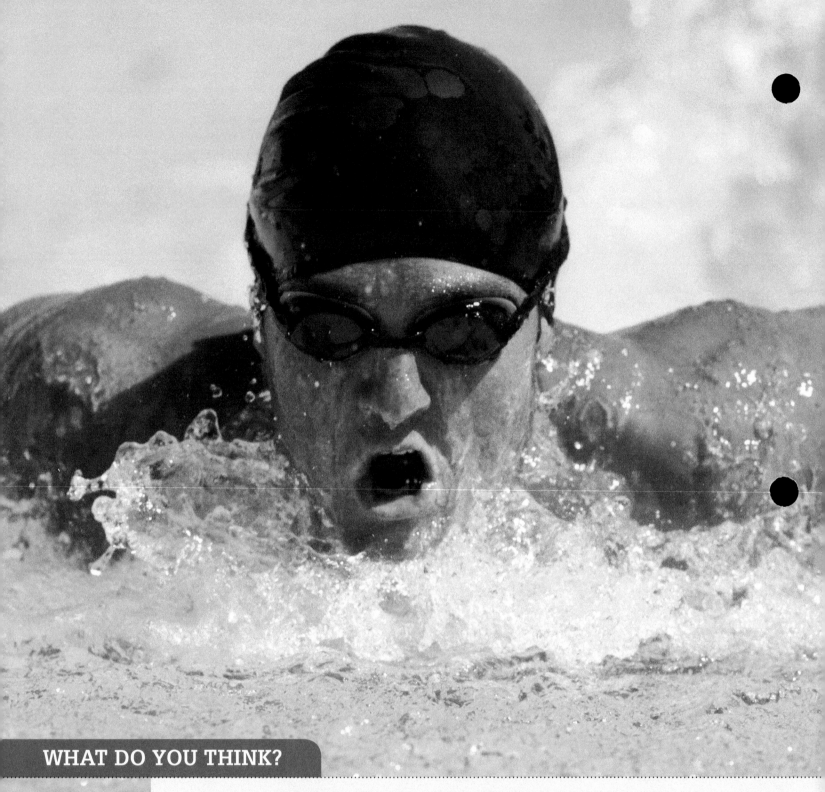

WHAT DO YOU THINK?

- How important is fitness for your overall health?
- Why do college students need to exercise?
- What would be an ideal workout?
- How can you protect yourself from exercise injuries?

© bikeriderlondon/Shutterstock.com

8

The Joy of Fitness

As a boy, Derek never thought about doing anything special to stay physically fit. He loved sports so much that he spent every free moment on a softball field or basketball court. He could sprint faster, jump higher, and hit a ball harder than any of his friends. In high school, Derek's life revolved around practices and games. He was a varsity athlete and a regional all-star.

Early in his first year in college, an injury sidelined Derek. Frustrated that he had to sit out the season, he gave up his rigorous training routine. As he became immersed in academics and other activities, Derek stopped going to the gym or working out on his own. Yet he continued to think of himself as an athlete in excellent physical condition.

When Derek went home for spring break, he joined his younger brothers on a neighborhood basketball court. While he wasn't surprised that his long shots were off, Derek was amazed by how quickly he got winded. In 15 minutes, he was panting for breath. "Getting old," one of his brothers joked. "Getting soft," the other teased. <

After reading this chapter, you should be able to:

8.1 Explain the relationship between the dimensions of health and physical fitness.

8.2 Summarize the health risks of inactivity and the need for physical exercise.

8.3 Outline current physical activity recommendations.

8.4 Discuss the overload, FITT, and reversibility principles of exercise.

8.5 Specify methods to improve cardiovascular fitness.

8.6 Explain the significance of muscular fitness.

8.7 Compare static and dynamic flexibility.

8.8 Summarize the benefits of mind–body approaches to physical fitness and wellness.

8.9 Identify the causes and treatments of low back pain.

8.10 Discuss the nutritional requirements of athletes.

8.11 Specify precautions for preventing exercise-related problems.

Fitness can enhance every dimension of your health—improving your mood and your mind as well as your body.

Often the college years represent a turning point in physical fitness. Like Derek, many other students, busy with classes and other commitments, devote less time to physical activity. However, your daily choices and habits can affect not only how you feel now but how long and how healthfully you'll live.

As you'll see in this chapter, exercise yields immediate rewards: It boosts energy, improves mood, soothes stress, improves sleep, and makes you look and feel better. In the long term, physical activity slows many of the changes associated with chronological aging, lowers the risk of serious chronic illnesses, and extends the lifespan.

This chapter can help you reap these rewards. It presents the latest activity recommendations, documents the benefits of exercise, describes types of exercise, and provides guidelines for getting into shape and exercising safely.

✓**check-in** How active are you: Very? Moderately? Not very? Not at all?

What Is Physical Fitness?

The simplest, most practical definition of **physical fitness** is the ability to respond to routine physical demands, with enough reserve energy to cope with a sudden challenge. You can consider yourself fit if you

- Meet your daily energy needs
- Can handle unexpected extra demands
- Are protecting yourself against potential health problems, such as heart disease

The five health-related components of physical fitness are these:

- **Cardiorespiratory fitness**, which refers to the ability of the heart to pump blood through the body efficiently. It is achieved through aerobic exercise—any activity, such as brisk walking or swimming, in which sufficient or excess oxygen is continually supplied to the body. In other words, aerobic exercise involves working out strenuously without pushing to the point of breathlessness.

- **Metabolic fitness**, which refers to reduced risk for diabetes and cardiovascular disease,

can be achieved through a moderate-intensity exercise program even with little or no improvement in cardiorespiratory fitness.

- **Muscular strength**, which refers to the force within muscles; it is measured by the absolute maximum weight that you can lift, push, or press in one effort. Strong muscles help keep the skeleton in proper alignment, improve posture, prevent back and leg aches, help in everyday lifting, and enhance athletic performance. Muscle mass increases along with strength, which makes for a healthier body composition and a higher metabolic rate.

- **Muscular endurance**, which is the ability to perform repeated muscular effort; it is measured by counting how many times you can lift, push, or press a given weight. Important for posture, muscular endurance helps in everyday work as well as in athletics and sports.

- **Flexibility**, which is the range of motion around specific joints—for example, the stretching you do to touch your toes or twist your torso. Flexibility depends on many factors: your age, gender, and posture; how muscular you are; and how much body fat you have. As children develop, their flexibility increases until adolescence. Then a gradual loss of joint mobility begins and continues throughout adult life. Both muscles and connective tissue, such as tendons and ligaments, shorten and become tighter if they are not consistently used through their full range of motion.

- **Body composition**, which refers to the relative amounts of fat and lean tissue (bone, muscle, organs, water) in the body. As discussed later in this chapter, a high proportion of body fat has serious health implications, including increased incidence of heart disease, high blood pressure, diabetes, stroke, gallbladder problems, back and joint problems, and some forms of cancer.

Physical conditioning (or training) refers to the gradual building up of the body to enhance cardiorespiratory, or aerobic, fitness; muscular strength; muscular endurance; flexibility; and a healthy body composition.

Functional fitness, which is gaining greater emphasis among professional trainers, refers to the performance of activities of daily living. Exercises that mimic job tasks or everyday movements can improve an individual's balance, coordination, strength, and endurance.

© Howard Sandler/Shutterstock.com

physical fitness The ability to respond to routine physical demands, with enough reserve energy to cope with a sudden challenge.

cardiorespiratory fitness The ability of the heart and blood vessels to circulate blood through the body efficiently.

✓ **check-in** How would you rate your functional fitness—your ability to meet the routine demands of daily living (walking stairs, lifting heavy objects, etc.)?

Athletic, or Performance-Related, Fitness

You may jog five miles, work out with weights, and start each day with a stretching routine. This doesn't quality you for the soccer team. Most sports, such as softball, tennis, and basketball, require additional skills, including

- **Agility,** the ability to change direction rapidly
- **Balance**, or equilibrium the ability to maintain a certain body position
- **Coordination,** the ability to integrate the movement of body parts to produce smooth, fluid movements
- **Power,** the product of force and speed
- **Reaction time,** the time required to respond to a stimulus
- **Speed,** or velocity, the ability to move rapidly

While many amateur and professional athletes are in superb overall condition, you do not need athletic skills to keep your body operating at maximum capacity throughout life.

Fitness and the Dimensions of Health

The concept of fitness is evolving. Rather than focusing only on aerobic or strength training, instructors, coaches, and consumers are pursuing a broader vision of total fitness that encompasses every dimension of health:

- **Physical:** As described later in this chapter, becoming fit reduces your risk of major diseases, increases energy and stamina, and may prolong your life.
- **Emotional:** Fitness lowers tension and anxiety, lifts depression, relieves stress, improves mood, and promotes a positive self-image.
- **Social:** Physical activities provide opportunities to meet new people and to work out with friends or family.
- **Intellectual:** Fit individuals report greater alertness, better concentration, more creativity, and improved personal health habits.
- **Occupational:** Fit employees miss fewer days of work, are more productive, and incur fewer medical costs.

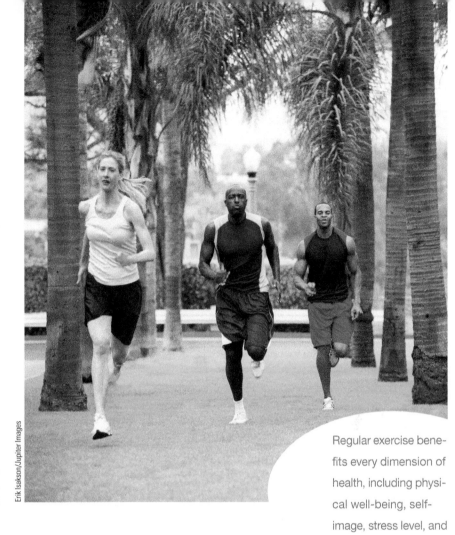

Erik Isakson/Jupiter Images

Regular exercise benefits every dimension of health, including physical well-being, self-image, stress level, and social relationships.

- **Spiritual:** Fitness fosters appreciation for the relationship between body and mind and may lead to greater realization of your potential.
- **Environmental:** Fit individuals often become more aware of their need for healthy air and food and develop a deeper appreciation of the physical world.

✓ **check-in** How does your fitness affect the various dimensions of health?

Working Out on Campus

Here is what we know about students' physical activity and fitness:

- Only about half of undergraduates meet the current recommendations for moderate or vigorous exercise (discussed later in this chapter).[1]
- Students who meet the vigorous physical activity recommendations report better mental health and less perceived stress compared to less active students.

metabolic fitness The reduction in risk for diabetes and cardiovascular disease, which can be achieved through a moderate-intensity exercise program.

muscular strength Physical power; the maximum weight one can lift, push, or press in one effort.

muscular endurance The ability to withstand the stress of continued physical exertion.

flexibility The range of motion allowed by one's joints; determined by the length of muscles, tendons, and ligaments attached to the joints.

body composition The relative amounts of fat and lean tissue (bone, muscle, organs, water) in the body.

functional fitness The ability to perform real-life activities, such as lifting a heavy suitcase.

SNAPSHOT: ON CAMPUS NOW

Student Bodies in Motion

College students reported the following behaviors within the past seven days:

Do moderate-intensity cardio or aerobic exercise for at least 30 minutes:

	Percent (%)		
	Male	Female	Average
0 days	22.5	22.1	22.3
1–4 days	54.4	57.6	56.5
5–7 days	23.1	20.3	21.2

✓**check-in** Did you engage in moderate-intensity aerobic exercise for at least 30 minutes in the last seven days? Or did you exercise vigorously for at least 20 minutes? How often do you exercise? Are you in better shape now than you were a year ago? Would you like to improve your

Do vigorous-intensity cardio or aerobic exercise for at least 20 minutes:

	Percent (%)		
	Male	Female	Average
0 days	33.1	38.8	36.9
1–2 days	30.9	30.0	30.0
3–7 days	36.1	31.2	32.3

fitness? Record your feelings on your fitness today and in the past in your online journal.

Source: American College Health Association. *American College Health Association–National College Health Assessment II: Reference Group Executive Summary, Spring 2014.* Hanover, MD: American College Health Association, 2014.

- College men are generally more active than women.
- Full-time students and those without jobs exercise more than part-time or employed students.
- Undergraduates living on campus are more active than those living off campus.
- Students living in fraternity or sorority housing engage in more exercise than those living in a house or an apartment.
- Single students report more days of vigorous workouts than married, divorced, or separated ones.
- Only 16 percent of students who are parents get the recommended levels of physical activity, compared with about half of those without children. (See Snapshot: On Campus Now.)

✓**check-in** Would you rate yourself as more, less, or about as active as other undergraduates?

As students progress from their first to fourth year of studies, they exercise less. The most drastic drop in physical activity occurs in the freshman year. As various studies have documented, physical fitness often declines, and levels of total cholesterol, harmful LDL (low-density lipoprotein) cholesterol, and fasting glucose (blood sugar) levels increase. (See Chapter 15 for a complete discussion of these risk factors for heart disease.)

In research on influences on students' health behaviors, peer pressure to exercise (for men more than women), and having an exercise partner, a flexible class schedule, access to fitness facilities, and a sense of being stressed all increase physical activity. College courses that require regular exercise in order to earn academic credit have proven effective in motivating students and in teaching them specific skills, such as how to monitor their heart rates.

The Perils of Inactivity

The greatest threat to your well-being is doing nothing. Inactivity

- Doubles the risk of diabetes and obesity
- Increases the risk of colon cancer, high blood pressure, **osteoporosis**, depression, and anxiety
- As a risk factor for heart disease, ranks as high as elevated cholesterol, high blood pressure, or cigarette smoking
- Doubles the likelihood of heart failure[2]

osteoporosis A condition in which the bones become increasingly soft and porous, making them susceptible to injury.

physical activity Any movement produced by the muscles that results in expenditure of energy.

exercise A type of physical activity that requires planned, structured, and repetitive bodily movement with the intent of improving one or more components of physical fitness.

- Leads to Sedentary Death Syndrome, which claims some 250,000 lives, accounting for 10 percent of all deaths in the United States every year

Obese Americans tend to be the least active. In a study of the diet and exercise patterns of nearly 2,600 adults ages 20 to 74, the average obese woman got only about an hour of exercise a year; obese men averaged 3.6 hours.[3] The one activity most Americans reported most often: sitting.

The greatest threat may come from television. Americans spend most of their leisure time watching television: on average, more than 30 hours a week. Compared with other sedentary activities, such as reading, writing, or driving, watching TV lowers metabolic rate, so people burn fewer calories.

√ **check-in** Did you know that trading two minutes of sitting for two minutes of a light-intensity activity like walking every hour can lower your risk of premature death by 33 percent?

Getting up and walking for two minutes every hour can reverse the negative effects of prolonged sitting. In a recent study, short bursts of activity—walking, going up and down stairs, doing household chores—boosted the longevity of people who are sedentary more than half of their day.[4]

Physical Activity and Exercise

Physical activity refers to any movement produced by the muscles that results in expenditure of energy (measured in calories). According to a study of more than 6,000 American adults, short stretches of physical activity, such as taking the stairs or walking several blocks, during the day can be as beneficial as a trip to the gym. An "active lifestyle" approach can be as effective as structured exercise in preventing hypertension and other cardiovascular risk factors.

√ **check-in** How do you build movement into your daily routine? By walking to class instead of taking the shuttle? Opting for the stairs rather than the elevator? Dancing during a study break?

Exercise is a type of physical activity that requires planned, structured, and repetitive bodily movement with the intent of improving one or more components of physical fitness. If exercise could be packed into a pill, it would be the single most widely prescribed and beneficial medicine in the nation. Why? Because nothing can do more to help your body function at its best.

Exercise Is Medicine

Declaring physical inactivity "the greatest public health problem of the 21st century," the American College of Sports Medicine (ACSM) has launched an "Exercise Is Medicine" global initiative involving health and fitness professionals, businesses, universities, government leaders, organizations of every kind, and "anyone who gets it" to start or renew an exercise program as "an investment in lifelong health."[4] As hundreds of studies over the last few decades have documented, exercise is indeed medicine.

√ **check-in** What can exercise do for you?
*Cut your risk of dying of breast cancer by about 50 percent
*Lower your risk of colon cancer by 60 percent
*Reduce your risk of Alzheimer's by about 40 percent
*Decrease your risk of heart disease and high blood pressure by about 40 percent
*Lower your risk of stroke by 27 percent[5]

The Benefits of Exercise

The benefits of exercise start *now*. As the latest scientific research demonstrates, the right types and amounts of exercise will lengthen your life, strengthen your brain, alter your waistline, and even clear debris from your body's cells.

As Figure 8.1 illustrates, exercise provides head-to-toe benefits:[6]

- You may live longer.

- Your heart muscles become stronger and pump blood more efficiently.

- Your heart rate and resting pulse slow down.

- Your blood pressure may drop slightly from its normal level.

- Your bones become denser, and the loss of calcium that normally occurs with age slows.

HEALTH NOW!

Excise Exercise Excuses

In your online journal, write down as many reasons as you can think of not to exercise. Then come up with quick excuse busters. Here are some ideas:

I can't afford a gym.
- Who needs a gym? You can get all the exercise you need on your own.
- Check out campus or community facilities.
- Walk or jog outdoors.
- Invest in inexpensive hand weights.

The school gym is always crowded.
- Always? Have you tried Sunday mornings, Friday evening at 7:00, Tuesdays at 3:00 p.m.? Ask the staff what times are quietest.
- If there are lines for the weight machines, use hand weights. If the treadmills are occupied, go to the outdoor track.
- Sign up for small-group training or classes to guarantee yourself a spot.

It's finals week.
- Break up study sessions with mini-workouts.
- Burn off tension with a jog.
- Unwind after studying with stretches, yoga, or Pilates.

I go to my dorm and just don't feel like leaving.
- Arrange to meet friends at the gym. If you know they're waiting, you'll go out even if it's rainy and cold.
- Sign up for a gym class during the day so that you don't have to make an extra trip.
- Recruit an exercise buddy so that the two of you can motivate each other to get moving.

Health Benefits of Physical Activity—A Review of the Strength of the Scientific Evidence

Strong Evidence

- Lower risk of early death
- Lower risk of coronary heart disease
- Lower risk of stroke
- Lower risk of high blood pressure
- Lower risk of adverse blood lipid profile
- Lower risk of type 2 diabetes
- Lower risk of metabolic syndrome
- Lower risk of colon cancer
- Lower risk of breast cancer
- Prevention of weight gain
- Weight loss, particularly when combined with reduced calorie intake
- Prevention of falls
- Reduced depression
- Better cognitive function (for older adults)

Moderate to Strong Evidence

- Better functional health (for older adults)
- Reduced abdominal obesity

Moderate Evidence

- Lower risk of hip fracture
- Lower risk of lung cancer
- Lower risk of endometrial cancer
- Weight maintenance after weight loss
- Increased bone density
- Improved sleep quality

Source: U.S. Department of Health and Human Services, www.hhs.gov

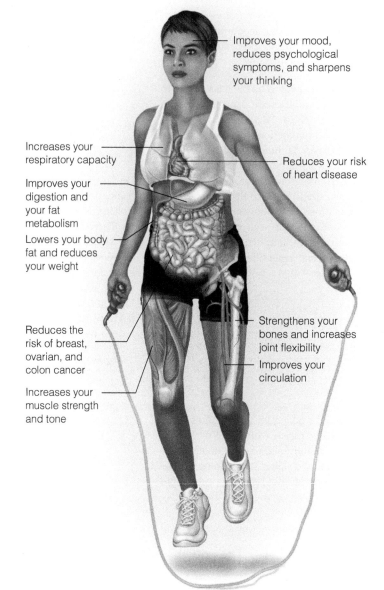

© Cengage Learning

......

FIGURE 8.1 The Benefits of Exercise

Regular physical activity enhances your overall physical and mental health and helps prevent disease.

- Your flexibility increases.
- Your digestive system works more efficiently.
- Your metabolism speeds up.
- Your lean body mass increases, so you burn more calories and body fat decreases.
- You become more sensitive to insulin (a great benefit for diabetics) and may lower the risk of developing diabetes.
- Because of increased clot-dissolving substances in the blood, you lessen the risk of strokes, heart attacks, and pulmonary embolisms (clots in the lungs).
- You reduce your likelihood of developing certain cancers.
- You lower levels of stress hormones like cortisol that can dampen resistance to disease.
- You increase the circulation of natural killer cells that fight off viruses and bacteria. Exercise also improves the body's response to the influenza vaccine, so it is more effective at keeping the virus at bay.

Longer Life In various studies, physical activity increased life expectancy by 1.3 to 5.5 years. The number of years you may be able to add to your life depends on your gender, age, and activity level. If you are a white, 20-year-old, active or somewhat active man, your estimated life expectancy would be about 2.4 years longer than that of your inactive peers. If you are a black, 20-year-old, active or somewhat active woman, you could gain an extra 5.5 years.

Even minutes count. A mere 10 minutes of physical activity may increase lifespans in adults by almost two years—even in those who are overweight.

Healthier Heart and Lungs Active individuals have about a 30 percent lower risk of cardiovascular disease than inactive ones. Regular physical activity makes blood less likely to clot and cause a stroke or heart attack. Sedentary people are about twice as likely to die of a heart attack as people who are physically active. Although rigorous exercise somewhat increases the risk of sudden cardiac death for men, regular physical activity lowers the overall danger, especially in women. (See Chapter 15 for a discussion of heart disease.)

Exercise also lowers levels of the indicators of increased risk of heart disease, such as high cholesterol. Exercise itself, even without weight loss, may reduce dangerous blood fats in obese individuals. It also lowers the risk of developing the prediabetic condition called metabolic syndrome, which if untreated can lead to type 2 diabetes and increase the risk of heart disease.

In women exercise lowers the risk of a fatal heart attack by slowing a rapid heart rate. The faster the resting heart rate (beats per minute), the greater the risk of dying from a heart attack in both sexes, although the risk is higher in women.

In addition to its effects on the heart, exercise makes the lungs more efficient. The lungs take in more oxygen, and their vital capacity (the maximum amount of air volume the lungs can take in and expel) increases, providing more energy for you to use.

Cardiorespiratory fitness declines more rapidly after age 45, but exercising regularly, maintaining a healthy weight, and not smoking can help maintain cardiorespiratory health throughout life. Even individuals with a genetic predisposition to cardiovascular disease can improve their cardiorespiratory fitness.

Protection against Cancer Physical activity may reduce the risk of several cancers, including breast, colon, endometrial, prostate, and possibly pancreatic as well as non-Hodgkin's lymphoma.[7] In addition to helping maintain a healthy body weight, exercise may help prevent cancer by regulating sex hormones, insulin, and prostaglandins and by enhancing the immune system.

In its most recent Nutrition and Physical Activity Guidelines, the American Cancer Society recommends the following:

- For adults, engaging in at least 150 minutes of moderate-intensity or 75 minutes of vigorous-intensity activity each week, preferably spread throughout the week

- For children and adolescents, engaging in at least one hour of moderately or vigorously intense activity at least three days a week

- Limiting sedentary behavior such as sitting, lying down, and watching television or other forms of screen-based entertainment

- Engaging in some physical activity above one's usual level—for example, taking the stairs rather than the elevator

According to the American Institute for Cancer Research, physical activity may lower the risk of colon cancer by 40 to 50 percent; the risk of breast, endometrial, and lung cancers by 30 to 40 percent; and the risk of prostate cancer by 10 to 30 percent. Along with a healthful diet and limited alcohol intake, regular exercise could prevent about 340,000 cancer cases a year.

The combination of excess weight and physical inactivity may account for one-quarter to one-third of all breast cancer cases. Regular, lifelong exercise may lower a woman's breast cancer risk by 20 percent, possibly by reducing weight and body mass and preventing metabolic syndrome and chronic inflammation (discussed in Chapter 15). Men who regularly get moderate exercise may have a lower risk of developing prostate cancer; those who do get the disease are less likely to have aggressive, fast-growing tumors.

Better Bones You may think that weak, brittle bones are a problem only for elderly people. However, 2 percent of college-age women have osteoporosis; another 15 percent have already sustained significant losses in bone density and are at high risk of osteoporosis.

The college women at greatest risk often are extremely skinny and maintain their low weights by dieting (often not eating calcium-rich dairy products) and by avoiding exercise so as not to increase their muscle mass. Depo-Provera, a method of birth control that consists of hormone injections every three months, also is associated with low bone density, especially with long-term use. (See Chapter 9 on contraception.)

Exercise during adolescence and young adulthood may prevent bone weakening and fractures in old age—particularly in individuals who continue to exercise as they grow older, as confirmed by a recent longitudinal study of professional baseball players.[8]

√ **check-in** Do you know the best exercises to boost bone density?

According to a study of college women, high-impact aerobics, such as Zumba, may offer the quickest route to building bone. Resistance exercises such as squats, leg presses, and calf presses were found to strengthen leg muscles but to have no effect on bone density. The American College of Sports Medicine (ACSM) recommends moderate- to high-intensity weight-bearing activities to maintain bone mass in adults.

Lower Weight According to the ACSM's statement on "appropriate physical activity intervention strategies for weight loss and prevention of weight regain," long-term weight loss requires 250 or more minutes (2 hours and 30 minutes) of moderately intense physical activity per week. Less exercise can prevent a gain greater than 3 percent of current weight but provides what the ACSM describes as "only modest" weight loss. In addition to aerobic workouts, the ACSM recommends resistance training to increase lean tissue and decrease fat.

For individuals on a diet, exercise provides extra benefits: Dieters who work out lose more fat than lean muscle tissue, which improves their body composition. Exercise also may help to control weight by suppressing appetite.

Better Mental Health and Functioning Exercise is an effective—but underused—treatment for mild to moderate depression and may help in treating other mental disorders. Regular, moderate exercise—such as walking, running, or lifting weights—three times a week has proved helpful for depression and anxiety disorders, including panic attacks. Exercise is as effective as medication in improving mood and also helps prevent relapse.

Lifelong fitness may protect the brain as we age. According to numerous long-term studies, physically fit adults perform better on cognitive tests than their less fit peers. Exercise may protect the aging brain by means of increased blood flow, improved development and survival of neurons, and decreased risk of heart and blood vessel diseases.[9]

Benefits for Students Unlike middle-aged and older individuals, traditional-age college students cite improved fitness as the number-one advantage that exercise offers, followed by improved appearance and muscle tone. Undergraduates who recognize the benefits of exercise are more likely to be physically active than those who focus on barriers to working out.

Your brain may also benefit. In research on more than 1.2 million men, strong cardiorespiratory fitness in young adulthood was associated with higher intelligence, better grades, and greater success in life. The reasons may be improved blood flow to the brain, diminished anxiety, enhanced mood, and less fatigue. In individuals under age 35, short bouts of moderate exercise—such as 10 to 40 minutes of cycling or running—may improve higher executive functions in your brain, enhancing your ability to focus attention and to control impulses.[10]

√ **check-in** Do you think fitness affects your academic performance?

Brighter Mood and Less Stress As a multinational study recently demonstrated, physical activity produces an unexpected positive psychological benefit: happiness (discussed in depth in Chapter 2). Compared to sedentary individuals, active people report higher levels of happiness—from 20 to 52 percent higher, depending on the exercise "dose." For men, vigorous exercise yielded the greatest happiness dividends; for women, moderate-intensity activities like walking were most likely to boost their moods.[11]

Exercise makes people feel good from the inside out in various ways, including

- Boosting mood
- Elevating self-esteem
- Increasing energy
- Reducing tension
- Relieving stress
- Improving concentration and alertness

During long workouts, some people experience what is called "runner's high," which may be the result of increased levels of mood-elevating brain chemicals called endorphins. Psychological improvements occur even after a 20-minute bout of exercise, regardless of how intensely you exercise.

✓**check-in** Don't worry: Get active—and happy! Tune into your mood before and after you engage in different activities.

Do you feel happier after a bicycle ride or a run? A swim or a stretch class?

Men and women of various ages in different countries report different responses, but around the world, moving makes people happier than staying still.

A More Active and Healthy Old Age

Exercise slows the changes that are associated with advancing age: loss of lean muscle tissue, increase in body fat, and decrease in work capacity. In addition to lowering the risk of heart disease and stroke, exercise helps older men and women retain the strength and mobility needed to live independently. Studies that followed competitive runners, cyclists, and swimmers from ages 40 to 81 found little evidence of deterioration in their musculature.

In a longitudinal study of mainly white, highly educated adults, those who were physically fit in middle age showed a lower risk of dementia later in life. Other research has shown that remaining physically active as you age may help protect parts of the brain related to memory and thinking from shrinking.

As a recent study of twins demonstrated, exercise increases the size of brain regions involved in balance and coordination, which in the long term could reduce the risk of falls in old age.[12] Even low-intensity activities can enhance mobility as well as cardiovascular health in older individuals.[13]

Enhanced Sexuality

By improving physical endurance, muscle tone, blood flow, and body composition, exercise improves sexual functioning. Simply burning 200 extra calories a day can significantly lower the risk of erectile dysfunction in sedentary men. Exercise also may increase sexual drive, activity, and sexual satisfaction in people of all ages.

More exercise may mean better sex—at least for men. In a recent study, men who engaged in the equivalent of 2 hours of strenuous exercise, 3.5 hours of moderate exercise, or 6 hours of light exercise a week reported higher sexual function, including their ability to have erections and orgasms and the quality and frequency of erections.[14]

Exercise Risks

Despite its many benefits, exercise can pose risks—and not just for those over age 40. Even young college athletes who seem in perfect health have collapsed and died while running and while playing sports such as football and basketball.

The most common cause is hypertrophic cardiomyopathy (HCM), a genetic disease that results in thickening or enlargement of the heart that affects up to 1 in 500 people. HCM accounts for 40 percent of all deaths on athletic fields in the United States. An average of 66 athletes younger than age 40 die each year from cardiac arrest in the United States.

HCM can be detected and treated. Medical experts urge screening for all young athletes, beginning in elementary school. However, screening results in a high number of false positives and has not proven to reduce young athlete deaths.

College students who play contact sports such as football may be at risk of a condition called chronic traumatic encephalopathy (CTE), the result of multiple mild head injuries. Initial symptoms include headache and difficulty paying attention. As the condition worsens, sufferers may face depression, outbursts of anger, short-term memory loss, and difficulty thinking and making decisions. The most severe forms can cause dementia, aggression, and difficulty finding words.

Concern is increasing about the long-term effects of injuries many elite college athletes suffered during their brief college sports careers. A recent study compared 232 male and female intercollegiate athletes and 225 men and women who didn't play high-level sports. By the time they reached ages 40 to 65, the former athletes were more than twice as likely to have physical problems that limited their daily activities as well as higher levels of depression, fatigue, and poor sleep than non-athletes.

✓**check-in** If you are a college athlete, what steps are you taking to protect your long-term health?

Physical Activity and Exercise   **213**

Physical Activity Guidelines for Americans

The U.S. Department of Health and Human Services *Physical Activity Guidelines for Americans*, based on the most significant research findings on the health benefits of physical activity, recognize that some activity is better than none. However, the *Guidelines* emphasize that more activity—consisting of both aerobic (endurance) and muscle-strengthening (resistance) physical activity—is more beneficial.

Here are the government's key recommendations:

- **All adults should avoid inactivity.** Some physical activity is better than none, and adults who participate in any amount of physical activity gain some health benefits.

- For substantial health benefits, **adults should do at least 150 minutes (2 hours and 30 minutes) a week** of moderate-intensity or 75 minutes (1 hour and 15 minutes) a week of vigorous-intensity aerobic physical activity or an equivalent combination of moderate- and vigorous-intensity aerobic activity. The ACSM recommends episodes of at least 10 minutes. However, new studies have found that physical activity for periods even briefer than 10 minutes may influence cardiometabolic risk. In an analysis of more than 2,000 volunteers, more than half met the guidelines of 150 minutes a week—but mostly in short bouts that lasted less than 10 minutes.

- For additional and more extensive health benefits, **adults should increase their aerobic physical activity to 300 minutes (5 hours)** a week of moderate-intensity or 150 minutes a week of vigorous-intensity aerobic physical activity or an equivalent combination of moderate- and vigorous-intensity activity. Additional health benefits are gained by engaging in physical activity beyond this amount.

- Adults should also do muscle-strengthening activities that are moderate or high intensity and involve all major muscle groups **on two or more days a week,** as these activities provide additional health benefits.

MET (metabolic equivalent of task) The amount of energy used at rest.

The ACSM and the American Heart Association (AHA) have released similar guidelines that call for the following:

- Moderately intense cardiorespiratory exercise 30 minutes a day, 5 days a week

or

- Vigorously intense cardiorespiratory exercise 20 minutes a day, 3 days a week

and

- 8 to 10 strength-training exercises, with 8 to 12 repetitions of each exercise, twice a week

According to the ACSM, moderate-intensity physical activity means working hard enough to raise your heart rate and break a sweat yet still being able to carry on a conversation. The 30-minute recommendation is for an average healthy adult to maintain health and reduce the risk for chronic disease.

✓**check-in** Do you exercise often and intensely enough to meet these guidelines?

How Much Exercise Is Enough?

In developing federal physical activity guidelines, experts considered dozens of studies and concluded that the "amount of physical activity necessary to produce health benefits cannot yet be identified with a high degree of precision." However, they did determine the minimum amount of exercise required for a significant lowering of the risk of premature dying: 500 MET minutes of exercise a week.

A single **MET (metabolic equivalent of task)** is the amount of energy a person uses at rest. Two METs represent twice the energy burned at rest; four METs, four times the energy used at rest; and so on. Walking at 3 miles per hour is a 3.3-MET activity, while running at 6 miles per hour is a 10-MET activity.

The Department of Health and Human Services defines moderate exercise as activities of between three and six METs, equivalent to about 45 to 64 percent of your maximum heart rate (discussed on page 217)—or, in simpler terms, activities during which you can carry on a conversation but cannot sing out loud. (See Table 8.1.)

The weekly minimum of 500 MET minutes of exercise does not mean 500 minutes of exercise.

Instead, 150 minutes a week (2.5 hours) of a moderate, three- to five-MET activity, such as walking, works out to be about 500 MET minutes. Half as much time (1.25 hours per week) spent on a six-plus-MET activity like easy jogging produces similar health effects. As a rule of thumb, 1 minute of vigorous-intensity activity is as beneficial as 2 minutes of moderate-intensity activity.

Are more METS better? To a certain extent, the answer is yes. Activity of 500 MET minutes a week substantially reduces the risk of premature death, but a significant reduction in breast cancer risk requires more METs. Exercise in the range of 500 to 1,000 MET minutes a week, experts generally agree, delivers substantial benefits.

✓**check-in** Do you get 500 MET minutes of exercise a week?

Your Exercise Prescription

For years, exercise has had what some call a "Goldilocks problem," with endless debate over how much is too much, too little, or just about the right amount. A recent large-scale, fourteen-year study of more than 661,000 people produced some answers, including the following[15]:

- Individuals who didn't exercise at all were at greatest risk of many diseases as well as of early death. Even a little exercise helped lower the likelihood of premature death.

- Individuals who got the recommended minimum of 150 minutes of moderate exercise per week significantly reduced their risk of dying (by 31 percent over a 14-year period) compared to those who didn't exercise.

- Individuals who tripled the recommended level of exercise, working out moderately (generally by walking) for 450 minutes per week (a little more than an hour per day) were even less likely to die prematurely.

- Those who engaged in 10 or more times the recommended amount of exercise did not gain any greater health benefits—but they also did not increase their risk of dying young.

Another study of more than 200,000 Australian adults found that moderate exercise, such as walking, for the recommended 150 minutes a week substantially reduced the risk of premature death. However, those who spent up to 30 percent of their weekly exercise time in vigorous activities gained an extra reduction in early

TABLE 8.1 Exercise Options

Vigorous activities take more effort than moderate ones. Here are just a few moderate and vigorous aerobic physical activities. Do these for 10 minutes or more at a time.

Moderate Activities (I can talk while I do them, but I can't sing.)	Vigorous Activities (I can only say a few words without stopping to catch my breath.)
• Ballroom and line dancing	• Aerobic dance
• Biking on level ground or with few hills	• Biking faster than 10 miles per hour
• Canoeing	• Fast dancing
• General gardening (raking, trimming shrubs)	• Heavy gardening (digging, hoeing)
• Sports where you catch and throw (baseball, softball, volleyball)	• Hiking uphill
• Tennis (doubles)	• Jumping rope
• Using your manual wheelchair	• Martial arts (such as karate)
• Using hand cyclers—also called ergometers	• Race walking, jogging, or running
• Walking briskly	• Sports with a lot of running (basketball, hockey, soccer)
• Water aerobics	• Swimming fast or swimming laps
	• Tennis (singles)
	• Zumba

© Cengage Learning

© Sean Nel/Shutterstock.com

mortality. The researchers' recommendation: Get at least 150 minutes of physical activity per week, including 20 to 30 minutes of vigorous exertion.[16]

In other research, higher-intensity exercise (such as walking on a treadmill) proved to be more effective than moderate activity (such as strolling) in lowering blood sugar and cardiovascular risks in middle-aged sedentary, obese individuals.[17]

The Principles of Exercise

Your body is literally what you make of it. Superbly designed for multiple uses, it adjusts to meet physical demands. If you need to sprint for a bus, your heart will speed up and pump more blood. Beyond such immediate, short-term adaptations, physical training can produce long-term changes in heart rate, oxygen consumption, and muscle strength and endurance. Although there are limits on the maximum levels of physical fitness and performance that any individual can

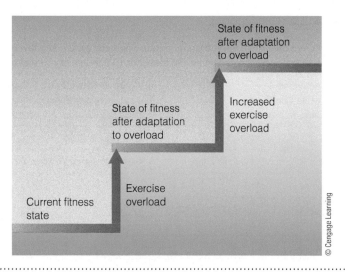

FIGURE 8.2 The Overload Principle

By increasing frequency, intensity, or duration, you will improve your level of fitness. Once your body adapts to (becomes comfortable with) the demands, you can again apply the overload principle to achieve a higher level of fitness.

achieve, regular exercise can produce improvements in everyone's baseline wellness and fitness.

The following principles of exercise are fundamental to any physical activity plan.

Overload Principle

The **overload principle** requires a person exercising to provide a greater stress or demand on the body than it's usually accustomed to handling. For any muscle, including the heart, to get stronger, it must work against a greater-than-normal resistance or challenge. To continue to improve, you need further increases in the demands—but not too much too quickly. **Progressive overloading**—gradually increasing physical challenges—provides the benefits of exercise without the risk of injuries (Figure 8.2).

Overloading is specific to each body part and to each component of fitness. Leg exercises develop only the lower limbs; arm exercises, only the upper limbs. This is why you need a comprehensive fitness plan that includes a variety of exercises to develop different parts of the body. If you play a particular sport, you also need training to develop sports-specific skills, such as a strong, efficient stroke in swimming.

√**check-in** Does your fitness program include exercises for different parts of the body?

overload principle The idea that for the body to get stronger, you must provide a greater stress or demand on the body than it is normally accustomed to handling.

progressive overloading Gradually increasing physical challenges once the body adapts to the stress placed upon it to produce maximum benefits.

FITT A formula that describes the frequency, intensity, type, and length of time for physical activity.

specificity principle The idea that each part of the body adapts to a particular type and amount of stress placed upon it.

FITT

Although low-intensity activity can enhance basic health, you need to work harder—that is, at a greater intensity—to improve fitness. Whatever exercise you do, there is a level, or threshold, at which fitness begins to improve; a target zone, where you can achieve maximum benefits; and an upper limit, at which potential risks outweigh any further benefits. The acronym **FITT** sums up the four dimensions of progressive overload: *frequency* (how often you exercise), *intensity* (how hard), *time* (how long), and *type* (specific activity).

Frequency To attain and maintain physical fitness, you need to exercise regularly, but the recommended frequency varies with different types of exercise and with an individual's fitness goals. Health officials urge Americans to engage in moderate-intensity aerobic activity most days and in resistance and flexibility training two or three days a week.

Intensity Exercise intensity varies with the type of exercise and with personal goals. To improve cardiorespiratory fitness, you need at a minimum to increase your heart rate to a target zone (the level that produces benefits). To develop muscular strength and endurance, you need to increase the amount of weight you lift or the resistance you work against and/or the number of repetitions. For enhanced flexibility, you need to stretch muscles beyond their normal length.

Time (Duration) The amount of time, or duration, of your workouts is also important, particularly for cardiorespiratory exercise. The ACSM recommends 30 to 45 minutes of aerobic exercise, preceded by 5 to 10 minutes of warm-up and followed by 5 to 10 minutes of stretching. However, experts have found similar health benefits from a single 30-minute session of moderate exercise as from several shorter sessions throughout the day. Duration and intensity are interlinked. If you're exercising at high intensity (biking or running at a brisk pace, for instance), you don't need to exercise as long as when you're working at lower intensity (walking or swimming at a moderate pace). For muscular strength and endurance and for flexibility, duration is defined by the number of sets or repetitions rather than total time.

Type (Specificity) The **specificity principle** refers to the body's adaptation to a particular type of activity or amount of stress placed on it.

Jogging, for instance, trains the heart and lungs to work more efficiently and strengthens certain leg muscles. However, it does not build upper body strength or enhance flexibility.

Reversibility Principle

The **reversibility principle** is the opposite of the overload principle. Just as the body adapts to greater physical demands, it also adjusts to lower levels. If you stop exercising, you can lose as much as 50 percent of your fitness improvements within two months. If you have to curtail your usual exercise routine because of a busy schedule, you can best maintain your fitness by keeping the intensity constant and reducing frequency or duration. The principle of reversibility is aptly summed up by the phrase "Use it or lose it."

Improving Cardiorespiratory Fitness

Cardiorespiratory endurance refers to the ability of the heart, lungs, and circulatory system to deliver oxygen to muscles working rhythmically over an extended period of time. Unlike muscular endurance (discussed later in this chapter), which is specific to individual muscles, cardiorespiratory endurance involves the entire body and can be aerobic or anaerobic.

- **Aerobic exercise**, which improves cardiorespiratory endurance, can take many forms, but all involve working strenuously without pushing to the point of breathlessness. A person who builds up good aerobic capacity can maintain long periods of physical activity without great fatigue.

- In **anaerobic exercise**, the amount of oxygen taken in by the body cannot meet the demands of the activity. This quickly creates an oxygen deficit that must be made up later. Anaerobic activities are high in intensity but short in duration, usually lasting only about 10 seconds to 2 minutes. An example is sprinting the quarter-mile, which leaves even the best-trained athletes gasping for air. In *nonaerobic exercise*, such as bowling, softball, or doubles tennis, there is frequent rest

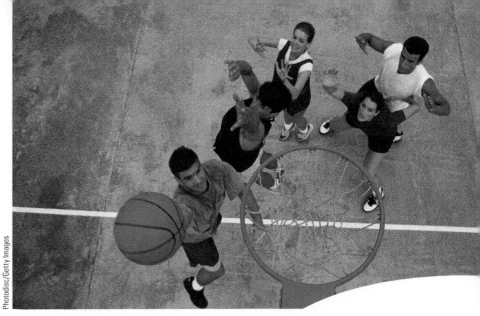

Group sports provide a fun alternative way to exercise, but an occasional game is no substitute for regular physical activity.

between activities. Because the body can take in all the oxygen it needs, the heart and lungs don't get much of a workout.

Monitoring Intensity

To use your pulse, or heart rate, as a guide, feel your pulse in the carotid artery in your neck. Slightly tilt your head back and to one side. Use your middle finger or forefinger, or both, to feel for your pulse. (Do not use your thumb; it has a beat of its own.) To determine your heart rate, count the number of pulses you feel for 10 seconds and multiply that number by six, or count for 30 seconds and multiply that number by two. Learn to recognize the pulsing of your heart when you're sitting or lying down. This is your **resting heart rate**.

Start taking your pulse during or immediately after exercise, when it's much more pronounced than when you're at rest. Three minutes after heavy exercise, take your pulse again. The closer that reading is to your resting heart rate, the better your condition. If it takes a long time for your pulse to recover and return to its resting level, your body's ability to handle physical stress is poor. As you continue working out, however, your pulse will return to normal much more quickly.

Target Heart Rate   You don't want to push yourself to your maximum heart rate. The ACSM recommends working at 50 to 85 percent, depending on your level of fitness, of that maximum to get cardiorespiratory benefits from your training. This range is called your **target heart rate**. If you don't exercise intensely enough to raise your

reversibility principle The idea that the physical benefits of exercise are lost through disuse or inactivity.

aerobic exercise Physical activity in which sufficient or excess oxygen is continually supplied to the body.

anaerobic exercise Physical activity in which the body develops an oxygen deficit.

resting heart rate The number of heartbeats per minute during inactivity.

target heart rate Fifty to 85 percent of the maximum heart rate; the heart rate at which one derives maximum cardiovascular benefit from aerobic exercise.

Rating of Perceived Exertion (RPE)	
0	Nothing at all
0.5	Extremely weak (just noticeable)
1	Very weak
2	Weak (light)
3	Moderate
4	Somewhat strong
5	Strong (heavy)
6	—
7	Very strong
8	—
9	—
10	Extremely strong (almost maximum)

4, 5 — Correlate to target heart rate

FIGURE 8.3 Revised Scale for Rating of Perceived Exertion (RPE)
You can learn to rate your exertion based on this scale.

Source: Original scale from G. Borg, "Psychophysical Bases of Perceived Exertion," *Medicine and Science in Sports and Exercise*, vol. 14, no. 5 (2003): pp. 377-381.

heart rate at least this high, your heart and lungs won't reap the most benefit from the workout. If you push too hard and exercise at or near your absolute maximum heart rate, you run the risk of placing too great a burden on your heart.

In order to find the best "zone" for your goals and activity, you must first know how to calculate your maximum heart rate. The following formula offers a rough baseline:

$$220 - \text{Age} = \text{Maximum heart rate (MHR)}$$

The ACSM recommends that for endurance training and general aerobic conditioning, you calculate 50 to 65 percent of your maximum heart rate if you're a beginner; 60 to 75 percent for intermediate-level exercisers; and 70 to 85 percent for established aerobic exercisers. For example, if you're a 45-year-old beginner with no known health issues, your maximum heart rate is approximately 175 beats a minute. Fifty to 65 percent of that maximum is 87 to 113 beats per minute.

Recent research has found a gender difference in heart rates. Young men tend to have a lower resting heart rate and a higher peak heart rate than women. Men's heart rates also rise more dramatically during exercise and return to normal more quickly.

Rating of Perceived Exertion (RPE) A self-assessment scale that rates symptoms of breathlessness and fatigue.

Your heart rate can also help you keep tabs on your progress: Measure your heart rate 15 to 60 minutes after exercising and compare these numbers over time as you get in better shape. The numbers decrease as your heart becomes stronger.

The Karvonen Formula The Karvonen formula is another mathematical formula for determining your target heart rate (HR) training zone. The formula uses maximum and resting heart rate with the desired training intensity to get a target heart rate:

$$\text{Target heart rate} = ((\text{Max HR} - \text{Resting HR}) \times \text{Intensity}) + \text{Resting HR}$$

Ideally, you should measure your resting and maximum heart rates for more accurate results. If the maximum heart rate cannot be measured directly, it can be roughly estimated using the traditional formula of 220 minus your age. You can also use an average value of 70 bpm (beats per minute) for your resting heart rate.

For example, if you are a 25-year-old male who has been exercising regularly, with a resting heart rate of 65, you would calculate your training heart rate for the intensity level of 70 percent, using the following formula:

$$220 - 25 \, (\text{age}) = 195$$
$$195 - 65 \, (\text{resting heart rate}) = 130$$
$$130 \times .70 \, (\text{percent of maximum}) + 65 \, (\text{resting heart rate}) = 156 \text{ beats per minute}$$

Rating of Perceived Exertion (RPE) Another option besides heart rate for monitoring your exercise intensity is the **Rating of Perceived Exertion (RPE)**, a self-assessment scale that rates symptoms of breathlessness and fatigue. You can use the RPE scale to describe your sensation of effort when exercising and gauge how hard you are working. The ACSM revised the original RPE scale to a range of 0 to 10 (Figure 8.3). Most exercisers should aim for a perceived exertion of "somewhat strong" or "strong," the equivalent of 4 or 5 on the RPE scale.

RPE is considered fairly reliable, but about 10 percent of the population tends to over- or underestimate their exertion. Your health or physical education instructor can help you learn to match what your body is feeling to the RPE scale. By paying attention to how you feel at different exercise intensities, you can learn to challenge yourself without risking your safety.

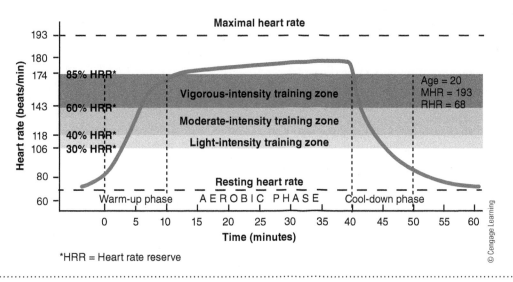

Maximal heart rate

Age = 20
MHR = 193
RHR = 68

85% HRR*

Vigorous-intensity training zone

60% HRR*

Moderate-intensity training zone

40% HRR*

Light-intensity training zone

30% HRR*

Resting heart rate

Warm-up phase   A E R O B I C   P H A S E   Cool-down phase

Heart rate (beats/min)

193
180
174
143
118
106
80
60

0   5   10   15   20   25   30   35   40   45   50   55   60

Time (minutes)

© Cengage Learning

*HRR = Heart rate reserve

FIGURE 8.4 Recommended Cardiorespiratory or Aerobic Training Pattern

Designing an Aerobic Workout

Whatever activity you choose, your aerobic workout should consist of several stages: a warm-up, an aerobic activity, and a cool-down. (See Figure 8.4.)

Warm-up   Just as you don't get in your car and immediately gun your engine to 60 miles per hour, you shouldn't do the same with your body. You need to prepare your cardiorespiratory system for a workout, speed up the blood flow to your lungs, and increase the temperature and elasticity of your muscles and connective tissue to avoid injury. After reviewing more than 350 scientific studies, the ACSM concluded that preparing for sports or exercise should involve a variety of activities and not be limited to stretching alone. Researchers found little to no relationship between stretching and injuries or postexercise pain. A better option is a combination of warm-up, strength training, and balance exercises.

√**check-in** How do you warm up before exercising?

Aerobic Activity   The two key components of this part of your workout are intensity and duration. As described in the previous section, you can use your target heart rate range to make sure you are working at the proper intensity. The current recommendation is to keep moving for 30 to 60 minutes, either in one session or several briefer sessions, each lasting at least 10 minutes.

Cool Down   After you've pushed your heart rate up to its target level and kept it there for a while, the worst thing you can do is slam on the brakes. If you come to a sudden stop, you put your heart at risk. When you stand or sit immediately after vigorous exercise, blood can pool in your legs. You need to keep moving at a slower pace to ensure an adequate supply of blood to your heart. Ideally, you should walk for 5 to 10 minutes at a comfortable pace before you end your workout session.

Your Long-Term Fitness Plan

One of the most common mistakes people make is to push too hard too fast. Often they end up injured or discouraged and quit entirely. If you are just starting an aerobic program, think of it as a series of phases: beginning, progression, and maintenance:

- **Beginning (4–6 weeks).** Start slow and low (in intensity). If you're walking, monitor your heart rate and aim for 55 percent of your maximum heart rate. Another good rule of thumb to make sure you're moving at the right pace: If you can sing as you walk, you're going too slow; if you can't talk, you're going too fast.

- **Progression (16–20 weeks).** Gradually increase the duration and/or intensity of your workouts. For instance, you might add five minutes every two weeks to your walking time. You also can gradually pick up your pace, using your target heart rate as your guide. Keep a log of your workouts so you can chart your progress until you reach your goal.

- **Maintenance (lifelong).** Once you've reached the stage of exercising for an hour every day, you may want to develop a repertoire of aerobic activities you enjoy. Combine or alternate activities to avoid monotony and keep up your enthusiasm (cross-training).

Aerobic Options

You have lots of choices for aerobic exercise, so experiment. Focus on one for a few weeks; alternate different activities on different days; try something new every month.

Stepping Out: Walk the Walk
Walking may reduce the risk factors for cardiorespiratory disease, such as insulin resistance, as much as vigorous activity does. Walking briskly three hours a week has proven as effective as an hour and a half a week in more vigorous activities, such as aerobics or running, in protecting women's hearts. Women engaging in either form of exercise have a rate of heart attacks 30 to 40 percent lower than that of sedentary women.

Walking also protects men's hearts, whether they're healthy or have had heart problems. Men who regularly engage in light exercise, including walking, have a significantly lower risk of death than their sedentary counterparts.

√**check-in** Do you track your steps with an app or monitor? If so, how many steps do you walk on an average day?

America on the Move
The typical adult averages about 5,310 steps; a child, from 11,000 to 13,000. According to the ACSM, college students who used a pedometer to count their daily steps took an average of 7,700 steps per day. This falls short of the 10,000 steps recommended as part of the national "America on the Move" program.

How far is 10,000 steps? The following statistics provide some guidance:

- The average person's stride length is approximately 2.5 feet.
- This means it takes just over 2,000 steps to walk 1 mile, and 10,000 steps is close to 5 miles.
- Brisk walking, according to researchers' calculations, translates into an average of 118 steps—116 for men, 121 for women—per minute.[18]

Why 10,000 steps? According to researchers' estimates, you take about 5,000 steps just to accomplish your daily tasks. Adding about 2,000 steps brings you to a level that can improve your health and wellness. Another 3,000 steps can help you lose excess pounds and prevent weight gain. People who walk at least 10,000 steps a day are more likely to have healthy weights. In addition, 10,000 steps generally translates into 30 minutes of activity, the minimum recommended by the U.S. Surgeon General.

Treadmills are good alternatives to outdoor walks—and not just in bad weather. They keep you moving at a certain pace, and they allow you to exercise in a climate-controlled, pollution-free environment—a definite plus for many city dwellers. Holding onto the handrails while walking on a treadmill reduces both heart rate and oxygen consumption, so you burn fewer calories. Slow the pace if necessary so you can let go of the handrails while working out.

Elliptical trainers are another aerobic option—with the additional benefit of being easier on the feet, knees, and other joints. In a study that compared the impact of walking on the ground, jogging on the ground, treadmill jogging, and elliptical exercise, elliptical training registered the lowest impact, followed by outdoor walking, treadmill jogging, and outdoor jogging.[19]

Jogging and Running
If you have been sedentary, it's best to launch a walking program before attempting to jog or run indoors or out. Start by walking for 15 to 20 minutes three times a week at a comfortable pace. Continue at this same level until you no longer feel sore or unduly fatigued the day after exercising. Then increase your walking time to 20 to 25 minutes, speeding up your pace as well.

When you can handle a brisk 25-minute walk, alternate fast walking with slow jogging. Begin each session walking and gradually increase the amount of time you spend jogging. If you feel breathless while jogging, slow down and walk. Continue to alternate in this manner until you can jog for 10 minutes without stopping. If you gradually increase your jogging time by 1 or 2 minutes with each workout, you'll slowly build up to 20 or 25 minutes per session. For optimal fitness, you should jog at least three times a week.

The difference between jogging and running is speed. You should be able to carry on a conversation with someone on a long jog or run; if you're too breathless to talk, you're pushing too hard.

If your goal is to enhance aerobic fitness, long, slow, distance running is best. If you want to improve your speed, try *interval training*—repeated hard runs over a certain distance, with intervals of relaxed jogging in between. Depending on what suits you and what your training goals are, you can vary the distance, duration, and number of fast runs, as well as the time and activity between them.

Other Aerobic Activities   Because variety is the spice of an active life, many people prefer different forms of aerobic exercise. All can provide many health benefits. Among the popular options:

- **Swimming:** For aerobic conditioning, you have to swim laps using the freestyle, butterfly, breaststroke, or backstroke. (The sidestroke is too easy.) You must also be a good enough swimmer to keep churning through the water for at least 20 minutes. Your heart will beat more slowly in water than on land, so your heart rate while swimming is not an accurate guide to exercise intensity. Try to keep up a steady pace that's fast enough to make you feel pleasantly tired, but not completely exhausted, by the time you get out of the pool.

- **Cycling:** Bicycling, indoors and out, can be an excellent cardiovascular conditioner, as well as an effective way to control weight—provided you aren't just along for the ride. If you coast down too many hills, you'll have to ride longer up hills or on level ground to get a good workout. An 18-speed bike can make pedaling too easy unless you choose gears carefully. To gain aerobic benefits, mountain bikers have to work hard enough to raise their heart rates to their target zone and keep up that intensity for at least 20 minutes.

- **Spinning:** Spinning is a cardiovascular workout for the whole body that utilizes a special stationary bicycle. Led by an instructor, a group of bikers listens to music, and a participant modifies his or her individual bike's resistance and his or her own pace according to the rhythm. An average spinning class lasts 45 minutes.

- **Cardio kick-boxing:** Also referred to as kick-boxing or boxing aerobics, this hybrid of boxing, martial arts, and aerobics offers an intense total-body workout. An hour of kick-boxing burns an average of 500 to 800 calories, compared to 300 to 400 calories in a typical step aerobics class.

- **Rowing:** Whether on water or a rowing machine, rowing provides excellent

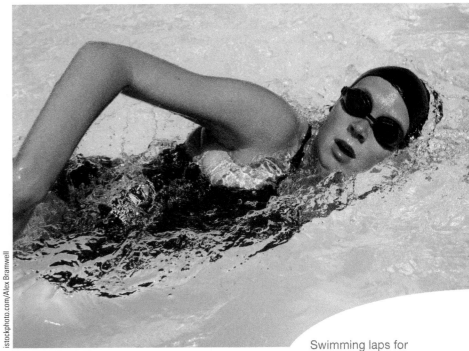

istockphoto.com/Alex Bramwell

Swimming laps for 20 minutes or longer at a steady pace is a good option for aerobic exercise.

aerobic exercise as well as working the upper and lower body and toning the shoulders, back, arms, and legs. Correct rowing techniques are important to avoid back injury.

YOUR STRATEGIES FOR CHANGE

The Right Way to Walk and Run

Here are some guidelines for putting your best foot forward, whether you are walking or running:

- **Take time to warm up.**

- **Maintain good posture.** Keep your back straight, your head up, and your eyes looking straight ahead. Hold your arms slightly away from your body—your elbows should be bent slightly so that your forearms are almost parallel to the ground.

- **Use the heel-to-toe method.** The heel of your leading foot should touch the ground before the ball or toes of that foot do. Push off the ball of your foot, and bend your knee as you raise your heel. You should be able to feel the action in your calf muscles.

- **Pump your arms back and forth.** This burns more calories and gives you an upper-body workout as well.

- **Do not walk or run on the balls of your feet**. This produces soreness in the calves because the muscles must contract for a longer time. Avoid running on hard surfaces and making sudden stops and turns.

- **End your walk or run with a cool-down period**. Let your pace become more leisurely for the last five minutes.

- **Skipping rope:** Essentially a form of stationary jogging with some extra arm action thrown in, skipping rope is excellent as both a heart conditioner and a way of losing weight. Always warm up before starting and cool down afterward.

- **Stair climbing:** You could run up the stairs in an office building or dormitory, but most people use stair-climbing machines available in home models and at gyms and health clubs.

- **Inline skating:** Inline skating can increase aerobic endurance and muscular strength and is less stressful on joints and bones than running or high-impact aerobics. Skaters can adjust the intensity of their workout by varying the terrain.

- **Tennis:** As with other sports, tennis can be an aerobic activity—depending on the number of players and their skill level. In general, a singles match requires more continuous exertion than playing doubles.

- **Zumba:** Zumba combines dance and aerobic elements with choreography that incorporates hip-hop, samba, salsa, merengue, mambo, martial arts, and belly dancing. Different types of classes target individuals of different ages and fitness levels. As many as 14 million people take weekly Zumba classes in more than 150 countries around the world.

Building Muscular Fitness

Although aerobic workouts condition your insides (heart, blood vessels, and lungs), they don't exercise many of the muscles that shape your outsides and provide power when you need it. Strength workouts are important because they enable muscles to work more efficiently and reliably. Conditioned muscles function more smoothly and contract somewhat more vigorously and with less effort. With exercise, muscle tissue becomes firmer and can withstand much more strain—the result of toughening the sheath protecting the muscle and developing more connective tissue within it (Figure 8.5).

The two dimensions of muscular fitness are strength and endurance:

- *Muscular strength* is the maximal force that a muscle or group of muscles can generate for one movement.

- *Muscular endurance* is the capacity to sustain repeated muscle actions.

Both are important. You need strength to hoist a shovelful of snow and endurance so you can keep shoveling the entire driveway.

Regardless of your age, muscular fitness matters. In a study that followed more than 1 million men ages 16 to 19 for 24 years, those who had low muscle strength in their teen years were at increased risk of early death from several major causes, including suicide, cancer, and cardiovascular illness. Those with high muscle strength were at significantly lower risk of early death from any cause, including cardiovascular disease and suicide. Low muscle strength, the researchers concluded, is "an emerging risk factor for major causes of death in young adulthood."

Muscle mass remains important throughout the lifespan. In older as well as younger adults, the greater the muscle mass, the lower the risk of death. Some researchers suggest that maximizing and maintaining muscles may be as important as weight or body mass index.[20]

There are no shortcuts to muscular fitness (see Consumer Alert, page 224). The latest research on fat-burning shows that the best way to reduce your body fat is to add muscle-strengthening exercise to your workouts. Muscle tissue is your very best calorie-burning tissue, and the more you have, the more calories you burn, even when you are resting. You don't have to become a serious body-builder. Using handheld weights (also called *free weights*) two or three times a week is enough. Just be sure you learn how to use them properly because you can tear or strain muscles if you don't practice the proper weight lifting techniques. As more people have begun to lift weights, injuries have soared.

A balanced workout regimen of muscle building and aerobic exercise does more for you than just burn fat. It gives you more endurance by promoting better distribution of oxygen to your tissues and increasing the blood flow to your heart.

Strength training has particular benefits for women: As numerous studies have documented, it makes their muscles stronger, their bodies leaner, and their bones more resistant to falls. In young women, it boosts self-esteem, body image, and emotional well-being. In middle-aged and older women, it enhances self-concept, boosts psychological health, and prevents weight gain.

Muscles at Work

Your muscles never stay the same. If you don't use them, they atrophy, weaken, or break down. If you use them rigorously and regularly, they

Strength workouts increase circulation

The heart's right half pumps oxygen-poor blood to capillary beds in lungs. There, O_2 diffuses into blood and CO_2 diffuses out. The oxygenated blood flows into the heart's left half where it is then pumped to capillary beds throughout the body.

Strength workouts build muscles

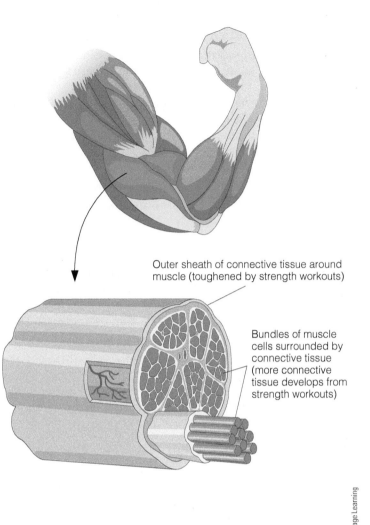

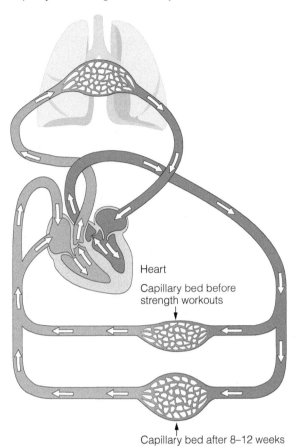

Heart

Capillary bed before strength workouts

Capillary bed after 8–12 weeks of strength workouts (extra capillaries develop, circulation increases)

Outer sheath of connective tissue around muscle (toughened by strength workouts)

Bundles of muscle cells surrounded by connective tissue (more connective tissue develops from strength workouts)

© Cengage Learning

FIGURE 8.5 Benefits of Strength Training on the Body
Strength training increases blood circulation to body tissues and develops muscles.

grow stronger. The only way to develop muscles is by demanding more of them than you usually do. This is called **overloading**. (Remember the overload principle?)

As you train, you have to gradually increase the number of repetitions or the amount of resistance and work the muscle to temporary fatigue. That's why it's important not to quit when your muscles start to tire. Progressive overload—steadily increasing the stress placed on the body—builds stronger muscles.

You need to exercise differently for strength than for endurance:

- *To develop strength*, do a few repetitions with heavy loads. As you increase the weight

your muscles must move, you increase your strength.

- *To increase endurance*, do many more repetitions with lighter loads. If your muscles are weak and you need to gain strength in your upper body, you may have to work for weeks to do a half-dozen regular push-ups. Then you can start building endurance by doing as many push-ups as you can before collapsing in exhaustion.

Muscles can do only two things: contract and relax. As they do so, skeletal muscles either pull on bones or stop pulling on bones. All exercise

overloading A method of physical training that involves increasing the number of repetitions or the amount of resistance gradually to work the muscle to temporary fatigue.

True **isokinetic** contraction is a constant-speed contraction. Isokinetic exercises require special machines that provide resistance to over-load muscles throughout the entire range of motion.

Designing a Muscle Workout

A workout with weights should exercise your body's primary muscle groups (Figure 8.6):

- *Deltoids* (shoulders)
- *Pectorals* (chest)
- *Triceps* and *biceps* (back and front of upper arms)
- *Quadriceps* and *hamstrings* (front and back of thighs)
- *Gluteus maximus* (buttocks)
- *Trapezius* and *rhomboids* (back)
- *Abdomen*

Various machines and free-weight routines focus on each muscle group, but the principle is always the same: Muscles contract as you raise and lower a weight, and you repeat the lift-and-lower routine until the muscle group is tired.

A weight-training program is made up of

- **Reps (or repetitions)**—Multiple performances of an exercise, such as lifting 50 pounds one time
- **Sets**—A *set* number of repetitions of the same movement, such as a set of 20 push-ups. You should allow your breath to return to normal before moving on to each new set. Although the ideal number of sets in a resistance-training program remains controversial, recent evidence suggests that multiple sets lead to additional benefits in short- and long-term training in young and middle-aged adults.

Maintaining proper breathing during weight training is crucial. To breathe correctly, inhale when muscles are relaxed and exhale when you push or lift. Don't ever hold your breath because oxygen flow helps prevent muscle fatigue and injury.

Free Weights vs. Machines

No one type of equipment—free weight or machine—has a clear advantage in terms of building fat-free body mass, enhancing strength and endurance, or improving a sport-specific skill. Each type offers benefits but also has drawbacks.

Free weights offer great versatility for strength training. With dumbbells, for example, you can perform a variety of exercises to work specific

---

isometric Of the same length; exercise in which muscles increase their tension without shortening in length, such as when pushing an immovable object.

isotonic Having the same tension or tone; exercise requiring the repetition of an action that creates tension, such as weight lifting or calisthenics.

isokinetic Having the same force; exercise with specialized equipment that provides resistance equal to the force applied by the user throughout the entire range of motion.

reps (or repetitions) In weight training, multiple performances of a movement or an exercise.

sets In weight training, multiples of repetitions of the same movement or exercise.

involves muscles pulling on bones across a joint. The movement that takes place depends on the structure of the joint and the position of the muscle attachments involved.

In an **isometric** contraction, the muscle applies force while maintaining an equal length. The muscle contracts and tries to shorten but cannot overcome the resistance. An example is pushing against an immovable object, like a wall, or tightening an abdominal muscle while sitting. The muscle contracts, but there is no movement. Push or pull against the immovable object, with each muscle contraction held for five to eight seconds; repeat 5 to 10 times daily.

An **isotonic** contraction involves movement, but the muscle tension remains the same. In an isotonic exercise, the muscle moves a moderate load several times, as in weight lifting or calisthenics. The best isotonic exercise for producing muscular strength involves high resistance and a low number of repetitions. On the other hand, you can develop the greatest flexibility, coordination, and endurance with isotonic exercises that incorporate lower resistance and frequent repetitions.

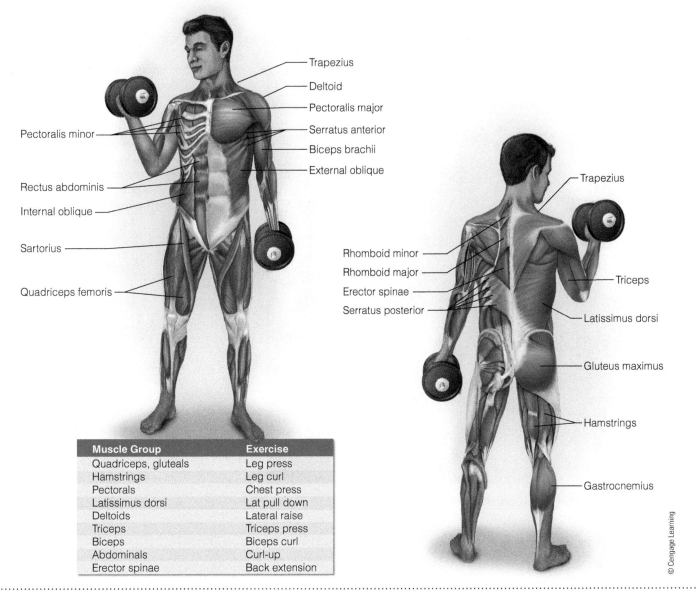

Muscle Group	Exercise
Quadriceps, gluteals	Leg press
Hamstrings	Leg curl
Pectorals	Chest press
Latissimus dorsi	Lat pull down
Deltoids	Lateral raise
Triceps	Triceps press
Biceps	Biceps curl
Abdominals	Curl-up
Erector spinae	Back extension

FIGURE 8.6 Primary Muscle Groups

Different exercises can strengthen and stretch different muscle groups.

muscle groups, such as the chest and shoulders. Machines, in contrast, are more limited; many allow only one exercise.

Strength-training machines have several advantages:

- They ensure correct movement for a lift, which helps protect against injury and prevent cheating when fatigue sets in.

- They isolate specific muscles, which is good for rehabilitating an injury or strengthening a specific body part.

- Because they offer high-tech options like varying resistance during the lifting motion, they can tax muscles in ways that a traditional barbell cannot.

Recovery

The ACSM recommends a minimum of 8 to 10 exercises involving the major muscle groups two to three days a week. Remember that your muscles need sufficient time to recover from a weight-training session. Never work a sore muscle because soreness may indicate that too-heavy weights have caused tiny tears in the fibers.

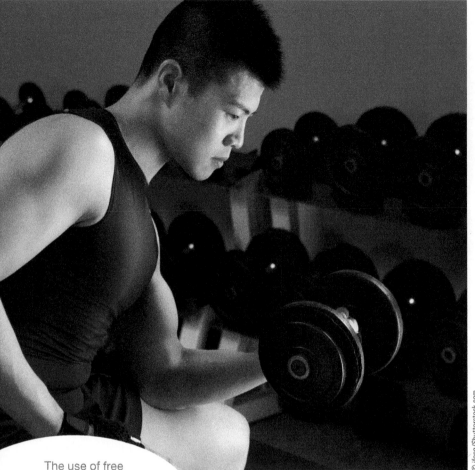

The use of free weights or strength-training machines can build muscle strength and endurance.

Allow no less than 48 hours, but no more than 96 hours, between training sessions, so your body can recover from the workout and you avoid overtraining. Workouts on consecutive days do more harm than good because the body can't recover that quickly. Strength training twice a week at greater intensity and for a longer duration can be as effective as working out three times a week. However, your muscles will begin to atrophy if you let more than three or four days pass without exercising them.

✓ **check-in** How often do you do strength training?

Core Strength Conditioning

"Core strength," a popular trend in exercise and fitness, refers to the ability of the muscles to support your spine and keep your body stable and balanced. The major muscles of your core include these:

- The transverse abdominis, the deepest of the abdominal muscles

- The external and internal obliques on the side and front of the abdomen around your waist

- The rectus abdominis, a long muscle that extends along the front of the abdomen

When you have good core stability, the muscles in your pelvis, low back, hips, and abdomen work in harmony. Strengthening all of your core muscles provides stability; improves posture, breathing, appearance, and balance; and protects you from injury. When your core is weak, you become more susceptible to low back pain and injury.

✓ **check-in** Do you do exercises to strengthen your core?

Muscle Dysmorphia

Also referred to as "bigorexia" or "reverse anorexia," **muscle dysmorphia** is a condition that primarily affects male bodybuilders. Convinced that they are too small or insufficiently muscular, they spend hours working out at the gym, invest large sums in exercise equipment, take various supplements including potentially harmful drugs, and obsess about their appearances.

Some researchers believe muscle dysmorphia is a form of body dysmorphic disorder; others view it as an eating disorder. Its primary characteristics are the following:

- Frequently giving up important social, occupational, or recreational activities because of a compulsive need to maintain a workout and diet regimen

- Avoiding situations that involve bodily exposure (such as swimming) or enduring them only with great distress

- Preoccupation with body size or musculature that causes significant distress or interferes with work, socializing, or other important aspects of daily life

- Continued exercise, diet, or use of performance-enhancing substances despite knowledge of their potential for physical or psychological harm

Drugs Used to Boost Athletic Performance

In recent years, revelations that many athletes have used performance-enhancing drugs have shaken the sports profession. Some sports stars

muscle dysmorphia A condition that affects mostly male bodybuilders in which they become obsessed with appearance and size of muscles.

have served time in prison. Others have had to end their careers and see their reputations forever tarnished.

The number of college athletes using or at least checking into performance-enhancing drugs is believed to be growing. Some feel the stakes are high enough to outweigh the risks, which include cancer, liver disease, blood diseases, severe arthritis, and sexual dysfunction.

✓check-in What do you think of sports doping among college and professional athletes?

Despite the hype, more than 7,500 scientific investigations have found that performance-enhancing drugs do not provide strength benefits. The drugs have been shown to increase lean body mass, heart rate, and metabolic rate, but these do not translate into improved performance.

Here's what we know—and don't know—about the most widely used performance boosters:

- **Anabolic steroids: Anabolic steroids** are synthetic derivatives of the male hormone testosterone that promote the growth of skeletal muscle and increase lean body mass. Taking them to improve athletic performance is illegal. Approximately 1 percent of college students have used steroids for nonmedical purposes. Anabolic steroids have been reported to increase lean muscle mass, strength, and ability to train longer and harder, but they pose serious health hazards, including the following:

  - They may cause liver tumors, jaundice (yellowish pigmentation of skin, tissues, and body fluids), fluid retention, high blood pressure, decreased immune function, and severe acne.

  - Men may experience shrinking of the testicles, reduced sperm count, infertility, baldness, and development of breasts. In men, side effects may be reversible once abuse stops.

  - Women may experience growth of facial hair, acne, changes in or cessation of the menstrual cycle, enlargement of the clitoris, and deepened voice. In women, these changes are irreversible.

  - In adolescents, steroids may bring about a premature halt in skeletal maturation.

  - Anabolic steroid abuse may lead to aggression and other psychiatric side effects, including maniclike symptoms leading to "'roid rage," or violent, even homicidal, episodes. Users may suffer from paranoid jealousy, extreme irritability, delusions, and impaired judgment stemming from feelings of invincibility. Stopping the drugs abruptly can lead to depression.

- **Androstenedione ("andro"):** This testosterone precursor is normally produced by the adrenal glands and gonads. Despite manufacturers' claims, studies have shown that supplemental androstenedione doesn't increase testosterone, and muscles don't get stronger with andro use. Andro has been classified as a controlled substance, and its use is illegal.

- **Creatine:** This amino acid, which is made by the body and stored predominantly in skeletal muscle, serves as a reservoir to replenish adenosine triphosphate (ATP), a substance involved in energy production. Some studies suggest that creatine may increase strength and endurance. Other effects on the body remain unknown.

  The Food and Drug Administration has warned consumers to consult a physician before taking creatine supplements. Creatine may cause dehydration and heat-related illnesses, reduced blood volume, and electrolyte imbalances. Some athletes drink quantities of water hoping to avoid such effects. However, many coaches forbid or discourage creatine use because its long-term effects remain unknown.

- **GBL (gamma butyrolactone):** This unapproved drug is marketed on the Internet and in some professional gyms as a muscle builder and performance enhancer. The Food and Drug Administration has warned consumers to avoid any products containing GBL, noting that they have been associated with at least one death and several incidents in which users became comatose or unconscious.

- **Ergogenic aids:** These substances, some of them very common, are used to enhance energy and provide athletes with a competitive advantage:

  - *Caffeine* (discussed in Chapter 11) may boost alertness in some people but cause jitteriness in others.

anabolic steroids Synthetic derivatives of the male hormone testosterone that promote the growth of skeletal muscle and increase lean body mass.

- *Baking soda* (sodium bicarbonate) is believed to delay fatigue by neutralizing lactic acid in the muscles. Its potential drawbacks include explosive diarrhea, abdominal cramps, bloating, and nausea.

- *Glycerol* is a natural element derived from fats. Some sports-drink manufacturers are testing formulations that include glycerol, which they claim can lower heart rate and stave off exhaustion in marathon events. Glycerol-induced hyperhydration (holding too much water in the blood) may be hazardous to health.

- **Human growth hormone and erythroprotein (EPO):** According to an analysis of all existing research, human growth hormone increases lean body mass but does not affect exercise capacity or aerobic endurance. Previous studies found no beneficial effect on aging in healthy older people. EPO is a hormone that increases red blood cell production and improves endurance. Side effects include blood clots, increased bone growth, increased cholesterol, heart disease, and impotence.

Becoming More Flexible

Flexibility is the characteristic of body tissues that determines the **range of motion** achievable without injury at a joint or group of joints. There are two types of flexibility:

- **Static flexibility**—the type most people think of as flexibility—refers to the ability to assume and maintain an extended position at one end point in a joint's range of motion. Static flexibility depends on many factors, including the structure of a joint and the tightness of the muscles, tendons, and ligaments attached to it.

- **Dynamic flexibility**, by comparison, involves movement. It is the ability to move a joint quickly and fluidly through its entire range of motion with little resistance. Dynamic flexibility is influenced by static flexibility but also depends on additional factors, such as strength, coordination, and resistance to movement.

range of motion The fullest extent of possible movement in a particular joint.

static flexibility The ability to assume and maintain an extended position at one end point in a joint's range of motion.

dynamic flexibility The ability to move a joint quickly and fluidly through its entire range of motion with little resistance.

Static flexibility in the hip joint determines whether you can do a split; dynamic flexibility is what would enable you to perform a split leap.

Genetics, age, gender, and body composition all influence how flexible you are. Girls and women tend to be more flexible than boys and men to a certain extent because of hormonal and anatomical differences. The way females and males use their muscles and the activities they engage in can also have an effect. Over time, the natural elasticity of muscles, tendons, and joints decreases in both genders, resulting in stiffness.

✓**check-in** How would you rate your flexibility?

The Benefits of Flexibility

Just as cardiorespiratory fitness benefits the heart and lungs and muscular fitness builds endurance and strength, a stretching program produces unique benefits, including enhancement of the ability of the respiratory, circulatory, and neuromuscular systems to cope with the stress and demands of our high-pressure world (Figure 8.7). Among the other benefits of flexibility are:

- **Prevention of injuries:** Strong, flexible muscles resist stress better than weak or inflexible ones. Adding flexibility to a training program for sports such as soccer, football, or tennis can reduce the rate of injuries by as much as 75 percent. However, stretching before a run has proven neither to prevent nor to cause injury.

- **Relief of muscle strain:** Muscles tighten as a result of stress or prolonged sitting. Stretching helps relieve this tension and enables you to work more effectively.

- **Relaxation:** Flexibility exercises reduce stress and mental strain, slow the rate of breathing, and reduce blood pressure.

- **Relief of soreness after exercise:** Many people develop delayed-onset muscle soreness (DOMS) one or two days after they work out. This may be the result of damage to the muscle fibers and supporting connective tissue.

- **Improved posture:** Bad posture can create tight, stressed muscles. If you slump in your chair, for instance, the muscles in the front of your chest may tighten, causing those in the upper spine to overstretch and become loose.

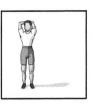

Triceps Stretch
1. Starting position: This exercise may be done while standing or seated. Reach both arms overhead, bend the right elbow, and grasp it with the left hand. The right hand should be pointing straight down the back.
2. Pull the elbow up and slightly back and hold for at least 20 seconds.
3. Repeat on the other side.

Deltoid Stretch—Rear
1. Starting position: Sit or stand with good posture. Cross the right arm across the front of the body at neck level. Grasp the elbow with the left hand while keeping the shoulders down and relaxed.
2. Press the elbow toward the neck and hold for at least 20 seconds.
3. Repeat on the other side.

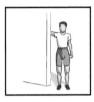

Chest Stretch
1. Starting position: Stand beneath a doorway. Bend the left arm and place the forearm against the wall with the elbow at shoulder height.
2. Rotate the body away from the arm and hold for at least 20 seconds.
3. Repeat on the other side.

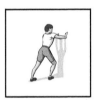

Calf Stretch—Wall
1. Starting position: Stand approximately two feet away from a wall and place hands on wall at about shoulder height. Place one foot at the base of the wall with the heel on the floor and toes against the wall.
2. Slowly straighten the knees and press the chest toward the wall to feel a stretch in the back of the lower leg.
3. Hold for at least 20 seconds and repeat on the other side.

Inner Thigh
1. Starting position: Stand with feet three or more feet apart and toes turning outward. Bend one knee and lunge to one side, being careful not to allow the knee to extend beyond the toes.
2. Keeping weight on bent leg, lift the toes of the extended leg to increase the stretch in the inner thigh. Keep torso upright and head lifted.
3. Hold for at least 20 seconds.

Quadriceps Stretch—Lying
1. Starting position: Lie on your side with your legs extended and your lower arm or hand supporting your head. Bend the top knee and grasp the top of the foot with your hand. Knees should be in alignment.
2. Press the top hip forward to feel a stretch along the front of the thigh.
3. Hold for at least 20 seconds and repeat on the other side.

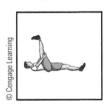

Hamstring Stretch—Lying
1. Starting position: Lie on your back with your legs extended. Lift one leg up and grasp behind the thigh or knee with both hands as you bring the knee to the chest.
2. Press the heel up toward the ceiling as you straighten the leg.
3. Hold for at least 20 seconds and repeat on the other side.

© Cengage Learning

FIGURE 8.7 Basic Stretching Program

Just doing a few minutes of stretching to your major muscle groups can yield many benefits. Here is a simple yet comprehensive program.

Stretching

When you stretch a muscle, you are primarily stretching the connective tissue. The stretch must be intense enough to increase the length of the connective tissue without tearing it.

Static stretching involves a gradual stretch held for a short time (10 to 30 seconds). A shorter stretch provides little benefit; a longer stretch does not provide additional benefits. Since a slow stretch provokes less of a reaction

static stretching A stretching technique in which a gradual stretch is held for a short time of 10 to 30 seconds.

YOUR STRATEGIES FOR PREVENTION

How to Avoid Stretching Injuries

- **Before you begin, increase your body temperature by slowly marching or running in place.** Sweat signals that you're ready to start stretching.

- **Don't force body parts beyond their normal range of motion.** Stretch to the point of tension, back off, and hold for 10 seconds to 1 minute.

- **Do a minimum of four repetitions of each stretch, with equal repetitions on each side.**

- **Don't hold your breath.** Continue breathing slowly and rhythmically throughout your stretching routine.

- **Don't attempt to stretch a weak or injured muscle.**

- **Start small.** Work the muscles of the smaller joints in the arms and legs first and then work the larger joints like the shoulders and hips.

- **Stretch individual muscles before you stretch a group of muscles; for instance, stretch the ankle, knee, and hip before doing a stretch that works all three at once.**

- **Don't make any quick, jerky movements while stretching.** Stretches should be gentle and smooth.

- **Certain positions can be harmful to the knees and low back.** In particular, avoid stretches that require deep knee bends or full squats because they can harm your knees and low back.

passive stretching A stretching technique in which an external force or resistance (your body, a partner, gravity, or a weight) helps the joints move through their range of motion.

active stretching A technique that involves stretching a muscle by contracting the opposing muscle.

dynamic stretching Stretching that increases the range of motion around a joint or group of joints by using active muscular effort, momentum, and speed.

ballistic stretching Rapid bouncing movements.

from the stretch receptors, the muscles can safely stretch farther than usual. Fitness experts most often recommend static stretching because it is both safe and effective.

An example of such a stretch is letting your hands slowly slide down the front of your legs (keeping your knees in a soft, unlocked position) until you reach your toes and holding this final position for several seconds before slowly straightening up. You should feel a pull, but not pain, during this stretch.

In **passive stretching**, your own body, a partner, gravity, or a weight serves as an external force or resistance to help your joints move through their range of motion. You can achieve a more intense stretch and a greater range of motion with passive stretching. There is a greater risk of injury, however, because the muscles themselves are not controlling the stretch.

Active stretching involves stretching a muscle by contracting the opposing muscle (the muscle on the opposite side of the limb). This method allows the muscle to be stretched farther with a low risk of injury.

Dynamic stretching increases the range of motion around a joint or group of joints by using active muscular effort, momentum, and speed.

Dynamic stretches, such as walking lunges and arm circles, are considered better alternatives to static stretching for gymnasts, dancers, figure skaters, divers, and hurdlers because they do not decrease muscle strength and power.

Ballistic stretching is characterized by rapid bouncing movements, such as a series of up-and-down bobs as you try again and again to touch your toes with your hands. These bounces can stretch the muscle fibers too far, causing the muscle to contract rather than stretch. They also can tear ligaments and weaken or rupture tendons, the strong fibrous cords that connect muscles to bones. The heightened activity to stretch receptors caused by the rapid stretches can continue for some time, possibly causing injuries during any physical activities that follow. Because of the potential dangers of ballistic stretching, fitness experts generally recommend against it.

Stretching and Warming Up

Warming up means getting the heart beating, breaking a sweat, and readying the body for more vigorous activity. Stretching is a specific activity intended to elongate the muscles and keep joints limber, not simply a prelude to a game of tennis or a 3-mile run. According to a review of recent studies, the value of stretching varies with different activities. While it does not prevent injuries from jogging, cycling, or swimming, stretching may be beneficial in sports, like soccer and football, that involve bouncing and jumping.

√**check-in** Did you know that one of the best times to stretch is after an aerobic workout?

After stretching, your muscles will be warm, more flexible, and less prone to injury. In addition, stretching after aerobic activity can help a fatigued muscle return to its normal resting length and may help reduce delayed-onset muscle soreness.

Stretching and Athletic Performance

Conventional wisdom holds that stretching improves athletic performance, but a review of the research finds that this isn't necessarily so. In some cases, active stretching can impede rather than improve performance in terms of muscle force and jumping height. Passive stretching prior to a sprint—a common practice—also has proved to reduce runners' speed. On the other hand, regular stretching can improve athletic performance in a variety of sports.

Pre-exercise stretching is generally unnecessary and may be counterproductive. Static stretching reduces strength in the stretched muscle especially in people who hold the stretch for 90 seconds or more.

A better choice is to warm up dynamically by moving the muscles that will be used in your workout. Jumping jacks and toy-soldier high leg kicks prepare muscles for many forms of exercise better than stretching.

Mind–Body Approaches

Yoga, Pilates, and t'ai chi—increasingly popular on campuses and throughout the country—can help reduce stress, enhance health and wellness, and improve physical fitness, including balance.

Yoga

One of the most ancient of mind–body practices, *yoga* comes from the Sanskrit word meaning "union." Traditionally associated with religion, yoga consists of various breathing and stretching exercises that unite all aspects of a person.

Yoga has grown more popular among Americans of all ages, with the greatest increase in adults ages 18 to 44.[21]

Once considered an exotic pursuit, yoga has gained acceptance as part of a comprehensive stress management and fitness program and scientific studies have demonstrated its benefits, which include the following:

- **Improved flexibility,** which may offer protection from back pain and injuries

- **Protection of joints** because yoga postures take joints through their full range of motion, providing a fresh supply of nutrients to joint cartilage

- **Stronger, denser bones** from yoga's weight-bearing postures

- **Enhanced circulation,** which also boosts the supply of oxygen throughout the body

- **Lower blood pressure**

- **Relief of stress-related symptoms** and anxiety

- **Lower blood sugar** in people with diabetes, which reduces the risk of complications

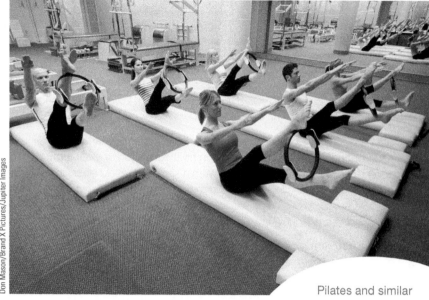

Don Mason/Brand X Pictures/Jupiter Images

Pilates and similar exercises strengthen the core muscles while also improving flexibility and joint mobility.

- **Reduced pain** in people with back problems, arthritis, carpal tunnel syndrome, fibromyalgia, and other chronic problems

- **Improved lung function** in people with asthma

- **Less inflammation, fatigue, and depression** in breast cancer survivors[22]

- Eased depression in pregnant women, serving as an alternative to antidepressants[23]

The best way to get started is to find a class that appeals to you and learn a few yoga poses and breathing techniques. Once you have mastered these, you can easily integrate yoga into your total fitness program.

The ACSM cautions that yoga should help, not hurt. To prevent injuries to your knees, back, neck, shoulders, wrists, or ankles, avoid forcing your body into difficult postures. Proper technique is essential to safety.

Pilates

Used by dancers for deep-body conditioning and injury rehabilitation, Pilates (pronounced Puh-lah-teez) was developed more than seven decades ago by German immigrant Joseph Pilates. Increasingly used to complement aerobics and weight training, Pilates exercises improve flexibility and joint mobility and strengthen the core by developing pelvic stability and abdominal control.

Pilates-trained instructors offer "mat" or "floor" classes that stress the stabilization and

YOUR STRATEGIES FOR PREVENTION

How to Protect Your Back

- **When standing, shift your weight from one foot to the other.** If possible, place one foot on a stool, step, or railing 4 to 6 inches off the ground. Hold in your stomach, tilt your pelvis toward your back, and tuck in your buttocks to provide crucial support for the low back.

- **Because sitting places more stress on the low back than standing, try to get up from your seat at least once an hour to stretch or walk around.** Whenever possible, sit in a straight chair with a firm back. Avoid slouching in overstuffed chairs or dangling your legs in midair. When driving, keep the seat forward so that your knees are raised to hip level; your right leg should not be fully extended. A small pillow or towel can help support your low back.

- **Sleep on a flat, firm mattress.** The best sleep position is on your side, with one or both knees bent at right angles to your torso. The pillow should keep your head in line with your body so that your neck isn't bent forward or to the side.

- **When lifting, bend at the knees, not from the waist.** Get close to the load. Tighten your stomach muscles but don't hold your breath. Let your leg muscles do the work.

strengthening of the back and abdominal muscles. Fitness centers also may offer training on Pilates equipment, primarily a device called the Reformer, a wooden contraption with various cables, pulleys, springs, and sliding boards attached that is used for a series of progressive range-of-motion exercises.

According to research from the ACSM, Pilates enhances flexibility and muscular endurance, particularly for intermediate and advanced practitioners, but its potential to increase cardiorespiratory fitness and reduce body weight is limited. The intensity of a Pilates workout increases from basic to intermediate to advanced levels, as does the number of calories burned. For intermediate practitioners, a 30-minute session burns 180 calories, with each additional quarter-hour burning another 90 calories. A single weekly session enhances flexibility but has little impact on body composition.

T'ai Chi

This ancient Chinese practice, designed to exercise body, mind, and spirit, gently works muscles, focuses concentration, and improves the flow of "qi" (often spelled "chi"), the vital life energy that sustains health. Popular with all ages, from children to seniors, t'ai chi is easy to learn and perform. Because of its focus on breathing and flowing gestures, t'ai chi is sometimes described as "meditation in motion."

Classes are available on campuses and in fitness centers, community centers, and some martial arts schools. According to recent research, t'ai chi enhances college students' self-assessed mental and physical well-being.

√**check-in** Have you ever tried mind–body approaches?

Keeping Your Back Healthy

Low back pain causes more disability than nearly 300 other conditions worldwide, according to new research, and nearly 1 in 10 people around the globe suffers from an aching low back.[24] Back pain strikes slightly more women than men and is most common between the ages of 20 and 55. You are at increased risk if you smoke or if you're overstressed, overweight, or out of shape. In most cases, the most effective treatment for low back pain, which usually is caused by degeneration of the lumbar spinal disks, is a combination of physical therapy and anti-inflammatory medication. According to a review of research on this common problem, 90 percent of patients with low back pain recover within three months and most within six weeks. One of the most effective ways to prevent or recover from back problems is to strengthen the core muscles.

Once bed rest was the primary treatment for back pain, but now doctors urge patients to avoid it. Even two to seven days of bed rest may provide little, if any, benefit. Acetaminophen (Tylenol) is the first-line therapy for pain relief. If it is not effective, doctors recommend nonsteroidal anti-inflammatory drugs, such as ibuprofen (Motrin or Advil). Muscle relaxants seem to be effective for a spasm in the low back. The sooner that back patients return to normal activity, the less pain medication they require and the less long-term disability they suffer. Fewer than 1 percent of patients with chronic low back pain benefit from surgery.

√**check-in** Have you ever experienced back pain?

Not all fitness equipment comes with a big price tag. Here are some affordable ways to expand and enhance a home workout:

- **Dumbbells.** You can purchase light weights to carry when walking and jogging to build and firm arm muscles. Training with heavier weights increases muscle strength and endurance, improves balance and body composition, and may reverse some bone loss. An adjustable dumbbell set allows you to add more weight as you build strength.

- **Stability balls.** A large inflatable rubber ball can be a fun, effective way of building core strength, improving posture, and increasing balance. When performing standard exercises like crunches and abdominal curls, the ball provides an additional challenge: maintaining a stable trunk throughout each exercise. You also can sit on the ball while working with hand weights to build core strength and balance. Introductory videos and DVDs are available for rental or purchase.

- **Resistance tubing.** Developed by physical therapists for rehabilitation after injuries, elastic bands and tubing come in different strengths, based on the thickness of the plastic. If you're a beginner, start with a thin band, particularly for the upper body. The lightweight, inexpensive, and easy-to-carry bands aren't particularly risky, but you should check for holes or worn spots, choose a smooth surface, maintain good posture, and perform the exercises in a slow, controlled manner.

Evaluating Fitness Products and Programs

As fitness has become a major industry in the United States, consumers have been bombarded with pitches for products that promise to do everything from whittle a waistline to build up biceps. As always, you have to ask questions and do your own research—whether you're buying basic exercise aids or joining a health club. Beware of any promise that sounds too good to be true. And keep in mind that nothing matters more than your own commitment.

Individuals who are overweight or obese, even when they believe in the benefits of exercise, often don't work out because they're self-conscious about sweating pounds off in a health club or public gym. If you feel self-conscious about joining a spinning class or swimming laps at the university pool, start with short walks or working with hand weights.

Exercise Equipment

Always try out equipment before buying it. If you decide to purchase a stationary bicycle, for instance, read all the product information. Ask someone in your physical education department or at a local gym for recommendations. Try out a bicycle at the gym. Any equipment you purchase should be safe and durable, but not necessarily expensive (see Health on a Budget).

Athletic Shoes

Footwear has come a long way from the days of canvas sneakers. With so many new materials and high-tech options, choosing the right shoe for working out can be confusing. The best shoes aren't necessarily the most expensive but the ones that fit you best. (See Figure 8.8.) Here are some basic guidelines:

- **Choose the right shoe for your sport.** If you're a walker or runner, you want maximum overall shock absorption for the foot, with extra cushioning in the heel and under the ball of the foot (the metatarsal area) to prevent pain, burning, and tenderness. If you also participate in other types of exercise, consider "cross-trainers," shoes that are flexible enough in the front for running but provide the side-to-side, or lateral, control you need for aerobics or tennis.

- **Check out the shoe.** A "slip-lasted" shoe, made by sewing together the upper like a moccasin and gluing it to the sole, is

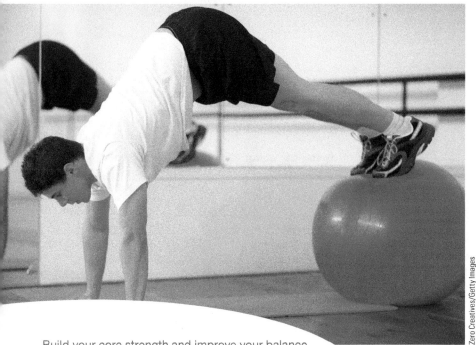

Build your core strength and improve your balance inexpensively with a stability ball. Maintaining appropriate air pressure is important—the exercise will become more difficult as pressure increases.

Zero Creatives/Getty Images

lightweight and flexible. A "board-lasted" shoe has a leather, nylon mesh, or canvas upper sewn to a cardboardlike material, which provides more support and control. A "combination-lasted" shoe offers the advantages of both and works well for a variety of foot types.

- **Shop late.** Try on shoes at the end of the day or after a workout, when your foot size is at its maximum (sometimes half a shoe size larger than in the morning).

- **Give your toes room.** Allow a half-inch, or the width of your index finger, between the end of your longest toe and the tip of the shoe. Try on both shoes. If one foot is larger than the other, buy the larger size.

- **Check the width.** A shoe should be as wide as possible across the forefoot without allowing the heel to slip. Lace up the shoe completely and walk or jog a few steps to make sure the shoes are comfortable.

- **Replace shoes when they lose their cushioning.** After about 300 to 500 miles of running or 300 hours of aerobic activity, your shoes are no longer absorbing the pounding and jarring of your sport. Don't put yourself at increased risk of knee and ankle injuries.

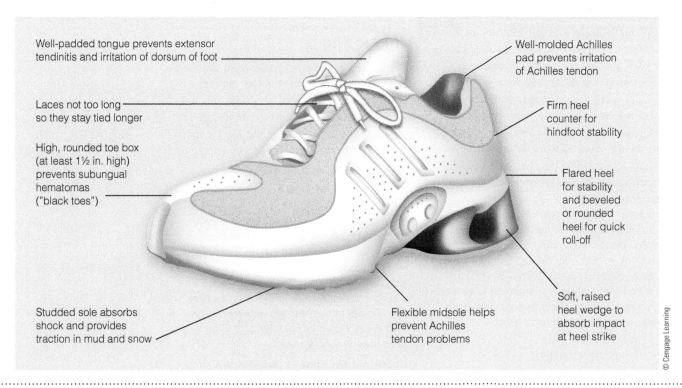

Well-padded tongue prevents extensor tendinitis and irritation of dorsum of foot

Laces not too long so they stay tied longer

High, rounded toe box (at least 1½ in. high) prevents subungual hematomas ("black toes")

Studded sole absorbs shock and provides traction in mud and snow

Well-molded Achilles pad prevents irritation of Achilles tendon

Firm heel counter for hindfoot stability

Flared heel for stability and beveled or rounded heel for quick roll-off

Flexible midsole helps prevent Achilles tendon problems

Soft, raised heel wedge to absorb impact at heel strike

© Cengage Learning

FIGURE 8.8 What to Look for When You Buy Running Shoes

Barefoot Running and Alternative Running Shoes

Some runners have shed conventional athletic shoes to run barefoot or in lightweight shoes. One theory behind this popular trend is that our shoeless ancestors may have used a different form for running, striking the ground with the forefoot near the ball of the foot rather than the heel. Running, whether "shod" or "unshod," involves different body mechanics, with barefoot running increasing work at the ankle and decreasing work at the knee.

"Minimalist" running shoes have a lower profile and greater sole flexibility and lack the motion control and heavy cushioning of conventional running shoes. However, it is not certain that these shoes replicate the mechanics of barefoot running so they may not produce similar potential benefits.

In theory, running barefoot or in minimalist shoes may reduce oxygen consumption and thereby improve distance running performance. However, this may be true only in runners who habitually have trained and competed unshod rather than in traditionally shod runners.[25]

Fitness Centers

√ **check-in** Are there recreational facilities on your own campus?

Is there a gym, running track, pool, basketball court, athletic fields? Are they crowded at certain times? Are they convenient? Are classes in Zumba or Pilates available? Try out a range of activities over the course of several weeks.

If you decide to join a private gym or health club, find out exactly what facilities and programs it offers. The club should be located close to home, campus, or work and should be open at convenient hours. Think about your schedule and when you'll have time to work out. Visit the club at the times you're most likely to use it.

A club should have facilities for a complete workout, including both aerobic and muscle workouts: exercycles, rowing machines, treadmills, stair-climbing machines, stationary bicycles, a running track, aerobics classes, a swimming pool, strength-training equipment, and, if it's what you're looking for, racquetball courts and a large gym for basketball and volleyball.

Find out whether all facilities are available to all members at all times. Some clubs reserve the pool for families only or kids' lessons at certain times. Ask if you can try out the club before joining. Find out what the membership includes. Will you end up paying extra for lockers, towels, classes, and the like? Are student discounts offered? Beware of long-term memberships; many clubs go out of business or change ownership often. Do the members seem to be significantly older or younger, or in much better or worse shape, than you are? Remember: You're more likely to work out regularly in a place, and with people, you like. In a study of undergraduates in university physical activity classes (such as spinning, aerobic water exercise, kickboxing, and aerobics), students reported greater effort, enjoyment, and commitment to future exercise and lower tension and anxiety about their physiques when they perceived the atmosphere in the class as caring and positive.

Sports Nutrition

In general, active people need the same basic nutrients as others and should follow the recommendations in Chapter 6. However, athletes in competitive sports—amateur as well as professional—may have increased energy requirements:

- Athletes generally do not need more protein; the exception may be those engaged in intense strength training. Like most other Americans, athletes typically consume more than the Recommended Daily Allowance for protein.

- Complex carbohydrates are essential in an athlete's diet. (See Chapter 5 for the best sources.)

- Including the right types of fat in the daily diet can actually improve athletic performance—not just by providing calories but by replenishing intramuscular fat stores (fat stored within the muscle and used to fuel extended exercise).

Not just *what* you eat but *when* you eat can affect your exercise performance. If you eat immediately prior to a workout, you may feel sluggish or develop nausea, cramping, or diarrhea. If you don't eat, you may feel weak, faint, or tired.

√ **check-in** Eat and run? Or run and eat?

Time your meals so that you exercise three to four hours after a large meal and one to two hours after a small one. After a workout, eat a meal containing both protein and carbohydrates within two hours to help your muscles recover and to replace fuel stores.

Water

Water, which we need more than any other nutrient, is especially important during exercise and exertion. Rather than wait until you're already somewhat dehydrated, you should be fully hydrated when you begin your activity or exercise and, depending on the duration and intensity of your workout, continue to replace fluids both during and afterward.

The ACSM recommends fluid intake before, during, and after exercise to regulate body temperature and replace body fluids lost through sweating. Failure to replace fluids during exercise can lead to dehydration, which can cause muscle fatigue, loss of coordination, heat exhaustion, and an elevation of body-core temperature to dangerously high levels. To avoid this danger, the ACSM advises the following:

- **Consume a nutritionally balanced diet and drink adequate fluids** in the 24 hours before an exercise event.

- **Drink about 17 ounces of fluid** about two hours before.

- **During exercise, start drinking early** and at regular intervals to replace all the water lost through sweating (i.e., body weight loss).

- **Drink fluids with carbohydrates and/ or electrolytes** for exercise lasting more than an hour. For shorter periods, there is little evidence of differences between drinking a carbohydrate–electrolyte drink and plain water.

Too much water during prolonged bouts of exercise, such as a marathon, can lead to *hyponatremia*, or water intoxication. This condition occurs when the body's sodium level falls below normal as a result of salt loss from sweat and dilution of sodium in the bloodstream by overdrinking. Symptoms of hyponatremia include nausea, vomiting, weakness, and, in severe cases, seizures, coma, and death.

....
✓**check-in** Do you pay attention to proper hydration when working out?
....

Sports Drinks

In its most recent position stand, the International Society of Sports Nutrition (ISSN) has noted that the primary nutrients in energy and sports drinks are carbohydrates and caffeine. Caffeine's effects, discussed in Chapters 6 and 12, have been well studied, but other ingredients added to energy and sports drinks have not been.

Consuming a high-carbohydrate, high-caffeine sports drink 10 to 60 minutes before exercise may improve mental focus, alertness, anaerobic performance, and endurance, but athletes should consider the effects on their metabolic health. Use of more than one serving a day, the ISSN stated, may lead to adverse effects. Individuals with cardiovascular, metabolic, liver, or neurologic disease who are taking medication should avoid all use of energy or sports drinks.

As noted earlier, water best meets the fluid needs of most athletes, but you have other choices. Nonfat milk may be more effective than even a soy protein beverage or sports drink such as Gatorade at burning fat and building lean muscle mass. Most sports drinks contain about 7 percent carbohydrate (about half the sugar of ordinary soft drinks). Less than 6 percent may not enhance performance; more than 8 percent could cause abdominal cramping, nausea, and diarrhea.

Sodium and other electrolytes in sports drinks help replace those lost during physical activity. However, most exercisers do not have to replace minerals lost in sweat immediately. A meal eaten within several hours does so soon enough.

Dietary Supplements

Athletes involved in heavy training may need more of several vitamins, such as thiamin, riboflavin, and vitamin B_6, which are involved in energy production. The best source, nutritionists advise, is vitamin-rich foods, such as fruits and vegetables.

Vitamin and mineral supplements, as discussed in Chapter 6, do not provide benefits to healthy, well-nourished individuals. Vitamin supplements marketed for athletes are poorly regulated, and some may be adulterated with banned substances, such as ephedrine.

Mineral deficiencies, such as too little iron in female athletes, can impair athletic performance. Women who exercise rigorously should undergo regular blood testing and, if needed, take iron supplements. In general, calcium, magnesium, iron, zinc, and copper supplements do not enhance sport performance in well-nourished athletes. Chromium, boron, and vanadium have no beneficial effects on body composition or muscular strength and endurance.

Taking salt pills does little to boost performance in endurance exercises. Researchers have found no difference between athletes taking additional salt and those given placebos.[26]

Energy Bars

Little scientific research has studied the benefits of the various types of energy bars, including their effects on blood glucose levels and athletic performance. One nutritional analysis found high-carbohydrate energy bars to be similar to candy bars in their impact on glucose—even though sugars composed 31 percent of the high-carbohydrate energy bar and 86 percent of the candy bar. In fact, the high-carbohydrate energy bar caused a more rapid peak in blood glucose followed by a sharper decline than did the candy bar. This effect may be desirable for athletes involved in short-duration events who want a quick increase in blood glucose.

Energy bars with a lower carbohydrate level produce a more moderate, sustained increase in blood glucose level, possibly because the protein and fat in a 40–30–30 bar diminish blood glucose response. These bars would be a better choice for athletes involved in endurance events. As an alternative, try fiber-rich whole foods, like nuts and fruit, that provide a steady release of energy.

√**check-in** Do you eat energy bars frequently?

Safe and Healthy Workouts

Whenever you work out, you don't want to risk becoming sore or injured. Starting slowly when you begin any new fitness activity is the smartest strategy. Keep a simple diary to record the time and duration of each workout. Get accustomed to an activity first and then begin to work harder or longer. In this way, you strengthen your musculoskeletal system so you're less likely to be injured, you lower the cardiorespiratory risk, and you build the exercise habit into your schedule.

To prevent exercise-related problems before they happen, use common sense and take appropriate precautions, including the following:

- **Get proper instruction** and, if necessary, advanced training from knowledgeable instructors.

- **Make sure you have good equipment** and keep it in good condition. Know how to check and do at least basic maintenance on the equipment yourself. Always check your equipment prior to each use (especially if you're renting it).

- **Always warm up before and cool down after** a workout.

- Rather than being sedentary all week and then training hard on weekends, try to stay active throughout the week and **don't overdo on weekends.**

- **Use reasonable protective measures,** including wearing a helmet when cycling or skating.

- For some sports, such as boating, **always go with a buddy.**

- **Take each outing seriously**—even if you've dived into this river a hundred times before, even if you know this mountain like you know your own backyard. Avoid the unknown under adverse conditions (for example, hiking unfamiliar terrain during poor weather or kayaking a new river when water levels are unusually high or low) or when accompanied by a beginner whose skills may not be as strong as yours.

- **Never combine alcohol or drugs with any workout or sport.**

√**check-in** Should you exercise outdoors on a smoggy day?

Although health professionals advise people to exercise in low-pollution areas such as parks, the health benefits of outdoor workouts appear to outweigh the potential harm of air pollution.[27]

Temperature

Prevention is the wisest approach to heat and cold problems. And knowing what can go wrong is part of that preventive approach.

Heat Cramps These muscle cramps are caused by profuse sweating and the consequent loss of electrolytes (salts). They occur most often during exercise in hot weather. Salty snacks and sports beverages like Gatorade can help, but be aware that sports drinks can be very high in calories. Salt tablets usually aren't necessary except in cases of extreme sweating.

Heat Syndromes More serious temperature-related conditions include heat exhaustion and heat stroke. These are most likely to occur when both temperature and humidity are high because sweat does not evaporate as quickly, preventing the body from releasing heat quickly. Other conditions that limit the body's ability to regulate temperature are old age, fever, obesity, dehydration, heart disease, poor circulation, sunburn, and drug and alcohol use. Some medicines that increase the risk include allergy medicines (antihistamines), some cough and cold medicines, blood pressure and heart medicines, diet pills, laxatives, and psychiatric medications.

Heat Exhaustion

Heat exhaustion is a mild form of heat-related illness that can be caused by exercise or hot weather. The signs of heat exhaustion are heavy sweating, paleness, muscle cramps, tiredness, weakness, dizziness, headache, nausea or vomiting, and/or fainting. Your pulse rate or heart rate may be fast and weak, and your breathing may be fast and shallow.

....
✓**check-in** Do you know what to do if you
....
think you may have heat exhaustion?
....

First of all, get out of the heat immediately. Rest in a cool, shady place and drink plenty of water or other fluids. Do *not* drink alcohol, which can make heat exhaustion worse. If you do not feel better within 30 minutes, seek medical attention. If left untreated, heat exhaustion may lead to a heat stroke.

Heat Stroke

A heat stroke can occur when the body temperature rises to 106 degrees Fahrenheit or higher within 10 to 15 minutes. A heat stroke is a medical emergency that can be fatal. The warning signs are extremely high temperature; red, hot, and dry skin; rapid, strong pulse; throbbing headache; dizziness; nausea; and confusion or unconsciousness.

If you think someone might have heat stroke, you should quickly take him or her to a cool, shady place and call a doctor. Remove unnecessary clothing and bathe or spray the victim with cool water. People with heat stroke may seem confused. They may have seizures or go into a coma.

Protecting Yourself from Cold

The tips of the toes, fingers, ears, nose, and chin and the cheeks are most vulnerable to exposure to high wind speeds and low temperatures, which can result in *frostnip*.

Because frostnip is painless, you may not even be aware that it is occurring. Watch for a sudden blanching or lightening of your skin. The best early treatment is warming the area with firm, steady pressure from a warm hand; blowing on it with hot breath; holding it against your body; or immersing it in warm (not hot) water. As the skin thaws, it becomes red and starts to tingle. Be careful to protect it from further damage. Don't rub the skin vigorously or with snow, as you could damage the tissue.

More severe is *frostbite*. There are two types of frostbite:

- *Superficial frostbite*, the freezing of the skin and tissues just below the skin, is characterized by a waxy look and firmness of the skin, although the tissue below is soft. Initial treatment should be to slowly rewarm the area. As the area thaws, it will be numb and bluish or purple, and blisters may form. Cover the area with a dry, sterile dressing and protect the skin from further exposure to cold. See a doctor for further treatment.

- *Deep frostbite*, the freezing of skin, muscle, and even bone requires medical treatment. It usually involves the tissues of the hands and feet, which appear pale and feel frozen. Keep the victim dry and as warm as possible on the way to a medical facility. Cover the frostbitten area with a dry, sterile dressing.

The center of the body may gradually cool at temperatures above, as well as below, freezing—usually in wet, windy weather. When body temperature falls below 95 degrees Fahrenheit, the body is incapable of rewarming itself because of the breakdown of the internal system that regulates its temperature. This state is known as **hypothermia**. The first sign of hypothermia is severe shivering. Then the victim becomes uncoordinated, drowsy, listless, and confused and is unable to speak properly. Symptoms become more severe as body temperature continues to drop, and coma or death can result.

Hypothermia requires emergency medical treatment. Try to prevent any further heat loss. Move the victim to a warm place, cover him or her with blankets, remove wet clothing, and replace it with dry garments. If the victim is conscious, administer warm liquids, not alcohol.

Here are ways to protect yourself in cold weather (or cold indoor gyms):

- Cover as much of your body as possible but don't overdress.

- Wear one layer less than you would if you were outside but not exercising.

- Don't use warm-up clothes made of waterproof material because they tend to trap heat and keep perspiration from evaporating.

- Make sure your clothes are loose enough to allow movement and exercise of the hands, feet, and other body parts, thereby maintaining proper circulation.

hypothermia An abnormally low body temperature; if not treated appropriately, coma or death could result.

- Choose dark colors that absorb heat.

- Because 40 percent or more of your body heat is lost through your head and neck, wear a hat, turtleneck, or scarf. Make sure you cover your hands and feet as well; mittens provide more warmth and protection than gloves.

- Warm up and cool down. Cold weather constricts muscles, so you need to allow enough time for proper stretching to warm up muscles before you exercise.

Exercise Injuries

According to the American Physical Therapy Association, the most common exercise-related injury sites are the knees, feet, back, and shoulders, followed by the ankles and hips. Types of injuries include the following:

- **Acute injuries**—sprains, bruises, and pulled muscles—result from sudden trauma, such as a fall or collision.

- **Overuse injuries**, on the other hand, result from overdoing a repetitive activity, such as running. When one particular joint is overstressed—such as a tennis player's elbow or a swimmer's shoulder—tendinitis, an inflammation at the point where the tendon meets the bone, can develop. Other overuse injuries include muscle strains and aches and stress fractures, which are hairline breaks in a bone, usually in the leg or foot.

The way a runner's foot strikes the ground can affect the risk of injury. In a study of college middle- and long-distance runners, about three in four experienced a moderate or severe injury each year, but those who habitually hit the ground with the rear of their foot had twice the rate of repetitive stress injuries as those who habitually hit with their forefoot.

✓**check-in** Have you ever suffered a sports-related injury?

Sooner or later, most active people do. Although most sports injuries are minor, they all require attention. Ignoring a problem or trying to push through the pain can lead to more serious complications.

PRICE   If you develop aches and pains beyond what you might expect from an activity, stop. Never push to the point of fatigue. If you do, you could end up with sprained or torn muscles. Figure 8.9 gives the PRICE prescription for coping with an exercise injury.

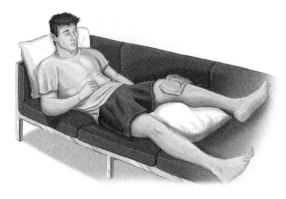

- **P**rotect the area with an elastic wrap, a sling, splint, cane, crutches, or an air cast.

- **R**est to promote tissue healing. Avoid activities that cause pain, swelling, or discomfort.

- **I**ce the area immediately, even if you're seeking medical help. (Don't put the ice pack directly on the skin.) Repeat every 2 or 3 hours while you're awake for the first 48 to 72 hours. Cold reduces pain, swelling, and inflammation in injured muscles, joints, and connecting tissues and may slow bleeding if a tear has occurred.

- **C**ompress the area with an elastic bandage until the swelling stops. Begin wrapping at the end farthest from your heart. Loosen the wrap if the pain increases, the area becomes numb, or swelling is occurring below the wrapped area.

- **E**levate the area above your heart, especially at night. Gravity helps reduce swelling by draining excess fluid.

- After 48 hours, if the swelling is gone, you may apply warmth or gentle heat, which improves the blood flow and speeds healing.

FIGURE 8.9 PRICE: How to Cope with an Exercise Injury

Overtraining About half of all people who start an exercise program drop out within six months. One common reason is that they **overtrain**, pushing themselves to work too intensely or too frequently. Signs of overdoing it include persistent muscle soreness, frequent injuries, unintended weight loss, nervousness, and inability to relax.

If you develop any of the symptoms of overtraining, reduce or stop your workout sessions temporarily. Make gradual increases in the intensity of your workouts. Allow 24 to 48 hours for recovery between workouts. Make sure you get adequate rest.

Exercise Addiction Excessive exercise can become a form of addiction, and "exercise dependence" is not uncommon among young men and women. Although most physically active college students work out at healthy levels, some exercise to an extent that could signal dependence.

acute injuries Physical injuries, such as sprains, bruises, and pulled muscles, which result from sudden traumas, such as falls or collisions.

overuse injuries Physical injuries to joints or muscles, such as strains, fractures, and tendinitis, which result from overdoing a repetitive activity.

overtrain Working muscles too intensely or too frequently, resulting in persistent muscle soreness, injuries, unintended weight loss, nervousness, and an inability to relax.

- How important is fitness for your overall health?
- Why do college students need to exercise?
- What would be an ideal workout?
- How can you protect yourself from exercise injuries?

THE POWER OF NOW!
Shaping Up

This chapter has given you the basic information you need to launch a fitness program. However, you're more likely to succeed if you create a plan and follow it. Check off these basic steps to help you determine where you are now and how to get to where you want to be.

____ Keep track of your progress in your online journal.

____ Set fitness goals. Do you have an overall conditioning goal, such as losing weight? Or do you have a training goal, such as preparing for a 5K race or trying out for the volleyball team? Break down your goal into smaller "step" goals that lead you toward it.

____ Think through your personal preferences. What are your physical strengths and weaknesses? Do you have good upper body strength but easily get winded? Do you have a stiff back? Do your allergies flare up when you exercise outdoors? By paying attention to your needs, likes, and dislikes, you can choose activities you enjoy—and are more likely to continue.

____ Schedule exercise into your daily routine. If you can, block out a half-hour for working out at the beginning of the day, between classes, or in the evening. Write it into your schedule as if it were a class or doctor's appointment. If you can't find 30 minutes, look for two 15-minute or three 10-minute slots that you can use for "mini-workouts." Once you've worked out a schedule, write it down. A written plan encourages you to stay on track.

____ Assemble your gear. Make sure you put your athletic shoes in your car or in the locker at the gym. Lay out the clothes you'll need to shoot hoops or play racquetball.

____ Start slowly. If you are just beginning regular activity or exercise, begin at a low level. If you have an injury, disability, or chronic health problem, be sure you get medical clearance from a physician.

____ Progress gradually. If you have not been physically active, begin by incorporating a few minutes of physical activity into each day, building up to 30 minutes or more of moderate-intensity activities. If you have been active but not as often or as intensely as recommended, become more consistent. Continue to increase the frequency, intensity, and duration of your workouts.

____ Take stock. After a few months of leading a more active life, take stock. Think of how much more energy you have at the end of the day. Ask yourself if you're feeling any less stressed, despite the push and pull of daily pressures. Focus on the unanticipated rewards of exercise. Savor the exhilaration of an autumn morning's walk; the thrill of feeling newly toughened muscles bend to your will; or the satisfaction of a long, smooth stretch after a stressful day. Enjoy the pure pleasure of living in the body you deserve.

What's Online

CENGAGE brain.com   Visit www.cengagebrain.com to access course materials for this text, including the Behavior Change Planner, interactive quizzes, and more.

Are You Ready to Become More Active?

Physical Activity Stages of Change Questionnaire

For each of the following questions, please circle Yes or No. Please be sure to read the questions carefully.

Physical activity or exercise includes activities such as walking briskly, jogging, bicycling, swimming, or any other activity in which the exertion is at least as intense as these activities.

1. I am currently physically active.   NO   YES

2. I intend to become more physically active in the next 6 months.   NO   YES

For activity to be regular, it must add up to a total of 30 minutes or more per day and be done at least 5 days per week. For example, you could take one 30-minute walk or take three 10-minute walks for a daily total of 30 minutes.

3. I currently engage in regular physical activity.   NO   YES

4. I have been regularly physically active for the past 6 months.   NO   YES

Scoring Algorithm	Question			
	1	**2**	**3**	**4**
Precontemplation	No	No		
Contemplation	No	Yes		
Preparation	Yes		No	
Action	Yes		Yes	No
Maintenance	Yes		Yes	Yes

Source: Adapted, with permission, from B.H. Marcus and L.H. Forsyth, 2003, *Motivating people to be physically active,* 2nd ed. (Champaign, IL: Human Kinetics), 168

MAKING THIS CHAPTER WORK FOR YOU

Review Questions

(LO 8.1) 1. _____ refers to the ability of the heart to pump blood through the body efficiently.
   a. Cardiorespiratory fitness
   b. Metabolic fitness
   c. Muscular endurance
   d. Muscular strength

(LO 8.1) 2. Which of the following is true of college students' fitness habits?
   a. College women are generally more active than men.
   b. Part-time or employed students exercise less than full-time students.
   c. Married students report more days of vigorous workouts than single students.
   d. Undergraduates living on campus are less active than those living off campus.

(LO 8.2) 3. Which of the following is a benefit of regular physical activity?
   a. Decreased bone mass
   b. Enlargement of the heart
   c. Reduced depression
   d. Difficulty sleeping

(LO 8.2) 4. Which of the following is a risk associated with exercise?
   a. Enlargement of the heart
   b. Increased tension
   c. Brittle bones
   d. Increased sensitivity to insulin

(LO 8.3) 5. Which of the following defines the metabolic equivalent of task (MET)?
   a. One MET is the energy needed to raise the temperature of one gram of water by one degree Celsius.
   b. One MET is the energy that animals derive from their food through cellular respiration.
   c. It is an individual's body mass divided by the square of his or her height.
   d. A single MET is the amount of energy a person uses at rest.

(LO 8.3) 6. The minimum amount of exercise required for a significant lowering of the risk of premature dying is _____ MET minutes of exercise a week.
   a. 1,000
   b. 150
   c. 500
   d. 1,500

(LO 8.4) 7. The _____ principle states that muscles must work against a greater-than-normal resistance in order to get stronger.
   a. reversibility
   b. overload
   c. variation
   d. Karvonen

(LO 8.4)   8. Hussain was an athlete throughout high school. However, he stopped exercising once he reached college, and his fitness levels dropped to half. This is an example of the _____ principle.
a. overload
b. reversibility
c. variation
d. specificity

(LO 8.5)   9. Which of the following is true of the aerobic activity spinning?
a. It is a hybrid of boxing, martial arts, and aerobics.
b. It combines dance and aerobic elements.
c. It is a cardiovascular workout for the whole body.
d. It involves mountain biking.

(LO 8.5)   10. _____ combines dance and aerobic elements with choreography that incorporates hip-hop, samba, salsa, merengue, mambo, martial arts, and belly dancing.
a. Yoga
b. Spinning
c. Zumba
d. Pilates

(LO 8.6)   11. In a(n) _____ contraction, the muscle applies force while maintaining an equal length.
a. isotonic
b. isometric
c. isokinetic
d. hypotonic

(LO 8.6)   12. Which of the following muscles form a part of the core?
a. Quadriceps
b. Deltoids
c. Pectorals
d. Obliques

(LO 8.7)   13. Which of the following is true of static flexibility?
a. It is the ability to move a joint quickly.
b. It depends on the structure of a joint and the tightness of the muscles.
c. It refers to the ability to move a joint fluidly through its entire range of motion.
d. It determines whether one can do a split leap.

(LO 8.7)   14. _____ stretching involves stretching a muscle by contracting the opposing muscle.
a. Passive
b. Active
c. Dynamic
d. Static

(LO 8.8)   15. Which of the following exercise routines employs a device called the Reformer?
a. Pilates
b. Yoga
c. T'ai chi
d. Zumba

(LO 8.8)   16. Which of the following Chinese practices is sometimes described as "meditation in motion"?
a. Shooto
b. Karate
c. T'ai chi
d. Jiu-jitsu

(LO 8.9)   17. One of the most effective treatments for back pain is _____.
a. surgery
b. inflammatory medication
c. bed rest
d. core muscle strengthening

(LO 8.9)   18. Which of the following groups of people is at increased risk for back pain?
a. Men
b. Children
c. Smokers
d. Teenagers

(LO 8.10)   19. Which of the following is true of athletes' nutritional requirements?
a. Complex carbohydrates are essential in their diet.
b. They have higher protein requirements than others, with the exception of those engaged in intense strength training.
c. Fat should be eliminated entirely from their diet.
d. They should eat immediately before a workout to avoid feeling weak or tired.

(LO 8.10)   20. Too much water during prolonged bouts of exercise can lead to _____, or water intoxication.
a. hyperthermia
b. hyponatremia
c. hypoxia
d. hypothermia

(LO 8.11)   21. _____ is a medical emergency that can be fatal and occurs when the body temperature rises to 106 degrees Fahrenheit or higher within 10 to 15 minutes.
a. Hypothermia
b. Heat exhaustion
c. Heat cramps
d. Heat stroke

(LO 8.11)   22. _____ is characterized by a waxy look and firmness of the skin, although the tissue below is soft.
a. Superficial frostbite
b. Deep frostbite
c. Hypothermia
d. Acrocyanosis

Answers to these questions can be found on page 623.

Critical Thinking Questions

1. Allison knows that exercise is good for her health, but she thinks that if she can keep her weight in check by going on a diet, her health will be fine. "I look good. I feel okay. Why should I bother with exercising?" she asks. What would be your response?

2. Your younger brother, Andre, is a part of his high school football team. The team practice began in July. You are aware that a couple players in his team recently suffered from heat-related problems. However, according to Andre, these players just weren't tough enough. What can you do to help your brother protect his health?

Additional Online Resources

www.acefitness.org
This website features information for the general public as well as for certified fitness trainers. The comprehensive site includes health and fitness news headlines, Fit Facts information sheets, a question-and-answer site, whole-body exercise workouts, daily fitness tips, discussion boards, newsletters, and information on ACE certification.

www.shapeamerica.org
The Society of Health and Physical Educators (SHAPE) provides legislative advocacy for healthy lifestyles through high-quality programs in health and physical education. The website features consumer news, career links, listing of graduate programs, research, and a link for the *International Electronic Journal of Health Education.*

www.shapeup.org/fitness/index.html
At this site, you can perform a battery of physical fitness assessments, including activity level, strength, flexibility, and an aerobic fitness test. You get started by entering your weight, height, age, and gender and then take a quick screen test to assess your physical readiness for physical activity. Your final results in each area will be based on your personal data.

Key Terms

The terms listed are used on the pages indicated. Definitions of the terms are in the glossary at the end of the book.

active stretching   230
acute injuries   239
aerobic exercise   217
anabolic steroids   227
anaerobic exercise   217
ballistic stretching   230
body composition   207
cardiorespiratory fitness   206
dynamic flexibility   228
dynamic stretching   230
exercise   208
FITT   216
flexibility   207
functional fitness   207
hypothermia   238
isokinetic   224
isometric   224
isotonic   224
MET (metabolic equivalent of task)   214
metabolic fitness   207
muscle dysmorphia   226
muscular endurance   207

muscular strength   207
osteoporosis   208
overload principle   216
overloading   223
overtrain   239
overuse injuries   239
passive stretching   230
physical activity   208
physical fitness   206
progressive overloading   216
range of motion   228
Rating of Perceived Exertion (RPE)   218
reps (or repetitions)   224
resting heart rate   217
reversibility principle   217
sets   224
specificity principle   216
static flexibility   228
static stretching   229
target heart rate   217

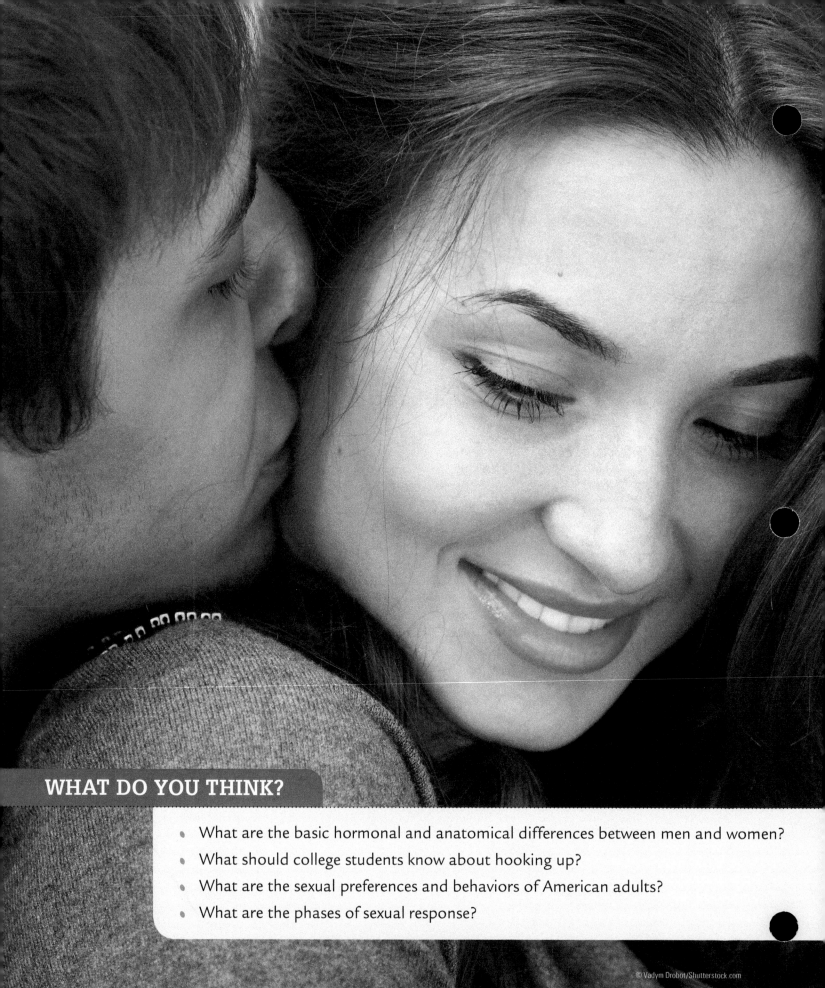

WHAT DO YOU THINK?

- What are the basic hormonal and anatomical differences between men and women?
- What should college students know about hooking up?
- What are the sexual preferences and behaviors of American adults?
- What are the phases of sexual response?

9

Sexual Health

Alex, several years older than the typical college freshman, usually doesn't think much about the age difference—until the conversation turns to sex. He understands his younger classmates' seemingly endless fascination with sex, but his perspective is different. As a teenager, he had plunged recklessly into dangerous territory of every type. Sex—casual and sometimes unprotected—was one of them.

"Looking back," Alex muses, "I feel lucky that I didn't end up a statistic." But he still regrets the irresponsible ways he acted—and the chronic sexually transmitted infection (STI) acquired along the way.

Now 28, Alex is a veteran of military service, a married man, and an expectant father. His enjoyment of sex hasn't faded; in many ways, it has deepened and become more gratifying. He now realizes that sexual choices have consequences and effects on one's own life and on other people. These are the lessons he hopes someday to pass on to his own children.

As Alex learned with time and experience, you are ultimately responsible for your sexual health and behavior. You make decisions that affect how you express your sexuality, how you respond sexually, and how you give and receive sexual pleasure. Yet most sexual activity involves another person. Therefore, your decisions about sex—more so than those you make about nutrition, drugs, or exercise—have important effects on other people. <

After reading this chapter, you should be able to:

9.1 Describe women's and men's sexual health, their sexual anatomy, and the role of sex hormones in the development of gender identities.

9.2 Specify the aspects of healthy sexual relationships that lead toward responsible sexuality.

9.3 Summarize some sexual practices engaged in by college students.

9.4 Discuss sexual diversity in human beings.

9.5 Outline the major types of sexual activity.

9.6 Describe the stages of sexual response in men and women.

9.7 Comment on sexual dysfunctions and their treatments in men and women.

9.8 Give three examples of atypical sexual behavior in men and women.

Sexual responsibility begins with learning about your body, your partner's body, your sexual development and preferences, and the health risks associated with sexual activity, including STIs. This chapter provides information and insight you can use in making decisions and choosing sexually responsible behaviors.

Sexual Health

Human **sexuality**—the quality of being sexual—is as rich, varied, and complex as life itself. Along with our **sex**, or biological maleness or femaleness, it is an integral part of who we are, how we see ourselves, and how we relate to others. Of all of our involvements with others, sexual **intimacy**, or physical closeness, can be the most rewarding. But while sexual expression and experience can provide intense joy, they also can involve great emotional turmoil.

Sexual health refers, by simplest definition, to "a state of optimal well-being related to sexuality throughout the lifespan."[1] The World Health Organization (WHO) describes it more comprehensively as "a state of physical, emotional, mental, and social well-being related to sexuality; it is not merely the absence of disease, dysfunction, or infirmity. Sexual health requires a positive and respectful approach to sexuality and sexual responses, as well as the possibility of having pleasurable and safe sexual experiences, free of coercion, discrimination, and violence."

The sexual health of college students, particularly those in the period termed "emerging adulthood" (ages 18–25), is at greater risk than that of the rest of the population. Less likely to use condoms or practice birth control, undergraduates in this age group face a greater likelihood of STIs and, if heterosexual, unwanted pregnancy.[2]

✓**check-in** Do you think of your sexual health as a personal responsibility or as the responsibility of your school?

According to a recent survey, college students view themselves as adults responsible for decisions related to their sexual health, but they also expect and want support from their schools. Students feel that their four-year schools should be responsible for providing access to resources, such as condoms and tests for STIs and pregnancy, but trust that undergraduates will take charge of their own sexual decisions.[3]

Those at two-year institutions want access to basic information such as pamphlets on sexual health topics and referrals to community resources. One student viewed his two year school as a place "mainly to learn, to get degrees and stuff like that, not to be tested [for STIs]." Some of those in urban settings appreciate the fact that the ability to use resources beyond the campus decreased their dependence on the institution.

Only about half of college students report receiving information from their school on human immunodeficiency virus (HIV) and other STIs; even fewer indicate that they received information on unintended pregnancy. One of the *Healthy People 2020* objectives (discussed in Chapter 1) is increasing the proportion of undergraduates given information on these topics by their institutions.

✓**check-in** How does your school compare? What types of sexual information have you received?

Sexuality and the Dimensions of Health

Our sexuality both affects and is affected by the various dimensions of health. Responsible sexuality and high-level sexual health contribute to the fullest possible functioning of body, mind, spirit, and social relationships. In turn, other aspects of health enhance our sexuality. Here are some examples:

- **Physical:** Safer sex practices reduce the risk of sexually transmitted infections that can threaten sexual health, physical health, and even survival. When our bodies are healthy and well, we feel better about ourselves, which enhances both self-esteem and healthy sexuality.

- **Emotional:** By acknowledging and respecting the intimacy of a sexual relationship, responsible sexuality builds trust and commitment. When our emotional health is high, we can better understand and cope with the complex feelings related to being sexual.

- **Social:** From dating to mating, we express and fulfill our sexual identities in the context of families, friends, and society as a whole. Having strong friendships, intimate relationships, and caring partnerships enables us to explore our sexuality in safe and healthy ways.

- **Intellectual:** Our most fulfilling relationships involve a meeting of minds as well as bodies. High-level intellectual health enables us to acquire and understand sexual information,

sexuality The behaviors, instincts, and attitudes associated with being sexual.

sex Maleness or femaleness, resulting from genetic, structural, and functional factors.

intimacy A state of closeness between two people, characterized by the desire and ability to share one's innermost thoughts and feelings with each other either verbally or nonverbally.

sexual health The integration of the physical, emotional, intellectual, social, and spiritual aspects of sexual being in ways that are positively enriching and that enhance personality, communication, and love.

analyze it critically, and make healthy sexual decisions.

- **Spiritual:** At its deepest, most fulfilling level, sexuality uplifts the soul by allowing us to connect to something greater than ourselves. Individuals who have developed their spirituality bring to their most intimate relationships an awareness and appreciation that lifts them beyond the physical.

- **Environmental:** Responsible sexuality makes people more aware of the impact of their decisions on others. Protecting yourself from sexual threats and creating a supportive environment in which to study and work are crucial to high-level health and to healthy sexuality.

....
√ **check-in** How do the various dimensions of health affect your sexuality?
....

Becoming Male or Female

Physiological maleness or femaleness, or biological sex, is indicated by the sex chromosomes, hormonal balance, and genital anatomy. **Gender** refers to the psychological and sociological, as well as the physical, aspects of being male or female. You are born with a certain *sexual identity* based on your sexual anatomy and appearance; you, your parents, and society mold your gender identity.

Are You an X or a Y?   Biologically, few absolute differences separate the sexes: Males alone can make sperm and contribute the chromosome that causes embryos to develop as males; females alone are born with sex cells (eggs, or ova), menstruate, give birth, and breast-feed babies. But the process of becoming male or female is a long and complex one.

In the beginning, all human embryos have undifferentiated sex organs. Only after several weeks do the sex organs differentiate, becoming either male or female *gonads* (testes or ovaries), the structures that produce the future reproductive cells of an individual. This initial differentiation process depends on genetic instructions in the form of the sex chromosomes, referred to as X and Y. If a Y (or male) chromosome is present in the embryo, about seven weeks after conception, it signals the sex organs to develop into testes. If a Y chromosome isn't present, an embryo begins developing ovaries in the eighth week. From this point on, the sex hormones produced by the gonads, not the chromosomes, play the crucial role in making a male or female.

How Hormones Work   In Greek, *hormone* means "set into motion"—and that's

exactly what our **hormones** do. These chemical messengers, produced by various organs in the body, including the sex organs, and carried to target structures by the bloodstream, arouse cells and organs to specific activities and influence the way we look, feel, develop, and behave.

The group of organs that produce hormones is referred to as the **endocrine system**. Except for the sex organs, males and females have identical endocrine systems. Directing the endocrine system is the hypothalamus, a pea-sized section of the brain. The pituitary gland, directly beneath the hypothalamus, turns the various glands on and off in response to messages from it.

The ovaries produce the sex hormones most crucial to women, **estrogen** and **progesterone**. The primary sex hormone in men is **testosterone**, which is produced by the testes and the adrenal glands. However, both men and women have small amounts of the hormones of the opposite sex. Estrogen, in fact, is crucial to male fertility and gives sperm what researchers describe as their "reproductive punch."

The sex hormones begin their work early in an embryo's development. As soon as the testes are formed, they start releasing testosterone, which stimulates the development of other structures, such as the penis. The absence of testosterone in an embryo causes female genitals to form. (If the testes of a genetic male don't produce testosterone, the fetus will develop female genitals. Similarly, if a genetic female is exposed to excessive testosterone, the fetus will have ovaries but will also develop male genitals.)

As puberty begins, the pituitary gland initiates the changes that transform boys into men and girls into women (Figure 9.1). When a boy is about 14 years old and a girl about 12, their brains stimulate the hypothalamus to secrete a hormone called gonadotropin-releasing hormone (GnRH). This substance causes the pituitary gland to release hormones called **gonadotropins**. These, in turn, stimulate the gonads to make sex hormones.

The gonadotropins are *follicle-stimulating hormone (FSH)* and *luteinizing hormone (LH)*. In girls, these hormones travel to the ovary and stimulate the production of estrogen. As estrogen increases, a girl's **secondary sex characteristics** develop. Her breasts become fuller, her external genitals enlarge, and fat is deposited on her hips and buttocks. Estrogen keeps her hair thick and skin smooth. She begins menstruating because she has begun ovulating, the process that prepares her body to conceive and carry a baby.

This process seems to be beginning earlier than in the past. Breast development, typically

gender Maleness or femaleness, as determined by a combination of anatomical and physiological factors, psychological factors, and learned behaviors.

hormones Substances released in the blood that regulate specific bodily functions.

endocrine system The group of ductless glands that produce hormones and secrete them directly into the blood for transport to target organs.

estrogen The female sex hormone that stimulates female secondary sex characteristics.

progesterone The female sex hormone that stimulates the uterus, preparing it for the arrival of a fertilized egg.

testosterone The male sex hormone that stimulates male secondary sex characteristics.

gonadotropins Gonad-stimulating hormones produced by the pituitary gland.

secondary sex characteristics Physical changes associated with maleness or femaleness, induced by the sex hormones.

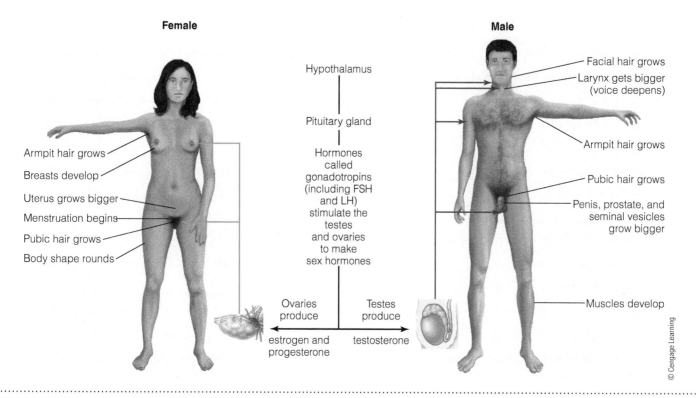

Female

- Armpit hair grows
- Breasts develop
- Uterus grows bigger
- Menstruation begins
- Pubic hair grows
- Body shape rounds

Hypothalamus

Pituitary gland

Hormones called gonadotropins (including FSH and LH) stimulate the testes and ovaries to make sex hormones

Ovaries produce

estrogen and progesterone

Testes produce

testosterone

Male

- Facial hair grows
- Larynx gets bigger (voice deepens)
- Armpit hair grows
- Pubic hair grows
- Penis, prostate, and seminal vesicles grow bigger
- Muscles develop

© Cengage Learning

FIGURE 9.1 Puberty

The body's endocrine system produces hormones that trigger body changes, including growth spurts, in boys and girls.

the first sign of puberty in girls, now starts at age 7 in about 10 percent of white girls, 23 percent of blacks, and 15 percent of Hispanics.

African American girls reach **menarche**—the term for first menstruation—at a mean age of 12.16 years; white girls, at 12.88 years. By comparison, a hundred years ago girls didn't reach menarche until the relatively ripe age of fifteen.

Improved nutrition and good health seem to be the primary factors. Girls today are bigger, taller, better fed, and more sedentary and have a higher percentage of body fat (one of the triggers of sexual maturation). They also grow up amid a host of environmental influences that may further speed development.

Cultural influences affect a girl's response to menarche. In a cross-cultural study of college students, the most common emotions expressed by American women at menarche were embarrassment, pride, and anxiety. Malaysian women cited fear, embarrassment, and worry. Lithuanian women described themselves as happy or scared, while Sudanese women cited fear, anxiety, embarrassment, and anger. On the positive side, the Lithuanian women reported feeling more valuable and believing they had entered the world of women.

American boys also are reaching puberty at earlier ages—at an average age of 9 for blacks and 10 for whites and Hispanics—up to two years earlier than in the past. Boys' gonadotropins stimulate

the testes to produce testosterone, which triggers the development of male secondary sex characteristics. Their voices deepen, hair grows on their faces and bodies, their penises become thicker and longer, and their muscles become stronger.

The sex hormones released during puberty change the growth pattern of childhood, so that a boy or girl may now spurt up four to six inches in a single year. The skeleton matures very rapidly until, at the end of puberty (usually around age 18), the growth centers at the ends of the bones close off. Estrogen halts bone growth in girls at an earlier age than in boys.

Sexual and Gender Identity It's a boy! It's a girl! These statements confer an instant identity on a newborn. However, in recent years, researchers have challenged such either/or distinctions as male or female, masculine or feminine, heterosexual or homosexual. Although most people have the biological characteristics of a male or a female, some possess some degree of both male and female reproductive structures. They are referred to as intersexual.

The continuum for gender identity ranges from extreme stereotypical masculine notions to extreme stereotypical feminine behaviors. Different cultures vary in defining what is masculine or feminine. Individuals who consider themselves androgynous choose not to conform to sexual

menarche The onset of menstruation at puberty.

stereotypes. **Androgyny** includes those who are "positively androgynous," combining positive attributes linked with both sexes—for example, feminine compassion and masculine independence—and individuals who are "negatively androgynous" and might show less desirable characteristics of each gender, such as feminine dependency and masculine assertiveness. (The gender spectrum is discussed on page 263.)

Women's Sexual Health

All women of childbearing age should undergo regular "health maintenance" exams to monitor their sexual and reproductive well-being, detect infections and other medical problems, and prevent unwanted pregnancy. The latest guidelines from government and specialty organizations advise the following services:[4]

- Counseling on contraception for women who do not want to get pregnant.

- Counseling on pre-pregnancy health care for women who are attempting to conceive.

- Counseling for all women who may become pregnant to take a daily folic acid supplement of 400 to 800 mcg.

- Counseling on reducing the risks of STIs.

- Screening of all women age 24 or younger for chlamydia.

- Screening of all women at high risk for chlamydia, gonorrhea, and syphilis and screening of all women for HIV.

- Initial screening for cervical cancer at age 21. (See Chapter 11 for more information on the subsequent timing of screening and co-testing for human papillomavirus [HPV].)

- Screening for domestic violence and sexual or reproductive coercion.

✓**check-in** If you are a woman, when was your last gynecological exam?

In the past, gynecologists recommended annual pelvic exams for all women age 21 and older. However, some physicians question the need for pelvic exams in women who do not have symptoms such as pelvic pain, menstrual problems, or vaginal discharge. Other less expensive and less invasive forms of testing can detect STIs, and an exam usually is not required before initiation of many forms of birth control.[5]

✓**check-in** If you are a woman, have you asked your doctor how often you need a pelvic exam?

Female Sexual Anatomy As illustrated in Figure 9.2a, the **mons pubis** is the rounded, fleshy area over the junction of the pubic bones. The folds of skin that form the outer lips of a woman's genital area are called the **labia majora**. They cover soft flaps of skin (inner lips) called the **labia minora**. The inner lips join at the top to form a hood over the **clitoris**, a small elongated erectile organ, and the most sensitive spot in the entire female genital area. Below the clitoris is the **urethral opening**, the outer opening of the thin tube that carries urine from the bladder. Below that is a larger opening, the mouth of the **vagina**, the canal that leads to the primary internal organs of reproduction. The **perineum** is the area between the vagina and the anus (the opening to the rectum and large intestine).

At the back of the vagina is the **cervix**, the opening to the womb, or **uterus** (see Figure 9.2b). The uterine walls are lined with a layer of tissue called the **endometrium**. The **ovaries**, about the size and shape of almonds, are located on either side of the uterus and contain egg cells called ova (singular, **ovum**). Extending outward and back from the upper uterus are the **fallopian tubes**, the canals that transport ova from the ovaries to the uterus. When an egg is released from an ovary, the fingerlike ends of the adjacent fallopian tube "catch" the egg and direct it into the tube.

Discharge and changes in odor normally occur in a healthy vagina. They typically fluctuate through the menstrual cycle, depending on hormone level. In the past, many women practiced douching, the introduction of a liquid into the vagina, to cleanse the vagina. However, particularly if done frequently, douching may increase the risk of pelvic inflammatory disease (discussed later in this chapter) and ectopic or out-of-uterus pregnancy.

The Menstrual Cycle The menstrual cycle begins in the brain with the production of gonadotropin-releasing hormone (GnRH) and then proceeds through the following steps:

- GnRH sets into motion the sequence of steps that lead to ovulation, the potential for conception, and, if conception doesn't occur, menstruation. The hypothalamus monitors hormone levels in the blood and sends messages to the pituitary gland to release follicle-stimulating hormone (FSH) and luteinizing hormone (LH).

- As shown in Figure 9.3, in the ovaries, these hormones stimulate the growth of a few of the immature eggs, or ova, stored in follicles

androgyny The expression of both masculine and feminine traits.

mons pubis The rounded, fleshy area over the junction of the female pubic bones.

labia majora The fleshy outer folds that border the female genital area.

labia minora The fleshy inner folds that border the female genital area.

clitoris A small erectile structure on the female, corresponding to the penis on the male.

urethral opening The outer opening of the thin tube that carries urine from the bladder.

vagina The canal leading from the exterior opening in the female genital area to the uterus.

perineum The area between the anus and vagina in the female and between the anus and scrotum in the male.

cervix The narrow, lower end of the uterus that opens into the vagina.

uterus The female organ that houses the developing fetus until birth.

endometrium The mucous membrane lining the uterus.

ovaries The female sex organs that produce egg cells, estrogen, and progesterone.

ovum (plural, ova) The female gamete (egg cell).

fallopian tubes The pair of channels that transport ova from the ovaries to the uterus; the usual site of fertilization.

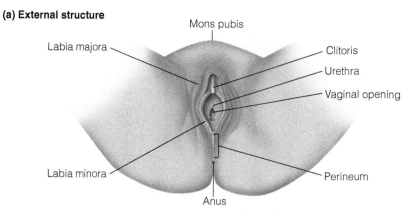

(a) External structure

Mons pubis

Labia majora

Clitoris

Urethra

Vaginal opening

Labia minora

Perineum

Anus

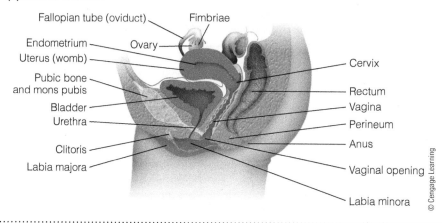

(b) Internal structure

Fallopian tube (oviduct)

Fimbriae

Endometrium

Ovary

Uterus (womb)

Pubic bone and mons pubis

Bladder

Urethra

Clitoris

Labia majora

Cervix

Rectum

Vagina

Perineum

Anus

Vaginal opening

Labia minora

© Cengage Learning

FIGURE 9.2 The Female Sex Organs and Reproductive Structures

---

ovulation The release of a mature ovum from an ovary approximately 14 days prior to the onset of menstruation.

corpus luteum A yellowish mass of tissue that is formed, immediately after ovulation, from the remaining cells of the follicle; it secretes estrogen and progesterone for the remainder of the menstrual cycle.

menstruation Discharge of blood from the vagina as a result of the shedding of the uterine lining at the end of the menstrual cycle.

premenstrual syndrome (PMS) A disorder that causes physical discomfort and psychological distress prior to a woman's menstrual period.

in every woman's body. Usually, only one ovum matures completely during each monthly cycle. As it does, it increases its production of the female sex hormone estrogen, which in turn triggers the release of a larger surge of LH.

- At midcycle, the increased LH hormone levels trigger **ovulation**, the release of the egg cell, or ovum, from the follicle. Estrogen levels drop, and the remaining cells of the follicle then enlarge, change character, and form the **corpus luteum**, or yellow body.

- In the second half of the menstrual cycle, the corpus luteum secretes estrogen and larger amounts of progesterone. The endometrium (uterine lining) is stimulated by progesterone to thicken and become more engorged with blood in preparation for nourishing an implanted, fertilized ovum.

- If the ovum is not fertilized, the corpus luteum disintegrates. As the level of progesterone drops, **menstruation** occurs; the uterine lining is shed during the course of a menstrual period.

- If the egg is fertilized and pregnancy occurs, the cells that eventually develop into the

placenta secrete *human chorionic gonadotropin (HCG)*, a messenger hormone that signals the pituitary not to start a new cycle. The corpus luteum then steps up its production of progesterone.

Many women experience physical or psychological changes, or both, during their monthly cycles. Usually the changes are minor, but more serious problems can occur.

Women's attitudes toward menstruation may reflect how positively or negatively they view their bodies in general.[6]

Premenstrual Syndrome

Women with **premenstrual syndrome (PMS)** experience bodily discomfort and emotional distress for up to two weeks, from ovulation until the onset of menstruation. As many as 75 percent of menstruating women report one or more premenstrual symptoms; 3 to 9 percent experience disabling, incapacitating symptoms.

Among the factors linked with premenstrual symptoms in college students are stress, sleep quality, and higher rates of psychological disorders.[7]

FIGURE 9.3 Menstrual Cycle

(a) In response to the hypothalamus, the pituitary gland releases the gonadotropins FSH and LH. Levels of FSH and LH stimulate the cycle (and in turn are affected by production of estrogen and progesterone).

(b) FSH does what its name says: it stimulates follicle development in the ovary. The follicle matures and ruptures, releasing an ovum (egg) into the fallopian tube.

(c) The follicle produces estrogen, and the corpus luteum produces estrogen and progesterone. The high level of estrogen at the middle of the cycle produces a surge of LH, which triggers ovulation.

(d) Estrogen and progesterone stimulate the endometrium, which becomes thicker and prepares to receive an implanted, fertilized egg. If a fertilized egg is deposited in the uterus, pregnancy begins. If the egg is not fertilized, progesterone production decreases, and the endometrium is shed (menstruation). At this point, both estrogen and progesterone levels have dropped, so the pituitary responds by producing FSH, and the cycle begins again.

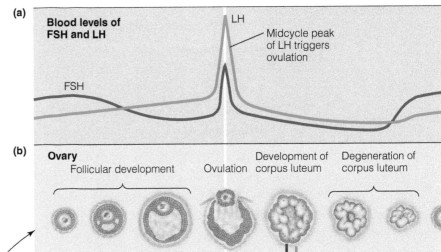

(a) **Blood levels of FSH and LH**

LH — Midcycle peak of LH triggers ovulation

FSH

(b) **Ovary**

Follicular development — Ovulation — Development of corpus luteum — Degeneration of corpus luteum

↓ Estrogen   Progesterone ↓   ↓ Estrogen

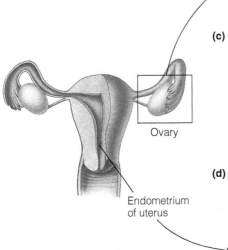

Ovary

Endometrium of uterus

(c) **Blood levels of estrogen and progesterone**

Estrogen   Progesterone

(d) **Uterus (endometrial lining)**

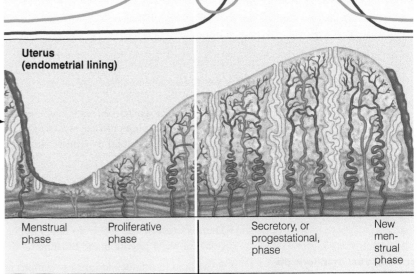

| **Uterine phases** | Menstrual phase | Proliferative phase | | Secretory, or progestational, phase | New menstrual phase |

| **Ovarian phases** | Follicular phase | | Ovulation | Luteal phase | New follicular phase |

Days of cycle: 0 2 4 6 8 10 12 14 16 18 20 22 24 26 28

Days of cycle

© Cengage Learning

Once dismissed as a psychological problem, PMS has been recognized as a very real physiological disorder that may be caused by various factors, including the following:

- A hormonal deficiency
- Abnormal levels of thyroid hormone
- An imbalance of estrogen and progesterone
- Social and environmental factors, particularly stress

The most common symptoms of PMS are

- Mood changes
- Anxiety
- Irritability
- Difficulty concentrating
- Forgetfulness
- Impaired judgment
- Tearfulness
- Digestive symptoms (diarrhea, bloating, constipation)
- Hot flashes
- Palpitations
- Dizziness
- Headache
- Fatigue
- Changes in appetite
- Cravings (usually for sweets or salt)
- Water retention
- Breast tenderness
- Insomnia[8]

√ **check-in** If you are a woman, have you experienced any of these symptoms of PMS?

For a diagnosis to be made, women must report troubling premenstrual symptoms in the days before menstruation in at least two successive menstrual cycles.

Treatments

Treatments for PMS depend on specific symptoms:

- Diuretics (drugs that speed up fluid elimination) for water retention and bloating
- Relaxation techniques for anxiety symptoms
- Sleep deprivation or the use of bright light to adjust a woman's circadian or daily rhythm
- Charting of cycles to identify vulnerable periods
- Low doses of medications known as *selective serotonin-reuptake inhibitors* (*SSRIs*), such as

fluoxetine (marketed as Prozac and Sarafem and in generic forms), for symptoms such as tension, depression, irritability, and mood swings, taken only during the premenstrual phase or daily throughout the month

- YAZ, a low-dose combination birth control pill made up of the hormones drospirenone and ethinyl estradiol, the only oral contraceptive approved by the FDA to treat emotional and physical premenstrual symptoms (see Chapter 10)
- A diet rich in calcium and vitamin D or supplements to decrease the severity of symptoms
- Cognitive-behavioral therapy, described in Chapter 3, which may be the most effective psychological approach

Other treatments with some reported success include exercise; lower caffeine, alcohol, salt, and sugar intake; acupuncture; and stress management techniques such as meditation or relaxation training.

Premenstrual Dysphoric Disorder

Premenstrual dysphoric disorder (PMDD), which is not related to PMS, occurs in an estimated 3 to 5 percent of all menstruating women. It is characterized by regular symptoms of depression (depressed mood, anxiety, mood swings, diminished interest or pleasure) as well as physical symptoms, such as changes in appetite, energy, weight, or sleep during the last week of the menstrual cycle.

Women with PMDD cannot function as usual at work, school, or home. They feel better a few days after menstruation begins. Certain birth control pills can help by stopping ovulation and stabilizing hormone fluctuations. SSRIs, which are often used to treat PMS, also are effective in relieving symptoms of PMDD. Some women may benefit from exercise, relaxation, or cognitive behavioral therapy.[9]

Menstrual Cramps

Dysmenorrhea is the medical name for the discomforts—abdominal cramps and pain, back and leg pain, diarrhea, tension, water retention, fatigue, and depression—that can occur during menstruation. About half of all menstruating women suffer from dysmenorrhea. The cause seems to be overproduction of bodily substances called prostaglandins, which typically rise during menstruation. Medications that inhibit prostaglandins can reduce menstrual pain, and exercise can also relieve cramps.

√ **check-in** If you are a woman, have you ever experienced dysmenorrhea?

premenstrual dysphoric disorder (PMDD) A disorder that causes symptoms of psychological depression during the last week of the menstrual cycle.

dysmenorrhea Painful menstruation.

Amenorrhea

Women may stop menstruating—a condition called **amenorrhea**—for a variety of reasons, including a hormonal disorder, drastic weight loss, strenuous exercise, or change in the environment. "Boarding-school amenorrhea" is common among young women who leave home for school. Distance running and strenuous exercise also can lead to amenorrhea. The reason may be a drop in body fat from the normal range of 18 to 22 percent to a range of 9 to 12 percent.

To be considered amenorrheic, a woman's menstrual cycle is typically absent for three or more consecutive months. Prolonged amenorrhea can have serious health consequences, including a loss of bone density that may lead to stress fractures or osteoporosis. Scientists have developed chemical mimics, or analogues, of GnRH—usually administered by nasal spray—that trigger ovulation in women who don't ovulate or menstruate normally.

Toxic Shock Syndrome

This rare, potentially deadly bacterial infection primarily strikes menstruating women under age 30 who use tampons. Both *Staphylococcus aureus* and group A *Streptococcus pyogenes* can produce **toxic shock syndrome (TSS)**. Symptoms include a high fever; a rash that leads to peeling of the skin on the fingers, toes, palms, and soles; dizziness; dangerously low blood pressure; and abnormalities in several organ systems (the digestive tract and the kidneys) and in the muscles and blood. Treatment usually consists of antibiotics and intense supportive care; intravenous administration of immunoglobulins that attack the toxins produced by these bacteria also may be beneficial.

Men's Sexual Health

Because the male reproductive system is simpler in many ways than the female, it is often ignored—especially by healthy young men. However, men should make regular self-exams (including checking the penis and testes, as described in Chapter 15) part of their routine.

Male Sexual Anatomy The visible parts of the male sexual anatomy are the **penis** and the **scrotum**, the pouch that contains the **testes** (Figure 9.4a). The testes manufacture testosterone, the hormone that stimulates the development of a male's secondary sex characteristics, and **sperm**, the male reproductive cells. Immature sperm are stored in the **epididymis**, a collection of coiled tubes adjacent to each testis.

The Penis The penis contains three hollow cylinders loosely covered with skin. The two major cylinders, the corpora cavernosa, extend side by side through the length of the penis. The third cylinder, the corpus spongiosum, surrounds the urethra, the channel for both seminal fluid and urine; see Figure 9.4b.

amenorrhea The absence or suppression of menstruation.

toxic shock syndrome (TSS) A disease characterized by fever, vomiting, diarrhea, and often shock, caused by a bacterium that releases toxic waste products into the bloodstream.

penis The male organ of sex and urination.

scrotum The external sac or pouch that holds the testes.

testes (singular, testis) The male sex organs that produce sperm and testosterone.

sperm The male gamete produced by the testes and transported outside the body through ejaculation.

epididymis The portion of the male duct system in which sperm mature.

A. External structure

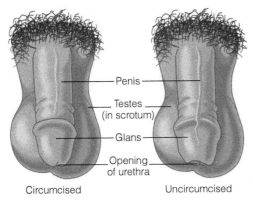

Penis
Testes (in scrotum)
Glans
Opening of urethra

Circumcised   Uncircumcised

B. Internal structure

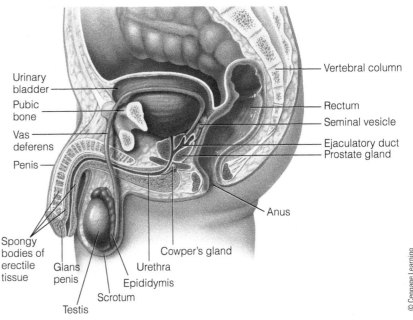

Urinary bladder
Pubic bone
Vas deferens
Penis
Vertebral column
Rectum
Seminal vesicle
Ejaculatory duct
Prostate gland
Anus
Spongy bodies of erectile tissue
Glans penis
Urethra
Cowper's gland
Epididymis
Scrotum
Testis

© Cengage Learning

FIGURE 9.4 Male Sex Organs and Reproductive Structures

Men of all ages may have concerns about the size of their penises. In a recent scholarly analysis entitled "Am I Normal?" researchers analyzed 20 studies of the penis size of more than 15,000 men around the world—all measured by physicians in clinical settings. The mean length of a flaccid penis was 3.6 inches; of both a stretched flaccid penis or an erect penis, about 5.2 inches. Penile lengths varied by 1 to 1.5 inches, and the analysis found no indications of size variability based on race.[10]

Does penis size matter? In surveys of heterosexual men and women, 85 percent of women typically report satisfaction with their partner's penis size, but only about 55 percent of the men say they are satisfied. Some men's anxiety is so distressing that they develop what therapists term "small penis anxiety" or "small penis disorder." Among those who consult physicians, almost all learn that their penises are within the normal size range. Fewer than 2 percent of men have a "micropenis," measuring two inches or less in flaccid state and less than 3.3 inches when stretched.[11]

Inside the body are several structures involved in the production of seminal fluid, or **semen**, the liquid in which sperm cells are carried out of the body during ejaculation. The **vas deferens** are two tubes that carry sperm from the epididymis into the **urethra**. The **seminal vesicles**, which make some of the seminal fluid, join with the vas deferens to form the **ejaculatory ducts**.

The **prostate gland** produces some of the seminal fluid, which it secretes into the urethra during ejaculation. The **Cowper's glands** are two pea-sized structures on either side of the urethra (just below where it emerges from the prostate gland) and connected to it via tiny ducts. When a man is sexually aroused, the Cowper's glands often secrete a fluid that appears as a droplet at the tip of the penis. This fluid is not semen, although it occasionally contains sperm.

Circumcision   In its natural state, the tip of the penis is covered by a fold of skin called the *foreskin*. About 60 percent of baby boys in the United States undergo **circumcision**, the surgical removal of the foreskin, for reasons that vary from religious traditions to preventive health measures.

The first federal guidelines affirmed that circumcision is a personal decision that may involve religious or cultural preferences. They concluded that, based on the scientific evidence, circumcision provides numerous health benefits that outweigh its risks, including the following:

- Reduction of 50 to 60 percent in the risk of getting HIV from an infected female partner

- Reduction of 30 percent or more in the risk of acquiring genital herpes and certain strains of human papillomavirus

- Lessened risk of urinary tract infections during infancy and of cancer of the penis in adulthood

✓ **check-in** If you are a man, have you been circumcised?

It also may lower a man's risk of prostate cancer. In an Australian study, uncircumcised boys and men were at significantly greater risk of infections of the kidney, bladder, and urethra. Female partners of circumcised men are less likely to develop bacterial vaginosis and *Trichomonas vaginalis* infection (discussed later in this chapter).

Additional health benefits of circumcision include the following:

- Lower risk of cancer of the penis (which is rare).

- Less risk of urinary tract infections during the first year of life. (An uncircumcised baby boy has a 1 in 100 chance of getting a urinary tract infection, compared with a 1 in 1,000 chance for a circumcised baby boy.)

- Prevention of foreskin infections and retraction.

- Easier genital hygiene.

Critics of circumcision emphasize the pain, bleeding, and risk of infections. In newborns, the estimated complication rate is 0.5 percent.[12]

Complications may include bleeding, infection, improper healing, or cutting the foreskin too long or too short. Analgesic creams or anesthetic shots are typically used to minimize discomfort. There is little consensus on what impact the presence or absence of a foreskin has on sexual function or satisfaction.

Responsible Sexuality

Most people grow up with a lot of myths and misconceptions about sex. (See this chapter's Self Survey: "How Much Do You Know about Sex?") Rather than rely on what peers say or what you've always thought was true, find out the facts.

✓ **check-in** How would you rate your knowledge about sex and sexuality?

semen The viscous whitish fluid that is the complete male ejaculate; a combination of sperm and secretions from the prostate gland, seminal vesicles, and other glands.

vas deferens Two tubes that carry sperm from the epididymis into the urethra.

urethra The canal through which urine from the bladder leaves the body; in the male, also serves as the channel for seminal fluid.

seminal vesicles Glands in the male reproductive system that produce the major portion of the fluid of semen.

ejaculatory ducts The canals connecting the seminal vesicles and vas deferens.

prostate gland A structure surrounding the male urethra that produces a secretion that helps liquefy the semen from the testes.

Cowper's glands Two small glands that discharge into the male urethra; also called bulbourethral glands.

circumcision The surgical removal of the foreskin of the penis.

This textbook is a good place to start expanding your sexual literacy. The student health center and the library can provide additional materials on sexual identity, orientation, behavior, and health, as well as on options for reducing your risk of acquiring sexually transmitted infections (discussed in Chapter 11) or becoming pregnant.

Creating a Sexually Healthy Relationship

A sexually healthy relationship, as defined by the Sexuality Information and Education Council of the United States (SIECUS), is based on shared values and has five characteristics; it is

- Consensual
- Nonexploitative
- Honest
- Mutually pleasurable
- Protected against unintended pregnancy and sexually transmitted infections

✓**check-in** If you are in a sexual relationship, does it have these five characteristics?

All individuals also have sexual rights, which include the right to the information, education, skills, support, and services they need to make responsible decisions about their sexuality, consistent with their own values, as well as the right to express their sexual orientation without violence or discrimination.

Communication is vital in a sexually healthy relationship, even though these discussions can be awkward. Yet if you have a need or a problem that relates to your partner, it is your responsibility to bring it up. (See Health on a Budget, p.256.)

Making Sexual Decisions

Sexual decision making should always take place within the context of an individual's values and perceptions of right and wrong behavior. Making responsible sexual decisions means considering all the possible consequences—including emotional consequences—of sexual behavior for both yourself and your partner. (See Health Now, page 257.)

Culture can influence sexual attitudes and activities through the messages young people receive. In a recent study, Latino college students described four types of messages from parents and friends:

- Sex is only for marriage (procreational).
- Sex is only appropriate in a loving relationship (relational).

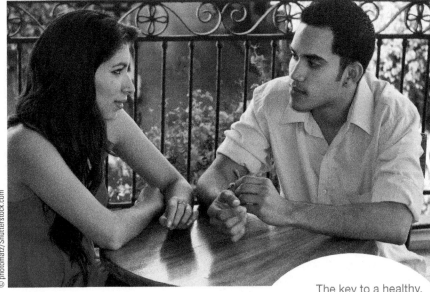

© photomatz/Shutterstock.com

The key to a healthy, happy sexual relationship is open, honest communication— even when you and your partner have different points of view.

- Sex is for pleasure (recreational).
- There is a gender-based double standard for male and female sexual behavior.

The students who received fewer procreational sex messages from parents and more recreational sex messages from friends reported higher levels of sexual exploration and assertiveness.[13]

✓**check-in** How would you describe the messages about sex you have received from parents and friends?

Prior to any sexual activity that involves a risk of sexually transmitted infection or pregnancy, both partners should talk about their prior sexual histories (including number of partners and exposure to STIs) and other high-risk behavior, such as the use of injection drugs. They should also discuss the issue of birth control and which methods might be best for them to use. If you know someone well enough to consider having sex with that person, you should be able to talk about such sensitive subjects. If a potential partner is unwilling to talk or hedges on crucial questions, you shouldn't be engaging in sex.

Here are some questions to consider as you think and talk about the significance of becoming sexually intimate with a partner:

- **What role do we want relationships and sex to have in our life at this time?**
- **What are my values and my potential partner's values as they pertain to**

Seven Secrets to a Good Sexual Relationship

The secret to a healthy, happy sexual relationship isn't a hot car or sexy outfit. It's the ability to communicate openly, honestly, and respectfully with your partner. Here are some specific suggestions:

- **Choose an appropriate time and place for an intimate discussion.** In a new relationship, talking in a public place, such as a park bench or a quiet table at a coffeehouse, can seem safer. If you're in an established relationship, choose a time when you can give each other complete attention and a setting in which you can both relax.

- **Ask open-ended questions that encourage a dialogue**—for instance, "How do you feel about . . . ?" or "What are your thoughts about . . . ?"

- **Listen actively rather than passively when your partner speaks.** Show that you're paying attention by nodding, smiling, and leaning forward. Paraphrase what he or she says to show you understand it fully.

- **Use "I" statements, such as "I really enjoy making love, but I'm so tired right now that I won't be a responsive partner.** Why don't we get the kids to bed early tomorrow so we can enjoy ourselves a little earlier?"

- **If you would like to try something different, say so.** Practice saying the words first if they embarrass you. If your partner feels uncomfortable, don't force the issue, but do try talking it through.

- **If you want to request changes or tackle a touchy topic, start with positive statements.** Let your partner know how much you enjoy having sex, and then express your desire to enjoy lovemaking more often or in different ways.

- **Encourage small changes.** If you want your partner to be less inhibited, start slowly, perhaps by suggesting sex in a different room or place.

sexual relationships? Does each of us believe that intercourse should be reserved for a permanent partnership or committed relationship?

- **Will a decision to engage in sex enhance my positive feelings about myself or my partner?** Does either of us have questions about sexual orientation or the kinds of people we are attracted to?

- **Do my partner and I both want to have sex?** Is my partner pressuring me in any way? Am I pressuring my partner? Am I making this decision for myself or for my partner?

- **Have my partner and I discussed our sexual histories and risk factors?** Have I spoken honestly about any STIs I've had in the past? Am I sure that neither my partner nor I have a sexually transmitted infection?

- **Have we taken precautions against unwanted pregnancy and STIs?**

Saying No to Sex

Whether couples are on a first date or have been married for years, each partner always has the right not to have sex. Unfortunately, "no" sometimes seems to mean different things to men and women.

The following strategies can help you assert yourself when saying no to sex:

- **Recognize your own values and feelings.** If you believe that sex is something

to be shared only by people who've already become close in other ways, be true to that belief.

- **Be direct.** Look the person in the eyes, keep your head up, and speak clearly and firmly.

- **Just say no.** Make it clear you're rejecting the offer, not the person. You don't owe anyone an explanation for what you want, but if you want to expand on your reasons, you might say, "I enjoy your company, and I'd like to do something together, but no," or "Thank you. I appreciate your interest, but no."

- **If you're still at a loss for words,** try these responses: "I like you a lot, but I'm not ready to have sex," "You're a great person, but sex isn't something I do to prove I like someone," or "I'd like to wait until I'm in a committed relationship to have sex."

- **If you're feeling pressured,** let your date know that you're uncomfortable. Be simple and direct. Watch out for emotional blackmail. If your date says, "If you really liked me, you'd want to make love," point out that if he or she really liked you, he or she wouldn't try to force you to do something you don't want to do.

- **If you're a woman, monitor your sexual signals.** Men impute more sexual meaning to gestures (such as casual touching) that women perceive as friendly and innocent.

- **Communicate your feelings** to your date sooner rather than later. It's far easier to say,

"I don't want to go to your apartment" than to fight off unwelcome advances once you're there.

- **Remember that if saying no to sex** puts an end to a relationship, it wasn't much of a relationship in the first place.

Sexual Behavior

From birth to death, we are sexual beings. Our sexual identities, needs, likes, and dislikes emerge in adolescence and become clearer as we enter adulthood, but we continue to change and evolve throughout our lives. In men, sexual interest is most intense at age 18; in women, it reaches a peak in the 30s. Although age brings changes in sexual responsiveness, we never outgrow our sexuality.

Sexuality may be timeless, but sexual behaviors change over time. According to a recent national survey of Americans aged 14 to 59, the sex lives of Americans born between 1980 and 1989 are quite different from those of Americans born in preceding decades. Among the key changes:

- Younger age for sexual initiation. The median age at first intercourse for today's "emerging adults" is 16.1 years for males and 16.2 years for females.

- The percentage of sexually active adolescents increases with age, from 13.1 percent of males and 12.5 percent of females at age 14 to more than 75 percent for both sexes at age 19.[14]

- More sexual partners. The median number of lifetime partners has risen to 8.8 for males and 5.3 for females.

- More women with same-sex partners. Among women ages 20 to 24, 14.9 percent report having had sex with another woman. The percentage of men having sex with men did not change over recent decades.

- Less of a gender gap in sexual activity. Female respondents report initiating sexual activity at about the same age as males. Men report more lifetime partners than women, but the difference has narrowed over time.[15]

Sexual Initiation: The First Time

According to a review of 35 longitudinal studies, most people have sex for the first time between the ages of 15 and 17, with 70 to 90 percent engaged in sexual behavior by age 18. First-time sexual experiences can affect a variety of health outcomes. For instance, individuals who use condoms during first intercourse are more likely to continue to do so.

The circumstances of losing one's virginity also have psychological effects. According to research, women who did not lose their virginity with a steady dating or committed partner have greater feelings of guilt and remain less comfortable with their sexuality and less sexually satisfied. Men generally have higher levels of physical and emotional satisfaction with their initial sexual experience and less anxiety and negativity than do women.

Sex on Campus

The last 40 years have brought dramatic changes in the nature and context of sexual activity among young adults. Once relatively rare, premarital sex has become common among both sexes.

College students see sexual activity as normal behavior for their peer group, but they tend to overestimate how much sex their peers are having. According to the American College Health Association National College Health Assessment, about 30 percent of undergraduates reported having no sexual partners within the last 12 months. Among sexually active students, the mean number of partners was two.[16] (See Snapshot: On Campus Now: The Sex Lives of College Students.)

In a study that compared young adults (ages 18 to 24) attending two-year colleges, four-year colleges, and no college, nonstudents were more likely than students to report multiple lifetime sexual partners and to report never using a condom. Undergraduates enrolled at two-year colleges were more likely than their counterparts at four-year schools to have had multiple partners and to have been tested for HIV.[17]

"Casual" sex, defined as any sexual experience outside a committed relationship, is common on college campuses, with estimates ranging from 14 to 64 percent among "emerging adults." At one Northeastern state college, 30 percent of undergraduates reported sexual intercourse with a stranger of brief acquaintance, while almost half engaged in some form of intimate physical interaction.[18] Students often define casual sex differently, depending on the nature of the sexual encounter (for instance, kissing versus intercourse), perceived intimacy, commitment level, and length of the acquaintance or relationship.

Hooking up

Hooking up has been defined as an experience "in which partners engage in physically intimate behaviors (such as kissing, oral sex, or sexual intercourse) without explicit expectation of future romantic commitment. Some students have

HEALTH NOW!

Developing Sexual Responsibility

The Sexuality Information and Education Council of the United States (SIECUS) has worked with nongovernmental organizations around the world to develop a consensus about the life behaviors of a sexually healthy and responsible adult. These include the following:

- Appreciating one's own body
- Seeking information about reproduction as needed
- Affirming that sexual development may or may not include reproduction or genital sexual experience
- Interacting with both genders in respectful and appropriate ways
- Affirming one's own sexual orientation and respecting the sexual orientation of others
- Expressing love and intimacy in appropriate ways
- Developing and maintaining meaningful relationships
- Avoiding exploitative or manipulative relationships
- Making informed choices about family options and lifestyles
- Enjoying and expressing one's sexuality throughout life
- Expressing one's sexuality in ways congruent with one's values
- Discriminating between life-enhancing sexual behaviors and those that are harmful to oneself and/or others

From the preceding list, choose three characteristics that you would like to improve in your intimate relationships. Why did you choose these three? Do they have special significance for you? How will you go about strengthening them? Do you have other goals for responsible sexuality? Record your reflections in your online journal.

SNAPSHOT: ON CAMPUS NOW

The Sex Lives of College Students

Students reporting having:

Oral sex within the past 30 days:

	Percent (%)		
	Male	Female	Average
No, have never done this sexual activity	25.8	28.0	27.3
No, have done this sexual activity but not in the past 30 days	28.3	26.7	27.3
Yes	45.9	45.3	45.5

Vaginal sex within the past 30 days:

	Percent (%)		
	Male	Female	Average
No, have never done this sexual activity	31.5	30.1	30.6
No, have done this sexual activity but not in the past 30 days	22.6	19.0	20.2
Yes	45.8	50.9	49.2

Most college students assume that their classmates are more sexually active than they are. As the preceding data indicate, a significant percentage have never had sexual intercourse. Those who are sexually active report a median of two partners. Do these statistics change your perception of sexual activity on campus? Do they have any influence on your own intimate relationships? Record your thoughts in your online journal.

Anal sex within the past 30 days:

	Percent (%)		
	Male	Female	Average
No, have never done this sexual activity	72.2	77.9	75.8
No, have done this sexual activity but not in the past 30 days	20.7	18.0	18.9
Yes	7	4.2	5.2

College students reporting having the following number of sexual partners (oral sex, vaginal or anal intercourse) within the past 12 months:

	Percent (%)		
	Male	Female	Average
None	29.8	29.5	29.6
1	41.4	45.5	44.0
2	9.9	10.2	10.1
3	6.3	6.1	6.2
4 or more	12.5	8.7	10.1

Source: American College Health Association. *American College Health Association–National College Health Assessment II: Reference Group Executive Summary, Spring 2014.* Hanover, MD: American College Health Association, 2014.

defined it more informally as "making out with no future" or "a one-time experience without any kind of responsibility to each other."[19] (See Chapter 5).

In studies of U.S. undergraduates, more than half—a range of 56 to 86 percent—have reported some form of hooking up. Although some report positive reactions and view hooking up as an opportunity for sexual exploration, it also involves potential risks, such as unprotected sex, unwanted sex, and emotional distress, including sexual regret, loss of self-respect, and embarrassment.[20]

The strongest predictors of hookups among students are prior hooking up, alcohol consumption, and situational factors that encourage hookups (such as spring break).

Pornography, discussed on page 264, may also play a role. According to recent research, more frequent viewing of pornography is associated with a higher incidence of hooking up and a greater number of unique hookup partners.[21]

College students hook up for a wide range of reasons: looking for sexual gratification and excitement, feeling happier and less lonely, conforming to what their peers seem to be doing, connecting with another person without making any commitment—and, conversely, increasing the likelihood of forming a committed relationship. Students' motives can influence the nature of a hookup and its consequences. Those who, for instance, want to make themselves feel less sad or lonely are more likely to engage in sex, often unprotected, with multiple partners. Women who are seeking greater intimacy are more likely to engage in oral sex or vaginal intercourse.[22]

In a recent analysis on two college campuses, students who reported at least one hookup in the previous year cited a range of motives (see Table 9.1). College men were more interested in hooking up, regardless of any specific motivator. However, the men were just as likely

hooking up An experience in which partners engage in intimate behaviors without explicit expectation of future romantic commitment.

as the women to view hooking up as a way of establishing an interpersonal relationship rather than just a quest for sexual gratification.[23]

✓**check-in** Have you ever hooked up? If so, what was your motivation?

Some earlier studies suggested that hookups were more likely to lead to psychological distress for women, who expressed greater guilt and regret and less enjoyment of sex, than men. However, a more recent, much larger analysis of almost 4,000 students ages 18 to 25 at 30 campuses came up with different results.

Among these undergraduates, 18.6 percent of the men and 7.4 percent of the women reported intercourse with someone they had known less than a week in the previous month. Both the male and female participants reported similar levels of psychological distress and diminished well-being. It may be that the students engaging in these hookups were impulsive risk-takers or may have hooked up to relieve feelings of depression or loneliness. In other words, they were distressed before engaging in casual sex. It may also be that men, just like women, hook up at least in part in the hope of finding a partner for a committed relationship—and feel disappointment and regret when that doesn't occur.[24]

Friends with Benefits

Like hookups, relationships between "friends with benefits" include varied sexual behaviors but occur between two individuals who have a friendship extending beyond a one-time sexual encounter. An estimated 45 to 50 percent of college students report engaging in a friends-with-benefits relationship in the preceding 12 months. A significant number also were involved in other sexual relationships, often with other friends.

The more committed that two partners felt to both the friendship and the sexual aspects of the relationship, the less likely they were to use condoms. Men were more likely to desire no change in such a relationship, while women preferred either going back to being "just friends" or moving into a committed romantic relationship.[25]

✓**check-in** Have you ever been in a "friends-with-benefits" relationship?

Choosing Sexual Partners

How do students choose partners (researchers sometimes use the term *targets*) for casual sex? Physical attraction may matter most. Men, according to numerous studies, are more likely to judge

TABLE 9.1 Why Do College Students Hook up?

Social-Sexual Motives
- It allows me to avoid being tied down to one person.
- It provides me with "friends with benefits."
- It provides me with sexual benefits without a committed relationship.
- It enables me to have multiple partners.

Social-Relationship Seeking Motives
- It's a way to find a relationship.
- It's the first step to forming a committed relationship.
- It can help me decide if I want something more serious with my hookup partner.

Enhancement Motives
- It's fun.
- It's sexually pleasurable.
- I'm attracted to the person.
- It's exciting.

Coping Motives
- It makes me feel good when I'm not feeling good about myself.
- It makes me feel attractive.
- It cheers me up when I'm in a bad mood.
- It helps me feel less lonely.

Conformity Motives
- I feel pressure from my friends to hook up.
- My friends will tease me if I don't.
- It helps me fit in.
- I feel I'll be left out if I don't.

Source: Kenney, Shannon R., et al. "Development and validation of the Hookup Motives Questionnaire (HMQ)." *Psychological assessment* 26.4 (2014): 1127.

an attractive woman as less risky because she looks healthy. Even when men acknowledge that an attractive woman has probably had more sexual encounters, including one-night stands, they still say they would have sex with her.

Women also see physically attractive men as more desirable short-term sexual partners than those who look less appealing. In a recent study, college women said they would be willing to have sex with a physically attractive man, even if he seemed more likely to have an STI and if the sexual encounter would be unprotected. The reasons, researchers theorize, may be that sexual arousal lowers inhibitions and impairs decision making or that "sociosexuality"—the willingness to engage in casual sexual encounters—decreases perception of risk.

Romantic Relationships

Most college students still engage in sex in the context of a romantic relationship. In one study

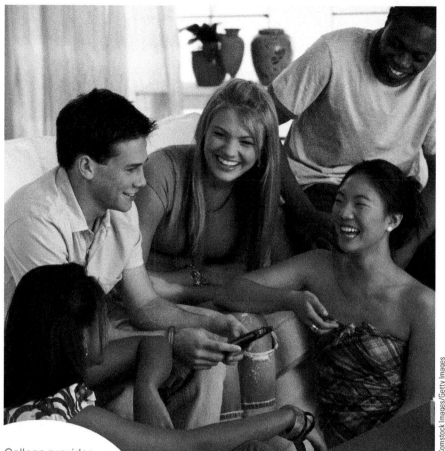

College provides opportunities for students of different backgrounds to form friendships that may or may not lead to more intimate relationships.

behaviors. Researchers raised concern about young Latina women, who have the highest teen birth rate in the United States (twice the national rate) and are at greater risk of sexually transmitted infections. Although Latinas represent about 10 percent of women over age 21, they account for 20 percent of female AIDS cases. Among college students and other populations, Latinas are more likely to engage in unprotected intercourse than women from other ethnic groups.

Acculturation—the process of adaptation that occurs when immigrants enter a new country—also affects sexual behavior. As Latina immigrants become more acculturated in the United States, some aspects of their sexual behavior become more Americanized; for instance, they become more likely to engage in nonmarital sexual activity and to have multiple partners. In a study of Cuban American college women, older, less religious, and U.S.-born Latinas were more likely to be sexually active and to engage in risky sexual behavior than other Latinas.

Sex in America

The average American adult reports having sex about once a week. However, 1 in 5 Americans has been celibate for at least a year, and 1 in 20 engages in sex at least every other day. Men report more sexual frequency than women—probably because more older women are widowed or do not have healthy partners.

Among married people, husbands and wives report having sex 58 to 59 times a year. If other differences between men and women are statistically controlled (such as sexual preference, age, and educational attainment), married women actually report a slightly higher frequency than men.

Sexual frequency peaks among those with some college education, then decreases among four-year college graduates, and declines even further among those with professional degrees. Americans who have attended graduate school are the least sexually active educational group in the population. These respondents may be more honest than others in reporting sexual activity, or they may be more precise in their definition of what counts as sex.

✓ **check-in** Do you think that sex makes people happier or healthier?

Researchers have concluded that the more sex a person has, the more likely he or she is to report

of first-year female undergraduates, romantic sexual encounters—including oral and vaginal sex—were approximately twice as common as hookup sex. "Although college students may report more hookups than first dates," researchers note, "they continue to develop romantic relationships—the most common context for sexual behavior." (See Chapter 5 for a more extensive discussion of dating on campus.)

The context of sexual activity can affect sexual enjoyment in both sexes. In a recent study, young adults who saw themselves in more-committed relationships reported enjoying their "partnered sex acts" more, on average, than those in less-committed relationships. However, there was no consistent association between sexual enjoyment and formal relationship status. The reasons may be that people who feel a commitment experience fewer inhibitions and less anxiety, are more motivated to invest time and energy in learning to please each other sexually, and communicate more successfully, ultimately providing each other with greater sexual satisfaction.

Ethnic Variations

As with other aspects of health, cultural, religious, and personal values affect students' sexual

having a happy life and marriage. This connection is stronger among women than among men. A second and more important predictor of sexual frequency is the feeling that one's life is exciting rather than routine or dull. As researchers have noted, "Increased sexual activity is one of the many benefits of having a positive attitude."

Sexual Diversity

Human beings are diverse in all ways, including sexual preferences and practices. Physiological, psychological, and social factors determine whether we are attracted to members of the same sex or the other sex. This attraction is our **sexual orientation**. **Heterosexual** is the term used for individuals whose primary orientation is toward members of the other sex. In virtually all cultures, some men and women are **homosexuals**, preferring partners of their own sex. The gender spectrum is discussed on page 263.

Heterosexuality

Heterosexuality, the most common sexual orientation, refers to sexual or romantic attraction between opposite sexes. The adjective *heterosexual* describes intimate relationships and/or sexual relations between a man and a woman. The term *straight* is used predominantly for self-identified heterosexuals of either sex. In his landmark research in the 1940s, Alfred Kinsey reported that while many men and women were exclusively heterosexual, a significant number (37 percent of men and 13 percent of women) had at least one adult sexual experience with a member of the same sex.

Bisexuality

Bisexuality—sexual attraction to both males and females—can develop at any point in one's life. Individuals may identify themselves as bisexual even if they don't behave bisexually. Some are *serial bisexuals*—that is, they are sexually involved with same-sex partners for a while and then with partners of the other sex or vice versa.

An estimated 7 to 9 million men, about twice the number thought to be exclusively homosexual, could be described as bisexual during some extended period of their lives. The largest group are married, rarely have sexual relations with women other than their wives, and have secret sexual involvements with men.

In a recent survey in the midwestern United States, behaviorally bisexual men were most likely to engage in vaginal intercourse and oral sex with both men and women, with similar reports of pleasure and arousal with male and female partners.[26]

YOUR STRATEGIES FOR PREVENTION

How to Stay Safe in the "Hookup Era"

- **Avoid drugs and excess alcohol.** Alcohol or drugs are involved in at least one-third of hookups—sometimes consumed on purpose to facilitate hooking up and sometimes the reason a hookup went farther than expected or wanted. When either or both partners drink too much, what starts off as a consensual hookup situation can get out of control and culminate in date rape (discussed in Chapter 18).

- **Plan ahead.** Think through a strategy for a situation that might lead to casual sex, whether it's deciding to leave with a friend at a certain hour or always carrying a condom if you get caught up in the heat of the moment.

- **Prepare for talking to a potential partner about safe sex.** Rehearse in your mind what you want—and need—to say to protect yourself. Inform yourself about condoms so you know how to use them correctly and can refute myths such as the assertion that they interfere with sexual pleasure (see Chapter 10).

- **Don't assume that "friends" who care about you are safe sexual partners.** They may not realize that they have an STI or may assume that they aren't infectious at the moment. Keep in mind that real friends look out for each other and take steps to ensure each other's well-being.

- **Don't let looks fool you.** Attractiveness may make someone desirable but tells you nothing about his or her sexual history and riskiness. Don't shut down your brain just because your body is aroused.

Bisexual men who try to keep their sexual relationships with men secret—often because they are married or living with a woman and do not consider themselves gay—have higher rates of mental disorders such as anxiety and depression.[27]

Fear of HIV infection has sparked concern about bisexuality, particularly among heterosexual women who worry about becoming involved with a bisexual man. About 20 to 30 percent of women with AIDS were infected by bisexual partners, and health officials note that bisexual men who hide their homosexual affairs could transmit HIV to many more women.

Homosexuality

Homosexuality—social, emotional, and sexual attraction to members of the same sex—exists in almost all cultures. Men and women attracted to same-sex partners are commonly referred to as *gays*; female homosexuals are also called *lesbians*.

Homosexuality threatens and upsets many people, perhaps because homosexuals are viewed as different, or perhaps because no one understands why some people are heterosexual and others homosexual. *Homophobia* has led to *gay bashing* (attacking homosexuals) in many communities, including college campuses.

sexual orientation The direction of an individual's sexual interest, either to members of the opposite sex or to members of the same sex.

heterosexual Primary sexual orientation toward members of the other sex.

homosexuals Those with primary sexual orientation toward members of the same sex.

bisexuality Sexually oriented toward both sexes.

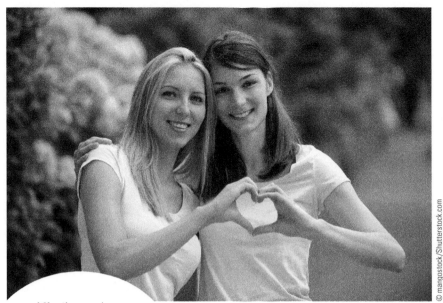

Affection and romance are significant for partners in same-sex as well as heterosexual relationships.

Different ethnic groups respond to homosexuality in different ways. To a greater extent than white homosexuals, gays and lesbians from ethnic groups tend to stay in the closet longer rather than risk alienation from their families and communities. Often they feel forced to choose between their gay and their ethnic identities.

Among men, more masculine gender identity and less spiritual meaning in life are associated with greater homophobia.[28] Young black men who have sex with men report greater gender role strain arising from conflict between homosexuality and rigid, often anti homosexual expectations of masculinity from their families, peers, and communities. As a result, they may feel greater psychological distress, try to camouflage their homosexuality, or attempt to prove their masculinity in ways that damage their self-esteem and increase social isolation.[29] Stigma may contribute to a phenomenon called "the down low" or DL, which refers to African American men who publicly present themselves as heterosexuals while secretly having sex with other men. This practice, which is neither new nor limited to African American men, can increase the risk of HIV infection in unsuspecting female partners.

Hispanic culture, with its emphasis on machismo, also has a very negative view of male homosexuality. Asian cultures, which tend to view an individual as a representative of his or her family, tend to view open declarations of sexual orientation as shaming the family and challenging their reputation and future.

Roots of Homosexuality Nobody knows what causes a person's sexual orientation. Research has discredited theories tracing homosexuality to troubled childhoods or abnormal psychological development. Sexual orientation probably emerges from a complex interaction that includes biological and environmental factors.

Coming Out Many young people have questions about their sexuality, but relatively few gay adolescents declare their homosexuality, or *come out*, while in a state of identity confusion. Many lesbian and bisexual women report that their first sexual experience occurred with a man (at the median age of 18) and that sex with a woman followed a few years later (at median age 21).

Most homosexual men and women progress through several stages:[30]

- **Stage 1: "I feel different from other kids . . ."** Many gay and lesbian teens say they sensed something "different" about themselves early in life, sometimes as far back as age 5. A boy may have liked to play house instead of sports, and vice versa for a girl. Patterns of social isolation from peers frequently start very young.

- **Stage 2: "I think I might be gay, but I'm not sure, and if I am, I'm not sure that I want to be . . ."** Many homosexual youngsters first realize that they are attracted to members of their own sex at puberty. A common response is to try to bury those feelings or to isolate themselves from other teens for fear of being exposed, or "outed."

- **Stage 3: "I accept the fact that I'm gay, but what's my family going to say?"** Homosexual men and women often do not accept their sexual orientation until their late teens or their 20s. Even then, they often fear their family's rejection or disapproval. As societal prejudice against gays and lesbians abates, boys and girls may arrive at this point somewhat earlier.

- **Stage 4: "I finally told my parents I'm gay."** In an online survey of nearly 2,000 gay and bisexual young people age 25 and under, the respondents were 16 the first time they revealed their sexuality to anyone, including their parents. Many homosexual teens don't begin to date until they're on their own— possibly on a campus or in a city with a sizable gay population. Only then do they begin having the experiences that straight kids encounter earlier in their sexual development.

Homosexuality on Campus In a study of almost 700 heterosexual students at six small liberal arts colleges, attitudes toward homosexuals and homosexuality varied, depending on students' membership in fraternities or sororities, sex-role attitudes, religion and religiosity, and contact with and knowledge of gays, lesbians, and bisexuals. The students most likely to be accepting were women, had less traditional sex-role attitudes, were less religious, attended colleges that did not have Greek social clubs, and had gay, lesbian, and/or bisexual friends.

√ **check-in** How would you describe attitudes about homosexuality on your campus?

The Gender Spectrum

Rather than divide all individuals into male or female and heterosexual, homosexual, or bisexual, experts in human sexuality have created a multidimensional gender spectrum that includes biology, gender identity, and gender expression. One person may be born female with two X chromosomes, identify as a woman, act feminine, and have sex with men; another may be born a chromosomal female, identify as a woman, act masculine, and have sex with both men and women or exclusively with women.

The **transgender** community includes individuals whose behaviors do not conform to commonly understood gender norms. These include the following:

- Transyouth (young people experiencing issues related to gender identity or expression)

- Transsexuals (who identify with a gender other than the one they were given at birth)

- Transwomen (a term for male-to-female transsexuals to signify that they are female with a male history)

- Transmen (a term for female- to-male transsexuals to signify they are male with a female history)

The terms *queer* and *gender queer* refer to a range of sexual orientations, gender behaviors, or ideologies. LGBTQQI is an acronym for lesbian, gay, bisexual, transgendered, queer/questioning, and intersex individuals. Sometimes an *A* is added for allies of these communities.

Transgender individuals may be happy with the biological sex in which they are born but enjoy dressing up and behaving like the other sex. Most do so for psychological and social pleasure rather than sexual gratification.

Some transsexuals feel trapped in the body of the wrong gender—a condition called *gender dysphoria*. In general, more men than women have this experience. Transsexualism is now viewed as a disorder that can be treated with sexual reassignment surgery. However, this intervention, which requires long psychological counseling, hormonal treatments, and complicated operations, remains controversial. Some studies report healthy postoperative functioning, while others note that many male and female transsexuals do not escape their psychological misery.

Transgender individuals face varied health risks, including unprotected sex, sexually transmitted diseases, and HIV infection. Violence, including rape, sexual abuse, physical abuse, and suicide, is a major threat.

Compared to heterosexual students, LGBT undergraduates experience multiple health inequities, including higher rates of being verbally and physically threatened and lower rates of condom use.[31] As noted in Chapter 18, they also are less to seek help after a sexual assault, primarily because "they thought they would be blamed."[32]

Sexual Activity

Part of learning about your own sexuality is having a clear understanding of human sexual behaviors. Understanding frees us from fear and anxiety so that we can accept ourselves and others as the natural sexual beings we all are.

Celibacy

A celibate person does not engage in sexual activity. Complete **celibacy** means that the person doesn't masturbate (stimulate himself or herself sexually) or engage in sexual activity with a partner. In partial celibacy, the person masturbates but doesn't have sexual contact with others. Many people decide to be celibate at certain times of their lives. Some don't have sex because of concerns about pregnancy or STIs; others haven't found a partner for a permanent, monogamous relationship. Many simply have other priorities, such as finishing school or starting a career, and realize that sex outside a committed relationship is a threat to their physical and psychological well-being.

Abstinence

The Centers for Disease Control and Prevention (CDC) defines **abstinence** as "refraining from sexual activities which involve vaginal, anal, and oral intercourse." The definition of abstinence remains a subject of debate and controversy, with

transgender Having a gender identity opposite one's biological sex.

celibacy Abstention from sexual activity; can be partial or complete, permanent or temporary.

abstinence Voluntarily refraining from sexual intercourse.

some emphasizing positive choices and others avoidance of specific behaviors. In reality, abstinence means different things to different people, cultures, and religious groups.

Increasing numbers of adolescents and young adults are choosing to remain virgins and abstain from sexual intercourse until they enter a permanent, committed, monogamous relationship. About 2.5 million teens have taken pledges to abstain from sex.

People who were sexually active in the past may choose abstinence because the risk of medical complications associated with STIs increases with the number of sexual partners a person has. Practicing abstinence is the safest, healthiest option for many. However, there is confusion about what it means to abstain, and individuals who think they are abstaining may still be engaging in behaviors that put them at risk for HIV and STIs. (See Chapter 10 for more on abstinence as a form of birth control.)

✓**check-in** What do you think are good reasons for abstaining from sex?

Among the reasons students give for abstaining are these:

- Remaining a virgin until you meet someone you love and see as a life partner
- Being true to your religious and moral values
- Getting to know a partner better
- Avoiding pregnancy
- Ensuring you're safe from sexually transmitted infections

Abstinence education programs, which received federal support and became widespread in American schools, have had little, if any, impact on teen sexual behavior.

Fantasy

The mind is the most powerful sex organ in the body, and erotic mental images can be sexually stimulating. Sexual fantasies can accompany sexual activity or be pleasurable in themselves.

Fantasies generally enhance sexual arousal, reduce anxiety, and boost sexual desire. They're also a way to anticipate and rehearse new sexual experiences, as well as to bolster a person's self-image and feelings of desirability. Part of what makes fantasies exciting is that they provide an opportunity for expressing forbidden desires, such as sex with a different partner or with a past lover.

Men and women have different types of sexy thoughts, with men's fantasies containing more explicit genital images and culminating in sexual acts more quickly than women's. In women's fantasies, emotional feelings play a greater role, and there is more kissing and caressing rather than genital contact. For many women, fantasy helps in reaching orgasm during intercourse; a loss of fantasy often is a sign of low sexual desire.

Fantasies lived out via the Internet are becoming more common but may also be harmful to psychological health. (See Consumer Alert.)

Pornography

The explosive growth of the Internet has made pornography more available, affordable, and accessible almost anywhere on computers and mobile devices. Although, as researchers put it, "the effects of pornography are probably not uniformly negative," a considerable amount of research suggests potentially negative impacts, including the following:

- Increased viewing of women as sex objects
- Increased aggression toward women
- Greater acceptance of rape
- Decreased sexual satisfaction within romantic relationships

 # CONSUMER ALERT

Safe Sex in Cyberspace

Sex is the number one word searched for online. About 15 percent of Americans logging onto the Internet visit sexually oriented sites. Most people who check out sex sites on the Internet do not suffer any negative impact, but be aware of some potential risks.

Facts to Know

- Men are the largest consumers of sexually explicit material and outnumber women by a ratio of six to one. However, while men look for visual erotica, women are more likely to visit chat rooms, which offer more interactions.

- While most individuals use their home computers when surfing the Internet for sex-related sites, one in ten has used a school computer. Some universities have strict policies barring such practices and may take punitive actions against students or employees who violate the rules.

Steps to Take

- **Limit time online.** Individuals who spend 11 hours or more a week online in sexual pursuits show signs of psychological distress and admit that their behavior interferes with some areas of their lives.

- **Be skeptical.** Most Internet surfers admit that they occasionally "pretend" about their age on the Internet. Most keep secret how much time they spend on sexual pursuits in cyberspace.

- **Monitor yourself for signs of compulsivity.** A small but significant number of users are at risk of a serious problem as a result of their heavy Internet use.

- **Don't do anything virtually that you wouldn't do in real life.** For instance, "sexting" a photo of yourself nude or partially nude to your boyfriend or girlfriend might seem funny and flirty at the time. But would you flash your body on the quad or at a mall? Remember that nothing remains totally private once it makes its way into cyberspace.

- Partner's feelings of betrayal
- More infidelity among college students in committed relationships
- Increased hooking up, with more risky behaviors (oral sex and intercourse rather than kissing and petting)
- Increased number of hookup partner.[33]

Another negative effect of pornography is its seemingly addictive nature. Therapists debate whether some individuals, usually men, develop a specific compulsion for pornography or whether their behavior is a manifestation of sexual addiction (discussed on page 273).[34] Yet those unable to curtail or limit their use of pornography can suffer intense psychological distress, including a deep sense of guilt and shame.[35]

Masturbation

Not everybody masturbates, but most people do. Kinsey estimated that 7 out of 10 women and 19 out of 20 men masturbate (and admit they do). Their reason is simple: It feels good. **Masturbation** produces the same physical responses as sexual activity with a partner and can be an enjoyable form of sexual release.

Masturbation has been described as immature; unsocial; tiring; frustrating; and a cause of hairy palms, warts, blemishes, and blindness. None of these myths is true. Sex educators recommend masturbation to adolescents as a means of releasing tension and becoming familiar with their sexual organs.

In a recent survey of college students, nearly all learned about masturbation through the media or from peers rather than from parents or teachers. Most of the women reported struggling with feelings of stigma and taboo and enjoying this pleasurable act. Most of the men saw masturbation as part of healthy sexual development.

Throughout adulthood, masturbation often is the primary sexual activity of individuals not involved in a sexual relationship and can be particularly useful when illness, absence, divorce, or death deprives a person of a partner. In a University of Chicago survey, about 25 percent of men and 9 percent of women said they masturbate at least once a week.

✓ **check-in** How do you compare with this statistic?

White men and women have a higher incidence of masturbation than African American men and women. Latina women have the lowest rate of masturbation, compared with Latino men, white men and women, and African American

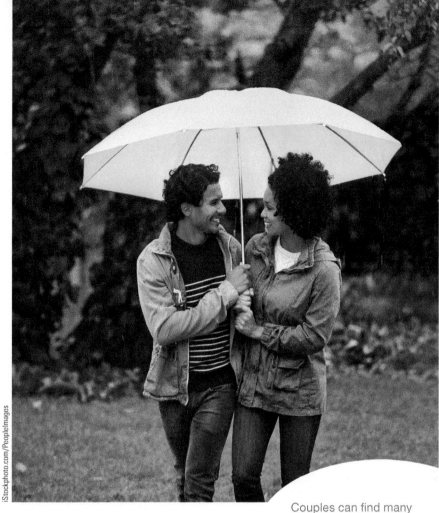

iStockphoto.com/PeopleImages

Couples can find many ways to express their affection for and delight in each other.

men and women. Individuals with a higher level of education are more likely to masturbate than those with less schooling, and people living with sexual partners masturbate more than those who live alone.

Nonpenetrative Sexual Activity (Outercourse)

Various pleasurable behaviors can lead to orgasm with little risk of pregnancy or sexually transmitted infection (also discussed in Chapter 11). The options for "outercourse" include kissing, hugging, and touching but do not involve genital-to-genital, mouth-to-genital, or insertive anal sexual contact.

A kiss can be just a kiss—a quick press of the lips—or it can lead to much more. Usually kissing is the first sexual activity that couples engage in, and even after years of sexual experimentation and sharing, it remains an enduring pleasure for partners.

Touching is a silent form of communication between friends and lovers. Although a touch to any part of the body can be thrilling, some areas, such as the breasts and genitals, are especially

masturbation Manual, (or nonmanual) self-stimulation of the genitals, often resulting in orgasm. erogenous Sexually sensitive.

sensitive. Stimulating these **erogenous** regions can lead to orgasm in both men and women. Though such forms of stimulation often accompany intercourse, more couples are gaining an appreciation of these activities as primary sources of sexual fulfillment—and as safer alternatives to intercourse.

Intercourse

Vaginal **intercourse**, or coitus, refers to the penetration of the vagina by the penis (Figure 9.5). This is the preferred form of sexual intimacy for most heterosexual couples, who may use a wide variety of positions. The most familiar position for intercourse in our society is the so-called missionary position, with the man on top, facing the woman. An alternative is the woman on top, either lying down or sitting upright. Other positions include lying side by side (either face-to-face or with the man behind the woman, his penis entering her vagina from the rear); lying with the man on top of the woman in a rear-entry position; and kneeling or standing (again, in either a face-to-face or rear-entry position). Many couples move into several different positions for intercourse during a single episode of lovemaking; others may have a personal favorite or may choose different positions at different times.

Sexual activity, including intercourse, is possible throughout a woman's menstrual cycle. However, some women prefer to avoid sex while menstruating because of uncomfortable physical symptoms, such as cramps, or concern about bleeding or messiness. Others use a diaphragm or cervical cap (see Chapter 10) to hold back menstrual flow. Since different cultures have different views on intercourse during a woman's period, partners should discuss their own feelings and try to respect each other's views. If they choose not to have intercourse, there are other gratifying forms of sexual activity.

Vaginal intercourse, like other forms of sexual activity involving an exchange of body fluids, carries a risk of sexually transmitted infections, including HIV infection. In many other parts of the world, in fact, heterosexual intercourse is the most common means of HIV transmission (see Chapter 11).

Oral Sex

The formal terms for oral sex are **cunnilingus**, which refers to oral stimulation of the woman's genitals, and **fellatio**, oral stimulation of the man's genitals. For many couples, oral sex is a regular part of their lovemaking. For others, it's an occasional experiment. Oral sex with a partner carrying a sexually transmitted infection, such as herpes or HIV infection, can lead to infection, so a condom should be used (with cunnilingus, a condom cut in half to lay flat can be used).

Anal Stimulation and Intercourse

Because the anus has many nerve endings, it can produce intense erotic responses. Stimulation of the anus by the fingers or mouth can be a source of sexual arousal; anal intercourse involves penile penetration of the anus. An estimated 25 percent of adults have experienced anal intercourse at least once. However, anal sex involves important health risks, such as damage to sensitive rectal tissues and the transmission of various intestinal infections, hepatitis, and STIs, including HIV.

Cultural Variations

While the biological mechanisms underlying human sexual arousal and response are essentially universal, the particular sexual stimuli or behaviors that people find arousing are greatly influenced by cultural conditioning. For example, in Western societies, where the emphasis during sexual activity tends to be heavily weighted toward achieving orgasm, genitally focused activities are frequently defined as optimally arousing. In contrast, devotees to Eastern Tantric traditions (where spirituality is interwoven with sexuality) often achieve optimal pleasure by emphasizing the sensual and spiritual aspects of shared intimacy rather than orgasmic release.

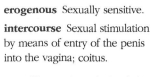

erogenous Sexually sensitive.

intercourse Sexual stimulation by means of entry of the penis into the vagina; coitus.

cunnilingus Sexual stimulation of a woman's genitals by means of oral manipulation.

fellatio Sexual stimulation of a man's genitals by means of oral manipulation.

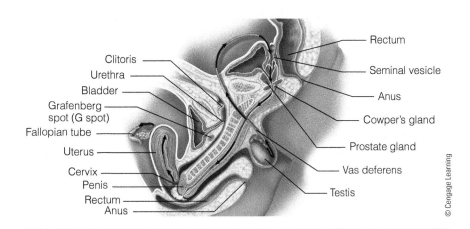

© Cengage Learning

FIGURE 9.5 A Cross-Sectional View of Sexual Intercourse

Sperm are formed in each of the testes and stored in the epididymis. When a man ejaculates, sperm carried in semen travel up the vas deferens. (The prostate gland and seminal vesicles contribute components of the semen.) The semen is expelled from the penis through the urethra and deposited in the vagina, near the cervix. During sexual excitement and orgasm in a woman, the upper end of the vagina enlarges and the uterus elevates. After orgasm, these organs return to their normal states, and the cervix descends into the pool of semen.

Kissing on the mouth, a universal source of sexual arousal in Western society, may be rare or absent in many other parts of the world. Certain North American Eskimo people and inhabitants of the Trobriand Islands would rather rub noses than lips, and among the Thonga of South Africa, kissing is viewed as odious behavior. The Hindu people of India are also disinclined to kiss because they believe such contact symbolically contaminates the act of sexual intercourse.

Oral sex (both cunnilingus and fellatio) is a common source of sexual arousal among island societies of the South Pacific, in industrialized nations of Asia, and in much of the Western world. In contrast, in Africa (with the exception of northern regions), such practices are likely to be viewed as unnatural or disgusting behavior.

Foreplay in general, whether it be oral sex, sensual touching, or passionate kissing, is subject to wide cultural variation. In some societies, most notably those with Eastern traditions, couples may strive to prolong intense states of sexual arousal for several hours. While varied patterns of foreplay are common in Western cultures, these activities often are of short duration as lovers move rapidly toward the "main event" of coitus. In still other societies, foreplay is either sharply curtailed or absent altogether. For example, the Lepcha farmers of the southeastern Himalayas limit foreplay to men briefly caressing their partners' breasts, and among the Irish inhabitants of Inis Beag, precoital sexual activity is reported to be limited to mouth kissing and rough fondling of the woman's lower body by her partner.

Sexual Response

Sexuality involves every part of you: mind and body, muscles and skin, glands and genitals. The pioneers in finding out exactly how human beings respond to sex were William Masters and Virginia Johnson, who first studied more than 800 individuals in their laboratory in the 1950s. They discovered that sexual response is a well-ordered sequence of events, so predictable it could be divided into four phases: excitement, plateau, orgasm, and resolution (Figure 9.6). In real life, individuals don't necessarily follow this well-ordered pattern. But the responses for both sexes are remarkably similar. And sexual response always follows the same sequence, whatever the means of stimulation.

Excitement

Stimulation is the first step: a touch, a look, a fantasy. In men, sexual stimuli set off a rush of blood to the genitals, filling the blood vessels in the penis. Because these vessels are wrapped in a thick sheath of tissue, the penis becomes erect. The testes lift.

Women respond to stimulation with vaginal lubrication within 10 to 20 seconds of exposure to sexual stimuli. The clitoris becomes larger, as do the vaginal lips (the labia), the nipples, and later the breasts. The vagina lengthens, and its inner two-thirds increase in size. The uterus lifts, further increasing the free space in the vagina.

Plateau

During this stage, the changes begun in the excitement stage continue and intensify. The penis further increases in both length and diameter. The outer one-third of the vagina swells. During intercourse, the vaginal muscles grasp the penis to increase stimulation for both partners. The upper two-thirds of the vagina become wider as the uterus moves up; eventually its diameter is 2½ to 3 inches.

Orgasm

Men and women have remarkably similar **orgasm** experiences. Both men and women typically have 3 to 12 pelvic muscle contractions approximately four-fifths of a second apart and lasting up to 60 seconds. Both undergo contractions and spasms of other muscles, as well as increases in breathing and pulse rates, and blood pressure. Both can sometimes have orgasms simply from kisses, stimulation of the breasts or other parts of the body, or fantasy alone.

The process of **ejaculation** (the discharge of semen by a male) requires two separate events. First, the vas deferens, the seminal vesicles, the prostate, and the upper portion of the urethra contract. The man perceives these subtle contractions deep in his pelvis just before the point of no return—which therapists refer to as the point of "ejaculatory inevitability." Then, seconds later, muscle contractions force semen out of the penis via the urethra.

Female orgasms follow several patterns. Some women experience a series of mini-orgasms—a response sometimes described as "skimming." Another pattern consists of rapid excitement and plateau stages, followed by a prolonged orgasm. This is the most frequent response to stimulation by a vibrator.

Female orgasms are primarily triggered by stimulating the clitoris. When stimulation reaches an adequate level, the vagina responds by contracting. Although it sometimes seems that vaginal stimulation alone can set off an orgasm, the clitoris is usually involved—at least indirectly during full penile penetration.

orgasm A series of contractions of the pelvic muscles occurring at the peak of sexual arousal.

ejaculation The expulsion of semen from the penis.

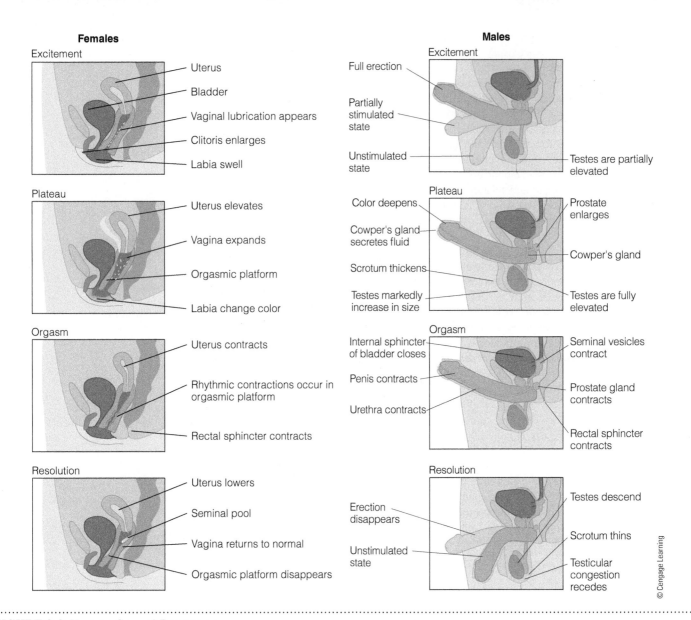

FIGURE 9.6 Human Sexual Response

The four stages of sexual response are excitement, plateau, orgasm, and resolution.

Some researchers have identified what they call the *Grafenberg* (or *G*) *spot* (or *area*) just behind the front wall of the vagina, between the cervix and the back of the pubic bone (see Figure 9.5). When this region is stimulated, women report various sensations, including slight discomfort, a brief feeling that they need to urinate, and increasing pleasure. Continued stimulation may result in an orgasm of great intensity, accompanied by ejaculation of fluid from the urethra. However, other researchers have failed to confirm the existence and importance of the G spot, and sex therapists disagree about its significance for a woman's sexual satisfaction.

As part of their sexual response, some women experience female ejaculation, the expulsion from the urethra of a fluid that is different from urine. Hundreds of studies over more than twenty years have confirmed this phenomenon and identified the chemical composition of the ejaculated fluid. G spot stimulation, orgasm, and female ejaculation are not always related. Some women report experiencing ejaculation with orgasm from clitoral stimulation; others experience ejaculation without orgasm.[36]

Is sexual satisfaction different for lesbians and heterosexual women? Not according to a recent study of married heterosexual women and lesbian/bisexual women in committed same-sex relationships. The same factors—the quality of the relationship, sexual functioning, social support, symptoms of depression—affected all the women's sexual satisfaction more than a partner's gender.

Resolution

The sexual organs of men and women return to their normal, nonexcited state during this final phase of sexual response. Heightened skin color quickly fades after orgasm, and the heart rate, blood pressure, and breathing rate soon return to normal. The clitoris also resumes its normal position and appearance very shortly thereafter, whereas the penis may remain somewhat erect for up to 30 minutes.

After orgasm, men typically enter a **refractory period**, during which they are incapable of another orgasm. The duration of this period varies from minutes to days, depending on age and the frequency of previous sexual activity. If either partner doesn't have an orgasm after becoming highly aroused, resolution may be much slower and may be accompanied by a sense of discomfort.

Other Models of Sexual Response

Since Masters and Johnson's pioneering work, other researchers have challenged and expanded their theories. Some argue that their model neglects the importance of desire in sexual response and that the plateau stage is virtually indistinguishable from excitement. Others note that arousal may come before desire, particularly for women who may not have spontaneous feelings of sexual desire.

As many experts have concluded, physiology alone can never explain the complexity of human sexual response. Desire, arousal, pleasure, and satisfaction are highly subjective. Positive feelings like trust and happiness enhance them. Negative emotions like anger and anxiety can undermine them. For women, sexual satisfaction cannot be defined, as it typically is for men, by whether or not they achieved orgasm.

Sexual Concerns

Many sexual concerns stem from myths and misinformation. There is no truth, for instance, behind these misconceptions: Men are always capable of erection, sex always involves intercourse, partners should experience simultaneous orgasms, or people who truly love each other always have satisfying sex lives.

Cultural and childhood influences can affect our attitudes toward sex. Even though America's traditionally puritanical values have eased, our society continues to convey mixed messages about sex. Some children, repeatedly warned of the evils of sex, never accept the sexual dimensions of their identity. Others—especially young boys—may be exposed to macho attitudes toward sex and feel a need to prove their virility. Young girls may feel confused by media messages that encourage them to look and act provocatively and a double standard that blames them for leading boys on. In addition, virtually everyone has individual worries. A woman may feel self-conscious about the shape of her breasts; a man may worry about the size of his penis; both partners may fear not pleasing the other.

The concept of sexual normalcy differs greatly in different times, cultures, or racial and ethnic groups. In certain times and places, only sex between a husband and wife has been deemed normal. In other circumstances, "normal" has been applied to any sexual behavior—alone or with others—that does not harm others or produce great anxiety and guilt. The following are some of the most common contemporary sexual concerns.

✓**check-in** What do you think is the most common sexual concern of people your age?

Safer Sex

Having sex is never completely safe; the only 100 percent risk-free sexual choice is abstinence. By choosing not to be sexually active with a partner, you can safeguard your physical health, your fertility, and your future.

For men and women who are sexually active, a mutually faithful sexual relationship with just one healthy partner is the safest option. For those not in such relationships, safer-sex practices are essential for reducing risks. See Chapter 10 for a complete discussion of safer sex.

Sexual Difficulties and Dysfunctions

SIECUS defines **sexual dysfunction** as the inability to react emotionally and/or physically to sexual stimulation in a way expected of the average healthy person or according to one's own standards. Sexual dysfunctions, which have a wide range of psychological and physiological origins, can affect different stages in the sexual response cycle. They are not all-or-nothing problems but vary considerably in how severe they are and how frequently they occur. In as many

refractory period The period of time following orgasm during which the male cannot experience another orgasm.

sexual dysfunction The inability to react emotionally and/or physically to sexual stimulation in a way expected of the average healthy person or according to one's own standards.

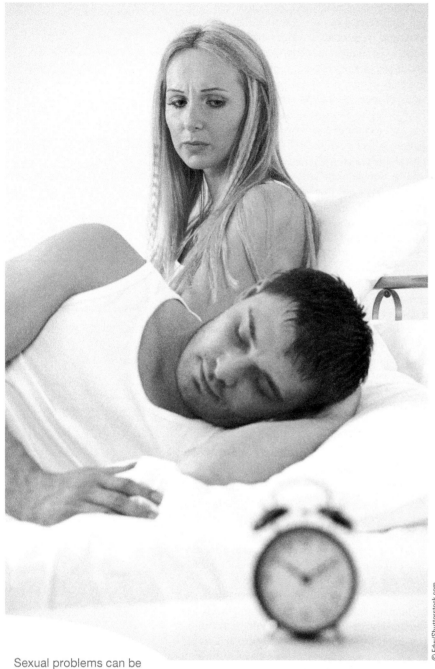

Sexual problems can be difficult for partners to talk about, but lack of communication can create tension and increase anxiety.

erectile dysfunction (ED) The consistent inability to maintain a penile erection sufficient for adequate sexual relations.

as one-third of people with sexual problems, the partner also has a sexual dysfunction.

Most men and women at one time or another experience some sort of sexual difficulty, but they tend to develop different types. The most common male sexual problems are early ejaculation, reported by 26 percent of men in a recent survey; erectile difficulties, reported by 23 percent; and lack of sexual interest, reported by 18 percent. The most common female problems are lack of sexual interest (reported by 33 percent), lubrication difficulties (reported by 22 percent), inability to reach orgasm (21 percent), and lack of sexual pleasure (20 percent).

Although sexual problems are common, fewer than 25 percent of men and women sought help from a health professional. Why don't more people seek help? Many are hesitant about bringing up the subject. Others are not informed about available treatments. Some are fatalistic and feel that nothing can help. Men are more likely to seek and receive treatment for sexual problems. Nevertheless, they find them very difficult to talk about and may delay or avoid seeking help.

Erectile Dysfunction (ED) An NIH consensus conference has defined **erectile dysfunction (ED)**, also referred to as *impotence,* as the consistent inability to maintain a penile erection sufficient for adequate sexual relations. Virtually all men are occasionally unable to achieve or maintain an erection because of fatigue, stress, alcohol, or drug use, but the incidence of erectile disorders increases with age. Recent research has overturned many common misconceptions about ED. Rather than a chronic condition that worsens with age, ED can be a temporary symptom that improves on its own much more commonly than was thought.[37]

Erectile dysfunction affects an estimated 18 million men—about 18 percent of those over age 20—in the United States. Only 5 percent of men between ages 20 and 40 report ED, which becomes more prevalent with age and illness. Both temporary and persistent ED over time can be an indicator of increased cardiovascular risk in men less than 50 years old.[38]

Psychological factors, such as anxiety about performance, may cause erectile dysfunction. But in as many as 80 percent of cases, the problem has physical origins. Diabetes and reactions to drugs—including an estimated 200 prescription medications—are the most frequent organic causes. Even cigarettes can create erection problems for men sensitive to nicotine.

Preventing Erectile Dysfunction "The way a man lives can affect the way he loves." This was the conclusion of Harvard's Health Professionals Follow-up Study, which found that healthy habits directly affect a man's risk of ED. Here are their key findings:

- **Smoking.** Men who smoke are twice as likely to develop ED as nonsmokers.

- **Exercise.** Men who exercise for 30 minutes or more a day are less likely to develop erectile dysfunction than sedentary men.

- **Obesity.** Overweight men are more likely to have ED, even after age, diabetes, exercise, and other risk factors are taken into account. For example, a man with a 42-inch waist is

© Edw/Shutterstock.com

50 percent more likely to be impotent than a man with a 32-inch waist.

- **Alcohol.** The effects of alcohol are complex: A man who averages one to two drinks a day is less likely to have erectile dysfunction than a nondrinker, but a man who drinks more will increase his risk of sexual dysfunction.

- **Cycling.** Sitting on a bicycle for a long time puts pressure on the perineum, the area between the genitals and anus. This pressure can harm nerves and temporarily block blood flow, causing tingling or numbness in the penis and eventually leading to ED. To prevent this problem
  - Wear padded biking shorts.
  - Raise the handlebars so you sit relatively upright, which shifts pressure from the perineum to the buttocks.
  - Use a wide, well-padded or gel-filled seat rather than a narrow one. Position the seat so you don't have to extend your legs fully at the bottom of your pedal stroke. Don't tilt the seat upward.
  - Shift position and take regular breaks during long rides.
  - If you feel tingling or numbness in the penis, stop riding for a week or two.

Lifestyle therapy has promise for erectile dysfunction, but men have to make changes early enough to prevent irreversible changes in the arteries and nerves required for normal sexual function.

Treating Erectile Dysfunction Men with erectile dysfunction can get help. If medication for a chronic medical problem is the culprit, a change in treatment may work. Treating underlying diseases, such as diabetes, may also help restore erectile function.

Millions of men, including about 1 percent of male undergraduates, have used the "erection pills": Viagra, Levitra, and Cialis. The three ED medications have similar success rates. In all, about 70 percent of men respond to the drugs, but the rates vary according to what is responsible for ED. About half of men with diabetes respond well, while 90 percent of those without an underlying disease benefit.

Because of their effects on the arteries, men with cardiovascular disease should try ED pills only with their doctors' supervision, and some cannot use them under any circumstances. Recent research has shown that erectile dysfunction drugs do not cause vision loss or abnormalities as once was thought. Some side effects include headache, facial flushing, nasal congestion, indigestion, and diarrhea.

Men can purchase ED drugs on the Internet, but they are taking a risk in using them without a legitimate medical evaluation. Other men turn to herbal remedies. The FDA warns that "all-natural" supplements may actually contain prescription-strength levels of Viagra that could be life-threatening for men with heart disease.

Erection drugs are not aphrodisiacs, but they can improve the erectile response to erotic stimulation. They correct impotence but do not enhance sexual performance. However, successful treatment correlates with greater emotional well-being. Wives of men treated for ED also report high levels of satisfaction with their sexual lives.

Orgasm Problems in Men About 20 percent of men complain of **premature ejaculation**, which is defined as ejaculating within 30 to 90 seconds of inserting the penis into the vagina, or after 10 to 15 thrusts. Another definition is that a premature ejaculator cannot control or delay his ejaculation long enough to satisfy a responsive partner at least half the time. By this definition, a man may be premature with some women but not with others.

To delay orgasm, men may try to think of baseball or other sports, but this just makes sex boring. Others may masturbate before intercourse, hoping to take advantage of the refractory period, during which they cannot ejaculate again. Others may bite their lips or dig their nails into their palms—although usually this just results in premature ejaculators with bloody lips and scarred palms. Topical anesthetics used to prevent climax dull pleasurable sensations for the woman as well as for the man.

Researchers are studying several medications, including clomipramine, SSRIs, and Viagra, in the treatment of premature ejaculation. The combination of medication and psychological and behavioral counseling seems most effective.

Men can learn to control their ejaculation by concentrating on their sexual responses rather than by trying to distract themselves or ignore their reactions. Some men find that they have greater control by lying on their backs with their partner on top, by relaxing during intercourse, and by communicating with their partner about when to stop or slow down movements.

Other techniques for delaying ejaculation include *stop-start*, in which a man learns to sense the feelings that precede ejaculation and stop his movements before the point of ejaculatory inevitability, allowing his arousal to subside slightly before restarting sexual activity. In the *squeeze technique*, a man's partner applies strong

premature ejaculation A sexual difficulty in which a man ejaculates so rapidly that his partner's satisfaction is impaired

pressure with the thumb on the frenum (the thin strip of skin that connects the glans to the shaft on the underside of the penis) and the second and third fingers on the top side of the penis, one above and one below the corona (rim of penile glans), until the man loses the urge to ejaculate.

Female Sexual Dysfunction The Urology Care Foundation classifies female sexual dysfunction into four categories: sexual desire disorders, arousal disorders, orgasmic disorders, and sexual pain disorders.

The most common sexual dysfunction in women is low or absent sexual desire, which peaks during midlife. Its causes may include biological, psychological, and social elements. Major risk factors are poor health, depression, certain medications, dissatisfaction with partner relationship, and a history of physical abuse, sexual abuse, or both. Treatment options include education and psychotherapy. While there are no FDA-approved medications to enhance female sexual desire, physicians may prescribe the antidepressant Bupropion or other agents.[39]

Many health professionals remain dubious about the "medicalization" of various patterns of female sexual response. A pill, whatever its nature, may not be the solution to many women's sexual concerns because psychology often is as important as or even more important than physiology. Effective therapy must address psychological problems in a sexual relationship as well as social constraints and inhibitions.

Some forms of female sexual dysfunction do respond to various therapies. These include **dyspareunia**, or pain during intercourse, and **vaginismus**, an extreme form of painful intercourse in which involuntary contractions of the muscles of the outer third of the vagina are so intense that they totally or partially close the vaginal opening. This problem often derives from a fear of being penetrated. Relaxation techniques, such as Kegel exercises (alternately tightening and relaxing the muscles of the pelvic floor), or the use of fingers or dilators to gradually open the vagina, can make penetration easier.

The female orgasm has long been a controversial sexual topic. According to recent estimates, about 90 percent of sexually active women have experienced orgasm, but only a much smaller percentage achieve orgasm through intercourse alone. Even fewer reach orgasm if intercourse isn't accompanied by direct stimulation of the clitoris. Is intercourse without orgasm a sexual problem? The best answer is that it is a problem if a woman wants to experience orgasm during intercourse but doesn't.

Many counseling programs urge women who have never had orgasms to masturbate. They are then encouraged to share with their partners what they've learned, communicating with words or gestures what is most pleasing to them. Some women want more than a single orgasm during intercourse. Partners can help by varying positions and experimenting with sexual techniques. However, in sexual response, more is not necessarily better, and the couple should keep in mind that no one else is counting.

Sex Therapy

Modern sex therapy, pioneered by Masters and Johnson in the 1960s, views sex as a natural, healthy behavior that enhances a couple's relationship. Their approach emphasizes education, communication, reduction of performance anxiety, and sexual exercises that enhance sexual intimacy.

Today most sex therapists, working either alone or with a partner, have modified Masters and Johnson's approach. Most see couples once a week for eight to ten weeks; the focus of therapy is on correcting dysfunctional behavior, not exploring underlying psychodynamics.

Contrary to common misconceptions, sex therapy does not involve conducting sexual activity in front of therapists. The therapist may review psychological and physiological aspects of sexual functioning and evaluate the couple's sexual attitudes and ability to communicate. The core of the program is the couple's "homework"—a series of exercises, carried out in private, that enhances their sensory awareness and improves nonverbal communication. These techniques have proved effective for couples regardless of their age or general health.

You and your partner should consider consulting a sex therapist if any of the following is true for you:

- Sex is painful or physically uncomfortable.
- You're having sex less and less frequently.
- You have a general fear of, or revulsion toward, sex.
- Your sexual pleasure is declining.
- Your sexual desire is diminishing.
- Your sexual problems are increasing in frequency or persisting for longer periods.

Drugs and Sex

Many recreational drugs, such as alcohol and marijuana, are believed to enhance sexual performance. However, none of the popular drugs touted as *aphrodisiacs*—including amphetamines, barbiturates, cantharides ("Spanish fly"), cocaine, LSD and other psychedelics, marijuana, amyl nitrite ("poppers"), and L-dopa (a medication used to

dyspareunia A sexual difficulty in which a woman experiences pain during sexual intercourse.

vaginismus A sexual difficulty in which a woman experiences painful spasms of the vagina during sexual intercourse.

treat Parkinson's disease)—is truly a sexual stimulant. In fact, these drugs often interfere with normal sexual response. Researchers are studying one drug that may truly enhance sexual performance: yohimbine hydrochloride, which is derived from the sap of the tropical yohimbe tree that grows in West Africa.

Because many psychiatric problems can lower sexual desire and affect sexual functioning, medications appropriate to the specific disorders can help. In addition, psychiatric drugs may be used as part of therapy. Drugs such as certain antidepressants may be used to prolong sexual response in conditions such as premature ejaculation.

Medications can also cause sexual difficulty. In men, drugs that are used to treat high blood pressure, anxiety, allergies, depression, muscle spasms, obesity, ulcers, irritable colon, and prostate cancer can cause impotence, breast enlargement, testicular swelling, priapism (persistent erection), loss of sexual desire, inability to ejaculate, and reduced sperm count. In women, they can diminish sexual desire, inhibit or delay orgasm, and cause breast swelling or secretions.

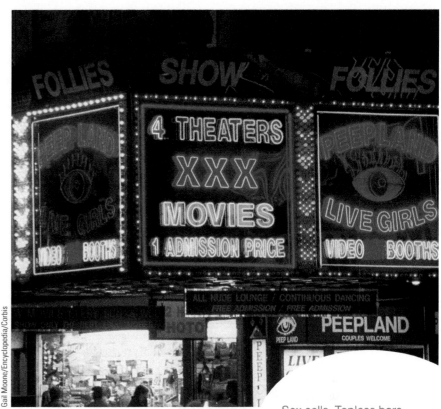

Gail Moone/Encyclopedia/Corbis

Sex sells. Topless bars and strip clubs are among the businesses that cater to those who enjoy sexual stimulation outside a loving relationship.

Atypical Behavior

Although sexual desire and response are universal, some individuals develop sexual appetites or engage in activities that are not typical sexual behaviors.

Sexual Addiction

Some men and women can get relief from their feelings of restlessness and worthlessness only through sex (either masturbation or with a partner). Once the sexual high ends, however, they're overwhelmed by the same negative feelings and driven, once more, to have sex.

Some therapists describe this problem as sexual addiction; others, as sexual compulsion. Professionals continue to debate exactly what this controversial condition is, how to diagnose it, and how to overcome it. However, most agree that for some people, sex is more than a normal pleasure: It is an overwhelming need that must be met, even at the cost of their careers and marriages.

Sex addicts can be heterosexual or homosexual, male or female. Their behaviors include masturbation, phone sex, reading or viewing pornography, attending strip shows, having affairs, engaging in anonymous sex with strangers or prostitutes, exhibitionism, voyeurism, child

molestation, incest, and rape. Many were physically and emotionally abused as children or have family members who abuse drugs or alcohol. They typically feel a loss of control and a compulsion for sexual activity, and they continue their unhealthy (and sometimes illegal) sexual behavior despite the dangers, including the risk of contracting STIs.

With help, sex addicts can deal with the shame that both triggers and follows sexual activity. Professional therapy may begin with a month of complete sexual abstinence, to break the cycle of compulsive sexual behavior. Several organizations, such as Sexaholics Anonymous and Sex Addicts Anonymous, offer support from people who share the same problem.

Sexual Deviations

Sexual deviations include the following:

- **Fetishism.** Obtaining sexual pleasure from an inanimate object or an asexual part of the body, such as the foot.

- **Transvestitism.** Becoming sexually aroused by wearing the clothing of the opposite sex.

- **Exhibitionism.** Exposing one's genitals to an unwilling observer.

- **Voyeurism.** Obtaining sexual gratification by observing people undressing or involved in sexual activity.

- **Sadism.** Becoming sexually aroused by inflicting physical or psychological pain.

- **Masochism.** Obtaining sexual gratification by suffering physical or psychological pain.

Another, increasingly common sexual variation, hypoxyphilia, involves attempts to enhance the pleasure of orgasm by reducing oxygen intake. Individuals who do so by tying a noose around the neck have accidentally killed themselves.

Psychiatrists distinguish between passive sexual deviancy, which doesn't involve actual contact with another, and aggressive deviancy. Most voyeurs and obscene phone callers don't seek physical contact with the objects of their sexual desire. These behaviors are performed predominantly, but not exclusively, by males.

The Business of Sex

Sex, without affection and individuality, becomes a product to be packaged, marketed, traded, bought, and sold. Two of the billion-dollar industries that treat sex as a commodity are prostitution and pornography.

Prostitution, described as the world's oldest profession, is a nationwide industry grossing more than $1 billion annually. In every state except Nevada (and in all but a few counties there), prostitution is illegal. Besides the threat of jail and fines, prostitutes and their clients face another danger: sexually transmitted infections, including HIV infection and hepatitis B.

Pornography is a multimedia industry—books, magazines, movies, the Internet, phone lines, and computer games are available to those who find sexually explicit material entertaining or exciting. Most laws against pornography are based on the assumption that such materials can set off uncontrollable, dangerous sexual urges, ranging from promiscuity to sexual violence. Research indicates that exposure to scenes of rape or other forms of sexual violence against women, or to scenes of degradation of women, does lead to tolerance of these hostile and brutal acts.

WHAT DID YOU DECIDE?

- What are the basic hormonal and anatomical differences between men and women?
- What should college students know about hooking up?
- What are the sexual preferences and behaviors of American adults?
- What are the phases of sexual response?

THE POWER OF NOW!
Being Sexually Responsible

We remain sexual beings throughout life. At different ages and stages, sexuality can take on different meanings. As you forge relationships and explore your sexuality, you may encounter difficult situations and unfamiliar feelings. But sex is never just about hormones and body parts. People describe the brain as the sexiest of our organs. Using your brain to make responsible sexual decisions leads to both a smarter and a more fulfilling sex life.

Which of the following characterize your behavior or the way you would want to behave in an intimate relationship?

_____ Communicate openly. If you or your partner cannot talk openly and honestly about your sexual histories and contraception, you should avoid having sex. For the sake of protecting your sexual health, you have to be willing to ask—and answer—questions that may seem embarrassing.

_____ Share responsibility in a sexual relationship. Both partners should be involved in protecting themselves and each other from STIs and, if heterosexual, unwanted pregnancy.

_____ Respect sexual privacy. Revealing sexual activities violates the trust between two partners. Bragging about a sexual conquest demeans everyone involved.

_____ Never sexually harass others. Pinches, pats, sexual comments or jokes, and suggestive gestures are offensive and disrespectful.

_____ Be considerate. A public display of sexual affection can be extremely embarrassing to others. Roommates, in particular, should be sensitive and discreet in their sexual behavior.

_____ Be prepared. If there's any possibility that you may be engaging in sex, be sure you have the means to protect yourself against unwanted pregnancy and sexually transmitted infections.

_____ In sexual situations, always think ahead. For the sake of safety, think about potential dangers—parking in an isolated area, going into a bedroom with someone you hardly know, and the like—and options to protect yourself.

_____ Be aware of your own and your partner's alcohol and drug intake. The use of such substances impairs judgment and reduces the ability to say no. While under their influence, you may engage in sexual behavior you'll later regret.

_____ Be sure sexual activity is consensual. Coercion can take many forms: physical, emotional, and verbal. All cause psychological damage and undermine trust and respect. At any point in a relationship, whether the couple is dating or married, either individual has the right to say no.

Source: Adapted from Robert Hatcher et al., *Sexual Etiquette 101 and More* (Atlanta, GA: Emory University School of Medicine, 2002).

What's Online

CENGAGE
brain.com

Visit www.cengagebrain.com to access course materials for this text, including the Behavior Change Planner, interactive quizzes, tutorials, and more.

self survey

How Much Do You Know about Sex?

Mark each of the following statements True or False:

1. **True** or **False**: Men and women have completely different sex hormones.

2. **True** or **False**: Premenstrual syndrome (PMS) is primarily a psychological problem.

3. **True** or **False**: Circumcision diminishes a man's sexual pleasure.

4. **True** or **False**: Sexual orientation may have a biological basis.

5. **True** or **False**: Masturbation is a sign of emotional immaturity.

6. **True** or **False**: Only homosexual men engage in anal intercourse.

7. **True** or **False**: Despite their awareness of AIDS, many college students do not practice safe sex.

8. **True** or **False**: After age 60, lovemaking is mainly a fond memory, not a regular pleasure of daily living.

9. **True** or **False**: Doctors advise against having intercourse during a woman's menstrual period.

10. **True** or **False**: Only men ejaculate.

11. **True** or **False**: It is possible to be infected with HIV during a single sexual encounter.

12. **True** or **False**: Impotence is always a sign of emotional or sexual problems in a relationship.

Scoring

1. **False.** Men and women have the same hormones, but in different amounts.

2. **False.** PMS has been recognized as a physiological disorder that may be caused by a hormonal deficiency, abnormal levels of thyroid hormone, or social and environmental factors such as stress.

3. **False.** Sex therapists have not been able to document differences in sensitivity to stimulation between circumcised and uncircumcised men.

4. **True** Researchers documented structural differences in the brains of homosexual men and women.

5. **False.** Throughout a person's life, masturbation can be a form of sexual release and pleasure.

6. **False.** As many as one in every four married couples under age 35 have reported that they occasionally engage in anal intercourse.

7. **True** In one recent study, more than a third of college students had engaged in vaginal or anal intercourse at least once in the previous year without using effective protection from conception or sexually transmitted infections (STIs).

8. **False.** More than a third of American married men and women older than 60 make love at least once a week, as do 10 percent of those older than 70.

9. **False.** There's no medical reason to avoid intercourse during a woman's menstrual period.

10. **False.** Some researchers say that stimulation of the Grafenberg spot in a woman's vagina may lead to a release of fluid from her urethra during orgasm.

11. **True** Although the risk increases with repeated sexual contact with an infected partner, an individual can contract HIV during a single sexual encounter.

12. **False.** Many erection difficulties have physical causes.

MAKING THIS CHAPTER WORK FOR YOU

Review Questions

(LO 9.1) 1. At its deepest and most fulfilling level, when sexuality uplifts the soul of an individual by allowing her or him to connect to something greater than her- or himself, the _____ aspect of sexuality is the focus.
   a. spiritual
   b. intellectual
   c. emotional
   d. environmental

(LO 9.1) 2. When an individual expresses and fulfills his or her sexual identities in the context of family and friends, the _____ aspect of sexuality is the focus.
   a. spiritual
   b. social
   c. emotional
   d. environmental

(LO 9.2) 3. Which of the following is a characteristic of sexually healthy relationships, according to the Sexuality Information and Education Council of the United States?
   a. It is open ended.
   b. It is exploitative.
   c. It is pleasurable to either of the sexual partners.
   d. It is protected against unintended pregnancy.

(LO 9.2) 4. Which of the following statements is true in the context of saying no to sex?
   a. It is important to prioritize the partner's feelings over one's own feelings and values.
   b. Men impute more sexual meaning to gestures than women.
   c. When declining sex, suggestive gestures are preferred over direct communication.
   d. Saying no to sex means the same for men and women.

(LO 9.3) 5. Which of the following is true of sexual behavior of young adults in college?
   a. Sexual interest peaks at age 18 in both men and women.
   b. Young adults who graduated from college report more lifetime sexual partners than those without a high school degree.
   c. College students report less conservative sex-related attitudes and behaviors than their non-college peers.
   d. Most college students still engage in sex in the context of a romantic relationship.

(LO 9.3) 6. Which of the following statements is true about sexual behaviors among young adults?
   a. An individual's sexual identity remains constant throughout his or her life.
   b. The average American teenager reports having sex at least once a week.
   c. College students, in general, prefer hookups over romantic relationships.
   d. The context of sexual activity affects sexual enjoyment in both sexes.

(LO 9.4) 7. _____ refers to sexual attraction to both males and females.
   a. Bisexuality
   b. Celibacy
   c. Heterosexuality
   d. Abstinence

(LO 9.4) 8. In the context of sexual diversity, the feeling of being trapped in the wrong body is known as _____.
   a. heterosexuality
   b. gender dysphoria
   c. toxic shock syndrome
   d. amenorrhea

(LO 9.5) 9. _____ means that a person doesn't masturbate or engage in sexual activity with a partner.
   a. Celibacy
   b. Abstinence
   c. Fantasy
   d. Outercourse

(LO 9.5) 10. _____ refers to oral stimulation of a woman's genitals.
   a. Cunnilingus
   b. Fellatio
   c. Circumcision
   d. Abstinence

(LO 9.6) 11. The process of discharge of semen by a male is known as _____.
   a. masturbation
   b. menstruation
   c. ejaculation
   d. circumcision

(LO 9.6) 12. After orgasm, men typically enter a(n) _____, during which they are incapable of another orgasm.
   a. abstinence period
   b. refractory period
   c. excitement stage
   d. plateau stage

(LO 9.7) 13. Sexual dysfunction is _____.
   a. having gender identity uncertainty
   b. wishing to have sex every day
   c. enjoying sex with both males and females
   d. the inability to react emotionally and/or physically to sexual stimulation in a way expected of an average healthy individual

(LO 9.7) 14. Certain otherwise healthy habits may increase a male's risk of erectile dysfunction. Which of the following might be a cause?
   a. Giving up smoking
   b. Cycling
   c. Maintaining a healthy weight
   d. Exercising regularly

(LO 9.8) 15. Which of the following is *not* considered a sexual deviation?
   a. Voyeurism
   b. Transvestitism
   c. Homosexuality
   d. Fetishism

(LO 9.8) 16. Common characteristics of sex addicts include which of the following?
   a. Having a fairly normal childhood
   b. Feelings of being in control
   c. Feelings of compulsion for sexual activity
   d. Having stable intimate relationships

Answers to these questions can be found on page 623.

Critical Thinking Questions

1. Have you come across an individual who displays expressions of alternate sexuality? If so, have you thought about the reasons, or what kind of alternate sexuality the individual displays? In the context of sexual diversity, think about the various types of sexualities other than heterosexuality into which individuals fall and analyze the risk factors of each category.

2. While engaging in sexual activity with a partner, have you ever thought about the risks of a sexually transmitted infection? Analyze the characteristics and risk factors of sexually transmitted diseases and evaluate where you and your partner stand.

3. Have you come across an individual who is infected with HIV? If so, what are the symptoms he or she displays?

Additional Online Resources

www.siecus.org
This website is sponsored by SIECUS, a national nonprofit organization that promotes comprehensive education about sexuality and advocates the right of all individuals of all sexual orientations to make responsible sexual choices. The site features a library of fact sheets and articles on a variety of sexuality topics and STIs designed for educators, adults, teens, parents, media, international audiences, and religious organizations.

www.hrc.org
The Human Rights Campaign is America's largest gay, lesbian, bisexual, and transgender civil rights organization. Its website features up-to-date information on issues related to gay rights and suggests courses of action to change government policies.

http://goaskalice.columbia.edu/
Sponsored by the health education and wellness program of the Columbia University Health Service, this site features educators' answers to questions on a wide variety of topics of concern to young people, including those related to sexual orientation and healthy sexuality.

www.nlm.nih.gov/medlineplus/sexualhealth.html
Here you can find trusted information on sexual health from MedlinePlus, a site maintained as a service of the U.S. National Library of Medicine and the National Institutes of Health (NIH).

Key Terms

The terms listed are used on the page indicated. Definitions of the terms are in the glossary at the end of the book.

abstinence   263

amenorrhea   253

androgyny   249

bisexuality   261

celibacy   263

cervix   249

circumcision   254

clitoris   249

corpus luteum   250

Cowper's glands   254

cunnilingus   266

dysmenorrhea   252

dyspareunia   272

ejaculation   267

ejaculatory ducts   254

endocrine system   247

endometrium   249

epididymis   253

erectile dysfunction (ED)   270

erogenous   266

estrogen   247

fallopian tubes   249

fellatio   266

gender   247

gonadotropins   247

heterosexual   261

homosexuals   261

hooking up   258

hormones   247

intercourse   266

intimacy   246

labia majora   249

labia minora   249

masturbation   263

menarche   248

menstruation   250

mons pubis   249

orgasm   267

ovaries   249

ovulation   250

ovum   249

penis   253

perineum   249

premature ejaculation   271

premenstrual dysphoric disorder (PMDD)   252

premenstrual syndrome (PMS)   250

progesterone   247

prostate gland   254

refractory period   269

scrotum   253

secondary sex characteristics   247

semen   254

seminal vesicles   254

sex   246

sexual dysfunction   269

sexual health   246

sexual orientation   261

sexuality   246

sperm   253

testes   253

testosterone   247

toxic shock syndrome (TSS)   253

transgender   263

urethra   254

urethral opening   249

uterus   249

vagina   249

vaginismus   272

vas deferens   254

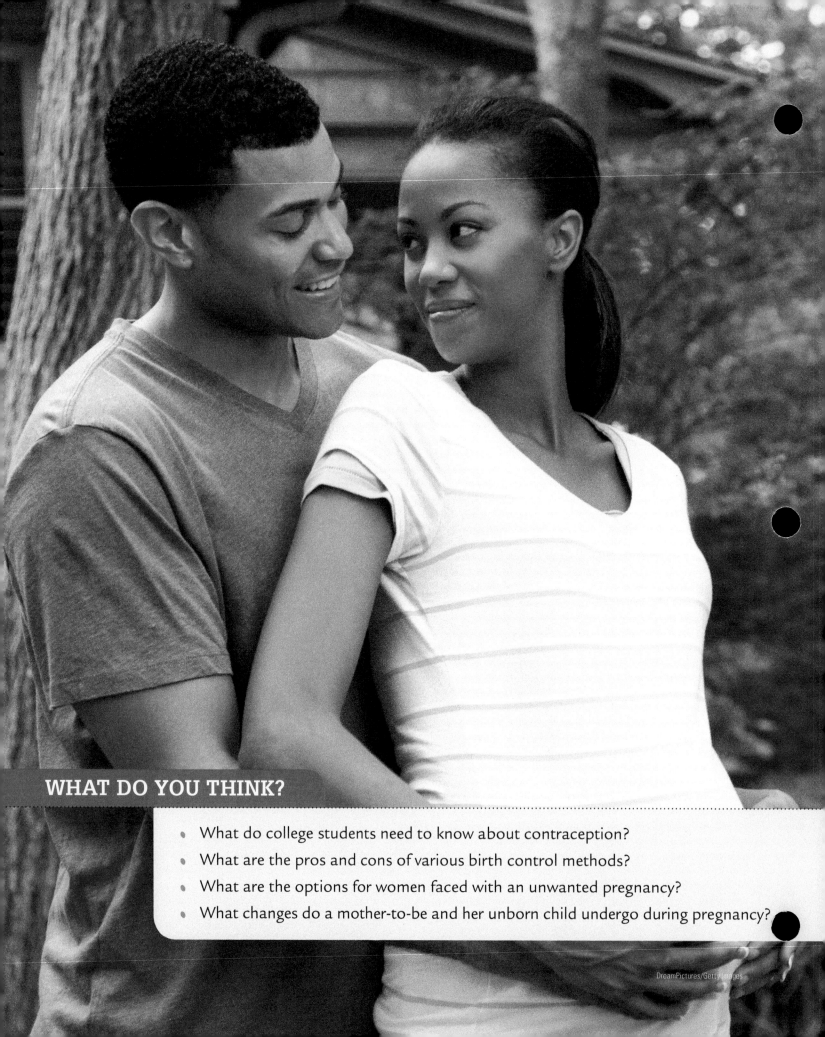

WHAT DO YOU THINK?

- What do college students need to know about contraception?
- What are the pros and cons of various birth control methods?
- What are the options for women faced with an unwanted pregnancy?
- What changes do a mother-to-be and her unborn child undergo during pregnancy?

DreamPictures/Getty Images

10

Reproductive Choices

Justin and Sara, second-year students at the same community college, can't remember a time when abortion was illegal, when AIDS wasn't a deadly threat, and when safe sex wasn't a concern of every sexually active individual. Yet even though they were aware of the risks and the realities involved, neither used contraception during every single sexual encounter. Then one of Justin's partners had a pregnancy scare. He decided never again to engage in unprotected sex. Sara had a different reality check:

At her regular physical, she learned that she had contracted chlamydia, the most common sexually transmitted infection in the United States.

"When we started dating," Sara recalls, "both of us felt that something was special about our relationship." Despite their mutual attraction, they decided to take every step toward intimacy slowly. Both considered and talked about their personal priorities and concerns. Even though it was awkward,

they also discussed their own sexual histories and underwent tests for STIs.

Looking toward a continuing committed relationship, they decided on not one but two forms of contraception: the birth control pill and a condom. In the future, they realized that they might switch to other forms of birth control or consider different options, including both marriage and parenthood.

After reading this chapter, you should be able to:

10.1 Explore issues that should be considered when choosing either to reproduce or not to reproduce.

10.2 Describe the process of conception from spermatogenesis to implantation.

10.3 Explain abstinence and nonpenetrative sexual activity.

10.4 Summarize the methods, benefits, risks, and incidences of contraception.

10.5 Describe the major types of contraceptives, their benefits, and their risks.

10.6 Outline the stages of pregnancy and childbirth.

10.7 Give examples of options available to childless couples.

As human beings, we have a unique power: the ability to choose to conceive or not to conceive. No other species on earth can separate sexual activity and pleasure from reproduction. However, simply not wanting to get pregnant is never enough to prevent conception, nor is wanting to have a child always enough to get pregnant. Both desires require individual decisions and actions.

This chapter provides information on conception, birth control, abortion, infertility, adoption, and the processes by which a new human life develops and enters the world. ◄

Reproductive Responsibility

Anyone who engages in vaginal intercourse must be willing to accept the consequences of that activity—the possibility of pregnancy and responsibility for the child who might be conceived—or take action to avoid those consequences.

The typical American woman who wants two children spends about five years pregnant or trying to become pregnant and three decades—more than three-quarters of her reproductive life—trying to avoid pregnancy. As many as half of pregnancies in the United States each year are unintended; most are the result of not using birth control.

If you are engaging in sexual activity that could lead to conception, you have to be realistic about your situation. This means assuming full responsibility for your reproductive ability, whether you're a man or a woman. The more you know about contraception, the more likely you are to use birth control.

In a survey of 1,800 unmarried young adults, aged 18 to 29 years, "doctors/nurses" were the most frequently used—and the most accurate—contraceptive information sources. Young women are more likely to rely on health-care professionals, whereas men are more likely to turn to friends, partners, the Internet, or the media.[1]

✓**check-in** Where do you turn for information on contraception?

While getting information is a crucial first step, communicating with your partner is equally important. Regardless of their age, couples who engage in honest, open conversations about contraception are more likely to use birth control consistently and correctly.[2]

Reproductive responsibility involves more than protection against pregnancy. Even on a woman's most fertile day of the month, her risk of becoming pregnant is less than half her risk of acquiring an STI from an infected partner (see Chapter 11). Yet the risk of an STI exists only with infected partners, whereas the risk of pregnancy exists with virtually all partners.[3]

The bottom line is that it takes two people to conceive a baby, and two people should be involved in deciding not to conceive a baby. In the process, they can also enhance their skills in communication, critical thinking, and negotiating.

✓**check-in** How do you take responsibility for your reproductive ability?

Conception

The equation for making a baby is quite simple: One sperm plus one egg equals one fertilized egg, which can develop into an infant. But the processes that affect or permit **conception** are quite complicated:

- The creation of sperm, or **spermatogenesis**, starts in the male at puberty, and the production of sperm is regulated by hormones.

- Sperm cells form in the seminiferous tubules of the testes and are passed into the epididymis, where they are stored until ejaculation.

- A single male ejaculation may contain 500 million sperm. Each sperm released into the vagina during intercourse moves on its own, propelling itself toward its target, an ovum.

- To reach its goal, the sperm must move through the acidic secretions of the vagina, enter the uterus, travel up the fallopian tube containing the ovum, then fuse with the nucleus of the egg (**fertilization**). Almost every sperm produced by a man in his lifetime fails to accomplish its mission.

- There are far fewer human egg cells than there are sperm cells. Each woman is born with her lifetime supply of ova, and between 300 and 500 eggs eventually mature and leave her ovaries during ovulation.

- As discussed in Chapter 9, every month, one or the other of the woman's ovaries releases

conception The merging of a sperm and an ovum.

spermatogenesis The process by which sperm cells are produced.

fertilization The fusion of sperm and egg nucleus.

zygote A fertilized egg.

blastocyst In embryonic development, a ball of cells with a surface layer and an inner cell mass.

implantation The embedding of the fertilized ovum in the uterine lining.

an ovum to the nearby fallopian tube. It travels through the fallopian tube until it reaches the uterus, a journey that takes three to four days.

- An unfertilized egg lives for about 24 to 36 hours, disintegrates, and during menstruation is expelled along with the uterine lining.

- Even if a sperm, which can survive in the female reproductive tract for two to five days, meets a ripe egg in a fallopian tube, its success is not ensured. A mature ovum releases the chemical allurin, which attracts the sperm. A sperm is able to penetrate the ovum's outer membrane because of a protein called fertilin. The egg then pulls the sperm inside toward its nucleus (Figure 10.1).

- The fertilized egg, called the **zygote**, travels down the fallopian tube, dividing to form a tiny clump of cells called a **blastocyst**. When it reaches the uterus, about a week after fertilization, it burrows into the endometrium, the lining of the uterus. This process is called **implantation**.

What are the chances that a single act of intercourse will result in pregnancy? It depends on a woman's menstrual cycle. If intercourse occurs within her fertile window (menstrual days 12 to 22), the odds of pregnancy can be as high as 25 percent, according to recently revised calculations.[4]

Abstinence and Nonpenetrative Sexual Activity

The contraceptive methods discussed in this chapter are designed to prevent pregnancy resulting from vaginal intercourse. Couples who choose abstinence make a very different decision—to abstain from vaginal intercourse and forms of nonpenetrative sexual activity that could result in conception (any in which ejaculation occurs near the vaginal opening).

People choose abstinence for various reasons, including the following:

- Waiting until they are ready for a sexual relationship

- Waiting until they find the "right" partner

- Respecting religious or moral values

- Enjoying friendships without sexual involvement

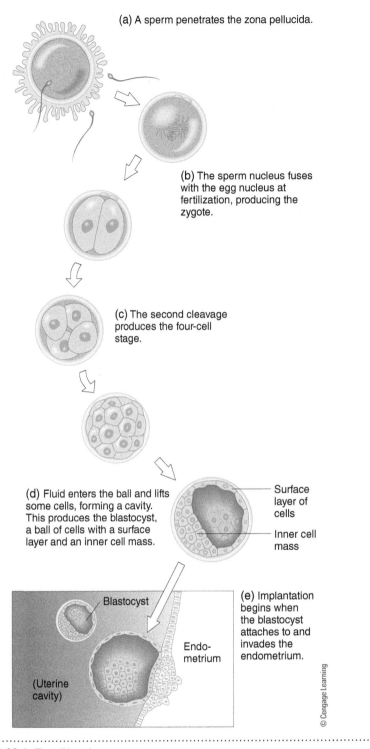

(a) A sperm penetrates the zona pellucida.

(b) The sperm nucleus fuses with the egg nucleus at fertilization, producing the zygote.

(c) The second cleavage produces the four-cell stage.

(d) Fluid enters the ball and lifts some cells, forming a cavity. This produces the blastocyst, a ball of cells with a surface layer and an inner cell mass.

Surface layer of cells

Inner cell mass

(e) Implantation begins when the blastocyst attaches to and invades the endometrium.

Blastocyst

Endo-metrium

(Uterine cavity)

© Cengage Learning

FIGURE 10.1 Fertilization

(a) The efforts of hundreds of sperm may allow one to penetrate the ovum's corona radiate, an outer layer of cells, and then the zona pellucida, a thick inner membrane. (b) The nuclei of the sperm and the egg cells merge, and the male and female chromosomes in the nuclei come together, forming a zygote. (c) The zygote divides into two cells, then four cells, and so on. (d) As fluid enters the ball, cells form a ball of cells called a blastocyst. (e) The blastocyst implants itself in the endometrium.

Contraception

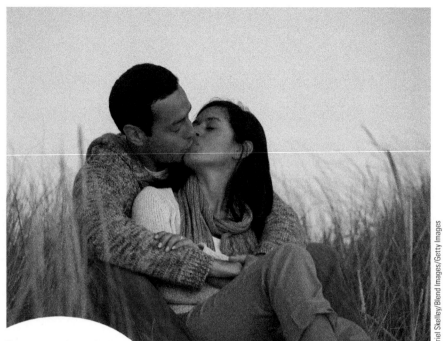

Some couples refrain from intercourse by engaging in outercourse, or intimacy that includes kissing and hugging.

Conception can be prevented by **contraception**. Some contraceptive methods prevent ovulation or implantation, and others block the sperm from reaching the egg. Some methods are temporary; others permanently alter one's fertility.

Contraception has an enormous impact on women's lives. According to the World Health Organization, 87 million women experience an unintended pregnancy every year. Many, particularly in low-income developing countries, face the risks of lower educational and job opportunities, disability, disease, and even death. The use of modern methods of contraception—condoms, intrauterine devices, oral and injectable contraceptives, implants, and sterilization—could prevent as many as four in five unwanted pregnancies every year.[5]

Even among educated women in developed countries, knowledge of conception and contraception is often limited, as a nationwide online survey of about 1,000 reproductive-age women in the United States showed. Younger women (ages 18 to 24) had less knowledge than older ones about conception and fertility and were often unaware that STIs, obesity, or irregular menstrual cycles could affect their ability to get pregnant.

✓**check-in** How would you rate your knowledge of conception and reproduction?

Some couples use withdrawal, or **coitus interruptus** (removal of the penis from the vagina before ejaculation), to prevent pregnancy, even though this is not a reliable form of birth control. About half the men who have tried coitus interruptus find it unsatisfactory, either because they cannot anticipate when they're going to ejaculate or because they cannot withdraw quickly enough. Also, the Cowper's glands, two pea-size structures located on each side of the urethra, often produce a fluid that appears as drops at the tip of the penis any time from arousal and erection to orgasm. This fluid can contain active sperm and, in infected men, human immunodeficiency virus (HIV).

Good decisions about birth control are based on sound information. Consult a physician or family-planning counselor if you have questions or want to know how certain methods might affect existing or familial medical conditions, such as high blood pressure or diabetes.

✓**check-in** How well informed are you about contraceptive options?

Table 10.1 presents your contraceptive choices. When you evaluate any contraceptive,

- Recovering from a breakup
- Preventing pregnancy and sexually transmitted infection

✓**check-in** What do you think are good reasons for choosing abstinence?

Practicing abstinence is the only form of birth control that is 100 percent effective and risk and cost free. It can also be a valid and valued lifestyle choice. A growing number of individuals, including some who have been sexually active in the past, are choosing abstinence until they establish a relationship with a long-term partner.

Abstinence offers special health benefits for women. Those who abstain until their 20s and engage in sex with fewer partners during their lifetime are less likely to get STIs, suffer infertility, or develop cervical cancer. However, there is a risk that people will abruptly end their abstinence without being prepared to protect themselves against pregnancy or infection.

Individuals who choose abstinence from vaginal intercourse often engage in activities sometimes called *outercourse*, such as kissing, hugging, sensual touching, and mutual masturbation. Pregnancy is possible if the man ejaculates near the vaginal opening because sperm can swim up the vagina and fallopian tubes to fertilize an egg. Outercourse may lower the risk of contracting sexually transmitted infections but does not eliminate the danger of transmission via a parasite or skin-to-skin contact.

contraception The prevention of conception; birth control.

coitus interruptus The removal of the penis from the vagina before ejaculation.

TABLE 10.1 Birth Control Guide

Methods	MD Visit Needed	How to Use It	Some Risks	Noncontraceptive Benefits
Sterilization surgery for women	yes	One-time procedure; nothing to do or remember	• Pain • Bleeding • Infection or other complications after surgery • Ectopic (tubal) pregnancy	Reduces risk of ovarian cancer
Surgical sterilization implant for women	yes	One-time procedure; nothing to do or remember	• Mild to moderate pain after insertion • Ectopic (tubal) pregnancy	Reduces risk of ovarian cancer
Sterilization surgery for men	yes	One-time procedure; nothing to do or remember	• Pain • Bleeding • Infection	Possible reduction in risk for prostate cancer
Implantable rod	yes	One-time procedure; nothing to do or remember	• Acne • Hair loss • Weight gain • Headache • Cysts of the ovaries • Upset stomach • Mood changes • Dizziness • Depression • Sore breasts	Can use while breast-feeding; reduced menstrual flow and cramping
IUD	yes	One-time procedure; nothing to do or remember	• Cramps • Lower interest in sexual activity • Bleeding • Pelvic inflammatory disease • Changes in your periods • Infertility • Tear or hole in the uterus	Decreased menstrual flow and cramping; can use while breast-feeding; reduced risk of endometrial cancer
Shot/injection	yes	Need a shot every 3 months	• Bone loss • Bleeding between periods • Weight gain • Breast tenderness • Headaches	
Oral contraceptives (combined pill): "the pill"	yes	Must swallow a pill every day	• Dizziness • High blood pressure • Nausea • Blood clots • Changes in your cycle (period) • Heart attack • Changes in your mood • Strokes • Weight gain	Decreases menstrual flow, cramping, PMS, acne, risk of ovarian and endometrial cancers, and the development of ovarian cysts

(Continued)

TABLE 10.1 Birth Control Guide (continued)

Methods	MD Visit Needed	How to Use It	Some Risks	Noncontraceptive Benefits
Oral contraceptives (progestin-only): "the pill"	yes	Must swallow a pill every day	• Irregular bleeding • Weight gain • Breast tenderness	May have similar noncontraceptive benefits as combined pills; reduction of uterine and ovarian cancer risk
Oral contraceptives (extended/continued use): "the pill"	yes	Must swallow a pill every day	• Risks are similar to other oral contraceptives • Bleeding • Spotting between periods	Four periods per year and fewer menstrual-related problems; may reduce uterine fibroids and endometriosis symptoms
Patch	yes	Must wear a patch every day	• Exposure to higher average levels of estrogen than most oral contraceptives	Decreases menstrual flow and cramping, PMS, acne, risk of ovarian and endometrial cancers, and the development of ovarian cysts
Vaginal contraceptive ring	yes	Must leave the ring in every day for 3 weeks	• Vaginal discharge • Swelling of the vagina • Irritation • Similar to oral contraceptives	Decreases menstrual flow and cramping, PMS, acne, risk of ovarian and endometrial cancers, and the development of ovarian cysts
Male condom	no	Must use every time you have sex; requires partner's cooperation	• Allergic reactions	Protects against STIs; delays premature ejaculation Except for abstinence, latex condoms are the best protection against HIV/AIDS and other STIs
Diaphragm with spermicide	yes	Must use every time you have sex	• Irritation • Urinary tract infection • Allergic reactions • Toxic shock	
Sponge with spermicide	no	Must use every time you have sex	• Irritation • Allergic reactions • Hard time removing • Toxic shock	Possible STI protection
Cervical cap with spermicide	yes	Must use every time you have sex	• Irritation • Allergic reactions • Abnormal Pap test • Toxic shock	
Female condom	no	Must use every time you have sex	• Irritation • Allergic reactions	Possible STI protection
Spermicide	no	Must use every time you have sex	• Irritation • Allergic reactions • Urinary tract infection	
Emergency Contraception (If your primary method of birth control fails)				
Emergency Contraceptives "The Morning-After Pill"	no	Must be used within 72 hours of unprotected sex It should not be used as a regular form of birth control	• Nausea • Vomiting • Abdominal pain • Fatigue • Headache	

Effectiveness of Family Planning Methods

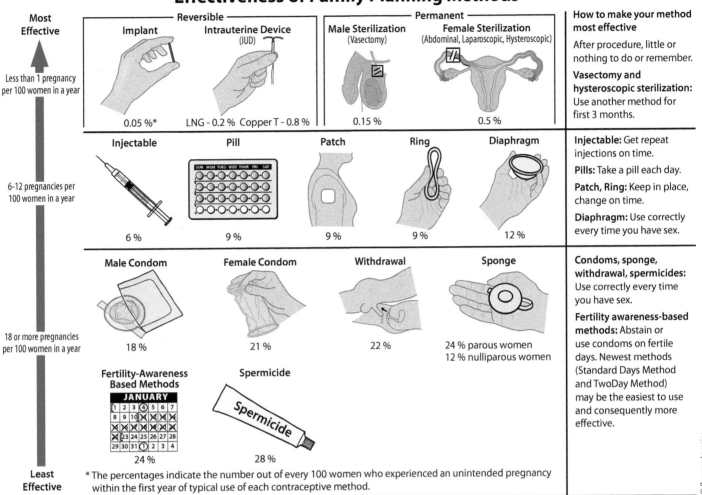

	Reversible		Permanent		How to make your method most effective

Most Effective

Less than 1 pregnancy per 100 women in a year

Implant — 0.05 %*

Intrauterine Device (IUD) — LNG - 0.2 % Copper T - 0.8 %

Male Sterilization (Vasectomy) — 0.15 %

Female Sterilization (Abdominal, Laparoscopic, Hysteroscopic) — 0.5 %

How to make your method most effective

After procedure, little or nothing to do or remember.

Vasectomy and hysteroscopic sterilization: Use another method for first 3 months.

6-12 pregnancies per 100 women in a year

Injectable — 6 %

Pill — 9 %

Patch — 9 %

Ring — 9 %

Diaphragm — 12 %

Injectable: Get repeat injections on time.

Pills: Take a pill each day.

Patch, Ring: Keep in place, change on time.

Diaphragm: Use correctly every time you have sex.

18 or more pregnancies per 100 women in a year

Male Condom — 18 %

Female Condom — 21 %

Withdrawal — 22 %

Sponge — 24 % parous women / 12 % nulliparous women

Fertility-Awareness Based Methods — 24 %

Spermicide — 28 %

Condoms, sponge, withdrawal, spermicides: Use correctly every time you have sex.

Fertility awareness-based methods: Abstain or use condoms on fertile days. Newest methods (Standard Days Method and TwoDay Method) may be the easiest to use and consequently more effective.

Least Effective

* The percentages indicate the number out of every 100 women who experienced an unintended pregnancy within the first year of typical use of each contraceptive method.

© Cengage Learning

FIGURE 10.2 Comparing Effectiveness of Birth Control Methods

Source: Public Domain. Centers for Disease Control and Prevention.

---

always consider its effectiveness (the likelihood that it will indeed prevent pregnancy). The **failure rate** refers to the number of pregnancies that occur per year for every 100 women using a particular method of birth control (see Figure 10.2).

Women or their partners may not use contraception consistently or correctly and thereby become pregnant without intending to do so. This is why researchers distinguish between "perfect" and "typical" use. The average probability of unintended pregnancy in one year of typical use is about 12 percent. Women under age 25 have higher rates of contraceptive failures during the first year of use than older women.

Hormonal methods (the pill, patch, ring, and injectable and implantable contraceptives) and the IUD are more effective in preventing

pregnancy.[6] A woman has a 1-in-15 chance of becoming pregnant within a year of typical use of a hormonal implant, compared with a 1-in-4 likelihood if she uses fertility awareness.

Women switch to different contraceptive methods for a variety of reasons, including changes in their life circumstances. In a common pattern, young women initially use condoms, begin a hormonal contraceptive in addition to condoms, and eventually discontinue condoms use, often because of their partners' negative attitude toward condom use.[7] (See Health Now on p. 288, for same criteria for choosing a form of contraceptive that works best for you.)

✓**check-in** What forms of contraception have you used or would you consider using?

failure rate The number of pregnancies that occur per year for every 100 women using a particular method of birth control.

HEALTH NOW!

Choosing a Contraceptive

You may choose different types of birth control at different stages of your life, or you may switch contraceptives for various reasons. (See Self Survey: Which Contraceptive Method Is Best for You?) You and your partner should always consider and discuss these factors:

- **Effectiveness:** Keep in mind that your own conscientiousness will play an important role. (See Figure 10.2.)

- **Suitability:** If you don't have sex very often, a contraceptive with many risks and side effects, such as the pill, may be a bad match for you.

- **Side effects:** Some complications related to contraceptives are serious health threats. Be sure to ask questions and gather information.

- **Safety:** The risks of certain contraceptives, such as the pill, may be too great to allow their use if, for example, you have high blood pressure.

- **Future fertility:** Some women don't return to regular menstrual cycles for six months to a year after discontinuing oral contraceptives.

- **Reduced risk of sexually transmitted infections:** Some forms of contraception, in particular barrier contraceptives and spermicides, help reduce the risk of transmission of some STIs. However, none provides complete protection.

What is your top priority for any form of birth control? Why? What is your top concern or source of hesitation? Record your reflections in your online journal.

The Benefits and Risks of Contraceptives

Using birth control is safer and healthier than not using it. According to the Population Reference Bureau, the use of contraceptives, including oral contraceptives, saves millions of lives each year. (see Table 10.2.)

Under the Affordable Care Act, insurance plans must cover all FDA-approved contraceptive methods, including birth control pills, shots, rings, implants, diaphragms, cervical caps, and sterilization. All costs are covered by monthly premiums, so there are no co-payments or deductibles.

If you have one of the following conditions, you should talk with your doctor about which types of contraceptive may increase your health risks:

- **High blood pressure (180/110 mmHg or higher):** Avoid birth control pills or injections containing estrogen, which may increase your risk of a heart attack or stroke.

TABLE 10.2 Noncontraceptive Benefits of Birth Control

Method	Benefits
Male sterilization	Possible reduction in prostate risk
Female sterilization	Reduces risk for ovarian cancer
Implanon	Reduced menstrual flow and cramping; can be used while breast-feeding
Mirena IUD	Decreases menstrual flow and cramping; reduced risk for endometrial cancer
ParaGard IUD	Reduced risk for endometrial cancer
Depo-Provera	Reduced menstrual flow and cramping; decreased risk for pelvic inflammatory disease (PID) and ovarian and endometrial cancers; can be used while breast-feeding
NuvaRing	Decreases menstrual flow and cramping, premenstrual syndrome (PMS), acne, ovarian and endometrial cancers, the development of ovarian cysts, uterine and breast fibroids, and PID
Ortho Evra Patch	Decreases menstrual flow and cramping, PMS, acne, ovarian and endometrial cancers, the development of ovarian cysts, uterine and breast fibroids, and PID
Combination birth control pill	Decreases menstrual flow and cramping, PMS, acne, ovarian and endometrial cancers, the development of ovarian cysts, uterine and breast fibroids, and pelvic inflammatory disease
Progestin-only birth control pill	May have similar contraceptive benefits as combination pills
Extended-use birth control pill	Four periods or less per year and fewer menstrual-related problems; may reduce uterine fibroids and endometriosis symptoms
Male condom	Protects against sexually transmitted infections (STIs); delays premature ejaculation
Female condom	Protects against STIs
Cervical barrier	Diaphragm may protect from cervical dysplasia
Contraceptive sponge	None
Fertility awareness methods	Can help a woman learn her cycle and eventually help in getting pregnant
Withdrawal	None
Spermicide	Provides lubrication
No method	n/a

Source: J. Carroll, *Sexuality Now,* 5th ed. (San Francisco, CA: Cengage Learning, 2014).

- **Episodes of depression:** Avoid products that contain progestin, such as Depo-Provera, the contraceptive implant, and the minipill. In some women with depression, progestin may worsen depressive symptoms. Also, check with your doctor if you are taking an antidepressant medication; it may affect or be affected by oral contraceptives and you may require a different dose.

- **Seizure disorder:** Avoid low-dose birth control pills. Some antiseizure medications, such as Dilantin, accelerate liver metabolism of all substances, including oral contraceptives, and make them less effective.

- **Ectopic pregnancy:** Avoid IUDs. Although IUDs do not cause ectopic pregnancies, if your fallopian tubes have been scarred by a previous ectopic gestation, you're more likely to have another ectopic pregnancy if you use an IUD.

- **Hepatitis:** Avoid birth control pills or injections containing estrogen, which is metabolized in the liver—an organ damaged by hepatitis.

You also have to recognize the specific risks associated with various methods of contraception. If you're a woman, the risks are chiefly yours. Various methods of birth control have side effects, although pregnancy and childbirth account for much higher rates of medical complications and deaths than any contraceptive. Most women never experience any serious complications, but it's important to be aware of potential risks.

Birth Control in America

Nearly all sexually experienced women use contraception at some point in their lifetimes. A recent statistical "snapshot" of current birth control in the United States reveals the following:

- Approximately 62 percent of women ages 15 to 44—some 37.6 million women—are using contraception.

- Non-Hispanic white women have the highest rates of use (65 percent); 58 percent of non-Hispanic black women and 57 percent of Hispanic women report birth control use.

- Current contraception use is higher among women ages 25 to 34 (67 percent) and 35 to 44 (70 percent) than among those between the ages of 15 and 24 (58 percent).

- The most commonly used contraceptive methods are birth control pills (16 percent),

female sterilization (16 percent), condoms (9 percent), and long-active reversible contraceptives (7 percent).[8]

Reproductive Coercion

Reproductive coercion refers to "behaviors intended to maintain power and control in a relationship" by someone who is, was, or wishes to be involved in an intimate or dating relationship.

In a study of almost a thousand female undergraduates at a large public university, nearly eight percent reported reproductive coercion, including the following:

- being told not to use any birth control

- being forced or pressured to become pregnant

- having partner say he would have a baby with someone else or leave if they did not get pregnant

- being hurt physically because they did not agree to get pregnant

- having partner refuse to pay for contraceptives

- having partner refuse to use, break, puncture, or remove a condom so they would get pregnant

- having birth control pills taken away[9]

As part of their regular screening exams, obstetrician-gynecologists now ask women if they have been the victims of reproductive coercion or any other form of intimate partner violence (discussed in Chapter 18).

Among the questions doctors suggest women ask themselves are the following:

- Is my partner respectful of my choices?

- Does my partner support my using birth control?

- Does my partner support my decisions about if or when I want to have more children?

Yes answers indicate a healthy approach to reproductive decision-making. Also ask

- Has my partner ever tried to pressure me to get pregnant or make me get pregnant?

- Has my partner ever hurt or threatened me because I didn't agree to get pregnant?

- If I've ever been pregnant, has my partner told me he would hurt me if I didn't do what he wanted with the pregnancy (in either direction—continuing the pregnancy or having an abortion)?

A yes to any of these questions indicates reproductive coercion. All women deserve to make their own decisions without being afraid. For information on where to turn for support, go to "Futures without Violence" at http://www.futureswithoutviolence.org. (See Chapter 18 for more on intimate partner violence.)

A Cross-Cultural Perspective

Culture, religion, gender roles, and folklore can affect birth control options and decisions. In countries that are predominantly Catholic, such as Ireland, Italy, and the Philippines, the church promotes fertility awareness and the rhythm method and condemns other contraceptive methods. Because Jewish law teaches men not to "spill their seed," methods that can cause damage to sperm, such as vasectomy, condoms, or spermicides, are less acceptable in Israel than oral contraceptives are.

According to the United Nations, 62.7 percent of women who are married or in a union use contraception. Worldwide, 8.8 percent use combination oral contraceptives; that percentage rises to 15.4 percent in more developed countries. More than 100 million women worldwide use combination oral contraceptives.

In an international study, women between the ages of 25 and 44 in five countries—the United States, England, Germany, Italy, and Spain—were most likely to rely on oral contraceptives (from 35 percent in Spain to 63 percent in Germany) and the male condom (20 percent in Germany to 47 percent in Spain).

In Japan, which has one of the lowest birthrates in the world, men are primarily responsible for birth control decisions. In Kenya, married couples view the use of a condom as an indicator of a husband's infidelity. In Scandinavian countries, where birth control is free and easily accessible, many women begin taking oral contraceptives before becoming sexually active.

Worldwide, sterilization is used by more people than any other birth control method. The intrauterine device (IUD) is the most commonly used reversible form of contraception. Among the countries with the highest usage rates are Turkey, China (where an IUD is often inserted immediately after a woman gives birth to her first child), Nigeria, England, Russia, and Korea.

Birth Control on Campus

In the ACHA's *National College Health Assessment*, 56.8 percent of students—54 percent of men and 58.6 percent of women—reported using contraception the last time they had vaginal intercourse. (See Snapshot: On Campus Now.)

Among students who had vaginal intercourse in the past 12 months, 14.9 percent reported that they or their partner had used emergency contraception (the morning-after pill), discussed later in this chapter, while 1.4 percent reported an unintended pregnancy.[10]

Even students who know and understand the risks associated with unprotected sex often do not take steps to prevent pregnancy or STIs. One reason is that many believe that "a known partner is a safe partner" and that sex with someone they know as a friend or have been dating for a while is safe.

✓**check-in** If you are sexually active, do you use condoms every time you engage in sex? Are you less likely to do so with a partner you know well?

Contraception Choices

Barrier Contraceptives

As their name implies, **barrier contraceptives** block the meeting of egg and sperm by means of a physical barrier (condom, sponge, diaphragm, cervical cap, or FemCap) or a chemical one (vaginal spermicide in jellies, foams, creams, suppositories, or film). As shown in Table 10.3 on page 292, they vary in effectiveness.

Nonprescription Barriers   The nonprescription barrier contraceptives include the male and female condom, the contraceptive sponge, and vaginal spermicides.

Condoms   Unlike other barrier contraceptives, **condoms** provide some protection against HIV infection and other STIs; spermicides, sponges, and films do not.

✓**check-in** Do you think condoms have a negative effect on sexual pleasure?

A recent study of 5,865 men and women ages 18 to 59 found that condoms do not detract from a sexual experience. Both genders, whether heterosexual or homosexual, described their most recent sexual experiences as highly arousing and pleasurable, regardless of whether they used condoms or engaged in oral, vaginal, or anal

barrier contraceptives Birth control devices that block the meeting of egg and sperm, either by physical barriers, such as condoms, diaphragms, or cervical caps, or by chemical barriers, such as spermicide, or both.

condoms Latex or polyurethane sheaths worn over the penis during sexual acts to prevent conception and/or the transmission of disease; the female condom lines the walls of the vagina.

SNAPSHOT: ON CAMPUS NOW

📷 Birth Control Choices of College Students

Contraceptive use reported by students or their partners the last time they had vaginal intercourse:

	Percent (%)		
	Male	Female	Total
Yes, used a method of contraception	54.0	58.5	56.8
Not applicable/Didn't use a method/Don't know	46.0	41.5	43.2

If YES to contraceptive use the last time student had vaginal intercourse, reported means of birth control used among college students or their partners to prevent pregnancy:

	Percent (%)		
	Male	Female	Total
Birth control pills (monthly or extended cycle)	64.4	61.4	62.4
Birth control shots	3.9	3.3	3.5
Birth control implants	3.2	2.5	2.8
Birth control patch	1.2	0.7	0.9
Vaginal ring	3.7	3.6	3.7
Intrauterine device	6.7	7.5	7.3
Male condom	66.6	59.5	61.8
Female condom	0.7	0.5	0.6
Diaphragm or cervical cap	0.6	0.2	0.4
Contraceptive sponge	0.5	0.2	0.3
Spermicide (foam, jelly, cream)	4.7	2.6	3.3
Fertility awareness (calendar, mucus, basal body temperature)	4.8	6.7	6.1
Withdrawal	27.4	30.3	29.3
Sterilization (hysterectomy, tubes tied, vasectomy)	2.2	2.4	2.3
Other method	2.5	1.8	2.0
Male condom use plus another method	**51.0**	**46.0**	**47.6**
Any two or more methods (excluding male condoms)	**28.6**	**29.5**	**29.1**

✓**check-in** If you engage in heterosexual intercourse, do you always use a form of birth control? If not, why not? If so, which type? How did you choose it? Did you discuss contraception with your sexual partner? Did you find this difficult? Write down your reflections in your online journal.

Source: American College Health Association. *American College Health Association–National College Health Assessment II: Reference Group Executive Summary, Spring 2014*. Hanover, MD: American College Health Association; 2014.

TABLE 10.3 How Effective Are Barrier Contraceptives?

Method	Number of women out of 100 who will become pregnant during the first year of typical use (when a method is used by the average person who does not always use the method correctly or consistently)
Diaphragm	12
Sponge	
Women who have not given birth	12
Women who have given birth	24
Cervical cap	
Women who have not given birth	13
Women who have given birth	23
Male condom	18
Female condom	21
Spermicide	28

Source: American Congress of Obstetricians and Gynecologists.

intercourse. The men in the study reported that condom use had no significant impact on the ease of their erections or their sexual pleasure.[11]

However, there can be issues related to condom fit or feel. The most common complaints from condom users include decreased sensation, lack of naturalness, condom size, decreased pleasure, and pain and discomfort.[12]

Advantages

- Effective when used correctly.
- Lowers a woman's risk of pelvic inflammatory disease (PID) and may protect against some urinary tract and genital infections.
- No side effects.
- No prescription required.
- Can be carried in a pocket or purse.
- Inexpensive.
- The female condom gives women more control in reducing their risk of pregnancy and STIs and does not require a prescription or medical appointment.
- No effect on a woman's natural hormones or fertility.
- The female condom can be inserted up to eight hours before sex.

Disadvantages

- Requires consistent and diligent use.
- Not 100 percent effective in preventing pregnancy or STIs.

- Risk of manufacturing defects, such as pin-size holes, and breaking or slipping off during intercourse.
- May inhibit sexual spontaneity.
- Users or partners may complain about odor, lubrication (too much or too little), feel, taste, difficulty opening the packages, and disposal.
- Some men complain of reduced penile sensitivity or cannot sustain an erection while putting on a condom.
- Some women complain that the female condom is difficult to use, squeaks, and looks odd.

Male Condom The male condom covers the erect penis and catches the ejaculate. This helps to prevent pregnancy and the exchange of bodily fluids for oral and anal sex in same and opposite sex partners (see Figure 10.3).

Among college and universities with health centers, about half provide free condoms.[13] At other schools, students may have limited access to condoms and may need to leave campus to buy condoms at convenience stores, pharmacies, or grocery stores.[14]

How It Works Most condoms are made of thin surgical latex or polyurethane. The polyurethane condom has proven to be not as effective as the latex condom for pregnancy prevention. However, polyurethane condoms may be a good option for those allergic to latex. Membrane condoms ("natural" or "sheepskin") are

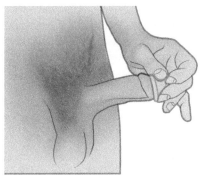
Pinch or twist the tip of the condom, leaving one-half inch at the tip to catch the semen.

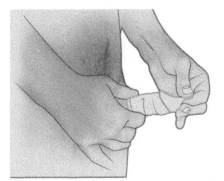
Holding the tip, unroll the condom.

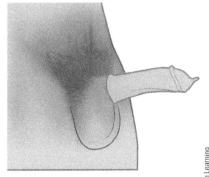
Unroll the condom until it reaches the pubic hairs.

© Cengage Learning

FIGURE 10.3 Male Condom

Condoms effectively reduce the risk of pregnancy as well as STIs if used consistently and correctly.

not recommended. Experts advise against use of condoms with nonoxynol-9, which may increase rather than lower the risk of sexual infections (see Chapter 11). Here are some additional guidelines for condom use:

- Before using a condom, check the expiration date and make sure it's soft and pliable.

- Do not tear open a packet with your teeth; you could puncture the condom.

- If it's yellow or sticky, throw the condom out.

- Don't check for leaks by blowing up a condom before using it; you may weaken or tear it.

- Put the condom on at the beginning of sexual activity, before genital contact occurs.

- Leave a little space at the top of the condom to catch the semen (see Figure 10.3).

- If a female partner is using a vaginal lubricant, it should be water based. Petroleum-based creams or jellies (such as petroleum jelly, baby oil, massage oil, vegetable oils, or oil-based hand lotions) can deteriorate latex.

- After ejaculation, hold the condom firmly against the penis so that it doesn't slip off or leak during withdrawal.

- Couples engaging in anal intercourse should use a water-based lubricant as well as a condom but should never assume that the condom will provide 100 percent protection from HIV infection or other STIs.

Effectiveness Although the theoretical effectiveness rate for condoms is 97 percent, the actual rate is only 80 to 85 percent. The condom can be torn during the manufacturing process or during use. Careless removal can also decrease the effectiveness of condoms.

The major reason that condoms have such a low actual effectiveness rate is that couples don't use them each and every time they have sex. Users who have little experience with condoms—who are young, single, or childless, or who engage in risky behaviors—are more likely to have condoms break.

Condoms are second only to the pill in popularity among college-age adults. Half of sexually active students report using condoms the last time they had vaginal intercourse.[15] (See Table 10.4.) College men give various reasons for not using a condom, including not having one available, a partner's objection, the belief that proposing its use could lead to problems between the couple, fear of irritation, and the belief that it doesn't feel natural. Comfort is also an issue. Men may be more likely to remove a condom that doesn't fit well.[16]

TABLE 10.4 Condoms on Campus

Using a condom or other protective barrier within the past 30 days (*mostly or always*):

	Percent (%)		
	Male	**Female**	**Average**
*Sexually active students reported**			
Oral sex	5.1	4.3	4.6
Vaginal intercourse	54.4	48.4	50.7
Anal intercourse	34.8	21.6	27.2

*Students responding "Never did this sexual activity" or "Have not done this during the past 30 days" were excluded from the analysis.

Source: American College Health Association. *American College Health Association–National College Health Assessment II: Reference Group Executive Summary, Spring 2014*. Hanover, MD: American College Health Association, 2014.

Female Condom The second-generation female condom, known as FC2, is a strong, thin, flexible nitrile sheath or pouch about 6.5 inches long, the same length as a male condom. It consists of a flexible polyurethane ring at the closed end of the pouch, the end that is inserted into the vagina, and a soft nitrite ring at the end that remains outside the vagina. There is a silicone-based lubricant on the inside of the condom; additional lubrication can be used.

How It Works As illustrated in Figure 10.4, a woman removes the condom and applicator from the wrapper and inserts the condom slowly by gently pushing the applicator toward the small of the back. When properly inserted, the outer ring should rest on the folds of skin around the vaginal opening, and the inner ring (the closed end) should fit against the cervix. The female condom may be placed up to eight hours before intercourse.

Effectiveness The female condom is about 75 to 82 percent effective with normal use; if it were used correctly during every occasion of intercourse, it is about 95 percent effective in preventing pregnancy. Female condoms can fail for the same reasons as male condoms, such as having a tear, not being put in place before the penis touches the vagina, and spilling the contents as the condom is being removed.

Friction of the female condom may reduce clitoral stimulation and lubrication, which may make intercourse less enjoyable, although lubricants may help. Some users have reported irritation and allergic reactions. A couple should not use a male and female condom together because friction between them can cause them to tear or bunch and should avoid petroleum-based lubricants such as Vaseline, which can break down latex.

Properly used, the female condom is considered as good as or better than the male condom for preventing infections, including HIV, because it is stronger and covers a slightly larger area. Female condoms may be more prone to slipping and other mechanical problems but are as effective as male condoms in blocking semen. The efficacy of female condoms increases with a woman's experience in using them.

Contraceptive Sponge The contraceptive sponge, which is made of soft polyurethane foam laced with spermicide, was sold as an over-the-counter contraceptive in the United States from 1983 to 1995, when it was withdrawn because of contamination problems at the manufacturing plant. It has returned to stores several times.

How It Works The contraceptive sponge acts as a barrier by blocking the entrance to the uterus and absorbing and deactivating sperm. Prior to inserting it in the vagina, moisten the sponge with water to activate the spermicide. Then fold it in half and insert deep into the vagina. Check to make sure it is covering the cervix. Intercourse can occur immediately or at any time during the next 24 hours. However, the sponge must remain in place for 6 hours after intercourse. To remove, gently pull the cloth loop or the tabs on the outside.

Advantages

- Does not require a prescription.
- Easy to carry and use.
- Can be inserted up to 24 hours before intercourse.
- Effective immediately if used correctly.
- No effect on fertility or a woman's natural hormones.

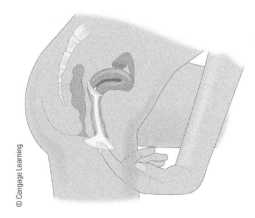
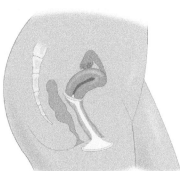
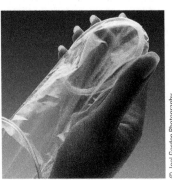

© Cengage Learning

© Joel Gordon Photography

FIGURE 10.4 Female Condom

No spermicide is used with the female condom. Like the male condom, this method does not require a prescription.

- Generally cannot be felt by a woman or her partner.

- Can be used by women who are breast-feeding for six weeks after childbirth.

Disadvantages

- May be difficult to remove.

- May be less effective in women who have had children.

- Does not provide reliable protection against STIs.

- Requires advance planning to place the sponge.

- Side effects include vaginal irritation and allergic reactions.

- Should not be used during menstruation.

- Slightly increased risk of toxic shock syndrome if left in place longer than 24–30 hours.

Vaginal Spermicides and Film The various forms of **vaginal spermicide** include chemical foams, creams, jellies, vaginal suppositories, gels, and film. Some creams and jellies are made for use with a diaphragm; others can be used alone. Several vaginal suppositories claim high effectiveness, but no American studies have confirmed these claims. In general, failure rates for vaginal suppositories are as high as 10 to 25 percent.

Frequent use of spermicides can increase the risk of getting HIV from an infected partner. They should be used only by those at low risk of HIV infection.

One widely used spermicide, nonoxynol-9, has proven to be less effective than once believed. It does not protect against many STIs, including HIV, chlamydia, and gonorrhea. Nonoxynol-9 also may increase the risk of infection with human papillomavirus (HPV) and with HIV. The Centers for Disease Control and Prevention has concluded that it is ineffective against HIV, and the World Health Organization describes it as only "moderately effective" for pregnancy prevention.

Vaginal contraceptive film (VCF), a thin 2-inch-square film laced with spermicide, is folded and inserted into the vagina, where it dissolves into a stay-in-place gel (see Figure 10.5). VCF, which can be used by people allergic to foams and jellies, is as effective as most spermicides.

How They Work Spermicides consist of a chemical that kills sperm and potential pathogens and an inert base, such as jelly, cream, foam, or film, that holds the spermicide close to the cervix. The jelly, cream, or foam spermicide is inserted into the vagina with an applicator or finger. Vaginal

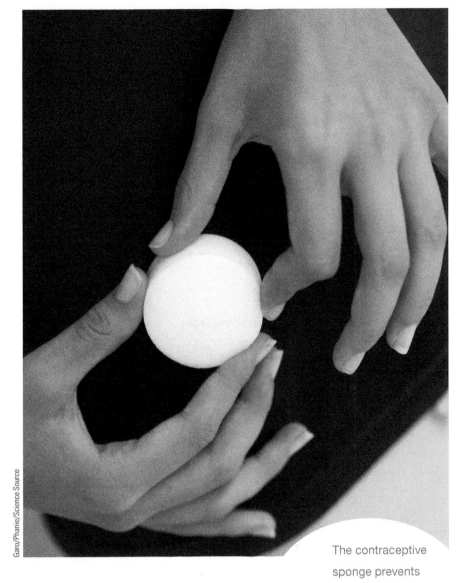

Garo/Phanie/Science Source

suppositories take about 20 minutes to dissolve and cover the vaginal walls. Follow package directions precisely.

You must apply additional spermicide or insert another VCF film before each additional intercourse. After sex, women should shower rather than bathe to prevent the spermicide from being rinsed out of the vagina, and they should not douche for at least six hours.

Advantages

- Easy to use.

- Effective if used with another form of contraception.

- Reduces the risk of some vaginal infections, PID, and STIs.

- No effect on a woman's natural hormones or fertility.

The contraceptive sponge prevents sperm from entering the uterus and is available without a prescription.

vaginal spermicide A substance that kills or neutralizes sperm, inserted into the vagina in the form of a foam, cream, jelly, suppository, or film.

vaginal contraceptive film (VCF) A small dissolvable sheet saturated with spermicide that can be inserted into the vagina and placed over the cervix.

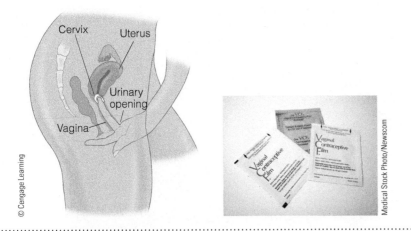

FIGURE 10.5 Vaginal Contraceptive Film

The effectiveness of this thin film, laced with spermicide, is similar to other spermicides.

Disadvantages

- When used alone, does not protect against STIs.

- Frequent use can increase risk of HIV from an infected partner.

- Insertion interrupts sexual spontaneity.

- May cause irritation.

- Some people cannot use foams or jellies because of an allergic reaction.

- Some users complain that spermicides are messy or interfere with oral–genital contact.

- Spermicidal suppositories that do not dissolve completely can feel gritty.

Prescription Barriers The prescription barrier contraceptives—the diaphragm, cervical cap, and FemCap, all used by women—are placed in the vagina with a spermicide. They do not protect against HIV infection and most STIs.

Diaphragm The **diaphragm** is a bowl-like rubber cup with a flexible rim that is inserted into the vagina to cover the cervix and prevent the passage of sperm into the uterus during sexual intercourse (see Figure 10.6).

When used with a spermicide, the diaphragm is both a physical and a chemical barrier to sperm. The effectiveness of the diaphragm in preventing pregnancy depends on strong motivation (to use it faithfully) and a precise understanding of its use. Without spermicide, the diaphragm is not effective.

How It Works Diaphragms are fitted and prescribed by a qualified health-care professional in diameter sizes ranging from 2 to 4 inches (50 to 105 millimeters). The diaphragm's main function is to serve as a container for a spermicidal (sperm-killing) foam or jelly, which is available at pharmacies without a prescription. A diaphragm should remain in the vagina for at least six hours after intercourse to ensure that all sperm are killed. If intercourse occurs again during this period, additional spermicide must be inserted with an applicator tube.

A sexually active woman should keep her diaphragm in the most accessible place—her purse, bedroom, or bathroom. Before every use, a diaphragm should be checked for tiny leaks (hold

diaphragm A bowl-like rubber cup with a flexible rim that is inserted into the vagina to cover the cervix and prevent the passage of sperm into the uterus during sexual intercourse; used with a spermicidal foam or jelly, it serves as both a chemical and a physical barrier to sperm.

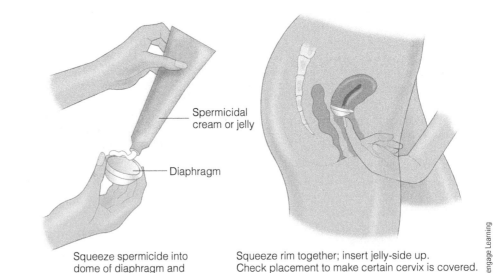

Spermicidal cream or jelly

Diaphragm

Squeeze spermicide into dome of diaphragm and around the rim.

Squeeze rim together; insert jelly-side up. Check placement to make certain cervix is covered.

FIGURE 10.6 Diaphragm

When used correctly and consistently with a spermicide, the diaphragm is effective in preventing pregnancy. It must be fitted by a health-care professional.

up to the light or place water in the dome). A health-care provider should check its fit and condition every year. Oil-based lubricants will deteriorate the latex of the diaphragm and should not be used.

Cervical Cap   Like the diaphragm, the **cervical cap** combined with spermicide serves as both a chemical and physical barrier blocking the path of the sperm to the uterus. The rubber or plastic cap is smaller and thicker than a diaphragm. It resembles a large thimble that fits snugly around the cervix and may work better for some women than others. It is about as effective as a diaphragm (see Figure 10.2 on page 287).

How It Works   The cervical cap is fitted by a qualified health-care professional. For use, a woman fills it one-third to two-thirds full with spermicide and inserts it by holding its edges together and sliding it into the vagina. The cup is then pressed onto the cervix. (Most women find it easiest to do so while squatting or in an upright sitting position.) The cap can be inserted up to 6 hours prior to intercourse and should not be removed for at least 6 hours afterward. It can be left in place up to 24 hours. Pulling on one side of the rim breaks the suction and allows easy removal. Oil-based lubricants should not be used with the cap because they can deteriorate the latex.

FemCap   The FemCap is a nonhormonal, latex-free barrier contraceptive that works with a spermicide (see Figure 10.7). The FemCap, designed to conform to the anatomy of the cervix and vagina, comes in three sizes. The smallest usually best suits women who have never been pregnant; the medium size, for women who have been pregnant but have not had a vaginal delivery; the largest, for those who have delivered a full-term baby vaginally.

How It Works   A prescription is required to purchase FemCap, and the woman selects the appropriate size. To use, a woman applies spermicide to the bowl of the FemCap (which goes over the cervix), to the outer brim, and to the groove that will face into the vagina. She inserts the squeezed, flattened cap into the vagina with the bowl facing upward. The FemCap must be pushed all the way in to cover the cervix completely and left in place at least six hours after intercourse.

Advantages

- Can be inserted up to six hours before sex.
- Doesn't interrupt sexual activity; can be inserted hours ahead of time.
- Usually not felt by either partner.
- Can easily be carried in pocket or purse.
- No effect on a woman's natural hormones or fertility.
- Cervical caps are an alternative for women who cannot use diaphragms or find them too messy.

Disadvantages

- Less effective than hormonal contraceptives.
- Available by prescription only.

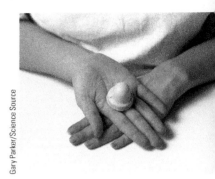

The cervical cap, preferred by some women, is about as effective as a diaphragm if used with a spermicide and inserted correctly.

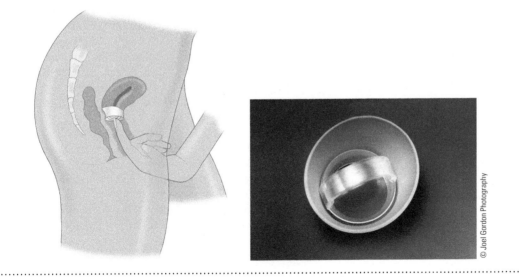

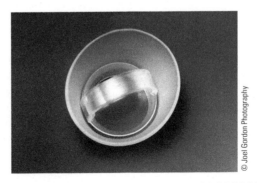

FIGURE 10.7 FemCap

The FemCap must be used with spermicide and correctly positioned to cover the cervix completely.

Source: Reproduced with permission from FemCap, Inc., and Alfred Shihata, MD.

cervical cap A thimble-size rubber or plastic cap that is inserted into the vagina to fit over the cervix and prevent the passage of sperm into the uterus during sexual intercourse; used with a spermicidal foam or jelly, it serves as both a chemical and a physical barrier to sperm.

- Requires advance planning or interruption of sexual activity to position the device before intercourse.

- May slip out of place during intercourse.

- May be uncomfortable for some women and their partners.

- Spermicidal foams, creams, and jellies may be messy, cause irritation, and detract from oral–genital sex.

- Some diaphragm users report bladder discomfort, urethral irritation, or recurrent cystitis.

- Some cap users find it difficult to insert and remove and uncomfortable to wear.

- Slightly increased risk of toxic shock syndrome.

Hormonal Contraceptives

In recent years, birth control methods made with synthetic hormones have become available in a variety of forms. Oral contraceptives, available for decades, are among the most well-researched of all medications. Other options for hormonal birth control include a skin patch, a vaginal ring, a three-month injection, and a three-year implant. All are extremely effective when used consistently and conscientiously. (See Table 10.5.)

Hormonal contraceptives can provide benefits beyond birth control, including the following:

- Regular menstrual cycles

- Reduction of menstrual pain and excess bleeding

- Treatment of premenstrual syndrome, polycystic ovarian syndrome, uterine fibroids, and endometriosis

- Prevention of menstrual migraines

- Decreased risk of endometrial cancer, ovarian cancer, and colorectal cancer

- Treatment of acne and excess facial hair

- Improved bone mineral density[17]

oral contraceptives Preparations of synthetic hormones that inhibit ovulation; also referred to as *birth control pills* or simply *the pill*.

monophasic pills Oral contraceptives that release synthetic estrogen and progestin at constant levels throughout the menstrual cycle.

TABLE 10.5 How Effective Are Hormonal Contraceptives?

The number of women out of 100 who will become pregnant during the first year of typical use (when a method is used by the average person who does not always use the method correctly or consistently) of each of these methods is as follows:

- Implant—The odds are lower than one in 100 women

- Injection—3 in 100 women will become pregnant

- Vaginal ring—8 in 100 women will become pregnant

- Skin patch—8 in 100 women will become pregnant

- Birth control pill—8 in 100 women will become pregnant

Source: American Congress of Obstetricians and Gynecologists.

Hormonal contraceptives do not protect against HIV infection and other STIs, so condoms and spermicides should also be used.

Oral Contraceptives The *pill*—the popular term for **oral contraceptives**—is the method of birth control preferred by unmarried women and by those under age 30, including college students. About one in five American women of childbearing age uses the pill. Women 18 to 24 years old are most likely to choose oral contraception. The American College of Obstetricians and Gynecologists (ACOG) has proposed that oral contraceptives be made available over the counter.[18]

Although many women incorrectly think that the risks of the pill are greater than those of pregnancy and childbirth, long-term studies show that oral contraceptive use does not increase mortality rates disease risks:

- Women who took the birth control pill beginning in the late 1960s lived longer than those never on the pill, according to a British study that followed more than 46,000 women for nearly four decades.

- The pill cuts women's risk of dying from colon cancer by 38 percent and from any other diseases by about 12 percent.

- Combination oral contraceptives significantly reduce the risk of ovarian and endometrial cancer.

- Oral contraceptives produce no increase in diabetes, multiple sclerosis, rheumatoid arthritis, or liver disease.

Combination Oral Contraceptives (COCs)
These pills consist of two hormones, synthetic estrogen and progestin, which play important roles in controlling ovulation and the menstrual cycle. The doses in today's oral contraceptives are much lower—less than one-fourth the amount of estrogen and one-twentieth the progestin in the original pill.

However, they may still increase cardiovascular risks for some women. They also appear to be less effective than those approved decades ago, with twice the failure rate of previous products. The reason seems to be lower doses of hormones that stop ovulation. Women on low-dose oral contraceptives should take their pills at the same time every day and follow their doctor's advice if they miss a dose. Oral contraceptives come in different forms:

- **Monophasic pills** release a constant dose of estrogen and progestin throughout a woman's menstrual cycle.

- **Multiphasic pills** mimic normal hormonal fluctuations of the natural menstrual cycle by providing different levels of estrogen and progesterone at different times of the month. Multiphasic pills reduce total hormonal dose and side effects.

Both monophasic and multiphasic pills block the release of hormones that would stimulate the process leading to ovulation. They also thicken and alter the cervical mucus, making it more hostile to sperm, and they make implantation of a fertilized egg in the uterine lining more difficult.

One combination pill, Yasmin, contains a unique progestin that works like a mild diuretic and prevents fluid retention. YAZ, a lower-dose 24-day version, can ease emotional and physical premenstrual symptoms (discussed in Chapter 9). Women who are taking potassium supplements, daily anti-inflammatory drugs, or heparin (a blood thinner) should talk with their doctor because of potentially dangerous drug interactions. Other pills offer different benefits, such as clearer skin and reduced facial hair, and less spotting.

Progestin-Only Pills   **Progestin-only pills**, also called **minipills**, contain only a small amount of progestin and no estrogen. They work somewhat differently than combination pills. Women taking minipills probably ovulate, at least occasionally. In those cycles, the pills prevent pregnancy by thickening cervical mucus, making it hard for sperm to penetrate, and by interfering with implantation of a fertilized egg.

The risk of heart disease and stroke is lower with progestin-only pills than with any combination pill. For this reason, they are a good choice for women over age 35 and others who cannot take estrogen-containing pills because of high blood pressure, diabetes, or clotting disorders. Because they do not affect the quality or quantity of breast milk, progestin-only pills often are recommended for nursing mothers, and they are recommended for smokers. Because progestin can affect mood and worsen the symptoms of depression, progestin-only pills are not recommended for women with a history of depression. Antiseizure medications, such as Dilantin, which accelerate liver metabolism, may make the minipill less effective.

Users of progestin-only pills have to be conscientious about taking these pills—not just every day, but at the same time every day. If you take a progestin-only pill three or more hours later than usual, use a backup method of contraception, such as a condom, for two days after you resume taking the pill.

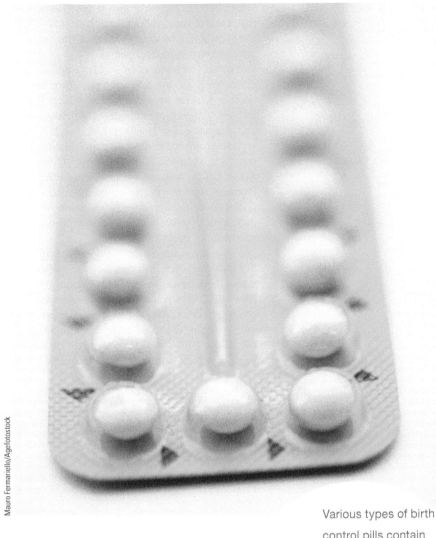

Mauro Fermariello/Agefotostock

✓**check-in** If you are a woman, have you ever used the pill?

Before Using Oral Contraceptives   Before starting the pill, a woman should undergo a physical examination that includes a blood pressure test, a breast exam, blood tests, and a urine sample. Let your doctor know about any personal or family incidence of high blood pressure or heart disease; diabetes; liver dysfunction; hepatitis; unusual menstrual history; severe depression; sickle-cell anemia; cancer of the breast, ovaries, or uterus; high cholesterol levels; or migraine headaches.

How They Work   Oral contraceptives usually come in 28-day packets: 21 of the pills contain the hormones, and 7 are "blanks," included so that the woman can take a pill every day, even during her menstrual period. If a woman forgets to take 1 pill, she should take it as soon as she

Various types of birth control pills contain different hormones and combinations of hormones.

multiphasic pills Oral contraceptives that release different levels of estrogen and progestin to mimic the hormonal fluctuations of the natural menstrual cycle.

minipills, progestin-only pills Oral contraceptives containing a small amount of progestin and no estrogen, which prevent contraception by making the mucus in the cervix so thick that sperm cannot enter the uterus.

remembers. However, if she forgets during the first week of her cycle or misses more than 1 pill, she should rely on another form of birth control until her next menstrual period.

Even if you experience no discomfort or side effects while on the pill, see a physician at least once a year for an examination, which should include a blood pressure test, a pelvic exam, and a breast exam. Notify your doctor at once if you develop severe abdominal pain, chest pain, coughing, shortness of breath, pain or tenderness in the calf or thigh, severe headaches, dizziness, faintness, muscle weakness or numbness, speech disturbance, blurred vision, a sensation of flashing lights, a breast lump, severe depression, or yellowing of your skin.

Generally, when a woman stops taking the pill, her menstrual cycle resumes the next month, but it may be irregular for the next couple months. However, 2 to 4 percent of pill users experience prolonged delays. Women who become pregnant during the first or second cycle after discontinuing use of the pill may be at greater risk of miscarriage; they also are more likely to conceive twins.

A Special Caution   Common antibiotics, including many of the ones prescribed for dental procedures or skin conditions, may lower the effectiveness of oral contraceptives, particularly low-dose birth control pills. Always ask a dentist or doctor who prescribes an antibiotic about its potential effect on your oral contraceptive, and check with your gynecologist or primary physician about using an additional nonhormonal means of contraception (such as a condom) to ensure protection against an unwanted pregnancy.

Other medicines and supplements that may make hormonal contraceptives less effective include St. John's wort, certain pills prescribed for yeast infections, certain HIV medications, and certain antiseizure medication. Body weight does not generally affect efficacy.

Advantages

- Extremely effective when taken consistently.
- Convenient.
- Moderately priced.
- Does not interrupt sexual activity.
- Reversible within three months of stopping the pill.
- Reduces the risk of benign breast lumps, ovarian cysts, iron-deficiency anemia, pelvic inflammatory disease, endometrial and ovarian cancer.
- May relieve painful menstruation.

Disadvantages

- In real life, rates of unintended pregnancies among pill users are as high as 2.8 percent in the first year of use and 5.7 percent after three years.
- Requires a prescription.
- Increases risk of cardiovascular problems, primarily for women over age 35 who smoke and those with high blood pressure or other health problems.
- Side effects vary with different brands but include spotting between periods, weight gain or loss, nausea and vomiting, breast tenderness, and decreased sex drive. Progestin-only pills may cause acne, body hair growth, and weight gain.
- Must be taken at the same time every day (especially critical with low-dose estrogen and progestin-only pills).
- No protection against STIs.
- Must use a secondary form of birth control for the initial seven days of use.

Extended-Use Pills   For years physicians have prescribed prolonged use of birth control pills to lessen the number of menstrual cycles for women with asthma, migraines, rashes, or other conditions that flare up during their periods. Eliminating periods eliminates symptoms, and having fewer cycles also may lower a woman's long-term risk of ovarian cancer. However, some women are wary of long-term hormone use or consider a lack of menstrual cycles unnatural.

Seasonale and Seasonique   Seasonale and Seasonique are prescription forms of oral contraception that prevent pregnancy as effectively as other birth control pills but produce only four menstrual periods a year.

How They Work   Unlike traditional birth control pills, women take "active" pills continuously for three months or 84 days. During this time, Seasonale prevents the uterine lining from thickening enough to produce a full menstrual period. Every three months, a woman takes 7 days of inactive pills to produce a "pill period," which may be lighter than a regular period. With Seasonique, women take a very low dose of estrogen for seven days to eliminate any symptoms of complete hormone withdrawal.

The chance of getting pregnant ranges from 5 percent with typical use to 1 percent with perfect use. For maximum effectiveness, each pill should be taken at the same time of day.

Advantages

- Fewer periods.
- Tri-monthly periods are usually lighter, with less blood flow.

Disadvantages

- Similar to those of other oral contraceptives in terms of health risks, costs, and side effects. Cigarette smoking increases these risks.
- No protection from STIs.
- More spotting and breakthrough bleeding than with a 28-day pill.
- Determining pregnancy is difficult without a monthly period.

Lybrel, the "No-Period" Pill Lybrel, described as a continuous contraceptive, works the same way as other combination hormonal birth control pills. However, women take the "365-day" pill every single day without interruption.

How It Works Like other oral contraceptives, Lybrel stops the body's monthly preparation for pregnancy by lowering the production of hormones that make pregnancy possible. However, it does not include the "week-off" of placebo pills that leads to vaginal bleeding. Most women resume menstruation within 90 days of stopping Lybrel.

Medical experts see no long-term risk in doing away with regular monthly periods, but the long-term safety of menstrual suppression is unknown.

Advantages

- No menstrual periods, cramps, or other symptoms.
- No need to stop taking pills or to switch to dummy pills for a week.
- Relief from menstruation-linked conditions such as endometriosis and menstrual migraine.

Disadvantages

- Spotting, which generally tapers off over the first year of use.
- Health risks similar to those of other combination pills.
- Determining pregnancy is difficult without a monthly period.
- Some women feel that eliminating periods is unnatural.

Contraceptive Patch The Ortho Evra birth control patch, the first transdermal (through

the skin) contraceptive, works like a combination pill but looks like a Band-Aid. Embedded in its adhesive layer are two hormones, a low-dose estrogen and a progestin. The contraceptive patch prevents pregnancy by delivering continuous levels of estrogen and progestin through the skin directly into the bloodstream so women are exposed to higher overall levels of estrogen, which may increase their risk of blood clots. The patch is waterproof and stays on in the shower, swimming pool, or hot tub.

How It Works A woman applies the 1¾-inch square to her back, upper arm, lower abdomen, or buttocks and changes it every seven days for three weeks. During the patch-free week, she experiences menstrual bleeding. A user should check every day to make sure the patch is still in place. If you don't replace a detached patch within 24 hours, use a backup method of contraception until your next period.

Advantages

- Good alternative for women who can't. remember, don't like, or have problems swallowing daily pills.
- Highly effective when used correctly.
- Does not interrupt sexual activity.
- Fewer side effects, such as nausea, breakthrough bleeding, and mood swings, than pills.
- Fertility returns quickly after you stop using it.

Disadvantages

- Must apply a new patch every week.
- Requires a prescription.
- No protection against STIs.
- Increases risk of blood clots, heart attack, and stroke, particularly for women who smoke or have certain health conditions. The risk of dying or suffering a survivable blood clot while using the patch is estimated to be about two times higher than with birth control pills. However, an FDA panel has concluded that the patch can be especially useful for younger women and those who have trouble taking a daily pill.
- Less effective in women who weigh more than 198 pounds.
- Some women report breast tenderness, headaches, bleeding between periods, upper respiratory infections, or self-consciousness wearing the patch.
- Contact lens wearers may experience vision changes.

Contraceptive hormones can be delivered through the skin with the patch.

- Five percent of women report that at least one patch slipped off; 2 percent report skin irritation.

- Must use another form of birth control for the initial seven days of use.

Contraceptive Vaginal Ring (CVR)

NuvaRing is a one-month combination hormonal ring. Progering, tested and approved in South America, is a three-month progesterone-releasing ring. Other longer-acting rings are under development.[19]

NuvaRing

The silver-dollar-size NuvaRing, a 2-inch ring made of flexible, transparent plastic, slowly emits the same hormones as oral contraceptives through the vaginal tissues (Figure 10.8). Smaller than the smallest diaphragm, it contains less estrogen than any pill. As effective as the pill, it provides a steady dose of hormones and causes fewer side effects. In a campus-based study, women were equally satisfied with birth control pills and with the vaginal ring, but were more likely to forget to take pills.

How It Works Unlike a diaphragm, the Nuva-Ring does not have to be exactly positioned within the vagina or used with a spermicide. The flexible, plastic 2-inch ring compresses so a woman can easily insert it. Each ring stays in place for three weeks and then is removed for the fourth week of the menstrual cycle.

If a NuvaRing pops out (uncommon but possible), it should be washed, dried, and replaced within three hours. If a longer time passes, users should rely on a backup form of birth control until the ring has been reinserted for a week and the medications have risen to protective levels again.

Advantages

- Under medical supervision, may be safer than birth control pills for women with mild hypertension or diabetes.

- Less likelihood of pill-related side effects, such as nausea, mood swings, spotting, and cramping.

- No need to remember a daily pill or weekly patch.

- Fertility returns quickly when ring is removed.

- Reduced pain during menstrual periods.

- May improve acne and reduce excess body hair.

- Can help prevent menstrual migraines

Disadvantages

- Slight increased risk of blood clots, heart attack, and stroke in women older than 35 who smoke 15 or more cigarettes a day or who have other cardiovascular risk factors.

- Some women do not feel comfortable placing and removing something inside their vagina.

- Possible side effects include vaginal discharge, irritation, infection, headaches, weight gain, and nausea.

- Cannot use oil-based vaginal medications for yeast infections while ring is in place.

- No protection against STIs.

Long-Acting Reversible Contraceptives

Long-acting reversible contraceptives (LARCs), which provide protection from pregnancy for an extended period without any action by users, include intrauterine devices (IUDs), injections, and implants. Their use has jumped five fold in the last decade, particularly among women who have had at least one child and those between ages 25 and 34. More than 7 percent of American women of child-bearing age are using LARCs.[20]

LARCs are cost effective and can save thousands of dollars for users over a five-year period compared to the cost of oral contraceptives and other birth control methods. Another advantage of these methods is that women do not have to remember to take a pill every day or insert a cap or diaphragm prior to sex. However, LARCs do not protect women from sexually transmitted infections.

long-acting reversible contraceptives (LARCs) Contraceptive devices that provide protection from pregnancy for an extended period without any action by users. Examples include intrauterine devices, injections, and implants.

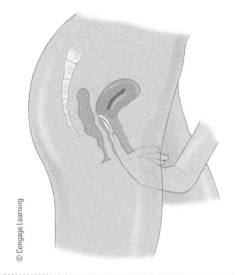
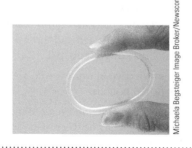

FIGURE 10.8 NuvaRing

The NuvaRing releases estrogen and progestin, preventing ovulation. The exact position of the NuvaRing in the vagina is not critical.

Intrauterine Device (IUD)   An **intrauterine device (IUD)** is a small piece of molded plastic, with a nylon string attached, that is inserted into the uterus through the cervix. It prevents pregnancy by interfering with implantation. Once widely used, IUDs became less popular after most brands were removed from the market because of serious complications such as pelvic infection and infertility.

The ParaGuard IUD, which contains copper, protects against pregnancy for 12 years. As confirmed in a recent study, neither copper IUDs nor those releasing levonorgestrel increase a woman's risk of breast cancer.

The Mirena intrauterine system consists of a T-shaped device inserted in the uterus by a physician. It releases a continuous low dose of progestin and provides five years of protection from pregnancy. Used in Europe, Asia, and Latin America for years, it is 99 percent effective.

Mirena is increasingly being used, not just for contraception, but as an alternative to hysterectomy for extremely heavy menstrual bleeding and as a treatment for problems such as iron-deficiency anemia.

How It Works   A physician must insert the IUD in a woman's uterus. In a five-year clinical trial, about 5 in every 100 women reported that an IUD had slipped out of the uterus. Users should check for the string that extends from the device through the vagina at least once a month.

Advantages

- Highly effective at preventing pregnancy.
- No need to think about contraception for five years.
- Allows sexual spontaneity; neither partner can feel it.
- Starts working immediately.
- New mothers can breast-feed while using it.
- Periods become shorter and lighter or stop altogether.
- Low incidence of side effects.
- Can be removed at any time.

Disadvantages

- Available sizes may be too large for some women, which can cause pain or embedment.[21]
- Spotting or breakthrough bleeding in first three to six months.
- No protection against STIs.
- Potential side effects include acne, headaches, nausea, breast tenderness, mood changes.

- Increased risk of benign ovarian cysts.
- May take up to a year for fertility to return after discontinuation.

Contraceptive Injection   A progestin-only contraceptive is available in the form of a birth control "shot" or injection. Depo-Provera or its newer form, Depo-subQ Provera, must be given every 12 weeks. Contraceptive injections provide no protection against HIV and other STIs.

Because of the risk of significant bone mineral loss, the FDA has recommended that women not use Depo-Provera for longer than two years. Although mineral loss is common and greater in the first year of use, most individuals regain bone density after discontinuing its use.

How It Works   One injection of this synthetic version of the natural hormone progesterone provides three months of contraceptive protection. This long-acting hormonal contraceptive raises levels of progesterone, thereby simulating pregnancy. The pituitary gland doesn't produce FSH and LH, which normally cause egg ripening and release. The endometrial lining of the uterus thins, preventing implantation of a fertilized egg.

Advantages

- Because it contains only progestin, it is safe for women who cannot take combination birth control pills.
- No risk of user error.
- No worry about buying, storing, or using contraceptives.
- No need to think about contraception for three months at a time.
- Possible protection against endometrial and ovarian cancer.
- Can be used by women who are breast-feeding.
- May decrease menstrual migraines.

Disadvantages

- Must visit a doctor or clinic every three months for injection.
- Menstrual cycles become irregular. After a year, 50 percent of women stop having periods.
- Potential side effects include decreased sex drive, depression, headaches, nervousness, dizziness, frequent urination, allergic reactions, hair loss, or increased hair growth.
- Increased weight gain, especially for obese women and teenage girls.
- No protection against STIs.
- May increase the risk of acquiring chlamydia and gonorrhea. compared with women not using a hormonal contraceptive.

intrauterine device (IUD)
A device inserted into the uterus through the cervix to prevent pregnancy by interfering with implantation.

- Delayed return of fertility.

- Long-term use may significantly reduce bone density, particularly for women who smoke, don't get enough calcium, and have never been pregnant.

Contraceptive Implant   This thin, flexible, plastic implant—about the size of a matchstick—is inserted under the skin of the upper arm to provide birth control that is 99 percent effective for up to three years. Easier to insert and remove than earlier implants (Norplant and Jadelle), Implanon has been used in other countries for years and is now available throughout the United States. Nexplanon is a newer version designed for easier insertion and removal.

How It Works Contraceptive implants work primarily by releasing progestin and suppressing ovulation. They also thicken cervical mucus, which inhibits sperm movement, inhibit the development and growth of the uterine lining, and limit secretion of progesterone during the second half of the menstrual cycle.

Advantages

- Can be used while breast-feeding.

- Can be used by women who cannot take estrogen.

- Provides continuous long-lasting birth control without sterilization.

- No medicine to take every day.

- Does not interfere with sexual foreplay.

- Ability to become pregnant returns quickly once implant is removed.

Disadvantages

- Irregular bleeding, especially in the first 6 to 12 months of use. Periods stop completely in one of three women after a year of use.

- Side effects include dizziness, acne, hair loss, headache, nausea, nervousness, pain at the insertion site, and weight gain.

- No protection against STIs.

- Change in appetite.

- Change in sex drive.

- Cysts on the ovaries.

- Depression, mood changes.

- Discoloring or scarring of the skin over the implant.

If implanted during the first five days of a woman's period, a contraceptive implant protects against pregnancy immediately. Otherwise, a woman needs to use some form of backup birth control for the first week after getting the implant.

Fertility Awareness Methods (FAMs)

Awareness of a woman's cyclic fertility can help in both contraception and conception. The different methods of birth control based on a woman's menstrual cycle are sometimes referred to as *natural family planning* or *fertility awareness methods*. New fertility monitors that use saliva to determine time of ovulation can improve the accuracy of these methods. There is no difference in the use of periodic abstinence by religious affiliation, importance of religion, or frequency of attendance at religious services.

Women's menstrual cycles vary greatly. To use one of the fertility awareness methods, a woman must know and understand her cycle. She should track her cycle for at least eight months—marking day one (the day bleeding begins) on a calendar and counting the length of each cycle. Figure 10.9 shows the days in a 28-day cycle

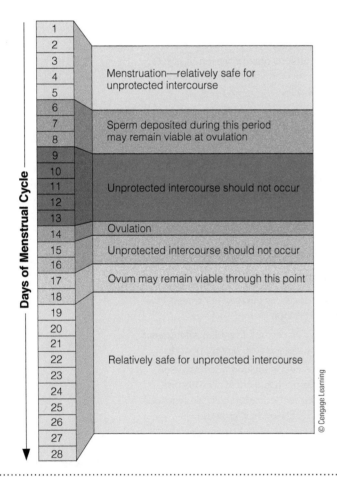

FIGURE 10.9 Safe and Unsafe Days

Events in the menstrual cycle determine the relatively safe days for avoiding pregnancy in unprotected intercourse.

when abstinence or other contraceptive methods would be necessary.

How It Works The calendar method, often called the **rhythm method**, is based on counting the woman's safe days based on her individual menstrual cycle. The basal-body-temperature method determines the safe days based on the woman's *basal body temperature*, which rises after ovulation. The cervical mucus method, also called the *ovulation method*, is based on observation of changes in the consistency of the woman's vaginal mucus throughout her menstrual cycle. The period of maximum fertility occurs when the mucus is smooth and slippery.

Advantages

- No expense.
- No side effects.
- No need for a prescription, medical visit, or fittings.
- Nothing to insert, swallow, or check.
- No effect on fertility.
- Complies with the teachings of the Roman Catholic Church.

Disadvantages

- Less reliable than other forms of birth control.
- Couples must abstain from vaginal intercourse eight to eleven days a month or use some form of contraception.
- Conscientious planning and scheduling are essential.
- May not work for women with irregular menstrual cycles.
- Some women find the mucus or temperature methods difficult to use.

Emergency Contraception

Emergency contraception (EC) is the use of a method of contraception to prevent unintended pregnancy after unprotected intercourse or the failure of another form of contraception, such as a condom breaking or slipping off. EC is available without a prescription. EC has proved extremely safe in almost all women.

The use of emergency contraception has more than doubled in recent years, particularly among women in their early 20s:

- Nearly one in four women between ages 20 and 24 who have ever had sex has used the morning-after pill.

- Among sexually active college women, 14.9 percent report having used emergency contraception in the past year.[22]
- Overall, one in nine sexually experienced women has used emergency contraception, including one in five never-married women, one in seven cohabiting women, and one in twenty currently or formerly married women.
- The most common reasons for using EC are unprotected sex and fear of contraceptive failure.[23]

✓**check-in** Have you or your partner ever used emergency contraception?

Emergency contraception provides a second chance to prevent pregnancy following unprotected sexual intercourse or contraceptive failure. The copper IUD is the most effective method for emergency contraception, but hormonal methods are often considered more convenient and acceptable. An IUD can safely be inserted on the same day it is prescribed without increasing the risk of infection.[24]

The progestin-only pill levonorgestrel, marketed as Plan B, Preven, One Step, or Next Choice, has proved more effective with fewer side effects than combination pills. Plan B morning-after pills are available without a prescription. Plan B, which should be taken within five days (120 hours) of unprotected sex, can reduce the risk of pregnancy up to 89 percent.

Most women can safely use emergency contraception pills (ECPs), even if they cannot use birth control pills as their regular method of birth control. (Although ECPs use the same hormones as birth control pills, not all brands of birth control pills can be used for emergency contraception.) Some women may experience spotting or a full menstrual period a few days after taking ECPs, depending on where they were in their cycle when they began therapy. Most women have their next period at the expected time.

As multiple studies have shown, increased access to EC does not increase sexual risk-taking or lead couples to abandon use of contraceptives.[25]

How It Works ECPs stop pregnancy in the same way as other hormonal contraceptives: They delay or inhibit ovulation, inhibit fertilization, or block implantation of a fertilized egg, depending on a woman's phase of the menstrual cycle.[26] They have no effect once a pregnancy has been established.

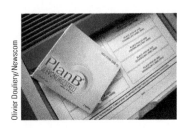

Emergency contraception can prevent unintended pregnancy after unprotected intercourse or when another form of contraception fails.

rhythm method A birth control method in which sexual intercourse is avoided during those days of the menstrual cycle in which fertilization is most likely to occur.

emergency contraception (EC) Types of oral contraceptive pills, usually taken within 72 hours after intercourse, that can prevent pregnancy.

Contraception Choices   **305**

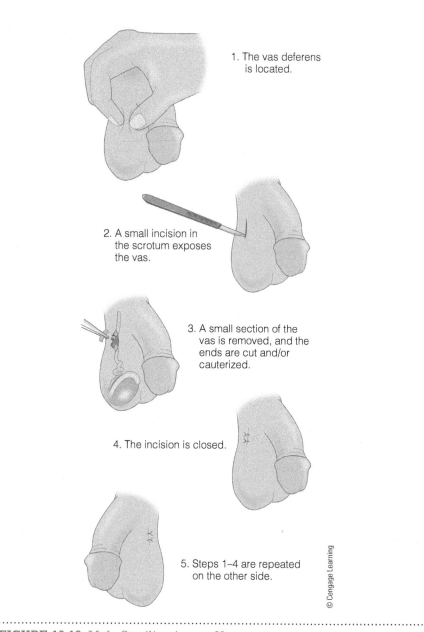

1. The vas deferens is located.

2. A small incision in the scrotum exposes the vas.

3. A small section of the vas is removed, and the ends are cut and/or cauterized.

4. The incision is closed.

5. Steps 1–4 are repeated on the other side.

© Cengage Learning

FIGURE 10.10 Male Sterilization, or Vasectomy

sterilization (surgery to end a person's reproductive capability). Each year an estimated 1 million men and women in the United States undergo sterilization procedures. Fewer than 25 percent ever seek reversal.

....
√**check-in** Would you consider sterilization as a contraceptive option?
....

Male Sterilization In men, the cutting of the vas deferens, the tube that carries sperm from one of the testes into the urethra for ejaculation, is called **vasectomy**. During the 15- or 20-minute office procedure, done under a local anesthetic, the doctor makes small incisions in the scrotum, lifts up each vas deferens, cuts it, and ties off the ends to block the flow of sperm (Figure 10.10). Sperm continue to form, but they are broken down and absorbed by the body.

The man usually experiences some local pain, swelling, and discoloration for about a week after the procedure. More serious complications, including the formation of a blood clot in the scrotum (which usually disappears without treatment), infection, and an inflammatory reaction, occur in a small percentage of cases.

Sometimes men want to reverse their vasectomies, usually because they want to have children with a new spouse. Although anyone who chooses to have a vasectomy should consider it permanent, surgical reversal (*vasovasostomy*), thanks to new microsurgical techniques, can restore fertility in more than 90 percent of vasectomized men, but it may take up to two years for fertility to return after vasectomy reversal.[27]

Female Sterilization Eleven million U.S. women ages 15 to 44 rely on tubal sterilization for contraception. An estimated 750,000 tubal sterilization procedures are performed each year in the United States. The average age of sterilization is about 30. Female sterilization procedures modify the fallopian tubes, which each month normally carry an egg from the ovaries to the uterus.

The two terms used to describe female sterilization are **tubal ligation** (the cutting or tying of the fallopian tubes) and **tubal occlusion** (the blocking of the tubes). The tubes may be cut or sealed with thread, a clamp, or a clip, or by electrical coagulation to prevent the passage of eggs from the ovaries (Figure 10.11). They also can be blocked with bands of silicone.

sterilization A surgical procedure to end a person's reproductive capability.

vasectomy A surgical sterilization procedure in which each vas deferens is cut and tied shut to stop the passage of sperm to the urethra for ejaculation.

tubal ligation The suturing or tying shut of the fallopian tubes to prevent pregnancy.

tubal occlusion The blocking of the fallopian tubes to prevent pregnancy.

ECPs may be moderately effective even if started between the third and fifth days (up to 120 hours) after unprotected sexual intercourse or contraceptive failure.

The morning-after pill also may be safe for use as a regular birth control method and may appeal to women who do not have sex regularly and who could use it before or after sex. However, it is not as effective as regular birth control pills, patches, or rings. The most common side effect is irregular bleeding.

Sterilization

The most popular method of birth control among married couples in the United States is

when abstinence or other contraceptive methods would be necessary.

How It Works The calendar method, often called the **rhythm method**, is based on counting the woman's safe days based on her individual menstrual cycle. The basal-body-temperature method determines the safe days based on the woman's *basal body temperature*, which rises after ovulation. The cervical mucus method, also called the *ovulation method*, is based on observation of changes in the consistency of the woman's vaginal mucus throughout her menstrual cycle. The period of maximum fertility occurs when the mucus is smooth and slippery.

Advantages

- No expense.
- No side effects.
- No need for a prescription, medical visit, or fittings.
- Nothing to insert, swallow, or check.
- No effect on fertility.
- Complies with the teachings of the Roman Catholic Church.

Disadvantages

- Less reliable than other forms of birth control.
- Couples must abstain from vaginal intercourse eight to eleven days a month or use some form of contraception.
- Conscientious planning and scheduling are essential.
- May not work for women with irregular menstrual cycles.
- Some women find the mucus or temperature methods difficult to use.

Emergency Contraception

Emergency contraception (EC) is the use of a method of contraception to prevent unintended pregnancy after unprotected intercourse or the failure of another form of contraception, such as a condom breaking or slipping off. EC is available without a prescription. EC has proved extremely safe in almost all women.

The use of emergency contraception has more than doubled in recent years, particularly among women in their early 20s:

- Nearly one in four women between ages 20 and 24 who have ever had sex has used the morning-after pill.

- Among sexually active college women, 14.9 percent report having used emergency contraception in the past year.[22]
- Overall, one in nine sexually experienced women has used emergency contraception, including one in five never-married women, one in seven cohabiting women, and one in twenty currently or formerly married women.
- The most common reasons for using EC are unprotected sex and fear of contraceptive failure.[23]

✓**check-in** Have you or your partner ever used emergency contraception?

Emergency contraception provides a second chance to prevent pregnancy following unprotected sexual intercourse or contraceptive failure. The copper IUD is the most effective method for emergency contraception, but hormonal methods are often considered more convenient and acceptable. An IUD can safely be inserted on the same day it is prescribed without increasing the risk of infection.[24]

The progestin-only pill levonorgestrel, marketed as Plan B, Preven, One Step, or Next Choice, has proved more effective with fewer side effects than combination pills. Plan B morning-after pills are available without a prescription. Plan B, which should be taken within five days (120 hours) of unprotected sex, can reduce the risk of pregnancy up to 89 percent.

Most women can safely use emergency contraception pills (ECPs), even if they cannot use birth control pills as their regular method of birth control. (Although ECPs use the same hormones as birth control pills, not all brands of birth control pills can be used for emergency contraception.) Some women may experience spotting or a full menstrual period a few days after taking ECPs, depending on where they were in their cycle when they began therapy. Most women have their next period at the expected time.

As multiple studies have shown, increased access to EC does not increase sexual risk-taking or lead couples to abandon use of contraceptives.[25]

How It Works ECPs stop pregnancy in the same way as other hormonal contraceptives: They delay or inhibit ovulation, inhibit fertilization, or block implantation of a fertilized egg, depending on a woman's phase of the menstrual cycle.[26] They have no effect once a pregnancy has been established.

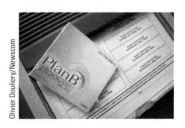
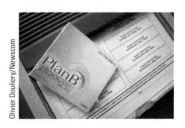Olivier Douliery/Newscom

Emergency contraception can prevent unintended pregnancy after unprotected intercourse or when another form of contraception fails.

rhythm method A birth control method in which sexual intercourse is avoided during those days of the menstrual cycle in which fertilization is most likely to occur.

emergency contraception (EC) Types of oral contraceptive pills, usually taken within 72 hours after intercourse, that can prevent pregnancy.

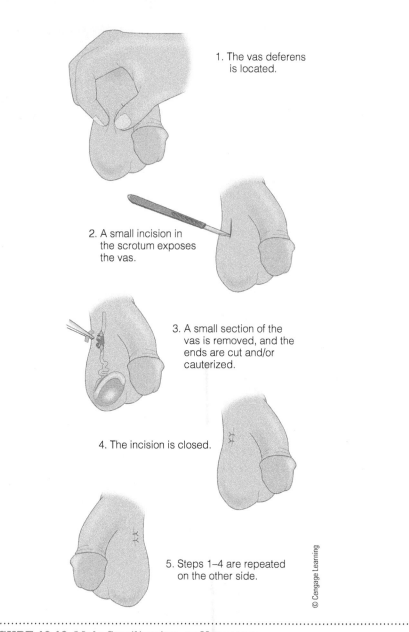

1. The vas deferens is located.

2. A small incision in the scrotum exposes the vas.

3. A small section of the vas is removed, and the ends are cut and/or cauterized.

4. The incision is closed.

5. Steps 1–4 are repeated on the other side.

© Cengage Learning

FIGURE 10.10 Male Sterilization, or Vasectomy

sterilization A surgical procedure to end a person's reproductive capability.

vasectomy A surgical sterilization procedure in which each vas deferens is cut and tied shut to stop the passage of sperm to the urethra for ejaculation.

tubal ligation The suturing or tying shut of the fallopian tubes to prevent pregnancy.

tubal occlusion The blocking of the fallopian tubes to prevent pregnancy.

ECPs may be moderately effective even if started between the third and fifth days (up to 120 hours) after unprotected sexual intercourse or contraceptive failure.

The morning-after pill also may be safe for use as a regular birth control method and may appeal to women who do not have sex regularly and who could use it before or after sex. However, it is not as effective as regular birth control pills, patches, or rings. The most common side effect is irregular bleeding.

Sterilization

The most popular method of birth control among married couples in the United States is sterilization (surgery to end a person's reproductive capability). Each year an estimated 1 million men and women in the United States undergo sterilization procedures. Fewer than 25 percent ever seek reversal.

√ **check-in** Would you consider sterilization as a contraceptive option?

Male Sterilization In men, the cutting of the vas deferens, the tube that carries sperm from one of the testes into the urethra for ejaculation, is called **vasectomy**. During the 15- or 20-minute office procedure, done under a local anesthetic, the doctor makes small incisions in the scrotum, lifts up each vas deferens, cuts it, and ties off the ends to block the flow of sperm (Figure 10.10). Sperm continue to form, but they are broken down and absorbed by the body.

The man usually experiences some local pain, swelling, and discoloration for about a week after the procedure. More serious complications, including the formation of a blood clot in the scrotum (which usually disappears without treatment), infection, and an inflammatory reaction, occur in a small percentage of cases.

Sometimes men want to reverse their vasectomies, usually because they want to have children with a new spouse. Although anyone who chooses to have a vasectomy should consider it permanent, surgical reversal (*vasovasostomy*), thanks to new microsurgical techniques, can restore fertility in more than 90 percent of vasectomized men, but it may take up to two years for fertility to return after vasectomy reversal.[27]

Female Sterilization Eleven million U.S. women ages 15 to 44 rely on tubal sterilization for contraception. An estimated 750,000 tubal sterilization procedures are performed each year in the United States. The average age of sterilization is about 30. Female sterilization procedures modify the fallopian tubes, which each month normally carry an egg from the ovaries to the uterus.

The two terms used to describe female sterilization are **tubal ligation** (the cutting or tying of the fallopian tubes) and **tubal occlusion** (the blocking of the tubes). The tubes may be cut or sealed with thread, a clamp, or a clip, or by electrical coagulation to prevent the passage of eggs from the ovaries (Figure 10.11). They also can be blocked with bands of silicone.

One of the common methods of tubal ligation or occlusion uses **laparoscopy**, commonly called *belly-button surgery* or *band-aid surgery*. This procedure is done on an outpatient basis and takes 15 to 30 minutes. A lighted tube called a laparoscope is inserted through a half-inch incision made right below the navel, giving the doctor a view of the fallopian tubes. Using surgical instruments that may be inserted through the laparoscope or through other tiny incisions, the doctor then cuts or seals the tubes, most commonly by electrical coagulation.

The cumulative failure rate of tubal sterilization is about 1.85 percent during a ten-year period. Complications include problems with anesthesia, hemorrhage, organ damage, and mortality.

Essure Essure involves placement of small, flexible microcoils into the fallopian tubes via the vagina by a physician. Unlike other methods, it does not require the risks of general anesthesia and surgery. The procedure itself does not require incisions and takes an average of about 35 minutes. Recovery occurs quickly; most women resume normal activities within 24 hours. For the first three months after insertion, women should use another form of contraception. An X-ray called a hysterosalpingogram must confirm that the inserts are correctly placed and the fallopian tubes are completely blocked.

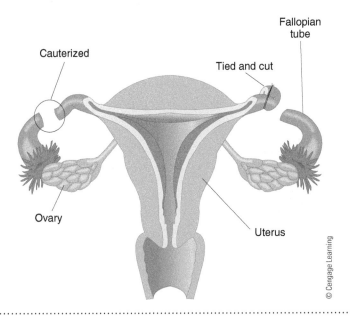

FIGURE 10.11 Female Sterilization, or Tubal Ligation

- Must use another form of birth control for first three months.
- Many long-term risks remain unknown, but there is no evidence of any link between vasectomy and prostate cancer.

Advantages

- Offers permanent protection against unwanted pregnancy.
- No effect on sex drive in men or women. Many couples report greater sexual activity and pleasure because they no longer have to worry about pregnancy or deal with contraceptives.
- Vasectomy and tubal ligation are performed as outpatient procedures, with a quick recovery time.
- Use of Essure requires no incision, so there's less discomfort and very rapid recovery. Essure may be an option for women with chronic health conditions, such as obesity, diabetes, or heart disease.

Disadvantages

- All procedures should be considered permanent and used only if both partners are certain they want no more children.
- No protection against STIs.

When Pregnancy Occurs

Unwanted Pregnancy

A woman faced with an unwanted pregnancy—often alone, unwed, and desperate—can find it extremely difficult to decide what to do. The political debate over the right to life almost always is secondary to practical and emotional matters, such as the quality of her relationship with the baby's father, their capacity to provide for the child, the impact on any children she already has, her age and health, and other important life issues.

Giving up the child for adoption is an option for women who do not feel abortion is right for them. Because the number of would-be adoptive parents greatly exceeds the number of available newborns, some women considering adoption may feel pressured by offers of money from couples eager to adopt. Others, particularly minority women, may feel cultural pressures to keep a child—regardless of their

laparoscopy A surgical sterilization procedure in which the fallopian tubes are observed with a laparoscope inserted through a small incision, and then cut or blocked.

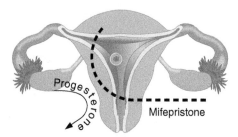

Step 1. Taken early in pregnancy, mifepristone blocks the action of progesterone and makes the body react as if it weren't pregnant.

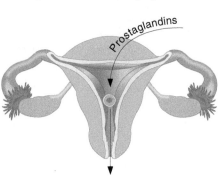

Step 2. Prostaglandins, taken two days later, cause the uterus to contract and the cervix to soften and dilate. As a result, the fertilized egg is expelled in 97 percent of cases.

© Cengage Learning

FIGURE 10.12 Medical Abortion

Mifepristone works by blocking the action of progesterone, a hormone produced by the ovaries that is necessary for the implantation and development of a fertilized egg.

age, economic situation, or ability to care for an infant.

Advocates of adoption reform are pressing for mandatory counseling for all pregnant women considering adoption (available now in agency-arranged, but not private, adoptions) and for extending the period of time during which a new mother can change her mind about giving up her child for adoption. (See the discussion of adoption on page 316.)

✓**check-in** Which alternatives would you consider if faced with an unplanned pregnancy?

medical abortion Method of ending a pregnancy within nine weeks of conception using hormonal medications that cause expulsion of the fertilized egg.

suction curettage A procedure in which the contents of the uterus are removed by means of suction and scraping.

Abortion

An *abortion* is a procedure that uses medicine or surgery to end a pregnancy. The number and rates of elective abortions have been declining since 2002 to all-time lows. About 730,000 elective abortions are performed every year—13.9 per 1,000 women ages 15 to 44.[28]

Women in their twenties account for the majority of abortions. Most take place early in gestation: nine in ten at less than 13 weeks' gestation and just 1 percent at 21 weeks' gestation. The complication rate for abortions is 2.1 percent, ranging from 1.3 percent for first-trimester aspiration abortions to 5.2 percent for medical abortions.[29]

Researchers have linked domestic violence with a greater likelihood of abortion.[30]

Claims that abortion increases the risk of breast cancer, based on retrospective studies that are less accurate because they rely on individuals' recall, have proved false. Research has found no correlation between the termination of a pregnancy, whether induced or spontaneous, and increased risk of breast cancer.

Medical Abortion The term **medical abortion** describes the use of drugs, also called *abortifacients*, to terminate a pregnancy. The abortion pill mifepristone (*Mifeprex*), formerly known as RU-486, is 97 percent effective in inducing abortion by blocking progesterone, the hormone that prepares the uterine lining for pregnancy. Two days after taking this compound, a woman takes a prostaglandin to increase uterine contractions. The uterine lining is expelled, along with the fertilized egg (Figure 10.12). Medical abortion accounts for about one in five abortions.

Women have compared the discomfort of this experience to severe menstrual cramps. Common side effects include excessive bleeding, nausea, fatigue, abdominal pain, and dizziness. About 1 woman in 100 requires a blood transfusion. The Food and Drug Administration has warned doctors about rare but deadly bloodstream infections in women using mifepristone. The rate of infection is about 1 in 100,000 uses, comparable to infection risks with surgical abortions and childbirth.

Medical abortion does not require anesthesia and can be performed very early in pregnancy. However, women experience more cramping and bleeding during medical abortion than during surgical abortion, and bleeding lasts for a longer period.

Other Abortion Methods About three-fourths of abortions performed in the United States today are surgical.[31] **Suction curettage**, usually done from 7 to 13 weeks after the last menstrual period, involves the gradual dilation (opening) of the cervix, often by inserting into the cervix one or more sticks of *laminaria* (a sterilized seaweed that absorbs moisture and expands, thus gradually stretching the cervix).

Some women feel pressure or cramping with the laminaria in place. Occasionally, the laminaria itself starts to bring on a miscarriage.

At the time of abortion, the laminaria is removed, and dilators are used to further enlarge the cervical opening, if needed. The physician inserts a suction tip into the cervix, and the uterine contents are drawn out via a vacuum system (Figure 10.13). A *curette* (a spoon-shaped surgical instrument used for scraping) is used to check for complete removal of the contents of the uterus. With suction curettage, the risks of complication are low. Major complications, such as perforation of the uterus, occur in fewer than 1 in 100 cases.

The Psychological Impact of Abortion

Abortion can have various psychological effects. As decades of research have shown, the primary emotion of women who have just had an abortion is relief. Although many women also express feelings of guilt or sadness, usually their anxiety levels drop to lower levels than immediately before the abortion.

Women who experienced violence, including rape, or high anxiety levels prior to becoming pregnant have more anxiety symptoms following an abortion. The best predictor of psychological well-being after abortion is a woman's emotional well-being prior to pregnancy. At highest risk are women who have had a psychiatric illness, such as an anxiety disorder or clinical depression, prior to an abortion, and those whose abortions occurred among complicated circumstances (such as a rape, or coercion by parents or a partner).

The vast majority of women manage to put the abortion into perspective as one of many life events.

In a two-year follow-up, women who underwent abortions had similar or lower levels of depression and anxiety than those who sought but were denied abortion. This finding, according to the researchers, refutes "the notion that abortion is a cause of mental health problems."[32]

The Politics of Abortion
Abortion is one of the most controversial political, religious, and ethical issues of our time. The issues of when life begins, a woman's right to choose, and an unborn child's right to survival are among the most divisive Americans face. Here is some background:

- Abortions were legal in the United States until the 1860s.

- For decades after that, women who decided to terminate unwanted pregnancies did so by attempting to abort on their own or by obtaining illegal abortions—often performed

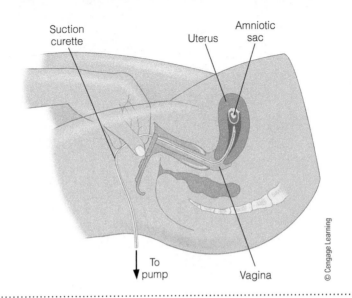

FIGURE 10.13 Suction Curettage

The contents of the uterus are extracted through the cervix with a vacuum apparatus.

by untrained individuals using unsanitary and unsafe procedures.

- In the late 1960s, some states changed their laws to make abortions legal.

- In 1973, the U.S. Supreme Court, following a 1970 ruling on the case of *Roe v. Wade* by the New York Supreme Court, said that an abortion in the first trimester of pregnancy was a decision between a woman and her physician and was protected by privacy laws.

- The court further ruled that abortion during the second trimester could be performed on the basis of health risks and that abortion during the final trimester could be performed only for the sake of the mother's health.

- The controversy over abortion has at times become violent: Physicians who perform abortions have been shot and killed; abortion clinics have been bombed, wounding and killing patients and staff members.

- The Supreme Court has upheld a federal law banning "partial-birth" abortions, a late-term procedure involving the removal of a fetus from the uterus and the collapsing of its skull. Pro-life groups hailed this ruling as a step toward the overthrow of *Roe v. Wade*.

- The debate over abortion continues to stir passionate emotions, with pro-life supporters arguing that life begins at conception and that abortion is therefore immoral, and pro-choice advocates countering that an individual woman should have the right to make decisions about her body and health.

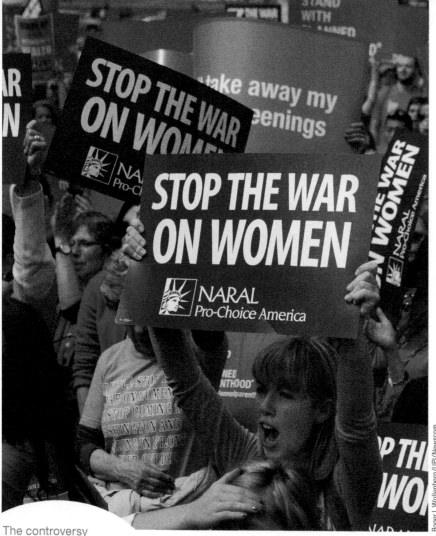

The controversy over abortion has triggered countless demonstrations and encounters between pro-choice and pro-life supporters.

24 weeks; others have no time limit. In recent years abortion has become more restrictive in terms of limits on timing, grounds, or methods in the United States, Russia, Hungary, and Poland.

Nicaragua and El Salvador have banned the practice outright. Romania has the world's highest abortion rate; three in four pregnancies are terminated. In the United States, Australia, Canada, Great Britain, and most of Western Europe, around 15 to 25 percent of pregnancies end in abortion.

Pregnancy

Pregnancy and birthrates in the United States have declined to the lowest rate ever recorded: 62.5 births per 1,000 women. According to the most recent statistics, total annual births number 3,932,181. Mothers' mean age at first birth is 26 year; 50.6 percent are unmarried.[34]

Pregnancy rates have fallen for women in their teens and 20s, while they have increased for women in their 30s. Despite a decline, the United States continues to have the highest teenage pregnancy rate in the developed word.[35]

Preconception Care The time *before* a child is conceived can be crucial in ensuring that an infant is born healthy, full-size, and full-term. The best chance for lowering the infant mortality rate and preventing birth defects is before pregnancy. **Preconception care**—the enhancement of a woman's health and well-being prior to conception in order to ensure a healthy pregnancy and baby—includes the following:

- Risk assessment (evaluation of medical, genetic, and lifestyle risks)

- Health promotion (such as teaching good nutrition)

- Interventions to reduce risk (such as treatment of infections and other diseases, assistance in quitting smoking or drug use, taking folic acid supplements to prevent pregnancy)

Home Pregnancy Tests Home pregnancy tests detect the presence of human chorionic gonadotropin (hCG), which is secreted as the fertilized egg implants in the uterus. If the concentration of hCG is high enough, a woman will test positive for pregnancy. If the test is done too early, the result will be a false negative. A follow-up test a week later can usually confirm a pregnancy. Although home pregnancy tests are 85 to 95 percent accurate, medical laboratory tests provide definitive confirmation of a pregnancy.

Although the majority of Americans continue to support abortion, many feel that it should be more restricted and difficult to obtain. Some states have required women to view ultrasounds, imposed waiting periods, cut funding for clinics, or banned abortions after 20 weeks.

As a result, the number of medical centers providing abortions has decreased, making it particularly difficult for low-income women to obtain abortions.[33]

✓**check-in** How do you view the politics of abortion?

A Cross-Cultural Perspective More than one in four pregnancies worldwide ends in abortion. Of the estimated 46 million global abortions, an estimated 20 million are illegal and lead to the death of about 70,000 women.

More than 50 countries now allow abortion up to at least the twelfth week of pregnancy. Some, such as Great Britain, permit it up to

preconception care Health care to prepare for pregnancy.

Prenatal Care   From the moment she learns she is pregnant, a woman must assume responsibility for the new life growing inside her. Fortunately, the same habits that maintain her good health also enhance her baby's well-being. These include a healthy diet, exercise, and avoidance of smoking and alcohol.

A Healthy Diet   Doctors have long recommended a well-balanced diet that provides a complete variety of key nutrients.[36] In addition, pregnant women should

- Make sure they are getting an adequate level of folic acid in order to prevent neural tube defects.

- Avoid soft unpasteurized cheeses to prevent Listeria infections, which can be harmful to a fetus.

- Eat a diet rich in fruit and vegetables, which provides an additional benefit: a lower risk of premature birth.[37]

- Increase their caloric intake to ensure adequate nutrition for the fetus but not put on so much weight that it increases the risks to their own health and their baby's.[38]

- Not avoid any specific foods unless they are allergic to them. Recent research suggests that eating nuts during pregnancy lowers a child's risk of having a nut allergy—as long as the mother is not allergic herself.[39]

Exercise   The proven benefits of light to moderate exercise during pregnancy include a greater sense of well-being, enhanced mood, shorter labor, fewer obstetric complications, and healthier infant birth weights.[40]

However, women should not exercise more strenuously than they did before pregnancy and should consult their doctors about any precautions they should take, particularly if working out on hot or smoggy days. They should also avoid certain high-risk activities, such as water-skiing, scuba diving, or contact sports.

Avoid Smoking and Smoke   As discussed in Chapter 14, smoking during pregnancy can put a growing fetus in jeopardy. Women who ever smoked during their reproductive years also are at risk for miscarriage, ectopic pregnancy, and still-births. According to a 40-year longitudinal study, the daughters of women who smoked while pregnant may be at higher risk for nicotine dependence.[41] Exposure to secondhand smoke puts a woman and her unborn child in jeopardy; the risk increased with the duration of her exposure.[42]

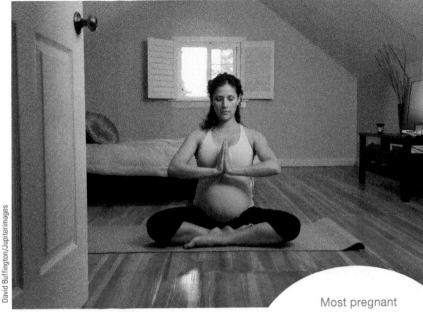

David Buffington/Jupiterimages

Most pregnant women benefit from mind-body practices and regular moderate exercise.

Don't Use Alcohol or Drugs   Alcohol, discussed in Chapter 13, and illegal drugs, discussed in Chapter 12, are clear threats to an unborn child.[43] However, even some common prescription drugs, such as acetaminophen[44] and antidepressants, can pose short- and long-term risks. A pregnant woman should discuss any medication with her doctor to weigh the risks and benefits. Recent research has shown that the widely used painkillers known as nonsteroidal anti-inflammatory drugs (NSAIDS) do not increase the risk of miscarriage.[45]

How a Woman's Body Changes during Pregnancy   The 40 weeks of pregnancy, divided into three-month periods called trimesters, transform a woman's body:

- At the beginning of pregnancy, the woman's uterus becomes slightly larger, and the cervix becomes softer and bluish due to increased blood flow.

- Progesterone and estrogen trigger changes in the milk glands and ducts in the breasts, which increase in size and feel somewhat tender.

- The pressure of the growing uterus against the bladder causes a more frequent need to urinate.

- As the pregnancy progresses, the woman's skin stretches as her body shape changes, her center of gravity changes as her abdomen protrudes, and her internal organs shift as the baby grows (Figure 10.14).

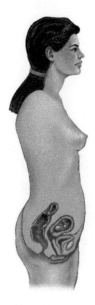
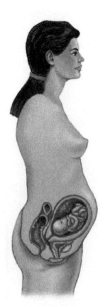
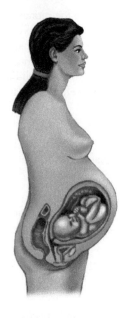

© Cengage Learning

First Trimester

Increased urination because of hormonal
  changes and the pressure of the enlarging
  uterus on the bladder.
Enlarged breasts as milk glands develop.
Darkening of the nipples and the area around them.
Nausea or vomiting, particularly in the morning,
  may occur.
Fatigue.
Increased vaginal secretions.
Pinching of the sciatic nerve, which runs from
  the buttocks down through the back of the legs,
  may occur as the pelvic bones widen and begin
  to separate.

Second Trimester

Thickening of the waist as the
  uterus grows.
Weight gain.
Increase in total blood volume.
Slight increase in size and change
  in position of the heart.
Darkening of the pigment around
  the nipple and from the navel to the pubic region.
Darkening of the face.
Increased salivation and perspiration.
Secretion of colostrum from the breasts.

Third Trimester

Increased urination because of
  pressure from the uterus.
Tightening of the uterine muscles
  (called Braxton-Hicks
  contractions).
Shortness of breath because of
  increased pressure by the uterus
  on the lungs and diaphragm.
Interrupted sleep because of the
  baby's movements or the need to urinate.
Descending ("dropping") of the baby's
  head into the pelvis about two to
  four weeks before birth.
Navel pushed out.

FIGURE 10.14 Physiological Changes of Pregnancy

embryo An organism in its early stage of development; in humans, the embryonic period lasts from the second to the eighth week of pregnancy.

amnion The innermost membrane of the sac enclosing the embryo or fetus.

fetus The human organism developing in the uterus from the ninth week until birth.

placenta An organ that develops after implantation and to which the embryo attaches, via the umbilical cord, for nourishment and waste removal.

ectopic pregnancy A pregnancy in which the fertilized egg has implanted itself outside the uterine cavity, usually in the fallopian tube.

How a Baby Grows   Silently and invisibly, over a nine-month period, a fertilized egg develops into a human being:

• When the zygote reaches the uterus, it's still smaller than the head of a pin.

• Once nestled into the spongy uterine lining, it becomes an **embryo**.

• The embryo takes on an elongated shape, rounded at one end. A sac called the **amnion** envelops it (see photo in Figure 10.15).

• As water and other small molecules cross the amniotic membrane, the embryo floats freely in the absorbed fluid, cushioned from shocks and bumps.

• At nine weeks the embryo is called a **fetus**.

• A special organ, the **placenta**, forms. Attached to the embryo by the umbilical cord, it supplies the growing baby with fluid and nutrients from the maternal bloodstream and carries waste back to the mother's body for disposal (Figure 10.15).

Complications of Pregnancy   In about 10 to 15 percent of all pregnancies, there is increased risk of some problem, such as a baby's failure to grow normally. The mother-to-be can also be at risk. Pregnancy-related mortality rates have risen in recent years to 16 deaths per 100,000 live births. The danger increases with age and varies with race, with Hispanic black women at the greatest risk.[46] *Perinatology*, or maternal-fetal medicine, focuses on the special needs of high-risk mothers and their unborn babies, including the following potential complications:

Ectopic Pregnancy   Any woman who is of childbearing age, has had intercourse, and feels abdominal pain with no reasonable cause may have an **ectopic pregnancy**, in which the fertilized egg remains in the fallopian tube instead of traveling to the uterus. Ectopic, or tubal, pregnancies have increased dramatically in recent years, now accounting for 2 percent of all reported pregnancies. Risk factors include chlamydia

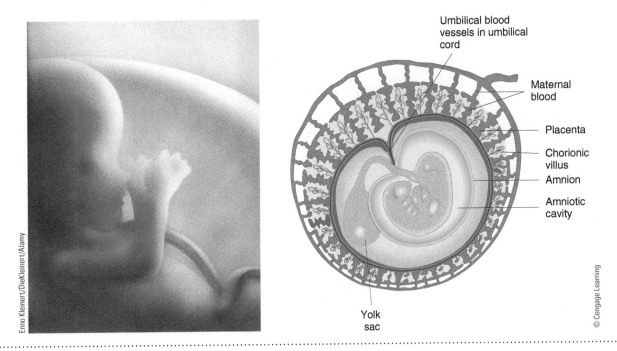

Umbilical blood
vessels in umbilical
cord

Maternal
blood

Placenta

Chorionic
villus

Amnion

Amniotic
cavity

Yolk
sac

Enno Kleinert/DieKleinert/Alamy

© Cengage Learning

FIGURE 10.15 The Placenta

The placenta supplies the growing embryo with fluid and nutrients from the maternal bloodstream and carries waste back for disposal.

(Chapter 11); previous pelvic surgery, particularly involving the fallopian tubes; pelvic inflammatory disease; infertility; and use of an IUD.

Miscarriage   About 10 to 20 percent of pregnancies end in **miscarriage**, or spontaneous abortion, before the twentieth week of gestation. Major genetic disorders may be responsible for 33 to 50 percent of pregnancy losses. The most common cause is an abnormal number of chromosomes. An estimated 70 to 90 percent of women who miscarry eventually become pregnant again.

Infections   The infectious disease most clearly linked to birth defects is **rubella** (German measles). All women should be vaccinated against this disease at least three months prior to conception to protect themselves and any children they may bear. The most common prenatal infection today is *cytomegalovirus*, which produces mild flu-like symptoms in adults but can cause brain damage, retardation, liver disease, cerebral palsy, hearing problems, and other malformations in unborn babies. STIs, such as syphilis, gonorrhea, and genital herpes, can be particularly dangerous during pregnancy if not recognized and treated.

Genetic Disorders   Every individual has an estimated four to six defective genes, but the chances of passing them on to a child are slim. Almost all are recessive, which means they are "masked" by a more influential dominant gene. The likelihood of a child inheriting the same faulty recessive gene from both parents is remote—unless the parents are so closely related that they have very similar genetic makeup.

The child of a parent with an abnormal dominant gene has a 50 percent likelihood of inheriting it. The most common of such defects are minor, such as the growth of an extra finger or toe. However, some single-gene defects can be fatal. Huntington's chorea, for example, is a degenerative disease that in the past was usually not diagnosed until midlife.

A mother's age has long been associated with increased risk of chromosomal disorders such as Down syndrome. More recently, research has linked a father's age of 45 or older to several neuro-psychiatric disorders, including autism spectrum disorder, attention-deficit/hyperactivity disorder, psychosis, bipolar disorders, and substance use problems.[47]

Premature Labor   Approximately 8 percent of all babies are born too soon (before the thirty-seventh week of pregnancy).[48] Prematurity is the main underlying cause of stillbirth and infant deaths within the first few weeks after birth. Bed rest, close monitoring, and, if necessary, medications for at-risk women can buy more time in the womb for their babies. The warning signs of **premature labor** include a dull, low backache; a feeling of tightness or pressure on the lower abdomen; and intestinal cramps, sometimes with diarrhea.

miscarriage A pregnancy that terminates before the twentieth week of gestation; also called spontaneous abortion.

rubella An infectious disease that may cause birth defects if contracted by a pregnant woman; also called German measles.

premature labor Labor that occurs after the twentieth week but before the thirty-seventh week of pregnancy.

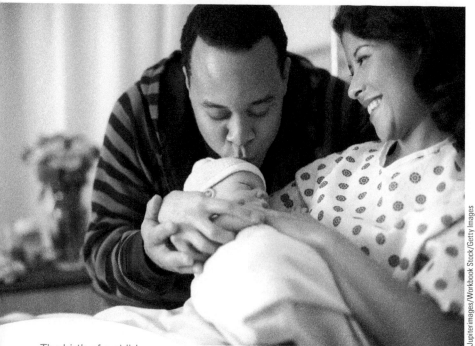

The birth of a child marks a new chapter in the life of a family.

Jupiterimages/Workbook Stock/Getty Images

Childbirth

Today parents can choose from many birthing options, including a birth attendant, who can be a physician or a nurse-midwife, and a birthing center, hospital, or home birth.

Preparing for Childbirth

Women who attend prenatal classes are less likely than others to undergo caesarean deliveries and more likely than others to breast-feed. They also tend to have fewer complications and require fewer medications. However, painkillers or anesthesia are always an option if labor is longer or more painful than expected. The lower body can be numbed with an *epidural block*, which involves injecting an anesthetic into the membrane around the spinal cord, or a spinal block, in which the injection goes directly into the spinal canal. General anesthesia is usually used only for emergency caesarean births.

Labor and Delivery

There are three stages of **labor**. The first starts with *effacement* (thinning) and *dilation* (opening up) of the cervix:

- Effacement is measured in percentages, and dilation in centimeters or finger-widths. Around this time, the amniotic sac of fluids usually breaks, a sign that the woman should call her doctor or midwife.

- The first contractions of the early, or *latent*, phase of labor are usually not uncomfortable; they last 15 to 30 seconds, occur every 15 to 30 minutes, and gradually increase in intensity and frequency.

- The most difficult contractions come after the cervix is dilated to about 8 centimeters, as the woman feels greater pressure from the fetus. The first stage ends when the cervix is completely dilated to a diameter of 10 centimeters (or five finger-widths) and the baby is ready to come down the birth canal. For women having their first baby, this first stage of labor averages 12 to 13 hours. Women having another child often experience shorter first-stage labor.

When the cervix is completely dilated, the second stage of labor occurs:

- The baby moves into the vagina, or birth canal, and out of the mother's body.

- As this stage begins, women who have gone through childbirth preparation training often feel a sense of relief from the acute pain of the transition phase and at the prospect of giving birth.

This second stage can take up to an hour or more. Strong contractions may last 60 to 90 seconds and occur every two to three minutes. As the baby's head descends, the mother feels an urge to push. By bearing down, she helps the baby complete its passage to the outside:

- As the baby's head appears, or *crowns*, the doctor may perform an *episiotomy*—an incision from the lower end of the vagina toward the anus to enlarge the vaginal opening. The purpose of the episiotomy is to prevent the baby's head from causing an irregular tear in the vagina, but routine episiotomies have been criticized as unnecessary.

- Usually the baby's head emerges first, then its shoulders, then its body. With each contraction, a new part is born. However, the baby can be in a more difficult position, facing up rather than down, or with the feet or buttocks first (a *breech birth*), and a caesarean birth may then be necessary.

In the third stage of labor, the uterus contracts firmly after the birth of the baby:

- Within about five minutes, the placenta separates from the uterine wall.

- The woman may bear down to help expel the placenta, or the doctor may exert gentle external pressure.

- If an episiotomy has been performed, the doctor sews up the incision. To help the uterus contract and return to its normal size, it may be massaged manually, or the baby may be put to the mother's breast to stimulate contraction of the uterus.

labor The process leading up to birth: effacement and dilation of the cervix; the movement of the baby into and through the birth canal, accompanied by strong contractions; and contraction of the uterus and expulsion of the placenta after the birth.

Caesarean Birth In a **caesarean delivery** (also referred to as a *caesarean section*, or *C-section*), the doctor lifts the baby out of the woman's body through an incision made in the lower abdomen and uterus. The most common reason for caesarean birth is *failure to progress*, a vague term indicating that labor has gone on too long and may put the baby or mother at risk. Other reasons include the baby's position (if feet or buttocks are first) and signs that the fetus is in danger.

Nearly one in three babies is delivered by this method, many in women who had a previous C-section. More than 95 percent are performed because of risk factors complicating labor or delivery.

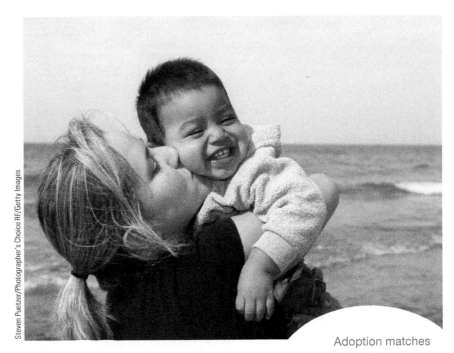

Steven Puetzer/Photographer's Choice RF/Getty Images

Other Conditions or Choices

Adoption matches would-be parents yearning for youngsters to love with infants or children who need loving homes.

Infertility

The World Health Organization defines **infertility** as the failure to conceive after one year of unprotected intercourse. Infertility affects one in six couples in the United States. Women between ages 35 and 44 are about twice as likely to have fertility problems as women ages 30 to 34.

Infertility is a problem of the couple, not of the individual man or woman. In 40 percent of cases, infertility is caused by female problems, in 40 percent by male problems, in 10 percent by a combination of male and female problems, and in 10 percent by unexplained causes.

In women, the most common causes of subfertility or infertility are age, abnormal menstrual patterns, suppression of ovulation, and blocked fallopian tubes. A woman's fertility peaks between ages 20 and 30 and then drops quickly: by 20 percent after 30, by 50 percent after 35, and by 95 percent after 40.

Male subfertility or infertility is usually linked to either the quantity or the quality of sperm, which may be inactive, misshapen, or insufficient (fewer than 20 million sperm per milliliter of semen in an ejaculation of 3 to 5 milliliters). Sometimes the problem is hormonal or a blockage of a sperm duct. Some men suffer from the inability to ejaculate normally, or from retrograde ejaculation, in which some of the semen travels in the wrong direction, back into the body of the male. Lifestyle factors, such as smoking, may also impair fertility.[49]

Infertility can have an enormous emotional impact. Many women long to experience pregnancy and childbirth and feel great loss if they cannot conceive. Women in their 30s and 40s fear that their biological clock is running out of time. Men may be confused and surprised by the intensity of their partner's emotions.

Options for Infertile Couples The odds of successful pregnancy range from 30 to 70 percent, depending on the specific cause of infertility. One result of successful infertility treatments has been a boom in multiple births, including quintuplets and sextuplets.

Artificial Insemination **Artificial insemination**—the introduction of viable sperm into the vagina by artificial means—is used primarily by couples in which the husband is infertile.

Assisted Reproductive Technology
An estimated 500,000 babies have been born in the United States through assisted reproductive technology (ART) since 1985. The most common ART procedure is *in vitro fertilization* (IVF), which removes the ova from a woman's ovary and places the woman's egg and her mate's sperm in a laboratory dish for fertilization. If the fertilized egg cell shows signs of development, within several days it is returned to the woman's uterus, the egg cell implants itself in the lining of the uterus, and the pregnancy continues as normal. ART accounts for slightly more than 1 percent of total U.S. births. One of the most common complications of ART is the birth of multiples.

caesarean delivery A surgical procedure in which an infant is delivered through an incision made in the abdominal wall and uterus.

infertility The inability to conceive a child.

artificial insemination The introduction of viable sperm into the vagina by artificial means for the purpose of inducing conception.

✓**check-in** Under what circumstances, if any, might you consider ART?

Adoption

Adoption matches would-be parents yearning for youngsters to love with infants or children who need loving homes. Couples interested in adoption can work with either public agencies or private counselors who contact obstetricians directly. Or they can contact organizations that arrange adoptions of children in need from other countries.

There are no reliable statistics on the annual number of adoptions in the United States, but census records indicate there are currently 1.6 million adopted children in the United States. Each year some 50,000 U.S. children become available for adoption—far fewer than the number of would-be parents looking for youngsters to adopt. An estimated 13 percent of adopted children are foreign born.

adoption The legal process for becoming the parent to a child of other biological parents.

Childfree by Choice

More women and men are deliberately choosing to remain "childfree." According to the limited data available, single childfree women tend to be better educated, more cosmopolitan, less religious, and more professional than those in the general population. In general, childfree women are high achievers, often in demanding careers, who describe their work as exciting and satisfying. Childfree couples are predominantly urban, well-educated, and upper middle class, with egalitarian and long-running marriages.

Their reasons for not having children are diverse: a desire to maintain their freedom and have more time with their partners, career ambitions, concern about overpopulation and the fate of the earth. Some women cite the hostile work environment for mothers and the inadequacy of day care. Others say they're disillusioned with the have-it-all hopes of baby boomers and believe in a have-most-of-it philosophy.

WHAT DID YOU DECIDE?

- What do college students need to know about contraception?
- What are the pros and cons of various birth control methods?
- What are the options for women faced with an unwanted pregnancy?
- What changes do a mother-to-be and her unborn child undergo during pregnancy?

THE POWER OF NOW!
Protecting Your Reproductive Health

The decisions you make about birth control can affect your reproductive health—and your partner's. Here are guidelines that can help prevent pregnancy and protect your reproductive well-being. Check those that you have used or think you will use in the future. Reflect on your choices in your online journal.

____ Abstinence. The only 100 percent safe and effective way to avoid unwanted pregnancy is not to engage in heterosexual intercourse.

____ Limiting sexual activity to outercourse or oral sex. You can engage in many sexual activities—kissing, hugging, touching, massage, oral–genital sex—without risking pregnancy.

____ Talking about birth control with any potential sex partner. If you are considering sexual intimacy with a person, you should feel comfortable enough to talk about contraception.

____ Knowing what doesn't work—and not relying on it. There are many misconceptions about ways to avoid getting pregnant, such as having sex in a standing position or during menstruation. Only the methods described in this chapter are reliable forms of birth control.

____ Talking with a health-care professional. A great deal of information and advice is available—in writing, from family planning counselors, and from physicians on the Internet. Check it out.

____ Choosing a contraceptive method that matches your personal habits and preferences. If you can't remember to take a pill every day, oral contraceptives aren't for you. If you're constantly forgetting where you put things, a diaphragm might not be a good choice.

____ Considering long-term implications. Since you may well wish to have children in the future, find out about the reversibility of various methods and possible effects on future fertility.

____ Resisting having sex without contraceptive protection "just this once." It only takes once—even the very first time—to get pregnant. Be wary of drugs and alcohol. They can impair your judgment and make you less conscientious about using birth control—or using it properly.

____ Using backup methods. If there's a possibility that a contraceptive method might not offer adequate protection (for instance, if it's been almost three months since your last injection of Depo-Provera), use an additional form of birth control.

____ Informing yourself about emergency contraception. Just in case a condom breaks or a diaphragm slips, find out about the availability of forms of after-intercourse contraception.

What's Online

 CENGAGE brain .com   Visit www.cengagebrain.com to access course materials for this text, including the Behavior Change Planner, interactive quizzes, tutorials, and more.

self survey

Which Contraceptive Method Is Best for You?

Answer Yes or No to each statement as it applies to you and, if appropriate, your partner.

1. You have high blood pressure or cardiovascular disease.
2. You smoke cigarettes.
3. You have a new sexual partner.
4. An unwanted pregnancy would be devastating to you.
5. You have a good memory.
6. You or your partner have multiple sexual partners.
7. You prefer a method with little or no bother.
8. You have heavy, crampy periods.
9. You need protection against STIs.
10. You are concerned about endometrial and ovarian cancer.
11. You are forgetful.
12. You need a method right away.
13. You're comfortable touching your own and your partner's genitals.
14. You have a cooperative partner.
15. You like a little extra vaginal lubrication.
16. You have sex at unpredictable times and places.
17. You are in a monogamous relationship and have at least one child.

Scoring:
Recommendations are based on Yes answers to the following numbered statements:

The combination pill: 4, 5, 6, 8, 10, 16

The progestin-only pill: 1, 2, 5, 7, 16

The patch: 4, 7, 8, 11, 16

The NuvaRing: 4, 7, 8, 11, 13, 16

Condoms: 1, 2, 3, 6, 9, 12, 13, 14

Depo-Provera: 1, 2, 4, 7, 11, 16

Diaphragm, cervical cap, or FemCap: 1, 2, 13, 14

Mirena IUD: 1, 2, 7, 8, 11, 13, 16, 17

Spermicides: 1, 2, 12, 13, 14, 15

Sponge: 1, 2, 12, 13

MAKING THIS CHAPTER WORK FOR YOU

Review Questions

(LO 10.1) 1. The percentage of unintended pregnancies in the U.S. is about _____.
   a. 75%
   b. 50%
   c. 25%
   d. 10%

(LO 10.1) 2. Among unmarried young adults, the most frequently used information source about contraceptives is _____.
   a. friends
   b. the Internet
   c. medical professionals
   d. magazines

(LO 10.2) 3. Fusion of a sperm with the nucleus of an egg is known as _____.
   a. ejaculation
   b. fertilization
   c. ovulation
   d. implantation

(LO 10.2) 4. A fertilized egg is called a(n) _____.
   a. zygote
   b. blastocyst
   c. fertilin
   d. allurin

(LO 10.3) 5. Which of the following is a reason people choose abstinence?
   a. They are in a hurry to be in a sexual relationship.
   b. They disregard moral and religious views.
   c. They are ready to get pregnant.
   d. They fear contracting a sexually transmitted infection.

(LO 10.3) 6. Which of the following statements is true of kissing?
   a. It is a form of outercourse.
   b. It results in pregnancy.
   c. It is the deepest form of physical contact.
   d. It results in the transfer of sperm.

(LO 10.4) 7. The most effective contraceptives for preventing pregnancy are _____.
   a. fertility awareness methods
   b. condoms
   c. sponges
   d. hormonal methods

(LO 10.4) 8. Removal of the penis from the vagina before ejaculation is known as _____.
   a. fertilization
   b. spermatogenesis
   c. coitus interruptus
   d. artificial insemination

(LO 10.5) 9. Which of the following is true about the use of contraceptives?
   a. Progestin checks depression in women.
   b. Birth control pills may increase the risk of heart attacks.
   c. Antiseizure medications slow down the liver metabolism of birth control pills.
   d. Birth control injections prevent the occurrence of strokes.

(LO 10.5) 10. Which of the following is an advantage of using a condom?
   a. It boosts sexual spontaneity.
   b. It is 100 percent effective in preventing STIs and pregnancies.
   c. It increases penile sensitivity.
   d. It is inexpensive.

(LO 10.6) 11. In the context of unwanted pregnancy, which of the following statements is true?
   a. Women faced with an unwanted pregnancy are often happily married.
   b. Minority women generally feel less cultural pressure to keep the child.
   c. Women faced with an unwanted pregnancy are often alone.
   d. The number of would-be adoptive parents is less than number of available newborns, so adoption is an unfavorable option.

(LO 10.6) 12. In the context of psychological impact of abortion, which of the following statements is true?
   a. The primary emotion of women following an abortion is stress.
   b. Women generally do not express feelings of guilt following an abortion.
   c. Women who were raped have low anxiety levels following an abortion.
   d. Research has documented no link between abortion and domestic violence.

(LO 10.7) 13. _____ is defined as the failure to conceive after one year of unprotected intercourse.
   a. Sterilization
   b. Infertility
   a. Miscarriage
   b. Abortion

(LO 10.7) 14. Which of the following is a contributing factor in the decision to live childfree?

   a. Indifference about the fate of Earth

   b. A desire to have more time with one's partner

   c. A belief in the have-it-all hopes of baby boomers

   d. Lack of career ambition

Answers to these questions can be found on page 623.

Critical Thinking Questions

1. Have you ever thought about the possibility of sexual abstinence in a relationship? If so, what are its benefits? How would it affect your satisfaction with the relationship?

2. In your personal view, how safe is abortion? Discuss the moral and political claims about abortion in your state.

Additional Online Resources

www.guttmacher.org
This site offers excellent resources on teen pregnancy rates and sexual health for teens and young adults, including discussions on contraceptives versus abstinence.

www.arhp.org
The Association of Reproductive Health Professionals (ARHP) calls its website "the ultimate resource offering comprehensive information and education on all reproductive health topics to healthcare professionals, policymakers, the media, and the public."

www.plannedparenthood.org
The website for the Planned Parenthood Federation of America offers a wealth of information on sexual and reproductive health, reproductive choices, methods of contraception, and reproductive policy.

Key Terms

The terms listed are used on the pages indicated. Definitions of the terms are in the glossary at the end of the book.

adoption 316

amnion 312

artificial insemination 315

barrier contraceptives 290

blastocyst 282

caesarean delivery 315

cervical cap 297

coitus interruptus 284

conception 282

condoms 290

contraception 284

diaphragm 296

ectopic pregnancy 312

embryo 312

emergency contraception (EC) 305

failure rate 287

fertilization 282

fetus 312

implantation 282

infertility 315

intrauterine device (IUD) 303

labor 314

laparoscopy 307

long-acting reversible contraceptives (LARCs) 302

medical abortion 308

minipills, progestin-only pills 299

miscarriage 313

monophasic pills 298

multiphasic pills 299

oral contraceptives 298

placenta 312

preconception care 310

premature labor 313

rhythm method 305

rubella 313

spermatogenesis 282

sterilization 306

suction curettage 308

tubal ligation 306

tubal occlusion 306

vaginal contraceptive film (VCF) 295

vaginal spermicide 295

vasectomy 306

zygote 282

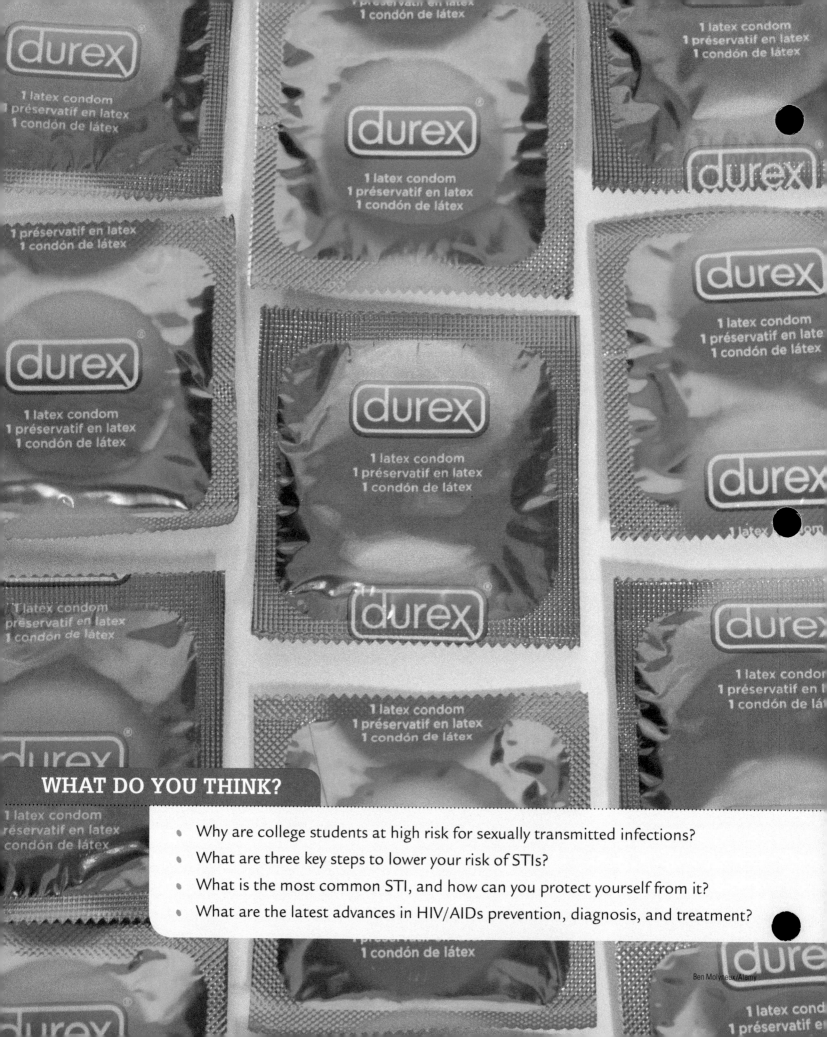

WHAT DO YOU THINK?

- Why are college students at high risk for sexually transmitted infections?
- What are three key steps to lower your risk of STIs?
- What is the most common STI, and how can you protect yourself from it?
- What are the latest advances in HIV/AIDs prevention, diagnosis, and treatment?

11

Lowering Your Risk of Sexually Transmitted Infections

"There's something I have to tell you." Stephanie knew, just by the sound of her boyfriend's voice, that the "something" wasn't good news.

"My herpes is back."

Stunned, Stephanie tried to absorb all the information packed into this short sentence: She'd had no idea that the man she'd been sleeping with for several months had a sexually transmitted infection (STI).

How did he get it? What else hadn't he told her about his past? What did he mean that it was "back"? Could she have caught it? And, finally, she asked the all-too-human question: How could this have happened to me?

By their very nature, infectious diseases take people by surprise. (See Chapter 16 for comprehensive coverage of infectious illnesses.) Some of today's most common and dangerous infectious illnesses spread primarily through sexual contact, and their incidence has skyrocketed. The federal government estimates that 65 million Americans have a sexually transmitted infection (STI). Each year more than 19 million people in the United States are diagnosed with an STI.[1] The odds of acquiring an STI in the course of a lifetime are one in four. These diseases cannot be prevented in the laboratory. Only you, by your behavior, can prevent and control them.

All human beings are sexual from birth to death. Whether you are male or female, single or married, straight, gay, lesbian, bisexual, or transgender, sexuality is a normal, natural part of your life. You are just as responsible for your sexual health as for any other aspect of your well-being. To safeguard your sexual health, you need to be aware of and protect yourself from sexually transmitted infections and diseases. ◀

After reading this chapter, you should be able to:

11.1 Identify the characteristics and risk factors of sexually transmitted infections and diseases.

11.2 Explain the factors that lead to a healthy sexual life.

11.3 Summarize the risk factors related to sexually transmitted infections among college students.

11.4 Discuss the nature, incidence, signs and symptoms, preventive measures, and treatments of common sexually transmitted diseases.

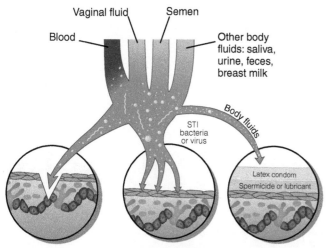

Tough outer skin
covers the outside of your body, including hands and lips. Viruses and bacteria enter when skin is chapped or through a hangnail, cut, scrape, sore, or needle puncture.

Fragile inner skin
lines the inside of your vagina or penis, anus, and mouth. Viruses and bacteria can enter through microscopic tears in the skin during sexual contact that involves movement or that lacks lubrication.

Barrier protection
Latex condoms prevent your partner's body fluids from entering your body. Spermicides kill many STI microbes and reduce friction so condoms are less likely to break.

© Cengage Learning

FIGURE 11.1 How STIs Spread

Most STIs are spread by viruses or bacteria carried in certain body fluids.

Sexually Transmitted Infections and Diseases

In medical terms, **sexually transmitted infection (STI)** refers to the presence of an infectious agent that can be passed from one sexual partner to another. In public health, this term is replacing **sexually transmitted disease (STD)** because sexual infections can be—and often are—transmitted by people who do not have symptoms. (See Chapter 16 for a complete discussion of infectious diseases.)

The federal government estimates that 65 million Americans have an STI. The odds of acquiring an STI in the course of a lifetime are one in four. These diseases cannot be prevented in a laboratory. Only you, by your behavior, can prevent and control them.

....
√**check-in** Do you consider yourself well informed about STIs and STDs?
....

sexually transmitted infection (STI) The presence in the human body of an infectious agent that can be passed from one sexual partner to another.

sexually transmitted disease (STD) A disease that is caused by a sexually transmitted infection that produces symptoms.

Remember, STIs can

- Last a lifetime
- Put stress on relationships
- Cause serious medical complications
- Impair fertility
- Cause birth defects
- Lead to major illness and death

Although each STI is distinct, they are all transmitted mainly through

- Direct sexual contact with someone's symptoms (like genital ulcers) or sexual contact with someone's infected semen, vaginal fluids, blood, and other body fluids
- Sharing contaminated needles through injectable drug use
- Maternal transfer (mother to fetus during pregnancy or childbirth)

All STI pathogens like dark, warm, moist body surfaces, particularly the mucous membranes that line the reproductive organs; they hate light, cold, and dryness. Figure 11.1 shows how STIs in body fluids spread from person to person and how a barrier can help prevent their entry. It is possible to catch or have more than one STI at a time. Curing one doesn't necessarily cure another, and treatments don't prevent another bout with the same STI.

Many STIs, including early HIV infection and gonorrhea in women, may not cause any symptoms. As a result, infected individuals may continue their usual sexual activity without realizing that they're jeopardizing another's well-being.

More Americans are infected with STIs now than at any other time in history. According to the Institute of Medicine, the odds of acquiring an STI during a lifetime are one in four. Almost half of STIs occur in young people ages 15 to 24.[2]

Within two years of having sex for the first time, half of teenage girls may acquire an STI. The three most common are chlamydia, gonorrhea, and trichomoniasis. (See Table 11.1 for a list and description of common sexually transmitted diseases.)

STI Risk Factors and Risk Continuum

Various factors put young people at risk of STIs, including the following:

- **A sexual partner who has an STI.**
- **A history of STIs.**

TABLE 11.1 Common Sexually Transmitted Infections (STIs)

STI	Transmission	Signs and Symptoms
Human papillomavirus (HPV) (genital warts) (pp. 328–330)	Spread primarily through vaginal, anal, or oral sex	Cauliflower-like growths in genital and rectal areas
Herpes simplex (pp. 330–331)	Genital herpes virus (HSV-2) transmitted by vaginal, anal, or oral sex. Oral herpes virus (HSV-1) transmitted primarily by kissing.	Small, painful red bumps (papules) to the genital region (genital herpes) or mouth (oral herpes). The papules become painful blisters that eventually rupture to form wet, open sores.
Chlamydia (pp. 331–332)	*Chlamydia trachomatis* bacterium transmitted primarily through sexual contact (can also be spread by fingers from one body site to another)	Men: Watery discharge; pain when urinating Women: Usually asymptomatic; sometimes a similar discharge to men's; leading cause of pelvic inflammatory disease (PID)
Gonorrhea ("clap") (pp. 333–334)	*Neisseria gonorrhoeae* bacterium ("gonococcus") spread through genital, oral-genital, or genital-anal contact	Men: Pus discharge from urethra; burning during urination Women: Usually asymptomatic; can lead to PID and sterility in both men and women
Nongonococcal urethritis (NGU) (p. 334)	Bacteria, most commonly transmitted through sexual intercourse	Men: Discharge from the penis and irritation during urination Women: Mild discharge of pus from the vagina but often no symptoms
Syphilis (pp. 334–335)	*Treponema pallidum* bacterium ("spirochete") transmitted from open lesions during genital, oral-genital, or genital-anal contact	Primary: Chancre Secondary: Rash Latent: Asymptomatic Late: Irreversible damage to central nervous system, cardiovascular system
Chancroid (p. 335)	*Haemophilus ducrevi* bacterium transmitted by sexual interaction	Men: Painful irregular chancre on penis Women: Chancre on labia
Pubic lice ("crabs") (p. 335)	*Phthirus pubis* spread easily through body contact or through shared clothing or bedding	Persistent itching; visible lice often located in pubic hair or other body hairs
HIV/AIDS (pp. 336–339)	HIV transmitted in blood and semen, primarily through sexual contact or needle sharing among injection drug users	Asymptomatic at first; opportunistic infections

© Cengage Learning 2015

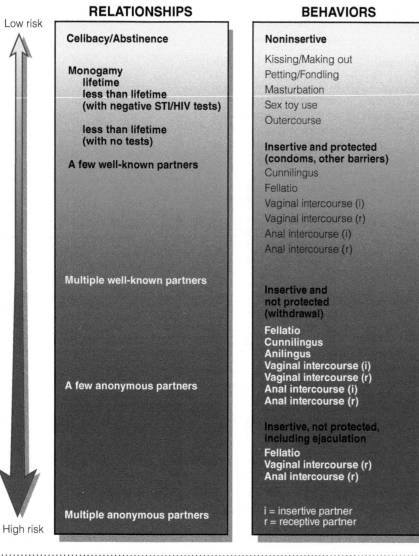

RELATIONSHIPS

Low risk ↑

Celibacy/Abstinence

Monogamy
  lifetime
  less than lifetime
  (with negative STI/HIV tests)

  less than lifetime
  (with no tests)

A few well-known partners

Multiple well-known partners

A few anonymous partners

Multiple anonymous partners

High risk ↓

© Cengage Learning

BEHAVIORS

Noninsertive
  Kissing/Making out
  Petting/Fondling
  Masturbation
  Sex toy use
  Outercourse

Insertive and protected
(condoms, other barriers)
  Cunnilingus
  Fellatio
  Vaginal intercourse (i)
  Vaginal intercourse (r)
  Anal intercourse (i)
  Anal intercourse (r)

Insertive and
not protected
(withdrawal)
  Fellatio
  Cunnilingus
  Anilingus
  Vaginal intercourse (i)
  Vaginal intercourse (r)
  Anal intercourse (i)
  Anal intercourse (r)

Insertive, not protected,
including ejaculation
  Fellatio
  Vaginal intercourse (r)
  Anal intercourse (r)

i = insertive partner
r = receptive partner

FIGURE 11.2 Continuum of Risk for Sexual Relationships and Behaviors
STI risks increase as relationships become less familiar and exclusive and as sexual activities become unprotected and receptive.

- **Feelings of invulnerability,** which lead to risk-taking behavior. Even when they are well informed of the risks, adolescents and young adults may remain unconvinced that anything bad can or will happen to them.

- **Multiple partners or a partner who has had more than one sexual partner.** Figure 11.2 illustrates how STI risks increase as relationships become less familiar and exclusive. In surveys of students, a significant number report having had four or more sexual partners during their lifetime. Individuals with more than one concurrent partner also are at greater risk.[3]

- **Meeting sex partners through the Internet.** Individuals who find sex partners online are more likely to report unprotected sex, higher rates of drug use in the past

12 months, more sexual partners, and failure to discuss sexual histories—all behaviors that increase the risk of STIs.[4]

- **Failure to use condoms.** Among those who reported having had sexual intercourse in the previous three months, fewer than half of the students reported condom use. Female undergraduates were less likely to insist on condom use over the course of their first year on campus.

- **Substance abuse.** Individuals who drink or use drugs are more likely to engage in sexually risky behaviors, including sex with partners whose health status and history they do not know, and unprotected intercourse. The more alcohol that college students drink or the more marijuana they use, the more likely they are to engage in risky sexual behavior.

- **Failure of a partner to be notified and treated.** Although physicians and health officials urge infected individuals to notify all their sexual partners, only an estimated 40 to 60 percent are notified and seek treatment.

- **Use of injection drugs or a sexual partner who uses them.**

The CDC has endorsed "expedited partner therapy" (giving medications to the infected person to give to partners) for cases of gonorrhea, chlamydia, or trichomoniasis. This approach is permissible or potentially allowable in most states but prohibited in Arkansas, Florida, Kentucky, Michigan, Ohio, Oklahoma, South Carolina, Vermont, and West Virginia.

✓**check-in** Are you at risk of getting an STI? Take the Self Survey "Assessing Your STI Risk."

The ABCs of Safer Sex

Making smart, healthy choices about sex is the key to preventing sexual illnesses. As you will discover in this chapter, there are many specific steps to take to safeguard your sexual health. However, the three key fundamentals are as simple as A, B, C.

A Is for *Abstain*

Abstinence from vaginal and anal intercourse and oral sex is free, available to everyone, extremely effective at preventing both pregnancy and sexually transmitted infections, and has no medical or hormonal side effects.

If you decide to abstain only from vaginal or anal penetration, remember that other sexual activity such as oral sex can also expose you to STIs. If you have oral sex, make it safer by using effective barrier methods such as condoms or latex dental dams. (A dental dam is a square piece of latex that can be stretched across the vulva or anus to prevent the transmission of STIs.) In the absence of barrier methods, men should avoid ejaculating in their partners' mouths. Also,

- Be aware of sores and discharge or unpleasant odors from your partner's genitals. These are signs to avoid oral sex.

- Don't floss or brush teeth before oral sex. It might tear the lining of the mouth, increasing exposure to viruses.

- Avoid aggressive and deep thrusting in oral sex, which can damage throat tissues and increase susceptibility for throat-based gonorrhea, herpes, and abrasions.

- Remember that oral sex can transmit various STIs, including HPV, herpes, gonorrhea, syphilis, and HIV.

B Is for *Be Faithful*

For men and women who are sexually active, a mutually faithful sexual relationship with just one healthy partner is the safest option. Women and men in a committed relationship don't need to worry about getting sexually transmitted infections if

- Neither partner ever had sex with anyone else.

- Neither partner ever shared needles.

- Neither partner currently has or ever had an STI.

If these criteria fail to apply, two partners should be sure that neither has an STI before giving up on safer-sex practices. Some infections, like HIV, may take years to develop symptoms. The only way to know is by being tested.

Of course, a committed relationship remains safe only as long as both partners remain committed. Most women who get HIV from having sex think they are their sex partners' only lover and never suspect that their partners' other lovers are men or women with HIV.

C Is for *Condoms*

Condoms are the only contraceptive that helps prevent both pregnancy and STIs when used properly and consistently. Male condoms reduce

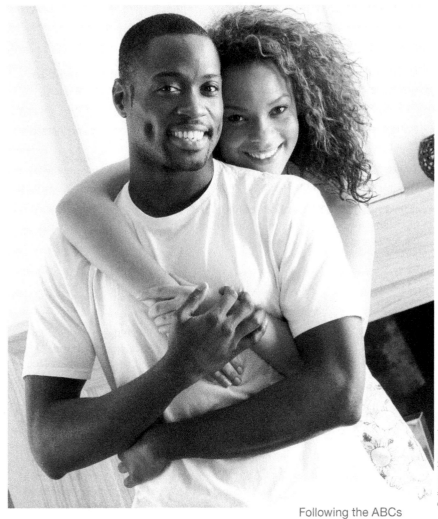

© oliveromg/shutterstock.com

Following the ABCs of safer sex—*Abstain, Be* Faithful, use Condoms—doesn't mean you can't have an intimate, loving relationship.

the risk of transmission of an STI by 50 to 80 percent. They are more effective against STIs transmitted by bodily fluids (chlamydia, gonorrhea, HIV, etc.) than those transmitted by skin-to-skin contact (HPV, syphilis, herpes, chancroid). Inexpensive and widely available in pharmacies, supermarkets, and convenience stores, condoms don't require a doctor visit or a prescription. According to a recent nationwide survey, condoms do not interfere with sexual enjoyment.[5] (See Chapter 10 for a comprehensive discussion of condoms.) Here are some essential guidelines to keep in mind:

- Most physicians recommend American-made latex condoms. Check the package for FDA approval.

- Also check the expiration (Exp) or manufacture (MFG) date on the box or individual package to make sure it is still safe to use the condom.

- Make sure the package and the condom appear in good condition. If the package does not state that the condoms are meant to prevent disease, they may not provide adequate

YOUR STRATEGIES FOR CHANGE

If You Have an STI

- **If you suspect that you have an STI, don't feel too embarrassed to get help through a physician's office or a clinic.** Treatment relieves discomfort, prevents complications, and halts the spread of the disease.

- **Following diagnosis, take oral medication** (which may be given instead of or in addition to shots) exactly as prescribed.

- **Try to figure out from whom you got the STI.** Be sure to inform that person, who may not be aware of the problem.

- **If you have an STI, never deceive a prospective partner about it.** Tell the truth—simply and clearly. Be sure your partner understands exactly what you have and what the risks are.

protection even if they are the most expensive ones on the shelf.

- Get the right size. Ill-fitting condoms lead to more problems with slippage and breakage, as well as diminished sexual pleasure. Men also may be more likely to remove a condom that doesn't fit well before sex.[6]

- Condoms can deteriorate if not stored properly since they are affected by both heat and light. Don't use a condom that has been stored in your back pocket, your wallet, or the glove compartment of your car. If a condom feels sticky or very dry, don't use it; the packaging has probably been damaged.

✓**check-in** If you are sexually active, did you or your partner use a condom the last time you had intercourse?

STIs and Gender

Both men and women can develop STIs, but their risks are not the same. Here is what you need to know about your risks. (See Health on a Budget for more ways of reducing risks of STIs.)

If You Are a Woman

- Keep in mind that your risk of getting an infection is greater than a man's. STIs can be transmitted through breaks in the mucous membranes, and women have more mucosal area exposed and experience more trauma to these tissues during sexual activity than men.

- Don't think you don't have to worry just because you have no symptoms. Symptoms of STIs also tend to be more "silent" in women, so they often go undetected and untreated, leading to potentially serious complications. For instance, pelvic inflammatory disease has no symptoms but puts you at risk of infertility and ectopic pregnancy.

- At your checkup, talk to your doctor about whether you should be tested for sexually transmitted infections. You need to ask for these tests, or else they won't be done.

If You Are a Man

- Involve your partner. Men are more likely to avoid common errors, such as removing condoms before sexual contact ends or slippage during withdrawal, when both partners mutually decide on their use.

- After potential exposure to an STI, give yourself a little extra protection by urinating and washing your genitals with an antibacterial soap.

- At your checkup, talk to your doctor about whether you should be tested for sexually transmitted infections. You need to ask for these tests, or else they won't be done.

Although it can be awkward to bring up the subject of condoms, don't let your embarrassment

HEALTH ON A BUDGET

Reducing Your Risk of STIs

- Abstain from sex until you are in a relationship with only one person, you are having sex only with each other, and each of you knows the other's health.

- Talk about STIs with every partner before you have sex.

- Learn as much as you can about each partner's past behavior, including sexual activity and drug use.

- Ask prospective partners if they have recently been tested for STIs.

- If you think you may have been exposed to an STI, get treatment.

- Do not inject illicit drugs.

- Do not put yourself in situations where sexual activity could occur when you are drunk or high because your judgment may be impaired.

🔘 Students and STIs

Students	Percent	Students	Percent
Vaccinated against HPV	68	Diagnosed with chlamydia	1.1
Tested for HIV infection	25.3	Diagnosed with genital herpes	0.7
Diagnosed with HPV	1.3	Diagnosed with PID	0.3

What have you done to protect yourself from STIs? Have you been vaccinated against HPV? Have you been tested for HIV (recommended for everyone over age 13)? The incidence of diagnosed STIs on campuses is low, but many individuals are not aware that they have these infections. Write down your feelings about how getting an STI might affect your health and your life in your online journal.

Source: American College Health Association, *American College Health Association-National College Health Assessment II: Reference Group Executive Summary Spring 2014.* Hanover, MD: American College Health Association, 2014.

put your health at risk. Discuss using a condom before having sex; don't wait until you're on the brink of a sexual encounter.

See Chapter 10 for instructions on condom use. Here are some additional guidelines:

- **Use a new condom** each and every time you engage in any form of intercourse.

- **Do not open the wrapper** of a condom with your teeth or long fingernails since this can weaken the condom or tear a hole in it.

- **Squeeze the air out of a condom** before putting it on.

- **Do not use spermicide containing nonoxynol-9.** Frequent use of nonoxynol-9 (N-9) may increase the risk of HIV by creating vaginal or rectal ulceration. N-9 does not offer protection from gonorrhea, chlamydia, or HIV. The FDA has required that products containing N-9 state that they do not protect against HIV and other STIs and may increase the risk of getting HIV from an infected partner.

- **If a condom fails** during vaginal or anal intercourse, remove it carefully. If you continue sexual activity, replace it with a new condom.

STIs on Campus

The college years are a prime time for contracting STIs. (See On Campus Now: Students and STIs.) Almost nine in ten undergraduates are sexually active, but only about half report that they used condoms most or all of the time they engaged in vaginal intercourse in the last 30 days. Fewer (27.2 percent) used condoms the last time they engaged in anal sex; only 4.6 percent used condoms for oral sex.[7]

Contracting STIs may increase the risk of being infected with HIV. Because college students have more opportunities to have different sexual partners and may use drugs and alcohol more often before sex, they are at greater risk.

About 60 percent of colleges with a student health center provide some STI testing and treatment.[8] However, in various studies, only 23 to 32 percent of students report that they've been tested for HIV or other STIs. The reasons may include shame, stigma, fear, denial, concern about social consequences, inaccurate beliefs about STIs, privacy concerns, and inconveniences, such as long waiting times.

What College Students Don't Know about STIs

"At my age, I know everything already and believe that my classmates do, too."

That's what an entering freshman said in a recent survey of students' sexual health knowledge. Many undergraduates say the same thing, yet often they think that they know more than they actually do. This is particularly true of STIs. Although they often can name common STIs, such as HIV, genital herpes, gonorrhea, and chlamydia, undergraduates are less familiar with human papilloma virus (HPV) and syphilis, the symptoms associated with STIs, and the ways in which STIs are transmitted or diagnosed. Many

Even though the conversation can be awkward and embarrassing, you need to talk honestly about any STI that you may have been exposed to or contracted. What you don't say can be hazardous to your partner's health. Here are some guidelines:

- **Talk before you become intimate.** A good way to start is simply by saying, "There is something we need to talk over first."

- **Be honest.** Don't downplay any potential risks.

- **Don't blame.** Even if you suspect that your partner was the source of your infection, focus on the need for medical attention.

- **Be sensitive to your partner's feelings.** Anger and resentment are common reactions when someone feels at risk. Try to listen without becoming defensive.

- **Seek medical attention.** Do not engage in sexual intimacies until you obtain a doctor's assurance that you are no longer contagious.

Even if you are not sexually active or have never had an STI, imagine yourself in this situation. What would be your biggest concern if you were the one with the STI? What would be your biggest concern if you were his or her partner? What do you think is the best possible way to deal with such circumstances? Record your thoughts in your online journal.

Source: Bacchus and Gamma Peer Education Network, www.smartersex.org.

human papillomavirus (HPV) A pathogen that causes genital warts and increases the risk of cervical cancer.

do not realize that STIs can exist without symptoms so they don't take steps to protect themselves or to avoid risky sexual behaviors. (See Table 11.2 for some facts about STIs.)

College students often report never using a condom or using condoms inconsistently during sex. The reasons may have more to do with emotions and attitude, according to recent research, than with availability or cost. Some fear that bringing up condom use might harm the relationship or cause embarrassment. Even if partners believe that condoms could help prevent an STI, those in or hoping for a long-term relationship report feeling that condoms are not necessary because they and their partners know each other well.[9] (See Health Now! for suggestions about how to tell a partner you have an STI.)

✓**check-in** Why do you think students don't use condoms consistently?

Common STIs and STDs

Human Papillomavirus (HPV)

Human papillomavirus (HPV) is the most common sexually transmitted infection. Of the 100 or more different strains, or types, of HPV, approximately 40 are sexually transmitted, and 15 have been identified as "oncogenic," or cancer causing.[10] Some "high-risk" HPV strains may lead to cancer of the cervix, vulva, vagina, anus, or penis. If transmitted via oral sex, they significantly increase the risk of mouth and throat cancers. The risk increases along with the number of oral sex partners. HPV-related cancers have increased in recent years.[11]

The "low-risk" types of HPV may cause changes in cervical cells that cause Pap test abnormalities or genital warts. Genital warts are single or multiple growths or bumps, sometimes shaped like cauliflower, that appear in the genital area.

Condoms provide only limited protection. Most people who become infected with HPV do not have any symptoms, and the infection clears on its own. However, HPV infection can cause cervical cancer in women and genital warts and other types of cancers in both sexes.

The primary risk factors for oral HPV infection include the following:

- Number of sex partners
- Smoking
- Heavy drinking
- Marijuana use[12]

✓**check-in** Do you consider yourself at risk for HPV infection?

Incidence Approximately 20 million people in the United States—almost 7 percent of those between ages 14 and 69—are currently infected with HPV, and 6.2 million Americans get a new HPV infection each year. Worldwide, more than 440 million individuals are infected with HPV.

As many as 80 percent of sexually active women acquire HPV by age 50. However, 44 percent of women ages 20 to 24 have HPV. Approximately 70 percent of sexually active women contract HPV, most within five years of their first sexual encounter.

Young women who engage in sexual intercourse at an early age are more likely than those with later sexual debuts to become infected with HPV. Their risk also increases if they are black, have multiple sexual partners or a history of a

TABLE 11.2 Did You Know? Some Facts about STDs

- Estimated number of Americans living with an STD: 65 million
- Number of new cases of STDs every year: 19 million
- Number of Americans who will get an STD in their lifetimes: 1 in 4
- Number of unsafe sexual contacts it takes to get an STD: 1
- Percentage of Americans who have herpes and do not know it: 35
- Seconds it takes for a new person to get genital herpes: 30 seconds
- Percentage of women living with chlamydia who do not know it: 75%
- Estimated cost of chlamydia in the U.S. each year: $2,000,000,000
- Average cost of antibiotic to treat a case of chlamydia: $15

Source: Centers for Disease Control

Kristoffer Tripplaar/Alamy

sexually transmitted infection, use drugs, or have partners with multiple sexual partners.[13] College-age women are among those at greatest risk of acquiring HPV infection. In various studies conducted in college health centers, 10 to 46 percent of female students (mean age 20 to 22) had positive HPV tests.

Men who have sex with men and men who have sex with both men and women have the highest rates of HPV. Men who have had more than 16 sex partners have about 3 times the HPV risk of those with fewer sex partners and are nearly 10 times more likely to contract a potentially cancer-causing strain. Once infected, men who have been circumcised are more likely to have their immune systems "clear" the virus. Circumcised men also are less likely to transmit the virus to female partners. HPV also has been linked to penile cancer.[14]

✓**check-in** Have you ever been tested for HPV?

HPV Vaccination   Two vaccines—Gardasil and Cervarix—are currently available to prevent cervical cancer in girls and young women. Both protect against HPV-16 and HPV-18, the two types of HPV that cause most cases of cervical cancer. Gardasil also protects against HPV-6 and HPV-11, which cause most cases of genital warts.

Gardasil is approved for females ages 9 to 26 to protect against cervical cancer and prevent genital warts and for males ages 9 to 26 to prevent genital warts. Cervarix, which does not protect against genital warts, is approved for females ages 10 to 26 to help prevent cervical cancer. Cervarix has not been approved for use in boys or men.

Federal authorities and the American Academy of Pediatrics recommends HPV vaccination for

- All girls and boys ages 11 or 12, with catch-up vaccinations for those ages 13 to 21.

- Women ages 13 through 26 who were not previously vaccinated.

- Men ages 13 through 21 who were not previously vaccinated; men ages 22 through 26 may also receive the vaccine.[15]

Initially, doctors had targeted girls because the vaccination is highly effective in preventing cervical cancer. However, other cancers linked to HPV, including anal cancer and some head and neck cancers, have been increasing, especially among men.

Either brand of the vaccine is given in three shots over a six-month period, with the second and third doses administered two and six months after the first dose. Compliance rates for receiving all three doses have been low.

Rates of HPV vaccination remain lower than for other routinely recommended immunizations. An estimated 57 percent of teenage girls and 35 percent of boys have initiated the three-dose series; significantly fewer have completed it.[16] One reason is concern that HPV vaccination might encourage teenagers to initiate sexual activity at earlier ages or to engage in riskier sexual behaviors.

However, several studies have confirmed that girls vaccinated against HPV are no more (and in some cases are less) likely than others to initiate sex or, if they already are sexually active, to have more partners or not use condoms during sex.[17] Follow-up studies have found no increases in STIs among vaccinated teens.[18]

Vaccination has proven effective in significantly lowering the incidence of genital warts[19] and the occurrence of precancerous cervical lesions.[20] Two doses of the HPV vaccine instead of the recommended three doses appears to provide some protection against genital warts.[21]

Adverse effects, reported in 6.2 percent of vaccinated patients, include the following:

- Fainting

- Itchiness

- Headache

- Nausea

- Blood clots

- Allergic reactions

This is considered within the normal range of a widespread vaccination program for young persons.

Although young women under age 25 are most likely to develop HPV, older women at risk for cervical cancer also can benefit from vaccination, according initial tests of the HPV vaccine in various age groups. If you are age 26 or older and have not been vaccinated, talk to your health care about the relative risks and benefits for you.[22]

HPV Vaccination on Campus   Sexually active young adults are at the highest risk of HPV infection. But according to a recent national analysis of some 40,000 female students ages 18 to 24 at schools around the country, fewer than half had not received the HPV vaccination. Among these women, similar percentages reported either not being in a relationship or being in a relationship but not living together. Fewer than 10% were living with a partner.[23] (See Consumer Alert.)

✓**check-in** Have you been vaccinated against HPV?

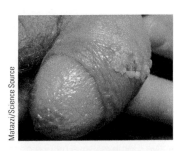
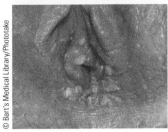

Matazzi/Science Source

© Bart's Medical Library/Phototake

Human papillomavirus, which causes genital warts, is the most common viral STI.

❗ CONSUMER ALERT

Should You Get the HPV Vaccine?

Some states are considering legislation to make HPV vaccination mandatory for all girls because the vaccine is most effective when given before a girl becomes sexually active. Some religious groups oppose mandatory immunization because they feel that vaccinating girls against an STI gives them the wrong message about sexual responsibility. Consumer advocates worry about the unknown long-term effects. Others feel that the decision should be made privately by parents, in consultation with their pediatricians. Vaccination is recommended for both sexes.

Facts to Know

- The HPV vaccines, which consist of three shots given over a six-month period, have been extensively tested worldwide and are considered safe. However, the long-term effects are not known.

- No one yet knows whether a booster shot or shots will be necessary.

- Adverse effects include fainting, nausea, headache, blood clots, allergic reactions, and death. The most common side effects are pain at the injection site and fever.

- An estimated 4,000 women die in the United States and about 274,000 women die internationally annually from cervical cancer. The National Cancer Institute estimates 11,300 new cases of cervical cancer each year.

Steps to Take

- Talk with your doctor if you are under age 26 or at risk for cervical cancer and have not yet been vaccinated.

- Check with your insurance provider. Vaccination costs about $400 for the three-shot series. Most insurance companies cover recommended vaccines.

- Do *not* get the HPV vaccine if you

  - Are pregnant

  - Have ever had a life-threatening allergic reaction to any component of HPV vaccine

  - Are moderately to severely ill at the time of vaccination

---

Signs and Symptoms   HPV lives in the skin or mucous membranes and usually causes no symptoms. Some people get visible genital warts or have precancerous changes in the cervix, vulva, anus, or penis. After contact with an infected individual, genital warts may appear within three weeks to 18 months, with an average period of about 3 months.

Most HPV infections are asymptomatic in men, who may unwittingly increase their partners' risk. Men who test positive for HPV typically report significantly more sex partners than those who do not. HPV may also cause genital warts in men and increase the risk of cancer of the penis.

HPV infection may invade the urethra and cause urinary obstruction and bleeding. It greatly increases a woman's risk of developing a precancerous condition called cervical *intraepithelial neoplasia*, which can lead to cervical cancer. Adolescent girls infected with HPV appear to be particularly vulnerable to developing cervical cancer.

It is not known if HPV itself causes cancer or acts in conjunction with cofactors (such as other infections, smoking, or suppressed immunity). A woman's risk of cervical cancer is strongly related to the number of her partner's current and lifetime female partners. Women are 5 to 11 times as likely to get cervical cancer if their steady sex partner has had 20 or more previous partners.

Diagnosis and Treatment   Most women are diagnosed with HPV after an abnormal Pap test or HPV DNA test. The results of HPV DNA testing can help health-care providers decide whether treatment is necessary to prevent or treat cervical cancer. (See Chapter 15 for a discussion of cervical cancer.) Warning signs for cervical cancer include irregular bleeding and unusual vaginal discharge. Precancerous cervical cells can be destroyed by laser surgery or freezing during a visit to a doctor's office.

No form of therapy has been shown to completely eradicate HPV, nor has any single treatment been uniformly effective in removing warts or preventing their recurrence. CDC guidelines suggest treatments that focus on the removal of visible warts—laser therapy, cryotherapy (freezing), and topical applications of podofilox, podophyllin, or trichloroacetic acid—and then eradication of the virus. At least 20 to 30 percent of treated individuals experience recurrence.

Genital Herpes

Herpes (from the Greek word that means "to creep") collectively describes some of the most common viral infections in humans. Characteristically, **herpes simplex** causes blisters on the skin or mucous membranes.

Herpes simplex exists in several varieties. *Herpes simplex virus 1* (*HSV-1*) can be transmitted by kissing and generally causes cold sores and fever blisters around the mouth. *Herpes simplex virus 2* (*HSV-2*) is sexually transmitted and may cause blisters on the penis, inside the vagina, on the cervix, in the pubic area, on the buttocks, on the thighs, or in the mouth and throat (transmitted via oral sex).

About one in five women and one in nine men have genital herpes. More than 80 percent do not realize they are infected.[24] HSV transmission occurs through close contact with mucous membranes or abraded skin. Condoms help prevent infection but aren't foolproof.

In the past, physicians viewed herpes as an episodic disease with the greatest risk of transmission during flare-up. But as recent research has documented, "classic herpes" that produces acute symptoms is not typical. For many people genital herpes is a chronic, nearly continuously active infection that may produce subtle, varied,

---

herpes simplex A condition caused by one of the herpes viruses and characterized by lesions of the skin or mucous membranes; herpes simplex virus 2 is sexually transmitted and causes genital blisters or sores.

and often-overlooked symptoms. Most cases are transmitted by sexual partners who are unaware of their infections or do not have symptoms at the time of transmission.

When herpes sores are present, the infected person is highly contagious and should avoid bringing the lesions into contact with someone else's body through touching, sexual interaction, or kissing. However, the herpes virus is present in genital secretions even when patients do not notice any signs of the disease, and people infected with genital herpes can spread it even between flare-ups, when they have no symptoms.[25]

A newborn can be infected with genital herpes while passing through the birth canal, and the frequency of mother-to-infant transmission seems to be increasing. Most infected infants develop typical skin sores, which can be cultured to confirm a herpes diagnosis. Some physicians recommend treatment with acyclovir. Because of the risk to the infant of severe damage and possible death, caesarean delivery may be advised for a woman with active herpes lesions.

Incidence

At least 50 million people in the United States have genital herpes, including 21 percent of women in the United States. Only a minority know they are affected, and many believe they could tell if a sexual partner were infected.[26] About 40 percent of new cases of genital herpes occur in young people ages 15 to 24.

Signs and Symptoms

Most people with genital herpes have no symptoms or very mild symptoms that go unnoticed or are not recognized as a sign of infection. The most common is a cluster of blistery sores, usually on the vagina, vulva, cervix, penis, buttocks, or anus. They may last several weeks and go away. They may return in weeks, months, or years

Other symptoms include blisters, burning feelings if urine flows over sores, inability to urinate if severe swelling of sores blocks the urethra, and itching and pain in the infected area. Severe first episodes of herpes may also cause swollen, tender lymph glands in the groin, throat, and under the arms; fever; chills; headache; and achy flu-like feelings.

The virus that causes herpes never entirely goes away; it retreats to nerves near the lower spinal cord, where it remains for the life of the host. Herpes sores can return without warning weeks, months, or even years after their first occurrence, often during menstruation or times of stress, or with sudden changes in body temperature. Of those who experience HSV recurrence, 10 to 35 percent do so frequently—that is, about six or more times a year. In most people, attacks diminish in frequency and severity over time.

√**check-in** Did you know that individuals can transmit genital herpes even when they don't have visible lesions?

Diagnosis and Treatment Testing for the herpes virus has become much more accurate. Several highly effective antiviral therapies not only reduce symptoms and heal herpes lesions but also, if taken continuously, significantly reduce the risk of transmission of the virus to sexual partners.

The three antiviral medications approved for the treatment of genital herpes are

- **Acyclovir:** The oldest antiviral medication for herpes, acyclovir is sold as a generic drug and under the brand name Zovirax. Available as an ointment and pill, acyclovir has been shown to be safe in persons who have used it continuously (every day) for as long as 10 years.

- **Valacyclovir:** Sold as Valtrex, this medication delivers acyclovir more efficiently so that the body absorbs more of the drug and medication can be taken fewer times during the day.

- **Famcyclovir:** Sold as Famvir, this drug utilizes penciclovir as its active ingredient to stop HSV. Like valacyclovir, it is well absorbed, persists for a long time in the body, and can be taken less frequently than acyclovir.

These antiviral medications are prescribed for initial and recurrent episodes of herpes. In episodic therapy, a person begins taking medication at the first sign of recurrence and continues for several days to hasten the healing or prevent a full outbreak from occurring. In suppressive therapy, people with genital herpes take antiviral medication daily to prevent symptoms. For individuals who have frequent recurrences (six or more per year), suppressive therapy can reduce the number of outbreaks by at least 75 percent. Suppressive therapy may also reduce asymptomatic shedding of HSV.

Various treatments—compresses made with cold water, skim milk, or warm salt water; ice packs; or a mild anesthetic cream—can relieve discomfort. Herpes sufferers should avoid heat, hot baths, and nylon underwear. Some physicians have used laser therapy to vaporize the lesions. Clinical trials of an experimental vaccine to protect people from herpes infections are under way.

Chlamydia

The most widespread sexually transmitted bacterium in the United States is *Chlamydia*

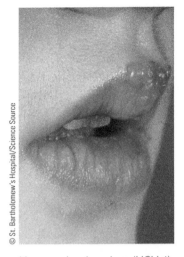
Herpes simplex virus (HSV-1) as a mouth sore.

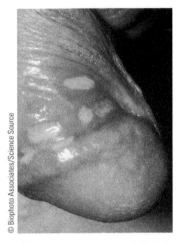
Herpes simplex virus (HSV-2) as a genital sore.

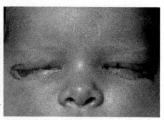

A baby exposed to chlamydial infection in the birth canal during delivery may develop an eye infection. Symptoms include a bloody discharge and swollen eyelids.

chlamydia A common sexually transmitted infection caused by bacteria known as Chlamydia trachomatis.

pelvic inflammatory disease (PID) An inflammation of the internal female genital tract, characterized by abdominal pain, fever, and tenderness of the cervix.

trachomatis, which causes more than a million cases of **chlamydia** each year, a number that continues to rise. Almost half of reported cases occur among sexually active young adults between ages 15 and 24. The use of condoms with spermicide can reduce, but not eliminate, the risk of chlamydial infection.

Incidence Some 1.4 million, or 1 in 25 Americans are infected with chlamydia. Chlamydia is much more prevalent in young black adults than in young white adults. However, this may be because black and Hispanic women are much more likely to be screened. Women have three times the rate of chlamydia as men. Chlamydial infections are more common in younger than in older women, and they also occur more often in both men and women with gonorrhea.

Those at greatest risk of chlamydial infection are individuals 25 years old or younger who engage in sex with more than one new partner within a two-month period and women who use birth control pills or other nonbarrier contraceptive methods. The U.S. Preventive Services Task Force recommends regular screening for chlamydia for all sexually active women under age 25.

The incidence of chlamydia is lower in older women, and screening is recommended only for those with multiple sexual partners, a history of STIs, or inconsistent use of condoms.[27]

✓**check-in** Have you ever been screened for chlamydia?

Signs and Symptoms As many as 75 percent of women and 50 percent of men with chlamydia have no symptoms or have symptoms so mild that they don't seek medical attention. Without treatment, up to 40 percent of cases of chlamydia can lead to pelvic inflammatory disease (PID), a serious infection of the woman's fallopian tubes that also can damage the ovaries and uterus. Also, women infected with chlamydia may have three to five times the risk of getting infected with HIV if exposed. Babies exposed to chlamydia in the birth canal during delivery can be born with pneumonia or with an eye infection called conjunctivitis, both of which can be dangerous unless treated early with antibiotics. Symptomless women who are screened and treated for chlamydial infection are almost 60 percent less likely than unscreened women to develop PID. Chlamydia may also be linked to cervical cancer.

When women have symptoms of chlamydia, they may experience

- Abdominal pain
- Abnormal vaginal discharge
- Bleeding between menstrual periods
- Cervical or rectal inflammation
- Low-grade fever
- Yellowish discharge from the cervix that may have a foul odor
- Vaginal bleeding after intercourse
- Painful intercourse
- Painful urination
- The urge to urinate more than usual

When men have symptoms of chlamydia, they may experience

- Pain or burning while urinating
- Pus or watery or milky discharge from the penis
- Swollen or tender testicles
- Rectal inflammation

Men often don't take these symptoms seriously because the symptoms may appear only early in the day and can be very mild.

Chlamydia, which can spread from a man's urethra to his testicles, can also cause a condition called epididymitis, which can cause sterility. Symptoms include fever, swelling, and extreme pain in the scrotum. Six percent of men with epididymitis develop reactive arthritis, which causes swelling and pain in the joints and can progress and become disabling.

In women and men, chlamydia may cause the rectum to itch and bleed. It can also result in a discharge and diarrhea. If it infects the eyes, it may cause redness, itching, and a discharge. If it infects the throat, it may cause soreness.

Diagnosis and Treatment Various antibiotics such as azithromycin and doxycycline kill *Chlamydia* bacteria. Some are taken in a single dose; others over several days. Both partners must be treated to avoid reinfections.

The CDC, in its most recent guidelines, recommends that all women with chlamydia be rescreened three to four months after treatment is completed. The reason is that reinfection, which often happens because a patient's sex partners were not treated, increases the risk of PID and other complications. Immediately treating the partners of people infected with gonorrhea or chlamydia can reduce rates of recurrence of these infections.

Pelvic Inflammatory Disease (PID)

Infection of a woman's fallopian tubes or uterus, called **pelvic inflammatory disease (PID)**, is not actually an STI but rather a complication of

STIs involving the uterus, oviducts, and/or ovaries.[28] Ten to 20 percent of initial episodes of PID lead to scarring and obstruction of the fallopian tubes severe enough to cause infertility. Other long-term complications are ectopic pregnancy and chronic pelvic pain. Smoking also may increase the likelihood of PID.

Two bacteria—*Gonococcus* (the culprit in gonorrhea) and *Chlamydia*—are responsible for one-half to one-third of all cases of PID. Other organisms are responsible for the remaining cases. Several studies have shown that women with PID are more likely to have used douches than those without the disease. Consistent condom use may decrease PID risk.

....
✓**check-in** Did you know that PID can
cause infertility in women?
....

Incidence   About one in every seven women of reproductive age has PID; half of all adult women may have had it. Each year, about 1 million new cases are reported.

Most cases of PID occur among women under age 25 who are sexually active. *Gonococcus*-caused cases tend to affect poor women; those caused by *Chlamydia* range across all income levels. One-third to one-half of all cases are transmitted sexually, and others have been traced to some IUDs that are no longer on the market.

Signs and Symptoms   PID is a silent disease that in half of all cases produces no noticeable symptoms as it progresses and causes scarring of the fallopian tubes. Early symptoms include

- Abdominal pain or tenderness
- Fever
- Vaginal discharge that may have a foul odor
- Painful intercourse or urination
- Irregular menstrual bleeding
- Rarely, pain in the right upper abdomen

Diagnosis and Treatment   Urine testing is a cost-effective method of detecting gonorrhea and chlamydia in young women and can prevent development of PID. For women with symptoms, a pelvic ultrasound can show whether fallopian tubes are enlarged or an abscess is present. Magnetic resonance imaging (MRI) also can establish a diagnosis of PID and detect other diseases that may be responsible for the symptoms. Treatment consists of antibiotic therapy, usually with at least two antibiotics effective against a wide range of bacteria. A woman's sex partner(s) also should be

treated to decrease the risk of reinfection, even if they have no symptoms. PID causes an estimated 15 to 30 percent of all cases of infertility every year and about half of all cases of ectopic pregnancy.

Gonorrhea

Gonorrhea (sometimes called "the clap") is one of the most common STIs in the United States.

Incidence   Some 330,000 new cases are reported annually. As with chlamydia, gonorrhea rates are higher in women, particularly those between ages 15 and 24, than in men. However, men having sex with men are also at risk.[29] Sexual contact, including oral sex, is the primary means of transmission. Gonorrhea has infected 106 of every 100,000 Americans.

Signs and Symptoms   Most men who have gonorrhea know it. Thick, yellow-white pus oozes from the penis, and urination causes a burning sensation. These symptoms usually develop two to nine days after the sexual contact that infected them. Men have a good reason to seek help: It hurts too much not to.

In men, untreated gonorrhea can spread to the prostate gland, testicles, bladder, and kidneys. Among the serious complications are urinary obstruction and sterility caused by blockage of the vas deferens (the excretory duct of the testis).

Women also may experience discharge and burning on urination. However, as many as 8 out of 10 infected women have no symptoms.

Gonococcus, the bacterium that causes gonorrhea, can live in the vagina, cervix, and fallopian tubes for months, even years, and continue to infect the woman's sexual partners. Approximately 5 percent of sexually active American women have positive gonorrhea cultures but are unaware that they are silent carriers.

If left untreated in men or women, gonorrhea spreads through the urinary-genital tract. In women, the inflammation travels from the vagina and cervix, through the uterus, to the fallopian tubes and ovaries. The pain and fever are similar to those caused by stomach upset, so a woman may dismiss the symptoms. Eventually these symptoms diminish, even though the disease spreads to the entire pelvis. Pus may ooze from the fallopian tubes or ovaries into the peritoneum (the lining of the abdominal cavity), sometimes causing serious inflammation. However, this, too, can subside in a few weeks.

Gonorrhea, the leading cause of sterility in women, can cause PID. In pregnant women, gonorrhea becomes a threat to the newborn. It can infect the infant's external genitals and can cause

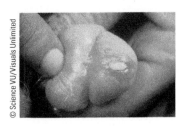

A cloudy discharge is symptomatic of gonorrhea.

gonorrhea A sexually transmitted infection caused by the bacterium *Neisseria gonorrhoeae*; symptoms include discharge from the penis; women are generally asymptomatic.

a serious form of conjunctivitis. As a preventive step, newborns may have penicillin dropped into their eyes at birth.

In both sexes, gonorrhea can develop into a serious, even fatal, bloodborne infection that can cause arthritis in the joints, attack the heart muscle and lining, cause meningitis, and attack the skin and other organs.

Diagnosis and Treatment Although a blood test has been developed for detecting gonorrhea, the tried-and-true method of diagnosis is still a microscopic analysis of cultures from the male's urethra, the female's cervix, and the throat and anus of both sexes.

Because gonorrhea often occurs along with chlamydia, practitioners often prescribe an agent effective against both, such as ofloxacin. Fluoroquinolones are no longer advised for use in its treatment. The CDC recommends a cephalosporin antibiotic plus azithromycin or doxycyline, but recommendations for treatment are rapidly evolving. A new strain of gonorrhea resistant to available antibiotics has emerged in North America. Antibiotics taken for other reasons may not affect or cure gonorrhea because of their dosage or type.

Nongonococcal Urethritis (NGU)

The term **nongonococcal urethritis (NGU)** refers to any inflammation of the urethra that is not caused by gonorrhea. NGU is the most common STI in men, accounting for 4 to 6 million visits to a physician every year. Three microorganisms—*Chlamydia trachomatis*, *Ureaplasma urealyticum*, and *Mycoplasma genitalium*—are the primary causes; the usual means of transmission is sexual intercourse. Other infectious agents, such as fungi or bacteria, allergic reactions to vaginal secretions, or irritation by soaps or contraceptive foams or gels also may lead to NGU.

In the United States, NGU is more common in men than gonococcal urethritis. The symptoms in men are similar to those of gonorrhea, including discharge from the penis (usually less than with gonorrhea) and mild burning during urination. Women frequently develop no symptoms or very mild itching, burning during urination, or discharge. Symptoms usually disappear after two or three weeks, but the infection may persist and cause cervicitis or PID in women and, in men, may spread to the prostate, epididymis, or both. Treatment usually consists of doxycycline or azithromycin and should be given to both sexual partners.

nongonococcal urethritis (NGU) Inflammation of the urethra caused by organisms other than the *Gonococcus* bacterium.

syphilis A sexually transmitted infection caused by the bacterium *Treponema pallidum* and characterized by early sores, a latent period, and a final period of life-threatening symptoms, including brain damage and heart failure.

Syphilis

A corkscrew-shaped, spiral bacterium called *Treponema pallidum* causes **syphilis**. This frail microbe dies in seconds if dried or chilled but grows quickly in the warm, moist tissues of the body, particularly in the mucous membranes of the genital tract. Entering the body through any tiny break in the skin, the germ burrows its way into the bloodstream. Sexual contact, including oral sex or intercourse, is a primary means of transmission. Genital ulcers caused by syphilis may increase the risk of HIV infection, while individuals with HIV may be more likely to develop syphilis.

Incidence The number of cases of syphilis in the United States has risen since 2012, with gay and bisexual men accounting for 75 percent of the increase. According to the CDC's most recent statistics, 5.5 per 100,000 Americans have syphilis, which can increase the risk of acquiring or transmitting HIV.[30]

Signs and Symptoms Syphilis has clearly identifiable stages:

- **Primary syphilis:** The first sign of syphilis is a lesion, or *chancre* (pronounced "shanker"), an open lump or crater the size of a dime or smaller, teeming with bacteria. The incubation period before its appearance ranges from 10 to 90 days; three to four weeks is average. The chancre appears exactly where the bacteria entered the body: in the mouth, throat, vagina, rectum, or penis. Any contact with the chancre is likely to result in infection.

- **Secondary syphilis:** Anywhere from 1 to 12 months after the chancre's appearance, secondary-stage symptoms may appear. Some people have no symptoms. Others develop a skin rash or a small, flat rash in moist regions on the skin; whitish patches on the mucous membranes of the mouth or throat; temporary baldness; low-grade fever; headache; swollen glands; or large, moist sores around the mouth and genitals. These sores are loaded with bacteria; contact with them, through kissing or intercourse, may transmit the infection. Symptoms may last for several days or several months. Even without treatment, symptoms eventually disappear as the syphilis microbes go into hiding.

- **Late and latent syphilis:** Although there are no signs or symptoms and no sores or rashes at this stage, the bacteria are invading various organs inside the body, including the heart and brain. For two to four years, there may be recurring infectious and highly contagious lesions of the skin or mucous membranes. However, syphilis loses its infectiousness as it progresses: After the first two years, a person rarely transmits syphilis through intercourse.

After four years, even congenital syphilis is rarely transmitted. Until this stage of the disease, however, a pregnant woman can pass syphilis to her unborn child. If the fetus is infected in its fourth month or earlier, it may be disfigured or even die. If infected late in pregnancy, the child may show no signs of infection for months or years after birth, but may then become disabled with the symptoms of tertiary syphilis.

- **Tertiary syphilis:** Ten to 20 years after the beginning of the latent stage, the most serious symptoms of syphilis emerge, generally in the organs in which the bacteria settled during latency. Syphilis that has progressed to this stage has become increasingly rare. Victims of tertiary syphilis may die of a ruptured aorta or of other heart damage, or may have progressive brain or spinal cord damage, eventually leading to blindness, insanity, or paralysis. About one-third of those who are not treated during the first three stages of syphilis enter the tertiary stage later in life.

Diagnosis and Treatment Health experts urge screening with a blood test for syphilis for everyone who seeks treatment for an STI, especially adolescents; for anyone using illegal drugs; and for the partners of those in these two groups. They also recommend that anyone diagnosed with syphilis be screened for other STIs and be counseled about voluntary testing for HIV.

Penicillin is the drug of choice for treating primary, secondary, and latent syphilis. The earlier treatment begins, the more effective it is. Those allergic to penicillin may be treated with doxycycline, ceftriaxone, or erythromycin. An added danger of not getting treatment for syphilis is an increased risk of HIV transmission.

Chancroid

A **chancroid** is a soft, painful sore or localized infection caused by the bacterium *Haemophilus ducrevi* and usually acquired through sexual contact. Half of the cases heal by themselves. In other cases, the infection may spread to the lymph glands near the chancroid, where large amounts of pus can accumulate and destroy much of the local tissue. The incidence of this STI, widely prevalent in Africa and tropical and semitropical regions, is rapidly increasing in the United States, with outbreaks in several states, including Louisiana, Texas, and New York. Chancroids, which may increase susceptibility to HIV infection, are believed to be a major factor

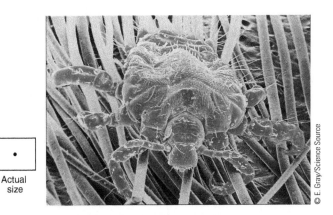

Actual size

© E. Gray/Science Source

in the heterosexual spread of HIV. This infection is treated with antibiotics (ceftriaxone, azithromycin, or erythromycin) and can be prevented by keeping the genitals clean and washing them with soap and water in case of possible exposure.

Pubic Lice and Scabies

These infections are sometimes, but not always, transmitted sexually. *Pubic lice* (or "crabs") are usually found in the pubic hair, although they can migrate to any hairy areas of the body. Lice lay eggs called nits that attach to the base of the hair shaft. Irritation from the lice may produce intense itching. Scratching to relieve the itching can produce sores. *Scabies* is caused by mites that burrow under the skin, where they lay eggs that hatch and undergo many changes in the course of their life cycle, producing great discomfort, including intense itching. Lice and scabies are treated with applications of permethrin cream and lindane shampoo to all the areas of the body where there are concentrations of body hair (genitals, armpits, scalp).

Trichomoniasis

An estimated 7.4 million new cases of this common curable STI appear each year in men and women. The cause is a single-celled protozoan parasite *Trichomonas vaginalis*, transmitted by vaginal intercourse or vulva-to-vulva contact with an infected partner. Women can acquire this disease from male or female partners; men usually contract it only from infected women.

Most men have no signs or symptoms; some experience irritation inside the penis, mild discharge, or slight burning on urination or ejaculation. Some women develop a frothy, yellow-green vaginal discharge with a strong odor and may experience discomfort during intercourse and urination as well as genital itching and irritation.

Diagnosis is based on a physical examination and a laboratory test. Treatment consists of a single dose of oral medication, either metronidazole or tinidazole. If untreated, an infected man, even if he has

chancroid A soft, painful sore or localized infection usually acquired through sexual contact.

Common STIs and STDs 335

never had symptoms or if his symptoms have gone away, can continue to infect or reinfect partners.

Bacterial Vaginosis

Bacterial vaginosis (BV), the most common vaginal infection in women ages 15 to 44, is caused by an imbalance of normal bacteria in the vagina. Having a new sex partner or multiple sex partners and douching can increase a woman's risk for getting BV. Although not considered an STD, BV increases vulnerability to STIs.

Women cannot get bacterial vaginosis from toilet seats, bedding, or swimming pools. The best ways to prevent BV are

• Not having sex

• Limiting the number of sex partners

• Not douching

Many women with BV do not have symptoms. Others may notice a thin white or gray vaginal discharge, odor, pain, itching, or burning in the vagina. Some women detect a strong fish-like odor, especially after sex; burning when urinating; or itching around the outside of the vagina.

Laboratory tests of vaginal fluid can determine if BV is present. Antibiotics can treat BV, although the infection may recur. Male sex partners of women diagnosed with BV generally do not need to be treated. However, BV may be transferred between female sex partners. Without treatment, BV increases the risk of various STIs, including chlamydia, gonorrhea, and HIV, and, in pregnant women, the risk of having a premature or low-birth-weight baby.

HIV and AIDS

Decades ago no one knew about **human immunodeficiency virus (HIV)**. No one had ever heard of **acquired immune deficiency syndrome (AIDS)**. Once seen as an epidemic affecting primarily gay men and injection drug users, AIDS has taken on very different forms.

Experts no longer think of AIDS as a single global health threat. Instead, many regions and countries are experiencing diverse epidemics. Sub-Saharan Africa has been the most affected region as measured by HIV/AIDS prevalence rates, followed by the Caribbean. Infection rates continue to rise in eastern Europe and Asia.

Incidence According to the most recent statistics, 34 million people are living with HIV/AIDS worldwide. Nearly 30 million have died.[31] The global HIV/AIDS prevalence rate (the percentage of people living with the disease) has leveled off, although the number of people living with the disease continues to increase. An estimated 2.5 million people become newly infected with HIV every year. Women comprise half of adults estimated to be living with HIV/AIDS worldwide. Young people account for approximately 40 percent of new HIV infections worldwide and a quarter of those in the United States.[32]

About 1.2 million people in the United States are living with HIV/AIDS, a number that has grown because those with the disease are living longer.[33] Someone in this country is infected every 9½ minutes. At highest risk are

• **Gay and bisexual men:** HIV infection rates have generally declined among gay and bisexual men, but new infections are on the rise among this group. An estimated 53% of new HIV infections occur in gay or bisexual men. Younger gay and bisexual men and those of color are at particularly high risk. One reason may be a misperception of risk. In a study of men engaging in behaviors such as unprotected anal sex, only 25 to 35 percent considered themselves high risk for infection.

• **Black Americans:** Although black Americans represent only 12 percent of the population, they account for 44 percent of new HIV infections. The rate of HIV diagnosis among black men is eight times that of whites, and the rate for black women is 19 times that of whites.[34]

Two percent of black Americans are HIV positive, higher than any other group. The AIDS diagnosis rate for blacks is more than nine times that for whites.

Only about one in three black Americans with the AIDS-causing virus have their infection under control.[35] Blacks have had the highest age-adjusted death rate due to HIV disease throughout most of the epidemic. The reasons for this discrepancy are complex and include a higher rate of other STDs in black communities, disparities in health care, and poverty.

• **Women:** In 1985 women represented 8 percent of AIDS diagnoses; now they account for 25 percent. According to CDC estimates, almost 280,000 women in the United States are living with HIV or AIDS. Black women make up about two-thirds of women diagnosed with AIDS, but the rate of new infections among black women has dropped. Latinos account for 18 percent of new infections in women.

Women are most likely to be infected through heterosexual sex, followed by injection drug use. Mother-to-child transmission of HIV has decreased dramatically because of the use of medicines that significantly reduce the risk of transmission from a woman to her baby.

At least one case of woman-to-woman infection has been documented. Although the

bacterial vaginosis (BV) A common vaginal infection caused by an imbalance of normal bacteria in the vagina.

human immunodeficiency virus (HIV) A virus that causes a spectrum of health problems, ranging from a symptomless infection to changes in the immune system, to the development of life-threatening diseases because of impaired immunity.

acquired immune deficiency syndrome (AIDS) The final stages of HIV infection, characterized by a variety of severe illnesses and decreased levels of certain immune cells.

risk is low, female sex partners can transmit HIV when bodily fluids such as menstrual blood and vaginal fluids come into contact with a cut, an abrasion, or a mucus membrane (the tissue lining the mouth and vagina).[36]

- **Young adults:** Teens and young adults under age 30 continue to be at risk. Those between ages 13 and 20 account for 34 percent of new HIV infections, the largest share of any age group. Most are infected sexually.

√**check-in** How do you rate your risk of HIV infection?

Reducing the Risk of HIV Transmission

HIV/AIDS can be so frightening that some people have exaggerated its dangers, whereas others understate them. The fact is that although no one is immune to HIV, you can reduce the risk if you abstain from sexual activity or remain in a monogamous relationship with an uninfected partner and if you do not inject drugs.

If you're not in a long-term monogamous relationship with a partner you're sure is safe and you're not willing to abstain from sex, there are things you can do to lower your risk of HIV infection. Remember that the risk of HIV transmission depends on sexual behavior, not sexual orientation. Among young men, the prevalence and frequency of sexual risk behaviors are similar regardless of sexual orientation, ethnicity, or age. Homosexual, heterosexual, and bisexual individuals all need to know about the kinds of sexual activity that increase their risk.

Sexual Transmission
Here's what you should know about sexual transmission of HIV:

- Casual contact does *not* spread HIV infection. You cannot get HIV infection from drinking from a water fountain, contact with a toilet seat, or touching an infected person.

- Compared to other viruses, HIV is extremely difficult to get.

- HIV can live in blood, semen, vaginal fluids, and breast milk.

- Many chemicals, including household bleach, alcohol, and hydrogen peroxide, can inactivate HIV.

- In studies of family members sharing dishes, food, clothing, and frequent hugs with people with HIV infection or AIDS, those who have contracted the virus have shared razor blades or toothbrushes or had other means of blood contact.

- You cannot tell visually whether a potential sexual partner has HIV. A blood test is needed

to detect the antibodies that the body produces to fight HIV, thus indicating infection. As noted in Chapter 9, circumcision greatly reduces the risk for HIV infection.

- HIV can be spread in semen and vaginal fluids during a single instance of anal, vaginal, or oral sexual contact between heterosexuals, bisexuals, or homosexuals. The risk increases with the number of sexual encounters with an infected partner.

- Teenage girls may be particularly vulnerable to HIV infection because the immature cervix is easily infected.

- Anal intercourse is an extremely high-risk behavior because HIV can enter the bloodstream through tiny breaks in the lining of the rectum. HIV transmission is much more likely to occur during unprotected anal intercourse than vaginal intercourse.

- Other behaviors that increase the risk of HIV infection include having multiple sexual partners, engaging in sex without condoms or virus-killing spermicides, having sexual contact with persons known to be at high risk (for example, prostitutes or injection drug users), and sharing injection equipment for drugs.

- Condom use significantly reduces the risk of HIV transmission (by as much as 78 percent).[37]

- Individuals are at greater risk if they have an active sexual infection. STIs, such as herpes, gonorrhea, and syphilis, facilitate transmission of HIV during vaginal or anal intercourse.

- No cases of HIV transmission by deep (French) kissing have been reported, but it could happen. Studies have found blood in the saliva of healthy people after kissing; other lab studies have found HIV in saliva. Social (dry) kissing is safe.

- Oral sex can lead to HIV transmission. The virus in any semen that enters the mouth could make its way into the bloodstream through tiny nicks or sores in the mouth. A man's risk in performing oral sex on a woman is smaller because an infected woman's genital fluids have much lower concentrations of HIV than does semen.

- HIV infection is not widespread among lesbians, although there have been documented cases of possible female-to-female HIV transmission. However, in each instance, one partner had had sex with a bisexual man or male injection drug user or had injected drugs herself.

Nonsexual Transmission
Efforts to prevent nonsexual forms of HIV transmission have been very effective. Screening the blood supply has

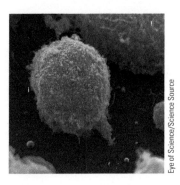

Electron micrograph of a white blood cell being attacked by HIV (light blue particles), the virus that causes AIDS.

reduced the rate of transfusion-associated HIV transmission by 99.9 percent. Treatment with antiretroviral drugs during pregnancy and birth has reduced transmission to newborns by about 90 percent in optimal conditions. HIV infections among injection drug users have fallen by half in the past decade.

Preventing HIV Infection   Behavioral methods, such as safer sex practices, remain the primary means of preventing transmission of HIV. (See Health on a Budget.) Among men having sex with men, effective treatment, which lowers the virus levels in the body, may be contributing to a decline in unrecognized HIV infection.[38]

Biological approaches may provide additional protection. In initial trials of "pre-exposure prophylaxis" (PrEP), a daily pill called Truvada, which combines two anti-HIV drugs, significantly reduced the risk of HIV transmission in high-risk men. The participants received condoms and intensive counseling on safe sex practices. An international study has shown that the medication doesn't lead people to stop using condoms or have more sex with more people.[39]

Recognizing and Treating HIV/AIDS
HIV infection refers to a spectrum of health problems that results from immunologic abnormalities caused by the virus when it enters the bloodstream. In theory, the body may be able to resist infection by HIV. In reality, in almost all cases, HIV destroys the cell-mediated immune system, particularly the CD4+ T-lymphocytes (also called *T4 helper cells*). The result is greatly increased susceptibility to various cancers and opportunistic infections (infections that take hold because of the reduced effectiveness of the immune system).

HIV triggers a state of all-out war within the immune system. Almost immediately following infection with HIV, the immune system responds aggressively by manufacturing enormous numbers of CD4+ cells. It eventually is overwhelmed, however, as the viral particles continue to replicate, or multiply. The intense war between HIV and the immune system indicates that the virus itself, not a breakdown in the immune system, is responsible for disease progression.

Shortly after becoming infected with HIV, individuals may experience a few days of flu-like symptoms, which most ignore or attribute to other viruses. Some people develop a more severe mononucleosis-type syndrome. After this stage, individuals may not develop any signs or symptoms of disease for a period ranging from weeks to more than 12 years.

HIV symptoms, which tend to increase in severity and number the longer the virus is in the body, may include any of the following:

- Swollen lymph nodes
- Fever, chills, and night sweats
- Diarrhea
- Weight loss
- Coughing and shortness of breath
- Persistent tiredness
- Skin sores
- Blurred vision and headaches
- Development of other infections, such as certain kinds of pneumonia

HIV infection is associated with a variety of HIV-related diseases, including different cancers and dangerous infections including tuberculosis. HIV-infected individuals may develop persistent generalized lymphadenopathy, enlargement of the lymph nodes at two or more different sites in the body. This condition typically persists for more than three months without any other illness to explain its occurrence. Diminished mental function may appear before other symptoms. Tests conducted on infected but apparently healthy men have revealed impaired coordination, problems in thinking, or abnormal brain scans. Psychological problems, including depression, anxiety, and stress, occur "in epidemic proportions" in individuals with HIV, according to recent research, and can affect their behavior (such as taking steps to prevent transmitting the virus) and treatment outcome.

HIV Testing   One in five Americans infected with HIV doesn't know it. An estimated one-third to nearly half of American teens and young adults with HIV delay treatment until their infection is advanced, putting them at risk for serious health problems.[40]

All HIV tests measure antibodies, cells produced by the body to fight HIV infection. A negative test indicates no exposure to HIV. It can take three to six months for the body to produce the telltale antibodies, however, so a negative result may not be accurate, depending on the timing of the test. Faster tests that can detect HIV earlier are under development.[41]

HIV testing can be either confidential or anonymous. In confidential testing, a person's name is recorded along with the test results, which are made available to medical personnel and, in 32 states, the state health department. In anonymous testing, no name is associated with the test results. Anonymous testing is available in 39 states.

The only home HIV test approved by the FDA, Home Access, is available in drugstores or online for $40 to $50. An individual draws a blood sample by pricking a finger and sends it to a laboratory, along with a personal identification number. Results are given over the phone by a trained counselor, usually within several days.

Newly developed blood tests can determine how recently a person was infected with HIV and distinguish between long-standing infections and those contracted within the previous four to six months.

Diagnosing AIDS   A diagnosis of AIDS applies to anyone with HIV whose immune system is severely impaired, as indicated by a CD4+ count of fewer than 200 cells per cubic millimeter of blood, compared to normal CD4+ cell counts in healthy people not infected with HIV of 800 to 1,200 per cubic millimeter of blood. In addition, AIDS is diagnosed in persons with HIV infection who experience recurrent pneumonia, invasive cervical cancer, or pulmonary tuberculosis.

People with AIDS also may experience persistent fever, diarrhea that persists for more than one month, or involuntary weight loss of more than 10 percent of normal body weight. Neurological disease—including dementia (confusion and impaired thinking) and other problems with thinking, speaking, movement, or sensation—may occur. Secondary infectious diseases that may develop in people with AIDS include *Pneumocystis carinii* pneumonia, tuberculosis, or oral candidiasis (thrush). Secondary cancers associated with HIV infection include Kaposi's sarcoma and cancer of the cervix.

Treatments   New forms of therapy have been remarkably effective in boosting levels of protective T cells and reducing *viral load*—the amount of HIV in the bloodstream. Starting HIV treatment early, before a patient's immune system is badly weakened, can dramatically improve survival. People with high viral loads are more likely to progress rapidly to AIDS than people with low levels of the virus.

The current "gold-standard" approach to combating HIV is known as ART (antiretroviral therapy), which dramatically reduces viral load but does not eradicate the virus. This complex regimen uses one of 250 different combinations of three or more antiretroviral drugs, often available in a single tablet. Treatment begins much earlier than in the past, even before moderate immune suppression. This benefits the individual patient and helps prevent HIV transmission to a sexual partner.

Early ART has shown promise in treating newborns with HIV infection but also causes serious complications.

Among the 40 million people living with HIV, there is only one confirmed cure: a patient who also developed cancer and underwent intensive chemotherapy, total body radiation, and bone marrow transplantation. A key challenge is that once HIV invades an individual's genome, it is extremely difficult to remove all HIV-infected cells, which—even with treatment—persist in the body for decades.[42]

- Why are college students at high risk for sexually transmitted infections?
- What are three key steps to lower your risk of STIs?
- What is the most common STI, and how can you protect yourself from it?
- What are the latest advances in HIV/AIDS prevention, diagnosis, and treatment?

THE POWER OF NOW!
Protecting Your Sexual Health

As with other aspects of your well-being, your sexual health depends on your choices and behaviors. Here are some basic guidelines:

____ Talk first. Get to know your partner. Before having sex, establish a committed relationship that allows trust and open communication. You should be able to discuss past sexual histories and any previous STIs or IV drug use. You should not feel coerced or forced into having sex.

____ Stay sober. Alcohol and drugs impair your judgment, make it harder to communicate clearly, and can lead to forgetting or failing to use condoms properly.

____ Practice safe sex. Avoid risky sex practices that can tear or break the skin, such as anal intercourse. Use latex condoms. Limit sexual partners.

____ Be honest. If you have an STI, like HPV or herpes, advise any prospective sexual partner. Allow him or her to decide what to do. If you mutually agree on engaging in sexual activity, use latex condoms and other protective measures.

____ Don't feel you have to have sex for fear of hurting someone's feelings or fear of being the "only one" who isn't doing it. If you don't want to have sex, be honest, discuss the reasons behind your decision with your partner, and stay true to you.

____ Respect everyone's right to make his or her own personal decision—including yours. There is no perfect point in a relationship where sex has to happen. If your partner tells you that he or she is not ready to have sex, respect this decision, discuss the reasons behind it, and be supportive.

____ Be prepared for a sex emergency. Consider carrying two condoms with you just in case one breaks or tears. Men and women are equally responsible for preventing STIs, and both should carry condoms.

____ Abstinence doesn't mean less affection. Practicing abstinence—the most effective way to protect against STIs—doesn't mean you can't have an intimate relationship with someone. It just means you don't have vaginal or anal intercourse or oral sex.

____ Make your sexual health a priority. Whether you are having sex or not, both men and women need regular check-ups to make sure they are sexually healthy. Get immunized against HPV.

What's Online

 CENGAGE Visit www.cengagebrain.com to access course materials for this text, including the Behavior Change Planner, interactive quizzes, and more.

Assessing Your STI Risk

This Self Survey looks at your risk of acquiring or transmitting any sexually transmitted infection.

STI Quiz

1. **True** or **False**: A person can have an STI and not know it.

2. **True** or **False**: It is normal for women to have some vaginal discharge.

3. **True** or **False**: Once you have had an STI and have been cured, you can't get it again.

4. **True** or **False**: HIV is mainly present in semen, blood, vaginal secretions, and breast milk.

5. **True** or **False**: Chlamydia and gonorrhea can cause pelvic inflammatory disease.

6. **True** or **False**: A pregnant woman who has an STI can pass the disease on to her baby.

7. **True** or **False**: Most STIs go away without treatment, if people wait long enough.

8. **True** or **False**: STIs that aren't cured early can cause sterility.

9. **True** or **False**: Birth control pills offer excellent protection from STIs.

10. **True** or **False**: Condoms can help prevent the spread of STIs.

11. **True** or **False**: If you know your partner, you can't get an STI.

12. **True** or **False**: Chlamydia is the most common bacterial STI.

13. **True** or **False**: A sexually active woman should get an annual Pap test from her doctor.

Scoring

1. **True** Some of the most common symptoms of an STI infection include abnormal discharge, painful urination, burning, and itching or tingling in the genital area, but it is important to remember that many women and men who have an STI often do not experience any symptoms at all. Chlamydia, for example, often has no symptoms.

2. **True** Normal vaginal discharge has several purposes: cleaning and moistening the vagina and helping to prevent and fight infections. Although it's normal for the color, texture, and amount of vaginal fluids to vary throughout a woman's menstrual cycle, some changes in discharge may indicate a problem.

   If you think you may have a problem, you should see a doctor as soon as possible. First, though, it helps to learn some of the differences between what is normal and abnormal vaginal discharge for you.

3. **False** Having an STI and being cured from it does not mean that your body now has a built-in immunity to the bacteria that causes the infection. You must protect yourself from becoming infected again by using a condom. Remember, it is your body!

4. **True** Although small traces of HIV can be found in tears, saliva, urine, and perspiration, extensive studies have shown that there is not enough of the virus or the virus is not strong enough to be transmitted. Only blood, semen, vaginal secretions, and breast milk have been proven to transmit the HIV virus and hepatitis B. HIV cannot be passed on by casual contact.

5. **True** Many different organisms can cause PID, but most cases are associated with gonorrhea and genital chlamydial infections, two very common STIs. Scientists have found that bacteria normally present in small numbers in the vagina and cervix also may play a role.

6. **True** STIs can be passed from a pregnant woman to the baby before, during, or after the baby's birth. Some STIs (like syphilis) cross the placenta and infect the baby while it is in the uterus (womb). Other STIs (like gonorrhea, chlamydia, hepatitis B, and genital herpes) can be transmitted from the mother to the baby during delivery as the baby passes through the birth canal. HIV can cross the placenta during pregnancy, infect the baby during the birth process, and unlike most other STIs, can infect the baby through breast-feeding.

7. **False** Even if symptoms appear to go away, the infected person will still have the infection and is able to pass the infection on to others until he or she gets treatment. STIs that aren't cured early can cause sterility.

8. **True** If the fallopian tubes are blocked at one or both ends, the egg can't travel through the tubes into the uterus. Blocked tubes may result from pelvic inflammatory disease, which is often caused by untreated STIs.

9. **False** The birth control pill does not protect against sexually transmitted infections. For those having sex, condoms must always be used along with birth control pills to protect against STIs. Abstinence (the decision to not have sex) is the only method that always prevents pregnancy and sexually transmitted infections.

10. **True** Most condoms are made of latex. Those made of lambskin may offer less protection against some sexually transmitted infections, including HIV, so use of latex condoms is recommended. For people who may have an allergic skin reaction to latex, both male and female condoms made of polyurethane are available.

When properly used, latex and plastic condoms are effective against most STIs. Condoms do not protect against infections spread from sores on the skin not covered by a condom (such as the base of the penis or scrotum).

11. **False** As stated in question number 1, a person can have an STI and not know it. If they can't tell, how can you?

12. **True** The U.S. Centers for Disease Control and Prevention estimates that more than 4 million new cases of chlamydia occur each year. The highest rates of chlamydial infection are in 15- to 19-year-old adolescents regardless of demographics or location.

13. **True** The Pap test is a way to find cell changes on the cervix. Abnormal cells may lead to cancer, so having a Pap test can find and treat them early, before they have time to progress to cancer.

Although Pap tests do not test for STIs, some STIs such as HPV (human papillomavirus infection) can cause abnormal Pap test results. Certain types of HPV are linked to cancer in both women and men.

Source: Material taken from The Bacchus Network™ Website, smartersex.org.

MAKING THIS CHAPTER WORK FOR YOU

Review Questions

(LO 11.1)   1. Which of the following is true of sexually transmitted infections?
   a. The odds of acquiring a sexually transmitted infection over a lifetime are low, at about 1 in 100.
   b. STIs cannot be transmitted unless the infected person displays symptoms at the time of sexual activity.
   c. Early HIV infections and gonorrhea in women may not be accompanied by any symptoms.
   d. STI pathogens prefer light, cold, and dry surfaces.

(LO 11.1)   2. Which of the following statements is true in the context of risk factors of sexually transmitted diseases?
   a. A person is safe as long as the partner shows no symptoms of a sexually transmitted infection.
   b. Multiple partners reduce the risk of a sexually transmitted infection.
   c. Failure to use condoms increases the risk of an infection.
   d. Substance abuse has a negligible contribution toward the risk associated with an infection.

(LO 11.2)   3. _____ are the only contraceptives that help prevent both pregnancy and STIs when used properly and consistently.
   a. Condoms
   b. Birth control pills
   c. Intrauterine devices
   d. Surgical sterilization methods

(LO 11.2)   4. Which of the following statements about sexually transmitted infections (STIs) is true?
   a. Symptoms of STIs tend to be more pronounced in women than in men.
   b. Women's risk of getting an infection is greater than that of men.
   c. Spermicides containing nonoxynol-9 protect from gonorrhea, chlamydia, and HIV.
   d. Pregnancy and fertility are unaffected by sexually transmitted infections.

(LO 11.3)   5. Of the 9 out of 10 college students who report they are sexually active, the percentage who say they use condoms is _____.
   a. about 50%
   b. about 75%
   c. about 25%
   d. almost none

(LO 11.3) 6. Students who don't consistently use condoms may be motivated by _____.
   a. cost
   b. availability
   c. lack of concern about contracting an STI
   d. fear of causing embarrassment

(LO 11.4) 7. Gardasil and Cervarix are vaccines available to prevent _____ in girls and young women.
   a. cervical cancer
   b. nongonococcal urethritis
   c. genital herpes
   d. pubic lice

(LO 11.4) 8. Which of the following is true of the incidence of HIV and AIDS?
   a. HIV infections are negligible in gay and bisexual men.
   b. The rate of HIV infections among black Americans is less than that in whites.
   c. Women are most likely to be affected through heterosexual sex.
   d. Young adults are least likely to contract an HIV infection.

Answers to these questions can be found on page 623.

Critical Thinking Questions

1. Have you come across an individual who displays expressions of alternate sexuality? If so, have you thought about the reasons for or what kind of alternate sexuality the individual displays? In the context of sexual diversity, think about the various types of sexualities other than heterosexuality in which individuals fall and analyze the risk factors of each category.
2. While engaging in sexual activity with a partner, have you ever thought about the risks of a sexually transmitted infection? Analyze the characteristics and risk factors of sexually transmitted diseases and evaluate where you and your partner stand.
3. Have you come across an individual who is infected with HIV? If so, what are the symptoms he displays?

Additional Online Resources

www.siecus.org
This website is sponsored by SIECUS, a national nonprofit organization that promotes comprehensive education about sexuality and advocates the right of all individuals of all sexual orientations to make responsible sexual choices. The site features a library of fact sheets and articles on a variety of sexuality topics and STIs designed for educators, adults, teens, parents, media, international audiences, and religious organizations.

www.hrc.org
The Human Rights Campaign is America's largest gay, lesbian, bisexual, and transgender civil rights organization. Its website features up-to-date information on issues related to gay rights and suggests courses of action to change government policies.

http://goaskalice.columbia.edu
Sponsored by the health education and wellness program of the Columbia University Health Service, this site features educators' answers to questions on a wide variety of topics of concern to young people, including those related to sexual orientation and healthy sexuality.

www.nlm.nih.gov/medlineplus/sexualhealth.html
Here you can find trusted information on sexual health from MedlinePlus, a site maintained as a service of the U.S. National Library of Medicine and the National Institutes of Health (NIH).

www.cdc.gov/std and www.cdc.gov/hiv
These sites at the CDC feature current information, fact sheets, treatment guides, surveillance, and statistics on sexually transmitted infections and HIV/AIDS.

www3.niaid.nih.gov/research/topics
This site, which is part of the National Institutes of Health, features research on STIs, including basic and clinical research and activities related to vaccine development.

http://hivinsite.ucsf.edu
This site, sponsored by the University of California San Francisco School of Medicine, provides statistics, education, prevention, and new developments related to HIV/AIDS.

Key Terms

The terms listed are used on the page indicated. Definitions of the terms are in the glossary at the end of the book.

acquired immune deficiency syndrome (AIDS) 336

bacterial vaginosis (BV) 336

chancroid 335

chlamydia 332

gonorrhea 333

herpes simplex 330

human immunodeficiency virus (HIV) 336

human papillomavirus (HPV) 328

nongonococcal urethritis (NGU) 334

pelvic inflammatory disease (PID) 332

sexually transmitted disease (STD) 322

sexually transmitted infection (STI) 322

syphilis 334

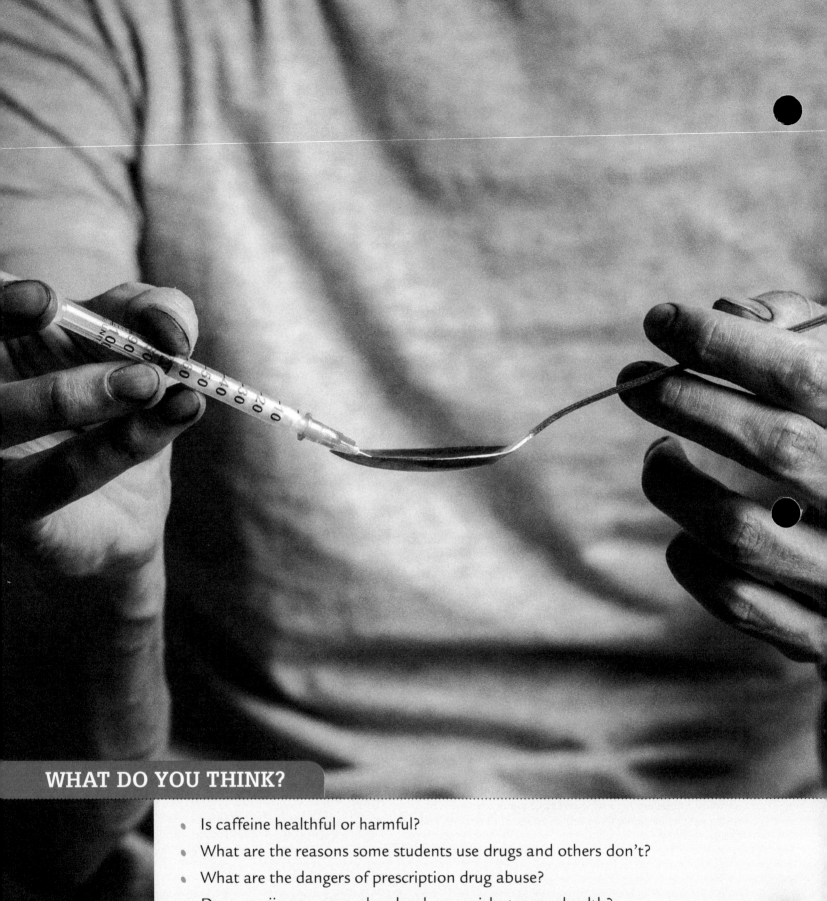

WHAT DO YOU THINK?

- Is caffeine healthful or harmful?
- What are the reasons some students use drugs and others don't?
- What are the dangers of prescription drug abuse?
- Does marijuana, even when legal, pose risks to your health?

12

Addictions

Jesse had too many papers to write and too little time to finish them. One of the guys in his fraternity suggested that he try a prescription stimulant a friend took for an attention-deficit disorder. The jolt felt like just what Jesse needed. During midterms he bought another prescription stimulant from a classmate. As finals approached, Jesse started hoarding stimulants from several people. He popped the final ones to rev up for the big end-of-school-year parties. Without realizing it, Jesse put himself at risk for drug-related problems—physical, psychological, and legal.

Although prescription drug abuse remains widespread on campuses, the drug scene across America may be changing. According to the most recent Monitoring the Future national survey, the use of many illicit drugs—MDMA (Ecstasy), inhalants, synthetic marijuana, the hallucinogen salvia, and the amphetamine-like stimulants known as bath salts—has declined among adolescents and young adults.[1] This is also true for college students—except for marijuana use, which has risen.[2] Nonetheless, according to the American College Health Association (ACHA), 61 percent of undergraduates report never having used marijuana; 66 percent have never used other drugs.[3]

After reading this chapter, you should be able to:

12.1 Explain how substance abuse and other self-destructive behaviors can affect health.

12.2 Discuss the ill effects of problem gambling and gambling disorder.

12.3 Outline the key indicators and effects of substance abuse on college campuses.

12.4 Summarize the effects that drugs have on the brain, body, and behavior.

12.5 Summarize the benefits and the adverse effects of caffeine.

12.6 Describe the harmful effects of inappropriate use of over-the-counter drugs and prescription drugs.

12.7 Identify the characteristics and consequences of substance use disorders.

12.8 Classify the characteristics and harmful effects of common drugs of abuse.

12.9 Explain how substance dependence and abuse can be treated.

(See Snapshot: On Campus Now Student Drug Use, on p. 350.)

Despite this decline, the toll of drug abuse remains high. Each year substance use contributes to more than 1,700 student deaths, 700,000 assaults, and almost 100,000 sexual attacks and rapes. Yet individuals who use drugs never think they will suffer such consequences.

They believe they are smart enough, strong enough, lucky enough not to get caught or hooked. However, addictions produce changes in an individual's body, brain, and behavior. In time their grip can outweigh everything else a person values and holds dearest.

This chapter provides information about and insights into how addictions start, why students use and abuse drugs, the nature and effect of drugs, and the most commonly used, misused, and abused drugs. It also offers practical strategies for preventing, recognizing the signs of, and seeking help for addictions. ◄

Addictive Behaviors: Risks and Rewards

College is a time when students want to experiment, enjoy, stretch, and take some risks. But there is a difference between the risks of experimenting with illicit drugs and the risks of forming a band or trying out for a team. One is an illegal activity that can get you in serious trouble in the short term and cause adverse health consequences in the long run. The others impart the thrill that comes with trying something new and mastering a challenge.

The majority of college students do not engage in addictive behaviors. One fundamental reason is that they have better things to do. "Substance-free reinforcement"—in simpler terms, a positive addiction to anything from rock climbing to snowboarding to zumba—can produce very real "highs," often for very little money.

Without passions to pursue, students are more likely to use and abuse multiple drugs. Such "polysubstance abuse" greatly increases their risk of physical, social, legal, and academic problems and pushes them deeper into drug involvement.[4]

As researchers have documented, the more that students use mind-altering substances, the less they engage in drug-free activities. This may be because substance abuse diminishes the brain's chemical response to other forms of pleasure. As a result, the delight of eating chocolate or the excitement of bungee-jumping fails to trigger the normal surge in dopamine, the brain's "feel-good" chemical. Instead chronic substance abusers develop anhedonia, an inability to experience pleasure.

Fortunately, this condition is reversible. When college students increase physical or creative activities, they often simultaneously reduce their drug and alcohol use, even without instruction to do so.[5] So the next time you're feeling bored, restless, anxious, frustrated, or overwhelmed, don't think a drug might offer a quick fix. Go for the longer-lasting, more fulfilling high of a positive addiction. (See "Health on a Budget," below.)

⑤ HEALTH ON A BUDGET

Develop a Positive Addiction

There is a crucial difference between a positive addiction and drug dependency: One is real, the other is chemical. With one, you're in control; with the other, drugs are.

Here are some examples:

- **If you feel a need for physical relaxation,** or if you want more energy or distraction from physical discomforts, you can turn to athletics, exercise (including walking and hiking), dance, or outdoor hobbies.

- **If you want to stimulate your senses,** enhance sexual stimulation, or magnify the sensations of sight, sound, and touch, train yourself to be more sensitive to nature and beauty. Take time to appreciate the sensations you experience when you're walking in the woods or embracing a person you love.

Through activities like sailing or sky-diving, you can literally fill up your senses without relying on chemicals.

- **If you want to escape mental boredom,** gain new understanding of the world around you, study better, experiment with your levels of awareness, or indulge your intellectual curiosity, you can challenge your mind through reading, classes, creative games, discussion groups, memory training, or travel.

- **If you're looking for kicks,** adventure, danger, and excitement, sign up for a wilderness survival course. Take up an adventurous sport, like hang gliding or rock climbing. Set a challenging professional or personal goal and direct your energies to meeting it.

✓**check-in** Are you taking risks that don't make sense and that don't add pleasure or passion to your life? Or are you taking risks that empower and inspire you?

Addictive Behaviors and the Dimensions of Health

Young adults have the highest rates of illicit drug use. Many do not realize that substance abuse and other self-destructive behaviors, such as gambling or compulsive eating, can affect every dimension of health. Some of the harmful effects are

- **Physical health:** Abuse of alcohol, tobacco, and drugs takes a toll on every organ system in the body, increasing the likelihood of disease, disability, and premature death. People who start using hard drugs, such as cocaine and amphetamines, as young adults and continue to use them in middle age have a five-fold increased risk of early death.

- **Psychological health:** Sometimes people begin abusing substances or engaging in addictive behavior as a way of "self-medicating" symptoms of anxiety or depression. However, alcohol and drugs provide only temporary relief. As abuse continues, shame and guilt increase, and coping with daily stressors becomes more difficult. Depression and anxiety are as likely to be consequences as causes of substance abuse.

- **Spiritual health:** Addictive behavior blocks the pursuit of meaning and inner fulfillment. As they rely more on a chemical or behavioral escape, individuals lose their sense of self and of connection with other people and with a Higher Power.

- **Social health:** Addictive behavior strains and, in time, severs ties to family, friends, colleagues, and classmates. The primary relationship in the life of alcoholics or addicts is with a behavior or a drug. As addicts withdraw from others, they become increasingly isolated.

- **Intellectual health:** The brain is one of the targets of alcohol and drugs. Under their influence, logic and reasoning break down. Impulses become more difficult to control. Judgment falters. Certain substances, such as Ecstasy, can lead to permanent changes in brain chemistry.

- **Environmental health:** The use of some substances, such as tobacco, directly harms the environment. Abusers of alcohol and drugs also pose indirect threats to others because their behavior can lead to injury and damage.

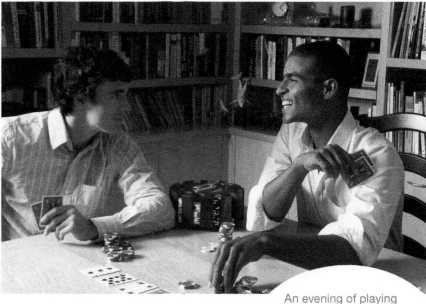

An evening of playing poker with friends can be a great way to relax. But for some college students, gambling can become addictive.

✓**check-in** Have alcohol or drugs affected any dimension of your health?

Gambling and Behavioral Addictions

Gambling disorder is the only "behavioral" addiction officially recognized as a psychiatric diagnosis. However, Internet use, video game playing, shopping, eating, and other behaviors also bear a resemblance to alcohol and drug dependence. Researchers are investigating their causes, characteristics, and impacts on psychological and physical well-being.[6]

Gambling is an act of risking a sum of money on the outcome of a game or an event that is determined by chance. Although most people who gamble limit the time and money they spend, some cross the line and lose control of their gambling "habit."[6]

Problem Gambling

The term *problem gambling* refers to all individuals with gambling-related problems, including mild or occasional ones. Here are some relevant key points:

- Problem gambling has become more common than alcohol dependence among American adults. Two factors associated with higher

gambling disorder Persistent and recurrent problematic gambling that leads to significant impairment or distress.

risk are male gender and lack of family engagement.[7]

- Levels of gambling, frequent gambling, and problem gambling increase during the teen years (even though underage gambling is illegal in most states), peak in the 20s and 30s, and decline after age 70.

- Men are more than twice as likely as women to be frequent gamblers and reach their highest gambling rates in their late teens.

- Whites are much more likely to report gambling in the past year than blacks or Asians, but both African Americans and Native Americans report higher levels of frequent gambling.

Gamblers typically progress through various stages:

- **Winning** In the winning phase, they feel empowered by their winnings and success.

- **Losing** Next comes the losing phase, during which gamblers try to win back their losses.

- **Desperation** During the desperation phase, a gambler may resort to illegal activity, including stealing, to continue gambling.

- **Giving up** In the giving-up phase, gamblers may desperately try to stay afloat in a game even though they realize they can't win.

Sports gamblers typically feel a sense of control because of their specialized knowledge of football, soccer, or other sports. However, professional gamblers are no more likely to correctly predict the outcome of a game or match than amateurs and laypeople.

Gambling Disorder

The American Psychiatric Association's *Diagnostic and Statistical Manual*, fifth edition (DSM-5), classifies persistent and recurrent problematic gambling that leads to significant impairment or distress as a gambling disorder, similar to other addictive disorders in its effects on brain and behavior. A diagnosis is made if individuals exhibit four or more of the following in a 12-month period:

- Need to gamble with increasing amounts of money to achieve excitement

- Becoming restless or irritable if they cut down or stop gambling

- Repeated unsuccessful attempts to control, reduce, or stop gambling

- Preoccupation with gambling

- Gambling when feeling guilty, anxious, or distressed

- After losing money, trying to recoup by "chasing" losses

- Lying to conceal the extent of gambling

- Putting a significant relationship, job, or opportunity in jeopardy because of gambling

- Reliance on others for money to relieve desperate financial situations caused by gambling.[8]

A gambling disorder can begin during adolescence or young adulthood but generally develops over the course of years. Many college students "grow out" of the disorder over time, although it remains a lifelong problem for some. Gambling disorders are more common among young men than among young women. Younger individuals prefer forms of gambling such as sports betting and Internet poker, whereas older adults are more likely to play slot machines or games of chance like bingo.

✓**check-in** Do you buy lottery or scratch tickets? Bet on sporting events? Play poker online? Go to casinos? Do you consider any or all of these forms of gambling?

Gambling on Campus

Gambling has become a more serious and widespread problem on college campuses. About half of students who gamble at least once a month experience significant problems related to their gambling, including poor academic performance, heavy alcohol consumption, illicit drug use, unprotected sex, and other risky behaviors. An estimated 3 to 6 percent of college students engage in "pathological gambling," which is characterized by "persistent and recurrent maladaptive gambling behavior."

Researchers have identified key indicators associated with "pathological" gambling:

- Gambling more than once a month

- Gambling more than two hours at a time

- Wagering more than 10 percent of monthly income

- A combination of parental gambling problems, gambling frequency, and psychological distress

College students who gamble say they do so for fun or excitement, to socialize, to win money, or to "just have something to do"— reasons similar to those of other adults who gamble. Simply having access to casino machines, ongoing card games, or Internet gambling sites increases the likelihood that students will gamble.

Researchers view problem or pathological gambling as an addiction that runs in families. Individuals predisposed to gambling because of their family history are more likely to develop a problem if they are regularly exposed to gambling. Alcoholism and drug abuse often occur along with gambling, leading to chaotic lives and greater health risks.

Risk Factors for Problem Gambling

Among young people (ages 16 to 25), the following behaviors indicate increased risk of problem gambling:

- Being male
- Gambling at an early age (as young as age 8)
- Having a big win early in one's gambling career
- Consistently chasing losses (betting more to recover money already lost)
- Gambling alone
- Feeling depressed before gambling
- Feeling excited and aroused during gambling
- Behaving irrationally during gambling
- Having poor grades at school
- Engaging in other addictive behaviors (smoking, drinking alcohol, illegal drug use)
- Lower socioeconomic class
- Parent with a gambling or other addiction problem
- A history of delinquency or stealing money to fund gambling
- Skipping class to go gambling

Drug Use on Campus

About 6 in 10 college students have never used marijuana or other illegal drugs (see Snapshot: On Campus Now). Yet substance abuse remains a serious health risk for the minority of undergraduates who do use drugs.

Drugs can threaten students' physical and psychological health as well as their academic futures. In a recent national survey, students who drank, smoked marijuana, or used other drugs were much more likely to drop out of high school. Pot smoking in particular was strongly linked with "discontinuous enrollment."[9]

College men are more likely to use drugs than women. For instance, four in ten college males reported marijuana use in the last year, compared with one in three college women. Also, 24 percent of men, compared with 16 percent of women, used an illicit drug other than marijuana. Nearly 9 percent of college men use marijuana daily or near daily, compared with 3 percent of women.[10]

Marijuana remains the most widely used illicit drug on campuses, but the nonmedical use of prescription drugs now outranks other forms of substance abuse. According to the ACHA survey, about 14 percent of college students report that they misused prescription drugs in the last year.[11]

✓**check-in** How widespread is drug use on your campus?

Why Students Don't Use Drugs

The majority of undergraduates do not use illegal drugs or abuse prescription drugs. What keeps them drug-free? Here are some important factors:

- **Lack of interest.** At one liberal arts college in the Northeast, eight in ten of the undergraduates who reported never taking prescription drugs for non-medical reasons said they simply had no interest in doing so.[12]
- **Timing of enrollment**. Students who enroll in college directly from high school show a greater increase in substance use than those who delay enrollment and enter college at an older age.[13]
- **Spirituality and religion:** The greater a student's religiousness or religiosity—terms that encompass prayer, attendance at religious services, and reading spiritual materials—the less likely the student is to use alcohol, illegal drugs, or tobacco. As a recent study showed, religiosity also lowers the likelihood of prescription drug abuse.[14]
- **Academic engagement:** Illicit drug use is much less common among students who actively participate in classes and feel connected with the subject matter.
- **Perceived harmfulness:** Students who perceive a great risk of harm from repeated or occasional use are the least likely to misuse medications.
- **Athletics:** Although male and female college athletes drink at higher rates than nonathletes,

SNAPSHOT: ON CAMPUS NOW

📷 Student Drug Use

Marijuana	Actual Use			Perceived Use		
Percent (%)	Male	Female	Total	Male	Female	Total
Never used	57.7	62.7	61.0	9.4	6.4	7.5
Used, but not in the past 30 days	20.6	21.0	20.7	10.4	8.0	8.8
Used 1–9 days	12.2	11.4	11.7	46.6	44.0	44.7
Used 10–29 days	5.7	3.2	4.1	24.4	30.0	28.0
Used all 30 days	3.9	1.8	2.6	9.3	11.7	10.9
Any use within the last 30 days	21.7	16.3	18.3	80.3	85.7	83.6

All other drugs combined*	Actual Use			Perceived Use		
Percent (%)	Male	Female	Total	Male	Female	Total
Never used	53.6	72.4	65.9	10.8	8.3	9.3
Used, but not in the past 30 days	25.2	18.2	20.5	15.9	14.3	14.8
Used 1–9 days	14.4	7.3	9.7	44.3	44.8	44.5
Used 10–29 days	3.1	1.3	2.0	18.8	21.2	20.4
Used all 30 days	3.7	0.8	1.9	10.1	11.4	11.0
Any use within the last 30 days	21.2	9.4	13.6	73.2	77.4	75.9

*Includes cigars, smokeless tobacco, cocaine, methamphetamine, other amphetamines, sedatives, hallucinogens, anabolic steroids, opiates, inhalants, MDMA, other designer drugs, other illegal drugs. (Excluding alcohol, cigarettes, tobacco from a water pipe, and marijuana).

Did you know that about 6 in 10 undergraduates have never used marijuana or illegal drugs? What has been your experience? If you are among the majority, what are the factors that have enabled you to say no to drugs? If you have used drugs, what were your reasons? What role do drugs now play in your life? What has been their impact? Write down your feelings about how drugs might affect your health and your life in your online journal.

Source: American College Health Association. *American College Health Association–National College Health Assessment II: Reference Group Executive Summary, Spring 2014.* Hanover, MD: American College Health Association 2014.

they are less likely to use illegal drugs. One exception is the use of anabolic steroids (discussed in Chapter 8), which college athletes use more than other students.

✓**check-in** What do you think is the best reason not to use drugs?

Why Students Use Drugs

Various factors influence which students use drugs, including the following:

- **Genetics and family history:** Some college students inherit a genetic or biological pre-disposition to substance abuse. Researchers have identified specific genes tied to all types

of addictions. Some genes associated with alcohol dependence are closely linked with addictions to marijuana, nicotine, cocaine, heroin, and other substances. Also, the risk for problem drinking and alcohol abuse is higher among children of substance abusers.

- **Parental attitudes and behavior:** Parents' concerns or expectations influence whether and how much most students drink, smoke, or use drugs. Those who perceive that their parents approve of their drinking, for instance, are more likely to report a drinking-related problem, such as memory loss or missing class.

✓**check-in** How would you describe your parents' attitudes toward alcohol and drugs?

- **Substance use in high school:** Many students start abusing drugs or alcohol well before getting to college. Misusing prescription drugs before age 16 increases the risk of a substance abuse disorder later in life.

- **Social norms:** College students tend to overestimate drug use on campus. In the American College Health Association National College Health Assessment survey, students reported believing that 7.5 percent of undergraduates had never used marijuana. In fact, 61 percent never had.[15]

- **Positive expectations:** Many students expect a drug to make them feel less stressed or anxious, more relaxed or confident, less shy or inhibited. Among students who use illicit drugs, many say that they do so to relieve stress.

- **Self-medication.** Some students take drugs to relieve depression or anxiety. Some abuse prescription medications, such as Adderall and Ritalin, because they mistakenly think these drugs will energize them to study longer or perform better.

- **Risk perception.** Individuals who view marijuana as not harmful, for instance, are more than nine times more likely to report having used the drug in the past.[16]

- **Mental health problems:** Students with feelings of hopelessness, sadness, depression, and anxiety as well as those with clinical mental disorders have higher rates of prescription drug abuse and illegal drug use. Students diagnosed with depression in the past school year have higher rates of marijuana, cocaine, alcohol, and tobacco use. Those with a history of ADHD (discussed in Chapter 3) are more likely to report having used marijuana and other illicit drugs, to begin use at a younger age, and to suffer higher levels of impairment.

- **Social influences:** More than 9 in 10 students who use illegal drugs were introduced to the habit through friends; most use drugs with friends. Sorority and fraternity members, who tend to socialize more often than their peers, are more likely to abuse prescription stimulants, but students who live off campus have higher rates of marijuana and cocaine use.

- **Alcohol use:** Often individuals engage in more than one risky behavior. Researchers have found that students who report binge drinking are much more likely than other students to report current or past use of marijuana, cocaine, or other illegal drugs.

- **Race/ethnicity:** In general, white students have higher levels of alcohol and drug use than do African American students. African American students at historically black colleges tend to have lower rates of alcohol and drug use than did either white or African American students at white schools. The reason may be that these colleges provide a greater sense of self-esteem, which helps prevent alcohol and drug use.

- **Sexual identity:** Gay, lesbian, and bisexual teens may rely on alcohol and marijuana to lessen social anxiety and boost self-confidence when they first come out. However, once they become more involved in the gay community, many are less likely to do so. Nonetheless, lesbians are significantly more likely than heterosexual women to use marijuana, Ecstasy, and other drugs. Gay and bisexual men are significantly less likely than heterosexual men to drink heavily but more likely to use drugs.

Understanding Drugs and Their Effects

A **drug** is a chemical substance that affects the way you feel and function. In some circumstances, taking a drug can help the body heal or relieve physical and mental distress. In others, taking a drug can distort reality, undermine well-being, and threaten survival.

No drug is completely safe; all drugs have multiple effects that vary greatly in different people at different times. Knowing how drugs affect the brain, body, and behavior is crucial to understanding their impact and making responsible decisions about their use:

- **Drug abuse** is a pattern of substance use resulting in negative consequences or impairment.

- **Drug dependence** is a pattern of continuing substance use despite cognitive, behavioral, and physical symptoms.

- **Drug misuse** is the taking of a drug for a purpose or by a person other than that for which it was intended or not taking the recommended doses.

- **Drug diversion** is the transfer of a medication from the individual to whom it was prescribed to another person.

All forms of drug use involve risk. Even medications that help cure illnesses or soothe

drug Any substance, other than food, that affects bodily functions and structures when taken into the body.

drug abuse The excessive use of a drug in a manner inconsistent with accepted medical practice.

drug dependence Continued substance use even when its use causes cognitive, behavioral, and physical symptoms.

drug misuse The use of a drug for a purpose (or person) other than that for which it was medically intended.

drug diversion The transfer of a drug from the person for whom it was prescribed to another individual.

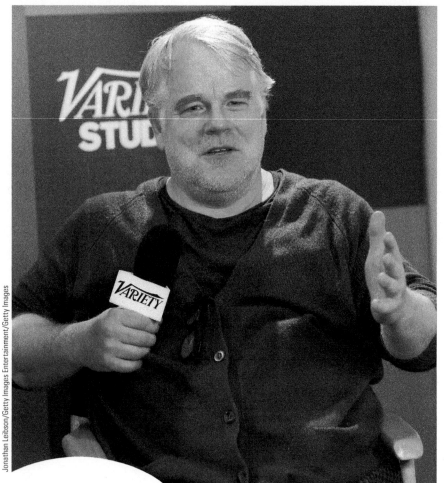

Jonathan Leibson/Getty Images Entertainment/Getty Images

Academy Award-winning actor Philip Seymour Hoffman died of "acute intoxication" with several drugs, including heroin, cocaine, benzodiazepines, and amphetamine.

intravenous Into a vein.

intramuscular Into or within a muscle.

subcutaneous Under the skin.

toxicity Poisonousness; the dosage level at which a drug becomes poisonous to the body, causing either temporary or permanent damage.

symptoms have side effects and can be misused. Some substances that millions of people use every day, such as caffeine, pose some health risks. Others—like the most commonly used drugs in our society, alcohol and tobacco—can lead to potentially life-threatening problems. With some illicit drugs, any form of use can be dangerous. Death rates related to drug overdose have tripled since 1990, with most of the increase tied to the growing abuse of prescription pain medications.

√ **check-in** Do you know of celebrities who died of drug overdoses? Do you personally know anyone who did?

Many factors determine the effects a drug has on an individual. These include how the drug enters the body, the dosage, the drug action, and the presence of other drugs in the body—as well as the physical and psychological makeup of the person taking the drug and the setting in which the drug is used.

Routes of Administration

Drugs can enter the body in a number of ways (Figure 12.1):

- **By swallowing:** The most common way of taking a drug is by swallowing a tablet, capsule, or liquid. However, drugs taken orally don't reach the bloodstream as quickly as drugs introduced into the body by other means and may not have any effect for 30 minutes or more.

- **By inhaling:** Drugs can enter the body through the lungs either by inhaling smoke—for example, from marijuana—or by inhaling gases, aerosol sprays, or fumes from solvents or other compounds that evaporate quickly. Young users of such inhalants, discussed later in this chapter, often soak a rag with fluid and press it over their nose. Or they may place inhalants in a plastic bag, put the bag over their nose and mouth, and take deep breaths—a practice called *huffing* that can produce serious, even fatal, consequences.

- **By injecting:** Drugs can be injected with a syringe subcutaneously (beneath the skin), intramuscularly (into muscle tissue, which is richly supplied with blood vessels), or intravenously (directly into a vein). **Intravenous** (IV) injection gets the drug into the bloodstream immediately (within seconds, in most cases); **intramuscular** injection, moderately fast (within a few minutes); and **subcutaneous** injection, more slowly (within 10 minutes).

Injecting drugs is extremely dangerous because many diseases, including hepatitis and infection with human immunodeficiency virus (HIV), can be transmitted by sharing contaminated needles. Injection-drug users who are HIV-positive are a major source of transmission of HIV among heterosexuals.

Dosage and Toxicity

The effects of any drug depend on the amount that an individual takes. Increasing the dose usually intensifies the effects produced by smaller doses. Also, the kind of effect may change at different dose levels. For example, low doses of barbiturates may relieve anxiety, while higher doses can induce sleep, loss of sensation, and even coma and death.

The dosage level at which a drug becomes poisonous to the body, causing either temporary or permanent damage, is called its **toxicity**. In most cases, drugs are eventually broken down in the liver by special body chemicals called *detoxification enzymes*.

Individual Differences

Each person responds differently to different drugs, depending on circumstances or setting. The enzymes in the body reduce the levels of drugs in the bloodstream; because there can be 80 variants of each enzyme, every person's body may react differently.

Often drugs intensify the emotional state a person is in. If you're feeling depressed, a drug may make you feel more depressed. A generalized physical problem, such as having the flu, may make your body more vulnerable to the effects of a drug. Genetic differences among individuals also may account for varying reactions.

Personality and psychological attitude play a role in drug effects. Each user's *mind-set*—his or her expectations or preconceptions about using the drug—affects the experience. Someone who takes a club drug (discussed further later in this chapter) to feel more "connected" may feel more sociable simply because that's what he or she expects.

Gender and Drugs

Beginning at a very early age, males and females show different patterns in drug use:

- Men generally encounter more opportunities to use drugs than women do.

- Given an opportunity to use drugs for the first time, both genders are equally likely to do so and to progress from initial use to dependence.

- Men and women are equally likely to become addicted to or dependent on cocaine, heroin, hallucinogens, tobacco, and inhalants.

- Women are more likely than men to become addicted to or dependent on sedatives and drugs designed to treat anxiety or sleeplessness.

- Men are more likely than women to abuse alcohol and marijuana.

- Male and female long-term cocaine users showed similar impairment in tests of concentration, memory, and academic achievement.

- Female cocaine users are more vulnerable to poor nutrition and below-average weight, depression, physical abuse, and, if pregnant, preterm labor or early delivery. Smoking marijuana, taking prescription painkillers, or using illegal drugs during pregnancy is associated with double or even triple the risk of stillbirth.[17]

Setting

The setting for drug use also influences its effects. Passing around a marijuana joint at a friend's is not a healthy or safe behavior, but the experience

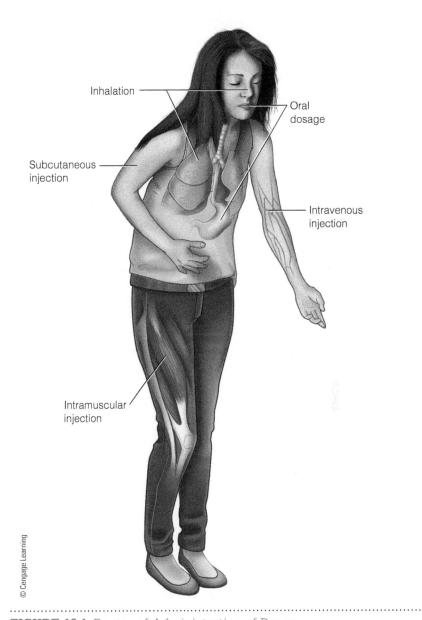

© Cengage Learning

FIGURE 12.1 Routes of Administration of Drugs

of going to a crack house is very different—and entails greater dangers.

Types of Action

A drug can act *locally*, as novocaine does to deaden pain in a tooth; *generally*, throughout a body system, as barbiturates do on the central nervous system; or *selectively*, as a drug does when it has a greater effect on one specific organ or system than on others, such as a spinal anesthetic. A drug that accumulates in the body because it's taken in faster than it can be metabolized and excreted is called *cumulative*; alcohol is such a drug.

Interaction with Other Drugs or Alcohol

A drug can interact with other drugs in four different ways:

- An **additive** interaction is one in which the resulting effect is equal to the sum of the effects of the different drugs used.

- A **synergistic** interaction is one in which the total effect of the two drugs taken together is greater than the sum of the effects the two drugs would have had if taken by themselves on separate occasions. Mixing barbiturates and alcohol, for example, has up to four times the depressant effect that either drug has alone.

- A drug can be **potentiating**—that is, one drug can increase the effect of another. Alcohol, for instance, can increase the drowsiness caused by antihistamines (antiallergy medications).

- Drugs can interact in an **antagonistic** fashion—that is, one drug can neutralize or block another drug with opposite effects. Tranquilizers, for example, may counter some of the nervousness and anxiety produced by cocaine.

The danger of mixing alcohol with other drugs cannot be emphasized too strongly. Alcohol and marijuana intensify each other's effects, making driving and many other activities extremely dangerous. Some people who have mixed sedatives or tranquilizers with alcohol never regained consciousness.

Caffeine and Its Effects

Caffeine, which has been drunk, chewed, and swallowed since the Stone Age, is the most widely used **psychoactive** (mind-affecting) drug in the world. Genetics may determine how much caffeine one craves. Scientists have identified the genes that drive people to consume more—or less—of this stimulant.

More than 85 percent of Americans consume caffeine. Coffee is our principal caffeine source, with Americans drinking an average of 3.5 cups a day. Coffee contains 100 to 150 milligrams of caffeine per cup; tea, 40 to 100 milligrams; cola, about 45 milligrams. Most medications that contain caffeine are one-third to one-half the strength of a cup of coffee. However, some, such as Excedrin, are very high in caffeine.

As a stimulant, caffeine relieves drowsiness, helps in the performance of repetitive tasks, and improves the capacity for work. Caffeine improves performance and endurance during prolonged, exhaustive exercise and, to a lesser degree, enhances short-term, high-intensity athletic performance. Additional benefits include improved concentration, reduced fatigue, and sharpened alertness.

You'll stay more alert, particularly if you are fighting sleep deprivation, if you spread your coffee consumption over the course of the day. For instance, rather than drinking two 8-ounce cups in the morning, try consuming smaller servings of an ounce or two during the course of the day.

In recent decades, some 19,000 studies have examined caffeine's impact on health. Their conclusion: For most people, caffeine poses few serious health risks. Drinking up to six cups a day of caffeinated or decaffeinated coffee won't shorten your lifespan and may convey some health benefits. Researchers have found no significant relationship between coffee and tea consumption and the risk of breast cancer or of miscarriage.[18]

More than 85 percent of Americans consume caffeine. Coffee is our principal caffeine source, with Americans drinking an average of 3.5 cups a day. Coffee contains 100 to 150 milligrams of caffeine per cup; tea, 40 to 100 milligrams; cola, about 45 milligrams. Most medications that contain caffeine are one-third to one-half the strength of a cup of coffee. However, some, such as Excedrin, are very high in caffeine. (See Table 12.1 for caffeine counts of various products.)

✓**check-in** Where do you get your coffee? It matters: A typical cup of coffee at home contains only 5 ounces of caffeine, but the smallest size available at most coffee shops contains 8 to 12 ounces, and larger ones even more.

As documented in numerous studies, caffeine can

- Relieve drowsiness
- Boost performance at repetitive tasks
- Improve memory for up to 14 hours after consumption[19]
- Improve performance and endurance during prolonged, exhaustive exercise
- Enhance, to a lesser degree, short-term, high-intensity athletic performance
- Sharpen concentration
- Reduce fatigue
- Increase alertness

additive Characterized by a combined effect that is equal to the sum of the individual effects.

synergistic Characterized by a combined effect that is greater than the sum of the individual effects.

potentiating Making more effective or powerful.

antagonistic Opposing or counteracting.

psychoactive Mind-affecting.

- Lower the risk of type 2 diabetes and cardio-vascular disease
- Possibly protect against Parkinson's disease, colon cancer, liver cirrhosis, gallstones, and stroke
- Possibly relieve migraines, boost mood, and prevent cavities
- Possibly lower the risk of endometrial cancer in women who drink four or more cups a day
- Possibly delay or protect against late-life cognitive impairment or decline, especially in women, although researchers describe the evidence to date as "inconclusive"[20]

Despite these positive findings, doctors advise pregnant women, heart patients, and those at risk for osteoporosis to limit or avoid coffee. Too much caffeine, particularly in high-powered energy drinks, can be dangerous for everyone and particularly harmful for children.[21] A single dose of 5 grams can be fatal.

√**check-in** If you normally drink a couple of 8-ounce cups of coffee in the morning, try smaller servings of an ounce or two during the course of the day. You'll feel more alert and less jittery.

Caffeine Intoxication

Doctors recommend that all adults limit their caffeine intake to 500 mg a day, with lesser amounts for those who have heart problems, high blood pressure, or trouble sleeping or who are taking medications. The recommended maximum for adolescents is 100 mg of caffeine a day. Ingesting more than 250 mg of caffeine may produce caffeine intoxication, which is diagnosed on the basis of five or more of the following signs and symptoms:

- Restlessness
- Nervousness
- Excitement
- Insomnia
- Flushed face
- Increased urination
- Digestive disturbances
- Muscle twitching
- Rambling thought or speech
- Rapid or irregular heart rate
- Periods of inexhaustibility
- Agitation

TABLE 12.1 Caffeine Content in Selected Soft Drinks and Energy Drinks

Drink	Company	Milligrams of Caffeine in 12 oz.
Soft Drinks		
JOLT	Wet Planet	72
Mountain Dew Code Red	PepsiCo	55
Mountain Dew	PepsiCo	55
Mello Yello	Coca-Cola	51
Diet Coke	Coca-Cola	45
Dr Pepper	Cadbury	41
Pepsi-Cola	PepsiCo	38
Energy Drinks		
Redline Power Rush	Vital Pharmaceuticals	1,680
JOLT Endurance Shot	Wet Planet	900
Cocaine Energy Drink	Redux Beverages	400
Blow (Energy Drink Mix)	Kingpin Concepts	360
Monster	Monster Beverage	120
Red Bull	Red Bull	116

© 2015 Cengage Learning

Jeffrey Blackler/Alamy

Higher doses may also produce ringing in the ears or flashes of light. Among the potentially life-threatening conditions that can result from caffeine intoxication are acute kidney injury, hepatitis, seizures, strokes, coronary artery spasms, and heart attack.

Caffeine withdrawal for those dependent on this substance can cause headaches and other neurological symptoms. Those who must cut back should taper off gradually. One approach is to mix regular and decaffeinated coffee, gradually decreasing the quantity of the former.

Caffeine-Containing Energy Drinks

Caffeine-containing energy drinks (CCEDs, in the scientific literature) have become extremely popular, especially in Western and Asian countries. These fortified beverages differ from soft or sports drinks in that they contain higher levels of caffeine—typically 500 mg or more—as well as sugars and dietary supplements. As consumption has increased, especially among adolescents and young adults, medical professionals have raised concerns about health impacts, including the following:

- Disrupted sleep
- Increased heart rate and blood pressure

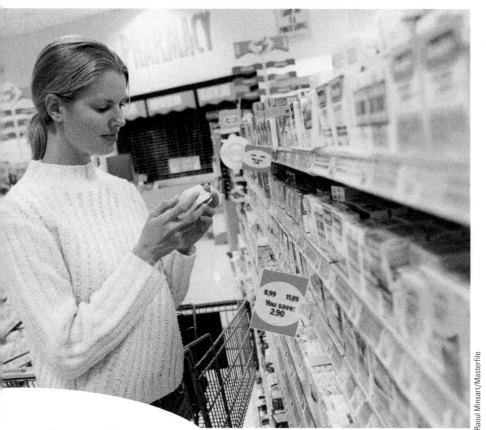

Always read the consumer-information label before using an over-the-counter drug.

Medications

As many as half of all patients take the wrong medications, in the wrong doses, at the wrong times, or in the wrong ways. Every year these inadvertent errors lead to an estimated 125,000 deaths and more than $8.5 billion in hospital costs. Mistakes occur among people of all ages, both genders, and every race, occupation, level of education, and personality type. Their number-one cause: not understanding directions.

Doctors occasionally make errors when it comes to prescription drugs. The most frequent are

- Over- or underdosing
- Omitting information from prescriptions
- Ordering the wrong dosage form (a pill instead of a liquid, for example)
- Not recognizing a patient's allergy to a drug

Over-the-Counter Drugs

More than half a million health products—remedies for everything from bad breath to bunions—are readily available without a doctor's prescription. This doesn't mean that they're necessarily safe or effective. Like other drugs, **over-the-counter (OTC)** medications can be used improperly, often simply because of a lack of education about proper use. Among those most often misused are the following:

- **Painkillers:** Federal regulators have issued warnings for many popular painkillers, including over-the-counter pills like Advil (ibuprofen) and Aleve (naproxen). Their labels cite risks to the heart, stomach, and skin. Tylenol (acetaminophen) and aspirin are generally considered safe for people with temporary pain like headaches and muscle aches. However, aspirin can cause stomach irritation and bleeding, and Tylenol, which is found in more than 600 over-the-counter and prescription medications, poses multiple dangers. (See Table 12.2 Acetaminophen Alert!)

- **Nasal sprays:** Nasal sprays relieve congestion by shrinking blood vessels in the nose. If they are used too often or for too many days in a row, the blood vessels widen instead of contracting, and the surrounding tissues become swollen, causing more congestion. To make the vessels shrink again, many people use more spray more often. The result can be permanent damage to nasal membranes, bleeding, infection, and partial or complete loss of smell.

- Overweight and obesity
- Heightened anxiety and tension
- Hallucinations (with the equivalent of seven or more cups of coffee a day)
- Dehydration
- Dental erosion
- Possible contribution to seizures or stroke[22]

Many of these drinks contain herbs that enhance the effects of caffeine and can interact with medication, causing harmful effects. Emergency department visits related to energy drinks have more than doubled in recent years.

Alcohol mixed with energy drinks—AmED in the medical literature—presents even greater dangers. About a third of college students report having consumed AmED in the past year.[23] Students mixing alcohol and caffeine engage in more high-risk drinking behaviors and are twice as likely to report being hurt or injured as those who don't. (See Chapter 13 for a comprehensive discussion on alcohol mixed with energy drinks.)

✓**check-in** Do you drink high-energy beverages? If so, do you know how much caffeine is in a single bottle or can?

over-the-counter (OTC)
Medications that can be obtained legally without a prescription from a medical professional.

- **Laxatives:** Believing that they must have one bowel movement a day (a common misconception), many people rely on laxatives. Brands that contain phenolphthalein irritate the lining of the intestines and cause muscles to contract or tighten, often making constipation worse rather than better. Bulk laxatives are less dangerous, but regular use is not advised. A high-fiber diet and more exercise are safer and more effective remedies for constipation.

- **Eye drops:** Eye drops make the blood vessels of the eye contract. However, as in the case of nasal sprays, with overuse (several times a day for several weeks), the blood vessels expand, making the eye look redder than before.

- **Sleep aids:** Although OTC sleeping pills are widely used, there has been little research on their use and possible risks. A national consensus panel on insomnia concluded that they are not effective and cause side effects such as morning-after grogginess. Medications like Tylenol PM and Excedrin PM combine a pain reliever with a sleep-inducing antihistamine, the same ingredient that people take for hay fever or cold symptoms. Although they make people drowsy, they can leave a groggy feeling the next day, and they dry out the nose and mouth.

- **Cough syrup:** Many of the "active" ingredients in over-the-counter cough preparations may be ineffective. Young people may chug cough syrup (called *roboing*, after the OTC medication Robitussin) because they think of dextromethorphan (DXM), a common ingredient in cough medicine, as a "poor man's version" of the popular drug Ecstasy.

✓**check-in** Which OTC painkillers have you used? Have you experienced any adverse effects?

Prescription Drugs

Like over-the-counter drugs, many prescribed medications aren't taken the way they should be; millions simply aren't taken at all. As many as 70 percent of adults have trouble understanding dosage information, and 30 percent can't read standard labels, according to the FDA, which has called for larger, clearer drug labeling.

The dangers of nonadherence (not properly taking prescription drugs) include

- recurrent infections
- serious medical complications
- emergency hospital treatment

TABLE 12.2 Acetaminophen Alert!

The FDA has issued the following guidelines for safe use of acetaminophen (www.fda.gov):

- Do not exceed 4,000 milligrams or 4 grams (the equivalent of eight 500-mg Tylenol Extra Strength pills) a day.
- Carefully read all labels for prescription and OTC medications and ask if any prescription medicine contains acetaminophen.
- Don't take more than one acetaminophen-containing product (including OTC medications) at the same time.
- Avoid drinking alcohol while taking acetaminophen.
- Stop taking acetaminophen and seek medical help immediately if you experience allergic reactions such as rash, itching, swelling of the face, and/or difficulty breathing.
- Seek medical help right away if you think you have taken more than the directed dosage of acetaminophen. Tylenol and other products containing acetaminophen account for 40 to 50 percent of all acute cases of liver failure, many resulting from unintentional overdose.
- Men younger than age 50 who take acetaminophen more than two times a week have roughly double the risk of hearing loss compared to men who do not. Men of similar ages who take ibuprofen (the main ingredient in Motrin or Advil) at least twice a week have a nearly two-thirds higher risk of hearing loss. Men who take aspirin twice a week have a one-third higher risk. However, the absolute risk of hearing loss remains small in young and middle-aged men.

Source: www.fda.gov

The drugs most likely to be taken incorrectly are those that treat problems with no obvious symptoms (such as high blood pressure), require complex dosage schedules, treat psychiatric disorders, or have unpleasant side effects.

The most common reason that college students fail to take medicines as directed is forgetting. Others are concerned about cost, or they stop when they feel better.

Physical Side Effects Most medications, taken correctly, cause only minor complications. No drug is entirely without side effects for all individuals taking it. Serious complications that may occur include heart failure, heart attack, seizures, kidney and liver failure, severe blood disorders, birth defects, blindness, memory problems, and allergic reactions. Overdoses of opioid painkillers now cause more deaths than heroin and cocaine combined—one fatality every 19 minutes, according to the CDC.

Allergic reactions to drugs are common. The drugs that most often provoke allergic responses are penicillin and other antibiotics (drugs used to treat infection). Aspirin, NSAIDs, sulfa drugs, barbiturates, anticonvulsants, insulin, and local anesthetics can also provoke allergic responses.

✓**check-in** Do you have any drug allergies? If so, what symptoms do they provoke?

Psychological Side Effects Dozens of drugs—both over-the-counter and prescription—can cause changes in the way people think, feel, and behave. Unfortunately, neither patients nor their physicians usually connect such symptoms with medications. Doctors may not even mention potential mental and emotional problems because they don't want to scare patients away from what otherwise may be a very effective treatment. What you don't know about a drug's effects on your mind *can* hurt you.

Among the medications most likely to cause psychiatric side effects are drugs for high blood pressure, heart disease, asthma, epilepsy, arthritis, Parkinson's disease, anxiety, insomnia, and depression. Some drugs—such as the powerful hormones called *corticosteroids*, used for asthma, autoimmune diseases, and cancer—can cause different psychiatric symptoms, depending on dosage and other factors. The older you are, the sicker you are, and the more medications you're taking, the greater your risk of developing some psychiatric side effects.

Drug Interactions OTC and prescription drugs can interact in a variety of ways. For example, mixing some cold medications with tranquilizers can cause drowsiness and coordination problems, thus making driving dangerous. Moreover, what you eat or drink can impair or completely wipe out the effectiveness of drugs or lead to unexpected effects on the body. For instance, aspirin takes 5 to 10 times as long to be absorbed when taken with food or shortly after a meal than when taken on an empty stomach. If tetracyclines encounter calcium in the stomach, they bind together and cancel each other out.

To avoid potentially dangerous interactions, do the following:

- Check the label(s) for any instructions on how or when to take a medication, such as "with a meal."

- If the directions say that you should take a drug on an empty stomach, take it at least one hour before eating or two or three hours after eating.

- Don't drink a hot beverage with a medication; the temperature may interfere with the effectiveness of the drug.

Drugs and Alcohol

About four in ten current drinkers in the United States take prescription drugs that interact with alcohol. Depending on the medication, the combination could cause side effects that range from drowsiness to depressed breathing and lower heart rate.[24]

Alcohol can change the rate of metabolism and the effects of many different drugs. Because it dilates the blood vessels, alcohol can add to the dizziness sometimes caused by drugs for high blood pressure, angina, or depression. Also, its irritating effects on the stomach can worsen stomach upset from aspirin, ibuprofen, and other anti-inflammatory drugs.

Generic Drugs The **generic** name is the chemical name for a drug. A specific drug may appear on the pharmacist's shelf under a variety of brand names, which tend to cost far more than the generic equivalent. About 75 percent of all prescriptions specify a brand name, but pharmacists may—and in some states must—switch to a generic drug unless the doctor specifically tells them not to. Prescriptions filled with generic drugs cost 20 to 85 percent less than their brand-name counterparts.

Generic drugs have the same active ingredients as brand-name prescriptions, but their fillers and binders, which can affect the absorption of a drug, may be different. For some serious illnesses, the generics may not be as effective; some experts recommend sticking with brand names for heart medications, psychiatric drugs, and anticonvulsant drugs (for epilepsy and other seizure disorders).

✓**check-in** Should you buy the generic version of a drug? Ask your physician if switching to a generic or from one generic to another might affect your condition in any way.

Buying Drugs Online Millions of people in the United States purchase prescription medications online. Although some websites fill only faxed prescriptions from medical doctors, others ignore or sidestep traditional regulations and safeguards.

Cyberspace distributors often ship pills across state lines without requiring a physical examination by a medical doctor. Instead, a "cyberdoc," who may or may not be qualified or up-to-date in a given specialty, reviews information submitted by a "patient." International pharmacies sometimes sell drugs that are not available or approved in the United States. And patients themselves use bulletin boards and other online resources to sell unused or unwanted medications to each other.

Many individuals turn to the Internet for "lifestyle" drugs such as pills for erectile dysfunction, weight control, and smoking cessation. Customers like the convenience and anonymity of buying drugs online. Although many people assume that drugs cost less on the

generic A consumer product with no brand name or registered trademark.

Internet, shipping costs tend to drive prices up to the same amount as or more than the price at a pharmacy.

The dangers of unregulated distribution of medications have alarmed government agencies and medical groups. The American Medical Association has declared it unethical for physicians to write prescriptions for people they've never met. The National Association of Boards of Pharmacy has developed a seal of approval to help customers determine which sites are legitimate. The FDA and other federal agencies, such as the Federal Trade Commission, which regulates advertising, are trying to find ways to impose some controls.

✓**check-in** Have you ever bought a medication online?

Consumers have to be wary. Ordering a drug like Accutane, an acne treatment, online may seem harmless. However, without close monitoring by a physician, you could develop complications, such as a bad reaction that aggravates hepatitis or inflames the pancreas.

Quality control is another concern. Counterfeit drugs, increasingly sold online, may do little, if any, good and could be harmful. Cyberspace pharmacies provide no information on how the drug was stored or whether its expiration date has passed. In addition, since importing medications without a prescription is against the law, you could find yourself in legal trouble.

Substance Use Disorders

People have been using psychoactive chemicals for centuries. Citizens of ancient Mesopotamia and Egypt used opium. More than 3,000 years ago, Hindus included cannabis products in religious ceremonies. For centuries the Inca in South America have chewed the leaves of the coca bush. Yet while drugs have existed in most societies, their use was usually limited to small groups. Today millions of people use drugs for a variety of reasons: to pick them up, bring them down, alter perceptions, or ease psychological pain.

The word **addiction**, as used by the general population, refers to the compulsive use of a substance, loss of control, negative consequences, and denial. The American Psychiatric Association defines a substance use disorder as "a cluster of cognitive, behavioral, and physiological symptoms indicating that the individual continues using the substance despite significant substance-related problems."[25] (See Health Now! Recognizing Substance Abuse.) A key characteristic is an underlying change in brain circuits that may persist beyond detoxification, particularly in individuals with severe disorders. These brain changes may result in repeated relapses and intense craving for the drug.

The characteristics of a substance use disorder include the following:

- Taking a substance in larger amounts or over a longer period than was originally intended
- A persistent desire to cut down or stop substance use
- Unsuccessful efforts to decrease or discontinue use
- A great deal of time given to obtaining the substance, using the substance, or recovering from its effects
- Cravings, which may be so strong that a user cannot think of anything else
- Failure to fulfill major obligations at work, school, or home because of substance use
- Recurrent substance use in physically hazardous situations[26]

Dependence

Substance users may develop **psychological dependence** and feel a strong craving for a drug because it produces pleasurable feelings or relieves stress and anxiety. **Physical dependence** occurs when a person develops *tolerance* to the effects of a drug and needs larger and larger doses to achieve intoxication or another desired effect. Individuals who are physically dependent and have a high tolerance to a drug may take amounts many times those that would produce intoxication or an overdose in someone who was not a regular user.

Men and women with a substance dependence disorder may use a drug to avoid or relieve withdrawal symptoms, or they may consume larger amounts of a drug or use it over a longer period than they'd originally intended.

Specific symptoms of dependence vary with particular drugs. Some drugs, such as marijuana, hallucinogens, and phencyclidine, do not cause withdrawal symptoms. The degree of dependence also varies. In mild cases, a person may function normally most of the time. In severe cases, the person's entire life may revolve around obtaining, using, and recuperating from the effects of a drug.

Individuals with drug dependence become intoxicated or high on a regular basis—whether

addiction A behavioral pattern characterized by compulsion, loss of control, and continued repetition of a behavior or an activity in spite of adverse consequences.

psychological dependence Emotional or mental attachment to the use of a drug.

physical dependence Physiological attachment to, and need for, a drug.

every day, every weekend, or several binges a year. They may try repeatedly to stop using a drug and yet fail, even though they realize that their drug use is interfering with their health, family life, relationships, and work.

Abuse

Some drug users do not develop the symptoms of tolerance and withdrawal that characterize dependence, yet they use drugs in ways that clearly have a harmful effect on them. These individuals are diagnosed as having a *psychoactive substance abuse disorder*. They continue to use drugs despite their awareness of persistent or repeated social, occupational, psychological, or physical problems related to drug use, or they use drugs in dangerous ways or situations (before driving, for instance).

Intoxication and Withdrawal

Intoxication refers to maladaptive behavioral, psychological, and physiologic changes that occur as a result of substance use. **Withdrawal** is the development of symptoms that cause significant psychological and physical distress when an individual reduces or stops drug use. (Intoxication and withdrawal from specific drugs are discussed later in this chapter.)

Polyabuse

Most users prefer a certain type of drug but also use several others; this behavior is called **polyabuse**. The average user who enters treatment is on five

different drugs. The more drugs anyone uses, the greater the chance of side effects, complications, and possibly life-threatening interactions.

Coexisting Conditions

Mental disorders and substance use disorders have a great deal of overlap. Many individuals with substance use disorders also have another psychiatric disorder, such as depression. Individuals with such *dual diagnoses* require careful evaluation and appropriate treatment for the complete range of complex and chronic difficulties they face. However, they can benefit from participation in 12 Step groups, like Double Trouble in Recovery, that provide treatment for both.

Causes of Substance Use Disorders

No one fully understands why some people develop drug dependence or abuse disorders, whereas others, who may experiment briefly with drugs, do not. Inherited body chemistry, genetic factors, and sensitivity to drugs may make some individuals more susceptible than others. These disorders may stem from many complex causes.

The Biology of Dependence Scientists now view drug dependence as a brain disease triggered by frequent use of drugs that change the biochemistry and anatomy of neurons and alter the way they work. A major breakthrough in understanding dependence has been the discovery that certain mood-altering substances and experiences—a puff of marijuana, a slug of whiskey, a snort of cocaine, a big win at blackjack—trigger a rise in a brain chemical called **dopamine**, which is associated with feelings of satisfaction and euphoria. This brain chemical or neurotransmitter is one of the crucial messengers that link nerve cells in the brain, and its level rises during any pleasurable experience, whether it be a loving hug or a taste of chocolate.

The mechanism governing the rise in dopamine levels is not the same for all drugs. Figure 12.2 shows the one for cocaine. Normally, after dopamine is released from the axon terminal of a neuron and activates dopamine receptors on the adjacent neuron, the dopamine is then transported back to its original neuron by "uptake pumps." Cocaine binds to the uptake pumps and prevents them from transporting dopamine back into the neuron terminal. So more dopamine builds up in the synapse and is free to activate more dopamine receptors.

intoxication Maladaptive behavioral, psychological, and physiologic changes that occur as a result of substance abuse.

withdrawal Development of symptoms that cause significant psychological and physical distress when an individual reduces or stops drug use.

polyabuse The misuse or abuse of more than one drug.

dopamine A brain chemical associated with feelings of satisfaction and euphoria.

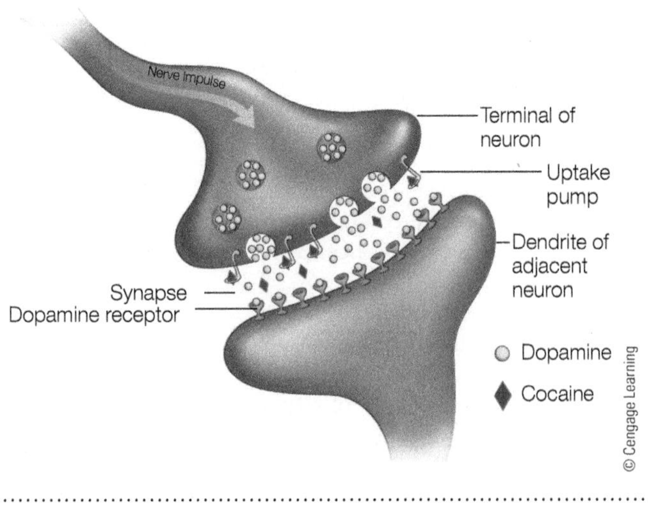

FIGURE 12.2 Dopamine Levels for Cocaine
Within the synapses between adjacent neurons, cocaine binds to the dopamine uptake pumps and thus allows the neurotransmitter dopamine to build up in the synapse and bind to more dopamine receptors.

The Psychology of Vulnerability Although scientists do not believe there is an addictive personality, certain individuals are at increased risk of drug dependence because of psychological factors, including

- Difficulty controlling impulses
- A lack of values that might constrain drug use (whether based in religion, family, or society)
- Low self-esteem
- Feelings of powerlessness
- Depression

The one psychological trait most often linked with drug use is denial. Young people in particular are absolutely convinced that they will never lose control or suffer in any way as a result of drug use.

People with mental illness such as depression, anxiety, schizophrenia, or bipolar disorder have an increased risk for substance use. Individuals may self-administer drugs to treat psychiatric symptoms; for example, they may take sedating drugs to suppress a panic attack. An estimated 8.4 million adults in the United States have both a mental and substance use disorder. However, only about 8 percent of people receive treatment for these problems.[27]

Users of illicit drugs are much more likely than the general population to think about suicide, according to the U.S. Substance Abuse and Mental Health Services Administration's (SAMHSA's) most recent National Survey on Drug Use and Health.

Drugged Driving

Driving under the influence of any substance that acts on the brain can impair motor skills, reaction time, and judgment. Some state laws define "drugged driving" as driving when a drug "renders the driver incapable of driving safely." Other states have "per se" laws, according to which it is illegal to operate a moving vehicle if there is any detectable level of a prohibited drug or its metabolites in a driver's blood.

According to the National Highway Traffic Safety Administration, more than 16 percent of weekend, nighttime drivers test positive for illegal, prescription, or over-the-counter medications. An estimated 10.5 million Americans over age 12 have reported driving under the influence of illicit drugs during the previous year. The rate of drugged driving is highest among young adults ages 18 to 25 (12.8 percent).

Prescription Drug Abuse

According to the most recent federal data, the "epidemic" of prescription painkiller abuse and

fatal overdoses may be starting to reverse course. After rising steadily until 2010, the rates of abuse have flattened or decreased nationwide.[28] About 5 percent of college students report use of Vicodin or OxyContin, down from 8 percent in previous years.[29]

Nonmedical use of any prescription medication remains highest among young adults between the ages of 18 and 25, compared with other age groups. Opioid painkillers (discussed later in this chapter) are the most widely misused prescription drugs.

Prescription Drugs on Campus

As many as 35 percent of college students have engaged in nonmedical use of prescription drugs.[30] The most widely used ones are pain medications, sedative or anxiety medications, sleeping medications, and stimulant medications.

Among painkillers, oxycodone—the active ingredient in OxyContin—and hydrocodone are the most widely used. OxyContin is favored by young males who like taking risks and prefer to inject or snort drugs to get high. Hydrocodone is more popular among women, older people, people who don't want to inject drugs, and those who prefer to deal with a doctor or friend instead of a drug dealer.[31]

College women use more antidepressants; college men, more painkillers and stimulants. (See Table 12.3.) In a study of undergraduates taking prescribed psychiatric medications, such as antidepressants and antianxiety drugs, a substantial proportion took larger or smaller quantities or took their medication more or less frequently than prescribed.

✓**check-in** Have you ever taken a medication that was not prescribed for you?

TABLE 12.3 Nonmedical Prescription Drug Use by College Students

Percentage of college students who reported using prescription drugs that were not prescribed to them within the past 12 months:

	Percent (%)		
	Male	Female	Average
Antidepressants	2.4	3.3	3
Erectile dysfunction drugs	1.1	0.8	0.9
Painkillers	6.9	5.7	6.2
Sedatives	3.5	3.6	3.6
Stimulants	9.6	7.6	8.3
Used one or more of the above	14.8	13.5	14

Source: American College Health Association, *American College Health Association–National College Health Assessment II: Reference Group Executive Summary, Spring 2014*. Hanover, MD: American College Health Association, 2014.

Mike Flippo/Shutterstock.com

Abuse of prescription medications on college campuses has increased in the last 15 years. Here is what we know about it:

- Only marijuana use is more widespread on campus than prescription drug abuse.

- College men have higher rates of prescription drug abuse than women.

- White and Hispanic undergraduates are significantly more likely to abuse medications than are African American and Asian students.

- Undergraduates who misuse or abuse prescription medications are much more likely to report heavy binge drinking and use of illicit drugs.

- College women who abuse prescription drugs are at increased risk for sexual victimization and assault.

Prescription Stimulants

Stimulants are among the most widely abused prescription drugs on campus, with as many as 17 percent of students reporting their misuse. The most common sources of these drugs are peers with prescriptions for the treatment of attention-deficit/hyperactivity disorder (ADHD), which affects an estimated 2 to 8 percent of undergraduates.[32]

Students who misuse stimulants are more likely to be

- male

- upperclassmen rather than freshmen or sophomores

- Caucasian

- from higher-income families

- members of fraternities and sororities[33]

The most common motives for misusing stimulants are academic, such as the following:

- to focus better while studying

- to improve study skills

- to stay awake to study longer

- to improve concentration[34]

Although students expect prescription stimulants to enhance learning and improve their grades, a meta-analysis of existing research found no scientific basis for this belief.[35] The lower a student's GPA, the greater the odds of stimulant misuse, which also is associated with skipping class and studying less than other students. Other reasons for stimulant misuse include wanting to get high, to prolong the effects of alcohol and other drugs, or to lose weight.

Students who misuse stimulants typically perceive them as relatively safe. Yet users report a range of adverse effects, including irritability, insomnia, headaches, and stomachaches. Frequent use has been linked with increased impulsivity, use of alcohol and other drugs, and risky behaviors, including unsafe sex and reckless driving.

Overdoses can cause delirium, confusion, aggressiveness, hallucinations, and psychotic symptoms. Combining stimulants with alcohol increases the likelihood of blackouts, accidents, and unprotected or unplanned sex. In individuals with certain cardiac conditions, stimulant medications can cause serious, even fatal, complications.[36]

Some universities are setting strict regulations for ADHD medications, including confirmation of the diagnosis through a medical evaluation and a formal written promise to submit to drug testing and not to share the pills.

Prescription Painkillers

About 5 percent of college students report use of Vicodin or OxyContin, down from 8 percent in previous years.[37] Students who are members of fraternities and sororities, who are enrolled at more competitive schools, who earn lower grade-point averages, and who engage in substance use and other risky behaviors are more likely to abuse these drugs. Smokers also are more prone to long-term prescription abuse.

As discussed later in this chapter, the rates of prescription opiate abuse have risen steadily, and some health officials view them as "heroin lite," a gateway to use of heroin.

Like other addictions, a prescription pain-killer "habit" is a treatable brain disease but not an easy habit to break. Recovery usually requires carefully supervised detoxification, appropriate medications (similar to those used for opioid dependence), behavioral therapy, and ongoing support.

√ check-in How widespread do you think prescription drug abuse is on your campus?

Common Drugs of Abuse

The common drugs of abuse fall within these categories: cannabinoids, herbal drugs, club drugs, stimulants, dissociative drugs, hallucinogens, opioids, and other compounds.

Cannabinoids

Marijuana (pot) and **hashish** (hash)—the most widely used illegal drugs—are derived from the cannabis plant and are classified as **cannabinoids**. The major psychoactive ingredient in both is *THC* (*delta-9-tetrahydrocannabinol*).

More than 100 million Americans have tried marijuana, the third most popular recreational drug in America (behind only alcohol and tobacco). According to government surveys, some 12 million Americans use cannabis; more than 1 million cannot control this use.

Marijuana has been and remains the illicit drug most widely used by college students. Five percent of undergraduates—one of every 11 males and one of every 34 females—report daily or near-daily use, the highest rate in about three decades.[38]

√ check-in Have you ever smoked marijuana?

Different types of marijuana have different percentages of THC. Because of careful cultivation, the strength of today's marijuana is much greater than that used in the 1960s and 1970s. Today a marijuana joint contains 150 mg of THC, compared to 10 mg in the 1960s.

Street Names: Marijuana: blunt, dope, ganja, grass, herb, joints, bud, Mary Jane, pot, reefer, green, trees, smoke, sinsemilla, skunk, weed. Hashish: boom, chronic, gangster, hash, hash oil, hemp

How Administered: Swallowed, smoked. Usually, marijuana is smoked in a joint (hand-rolled cigarette) or pipe; it may also be eaten as an ingredient in other foods (as when baked in brownies), though with a less predictable effect.

How Users Feel: The circumstances in which marijuana is smoked, the communal aspects of its use, and the user's experience all can affect the way a marijuana-induced high feels.

In low to moderate doses, marijuana typically creates

- A mild sense of euphoria.
- Slowed thinking and reaction time.
- A dreamy sort of self-absorption.
- Confusion.
- Some impairment in thinking and communicating.
- Heightened sensations of color, sound, and other stimuli.
- Impaired balance and coordination.
- Increased pulse rate, bloodshot eyes, and dry mouth and throat.
- Slowed reaction times.
- Impaired motor skills.
- Increased appetite and diminished short-term memory.

Some users—particularly those smoking marijuana for the first time or taking a high dose in an unpleasant or unfamiliar setting—experience acute anxiety, which may be accompanied by a panicky fear of losing control. They may believe that their companions are ridiculing or threatening them and experience a panic attack, a state of intense terror.

All the reactions experienced with low doses are intensified with higher doses, leading to sensory distortion and, in the case of hashish, vivid hallucinations and LSD-like, psychedelic reactions.

The sense of being stoned peaks within half an hour and usually lasts about 3 hours. Even when alterations in perception seem slight, it is not safe to drive a car for as long as 4 to 6 hours after smoking a single joint. The drug remains in the body's fat cells 50 hours or more after use, so people may experience psychoactive effects for several days after use. Drug tests may produce positive results for days or weeks after last use.

Risks and Potential Health Consequences: Marijuana produces a range of effects in different organs (see Figure 12.3 for a summary):

Brain

- Problems with memory and learning.
- Distorted perceptions.
- Difficulty thinking and solving problems.

marijuana The drug derived from the cannabis plant, containing the psychoactive ingredient THC, which causes a mild sense of euphoria when inhaled or eaten.

hashish A concentrated form of a drug derived from the cannabis plant that contains the psychoactive ingredient THC, which causes a sense of euphoria when inhaled or eaten.

cannabinoids A group of closely related compounds that include cannabinol and the active constituents of cannabis (marijuana).

Negative Long-Term Effects

Brain and central nervous system ————
- Causes brain abnormalities
- Dulls sensory and cognitive skills
- Impairs short-term memory
- Alters motor coordination
- Causes changes in brain chemistry
- Leads to difficulty in concentration, attention to detail, and learning new complex information
- Increases risk of stroke
- Increases risk of psychotic symptoms
- Causes disturbed sleep

Cardiovascular system ————
- Increases heart rate
- Increases blood pressure
- Decreases blood flow to the limbs

Respiratory system ————
- Damages the lungs (50% more tar than tobacco)
- May cause lung cancer
- May damage throat from inhalation

Reproductive system ————
- In women, may impair ovulation and cause fetal abnormalities if used during pregnancy
- In men, may suppress sexual functioning and may reduce the number, quality, and motility of sperm, possibly affecting fertility

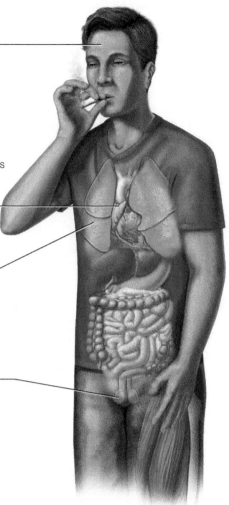

© Cengage Learning

FIGURE 12.3 Impact of Marijuana

Marijuana has negative long-term effects on many systems of the body.

- Loss of coordination.
- Increased anxiety.
- Panic attacks.
- Impaired verbal fluency, memory, and coordination.
- Disrupted sleep.
- Impaired brain development in adolescents and young adults.[39]
- Psychotic symptoms (particularly in young users).[40]
- Double the risk of stroke in young adults, even in those with no other risk factors.[41]
- Significant brain abnormalities, including shrinkage of key structures involved in memory, learning, and emotion, that can lead to memory loss, difficulty learning new information, and psychotic symptoms. Younger users seem most susceptible.[42]

- Cognitive impairment. Marijuana lowers performance in tests measuring memory, attention, reaction time, tracking, and motor function. The effects depend on the dose and are highest in the first hour after smoking marijuana and after one to two hours of oral intake. Frequent or heavy users show greater impairment than those who smoked marijuana an average of once a month.[43]
- Psychological symptoms. Some users experience feelings of anxiety and/or paranoia, with hallucinations and other psychotic symptoms that may last for minutes, hours, or, in some cases, days. Studies have also linked marijuana use with an earlier age of onset and increased incidence of schizophrenia and other psychiatric disorders (discussed in Chapter 3).[44]

Lungs

- Effects similar to those of smoking tobacco, although long-term effects on pulmonary function may vary.
- Frequent respiratory infections.
- Chronic bronchitis.
- Emphysema.

Heart

- Heart attacks and sudden death, even in healthy persons, shortly after smoking marijuana.
- Risk of elevated blood pressure and decreased oxygen supply to the heart muscle.
- If combined with cocaine, potentially deadly increases in heart rate and blood pressure.

Pregnancy

- Lower birth weight.
- More health problems after birth.
- Impaired motor development in nursing infants whose mothers smoke pot.
- **Cancer.** Marijuana smoke contains known cancer-causing chemicals. Some studies have suggested a link with cancers of the head and neck, lungs, and testicles, but most of the subjects also smoked tobacco, so the findings are inconclusive.[45]
- **Motor vehicle accidents.** Several states have reported increases of fatal crashes among drivers who tested positive for marijuana after the drug was legalized.[46]

Medical Marijuana A growing number of states have passed voter referenda or legislative actions making marijuana available to smoke for a variety of medical conditions upon a doctor's recommendation. There is limited scientific evidence supporting the use of cannabis or cannaboid drugs as a medical therapy. A recent comprehensive meta-analysis of clinical trials of medical marijuana found some benefits for relieving nausea and vomiting related to chemotherapy, specific pain syndromes, and spasticity from multiple sclerosis. However, research has shown little or weak evidence for the use of marijuana in treating conditions such as hepatitis C, Crohn disease, Parkinson disease, or Tourette syndrome. Common adverse effects among patients treated with marijuana included dizziness, dry mouth, nausea, fatigue, sleepiness, euphoria, vomiting, disorientation, drowsiness, confusion, loss of balance, and hallucinations. There is also a risk of dependence.[47]

Legalized Marijuana
Residents of nearly 30 states are considering or have voted to remove criminal and civil penalties for the adult possession of up to 1 ounce of cannabis. However, the possession and sale of marijuana remain illegal under federal law.

Medical scientists and policy experts are monitoring the effects of marijuana decriminalization on health, safety, crime, and other dimensions of daily life, but the impact is not yet clear. Some see legalized marijuana as no more (or less) perilous than alcohol; others fear that legalization will increase use by young people under age 21, marijuana-related accidents, and serious health consequences.[48]

The American Academy of Pediatrics has officially opposed legalizing marijuana because greater access may lead to increased use by teens and increased risks to them including

• Impaired memory and concentration

• Interference with learning

• Lower odds of completing high school or obtaining a college degree

• Impaired motor control, coordination, and judgment, which may contribute to unintentional deaths and injuries

• Psychological problems, poorer lung health, and a higher likelihood of drug dependence in adulthood.[49]

....
√**check-in** Do you think marijuana should be legalized?
....

Dependence
Although marijuana is less addictive than heroin or tobacco, it can cause dependence. One in six of those who start smoking pot at younger ages may become addicted. Young users also show significant impairment in brain development and functioning. Marijuana also increases the risk of respiratory problems, stroke, and cancer in users of all ages.

Withdrawal
Marijuana users can develop a compulsive, often uncontrollable craving for the drug. Stopping after long-term marijuana use can produce *marijuana withdrawal syndrome*, which is characterized by insomnia, restlessness, loss of appetite, and irritability. People who smoke marijuana daily for many years may become aggressive after they stop using it and may relapse to prevent aggression and other symptoms.

Herbal Drugs

Salvia
Salvia (*Salvia divinorum*) is an herb grown in southern Mexico and Central and South America. Its main active ingredient, salvinorin A, activates kappa opioid receptors that differ from those activated by the more commonly known opioids, such as heroin and morphine. Its use has fallen to 1 percent of students.[50]

Street Name: diviner's sage

How Administered: Traditionally ingested by chewing fresh leaves or drinking their extracted juices, *S. divinorum* when dried can also be smoked as a joint, in a water pipe, or vaporized and inhaled.

How Users Feel

• Hallucinations or "psychotomimetic" episodes (a transient experience that mimics a psychosis) that occur in less than a minute and last less than 30 minutes.

• Emotional swings.

• Laughter and euphoria.

• Feelings of detachment.

Risks and Potential Health Consequences

• Psychedelic-like changes in visual perception.

• Mood changes.

• Dizziness.

• Slurred speech, emotional swings, and a greatly altered perception of external reality and the self.

The long-term effects of salvia abuse have not been investigated systematically.[51]

Khat
For centuries people in East Africa and the Arabian peninsula consumed the fresh young

salvia An herb with hallucinogenic properties when smoked or inhaled.

leaves of the *Catha edulis* shrub in ways similar to our drinking coffee. Its active ingredients are two controlled substances, cathinone and cathine.

Street Names: kat, catha, chat, Abyssinian tea

How Administered: Chewed

How Users Feel

- Less fatigue.
- More energy.
- Reduced appetite.

Risks and Potential Health Consequences

- Increased risk of death and stroke in those with heart disease.
- With compulsive use, manic behavior, grandiose illusions, paranoia, and hallucinations.

Synthetic Designer Drugs

New, unregulated psychoactive substances, often referred to as **designer drugs**, include marijuana-like smoking blends frequently branded as "K2" or "Spice," designer stimulant preparations of powders generally termed "bath salts," and various tablets or capsules frequently described as "party pills" or "research chemicals." Their use on college campuses has fallen in recent years.[52]

✓**check-in** Do you think that synthetic drugs are widely used on your campus?

These compounds, many available legally via the Internet, may be sold as bath salts, plant food, insecticides, chicken feed, and research chemicals, often labeled "not for human consumption." Some are highly toxic industrial chemicals with potentially life-threatening adverse effects.

Specific agents include methoxetamine, sold on the Internet as "legal ketamine"; piperazine derivatives, amphetamine-like compounds known as BZP, TMFPP, or "legal Ecstasy"; and Kratom, a legal plant product derived from a Southeast Asian tree with opium-like effects, as well as the drugs described in the following sections.[53]

Synthetic Marijuana Synthetic versions of the active ingredient in marijuana, developed for medical use, act on the brain like the THC in smoked marijuana but eliminate the need to inhale harmful chemicals. Various herbal

mixtures, marketed as safe and legal alternatives to pot and labeled "not for human consumption," contain dried, shredded plant material and chemical additives. The majority of users are young men in their teens.[54] One in nine high school seniors reported use of K2 or Spice in the previous year,[55] and U.S. poison control centers have experienced an exponential increase in telephone calls regarding synthetic marijuana.[56]

Street Names: Spice, K2, fake weed, Yucatan fire, skunk, moon rocks

How Administered: Some Spice products are sold as incense, but they are mainly smoked or drunk in an herbal infusion.

How Users Feel

- Elevated mood.
- Relaxation.
- Altered perception.
- Effects similar to those of marijuana but in some cases much more intense.

Risks and Potential Health Consequences

- Dilated pupils.
- Agitation.
- Extreme nervousness.
- Nausea and vomiting.
- Fast heartbeat.
- Elevated blood pressure.
- Tremors.
- Seizures.
- Acute, potentially fatal kidney failure.[57]

Users of synthetic marijuana have required emergency treatment for reactions such as paranoia, anxiety, agitation, high blood pressure, profuse sweating, palpitations, elevated heart rate, dizziness, slowed speech, confusion, muscle rigidity, and catatonia (an inability to respond to verbal or physical stimulation).

✓**check-in** Do you know anyone who has had an adverse reaction to synthetic marijuana?

Synthetic Cathinone "Bath salts" are a new family of drugs that contain one or more synthetic chemicals related to **cathinone**, an amphetamine-like stimulant found naturally in the khat plant. They should not be confused with products like Epsom salts, which have no drug-like properties. The majority of users are young

designer drugs Illegally manufactured psychoactive drugs that have dangerous physical and psychological effects.

cathinone An amphetamine-like stimulant derived from the khat plant.

366   CHAPTER 12 • Addictions

men, most often between ages 20 and 29.[58] Bath salts are usually a white or brown crystalline powder in small plastic or foil packages labeled "not for human consumption," may be labeled as "plant food"—or, more recently, as "jewelry cleaner" or "phone screen cleaner"—and sold online and in drug product stores under a variety of brand names.

Street Names: bath salts and brand names such as Ivory Wave, Bloom, Cloud Nine, Lunar Wave, Vanilla Sky, White Lightning, and Scarface

How Administered: Typically swallowed, inhaled, or injected; the worst dangers are associated with snorting or needle injection. Bath salts contain various amphetamine-like chemicals, such as methylenedioxypyrovalerone (MDPV), mephedrone, and pyrovalerone.

How Users Feel

- Intense stimulation.
- Alertness.
- Euphoria.
- Increased sociability.
- Heightened sex drive.

Risks and Possible Health Consequences
The most common synthetic cathinone found in the blood and urine of patients admitted to emergency departments after taking bath salts raises brain dopamine in the same way as cocaine but is at least 10 times stronger.[59]

- Paranoia.
- Agitation.
- Hallucinations.
- Panic attacks.
- Break with reality.
- Violent behavior.
- Heart problems (such as racing heart, high blood pressure, and chest pains) and symptoms like paranoia, hallucinations, and panic attacks.

Patients with the syndrome known as "excited delirium" from taking bath salts also may have dehydration, breakdown of skeletal muscle tissue, and kidney failure. Intoxication has caused death in several instances. A common cause of death is suicide. Those who survive suicide attempts may suffer long-term psychiatric symptoms.

Club Drugs

A variety of drugs—MDMA, GHB, GBL, ketamine, fentanyl, Rohypnol, and nitrites—called

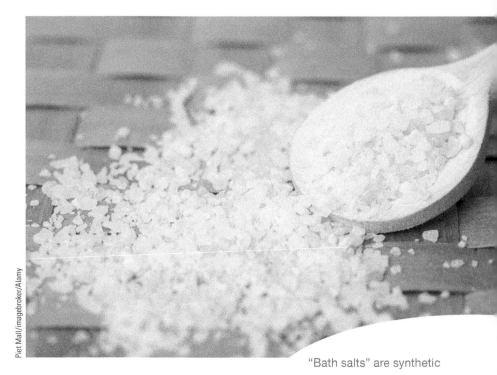

Piet Mall/imagebroker/Alamy

"club drugs"—first became popular among teens and young adults at nightclubs, bars, and raves, night-long dances often held in warehouses or other unusual settings. Their use by teenagers has been dropping in recent years.

How Users Feel: Young people may take club drugs to relax, energize, and enhance their social interactions, but a large number also experience negative consequences. As many as three in four report side effects such as these:

- Profuse sweating.
- Hot and cold flashes.
- Tingling or numbness.
- Blurred vision.
- Trouble sleeping.
- Hallucinations.
- Depression.
- Confusion.
- Anxiety.
- Irritability.
- Paranoia.
- Loss of libido (sex drive).
- Difficulty with their usual daily activities.
- Financial and work troubles.

Ecstasy **Ecstasy (MDMA)** is the most common street name for methylenedioxymethamphetamine, a synthetic compound with both

"Bath salts" are synthetic stimulants, often sold legally, that can cause dangerous physical and psychological effects.

club drugs A variety of drugs including MDMA, GHB, GBL, ketamine, fentanyl, Rohypnol, and nitrites that first became popular at nightclubs, bars, and raves.

Ecstasy (MDMA) A synthetic compound, also known as methylenedioxymethamphetamine, that is similar in structure to methamphetamine and has both stimulant and hallucinogenic effects.

stimulant and mildly hallucinogenic properties that belongs to a family of drugs called *enactogens*, which literally means "touching within."

According to various studies, students who take Ecstasy are more likely to use marijuana, binge-drink, smoke cigarettes, have multiple sexual partners, spend more time socializing with friends and less time studying, and consider parties important and religion less important.

Medical emergencies related to the drug have increased 75 percent in recent years. Most Ecstasy users requiring emergency care were between ages 18 and 29.

Street Names: E, XTC, X, hug, beans, love drug

How Administered: Although it can be smoked, inhaled (snorted), or injected, Ecstasy is almost always taken as a pill or tablet. Its effects begin in 45 minutes and last for three to six hours. Ecstasy pills often contain a variety of other chemicals that increase the danger to users.

How Users Feel:

- Relaxation and euphoria.

- Sense of connectedness with others. In some settings, they reveal intimate details of their lives (which they may later regret); in other settings, they join in collective rejoicing.

- Enhanced sensory experience.

- In rare cases, visual distortions, sudden mood changes, or psychotic reactions.

- In regular users, depression and anxiety the week after taking MDMA.

The psychological effects of Ecstasy become less intriguing with repeated use, and the physical side effects become more uncomfortable.

Risks and Potential Health Consequences: Ecstasy is more likely than other stimulants, such as methamphetamine, to kill young, healthy people between the ages of 16 and 24 who are not known to be regular drug users. Researchers theorize that young people's brains, which are still developing in late adolescence and early adulthood, may be more vulnerable to the effects of the drug.

Ecstasy poses risks similar to those of cocaine and amphetamines, including

- Confusion.
- Depression.
- Sleep problems.
- Drug craving.
- Severe anxiety.

- Paranoia.
- Muscle tension.
- Involuntary teeth clenching.
- Nausea and vomiting.
- Dizziness.
- Blurred vision.
- Rapid eye movement.
- Faintness.
- Chills.
- Sweating.
- Increases in heart rate and blood pressure, which pose a special risk for people with circulatory or heart disease.
- When combined with extended physical exertion, like dancing, hyperthermia (severe overheating), severe dehydration, serious increases in blood pressure, stroke, and heart attack.
- Without sufficient water, dehydration and heat stroke, which can be fatal. Individuals with high blood pressure, heart trouble, or liver or kidney disease are in the greatest danger.
- Fatal damage and death when users drink large amounts of water to counteract a drug-induced hyperthermia.
- Acute hepatitis, which can lead to liver failure. Even after liver transplantation, the mortality rate for individuals with this condition is 50 percent.
- If combined with the antidepressants known as SSRIs (see Chapter 2), which modulate the mood-altering brain chemical serotonin, jaw clenching, nausea, tremors, and, in extreme cases, potentially fatal elevations in body temperature.
- Although not a sexual stimulant (if anything, MDMA has the opposite effect), strong feelings of intimacy that may lead to risky sexual behavior.
- Risks to a developing fetus, including a greater likelihood of heart and skeletal abnormalities and long-term learning and memory impairments in children born to women who used MDMA during pregnancy.

....
✓**check-in** Do you think that Ecstasy is
....
widely used on your campus?
....

Herbal Ecstasy   Herbal Ecstasy, also known as herbal bliss, cloud 9, and herbal X, is a mixture of stimulants such as ephedrine, pseudoephedrine, and caffeine. Sold in tablet or capsule form as a "natural" and safe alternative to Ecstasy, its ingredients vary greatly. Herbal Ecstasy can have dangerous and unpleasant side effects, including stroke, heart irregularities, and a disfiguring skin condition.

GHB and GBL

Once sold in health-food stores for its muscle-building and alleged fat-burning properties, **gamma hydroxybutyrate** (**GHB**, G, Georgia home boy, grievous bodily harm, liquid ecstasy) was banned because of its effects on the brain and nervous system. The main ingredient is **GBL** (**gamma butyrolactone**), an industrial solvent often used to strip floors, which converts into GHB once ingested. GHB acts as a sedative while producing feelings of euphoria and heightened sexuality. Because of its amnesic properties, GHB has been used as a "date rape" drug, similar to Rohypnol. Alcohol intensifies its effects, which typically last up to four hours.

Large doses can cause someone to pass out in 15 minutes and fall into a coma within half an hour. Death can occur. Other side effects include nausea, amnesia, hallucinations, decreased heart rate, convulsions, and sometimes blackouts. Long-term use at high doses can lead to a withdrawal reaction: rapid heartbeat, tremor, insomnia, anxiety, and occasionally hallucinations that last a few days to a week.

GHB is addictive. Users who attempt to quit may experience significant withdrawal symptoms, including anxiety, tremors, and insomnia. Most symptoms decrease within one to two weeks of cessation, but severe psychological effects can last for weeks to months.

Nitrites

Nitrites (amyl, butyl, and isobutyl nitrite) are clear, amber-colored liquids that have had a history of abuse for more than three decades, especially in gay and bisexual men. Popular in dance clubs, they are used recreationally for a high feeling, a slowed sense of time, a carefree sense of well-being, and intensified sexual experiences.

Sold in small glass ampules containing individual doses, nitrites are usually inhaled and rapidly absorbed into the bloodstream. Users feel their physiological and psychological impact in seconds. Acute adverse effects include headache, dizziness, a drop in blood pressure, changes in heart rate, increased pressure within the eye, and skin flushing. Some individuals develop respiratory irritation and cough, sneezing, or difficulty breathing. Chronic use can lead to crusty skin lesions and chemical burns around the nose, mouth, and lips.

Stimulants

Central nervous system **stimulants** are drugs that increase activity in some portion of the brain or spinal cord. Some stimulants increase motor activity and enhance mental alertness, and some combat mental fatigue. Amphetamine, methamphetamine, caffeine, cocaine, and khat are stimulants. Stimulant medications are used to treat conditions such as ADHD. As discussed in Chapter 6, some college students abuse stimulants in order to lose weight.

Amphetamine

Amphetamines—benzedrine, dextroamphetamin, methamphetamine, Desoxyn, and related *uppers* such as the prescription drugs methylphenidate (Ritalin), pemoline (Cylert), and phenmetrazine (Preludin)—trigger the release of epinephrine (adrenaline), which stimulates the central nervous system. They were once widely prescribed for weight control because they suppress appetite, but they have emerged as a global danger.

Street Names: bennies, dex, meth, speed, crank, copilots

How Administered: Taken orally or injected

How Users Feel

- Hyper-alert and energetic.
- Confident in one's ability to think clearly and to perform any task exceptionally well—although amphetamines do not, in fact, significantly boost performance or thinking.
- Wired: talkative, excited, restless, irritable, anxious, moody.

If taken intravenously, a rush of elation and confidence, as well as adverse effects, including

- Confusion.
- Rambling or incoherent speech.
- Anxiety.
- Headache.
- Palpitations.
- Paranoia.
- Increased sexual interest.
- Unusual perceptions, such as ringing in the ears, a sensation of insects crawling on the skin, or hearing one's name called.

Risks and Possible Health Consequences

- Dependence with episodic or daily use.
- Bingeing—taking high doses over a period of several days—can lead to an extremely intense and unpleasant *crash*, characterized by a craving for the drug, shakiness, irritability, anxiety, and depression.

GHB (gamma hydroxybutyrate) A brain messenger chemical that stimulates the release of human growth hormone; commonly abused for its high and its alleged ability to trim fat and build muscles. Also known as "blue nitro" or the "date rape drug."

GBL (gamma butyrolactone) The main ingredient in gamma hydroxybutyrate (GHB); once ingested, GBL converts to GHB and can cause the ingestor to lose consciousness.

stimulants Agents, such as drugs, that temporarily relieve drowsiness, help in the performance of repetitive tasks, and improve capacity for work.

amphetamines Any of a class of stimulants that trigger the release of epinephrine, which stimulates the central nervous system; users experience a state of hyper-alertness and energy, followed by a crash as the drug wears off.

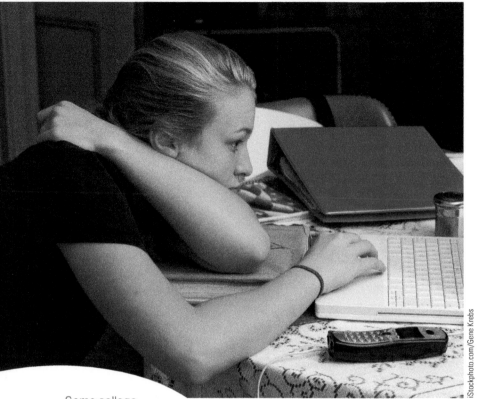

Some college students try stimulants to stay alert while cramming for exams, but these medications do not improve academic performance and can cause harmful effects.

Amphetamine intoxication can lead to:

- Feelings of grandiosity, anxiety, tension, hypervigilance, anger, social hypersensitivity, fighting, jitteriness or agitation, paranoia, and impaired judgment in social or occupational functioning.

- Increased heart rate, dilated pupils, elevated blood pressure, perspiration or chills, and nausea or vomiting.

- Less frequent effects, such as speeding up or slowing down of physical movement; muscular weakness; impaired breathing, chest pain, heart arrhythmia; confusion, seizures, impaired movements or muscle tone; or even coma.

- In high doses, a rapid or irregular heartbeat, tremors, loss of coordination, and collapse.

The long-term effects of amphetamine abuse include

- Malnutrition.
- Skin disorders.
- Ulcers.
- Insomnia.
- Depression.
- Vitamin deficiencies.

- Brain damage that results in speech and thought disturbances.

- Impaired concentration or memory.

- Sexual dysfunction.

- Withdrawal, characterized by fatigue, disturbing dreams, much more or less sleep than usual, increased appetite, and speeding up or slowing down of physical movements. Depression and irritability may persist for months.

- Significantly increased risk of suicide.[60]

✓**check-in** Do you think many students on your campus have tried stimulants?

Methamphetamine Methamphetamine, an addictive stimulant that is less expensive and possibly more addictive than cocaine or heroin, has become America's leading problem drug. More than 12 million Americans have tried methamphetamine, and 1.5 million are regular users, according to federal estimates. The estimated annual economic cost of methamphetamine is $23.4 billion.

Made in illegal laboratories, methamphetamine is chemically related to amphetamine, but its effects on the central nervous system are greater. The release of large amounts of dopamine creates a sensation of euphoria, increased self-esteem, and alertness. Users also report a marked increase in sexual appetite, which often leads to risky sexual behaviors while under the drug's influence.

Street Names: speed, crystal, fire, glass, meth, and chalk. Methamphetamine hydrochloride, clear chunky crystals resembling ice that can be inhaled by smoking, is called ice, crystal, glass, and tina.

How Administered: Snorted, smoked, injected, or ingested orally

How Users Feel

- Smoking or injection causes an intense pleasurable sensation, called a rush or flash, that lasts only a few minutes.

- Oral or intranasal use produces a high but not a rush.

Risks and Possible Health Consequences: Users may become addicted quickly, using more methamphetamine more and more frequently. Despair and suicidal thinking can develop when the stimulant effect wears off.

Even small amounts of methamphetamine can increase wakefulness and physical activity, depress

iStockphoto.com/Gene Krebs

appetite, and raise body temperature. Other effects on the central nervous system include

- Irritability.

- Insomnia.

- Confusion.

- Aggressive behavior.

- Tremors.

- Convulsions.

- Anxiety.

- Paranoia.

- Intellectual impairment.

- Anxiety.

- Depression.

- Increased heart rate and blood pressure.

- Irreversible damage to blood vessels in the brain, producing strokes.

- Damage to the frontal cortex of developing teen brains.[61]

- Respiratory problems.

- Irregular heartbeat.

- Extreme loss of appetite and weight.

- Elevated body (and probably brain) temperature, sometimes resulting in convulsions and high fevers that can be fatal.

- Inability to cope with everyday problems.

- High risk of psychotic symptoms, such as hallucinations and delusions that may persist for months or years after use stops.

- "Meth mouth," with teeth turning a grayish-brown, twisting, falling out, and taking on a peculiar texture. About 40 percent of meth users have serious dental problems.

- Risky sex. Meth has been linked to an increase in unsafe practices, including needle sharing with partners, which has led to a spike in HIV and hepatitis C infections in gay communities.

- Abnormalities in brain regions associated with selective attention and in those associated with memory. The brain may recover somewhat after months of abstinence, but problems often remain.

- With long-term use, changes in brain chemistry that may lead to compulsive drug-seeking and that make addiction especially hard to overcome.

- Significantly increased risk of Parkinson's disease.[62]

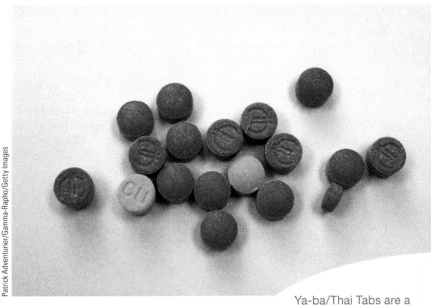

Patrick Adventurier/Gamma-Rapho/Getty Images

Ya-ba/Thai Tabs are a powerful form of meth-amphetamine that tastes sweet.

- Even after stopping use, chronic apathy and anhedonia (inability to experience pleasure).

The Toll on Society: Law enforcement officials consider methamphetamine their biggest drug problem. Meth addicts are pouring into prisons and recovery centers at an ever-increasing rate. "Meth babies" are crowding the foster-care system. Meth-making operations, which have been uncovered in all 50 states, involve the release of poisonous gases and toxic waste that is often dumped down household drains, in backyards, or by the side of the road. The cost of cleaning up the environmental impacts of meth is a growing problem for many communities.

Over-the-counter cold medicines (ephedrine and pseudoephedrine) are commonly used in meth production, which is one reason for federal and state restrictions on their sale.

√ **check-in** Do you believe that methamphetamine can be a threat to a neighborhood or community?

Withdrawal: Methamphetamine addiction is difficult to treat. As with cocaine, coming off methamphetamine causes intense distress, so users often seek out the drug to relieve their pain. Treatment usually requires the intervention of the patient's family as well as a substance abuse specialist team experienced in treating individuals with methamphetamine addiction.

Standard substance abuse treatment methods such as education, behavior therapy, individual and family counseling, and support groups may be effective for some. Methamphetamine abusers often use other illicit drugs as well, a problem

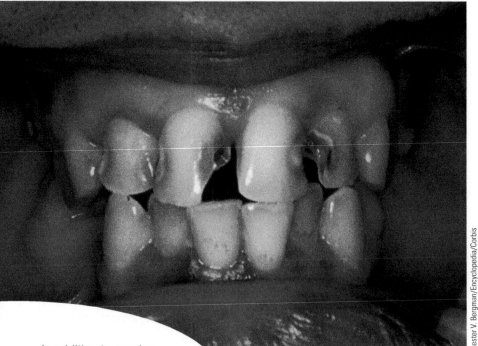

In addition to causing respiratory problems, brain damage, and mental impairment, methamphetamine damages teeth. This is how "meth mouth" looks.

Lester V. Bergman/Encyclopedia/Corbis

that can be addressed as part of a comprehensive program.

Cocaine

Cocaine is a white crystalline powder extracted from the leaves of the South American coca plant.

Street Names: coke, snow, lady

How Administered: Usually mixed with various sugars and local anesthetics like lidocaine and procaine, cocaine powder is generally inhaled. When sniffed or snorted, cocaine anesthetizes the nerve endings in the nose and relaxes the lung's bronchial muscles.

Cocaine can be dissolved in water and injected intravenously. The drug is rapidly metabolized by the liver, so the high is relatively brief, typically lasting only about 20 minutes. This means that users commonly inject the drug repeatedly, increasing the risk of infection and damage to their veins.

Cocaine alkaloid, or *freebase*, is obtained by removing the hydrochloride salt from cocaine powder. *Freebasing* is smoking the fumes of the alkaloid form of cocaine. *Crack*, pharmacologically identical to freebase, is a cheap, easy-to-use, widely available, smokeable, and potent form of cocaine named for the popping sound it makes when burned. Because it is absorbed rapidly into the bloodstream and large doses reach the brain very quickly, it is particularly dangerous. However, its low price and easy availability have made it a common drug of abuse in poor urban areas.

cocaine A white crystalline powder extracted from the leaves of the coca plant that stimulates the central nervous system and produces a brief period of euphoria followed by a depression.

How Users Feel: A powerful stimulant to the central nervous system, cocaine targets several chemical sites in the brain, producing

- Feelings of soaring well-being.
- Boundless energy.
- Restlessness and anxiety, although users feel that they have enormous physical and mental ability.

After a brief period of euphoria, users slump into a depression. They often go on cocaine binges, lasting from a few hours to several days, and consume large quantities of cocaine.

With crack, dependence develops quickly. As soon as crack users come down from one high, they want more crack. Whereas heroin addicts may shoot up several times a day, crack addicts need another hit within minutes. Thus, a crack habit can quickly become more expensive than heroin addiction.

✓**check-in** What is your impression of the dangers of crack cocaine?

Risks and Potential Health Consequences: Cocaine dependence is an easy habit to acquire. With repeated use, the brain becomes tolerant of the drug's stimulant effects, and users must take more of it to get high. Those who smoke or inject cocaine can develop dependence within weeks. Those who sniff cocaine may not become dependent on the drug for months or years. It is thought that 5 to 20 percent of all coke users—a group as large as the estimated total number of heroin addicts—are dependent on the drug.

The physical effects of acute cocaine intoxication include the following:

- Dilated pupils.
- Elevated or lowered blood pressure.
- Perspiration or chills.
- Nausea and vomiting.
- Speeding up or slowing down of physical activity.
- Muscular weakness.
- Impaired breathing.
- Chest pain.
- Impaired movements or muscle tone.
- With prolonged snorting, ulceration of the mucous membrane of the nose and damage to the nasal septum (the membrane between the nostrils) severe enough to cause it to collapse.
- Sexual side effects. At low doses, delayed orgasm and heightened sensory awareness.

With regular use, problems maintaining erections and ejaculating, low sperm counts, less active sperm, more abnormal sperm than in nonusers. Both male and female chronic cocaine users tend to lose interest in sex and have difficulty reaching orgasm.

- Increased risk of stroke, bleeding in the brain, and potentially fatal brain seizures.

- Psychiatric or neurological complications with repeated or high doses, including impaired judgment, hyperactivity, nonstop babbling, feelings of suspicion and paranoia, and violent behavior (Figure 12.4). The brain never learns to tolerate cocaine's negative effects; users may become incoherent and paranoid and may experience unusual sensations, such as ringing in their ears, feeling insects crawling on the skin, or hearing their name called.

- Damage to the liver and lungs in freebasers. Smoking crack causes bronchitis and may promote the transmission of HIV through burned and bleeding lips. Some smokers have died of respiratory complications, such as pulmonary edema (buildup of fluid in the lungs).

- Rapid rise in heart rate and blood pressure, which can trigger the symptoms of a heart attack in young people.

- Other cardiac complications, including arrhythmia (disruption of heart rhythm), angina (chest pain), and acute myocardial infarction (heart attack).

- Dangers to pregnant women and their babies, including miscarriages, developmental disorders, and life-threatening complications during birth. Reduced fetal oxygen supply may interfere with the development of the fetus's nervous system.

- Greatly increased risk of suicide.[63]

The combination of alcohol and cocaine is particularly lethal. The liver combines the two agents and manufactures cocaethylene, which intensifies cocaine's euphoric effects, while possibly increasing the risk of sudden death. Cocaine users who inject the drug and share needles put themselves at risk for another potentially lethal problem: HIV infection.

Withdrawal: When addicted individuals stop using cocaine, they often become depressed. This may lead to further cocaine use to alleviate depression. Other symptoms of cocaine withdrawal include

- Fatigue.
- Vivid and disturbing dreams.

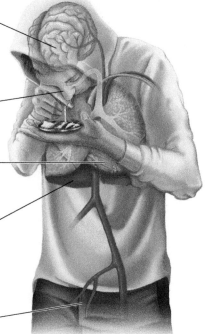

Central nervous system
- Repeated use or high dosages may cause severe psychological problems
- Suppresses desire for food, sex, and sleep
- Can cause strokes, seizures, and neurological damage

Nose
- Damages mucous membrane

Cardiovascular system
- Increases blood pressure by constricting blood vessels
- Causes irregular heartbeat
- Damages heart tissue

Respiratory system
- Freebasing causes lung damage
- Overdose can lead to respiratory arrest

Reproductive system
- In men, affects ability to maintain erections and ejaculate; also causes sperm abnormalities
- In women, may affect ability to carry pregnancy to term

© Cengage Learning

FIGURE 12.4 Some Effects of Cocaine on the Body

- Excessive or inadequate sleep.
- Irritability.
- Increased appetite.
- Physical slowing down or speeding up.

The initial crash may last one to three days after cutting down or stopping heavy use of cocaine. Some individuals become violent, paranoid, and suicidal.

Withdrawal symptoms usually reach a peak two to four days after cutting down or stopping heavy use of cocaine, although depression, anxiety, irritability, lack of pleasure in usual activities, and low-level cravings may continue for weeks. As memories of the crash fade, the desire for cocaine intensifies. For many weeks after stopping, individuals may feel an intense craving for the drug.

Treatment: Overcoming an addiction to cocaine or another stimulant drug can be challenging. Among the behavioral approaches that have shown the greatest success are

- Cognitive-behavioral therapy (CBT), which helps patients recognize and avoid drug triggers and learn new ways of coping with them.

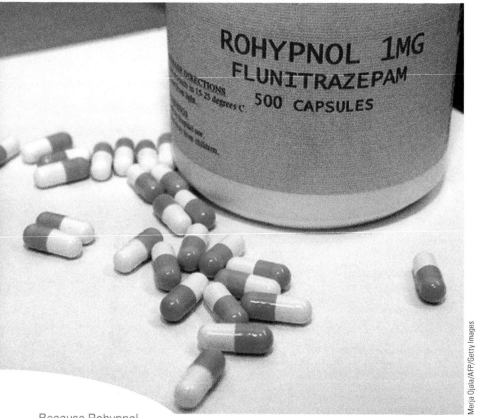

Because Rohypnol is colorless, tasteless, and odorless, it can be added to beverages without your knowledge.

Merja Ojala/AFP/Getty Images

- Contingency management, which uses tangible rewards, such as vouchers for movies, to encourage abstinence.
- The Matrix Model, which combines a 12 Step program, behavioral therapy, family education, and individual counseling.

The FDA has not approved any medications for addictions to cocaine and other stimulants, but several drugs have shown promise. These include Antabuse, widely used for alcohol dependence; the muscle relaxant baclofen (Lioresal); the anticonvulsant topiramate (Topamax); and the stimulant modafinil (Provigil), used to treat narcolepsy.

Depressants

Depressants depress the central nervous system, reduce activity, and induce relaxation, drowsiness, or sleep. They include the benzodiazepines and the barbiturates, the opioids, and alcohol.

Benzodiazepines and Barbiturates

These depressants are the sedative-hypnotics, also known as anxiolytic or antianxiety drugs. They include chlordiazepoxide (Librium), diazepam (Valium), oxazepam (Serax), lorazepam (Ativan), flurazepam (Dalmane), and alprazolam (Xanax). Benzodiazepines and barbiturates are most often prescribed for tension, muscular strain, sleep problems, anxiety, panic attacks, and anesthesia. They also are used to treat alcohol withdrawal.

Benzodiazepine sleeping pills have largely replaced the **barbiturates**, which were used medically in the past for inducing relaxation and sleep, relieving tension, and treating epileptic seizures. These drugs are usually taken by mouth in tablet, capsule, or liquid form. When used as a general anesthetic, benzodiazepines are administered intravenously. They differ widely in their mechanism of action, absorption rate, and metabolism, but all produce similar intoxication and withdrawal symptoms.

Rohypnol, a trade name for flunitrazepam—called roofies, rophie, roche, or the forget-me pill—is one of the benzodiazepines that has been of particular concern for the past few years because of its abuse in date rape. When mixed with alcohol, Rohypnol, which is flavorless and odorless, can incapacitate victims and prevent them from resisting sexual assault. It produces "anterograde amnesia," which means individuals may not remember events they experienced while under the effects of the drug. Other adverse effects include the following:

- Decreased blood pressure.
- Drowsiness.
- Visual disturbances.
- Dizziness.
- Confusion.
- Urinary retention.
- Digestive problems.

Rohypnol may be lethal when mixed with alcohol or other depressants.

How Users Feel

- Reduced or relieved tension with low doses.
- Loosening of sexual or aggressive inhibitions with increasing doses.
- Rapid mood changes.
- Impaired judgment.
- Impaired social or occupational functioning.

Risks and Potential Health Consequences:
All sedative-hypnotic drugs can produce physical and psychological dependence within two to four weeks. A complication specific to sedatives is *cross-tolerance* (cross-addiction), which occurs when users develop tolerance for one sedative or become dependent on it and develop tolerance for other sedatives as well.

benzodiazepine An antianxiety drug that depresses the central nervous system, reduces activity, and induces relaxation, drowsiness, or sleep; often prescribed to relieve tension, muscular strain, sleep problems, anxiety, and panic attacks; also used as an anesthetic and in the treatment of alcohol withdrawal.

barbiturates Antianxiety drugs that depress the central nervous system, reduce activity, and induce relaxation, drowsiness, or sleep; often prescribed to relieve tension and treat epileptic seizures or as a general anesthetic.

Intoxication with these drugs can produce

- Changes in mood or behavior, such as inappropriate sexual or aggressive acts.
- Mood swings.
- Impaired judgment.
- Slurred speech.
- Poor coordination.
- Unsteady gait.
- Involuntary eye movements.
- Impaired attention or memory.
- Stupor or coma.

Sedative-hypnotic drugs and alcohol together have a synergistic effect that can be dangerous or even lethal. For example, an individual's driving ability, already impaired by alcohol, will be made even worse, increasing the risk of an accident. Alcohol in combination with sedative-hypnotics leads to respiratory depression and may result in respiratory arrest and death.

Withdrawal: Regular users of any of these drugs who become physically dependent should not try to cut down or quit on their own. If they try to quit suddenly, they run the risk of seizures, coma, and death.

Withdrawal from sedative-hypnotic drugs may range from relatively mild discomfort to a severe syndrome with grand mal seizures, depending on the degree of dependence. Symptoms include

- Malaise or weakness.
- Sweating.
- Rapid pulse.
- Coarse tremors (of the hands, tongue, or eyelids).
- Insomnia.
- Nausea or vomiting.
- Temporary hallucinations or illusions.
- Physical restlessness.
- Anxiety or irritability.
- Grand mal seizures.

Withdrawal may begin within two to three days after stopping drug use, and symptoms may persist for many weeks.

Opioids

The **opioids** include opium and its derivatives (morphine, codeine, and heroin) and synthetic drugs that have similar sleep-inducing and pain-relieving properties. The opioids come from a resin taken from the seedpod of the Asian

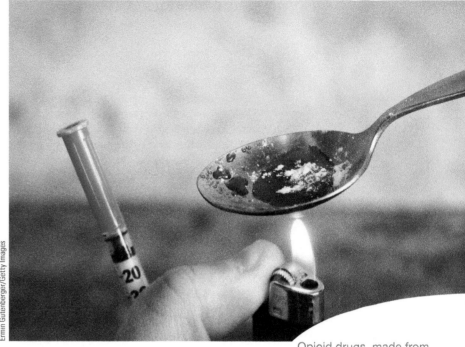

Ermin Gutenberger/Getty Images

Opioid drugs, made from the Asian poppy, come in both legal and illegal forms. All are highly addictive.

poppy. Synthetic opioids, such as meperidine (Demerol), methadone, and propoxyphene (Darvon), are synthesized in a chemical laboratory. Whether natural or synthetic, these drugs are powerful *narcotics*, or painkillers.

Heroin is the most widely abused opioid in this country, with an estimated 600,000 heroin addicts. Male addicts outnumber female addicts by three to one. Among people ages 18 to 25, the percentage of heroin users who inject the drug has doubled in the past decade. Nearly 80 percent of people who recently started using heroin had previously used prescription pain relievers illegally, according to the U.S. Substance Abuse and Mental Health Services Administration.[64]

Street Names: horse, junk, smack, or downtown

How Administered: Heroin users typically inject the drug into their veins. However, individuals who experiment with recreational drugs often prefer *skin-popping* (subcutaneous injection) rather than *mainlining* (intravenous injection); they also may snort heroin as a powder or dissolve it and inhale the vapors. To try to avoid addiction, some users begin by *chipping*, taking small or intermittent doses. Regardless of the method of administration, tolerance can develop rapidly.

Morphine, used as a painkiller and anesthetic, acts primarily on the central nervous system, eyes, and digestive tract. By producing mental clouding, drowsiness, and euphoria, it does not decrease the physical sensation of pain as much as it alters a

opioids Drugs that have sleep-inducing and pain-relieving properties, including opium and its derivatives and nonopioid, synthetic drugs.

person's awareness of the pain; in effect, the morphine user no longer cares about the pain.

How Users Feel: All opioids relax the user. When injected, they can produce an immediate rush (high) that lasts 10 to 30 minutes. For two to six hours thereafter, users may feel indifferent, lethargic, and drowsy; they may slur their words and have problems paying attention, remembering, and going about their normal routine. The primary attractions of heroin are the euphoria and pain relief it produces. However, some people experience very unpleasant feelings, such as anxiety and fear. Other effects include

- A sensation of warmth or heaviness.
- Dry mouth.
- Facial flushing.
- Nausea and vomiting (particularly in first-time users).

Risks and Potential Health Consequences: Addiction is common. Almost all regular users of opioids rapidly develop drug dependence, which can lead to lethargy, weight loss, loss of sex drive, and the continual effort to avoid withdrawal symptoms through repeated drug administration. Users continue taking opioids as much to avoid the discomfort of withdrawal, a classic sign of opioid addiction, as to experience pleasure. In addition, they experience the following:

- Anxiety.
- Insomnia.
- Restlessness.
- Craving for the drug.
- Constricted pupils (although pupils may dilate from a severe overdose).
- Drowsiness.
- Slurred speech.
- Impaired attention or memory.
- In pregnant women, increased risk of miscarriage, stillbirth, or low birth weight. Babies born to addicted mothers experience withdrawal symptoms after birth.

Morphine affects blood pressure, heart rate, and blood circulation in the brain. Both morphine and heroin slow down the respiratory system; overdoses can cause fatal respiratory arrest.

Over time, users who inject opioids may develop infections of the heart lining and valves, skin abscesses, and lung congestion. Infections from unsterile solutions, syringes, and shared needles can lead to hepatitis, tetanus, liver disease, and HIV. Depression is common and may

be both an antecedent and a risk factor for needle sharing.

Heroin overdose deaths have skyrocketed in recent years, quadrupling since 2000.[65]

Withdrawal: If a regular user stops taking an opioid, withdrawal begins within 6 to 12 hours. The intensity of the symptoms depends on the degree of the addiction; they may grow stronger for 24 to 72 hours and gradually subside over a period of 7 to 14 days, though some symptoms, such as insomnia, may persist for several months. Individuals may develop craving for an opioid, irritability, nausea or vomiting, muscle aches, runny nose or eyes, dilated pupils, sweating, diarrhea, yawning, fever, and insomnia. Opioid withdrawal usually is not life-threatening.

✓**check-in** Do you view opiate addicts as different from other drug users?

Hallucinogens

The drugs known as **hallucinogens** produce vivid and unusual changes in thought, feeling, and perception. Hallucinogens do not produce dependence in the same way as cocaine or heroin. Individuals who have an unpleasant experience after trying a hallucinogen may stop using the drug completely without suffering withdrawal symptoms. Others continue regular or occasional use because they enjoy the effects.

LSD (lysergic acid diethylamide commonly known as acid) was initially developed as a tool to explore mental illness. It became popular in the 1960s and resurfaced among teenagers in the 1990s. LSD is taken orally, either blotted onto pieces of paper that are held in the mouth or chewed along with another substance, such as a sugar cube. Peyote (whose active ingredient is mescaline) is another hallucinogen, but it is much less commonly used in this country.

Dissociative Drugs

Drugs such as PCP (phencyclidine) and ketamine, initially developed as general anesthetics for surgery, distort perceptions of sight and sound and produce feelings of dissociation or detachment from the environment and self. They alter distribution of the neurotransmitter glutamate, which is involved in perception of pain, responses to the environment, and memory, in the brain.

Because these mind-altering effects are not hallucinations, scientists refer to PCP and ketamine as "dissociative anesthetics." High doses of dextromethorphan, a widely available cough

hallucinogens Drugs that cause hallucinations.

LSD (lysergic acid diethylamide) A synthetic psychoactive substance originally developed to explore mental illness.

suppressant, and the herb salvia can produce effects similar to those of PCP and ketamine.

Ketamine

Ketamine—called K, Special-K, and vitamin K—is an anesthetic used by veterinarians. When cooked, dried, and ground into powder for snorting, ketamine blocks chemical messengers in the brain that carry sensory input. As a result, the brain fills the void with hallucinations. Users may report an "out-of-body" experience, with distorted perceptions of time and space. The effects typically begin within 30 minutes and last for approximately two hours.

Ketamine has become common in clubs and has been used as a date rape drug. Low doses can cause

- Impaired attention and memory.
- Anxiety.
- Agitation.
- Paranoia.
- Vomiting.

Higher doses can cause

- Delirium.
- Amnesia.
- Impaired motor function.
- High blood pressure.
- Depression.
- Potentially deadly breathing problems.

Repeated ketamine use can be addictive, and even a single use can occasionally produce audio-visual "flashbacks," similar to those described by phencyclidine (PCP) users, and long-term memory loss.

PCP

PCP (phencyclidine, brand name Sernyl; street names angel dust, peace pill, lovely, and green) is an illicit drug manufactured as a tablet, capsule, liquid, flake, spray, or crystal-like white powder that can be swallowed, smoked, sniffed, or injected. Sometimes it is sprinkled on crack, marijuana, tobacco, or parsley and smoked. A fine-powdered form of PCP can be snorted or injected.

PCP use peaked in the 1970s, but it remains a popular drug of abuse in both inner-city ghettos and suburban high schools. Users often think that the PCP they take together with another illegal psychoactive substance, such as amphetamines, coke, or hallucinogens, is responsible for the highs they feel, so they seek it out specifically.

The effects of PCP are utterly unpredictable. It may trigger violent behavior or irreversible psychosis the first time it is used, or the twentieth time, or never. In low doses, PCP produces changes similar to those produced by other psychoactive drugs, including

- Hallucinations.
- Euphoria.
- Feelings of emptiness or numbness.

Higher doses may produce

- A stupor that lasts several days.
- Increased heart rate and blood pressure.
- Skin flushing.
- Sweating.
- Dizziness.
- Numbness.

Some people experience repetitive motor movements (such as facial grimacing), hallucinations, and paranoia. Suicide is a definite risk. Intoxication typically lasts 4 to 6 hours, but some effects can linger for several days. Delirium may occur within 24 hours of taking PCP or after recovery from an overdose and can last as long as a week.

Inhalants

Inhalants, or *deleriants*, are chemicals that produce vapors with psychoactive effects. The most commonly abused inhalants are solvents, aerosols, model-airplane glue, cleaning fluids, and petroleum products like kerosene and butane. Some anesthetics and nitrous oxide (laughing gas) are also abused.

✓ **check-in** Do you know anyone who experimented with inhalants when they were younger?

Only alcohol is a more widely used intoxicant among preteens and teens. Young people who have been treated for mental health problems, have a history of foster care, or already abuse other drugs have an increased risk of abusing or becoming dependent on inhalants. In addition, adolescents who first begin using inhalants at an early age are more likely to become dependent on them. Approximately 11 percent of adolescents nationwide report having used inhalants in their lifetime. Many report coexisting multiple drug abuse and dependence, mental health treatment, and delinquent behaviors.

Inhalants very rapidly reach the lungs, bloodstream, and other parts of the body. At low doses, users may feel slightly stimulated; at higher doses, they may feel less inhibited.

PCP (phencyclidine) A synthetic psychoactive substance that produces effects similar to those of other psychoactive drugs when swallowed, smoked, sniffed, or injected and also may trigger unpredictable behavioral changes.

inhalants Substances that produce vapors having psychoactive effects when sniffed.

Intoxication often occurs within five minutes and can last more than an hour. Inhalant users do not report the intense rush associated with other drugs, nor do they experience the perceptual changes associated with LSD. However, inhalants interfere with thinking and impulse control, so users may act in dangerous or destructive ways.

Often there are visible external signs of use:

• A rash around the nose and mouth.

• Breath odors.

• Residue on the face, hands, and clothing.

• Redness, swelling, and tearing of the eyes.

• Irritation of the throat, lungs, and nose that leads to coughing and gagging.

• Nausea and headache.

Regular use of inhalants leads to tolerance, so the sniffer needs more and more to attain the desired effects. Younger children who use inhalants several times a week may develop dependence. Older users who become dependent may use the drugs many times a day.

Although some young people believe inhalants are safe, this is far from true. Inhalation of butane from cigarette lighters displaces oxygen in the lungs, causing suffocation. Users also can suffocate while covering their heads with a plastic bag to inhale a substance or from inhaling vomit into their lungs while high. The effects of inhalants are unpredictable, and even a single episode can trigger asphyxiation or cardiac arrhythmia, leading to disability or death. Abusers also can develop difficulties with memory and abstract reasoning, problems with coordination, and uncontrollable movements of the extremities.

Treating Substance Dependence and Abuse

An estimated 6.1 million Americans are in need of drug treatment, but the majority—some 5 million—never get treatment. The most difficult step for a drug user is to admit that he or she *is* in fact an addict. If drug abusers are not forced to deal with their problem through some unexpected trauma, such as being fired or going bankrupt, those who care—family, friends, coworkers, doctors—may have to confront them and insist that they do

something about their addiction. Often such an *intervention* can be the turning point for an addict and his or her family. Treatment has proved equally successful for young people and for older adults.

Undergraduates who enter substance abuse treatment programs are more likely to complete them successfully than nonstudents, often in a shorter period. The reason may be that academics provides a source of external goals and optimism that improves motivation to change and enhances a sense of urgency to complete treatment.[66]

✓**check-in** Do you know anyone who has been treated for substance abuse?

Treatment may take place in an outpatient setting, a residential facility, or a hospital. Increasingly, treatment thereafter is tailored to address coexisting or dual diagnoses. A personal treatment plan may consist of individual psychotherapy, marital and family therapy, medication, and behavior therapy. Once an individual has made the decision to seek help for substance abuse, the first step usually is detoxification, which involves clearing the drug from the body.

Antiaddiction medications that target neurotransmitters in the brain are becoming safer and more effective. With treatment, substance abusers are less prone to relapse. If they do return to drug use, their relapses tend to be shorter and less frequent.

The aim of chemical dependence treatment is to help individuals establish and maintain their recovery from alcohol and drugs of abuse. Recovery is a dynamic process of personal growth and healing in which the drug user makes the transition from a lifestyle of active substance use to a drug-free lifestyle.

Principles of Drug Addiction Treatment

Decades of scientific research have shown that treatment can help drug-addicted individuals stop drug use, avoid relapse, and successfully recover their lives. Based on this research, the National Institute on Drug Abuse (NIDA) has developed fundamental principles that characterize effect drug abuse treatment. They include the following:

• Addiction is a complex but treatable disease that affects brain function and behavior.

• No single treatment is appropriate for everyone.

• Treatment needs to be readily available.

• Effective treatment attends to multiple needs of an individual, not just his or her drug abuse.

- Remaining in treatment for an adequate period of time is critical.

- Counseling—individual and/or group—and other behavioral therapies are the most commonly used forms of drug abuse treatment.

- Medications are an important element of treatment for many patients, especially when combined with counseling and other behavioral therapies.

- Many drug-addicted individuals also have other mental disorders.

- Medically assisted detoxification is only the first stage of addiction treatment and by itself does little to change the long-term drug abuse.

- Treatment does not need to be voluntary to be effective.

- Drug use during treatment must be monitored continuously, as lapses during treatment do occur.

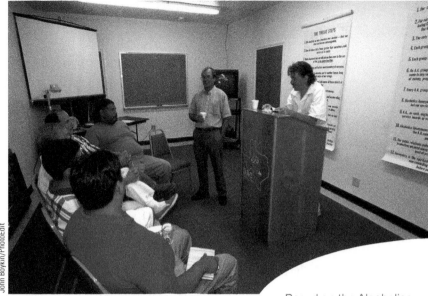

John Boykin/PhotoEdit

12 Step Programs

Since its founding in 1935, Alcoholics Anonymous (AA)—the oldest, largest, and most successful self-help program in the world—has spawned a worldwide movement. As many as 200 different recovery programs are based on the spiritual **12 Step program** of AA. Participation in 12 Step programs for drug abusers, such as Substance Anonymous, Narcotics Anonymous, and Cocaine Anonymous, is of fundamental importance in promoting and maintaining long-term abstinence.

The basic precept of 12 Step programs is that members have been powerless when it comes to controlling their addictive behavior on their own. These programs don't recruit members. The desire to stop must come from the individual, who can call the number of a 12 Step program, listed in the telephone book, and find out when and where the next nearby meeting will be held. A representative may offer to send someone to the caller's house to talk about the problem and to escort him or her to the next meeting.

Meetings of various 12 Step programs are held daily in almost every city in the country. (Some chapters, whose members often include disabled individuals or those in remote areas, meet via Internet chat rooms or electronic bulletin boards.) There are no dues or fees for membership. Many individuals belong to several programs because they have several problems, such as alcoholism, substance abuse, and pathological gambling. All these programs have only one requirement for membership: a desire to stop an addictive behavior.

Relapse Prevention

The most common clinical course for substance abuse disorders involves a pattern of multiple relapses over the course of a lifespan. It is important for individuals with these problems and their families to recognize this fact. When relapses occur, they should be viewed as neither a mark of defeat nor evidence of moral weakness. While painful, relapses do not erase the progress that has been achieved and ultimately may strengthen self-understanding. They can serve as reminders of potential pitfalls to avoid in the future.

One key to preventing relapse is learning to avoid obvious cues and associations that can set off intense cravings. This means staying away from the people and places linked with past drug use.

Some therapists use conditioning techniques to give former users a sense of control over their urge to use the drug. The theory behind this approach, which is called *extinction* of conditioned behavior, is that with repeated exposure—for example, to videotapes of dealers selling crack cocaine—the arousal and craving will diminish. While this technique by itself cannot ward off relapses, it does seem to enhance the overall effectiveness of other therapies.

As therapists emphasize, every lapse does not have to lead to a full-blown relapse. Users can turn to the skills acquired in treatment—calling people for support and going to meetings—to avoid a major relapse. Ultimately, users must learn much more than how to avoid temptation; they must examine their entire view of the world and learn new ways to live in it without turning to drugs. This is the underlying goal of the recovery process.

Based on the Alcoholics Anonymous model, "12 Step" programs have helped many people overcome addiction. The one requirement for membership is a desire to end a pattern of addictive behavior.

12 Step program Self-help group program based on the principles of Alcoholics Anonymous.

- Is caffeine healthful or harmful?
- What are the reasons some students use drugs and others don't?
- What are the dangers of prescription drug abuse?
- Does marijuana, even when legal, pose risks to your health?

THE POWER OF NOW!

Choosing an Addiction-Free Lifestyle

People with substance abuse disorders and addictive behaviors lose control of their choices and their lives. Their compulsion to gamble or to use a drug seems irresistible. You, in contrast, have a choice. You can create a life and a lifestyle with no need and no room for reliance on a substance or a self-destructive behavior. Check those that you have already implemented. Are there others you plan to incorporate into your life? In your online journal, discuss the ways in which you are creating an addiction-free lifestyle.

____ Set goals for yourself. Think about who you want to become, what you'd like to do, the future you wish for yourself. Focus on what it will take—years of education, perhaps, or specialized training—to achieve these goals. Understand that drugs can only get in the way and diminish your potential.

____ Participate in drug-free activities. If you're bored or unfocused, drugs may appeal to you simply as something to do.

Take charge of your time. Play a sport. Work out at the gym. Join a club. Volunteer. Start a blog.

____ Educate yourself. Much of the information that young people hear from friends, particularly drug-using friends, is incorrect. Drugs that are used as medicines are not safe for recreational use. The fact that many people at a party or club are having fun doesn't mean that some aren't endangering their brains and their lives by taking club drugs.

____ Choose friends who have a future. The world of drug users shrinks. Nothing matters more than the next hit, the next high, the next fix. Losing all sense of tomorrow, they focus on getting through the day, with the help of drugs. Are these the people you want to spend time with? Choose friends who can broaden your world with new ideas, ambitious plans, and great dreams for tomorrow.

What's Online

CENGAGE brain .com   Visit www.cengagebrain.com to access course materials for this text, including the Behavior Change Planner, interactive quizzes, and more.

self survey

Do You Have a Substance Use Disorder?

Check the statements that apply to you.

- Use more of an illegal drug or a prescription medication or use a drug for a longer period of time than you desire or intend. ____

- Try, repeatedly and unsuccessfully, to cut down or control drug use. ____

- Spend a great deal of time doing whatever is necessary in order to get drugs, taking them, or recovering from their use. ____

- Are so high or feel so bad after drug use that you often cannot work or fulfill other responsibilities. ____

- Give up or cut back on important social, work, or recreational activities because of drug use. ____

- Continue to use drugs even though you realize that they are causing or worsening physical or mental problems. ____

- Use a lot more of a drug in order to achieve a "high" or desired effect or feel fewer such effects than in the past. ____

- Use drugs in dangerous ways or situations. ____

- Have repeated drug-related legal problems, such as arrests for possession. ____

- Continue to use drugs, even though the drug causes or worsens social or personal problems, such as arguments with a spouse. ____

- Develop hand tremors or other withdrawal symptoms if you cut down or stop drug use. ____

- Take drugs to relieve or avoid withdrawal symptoms. ____

The more blanks that you (or someone close to you) checks, the more reason you have to be concerned about drug use. The most difficult step for anyone with a substance use disorder is to admit that he or she has a problem. Sometimes a drug-related crisis, such as being arrested or fired, forces individuals to acknowledge the impact of drugs. If not, those who care—family, friends, boss, physician—may have to confront them and insist that they do something about it. This confrontation, planned beforehand, is called an *intervention* and can be the turning point for drug users and their families.

MAKING THIS CHAPTER WORK FOR YOU

Review Questions

(LO 12.1) 1. Which of the following statements is true in the context of risky addictive behaviors among adults?
   a. Women are more likely to indulge in risky behaviors than men.
   b. Non-Hispanic white males are least likely to indulge in substance abuse.
   c. The vast majority of college students do not engage in addictive behaviors.
   d. There are no promising treatments for addictions.

(LO 12.1) 2. As neuroscientists have shown, the brain's "reward center" responds to both pleasurable and exciting experiences, such as eating chocolate or bungee-jumping, by producing _____, a "feel good" chemical in the brain.
   a. acetaminophen
   b. dopamine
   c. serotonin
   d. amphetamine

(LO 12.2) 3. Which of the following statements is true about problem gambling?
   a. A gambling disorder does not affect the brain and behavior.
   b. Pathological gambling is viewed as an addiction that runs in families.
   c. Individuals who have high academic grades are most likely to exhibit problem gambling.
   d. Having access to casino machines, ongoing card games, or Internet gambling sites does not increase the likelihood that students will gamble.

(LO 12.2) 4. Which of the following behaviors indicates an increased risk of problem gambling?
   a. Being very spiritual
   b. Feeling depressed during gambling
   c. Belonging to a high socioeconomic class
   d. Gambling at an early age

(LO 12.3) 5. _____ is the most widely used illicit drug on campuses.
   a. Marijuana
   b. Ritalin
   c. Adderall
   d. Tylenol

(LO 12.3) 6. Which of the following factors can influence students to use drugs?
   a. Reading spiritual material
   b. Participating actively in class activities
   c. Understanding the risks associated with drug usage
   d. Consuming alcohol

(LO 12.4) 7. Drug _____ is a pattern of continuing substance use despite cognitive, behavioral, and physical symptoms.
   a. misuse
   b. diversion
   c. dependence
   d. overdose

(LO 12.4)   8. The dosage level at which a drug becomes poisonous to the body, causing either temporary or permanent damage, is called its _____.
   a. toxicity
   b. tonicity
   c. osmolarity
   d. salubrity

(LO 12.5)   9. Which of the following statements is true about caffeine?
   a. It increases fatigue even when taken in very small amounts.
   b. It provides relief from anxiety and digestive disturbances.
   c. It lowers the risk of cardiovascular disease.
   d. It increases the risk of type 2 diabetes.

(LO 12.5) 10. Which of the following statements is true in the context of caffeine intoxication?
   a. Students who consume high-caffeine energy drinks are less likely to consume alcohol.
   b. The recommended maximum dosage for adolescents is 500 mg of caffeine a day.
   c. Ingesting 50 mg of caffeine produces serious caffeine intoxication.
   d. A single dose of 5 grams of caffeine can be fatal.

(LO 12.6) 11. Psychological side effects of over-the-counter and prescription drugs _____.
   a. do not include mental or emotional problems
   b. decrease as people get older
   c. can include changes in the way people think, feel, and behave
   d. remain the same irrespective of its dosage

(LO 12.6) 12. Which of the following is an over-the-counter painkiller that poses multiple dangers?
   a. Phenolphthalein
   b. Acetaminophen
   c. Oxycodone
   d. Robitussin

(LO 12.7) 13. _____ occurs when a person develops tolerance to the effects of a drug and needs larger and larger doses to achieve intoxication or another desired effect.
   a. Drug diversion
   b. Drug interaction
   c. Physical dependence
   d. Allergy

(LO 12.7) 14. Which of the following is a characteristic of substance use disorder?
   a. A persistent desire to cut down or stop substance use
   b. Developing intolerance toward the substance
   c. Adhering to prescribed medications
   d. Absence of cravings and withdrawal symptoms

(LO 12.8) 15. Which of the following is an herbal drug?
   a. K2
   b. Tylenol
   c. Acetaminophen
   d. Khat

(LO 12.8) 16. Which of the following is an example of a stimulant?
   a. Tylenol
   b. Phenolphthalein
   c. Aspirin
   d. Amphetamine

(LO 12.9) 17. Which of the following is a principle of drug addiction treatment?
   a. One single treatment is appropriate for everyone.
   b. Addiction does not affect brain functioning and behavior.
   c. Many drug-addicted individuals have other mental disorders.
   d. Treatment needs to be voluntary in order to be effective.

(LO 12.9) 18. Which of the following statements is true in the context of preventing relapses of substance abuse?
   a. Relapses should be considered evidence of moral weakness.
   b. Every lapse eventually leads to a full-blown relapse.
   c. The ultimate goal of treatment is learning how to avoid temptation.
   d. Relapses do not in any way affect the progress that has been achieved.

Answers to these questions can be found on page 623.

Critical Thinking Questions

1. Assume that your friend is using amphetamines to keep her energy levels high so that she can continue to attend school full time and hold a job to pay her school expenses. You fear that she is developing a substance use disorder. What can you do to help her realize the dangers of her behavior? What resources are available at your school or in your community to help her deal with both her drug problem and her financial needs?

2. Some people oppose any kind of government regulations on the Internet. How do you feel about this issue? How would you address the problems associated with distributing drugs online, including the sale of counterfeit drugs?

Additional Online Resources

www.drugabuse.gov
This government site—a virtual clearinghouse of information for students, parents, teachers, researchers, and health professionals—features current treatment and research, as well as a comprehensive database on common drugs of abuse. The science of drug abuse and addictions is discussed, with a focus on the major illegal drugs in use, with additional resources on drug testing, treatment research, and trends/statistics.

www.drugfree.org
This site features current resources and photographs on a wide spectrum of drugs, including performance-enhancing drugs, club drugs, and commonly abused prescription drugs. The drug guide even allows you to search for a drug by using its slang name.

www.drugabuse.gov/drugs-abuse/club-drugs
This site is a service of the National Institute on Drug Abuse to provide information on club drugs.

http://phoenixhouse.org
Facts on Tap is one of the programs of Phoenix House, the largest nonprofit alcohol and drug abuse treatment and prevention facility in the United States.

Key Terms

The terms listed are used on the pages indicated. Definitions of the terms are in the Glossary at the end of the book.

addiction 359

additive 354

amphetamines 369

antagonistic 354

barbiturates 374

benzodiazepine 374

cannabinoids 363

cathinone 366

club drugs 367

cocaine 372

designer drugs 366

dopamine 360

drug 351

drug abuse 351

drug dependence 351

drug diversion 351

drug misuse 351

Ecstasy (MDMA) 367

gambling disorder 347

generic 358

GHB (gamma hydroxy-butyrate) 369

GBL (gamma butyrol-actone) 369

hallucinogens 376

hashish 363

inhalants 377

intoxication 360

intramuscular 352

intravenous 352

LSD (lysergic acid diethylamide) 376

marijuana 363

opioids 375

over-the-counter (OTC) 356

PCP (phencyclidine) 377

physical dependence 359

polyabuse 360

potentiating 354

psychoactive 354

psychological dependence 359

salvia 365

stimulants 369

subcutaneous 352

synergistic 354

toxicity 352

12 Step program 379

withdrawal 360

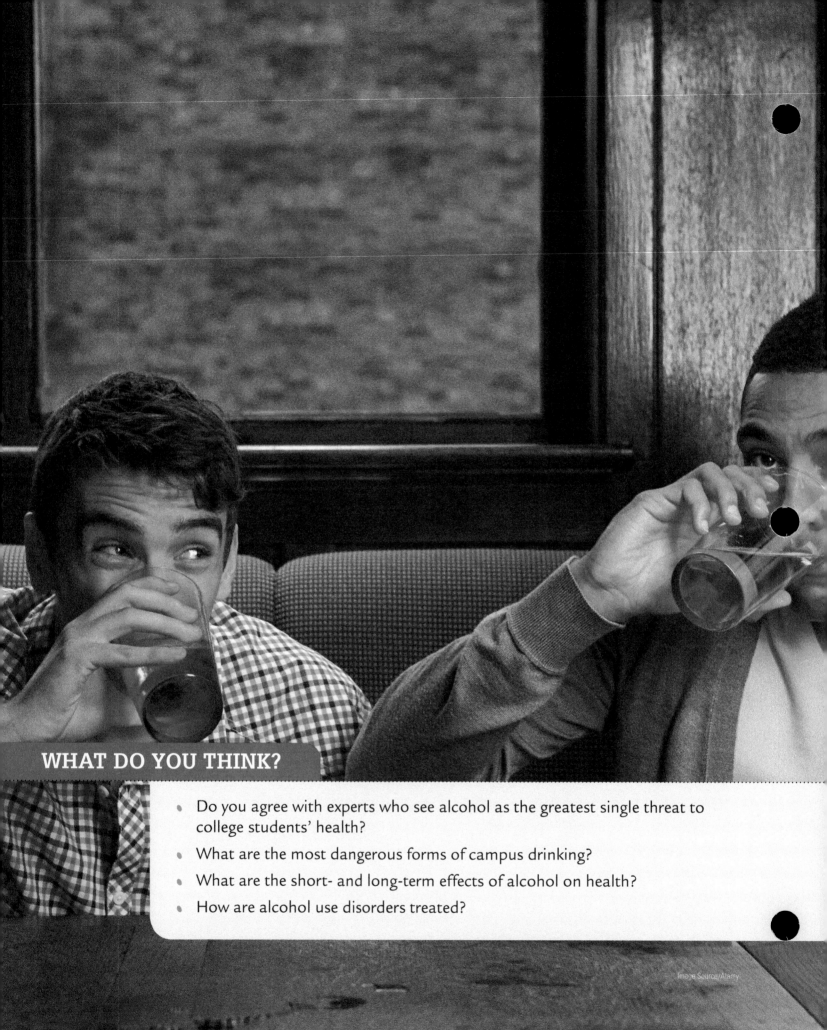

WHAT DO YOU THINK?

- Do you agree with experts who see alcohol as the greatest single threat to college students' health?
- What are the most dangerous forms of campus drinking?
- What are the short- and long-term effects of alcohol on health?
- How are alcohol use disorders treated?

Image Source/Alamy

13

Alcohol

At first glance the Friday night get-together looks like any other college party. Music booms. Clusters of undergraduates, plastic cups in hand, chat and laugh. A few couples dance. But there is one crucial difference: no alcohol. At hundreds of campuses across the United States—including some infamous "party schools"—students are finding ways to get together and have a good time without getting drunk, high, or wasted.

Katie, a third-year student at a large state university, couldn't imagine partying without alcohol. "In my freshman year, I carried a flask so I could take a few swigs and loosen up before going out," she recalls. Most evenings ended the same way—with her throwing up in some bushes on the way back to her dorm.

"It all got old—the drunk guys, the groping, the crazy fights, the hangovers," she says. With the help of a campus counseling program, she got sober. "For a while, I'd just hole up in my room and stream videos on weekends. Everyone else was out drinking."

Not everyone, she discovered. Through national organizations like the Collegiate Recovery Program and smaller campus groups, she found other students in various stages of recovery. Just sharing her story with them helped. But what she's enjoyed most is an entirely new social life.

"My old friends ask, 'How can you have fun in college without alcohol?' My answer is 'Easy,'" Katie says before summing up recent alcohol-free adventures: hikes, bike rides, tailgates, volleyball games, dances, film screenings, evenings at trendy

After reading this chapter, you should be able to:

13.1 Outline the patterns of alcohol consumption among different populations in America.

13.2 Discuss the patterns, reasons, and perils of drinking on campus.

13.3 Describe the characteristics of alcohol and its effects on human health.

13.4 Explain how alcohol is associated with serious health risks and disorders.

13.5 Review racial, ethnic, and gender differences in alcohol-related risks.

13.6 Examine the health consequences of alcohol-related disorders.

13.7 Discuss the various treatments for alcohol disorders.

"dry" bars that offer live music and cool nonalcoholic drinks. Some campuses offer special alcohol-free facilities that include flat-screen TVs, pool and ping-pong tables, and even "Clean Break" trips during spring vacation.

Although alcohol-free zones and opportunities are becoming more common, most college students still drink—the majority in ways that don't jeopardize their health or their futures. However, a recent surge of alcohol-linked sexual assaults and violence has triggered renewed focus on the negative, sometimes tragic consequences of excessive campus drinking. Universities are banning liquor at many campus events. Local police in many communities are cracking down on underage drinkers. And more students like Katie are choosing not to let alcohol take control of their lives.

Even if you never drink to excess, you live with the consequences of others' drinking. That's why it's important for everyone to know about the very real dangers of alcohol abuse. This chapter provides information that can help you understand, avoid, and change behaviors that could destroy your health, happiness, and life. <

Drinking in America

Although many Americans drink alcohol, most do not misuse or abuse it. According to the most recent statistics available from the National Institute on Alcohol Abuse and Alcoholism,

- 88 percent of Americans ages 18 or older report that they drank alcohol at some point in their lifetime.

- 71 percent report alcohol use in the last year.

- 56 percent report drinking in the last month.

- 25 percent report that they engaged in binge drinking in the last month (five or more drinks on one occasion for men; four for women).

- 7.2 percent report heavy drinking (five or more drinks on an occasion on five or more occasions per month) in the last month.[1]

Alcohol is the third leading preventable cause of death in the United States. No medical conditions other than heart disease cause more disability and premature death than alcohol-related problems. No mental or medical disorders touch the lives of more families. No other form of disability costs individuals, employers, and the government more for treatment, injuries, reduced worker productivity, and property damage. The costs in emotional pain and in lost and shattered lives because of irresponsible drinking are beyond measure.

Here are the most recent statistics on alcohol's toll:

- Nearly 88,000 people (62,000 men and 26,000 women) die from alcohol-related causes each year in the United States.

- Alcohol-impaired driving accounts for 10,322 deaths each year, about a third of all driving fatalities.

- Alcohol contributes to more than 200 diseases and injury-related health conditions.

- Globally, alcohol consumption is the fifth-leading risk factor for premature death and disability and leads to 3.3 million deaths annually.[2]

Why People Don't Drink

More Americans are choosing not to drink, and alcohol consumption is at its lowest level in decades. About a quarter of adults—31 percent of women and 18 percent of men—report drinking no alcohol in the past year.

With fewer people drinking alcohol, nonalcoholic beverages have grown in popularity. They appeal to drivers, boaters, individuals with health problems that could worsen with alcohol, older individuals who can't tolerate alcohol, anyone taking medicines that interact with alcohol (including antibiotics, antidepressants, and muscle relaxers), and everyone interested in limiting alcohol intake. Under federal law, these drinks can contain some alcohol but a much smaller amount than regular beer or wine. Nonalcoholic beers and wines on the market also are lower in calories than alcoholic varieties.

Certain people should not drink at all. These include the following:

- Anyone younger than age 21. Underage drinking (discussed later in this chapter) poses many medical, behavioral, and legal dangers.

- Anyone who plans to drive, operate motorized equipment, or engage in other activities that require alertness and skill (including sports and recreational activities).

- Women who are pregnant or trying to become pregnant.

- Individuals taking certain over-the-counter or prescription medications.
- People with medical conditions that can be made worse by drinking.
- Recovering alcoholics.

✓**check-in** Have you ever had an alcoholic drink? If so, how old were you when you had your first drink?

Why People Drink

The most common reason people drink alcohol is to relax. Because it depresses the central nervous system, alcohol can make people feel less tense. Some psychologists theorize that men engage in *confirmatory drinking*; that is, they drink to reinforce the image of masculinity associated with alcohol consumption. Both genders may engage in *compensatory drinking*, consuming alcohol to heighten their sense of masculinity or femininity.

Here are some other reasons men and women drink:

- **Social ease.** When people use alcohol, they may seem bolder, wittier, sexier. At the same time, they become more relaxed and seem to enjoy each other's company more. Because alcohol lowers inhibitions, some people see it as a prelude to seduction.
- **Role models.** Athletes, some of the biggest celebrities in our country, have a long history of appearing in commercials for alcohol. Many advertisements feature glamorous men and women holding or sipping alcoholic beverages.
- **Advertising.** Brewers and beer distributors spend many millions of dollars every year promoting this message: If you want to have fun, have a drink. Young people may be especially responsive to such sales pitches.
- **Relationship issues.** Single, separated, or divorced men and women drink more and drink more often than married ones.
- **Childhood traumas.** Female alcoholics often report that they were physically or sexually abused as children or suffered great distress because of poverty or a parent's death. Individuals being treated for alcoholism are likely to have experienced sexual, physical, or emotional abuse as well as physical or emotional neglect.
- **Unemployment.** Individuals who lose their jobs, according to recent research, are at increased risk of alcohol use and misuse, including more daily consumption and more binge-drinking episodes.[3]

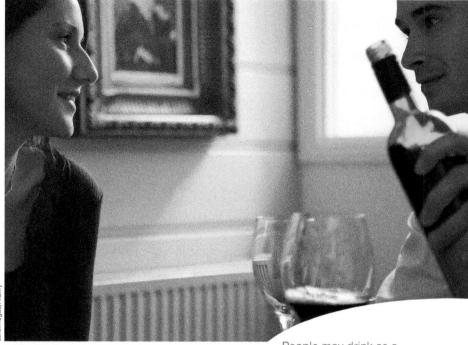

ableimages/Alamy

People may drink as a way to feel more at ease in social situations.

Individuals with drinking problems often turn to alcohol for other reasons, including

- **Psychological factors.** Both men and women may drink to compensate for feelings of inadequacy. Yet women who tend to ruminate or mull over bad feelings may find that alcohol increases this tendency and makes them feel more distressed.
- **Self-medication.** More so than men, some women feel it's permissible to use alcohol as if it were a medicine. As long as they're taking it for a reason, it seems acceptable to them.
- **Depression.** Women are more likely than men to be depressed prior to drinking and to suffer from both depression and a drinking problem at the same time.
- **Inherited susceptibility.** In both women and men, genetics accounts for 50 to 60 percent of a person's vulnerability to a serious drinking problem.
- **Long work hours.** According to an analysis of 36 studies, employees who work 55 hours or more a week are more likely than those working 40 hours or less to drink heavily—and thereby increase their risk of sleep problems, occupational injuries, depression, anxiety, cardiovascular disease, and alcohol-related medical conditions.[4]

✓**check-in** If you drink alcohol, when and why do you drink?

How Much Do Americans Drink?

On average the adult population consumes almost 100 calories per day from alcoholic beverages. However, on any given day, the majority of Americans—67 percent of men and 82 percent of women—do not drink any alcohol. Of those who do drink, 18 percent of men and 10 percent of women drink within the recommended amounts (two drinks for men and one for women). However, almost 20 percent of men and 6 percent of women consume more than 300 calories from alcoholic beverages, which is equivalent to two or more 12-ounce beers, more than 2½ glasses of wine, or more than 4.5 ounces of spirits.[5]

On average, men ages 20 to 39 consume the greatest number of calories—174 per day—from alcoholic beverages. Men of all ages consume more alcohol than women, with younger men consuming more than older men. A larger percentage of men than women drink beer; a larger percentage of women than men drink wine. There are no significant racial or ethnic differences in the average calories per day from alcoholic beverages.[6]

Drinking on Campus

Young adults are the most frequent users of alcohol in the United States. The highest proportion of heavy drinkers and individuals with diagnosable alcohol abuse disorders are 18 to 25 years old. College students consume more alcohol more often and more dangerously than nonstudents the same age. (See Snapshot: On Campus Now.)

According to the NIAAA,

- 60 percent of college students ages 18 to 22 report drinking alcohol in the last month.

- 40 percent engaged in binge drinking in the last month.

- 14 percent engaged in heavy drinking in the last month.[7]

Many health experts consider the abuse of alcohol the primary health concern for college students. Here are some reasons:

- 1,825 students between the ages of 18 and 24 die from alcohol-related unintentional injuries, including motor vehicle crashes.

- 696,000 students are assaulted by another student who has been drinking.

- 97,000 students experience alcohol-related sexual assault or date rape.

- About one in five students meet the diagnostic criteria for an alcohol use disorder (discussed later in this chapter).

- About one in four students report academic consequences from drinking, including missing class, falling behind on assignments, doing poorly on exams or papers, and getting lower grades overall.[8]

- Nearly 160,000 freshmen drop out of college after their first year for alcohol- or drug-related reasons, according to the Core Institute, which surveys drinking practices on campuses.

- Although the percentage of students who drink hasn't changed much over the years, drinking on campus has. At many schools, students' social lives revolve around parties, games, and bar crawls. More students drink simply to get drunk and drink a lot in each drinking episode.

- About one-third of students increase alcohol use and encounter more related problems throughout the college years, one-third do not change previous patterns, and one-third decrease drinking.

- More college women drink now than in the past, and they drink more than in the past. In the American College Health Association (ACHA) survey, 64 percent of female students reported drinking four drinks or less the last time they partied or socialized; 36 percent drank five or more.[9] College women who drink are at greatly increased risk of unwanted sexual activity. In one study more than one in five reported some type of sexual assault.

- Binge drinking (discussed later in this chapter) has been linked with lower grades, poorer performance on memory tests, and higher levels of both depression and anxiety.

- College men drink more, more often, and more intensely than college women. They report consuming almost six drinks the last time they partied or socialized; 29 percent drank six or more.[10]

- Caucasians drink more than African or Asian Americans.

- Female Hispanic students are more likely to report alcohol use than males.[11]

- Fraternity and sorority members, athletes, and vigorous exercisers use more alcohol more often than other students.

SNAPSHOT: ON CAMPUS NOW

📷 Student Drinking

Alcohol Consumption		Percent (%)					
		Actual Use			Perceived Use		
	Percent (%)	Male	Female	Total	Male	Female	Total
Never used		20.9	19.5	20.1	4.2	2.5	3.2
Used, but not in the last 30 days		12.3	13.5	13.1	2.3	1.6	1.8
Used 1–9 days		47.5	52.9	50.8	41.6	35.5	37.6
Used 10–29 days		17.6	13.5	14.9	40.3	46.5	44.2
Used all 30 days		1.7	0.6	1.0	11.7	13.9	13.2
Any use within the last 30 days		66.8	67.0	66.8	93.5	95.9	94.9

As the figures above show, most undergraduates over-estimate the number of students who drink—and drink frequently—and underestimate the number who don't drink often or at all. How do your perceptions and actual behavior compare? What role does alcohol play in your life? Describe its impact on you, your choices, and your behavior in your online journal.

Source: American College Health Association, *American College Health Association-National College Health Assessment II: Reference Group Executive Summary Spring 2014*. Hanover, MD: American College Health Association, 2014.

• The students who drink the least are those attending two-year institutions, religious schools, commuter schools, and historically black colleges and universities. (See "Health on a Budget" for ways to drink less.)

✓**check-in** How widespread is drinking on your campus?

Why Students Don't Drink

According to the American College Health Association, 20 percent of students report never using alcohol. African American students are more likely than white undergraduates to abstain and to report never having had an alcoholic drink or not having a drink in the past 30 days. They also drink less frequently and consume fewer drinks per occasion than whites.

Students who don't drink give various reasons for their choice, including these:

• Under age 21

• No access to alcohol

• Parental or peer pressure

• Cost

• Dislike for the taste

• Spiritual and religious values. In a recent study of more than 1,100 undergraduates, students who placed high importance on religion consumed less alcohol even when in an environment where drinking was the norm.[12]

✓**check-in** Do you choose not to drink? If so, why?

Why Students Drink

Undergraduates have always turned to alcohol for the same reasons. Away from home, often for the first time, many are excited by and apprehensive about their newfound independence. Social motives are the most common reason for drinking—and for problem drinking—on campus.[13] When new pressures seem overwhelming, when they feel awkward or insecure, when they just want to let loose and have a good time, they reach for a drink.

The following list summarizes key influences on student drinking.

• **Social norms.** Compared with other factors, such as race, gender, year in school, and fraternity/sorority membership, social norms (discussed in Chapter 1) have the strongest association with how much college students drink. Students' perceptions of how much their peers, particularly those closest to them, drink have more influence on their own drinking than do parents or resident advisors. However, students generally overestimate how much and how often their classmates drink.

• **Coping.** Students turn to alcohol to cope with everyday problems and personal issues. Those with symptoms of depression who lack skills to cope with daily problems, particularly

Drink Less, Save More

Yet another good reason to control how much you drink is economic. The less spending money that college students have, the less they drink—and the less likely they are to get drunk and to suffer alcohol-related negative consequences. Here are some simple ways to spend less on alcohol:

- **Pace yourself.** Start with a soft drink and have a non-alcoholic drink every second or third drink.

- **Stay busy.** You will drink less if you play pool or dance rather than just sit and drink.

- **Try low-alcohol alternatives,** such as light beers and low- or no-alcohol wines.

- **Have alcohol-free days.** Don't drink at all at least two days a week.

- **Drink slowly.** Take sips and not gulps. Put your glass down between sips.

- **Avoid salty snacks.** Salty foods like chips or nuts make you thirsty, and then you drink more.

- **Have one drink at a time.** Don't let people top up your drinks. It makes it harder to keep track of how much alcohol you're consuming.

males, are more likely to drink than others, as are those who feel anxious, angry, hostile, nervous, guilty, or ashamed.[14]

- **Party schools.** Colleges and universities in the Northeast, those with a strong Greek system, and those where athletics predominate have higher drinking rates than others. Students who never join or who drop out of a fraternity or sorority report less risky drinking behavior than those who go Greek.

- **Living arrangements.** Drinking rates are highest among students living in fraternity and sorority houses, followed by those in on-campus housing (dormitories, residence halls) and off-campus apartments or houses. Study-abroad students are at risk for increased and problematic drinking behavior.[15] Undergraduates living at home with their families drink the least.

- **Weekends and special occasions.** Students drink more heavily on weekends and holidays than on typical weekdays. The highest drinking days vary on different campuses but include Halloween, New Year's Eve, Mardi Gras, and St. Patrick's Day.[16] Alcohol consumption typically soars on big-game days for various sports, when a significant number of students engage in "extreme ritualistic alcohol consumption," defined as consuming 10 or more drinks on the same day for a male and 8 or more for a female.

- **Spring break.** Annual excursions devoted to nonstop partying with thousands of other young people have become notorious for extreme drinking.[17] Frequent consequences include intoxication, alcohol poisoning, accidents, and risky sexual behavior (see Chapter 8). Students who overestimate

their peers' alcohol consumption during spring break drink more; those traveling with friends engage in unprotected sex more often than those with their romantic partners.[18]

- **Participation in sports.** College athletes, who drink more often and more heavily than nonathletes, may be at greater risk because many are younger than 21, belong to Greek organizations, have lower GPAs, or spend more time socializing than other students. Intramural athletes drink more, binge-drink more often, and experience more alcohol-related consequences than varsity or club athletes or nonathletes.[19]

- **Parental attitudes.** Students who believe that their parents approve of drinking are more likely to drink and to report having a drinking-related problem. Those whose parents communicate clear zero-tolerance messages about alcohol drink less, drink less frequently, and use more strategies to avoid serious hazards related to drinking.[20]

- **First-year transition.** Some students who drank less in high school than classmates who weren't headed for college start drinking, and drinking heavily, in college—often during their first six weeks on campus and peaking during school breaks. Those who report poor adjustment to college are more likely to engage in risky drinking behaviors and suffer their consequences. Alcohol consumption declines over the course of an undergraduate education, but a substantial number of students continue to drink heavily through their third year.

- **Victimization.** Students who have experienced recent sexual victimization, are at increased risk of drinking and particularly binge drinking. Cyberbullying also increases problem drinking—but more so for the bullies than the bullied.[21] Risky drinking, including bingeing, in itself increases the risk of sexual victimization.[22]

- **Trauma and abuse.** Students who experienced childhood abuse[23] or recent trauma[24] may self-medicate with alcohol, which may make them more susceptible to alcohol-related problems.

- **Discrimination.** In a study of undergraduates at a historically African American college, male students (but not females) who reported higher lifetime discrimination and a negative mood engaged in more nonsocial drinking. The reason, researchers theorize, may be "the cumulative impact of racial discrimination."[25]

- **Alcohol-related cues.** In one recent study, some male students drank more while watching movies that portray actors drinking.[26] Taking a drink every time television or movie actors curse or say certain phrases—a popular viewing game—also boosts students' alcohol consumption.

High-Risk Drinking on Campus

The most common types of undergraduate high-risk drinking are binge-drinking, bingeing combined with disordered eating, predrinking, underage drinking, and consumption of caffeinated alcoholic beverages.

Binge Drinking According to the National Institute of Alcohol Abuse and Alcoholism, a **binge** is a pattern of drinking alcohol that brings blood-alcohol concentration (BAC) (discussed later in this chapter) to 0.08 gram-percent or above. For a typical adult man, this pattern corresponds to consuming five or more drinks in about two hours; for a woman, four or more drinks.

Colleges vary widely in their binge-drinking rates—from 1 percent to more than 70 percent. The federal government has set a goal of cutting in half the current binge-drinking rate of 40 percent among college students for *Healthy People 2020*.

√**check-in** Is binge-drinking common on your campus?

Who Binge-Drinks in College? An estimated 4 in 10 college students drink at binge levels or greater. They consume 91 percent of all alcohol that undergraduates report drinking. (See Table 13.1.) Hundreds of studies have created a portrait of who binge drinkers are and how they differ from others:

- Binge drinkers are more likely to be male than female, although one in three women—up from one in four—reports binge-drinking.[27]

- They are more likely to be white than any other ethnic or racial group. (African American women are least likely to be binge drinkers.)

- Most are under age 24.

- More binge drinkers are enrolled in four-year colleges than in two-year ones.

- Binge drinkers tend to be residents of states with fewer alcohol control policies.

- Binge drinkers tend to be involved in athletics and socialize frequently.

- They tend to be in a fraternity or sorority.

- They are dissatisfied with their bodies, not prone to exercise, eat poorly, and go on unhealthy diets.

- Binge drinkers tend to be behind in schoolwork or miss class.

- They are often users of other substances, including nicotine, marijuana, cocaine, and LSD.

TABLE 13.1 Binge Drinking on Campus

Reported number of drinks consumed the last time students "partied" or socialized. Only students reporting one or more drinks were included.

Number of Drinks*	Percent (%)	Male	Female	Total
4 or fewer		44.2	64.0	57.2
5		10.4	12.5	11.7
6		9.6	8.8	9.0
7 or more		35.8	14.7	22.0

Reported number of times college students consumed five or more drinks in a sitting within the last two weeks:

	Percent (%)	Male	Female	Total
N/A don't drink		22.1	20.7	21.3
None		35.5	48.7	44.1
1–2 times		25.7	22.1	23.3
3–5 times		13.1	7.3	9.3
6 or more times		3.6	1.1	2.0

Source: American College Health Association, *American College Health Association-National College Health Assessment II: Reference Group Executive Summary Spring 2014.* Hanover MD: American College Health Association, 2014.

binge For a man, having five or more alcoholic drinks at a single sitting; for a woman, having four drinks or more at a single sitting.

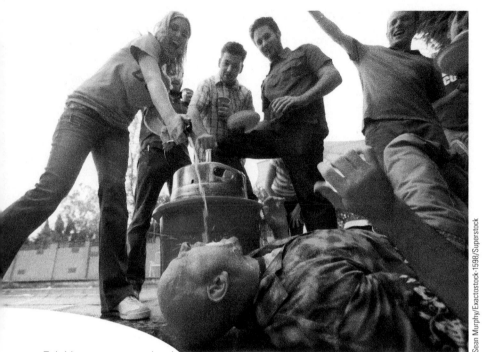
Drinking games can lead to extreme intoxication, alcohol-related injuries, and alcohol poisoning.

- **Early access to alcohol.** Places with lower drinking ages are associated with more frequent binge episodes.[28]

- **Campus environment.** Students tend to binge-drink at the beginning of the school year and then cut back as the semester progresses and academic demands increase. Binge drinking also peaks following exam times, during home football weekends, and during spring break.

- **Drinking games.** Two-thirds of college students engage in drinking games—such as beer pong or "Beirut"—that involve binge drinking. Although these games vary in many ways, all share a common theme: becoming intoxicated in a short period of time. Men are more likely to participate than women and to consume larger amounts of alcohol, often six drinks or more.[29] Drinking game players who don't monitor or regulate how much they're drinking are at risk of extreme intoxication, alcohol-related injuries, and alcohol poisoning.

✓**check-in** Have you ever played drinking games?

- Binge drinkers are likely to be injured or hurt, to engage in unplanned or unprotected sexual activity, or to get in trouble with campus police.

Why Students Binge-Drink Young people who came from, socialized within, or were exposed to "wet" environments—settings in which alcohol is cheap and accessible and drinking is prevalent—are most likely to engage in binge drinking. Students who report drinking at least once a month during their final year of high school are more likely to binge-drink in college than those who drank less frequently in high school.

The factors that most influence students to binge-drink are the following:

- **Low price for alcohol.** Beer, which is cheap and easy to obtain, is the beverage of choice among binge drinkers.

- **Easy access to alcohol.** In one study, the density of alcohol outlets (such as bars) near campus affected the drinking of students.

- **Proximity to other binge drinkers.** Students who attend a school or live in a residence with many binge drinkers tend to become binge drinkers themselves.

- **Peer pressure.** Those who believe that close friends are likely to binge end up bingeing themselves.

- **Family attitudes.** Students whose parents who drank or did not disapprove of their children drinking are more likely to binge.

predrinking Consuming alcoholic beverages, usually with friends, before going out to bars or parties; also called pregaming, preloading, or front-loading.

Binge Drinking and Disordered Eating
The combination of two risky behaviors—disordered eating and heavy drinking—poses special dangers to students. As discussed in Chapter 7, disordered eating can range from excessive concern about weight to binge eating to extreme weight-control methods, such as purging. White women report more binge drinking, alcohol-related problems, disordered eating, and symptoms of anorexia nervosa or bulimia nervosa than nonwhite female students.[30] In women, the combination of these behaviors increases the risk of many negative consequences, including blackouts, unintended sexual activity, and forced sexual intercourse.

Some students restrict calories from food prior to planned drinking—some to avoid weight gain and others to enhance the effects of alcohol. The popular media have created the term "drunk-orexia" to describe this risky behavior, but it is not an official psychiatric term.

Predrinking/Pregaming Drinking before going out has become increasingly common on college campuses, where **predrinking** (also called prepartying, prefunking, pregaming, preloading, or front-loading) is announced and celebrated in text messages, e-mails, blogs, YouTube videos, and Facebook posts.

In various studies, a greater proportion of white than Hispanic/Latino, African American, and Pacific Islander American students reported prepartying in the previous month. Within both genders and all ethnic groups, prepartyers consumed more drinks per week and experienced a higher number of alcohol-related consequences than non-prepartyers.[31]

Predrinkers consistently report much higher alcohol consumption during the evening and more negative consequences, such as getting into fights, being arrested, or being referred to a university's mandatory alcohol intervention program.

Why Is Predrinking Popular?
College students predrink for a variety of reasons, including the following:

- **Economy.** Many say they want to avoid paying for expensive drinks at a bar, although most end up drinking at least as much when they're out as they do when they don't predrink.

- **Intoxication.** A growing number of students seem to want to get drunk as quickly as possible or to do so early in case alcohol isn't available later.

- **Socializing.** Predrinking gives students a chance to chat with their friends, which often isn't possible in noisy, crowded clubs or bars.

- **Hooking up with a partner for the evening.**

- **Anxiety reduction.** By drinking before meeting strangers, students say they feel less shy or self-conscious.

- **Group bonding.** Young men may use predrinking as what one researcher calls "a collective ritual of confidence building to prepare themselves for subsequent interactions with the opposite sex."

The Perils of Predrinking
When students get together to drink before a game or a night out, they usually consume large quantities of alcohol quite rapidly. In part that's because they're drinking in places without restraints on how much they can drink. Various studies have shown that students drink more and have higher blood-alcohol concentrations on days when they predrink. They also are at greater risk of blackouts, passing out, hangovers, and alcohol poisoning.

In addition to drinking more alcohol, predrinkers are more likely to use other drugs, such as marijuana and cocaine. The combined effects of these substances further increase the risks of injury, violence, or victimization.

✓**check-in** Have you ever engaged in predrinking?

Underage Drinking on Campus
About one in four people between ages 12 and 20 report drinking alcohol in the last month.[32]

Students under age 21 drink less often than older students but tend to drink more heavily and to experience more negative alcohol-related consequences. More underage students report drinking "to get drunk" and drinking at binge levels when they consumed alcohol.

Underage college students are most likely to drink if they can easily obtain cheap alcohol, especially beer. They tend to drink in private settings, such as dorms and fraternity parties, and to experience negative drinking-related consequences, such as doing something they regretted, forgetting where they were or what they did, causing property damage, getting into trouble with police, and being hurt or injured. The drinking behavior of underage students also depends on their living arrangements. Those in controlled settings, such as their parents' home or a substance-free dorm, are less likely to binge-drink. Students living in fraternities or sororities are most likely to binge-drink, regardless of age.

A number of university chancellors and presidents have signed a public statement calling for informed, dispassionate discussion of the *Amethyst Initiative*, a proposal that supports a series of educational and policy-level efforts to enable 18- to 20-year-old adults to purchase, possess, and consume alcoholic beverages at their own discretion. Opponents note that the minimum legal drinking age of 21 has reduced alcohol-related deaths, injuries, and traffic crashes.

According to recent research, underage drinkers are at increased risk because various factors inhibit their ability to drink responsibly, including less self-efficacy and lower intentions to engage in responsible drinking behaviors.[33]

✓**check-in** What do you think the minimum legal drinking age should be?

Alcohol Mixed with Energy Drinks (AmED)
AmED (alcohol mixed with energy drinks) in the medical literature—refers to any combination of alcohol with caffeine and other stimulants.

Premixed beverages, often malt- or distilled spirits–based, usually have a higher alcohol content (5 to 12 percent) than beer (4 to 5 percent). Some states classify them as liquor, thereby limiting the locations where they can be sold.

AmED (alcohol mixed with energy drinks) Any combination of alcohol with caffeine and other stimulants.

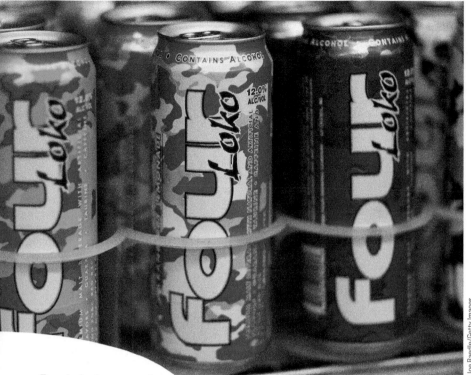

Four Loko is among the energy drinks combining caffeine and alcohol that have been banned at certain colleges.

According to a review of more than 60 studies of energy drinks mixed with alcohol on campus, AmED

- Lead to more alcohol consumption and more alcohol-related harm[34]
- Increase stimulation and alertness and offset fatigue from drinking
- Boost the desire to keep drinking
- Do not change blood alcohol concentration (BAC)
- Do not reverse alcohol-induced impairment of reaction time, coordination, and focused attention[35]

Like the energy drinks discussed in Chapters 6 and 12, AmED have surged in popularity among teens and young adults. The FDA has banned some premixed AmED, but young people continue to combine energy drinks like Red Bull with vodka or other forms of alcohol.

AmED users are most likely to be younger men who score higher on measures of risk-taking propensity.[36] In a recent study of college students, most had neutral or negative views of AmED. The most frequent users had positive expectations, such as being able to party longer.[37]

The caffeine in these drinks may mask the depressant effects of alcohol, but it has no effect on the liver's metabolism of alcohol and thus does not reduce blood-alcohol concentrations or reduce alcohol-related risks.[38]

Various studies have linked AmED use to risky behaviors on campus, including these:

- Unprotected sex and sex under the influence of drugs or alcohol[39]
- More high-risk drinking behaviors, such as consuming large amounts of alcohol[40]
- Increased danger of becoming alcohol dependent
- Double the likelihood of being hurt or injured compared with those who don't consume AmED

✓**check-in** Have you ever had an alcoholic energy drink?

Defensive Drinking In the most recent ACHA survey, the vast majority of students— 97.5 percent—report using at least one behavioral strategy to control their drinking and prevent alcohol-related problems.[41] The most popular strategies are the following:

- Staying with the same group of friends throughout an event
- Choosing a designated driver
- Eating before and/or while drinking
- Sticking with only one form of alcohol
- Deciding in advance not to exceed a set number of drinks

The more that students rely on protective behavioral strategies, the less alcohol they consume and the fewer alcohol-related problems they encounter. (For additional strategies, see Health on a Budget on p. 390.)

✓**check-in** What, if any, defensive strategies have you used to control your drinking?

Why Students Stop Drinking

Only 1 percent of students ages 18 to 24 receive treatment for alcohol or drug abuse. Nonetheless, as many as 22 percent of alcohol-abusing college students "spontaneously" reduce their drinking as they progress through college. Unlike older adults, who often hit bottom before they change their drinking behaviors, many college students go through a gradual process of reduced drinking. Researchers refer to this behavioral change as early cessation, natural reduction, natural recovery, or spontaneous recovery.

As with other behavioral changes, individuals must be ready to change their drinking patterns.

In one study, students who binged frequently, who experienced more alcohol-related interpersonal and academic problems, who did not also use marijuana, and who lived in a residence hall where binge drinking was the norm showed a greater readiness to change.

Why do students say they stop heavy drinking? Here are some common responses:

- "It was just getting old."
- Vomiting.
- Urinating in hallways.
- Being physically fondled.
- Sexual assault.
- Violence.
- Accidents.
- Injuries.
- Unprotected intercourse.
- Emergency room visits.
- Vicarious experiences, such as a roommate's arrest for driving under the influence or a sorority sister's date rape.

Psychologists have found that students "mature out" of heavy drinking as they become less impulsive and develop healthier coping behaviors. Several interventions have proven effective in reducing alcohol consumption and alcohol-related problems on college campuses.[42] They include getting personalized feedback about drinking habits, learning moderation strategies, challenging expectations, identifying risky situations, and setting goals for responsible drinking.[43]

√**check-in** Has your attitude toward drinking changed since you entered college?

Alcohol-Related Problems on Campus

As many as 10 to 30 percent of college students experience some negative consequences of drinking. In the ACHA's National College Health Assessment, 36.5 percent of students who drank did something they later regretted; 32.3 percent forgot who they were with or what they did. Men were more likely than women to injure themselves, have unprotected sex, or physically injure another person. Women were more likely to have someone use force or threat of force to have sex with them. (See Table 13.2.) Students who drink heavily also are much more likely to abuse prescription drugs (see Chapter 12).

TABLE 13.2 Consequences of Drinking

College students who drank alcohol reported experiencing the following in the past 12 months when drinking alcohol:

Percent (%)	Male	Female	Total
Did something you later regretted	36.5	36.6	36.5
Forgot where you were or what you did	34.0	31.5	32.3
Got in trouble with the police	4.2	2.3	3.0
Someone had sex with you without your consent	1.2	2.6	2.1
Had sex with someone without their consent	0.6	0.5	0.6
Had unprotected sex	22.3	19.4	20.4
Physically injured yourself	16.2	14.2	14.9
Physically injured another person	2.9	1.3	2.5
Seriously considered suicide	2.6	2.4	2.5
Reported one or more of the above	55.3	52.5	53.4

*Students responding "N/A, don't drink." were excluded from this analysis.
Source: American College Health Association. *American College Health Association-National College Health Assessment II: Reference Group Executive Summary Spring 2014.* Hanover, MD: American College Health Association, 2014.

Consequences of Drinking Among the other problems linked to drinking are

- **Atypical behavior.** Under the influence of alcohol, students behave in ways they normally wouldn't. Some sext or post comments and photos they later regret on social media.[44] Male heavy drinkers are more prone to behave in ways that are considered "antisocial," or contrary to the standards of our society, such as forcing or trying to force unwanted sexual contact, driving drunk, exposing themselves, or having sex with a stranger.

- **Academic problems.** The more that students drink, the more likely they are to fall behind in schoolwork, miss classes, have lower GPAs, and face suspensions. In general, students with an A average have 3 to 4 drinks per week, while students with D or F averages drink almost 10 drinks a week. (See Figure 13.1.)

- **Risky sexual behavior.** About one in five college students reports engaging in unplanned sexual activity, including having sex with someone they just met and having unprotected sex.

- **Sexual assault.** In a recent survey, almost 20 percent of undergraduate women reported some type of completed sexual assault since entering college. Most occurred after women voluntarily consumed alcohol; a few occurred after they were unknowingly given a drug in their drinks.

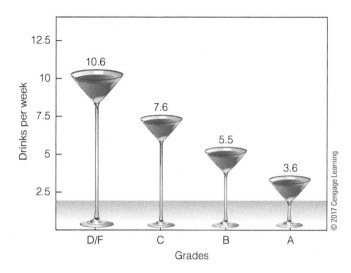

FIGURE 13.1 Alcohol and Academic Success

- **Intimate partner violence.** Each year an estimated 80 percent of college men perpetrate psychological aggression; 20 to 30 percent, physical aggression; and 15 to 20 percent, sexual aggression against a dating partner. Heavy drinking increases the likelihood of all three forms, especially physical violence.[45] Alcohol increases the likelihood that women will be either perpetrators or victims of partner aggression.[46]

- **Unintentional injury.** More than 30 percent of college drinkers have been injured as a result of drinking. They also are more likely to cause injury to others, to have a car accident, and to suffer burns or a fall serious enough to require medical attention. The costs of emergency treatment for alcohol-related injuries can be more than half a million dollars a year at schools with 40,000 or more students.

- **Consequences beyond college.** Alcohol-related convictions, including carrying a false I.D. or driving under the influence of alcohol, remain on an individual's criminal record and could affect a student's graduate school and professional opportunities.

- **Illness and death.** Many students suffer short-term health consequences of drinking, such as headaches and hangovers. Heavy alcohol use in college students is associated with immunological problems and digestive and upper respiratory disorders. Even moderate drinking can contribute to infertility in women. Longer-term consequences of heavy drinking include liver disease, stroke, heart disease, and certain types of cancer. About 300,000 of today's college students will eventually die from alcohol-related causes,

including drunk-driving accidents, cirrhosis of the liver, various cancers, and heart disease.

✓**check-in** Have you experienced any alcohol-related problems on campus?

Drinking and Driving Drunk driving is the most frequently committed crime in the United States. In the ACHA survey, 21.2 percent of students reported driving after having had any alcohol; 2.2 percent reported driving after five or more drinks.[47] Traditional-age undergraduates typically are more likely to drink and drive as they get older, with the biggest jump between ages 21 and 23.

Alcohol impairs driving-related skills regardless of the age of the driver or the time of day it is consumed. However, younger students who drink and drive are at greatest risk:

- Underage drinkers are more likely to drive after drinking, to ride with intoxicated drivers, and to be injured after drinking—at least in part because they believe that people can drive safely and legally after drinking.

- More young women than ever before are driving drunk and getting into fatal car accidents. More young women than men involved in deadly crashes had high blood-alcohol levels, according to a recent analysis of data from the National Highway Traffic Safety Administration.

- Of the 5,000 alcohol-related deaths among 18- to 24-year-olds, 80 percent were caused by alcohol-related traffic accidents. A young person dies in an alcohol-related traffic crash an average of once every three hours.

Since states began setting the legal drinking age at 21, the National Highway Traffic Safety Administration estimates that more than 26,000 lives have been saved. Safety groups, such as MADD (Mothers Against Drunk Driving) and SADD (Students Against Destructive Decisions) attribute the decline in alcohol-related deaths to enforcement tools like sobriety checkpoints and to the states' adoption of a uniform drunken-driving standard of a BAC of 0.08 percent. Since courts have held establishments that serve alcohol liable for the consequences of allowing drunk customers to drive, many bars and restaurants have joined the campaign against drunk driving.

✓**check-in** Do you always designate a driver who won't drink at all? Do you never get behind the wheel if you've had more than two drinks within two hours? Do you never allow intoxicated friends to drive home?

Secondhand Drinking Problems Heavy alcohol use can endanger both drinkers and others. Secondhand problems caused by other's alcohol use include

- Loss of sleep

- Interruption of studies

- Assaults

- Vandalism

- Unwanted sexual advances

Students living on campuses with high rates of binge drinking are two or more times as likely to experience these secondhand effects as those living on campuses with low rates. In one study, nearly three-quarters of campus rapes happened when the victims were so intoxicated that they were unable to consent or refuse.

How Schools Are Sobering Up

As alcohol-related deaths, assaults, and rapes have gained greater attention, colleges and universities have expanded alcohol education programs and toughened alcohol policies. Some schools have banned hard liquor on campus or alcohol at any university-sponsored events.

Many schools require incoming students to attend an alcohol awareness class, watch educational videos, or take online quizzes about appropriate alcohol use. These one-time interventions do work—at least temporarily. In one recent study, 8 in 10 students drank less a month after participating in a program, but the effects tended to wear off as the school year progressed. The courses were especially effective for women and younger, inexperienced drinkers, but for about 10 percent of the students—mostly men involved in Greek life—the educational classes had no impact on drinking behavior.[48]

University alcohol policies include campus alcohol bans, lack of alcohol at university-sponsored events, prohibition of beer kegs, limits on the maximum number of drinks served per student, and dry sorority and fraternity initiation activities. Studies suggest that students who attend schools that ban alcohol are less likely to engage in heavy binge drinking, more likely to abstain from using alcohol, and less likely to experience the secondhand effects of drinking.

Students who violate campus alcohol policies or who engage in underage drinking often must go through mandated programs, such as the following:

- Brief motivational interventions (BMIs), in which specially trained counselors use a nonjudgmental, supportive approach to help

boost students' ability to change their drinking behavior[49]

- Mindfulness training (discussed in Chapter 4), which has proven effective in reducing binge episodes and harmful alcohol-related consequences[50]

- Executive function training, which builds students' planning and organizational skills[51]

- Computerized interventions, which have helped high-risk or "hazardous" drinkers reduce the frequency and quantity of their alcohol use[52]

√**check-in Do** you know your school's alcohol policies?

Understanding Alcohol

Pure alcohol is a colorless liquid obtained through the fermentation of a liquid containing sugar. **Ethyl alcohol**, or *ethanol*, is the type of alcohol in alcoholic beverages.

Hospitals have reported cases of alcohol poisoning, some fatal, after consumption of hand sanitizers, such as Purell, which contain 60 percent ethyl alcohol. Some people drink it straight as a "Purell shot," and others use salt to separate the ethyl alcohol from the glycerin in the gel.[53] Another type—methyl, or wood, alcohol—is a poison that should never be drunk.

Any liquid containing 0.5 to 80 percent ethyl alcohol by volume is an alcoholic beverage. However, different drinks contain different amounts of alcohol. The types of alcohol consumed vary around the world. Beer accounts for most of the alcohol consumed in the United States. People in southern European countries such as France, Spain, Italy, and Portugal prefer wine.

Do you know what a "drink" is? Most students—particularly freshmen, sophomores, and women—don't. In one experiment undergraduates defined a "drink" as one serving, regardless of how big it was or how much alcohol it contained. In fact, one standard drink can be any of the following:

- **One bottle or can** (12 ounces) of beer, which is 5 percent alcohol

- **One glass** (4 or 5 ounces) of table wine, such as burgundy, which is 12 percent alcohol

- **One small glass** (2½ ounces) of fortified wine, which is 20 percent alcohol

ethyl alcohol The intoxicating agent in alcoholic beverages; also called ethanol.

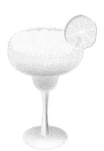

Margarita:

1 1/2 oz. tequila (80 proof) = 1.5 oz. × 40 percent alcohol = 0.6 oz. alcohol

3/4 oz. triple sec (60 proof) = 0.75 oz. × 30 percent alcohol = 0.23 oz. alcohol

Splash of sour mix   0.83 oz. alcohol = 1 1/2 drinks

Dash of lime juice

Salt for the rim

Malt liquor:

16 oz. × 6.4 percent alcohol = 1 oz. alcohol = 2 drinks

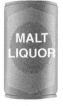

MALT LIQUOR

FIGURE 13.2 How Many Standard Drinks Are You Drinking?

- **One shot** (1 ounce) of distilled spirits (such as whiskey, vodka, or rum), which is 50 percent alcohol

All of these drinks contain close to the same amount of alcohol—that is, if the number of ounces in each drink is multiplied by the percentage of alcohol, each drink contains the equivalent of approximately ½ ounce of 100 percent ethyl alcohol.

Drinks at college parties vary greatly in their alcoholic content. It may be impossible for students to monitor their alcohol intake simply by counting the number of drinks they consume. In one study, when asked to pour a liquid into cups of various sizes to reflect what they perceived to be one beer, one shot, or the amount of liquor in one mixed drink, undergraduates overpoured beer by 25 percent, shots by 26 percent, and mixed drinks by 80 percent.

The words *bottle* and *glass* also can be deceiving:

- Drinking a 16-ounce bottle of malt liquor, which is 6.4 percent alcohol, is not the same as drinking a 12-ounce glass of light beer (3.2 percent alcohol): The malt liquor contains 1 ounce of alcohol and is the equivalent of two drinks.

- Two bottles of high-alcohol wines (such as Cisco), packaged to resemble much less powerful wine coolers, can lead to alcohol poisoning, especially in those who weigh less than 150 pounds.

With distilled spirits (such as bourbon, scotch, vodka, gin, and rum), alcohol content is expressed in terms of **proof**, a number that is twice the percentage of alcohol—for example, 100-proof bourbon is 50 percent alcohol, and 80-proof gin is 40 percent alcohol. Many mixed drinks are equivalent to one and a half or two standard drinks; for instance, see the margarita in Figure 13.2.

In a recent study, 18 percent of college students overestimated and 10 percent underestimated their alcohol consumption. Students in both groups were more likely to experience more negative consequences of drinking than those who made accurate estimations.[54]

✓**check-in** Do you think you can estimate how much you've drunk?

Blood-Alcohol Concentration

The amount of alcohol in your blood at any given time is your **blood-alcohol concentration (BAC)**. It is expressed in terms of the percentage of alcohol in the blood and is often measured from breath or urine samples.

Law enforcement officers use BAC to determine whether a driver is legally drunk. All the states have followed the recommendation of the federal Department of Transportation to set 0.08 percent—the BAC that a 150-pound man would have after consuming about three mixed drinks within an hour—as the threshold at which a person can be cited for drunk driving (Figure 13.3).

Using a formula for blood-alcohol concentration developed by highway transportation officials, researchers calculate that when college students drink, their typical BAC is 0.079, dangerously close to the legal limit.

A BAC of 0.05 percent indicates approximately 5 parts alcohol to 10,000 parts other blood components. Most people reach this level after consuming one or two drinks and experience all the positive sensations of drinking—relaxation, euphoria, and well-being—without feeling intoxicated. If they continue to drink past the 0.05 percent BAC level, they start feeling worse rather than better, gradually losing control of speech, balance,

proof The alcoholic strength of a distilled spirit, expressed as twice the percentage of alcohol present.

blood-alcohol concentration (BAC) The amount of alcohol in the blood, expressed as a percentage.

FIGURE 13.3 Alcohol Impairment
Chart

Source: Adapted from data supplied by the Pennsylvania
Liquor Control Board.

Men	Approximate blood alcohol percentage								
	Body weight in pounds								
Drinks	100	120	140	160	180	200	220	240	
0	.00	.00	.00	.00	.00	.00	.00	.00	Only safe driving limit
1	.04	.03	.03	.02	.02	.02	.02	.02	Impairment begins
2	.08	.06	.05	.05	.04	.04	.03	.03	Driving skills significantly affected
3	.11	.09	.08	.07	.06	.06	.05	.05	
4	.15	.12	.11	.09	.08	.08	.07	.06	Possible criminal penalties
5	.19	.16	.13	.12	.11	.09	.09	.08	
6	.23	.19	.16	.14	.13	.11	.10	.09	
7	.26	.22	.19	.16	.15	.13	.12	.11	
8	.30	.25	.21	.19	.17	.15	.14	.13	Legally intoxicated
9	.34	.28	.24	.21	.19	.17	.15	.14	Criminal penalties
10	.38	.31	.27	.23	.21	.19	.17	.16	

Subtract 0.01 percent for each 40 minutes of drinking.
One drink is 1.25 oz. of 80 proof liquor, 12 oz. of beer, or 5 oz. of table wine.

Women	Approximate blood alcohol percentage									
	Body weight in pounds									
Drinks	90	100	120	140	160	180	200	220	240	
0	.00	.00	.00	.00	.00	.00	.00	.00	.00	Only safe driving limit
1	.05	.05	.04	.03	.03	.03	.02	.02	.02	Impairment begins
2	.10	.09	.08	.07	.06	.05	.05	.04	.04	Driving skills significantly affected
3	.15	.14	.11	.10	.09	.08	.07	.06	.06	
4	.20	.18	.15	.13	.11	.10	.09	.08	.08	Possible criminal penalties
5	.25	.23	.19	.16	.14	.13	.11	.10	.09	
6	.30	.27	.23	.19	.17	.15	.14	.12	.11	
7	.35	.32	.27	.23	.20	.18	.16	.14	.13	
8	.40	.36	.30	.26	.23	.20	.18	.17	.15	Legally intoxicated
9	.45	.41	.34	.29	.26	.23	.20	.19	.17	Criminal penalties
10	.51	.45	.38	.32	.28	.25	.23	.21	.19	

Subtract 0.01 percent for each 40 minutes of drinking.
One drink is 1.25 oz. of 80 proof liquor, 12 oz. of beer, or 5 oz. of table wine.

.01–.06 BAC	.06–.10 BAC	.11–.20 BAC	.21–.29 BAC	.30–.39 BAC	.40+ BAC
Relaxation, sense of well-being, loss of inhibition, lowered alertness Some impact on thought, judgment, coordination, concentration	Blunted feelings, disinhibition, extroversion, reduced sexual pleasure Impaired reflexes, reasoning, depth perception, distance acuity, peripheral vision, glare recovery	Emotional swings, anger, sadness, boisterous Impaired reaction time, gross motor control, staggering, slurred speech	Stupor, impaired sensations Severe motor impairment, memory blackouts	Not responsive, slowed heart rate, breathing, risk of death	Not responsive, death

and emotions. At a BAC of 0.2 percent, they may pass out. At a BAC of 0.3 percent, they could lapse into a coma; at 0.4 percent, they could die.

Many factors affect your BAC and response to alcohol, including the following:

- **How much and how quickly you drink.** The more alcohol you put into your body, the higher your BAC. If you chug drink after drink, your liver, which metabolizes about ½ ounce of alcohol an hour, won't be able to keep up—and your BAC will soar.

- **What you're drinking.** The stronger the drink, the faster and harder the alcohol hits. Straight shots of liquor and cocktails such as martinis get alcohol into your bloodstream faster than beer or table wine. Beer and wine not only contain lower concentrations of alcohol but also contain nonalcoholic substances that slow the rate of **absorption** (passage of the alcohol into your body tissues).

- **Mixers.** Carbon dioxide—whether in champagne, ginger ale, or a cola—whisks alcohol into your bloodstream. Also, the alcohol in warm drinks—such as a hot rum toddy or warmed sake—moves into your bloodstream more quickly than the alcohol in chilled wine or scotch on the rocks. Mixing alcohol with a diet soft drink causes higher alcohol concentrations, as measured by breath analysis, in both women and men, compared to mixing alcohol with a nondiet beverage.[55]

- **Your size.** If you're a large person (whether due to fat or to muscle), you'll get drunk more slowly than someone smaller who's drinking the same amount of alcohol at the same rate. Heavier individuals have a larger water volume, which dilutes the alcohol they drink.

- **Your gender.** Women have lower quantities of a stomach enzyme that neutralizes alcohol, so one drink for a woman has the impact that two drinks have for a man. Hormone levels also affect the impact of alcohol. Women are more sensitive to alcohol just before menstruation, and birth control pills and other forms of estrogen can intensify alcohol's impact.

- **Your age.** The same amount of alcohol produces higher BACs in older drinkers, who have lower volumes of body water to dilute the alcohol than younger drinkers do. People over 50 may become impaired after only one or two drinks.

- **Your race.** Many members of certain ethnic groups, including Asians and Native Americans, are unable to break down alcohol as quickly as Caucasians. This can result in higher BACs, as well as uncomfortable reactions, such as flushing and nausea, when they drink.

- **Other drugs.** Some common medications—including aspirin, acetaminophen (Tylenol), and ulcer medications—can cause blood-alcohol levels to increase more rapidly. Individuals taking these drugs can be over the legal limit for blood-alcohol concentration after as little as a single drink.

- **Family history of alcoholism.** Some children of alcoholics don't develop any of the usual behavioral symptoms that indicate someone is drinking too much. It's not known whether this behavior is genetically caused or is a result of growing up with an alcoholic.

- **Eating.** Food slows the absorption of alcohol by diluting it, by covering some of the membranes through which alcohol would be absorbed, and by prolonging the time the stomach takes to empty. Eating while consuming alcohol can reduce alcohol concentrations in breath by 20 to 57 percent.[56]

- **Expectations.** In various experiments, volunteers who believed they were given alcoholic beverages but were actually given nonalcoholic drinks acted as if they were guzzling the real thing and became more talkative, relaxed, and sexually stimulated.

- **Physical tolerance.** If you drink regularly, your brain becomes accustomed to a certain level of alcohol. You may be able to look and behave in a seemingly normal fashion, even though you drink as much as would normally intoxicate someone your size. However, your driving ability and judgment will still be impaired.

Once you develop tolerance, you may drink more to get the desired effects from alcohol. In some people, this can lead to abuse and alcoholism. On the other hand, after years of drinking, some people become exquisitely sensitive to alcohol. Such reverse tolerance means that they can become intoxicated after drinking only a small amount of alcohol.

✓**check-in** Which of the above factors may influence your BAC when you drink?

Moderate Alcohol Use

Many people describe themselves as "light" or "moderate" drinkers. However, these are not scientific terms. It is more precise to think in terms of the amount of alcohol that seems safe for most people. The federal government's Dietary Guidelines for Americans recommend no more than

absorption The passage of substances into or across membranes or tissues.

one drink a day for women and no more than two drinks a day for men. The American Heart Association (AHA) advises that alcohol account for no more than 15 percent of the total calories consumed by an individual every day, up to an absolute maximum of 1.75 ounces of alcohol a day—the equivalent of three beers, two mixed drinks, or three and a half glasses of wine.

Even "light" drinkers can experience alcohol-related problems. As a recent study showed, all drinkers are at risk for hangovers, memory loss, nausea, vomiting, passing out, and other alcohol-induced conditions when they drink greater amounts of alcohol. However, lighter drinkers experience such consequences with an average of three drinks, while heavier drinkers do so at higher doses.[57]

Moderate alcohol use has been linked with some positive health benefits, including lower risks of heart disease. In addition, middle-aged women who report light to moderate drinking are less likely to put on excessive weight over time. However, even occasional binges of four to five drinks a day can undo alcohol's positive effects.

The benefits of alcohol also are related to age. Below age 40 drinking at all levels is associated with an increased risk of death. Among people older than 50 or 60, moderate drinkers have the lowest risk of death.

Using a mathematical model, researchers have determined that alcohol-related problems occur at every drinking level, including just two drinks, but increase fivefold at three drinks and more gradually thereafter. Individuals who drink heavily have a higher mortality rate than those who have two or fewer drinks a day. However, the boundary between moderate and heavy drinking isn't the same for everyone. For some people, the upper limit of safety is zero: Once they start, they can't stop.

✓**check-in** If you drink, do you consider yourself a moderate drinker?

Alcohol Intoxication

If you drink too much, the immediate consequence is that you get drunk—or, more precisely, intoxicated. Alcohol intoxication, which can range from mild inebriation to loss of consciousness, is characterized by at least one of the following signs: slurred speech, poor coordination, unsteady gait, abnormal eye movements, impaired attention or memory, stupor, or coma.

Medical risks of intoxication include falls, hypothermia in cold climates, and increased risk of infections because of suppressed immune function. Time and a protective environment are the recommended treatments for alcohol intoxication.

✓**check-in** Do you know how best to help someone who's intoxicated?

To help an intoxicated person, follow these guidelines:

- Continually monitor him or her.
- If the person is "out," check breathing and wake the person often to be sure he or she is not unconscious.
- Do not force him or her to walk or move around.
- Do not allow him or her to drive a car or ride a bicycle.
- Do not give him or her food, liquid (including coffee), medicines, or drugs to "sober up."
- Do not give him or her a cold shower; the shock of the cold could cause unconsciousness.

Alcohol Poisoning

In large enough doses, alcohol can and does kill. According to the CDC, alcohol poisoning kills more than 2,200 Americans a year—an average of six people a day. About three in four are men, most often between the ages of 35 and 64.[58]

Alcohol depresses nerves that control involuntary actions, such as breathing and the gag reflex (which prevents choking). A fatal dose of alcohol will eventually suppress these functions. Because alcohol irritates the stomach, people who drink an excessive amount often vomit. If intoxication has led to a loss of consciousness, a drinker is in danger of choking on vomit, which can cause death by asphyxiation. Blood-alcohol concentration can rise even after a drinker has passed out because alcohol in the stomach and intestine continues to enter the bloodstream and circulate throughout the body.

The signs of alcohol poisoning include

- Mental confusion, stupor, coma, or inability to be roused
- Vomiting
- Seizures
- Slow breathing (fewer than eight breaths per minute)
- Irregular breathing (10 seconds or more between breaths)
- Hypothermia (low body temperature), bluish skin color, paleness

Alcohol poisoning is a medical emergency requiring immediate treatment. Black coffee, a cold shower, and letting a person "sleep it off" do not help. Without medical treatment, breathing slows, becomes irregular, or stops. The heart beats irregularly. Body temperature falls, which can cause cardiac arrest. Blood sugar plummets, which can lead to seizures. Vomiting creates severe dehydration, which can cause seizures, permanent brain damage, or death. Even if the victim lives, an alcohol overdose can result in irreversible brain damage.

✓**check-in** Do you know what to do if you suspect alcohol poisoning? Call 911 immediately for help.

The Impact of Alcohol on the Body

Unlike food or drugs in tablet form, alcohol is directly and quickly absorbed into the bloodstream through the stomach walls and upper intestine. The alcohol in a typical drink reaches the bloodstream in 15 minutes and rises to its peak concentration in about an hour. The bloodstream carries the alcohol to the liver, heart, and brain (Figure 13.4).

Most of the alcohol you drink can leave your body only after metabolism by the liver, which converts about 95 percent of the alcohol to carbon dioxide and water. The other 5 percent is excreted unchanged, mainly through urination, respiration, and perspiration.

Alcohol is a diuretic, a drug that speeds up the elimination of fluid from the body, so it's a good idea to drink water when you drink alcohol to maintain your fluid balance. Also, alcohol lowers body temperature, so you should never drink in an attempt to get or stay warm.

Digestive System

Alcohol first reaches the stomach, where it is partially broken down. The remaining alcohol is absorbed easily through the stomach tissue into the bloodstream. In the stomach, alcohol triggers the secretion of acids, which irritate the stomach

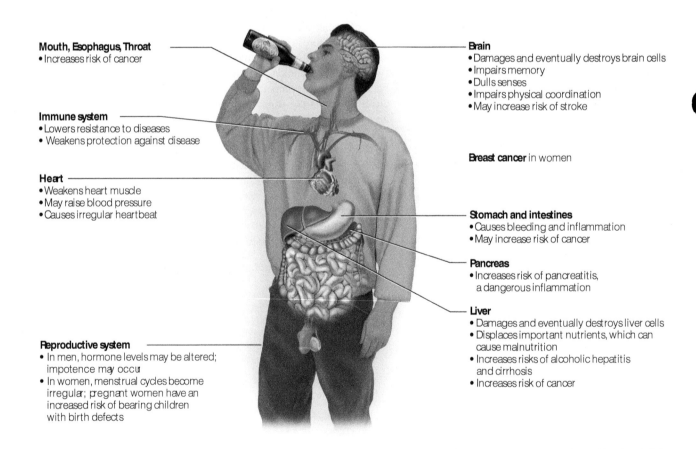

Mouth, Esophagus, Throat
• Increases risk of cancer

Immune system
• Lowers resistance to diseases
• Weakens protection against disease

Heart
• Weakens heart muscle
• May raise blood pressure
• Causes irregular heartbeat

Reproductive system
• In men, hormone levels may be altered; impotence may occur
• In women, menstrual cycles become irregular; pregnant women have an increased risk of bearing children with birth defects

Brain
• Damages and eventually destroys brain cells
• Impairs memory
• Dulls senses
• Impairs physical coordination
• May increase risk of stroke

Breast cancer in women

Stomach and intestines
• Causes bleeding and inflammation
• May increase risk of cancer

Pancreas
• Increases risk of pancreatitis, a dangerous inflammation

Liver
• Damages and eventually destroys liver cells
• Displaces important nutrients, which can cause malnutrition
• Increases risks of alcoholic hepatitis and cirrhosis
• Increases risk of cancer

FIGURE 13.4 The Effects of Alcohol Abuse on the Body

Alcohol has a major effect on the brain, damaging brain cells, impairing judgment and perceptions, and often leading to accidents and altercations. Alcohol also damages the digestive system, especially the liver.

Source: National Institute on Alcohol Abuse and Alcoholism

lining. Excessive drinking at one sitting may result in nausea; chronic drinking may result in peptic ulcers (breaks in the stomach lining) and bleeding from the stomach lining.

The alcohol in the bloodstream eventually reaches the liver. The liver, which bears the major responsibility of fat metabolism in the body, converts this excess alcohol to fat. After a few weeks of four or five drinks a day, liver cells start to accumulate fat. Alcohol also stimulates liver cells to attract white blood cells, which normally travel throughout the bloodstream, engulfing harmful substances and wastes. If white blood cells begin to invade body tissue, such as the liver, they can cause irreversible damage. More than 2 million Americans have alcohol-related liver diseases, such as alcoholic hepatitis and cirrhosis of the liver.

Frequency of drinking, as well as quantity of alcohol, may increase the likelihood of liver cirrhosis. In a recent study, drinking every day raised the risk more than less frequent drinking.[59]

Weight and Waists

At 7 calories per gram, alcohol has nearly as many calories as fat (9 calories per gram) and significantly more than carbohydrates or protein (which have 4 calories per gram). Since a standard drink contains 12 to 15 grams of alcohol, the alcohol in a single drink adds about 100 calories to your daily intake. A glass of wine contains as many calories as some candy bars; you would have to walk a mile to burn them off. In addition to being a calorie-dense food, alcohol stimulates the appetite, so you're likely to eat more. Obesity plus daily drinking boosts the risks of liver disease in men and women.

Cardiorespiratory System

Alcohol gets mixed reviews regarding its effects on the cardiorespiratory system. Several studies have shown that people who drink moderate amounts of alcohol have lower mortality rates after a heart attack as well as a lower risk of heart attack compared to abstainers and heavy drinkers.

However, some cardiologists contend that the benefits of moderate drinking may be overstated, especially because of alcohol's contribution to the epidemic of obesity around the world. Heavier drinking triggers the release of harmful oxygen molecules called free radicals, which can increase the risks of heart disease, stroke, and cirrhosis of the liver. Alcohol use can weaken the heart muscle directly, causing a disorder called cardiomyopathy. The combined use of alcohol and other drugs, including tobacco and cocaine, greatly increases the likelihood of damage to the heart.

Cancer

Overall past and current drinking may contribute to about 10 percent of all cancer cases in men and 3 percent in women. Alcohol consumption has been specifically implicated as a cause of cancers of the oral cavity, pharynx, larynx, esophagus, liver, colon-rectum, pancreas, and female breast.

According to a recent analysis, alcohol use accounts for approximately 3.5 percent of cancer deaths, or about 1 in 30, each year in the United States. Each alcohol-attributable cancer death results in about 18 years of potential life lost. Although cancer deaths are more common among persons who consume an average of three drinks or more per day, approximately 30 percent of deaths occur among people who drink less than three drinks per day. About 15 percent of breast cancer deaths among women in the United States may be attributable to alcohol consumption.[60]

Alcohol may make women more vulnerable to cancer by increasing estrogen levels. Health officials recommend that women should not exceed one drink a day, and those at an elevated risk for breast cancer, perhaps because of family history, should avoid alcohol or consume alcohol only occasionally.

Brain and Behavior

At first when you drink, you feel up. In low dosages, alcohol affects the regions of the brain that inhibit or control behavior, so you feel looser and act in ways you might not otherwise act. However, you also experience losses of concentration, memory, judgment, and fine motor control, and you have mood swings and emotional outbursts.

Moderate amounts of alcohol can have disturbing effects on perception and judgment, including the following:

- **Impaired perceptions.** You're less able to adjust your eyes to bright lights or to distinguish between sounds or judge their direction well.

- **Dulled smell and taste.** Alcohol may cause some vitamin deficiencies, and the poor eating habits of heavy drinkers result in further nutrition problems.

- **Diminished sensation.** On a freezing winter night, you may walk outside without a coat and not feel the cold.

- **Altered sense of space.** You may not realize, for instance, that you have been in one place for several hours.

- **Impaired motor skills.** Writing, typing, driving, and other abilities involving your muscles are impaired. This is why law enforcement officers sometimes ask suspected drunk

CONSUMER ALERT

Alcohol and Drug Interactions

Drug	Possible Effects of Interaction
Allergy, cold, flu medicines (Allegra, Benadryl, Claritin, Dimetapp, Sudafed, Tylenol Cold & Flu)	Drowsiness, dizziness, increased risk for overdose
Analgesics (painkillers)	
Narcotic (Codeine, Demerol, Percodan, Vicodin)	Increase in central nervous system depression, possibly leading to respiratory failure and death
Non-narcotic (aspirin, acetaminophen, ibuprofen)	Irritation of stomach resulting in bleeding and increased susceptibility to liver damage
Antabuse (disulfiram: an aid to quit drinking)	Nausea, vomiting, headache, high blood pressure, and erratic heartbeat
Antianxiety drugs (Valium, Librium, Ativan, Xanax)	Increase in central nervous system depression; decreased alertness and impaired judgment
Antidepressants (Prozac, Zoloft, Celexa, Lexapro, Paxil, Wellbutrin, Luvox, and others)	Increase in central nervous system depression; certain antidepressants in combination with red wine could cause a sudden increase in blood pressure
Antihistamines (Actifed, Dimetapp, and other cold medications)	Increase in drowsiness; decrease in ability to drive
Antibiotics	Nausea, vomiting, headache; some medications rendered less effective
Central nervous system stimulants (caffeine, Dexedrine, Ritalin)	Stimulant effects of these drugs may reverse depressant effect of alcohol but do not decrease its intoxicating effects
Cocaine	Intensification of cocaine's effects; increased risk of sudden death
Sedatives (Dalmane, Nembutal, Quaalude)	Increase in central nervous system depression, possibly leading to coma, respiratory failure, and death

drivers to touch their noses with a finger or to walk a straight line.

- **Sleep problems.** Even a single drink can increase snoring in normal sleepers and worsen sleep apnea in those with this disorder.[61] Among young adults, binge drinking increases the frequency and severity of sleep problems.[62]

- **Impaired sexual performance.** While drinking may increase your interest in sex, it may also impair sexual response, especially a man's ability to achieve or maintain an erection. As Shakespeare wrote, "It provokes the desire, but it takes away the performance."

- **Less impulse control.** As high-resolution neuroimaging scans have shown, chronic alcohol misuse damages white matter in areas of the brain that are involved in the brain's reward system. These networks are essential for controlling impulsive behavior and drinking. Longer and heavier alcohol abuse is associated with greater damage.[63]

√**check-in** Have you ever experienced any of these alcohol-induced effects?

Heavy alcohol use may pose special dangers to the brains of drinkers at both ends of the age spectrum. Adolescents who drink regularly show impairments in their neurological and cognitive functioning. Elderly people who drink heavily appear to have more brain shrinkage, or atrophy, than those who drink lightly or not at all. In general, moderate drinkers have healthier brains and a lower risk of dementia than those who don't drink and those who drink to excess.

Interaction with Other Drugs

Alcohol can interact with other drugs—prescription and nonprescription, legal and illegal. Of the 100 most frequently prescribed drugs, more than half contain at least one ingredient that interacts adversely with alcohol. Because alcohol and other psychoactive drugs may work on the same areas of the brain, their combination can produce an effect much greater than that expected of either drug by itself. For example, the liver combines alcohol and cocaine to produce cocaethylene, which intensifies the drug's effects and may increase the risk of sudden death. Alcohol is particularly dangerous when combined with other depressants and antianxiety medications. (See Consumer Alert.)

Immune System

Chronic alcohol use can inhibit the production of both white blood cells, which fight off infections, and red blood cells, which carry oxygen to all the organs and tissues of the body. Alcohol may increase the risk of infection with human immunodeficiency virus (HIV) by altering the judgment of users so that they more readily engage in activities such as unsafe sex that put them in danger. If you drink when you have a cold or the flu, alcohol interferes with the body's ability to recover. It also increases the chance of bacterial pneumonia in flu sufferers.

Increased Risk of Dying

Alcohol kills. Drinking, which claims 100,000 lives each year, is the third leading cause of death after tobacco and improper diet and lack of exercise:

- The leading alcohol-related cause of death is injury. Alcohol plays a role in almost half of all traffic fatalities, half of all homicides, and a quarter of all suicides.

- The second leading cause of alcohol-related deaths is cirrhosis of the liver, a chronic disease that causes extensive scarring and irreversible damage.

- As many as half of patients admitted to hospitals and 15 percent of those making office visits seek or need medical care because of direct or indirect effects of alcohol.

- Young drinkers—teens and those in their early 20s—are at highest risk of dying from injuries, mostly car accidents.

- Drinkers over age 50 face the greatest danger of premature death from cirrhosis of the liver, hepatitis, and other alcohol-linked illnesses.

Most studies of the relationship between alcohol consumption and death from all causes show that moderate drinkers—those who consume approximately seven drinks per week—have a lower risk of death than abstainers, while heavy drinkers have a higher risk than either group. In one 10-year study, never-drinkers showed no elevated risk of dying, while consistent heavier drinkers were at higher risk than other men of dying of any cause.

Alcohol, Gender, and Race

Experts in alcohol treatment are increasingly recognizing racial and ethnic differences in risk factors for drinking problems, patterns of drinking, and most effective types of treatment.

Gender

In general, men drink more frequently than women, consume a larger quantity of alcohol per drinking occasion, and report more problems related to drinking. More than half of women drink. Compared to men, women drink alone more often, binge less, have more regular drinking patterns, and drink smaller quantities than men.

The bodies of men and women respond to alcohol in different ways:

- Because they have a far smaller quantity of a protective enzyme in the stomach to break down alcohol before it's absorbed into the

TABLE 13.3 How Alcohol Discriminates

	Women ♀	Men ♂
Ability to dilute alcohol	Average total body water: 52%	Average total body water: 61%
Ability to metabolize alcohol	Women have a smaller quantity of dehydrogenase, an enzyme that breaks down alcohol.	Men have a larger quantity of dehydrogenase, which allows them to more quickly break down the alcohol they take in.
Monthly fluctuations	Premenstrual hormonal changes cause intoxication to set in faster during the days right before a woman gets her period.	Their susceptibility to getting drunk does not fluctuate dramatically at certain times of the month.
Estrogen levels	Alcohol increases estrogen levels. Birth control pills and other medicines containing estrogen increase intoxication.	Alcohol also increases estrogen levels in men. Chronic alcoholism has been associated with loss of body hair and muscle mass, development of swollen breasts and shrunken testicles, and impotence.

© Cengage Learning 2015

bloodstream, women absorb about 30 percent more alcohol into their bloodstream than men—see Table 13.3. The alcohol travels through the blood to the brain, so women become intoxicated much more quickly.

- Because there's more alcohol in the bloodstream to break down, the liver may also be adversely affected. In alcoholic women, the stomach seems to completely stop digesting alcohol, which may explain why female alcoholics are more likely to suffer liver damage than men.

- Nearly 14 million American women—one in eight—binge drink about three times a month, averaging about six drinks per binge. The risks to girls and women include injuries, sexual assault, chronic diseases, unintended pregnancy, learning and memory problems, and alcohol dependence.[64]

- An estimated 15 percent of women drink alcohol while pregnant, most having one drink or less per day. Even light consumption of alcohol can lead to **fetal alcohol effects (FAE)**: low birth weight, irritability as newborns, and permanent mental impairment. Drinking in the latter part of the first trimester may be most likely to cause the physical characteristics typical of FAE. A few drinking binges of four or more drinks a day during pregnancy may significantly increase the risk of childhood mental health and learning problems.

fetal alcohol effects (FAE)
Milder forms of FAS, including low birth weight, irritability as newborns, and permanent mental impairment as a result of the mother's alcohol consumption during pregnancy.

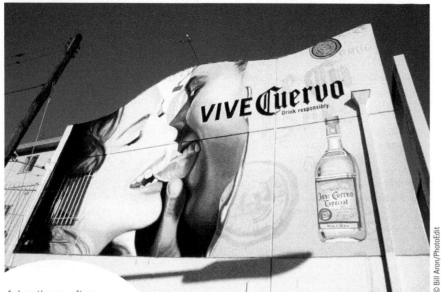

Advertisers often target particular types of alcohol to different ethnic communities.

© Bill Aron/PhotoEdit

- One of every 750 newborns has a cluster of physical and mental defects called **fetal alcohol syndrome (FAS)**: small head, abnormal facial features, jitters, poor muscle tone, sleep disorders, sluggish motor development, failure to thrive, short stature, delayed speech, mental retardation, and hyperactivity.

- Alcohol interferes with male sexual function and fertility through direct effects on testosterone and the testicles. In half of alcoholic men, increased levels of female hormones lead to breast enlargement and a feminine pubic hair pattern. Damage to the nerves in the penis by heavy drinking can lead to impotence. In women who drink heavily, a drop in female hormone production may cause menstrual irregularity and infertility.

Race

African American Community

Overall, African Americans consume less alcohol per person than whites, yet twice as many blacks die of cirrhosis of the liver each year. In some cities, the rate of cirrhosis is 10 times higher among African American men than among white men. Alcohol also contributes to high rates of hypertension, esophageal cancer, and homicide among African American men.

Hispanic Community

The various Hispanic cultures tend to discourage any drinking by women but encourage heavy drinking by men as part of machismo, or feelings of manhood. Hispanic men have higher rates of alcohol use and abuse than the general population and suffer a high rate of cirrhosis. Moreover, American-born Hispanic men drink more than those born in other countries.

Few Hispanics with severe alcohol problems enter treatment, partly because of a lack of information, language barriers, and poor community-based services. Hispanic families generally try to resolve problems themselves, and their cultural values discourage the sharing of intimate personal stories, which characterizes Alcoholics Anonymous and other support groups. Churches often provide the most effective forms of help.

Native American Community

European settlers introduced alcohol to Native Americans. Because of the societal and physical problems resulting from excessive drinking, at the request of tribal leaders, the U.S. Congress in 1832 prohibited the use of alcohol by Native Americans. Many reservations still ban alcohol use, so Native Americans who want to drink may have to travel long distances to obtain alcohol, which may contribute to the high death rate from hypothermia and pedestrian and motor-vehicle accidents among Native Americans. (Injuries are the leading cause of death among this group.)

Certainly, not all Native Americans drink, and not all who drink do so to excess. However, they have three times the general population's rate of alcohol-related injury and illness. Cirrhosis of the liver is the fourth leading cause of death among this cultural group. While many Native American women don't drink, those who do have high rates of alcohol-related problems, which affect both them and their children. Their rate of cirrhosis of the liver is 36 times that of white women. In some tribes, 10.5 out of every 1,000 newborns have fetal alcohol syndrome, compared with 1 to 3 out of 1,000 in the general population.

Asian American Community

Asian Americans tend to drink very little or not at all, in part because of an inborn physiological reaction to alcohol that causes facial flushing, rapid heart rate, lowered blood pressure, nausea, vomiting, and other symptoms. A very high percentage of women of all Asian American nationalities abstain completely. Some sociologists have expressed concern, however, that as Asian Americans become more assimilated into American culture, they'll drink more—and possibly suffer very adverse effects from alcohol.

✓**check-in** Are you at higher risk of alcohol-related consequences because of your gender or race?

fetal alcohol syndrome (FAS) A cluster of physical and mental defects in the newborn, including low birth weight, smaller-than-normal head circumference, intrauterine growth retardation, and permanent mental impairment caused by the mother's alcohol consumption during pregnancy.

Alcohol Use Disorders

As many as one in six adults in the United States may have a problem with drinking, which means, by the simplest definition, that they use alcohol in any way that creates difficulties, potential difficulties, or health risks. Like alcoholics, problem drinkers are individuals whose lives are in some way impaired by their drinking. The only difference is degree. Alcohol becomes a problem, and a person becomes an alcoholic, when the drinker can't "take it or leave it." He or she spends more and more time anticipating the next drink, planning when and where to get it, buying and hiding alcohol, and covering up secret drinking.

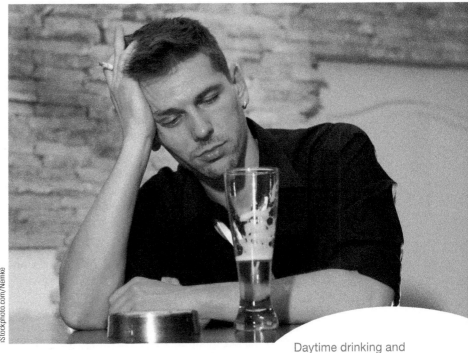

iStockphoto.com/Nemke

Alcohol Use Disorder

Approximately 17 million adults—an estimated 7.2 percent of Americans over 18, 9.9 percent of men and 4.6 percent of women—have an **alcohol use disorder**. The prevalence of this problem is greatest among individuals ages 18 to 29 but declines over the lifetime.[65]

In its most recent *Diagnostic and Statistical Manual (DSM-5)*, the American Psychiatric Association defines an alcohol use disorder as a problematic pattern of alcohol use leading to significant impairment or distress and characterized by at least two of the following:

- Drinking larger amounts of alcohol or drinking for a longer time than intended

- A strong urge or craving to use alcohol

- Persistent desire or unsuccessful efforts to cut down or control alcohol use

- Spending a great deal of time obtaining or using alcohol or recovering from its effects

- Use of alcohol in physically hazardous situations

- Continued alcohol use despite social, interpersonal, or occupational problems caused by drinking

- **Tolerance**, as defined by a need for markedly increased amounts of alcohol to achieve the desired effect or a markedly diminished effect with continued use of the same amount of alcohol

- **Withdrawal**, including symptoms such as sweating, rapid pulse, increased hand tremors, insomnia, nausea or vomiting, temporary hallucinations or illusions, physical agitation or restlessness, anxiety, or seizures.[66]

Alcoholism, as defined by the National Council on Alcoholism and Drug Dependence and the American Society of Addiction Medicine, is a primary, chronic disease whose development and manifestations are influenced by genetic, psychosocial, and environmental factors. The disease is often progressive and fatal. Its characteristics include an inability to control drinking; a preoccupation with alcohol; continued use of alcohol despite adverse consequences; and distorted thinking, most notably denial. Like other diseases, alcoholism is not simply a matter of insufficient willpower but a complex problem that causes many symptoms and can have serious consequences yet can improve with treatment.

Causes Although the exact cause of alcohol use disorders is not known, certain factors—including biochemical imbalances in the brain, heredity, cultural acceptability, and stress—all seem to play a role. They include the following:

- **Genetics.** Scientists have not yet identified conclusively a specific gene that puts people at risk for alcoholism. However, epidemiological studies have shown evidence of heredity's role. Studies of twins suggest that heredity accounts for two-thirds of the risk of becoming alcoholic in both men and women.

- **Parental alcoholism.** According to researchers, alcoholism is four to five times more common among the children of alcoholics, who

Daytime drinking and drinking alone can be signs of a serious problem, even though the drinker may otherwise appear to be in control.

alcohol use disorder
Problematic pattern of alcohol use leading to significant impairment or distress.

tolerance A need for markedly increased amounts of alcohol or a drug to achieve the desired effect or a markedly diminished effect with continued use of a substance.

withdrawal Development of symptoms, such as sweating, rapid pulse, tremor, nausea, vomiting, temporary hallucinations, physical agitation, anxiety, or seizures, when substance use is stopped.

alcoholism A chronic, progressive, potentially fatal disease characterized by impaired control of drinking; a preoccupation with alcohol; continued use of alcohol despite adverse consequences; and distorted thinking, most notably denial.

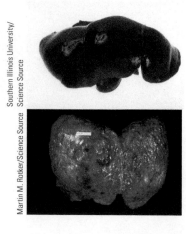

Southern Illinois University/ Science Source

Martin M. Rotker/Science Source

A normal liver (top) compared to one with cirrhosis.

detoxification The supervised removal of a poisonous or harmful substance (such as a drug) from the body; a therapy for alcoholics in which they are denied alcohol in a controlled environment.

may be influenced by the behavior they see in their parents.

✓**check-in** Do you have a family history of alcohol use disorders?

- **Drug abuse.** Alcoholism is associated with the abuse of other psychoactive drugs, including marijuana, cocaine, heroin, amphetamines, and various antianxiety medications.

- **Stress and traumatic experiences.** Many people start drinking heavily as a way of coping with psychological problems.

Medical Complications

As previously discussed, excessive alcohol use adversely affects virtually every organ system in the body, including the brain, the digestive tract, the heart, muscles, blood, and hormones (see Figure 12.4). In addition, because alcohol interacts with many drugs, it can increase the risk of potentially lethal overdoses and harmful interactions. A summary of the major risks and complications follows:[67]

- **Liver disease.** Chronic heavy drinking can lead to alcoholic hepatitis (inflammation and destruction of liver cells) and, in the 15 percent of people who continue drinking beyond this stage, cirrhosis (irreversible scarring and destruction of liver cells). The liver eventually may fail completely, resulting in coma and death.

- **Cardiorespiratory disease.** Heavy drinking can weaken the heart muscle (causing cardiac myopathy), elevate blood pressure, and increase the risk of stroke.

- **Cancer.** Heavy alcohol use may contribute to cancer of the liver, stomach, and colon, as well as malignant melanoma, a deadly form of skin cancer.

- **Brain damage.** Long-term heavy drinkers may suffer memory loss and be unable to think abstractly, recall names of common objects, and follow simple instructions. Chronic brain damage resulting from alcohol consumption is second only to Alzheimer's disease as a cause of cognitive deterioration in adults.

- **Vitamin deficiencies.** Alcoholism is associated with vitamin deficiencies, especially of thiamin (B_1). Lack of thiamin may result in Wernicke-Korsakoff syndrome, which is characterized by disorientation, memory failure, hallucinations, and jerky eye movements, and it can be disabling enough to require lifelong custodial care.

- **Digestive problems.** Alcohol triggers the secretion of acids in the stomach that irritate the mucous lining and cause gastritis. Chronic drinking may result in peptic ulcers (breaks in the stomach lining) and bleeding from the stomach lining.

Alcoholism Treatments

Of the 17 million adults in the United States who have alcohol use disorders, only an estimated 8 percent minority ever undergo treatment for alcohol-related problems.[68] Until recent years, the only options for professional alcohol treatment were, as one expert puts it, "intensive, extensive, and expensive," such as residential programs at hospitals or specialized treatment centers.

Individuals whose drinking could be hazardous to their health may choose from a variety of approaches, including medication, behavioral therapy, or both. There is no one path to sobriety. A wide variety of treatments may offer help and hope to those with alcohol-related problems. Men and women who have remained sober for more than a decade credit a variety of approaches, including Alcoholics Anonymous (AA), individual psychotherapy, and other groups, such as Women for Sobriety.

Detoxification The first phase of treatment for alcohol dependence focuses on **detoxification**, the gradual withdrawal of alcohol from the body. For 90 to 95 percent of alcoholics, withdrawal symptoms are mild to moderate.

YOUR STRATEGIES FOR PREVENTION

How to Recognize the Warning Signs of Alcoholism

- Experiencing the following symptoms after drinking: frequent headaches, nausea, stomach pain, heartburn, gas, fatigue, weakness, muscle cramps, irregular or rapid heartbeats

- Needing a drink in the morning to start the day

- Denying any problem with alcohol

- Doing things while drinking that are regretted afterward

- Experiencing dramatic mood swings, from anger to laughter to anxiety

- Having sleep problems

- Experiencing depression and paranoia

- Forgetting what happened during a drinking episode

- Changing brands or going on the wagon to control drinking

- Having five or more drinks a day

They include sweating; rapid pulse; elevated blood pressure; hand tremor; insomnia; nausea or vomiting; malaise or weakness; anxiety; depressed mood or irritability; headache; and temporary hallucinations or illusions. Withdrawal can be life-threatening when accompanied by medical problems, such as grand mal seizures, pneumonia, liver failure, or gastrointestinal bleeding. The standard treatment is a safer sedative, such as Valium or Ativan, with a gradual reduction in the dose.

Alcohol withdrawal delirium, commonly known as **delirium tremens (DTs)** is most common in chronic heavy drinkers who also suffer from a physical illness, fatigue, depression, or malnutrition. Delirium tremens are characterized by agitated behavior, delusions, rapid heart rate, sweating, vivid hallucinations, trembling hands, and fever. The symptoms usually appear over several days after heavy drinking stops. Individuals frequently report terrifying visual hallucinations, such as seeing insects all over their bodies. With treatment, most cases subside after several days, although delirium tremens has been known to last as long as four or five weeks. In some cases, complications such as infections or heart arrhythmias prove fatal.

Medications The most widely prescribed medications for alcoholism recovery include the following:

- Disulfiram (Antabuse), in use for more than 50 years, causes unpleasant effects when even small amounts of alcohol are consumed. These include flushing of the face, headache, nausea, vomiting, chest pain, weakness, blurred vision, mental confusion, sweating, choking, breathing difficulty, and anxiety. These effects begin about 10 minutes after alcohol enters the body and last for an hour or more.

- Acamprosate (Campra), combined with counseling and social support, helps the brains of people who have drunk large amounts of alcohol work normally again. Acamprosate does not prevent withdrawal symptoms and has not been shown to work in people who have not stopped drinking alcohol or who also abuse substances such as street drugs or prescription medications.

- Naltrexone (Revia, Decade, Vivitrol) reduces cravings, perhaps by blocking the normal pleasurable reaction of the part of the brain that reacts to alcohol or opioids.

Anticraving drugs are associated with a reduction in return to drinking, but long-term follow-ups have shown that their benefits are "only modestly greater than those of placebo."[69]

Inpatient or Residential Treatment In the past, 28-day treatment programs in a medical or psychiatric hospital or a residential facility were the cornerstone of early recovery treatment. According to outcome studies, inpatient treatment was effective, with as many as 70 percent of "graduates" remaining abstinent or stable, nonproblem drinkers for five years after. However, because of cost pressures from the insurance industry, the length of stay has been reduced, and there's been increasing emphasis on outpatient care.

Outpatient Treatment Outpatient treatment may involve group therapy, individual supportive therapy, marital or family therapy, regular attendance at Alcoholics Anonymous (AA) or another support group, brief interventions, and relapse prevention. According to outcome studies, intensive outpatient treatment at a day hospital (with individuals returning home every evening) are as effective as inpatient care. Outpatient therapy continues for at least a year, but many individuals continue to participate in outpatient programs for the rest of their lives.

Behavioral Therapies The goals of behavioral therapies are to increase motivation to abstain, enhance coping skills, facilitate self-change, and deal with adverse effects:

- Cognitive behavioral therapy (CBT) identifies high-risk situations that trigger relapse and uses cognitive and behavioral techniques to help recovering alcoholics deal with stressful experiences.

- Computer-based training reinforces the lessons of CBT.

- Brief behavioral interventions provide personalized feedback to help reduce harmful drinking practices

- Facilitated self-change focuses on goal-setting, self-monitoring, and problem-solving skills.[70]

Moderation Training Highly controversial, this approach uses cognitive-behavioral techniques, such as keeping a diary to chart drinking patterns and learning "consumption management" techniques, such as never having more than one drink an hour.

Treatment programs in other countries, such as Great Britain and Canada, have long offered moderation training for problem drinkers who consume too much alcohol. However, most experts agree that the best—and perhaps

delirium tremens (DTs) The delusions, hallucinations, and agitated behavior following withdrawal from long-term chronic alcohol abuse.

only—hope for recovery for chronic alcoholics who are physically dependent on alcohol is complete abstinence.

··
✓ **check-in Do** you think it is possible for
··
individuals with an alcohol use disorder to
··
learn to drink moderately? Why or why not?
··

12 Step Self-Help Programs The best-known and most commonly used self-help program for alcohol problems is Alcoholics Anonymous (AA), which was founded more than 60 years ago and which has grown into an international organization that includes 2 million members and 185,000 groups worldwide. Acknowledging the power of alcohol, AA offers support from others struggling with the same illness, from a sponsor available at any time of the day or night, and from fellowship meetings that are held every day of the year. Because anonymity is a key part of AA, it has been difficult for researchers to study its success, but it is generally believed to be a highly effective means of overcoming alcoholism and maintaining abstinence. Its 12 steps, which emphasize honesty, sobriety, and acknowledgment of a "higher power," have become the model for self-help groups for other addictive behaviors, including drug abuse (discussed in Chapter 12) and compulsive eating.

The average age of entry into AA is 30; about 60 percent of the members are men. Members encompass a wide range of ages, occupations, nationalities, and socioeconomic classes. People generally attend 12 Step meetings every day when they first begin recovery; most programs recommend 90 meetings in 90 days. Many people taper off to one or two meetings a week as their recovery progresses. No one knows exactly how 12 Step programs help people break out of addictions. Some individuals stop their drinking, or other destructive behavior, simply on the basis of the information they get at meetings. Others bond to the group and use it as a social support and refuge while they explore and release their inner feelings—a process similar to what happens in psychotherapy.

Many individuals recovering from substance abuse—as many as one in ten Americans, by some estimates—will attend a 12 Step meeting in their lifetime. For many with alcohol-related problems, AA is the first and only treatment they receive. Does AA work? Some studies have found that fewer than 1 in 30 people remain in AA after one year, although this may be because many are coerced to make their initial visits. However, continued AA attendance is modestly associated with abstinence and improved social functioning. According to the "helper theory principle,"

when people with a condition help others with a similar problem, they also help themselves. This principle, fundamental to AA, may contribute to their continuing sobriety.

Spirituality is another key and controversial component of AA, with 11 of its 12 steps explicitly referring to the importance of God or a higher power for recovery. Yet both spiritually oriented and atheistic individuals benefit equally from AA programs. In a ten-year study, individuals involved with AA reported significantly larger gains in religious practices, such as prayer, compared with those without such exposure. Individuals who maintain consistent AA membership reported the greatest increases in "God consciousness" and religious practices.

Harm Reduction Therapy This controversial approach aims to help substance abusers reduce the negative impact of alcohol or drugs on their lives. Its fundamental principles include the following:

- While absolute abstinence may be preferable for many or most substance abusers, very few achieve it. Even these few will take time to reach this point and may relapse periodically.

- The field of medicine accepts and practices other types of treatments that preserve health and well-being even when people fail to comply with all recommended behaviors.

- Therapists cannot make judgments for clients, even though they should present accurate information and may even express their own beliefs.

- There are many shades of improvement in every kind of therapy. If a certain level of improvement is all a person is capable of reaching, that person should be encouraged.

Alternatives to AA Secular Organizations for Sobriety (SOS) was founded in 1986 as an alternative for people who couldn't accept the spirituality of AA. Like AA, SOS holds confidential meetings, celebrates sobriety anniversaries, and views recovery as a one-day-at-a-time process.

Rational Recovery, which also emphasizes anonymity and total abstinence, focuses on the self rather than spirituality. Members use reason instead of prayer and learn to control the impulse to drink by learning how to control the emotions that lead them to drink.

Recovery

Recovery from alcoholism is a lifelong process of personal growth and healing. The first two years are the most difficult, and relapses are extremely common. By some estimates, more than 90 percent of those recovering from substance use will use alcohol or drugs in any one 12-month period after treatment. However, approximately 70 percent of those who get formal treatment stop drinking for prolonged periods. Even without treatment, 30 percent of alcoholics are able to stop drinking for long periods. Those most likely to remain sober after treatment have the most to lose by continuing to drink: they tend to be employed, married, and upper-middle class. Recovering alcoholics who help other alcoholics stay sober are better able to maintain their own sobriety.

Most recovering alcoholics experience urges to drink, especially during early recovery when they are likely to feel considerable stress. These urges are a natural consequence of years of drinking and diminish with time. Mood swings are common during recovery, and individuals typically describe themselves as alternately feeling relieved or elated and then discouraged or tearful. Such disconcerting ups and downs also decrease over time. Patience—learning to take "one day at a time"—is crucial.

Increasingly, treatment programs focus on **relapse prevention**, which includes the development of coping strategies and learning techniques that make it easier to live with alcohol cravings and rehearsal of various ways of saying "no" to offers of a drink. According to outcomes research, social skills training—a combination of stress management therapy, assertiveness and communication skills training, behavioral self-control training, and behavioral marital therapy—has proved effective in decreasing the duration and severity of relapses after one year in a group of alcoholics. A new approach to relapse behavior, Mindfulness-Based Relapse Prevention, teaches clients meditation techniques as a way of coping with cravings and high-risk relapse situations.

Alcoholism's Impact on Relationships

Alcoholism shatters families and creates unhealthy patterns of communicating and relating. Separation and divorce rates are high among alcoholics.

Having a heavy drinker—a friend, family member, or colleague—in your life can put your own health and well-being at risk. In a recent study, those linked with a heavy drinker reported more symptoms such as chronic pain, anxiety, and depression.

Growing Up with an Alcoholic Parent

More than 10 percent of children in the United States are living with a parent with an alcohol problem.[71] Parental alcoholism increases the likelihood of childhood ADHD, conduct disorder, and anxiety disorders. The experience often leads youngsters to play certain roles: The adjuster or "lost child" does whatever the parent says. The responsible child, or "family hero," typically takes over many household tasks and responsibilities. The acting-out child, or "scapegoat," shows his or her anger early in life by causing problems at home or in school and taking on the role of troublemaker. The "mascot" disrupts tense situations by focusing attention on himself or herself, often by clowning. Regardless of which roles they assume, the children of alcoholics are prone to learning disabilities, eating disorders, and addictive behavior.

Numerous studies have linked parental drinking to child abuse and neglect. Children of women who are problem drinkers have twice the risk of serious injury as children of mothers who don't drink. Children with two parents who are problem drinkers are at even higher risk. As teenagers, children of alcoholics are more likely to report early sexual intercourse and face a greater risk of adolescent pregnancy.

Adult Children of Alcoholics

Growing up with an alcoholic parent can have a long-lasting effect. Adult children of alcoholics are at risk for many problems. Some try to fill the emptiness inside with alcohol, drugs, or addictive habits. Others find themselves caught up in destructive relationships that repeat the patterns of their childhood. They are likely to have difficulty solving problems, identifying and expressing their feelings, trusting others, and being intimate. In addition to their own increased risk of addictive behavior, they are likely to marry individuals with some form of addiction and keep on playing out the roles of their childhood. They may feel inadequate, not know how to set limits or recognize normal behavior, be perfectionistic, and want to control all aspects of their lives. However, not

relapse prevention An alcohol recovery treatment method that focuses on social skills training to develop ways of preventing or minimizing a relapse.

all adult children are alike or necessarily suffer from psychological problems or face an increased risk of substance abuse themselves.

Because the impact of alcoholism can be so enduring, support groups—such as Adult Children of Alcoholics, Children of Alcoholics, and Adult Children of Dysfunctional Families—have spread throughout the country in the last decade. These organizations provide adult children of alcoholics a mutually supportive group setting in which to discuss their childhood experiences with alcoholic parents and the emotional consequences they carry into adult life. Through such groups or other forms of therapy, individuals may learn to move beyond anger and blame, see the part they themselves play in their current state of unhappiness, and create a future that is healthier and happier than their past. (See Health Now!)

WHAT DID YOU DECIDE?

- Do you agree with experts who see alcohol as the greatest single threat to college students' health?
- What are the most dangerous forms of campus drinking?
- What are the short-and long-term effects of alcohol on health?
- How are alcohol disorders treated?

THE POWER OF NOW!

Take Charge of Alcohol

If you use alcohol, develop a defensive drinking program. Check the steps that you have taken or will take in the future to stay in control of your alcohol intake.

____ Finding alternative ways to soothe stress. Daily sessions of meditation have proven effective in helping high-risk student drinkers relax.

____ Setting a limit on how many drinks you're going to have ahead of time—and sticking to it.

____ When you're mixing a drink, measuring the alcohol.

____ Alternating nonalcoholic and alcoholic drinks.

____ Drinking slowly; not guzzling.

____ Eating before and while drinking.

____ Avoiding tasks that require skilled reactions during or after drinking.

____ Not encouraging or reinforcing others' irresponsible behavior.

____ Checking out community resources. Are there chapters of AA and Al-Anon on campus? Find out more about the BACCHUS (Boosting Alcohol Consciousness Concerning the Health of University Students) network, including programs in your area. Do these groups offer volunteer opportunities that interest you?

____ Talking to your dormmates, fraternity brothers, sorority sisters, or roommates about steps you could take collectively, such as restricting drinking in rooms or setting up a "Seize the Keys" policy to prevent drunk driving.

What's Online

CENGAGE brain.com Visit www.cengagebrain.com to access course materials for this text, including the Behavior Change Planner, interactive quizzes, and more.

self survey

Do You Have a Drinking Problem?

This self-assessment, the Michigan Alcoholism Screening Test (MAST), is widely used to identify potential problems. This test screens for the major psychological, sociological, and physiological consequences of alcoholism.
Answer Yes or No to the following questions, and add up the points shown in the right column for your answers.

		Yes	No	Points
1.	Do you enjoy a drink now and then?	_____	_____	(0 for either)
2.	Do you think that you're a normal drinker? (By normal, we mean that you drink less than or as much as most other people.)	_____	_____	(2 for no)
3.	Have you ever awakened the morning after some drinking the night before and found that you couldn't remember part of the evening?	_____	_____	(2 for yes)
4.	Does your wife, husband, a parent, or other near relative ever worry or complain about your drinking?	_____	_____	(1 for yes)
5.	Can you stop drinking without a struggle after one or two drinks?	_____	_____	(2 for no)
6.	Do you ever feel guilty about your drinking?	_____	_____	(1 for yes)
7.	Do friends or relatives think that you're a normal drinker?	_____	_____	(2 for no)
8.	Do you ever try to limit your drinking to certain times of the day or to certain places?	_____	_____	(0 for either)
9.	Have you ever attended a meeting of Alcoholics Anonymous?	_____	_____	(2 for yes)
10.	Have you ever gotten into physical fights when drinking?	_____	_____	(1 for yes)
11.	Has your drinking ever created problems for you and your wife, husband, a parent, or other relative?	_____	_____	(2 for yes)
12.	Have your wife, husband, or other family members ever gone to anyone for help about your drinking?	_____	_____	(2 for yes)
13.	Have you ever lost friends because of your drinking?	_____	_____	(2 for yes)
14.	Have you ever gotten into trouble at work or school because of your drinking?	_____	_____	(2 for yes)
15.	Have you ever lost a job because of your drinking?	_____	_____	(2 for yes)
16.	Have you ever neglected your obligations, your family, or your work for two or more days in a row because of drinking?	_____	_____	(2 for yes)
17.	Do you drink before noon fairly often?	_____	_____	(1 for yes)
18.	Have you ever been told you have liver trouble? Cirrhosis?	_____	_____	(2 for yes)
19.	After heavy drinking, have you ever had delirium tremens (DTs) or severe shaking, or heard voices or seen things that weren't actually there?	_____	_____	(2 for yes*)

20. Have you ever gone to anyone for help about your drinking? _____ _____ (5 for yes)

21. Have you ever been in a hospital because of your drinking? _____ _____ (5 for yes)

22. Have you ever been a patient in a psychiatric hospital or on a psychiatric ward of a general hospital where drinking was part of the problem that resulted in hospitalization? _____ _____ (2 for yes)

23. Have you ever been seen at a psychiatric or mental health clinic or gone to any doctor, social worker, or clergyman for help with any emotional problem where drinking was part of the problem? _____ _____ (2 for yes)

24. Have you ever been arrested for drunk driving, driving while intoxicated, or driving under the influence of alcoholic beverages? _____ _____ (2 for yes)

25. Have you ever been arrested, or taken into custody, even for a few hours, because of drunken behavior? _____ _____ (2 for yes)

(If Yes, how many times?) _____ **

*Five points for delirium tremens
**Two points for each arrest

Scoring

In general, five or more points places you in an alcoholic category; four points suggests alcoholism; three or fewer points indicates that you're *not* an alcoholic.

MAKING THIS CHAPTER WORK FOR YOU

Review Questions

(LO 13.1)   1. Which of the following statements is true about alcohol consumption in America?
   a. White men and women are less likely to drink than other adults.
   b. Married men and women are more likely to drink than their single or divorced counterparts.
   c. Nonstudents consume more alcohol and more often than college students of the same age.
   d. More Americans are choosing not to drink, and alcohol consumption is at its lowest level in decades.

(LO 13.1)   2. The most common reason people drink alcohol is to _____.
   a. appear older than they look
   b. feel less tense
   c. treat medical conditions
   d. engage in skilled activities

(LO 13.2)   3. Which of the following statements is true in the context of alcohol consumption on campuses?
   a. More college women drink now, and they drink more than they did in the past.
   b. College women drink more, more often, and more intensely than men.
   c. The percentage of students who drink has reduced considerably over the years.
   d. The students who drink the most are those attending two-year institutions.

(LO 13.2)   4. Which of the following statements is true in the context of influences on student drinking?
   a. Students with symptoms of depression are least likely to report risky drinking behavior.
   b. Students who never join a fraternity or sorority report less risky drinking behavior.
   c. Students who live in on-campus housing drink the least.
   d. Students with parents who communicate zero-tolerance messages to alcohol drink the most.

(LO 13.3)   5. _____ is a type of alcohol found in alcoholic beverages.
   a. Ethanol
   b. Phenolphthalein
   c. Tylenol
   d. Acetaminophen

(LO 13.3)   6. Which of the following statements is true in the context of blood-alcohol concentration?
   a. Martinis get alcohol into the bloodstream faster than beer or table wine.
   b. Chilled alcohol moves more quickly into the bloodstream than warm alcohol.
   c. Alcohol moves slower into the bloodstream when it is mixed with carbon dioxide.
   d. One drink for a man has the impact that two drinks have for a woman.

(LO 13.4)   7. Which of the following statements is true in the context of alcohol's impact on the body?
   a. Alcohol slows down the elimination of fluid from the body.
   b. Alcohol lowers the body temperature.
   c. Alcohol strengthens the heart muscle and decreases the risk of heart diseases.
   d. Alcohol reduces appetite.

(LO 13.4)   8. The leading alcohol-related cause of death is _____.
   a. old age
   b. liver dysfunction
   c. hepatitis
   d. injury

(LO 13.5)   9. Which of the following statements is true about gender differences in alcohol consumption?
   a. Women tend to have more irregular patterns of drinking than men.
   b. Women alcoholics are less likely to suffer from liver damage than men.
   c. Women absorb about 30 percent more alcohol into their bloodstream than men.
   d. Women have a higher amount of a stomach enzyme that helps digest alcohol than men.

(LO 13.5) 10. Which of the following statements is true about racial factors associated with alcohol consumption?
  a. Cases of cirrhosis of the liver among African Americans are extremely rare compared cases among whites.
  b. Hispanic men suffer from a low rate of cirrhosis of the liver.
  c. American-born Hispanic men drink less than those born in other countries.
  d. Native Americans have three times the general population's rate of alcohol-related injury.

(LO 13.6) 11. _____ is defined by a need for markedly increased amounts of alcohol or a drug to achieve the desired effect or a markedly diminished effect with continued use of a substance.
  a. Tolerance
  b. Withdrawal
  c. Allergy
  d. Hypersensitivity

(LO 13.6) 12. Which of the following statements is true about alcoholism?
  a. It is caused only by insufficient will power.
  b. It can seldom be fatal.
  c. It can be influenced by heredity.
  d. It has not been reported among women.

(LO 13.7) 13. Children of alcoholic parents may assume one of several roles. Which of the following is NOT a typical role?
  a. family hero
  b. mascot
  c. baby
  d. scapegoat

(LO 13.7) 14. Adult children of alcoholics are at risk for many problems, including _____.
  a. higher incidence of heart disease
  b. overachiever syndrome
  c. higher incidence of falls and other accidents
  d. higher incidence of alcohol and/or drug abuse

Answers to these questions can be found on page 623.

Critical Thinking

1. Driving home from a friend's twenty-first birthday party, 18-year-old Rick has had too much to drink. As he crosses the dividing line on the two-lane road, the driver of an oncoming car—a young mother with two young children in the backseat—swerves to avoid an accident. She hits a concrete wall and dies instantly, but her children survive. Rick has no record of drunk driving. Should he go to prison? Is he guilty of manslaughter? How would you feel if you were the victim's husband? If you were Rick's friend?

2. Have you ever been around people who have been intoxicated when you have been sober? What did you think of their behavior? Were they fun to be around? Was the experience not particularly enjoyable, boring, or difficult in some way? Have you ever been intoxicated? How do you behave when you are drunk? Do you find the experience enjoyable? What do the people around you think of your actions when you are drunk?

3. What effects has alcohol use had in your life? Try making a list of the positive and negative effects your own alcohol use has had. Be specific. If you continue to drink at your current rate, what positive and negative effects do you think it will have on your future? What effects have other people's drinking had on your life? List family members and friends who drink regularly and how their drinking has affected you.

Additional Online Resources

http://www.phoenixhouse.org/
This excellent site is geared to college students. Sections include Alcohol & Student Life, Alcohol & Sex, and Alcohol & Your Body.

www.collegedrinkingprevention.gov
This website, sponsored by the National Institute on Alcohol Abuse and Alcoholism, focuses on the college alcohol culture with information for students, parents, college health administrators, and more. The site also features information about alcohol abuse prevention, college alcohol policies, research topics, and factual information about the consequences of alcohol abuse and alcoholism.

http://al-anon.alateen.org/
This site provides information and referrals to local Al-Anon and Alateen groups. It also includes a self-quiz to determine if you are affected by someone who has an alcohol problem.

http://nacoa.org/
This association provides information about and for children of alcoholics. The website contains numerous links to relevant support groups.

www.niaaa.nih.gov/alcohol-health/special-population -co-occuring-disorders/college-drinking
The problem with college drinking is not necessarily the drinking itself, but the negative conquences that result from excessive drinking. This website, sponsored by the National Institute on Alcohol Abuse and Alcoholism, outlines the widespread impacts of college drinking.

Key Terms

The terms listed are used on the page indicated. Definitions of the terms are in the glossary at the end of the book.

absorption   400
alcohol use disorder   407
alcoholism   407
(AmED) alcohol mixed with energy drinks   393
binge   391
blood-alcohol concentration (BAC)   398
delirium tremens (DTs)   409
detoxification   408

ethyl alcohol   397
fetal alcohol effects (FAE)   405
fetal alcohol syndrome (FAS)   406
predrinking   392
proof   398
relapse prevention   411
tolerance   407
withdrawal   407

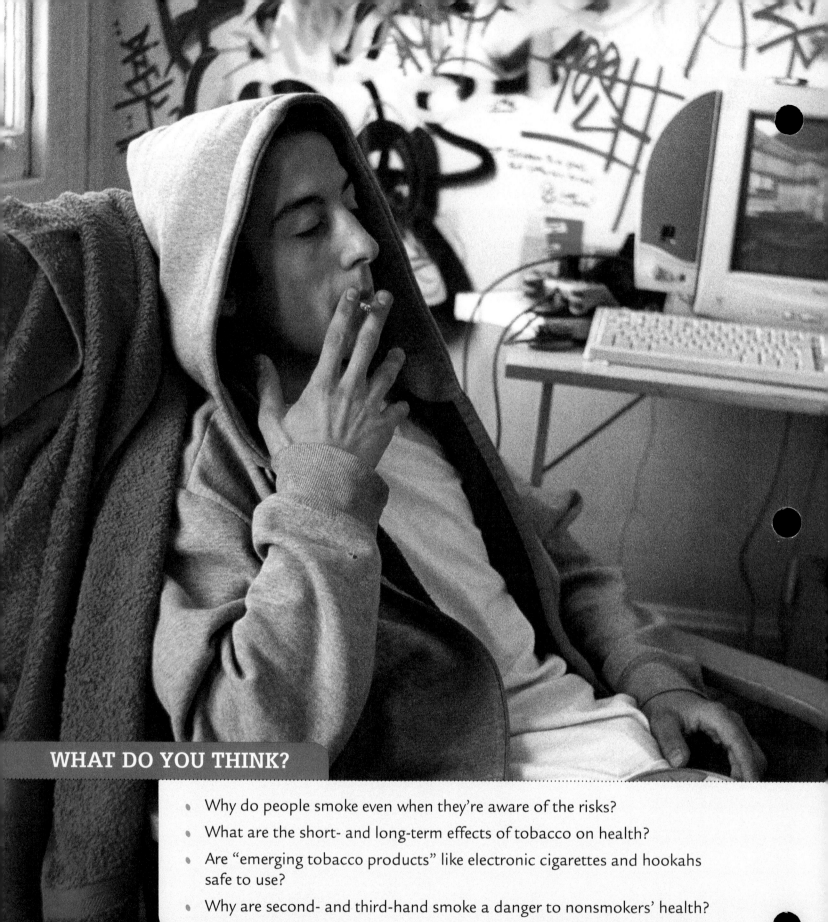

WHAT DO YOU THINK?

- Why do people smoke even when they're aware of the risks?
- What are the short- and long-term effects of tobacco on health?
- Are "emerging tobacco products" like electronic cigarettes and hookahs safe to use?
- Why are second- and third-hand smoke a danger to nonsmokers' health?

14

Tobacco

" **C**igarettes are bad for you."

J. T. had heard this message for as long as he could remember. His dad blamed his chronic respiratory problems on the cigarettes he had tried to quit a dozen times. His mother told him that cigarettes caused his grandfather's premature death. But the electronic cigarette a high school friend offered J. T. didn't look like a regular cigarette. No trace of tobacco. No stained fingers. No stale breath. And "vaping" (inhaling the vapor produced by e-cigarettes) seemed cool.

After starting college J. T. regularly joined some new friends passing around a hookah (water pipe).

Once again, it didn't seem the same as smoking cigarettes. He never realized that he was actually inhaling more nicotine. He never thought he would start smoking conventional cigarettes—first as a "social smoker," then as a daily one. At his girlfriend's insistence, J. T. agreed to quit—but relapsed time and again. Now he finds himself saying the same words he heard so often from his father: "I just wish I'd never started in the first place." <

After reading this chapter, you should be able to:

14.1 Compare the patterns of tobacco consumption among the populations in America.

14.2 Outline the patterns of tobacco consumption among different groups of students.

14.3 Discuss gender, racial, and ethnic differences in tobacco consumption.

14.4 Identify immediate effects of tobacco consumption on body and brain functions.

14.5 Evaluate the serious health risks and dangers associated with cigarette smoking.

14.6 Give examples of emerging tobacco products and their health risks.

14.7 Review the health risks posed by different forms of tobacco.

14.8 Compare the different ways of quitting to show advantages and disadvantages of each.

14.9 Analyze the harmful effects of environmental tobacco smoke on health.

J. T. is typical of a new generation of tobacco users. In the past, teenagers were most likely to take their first puff of tobacco from a cigarette. Now e-cigarettes and water pipes have become a common entry into tobacco use.[1] Among high school seniors in a recent nationwide survey, 7 percent reported smoking cigarettes—a substantial drop from five years ago—while 16 percent said they had used e-cigarettes.[2] Among college students, 12 percent smoked cigarettes within the last 30 days, while about 9 percent used a hookah.[3]

There is no risk-free method of using tobacco. Any exposure to tobacco smoke can cause both immediate and long-term damage to the body. Tobacco continues to kill more people than AIDS, alcohol, drug abuse, car crashes, murders, suicides, and fires combined. According to the Centers for Disease Control (CDC), more than 480,000 Americans die each year from smoking or exposure to secondhand smoke, while 16 million suffer from smoking-related illnesses.[4]

This chapter discusses smoking around the world, in America, and on campus. It provides information on tobacco products, the effects of tobacco on the body, tobacco dependence, quitting smoking, and environmental tobacco smoke. This information may help you to breathe easier today—and may help ensure cleaner air for others to breathe tomorrow.

✓**check-in** Did you know that if you smoke and are under age 35, you can add ten years to your life span by quitting?

Smoking in America

Health officials look back on the popularity of smoking in the 20th century as one of the "greatest public health catastrophes" and the cause of millions of preventable deaths. More than ten times as many U.S. citizens have died prematurely from cigarette smoking than in all the wars fought in the history of the United States.[5]

The tide against smoking turned in 1964, with publication of the landmark surgeon general's report on smoking and health. Since then, smoking rates have fallen from 42 to 18 percent of adults over age 18, but tobacco has killed more than 20 million Americans, including 2.5 million nonsmokers exposed to secondhand smoke (see page 435) and 100,000 babies who died of Sudden Infant Death Syndrome (SIDS) or complications, such as prematurity, linked to parental smoking. (See "Health on a Budget," below)

According to the Centers for Disease Control (CDC)[6]:

- 42 million men and women currently smoke.

- American Indians and Alaska Natives have the highest smoking rates, while Asians and Hispanics have the lowest. Individuals with undergraduate and graduate degrees are least likely to smoke.

⑤HEALTH ON A BUDGET

The Toll of Tobacco

Whether or not you smoke, you indirectly pay the price of tobacco use around the world:

Global economic cost	$500 billion
U.S. economic cost	$193 billion
Annual global number of tobacco-caused deaths	6 million
Annual number of premature deaths due to tobacco in the U.S.	443,000
Property damage in fires caused by smoking, globally	$27 billion
Injuries in fires caused by smoking, globally	60,000
Deaths in fires caused by smoking, globally	17,300
Deaths caused by secondhand smoke in the U.S.	3,000

Source: www.tobaccoatlas.org

- Smoking rates vary in different regions. The West has the fewest smokers (about 14 percent); the Midwest, the most (21 percent).
- Smoking rates are highest among the poor; the mentally ill; drug and alcohol abusers; the disabled; and lesbian, gay, bisexual, and transgender persons.[7]

✓**check-in** Have you ever smoked? If so, when did you start?

Why People Smoke

One of the key factors linked with the onset of a smoking habit is being young. Smoking a single cigarette before age 11 increases the odds of becoming dependent on nicotine. According to a recent poll, nearly 90 percent of adults who smoke report that, if they had it to do over again, they would not have started. In order to help adolescents avoid that regret as well as smoking's many dangers, some legislators have proposed raising the minimum legal age for purchasing tobacco products to 21.

✓**check-in** Do you think the minimal legal age for buying tobacco products should be raised to 21?

Factors other than age that are associated with reasons for smoking include the following

Limited Education   People who have graduated from college are much less likely to smoke than those with fewer than 12 years of education. An individual with 8 years or less of education is 11 times more likely to smoke than someone with postgraduate training.

Underestimation of Risks   Most people are aware that an enormous health risk is associated with smoking, but many don't know exactly what that risk is or how it might affect them. Young people who think the health risks of smoking are fairly low are more likely than their peers to start smoking.

Adolescent Experimentation and Rebellion   For teenagers, smoking may be a coping mechanism for dealing with boredom and frustration; a marker of the transition into high school or college; a bid for adult status or a way of gaining admission to a peer group. Adolescents may smoke as a means of gaining social acceptance or to self-medicate when they feel helpless, lonely, or depressed.

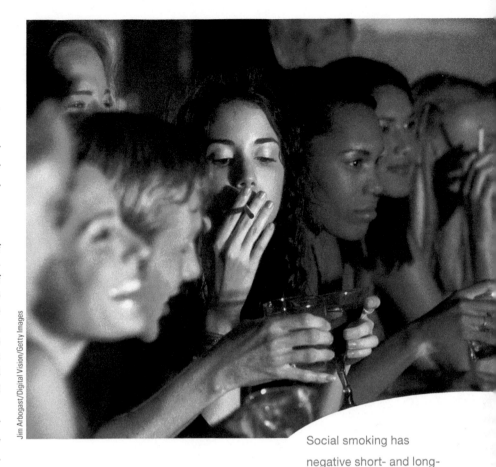

Jim Arbogast/Digital Vision/Getty Images

Social smoking has negative short- and long-term health effects and can lead to dependence.

Stress   In studies that have analyzed the impact of life stressors, depression, emotional support, marital status, and income, researchers have concluded that an individual with a high stress level is significantly more likely than a person with low stress to be a smoker.

Parent Role Models   Children who start smoking are 50 percent more likely than youngsters who don't smoke to have at least one smoker in their family. A mother who smokes seems to be a particularly strong influence in making smoking seem acceptable. The majority of youngsters who smoke say that their parents also smoke and are aware of their own tobacco use.

✓**check-in** Do your parents smoke? Did they smoke when you were growing up?

Addiction   Nicotine addiction is as strong as or stronger than addiction to drugs such as cocaine and heroin. The first symptoms of nicotine addiction can begin within a few days of starting to smoke and after just a few cigarettes, particularly in teenagers. (See Self Survey: "Are You Addicted to Nicotine?")

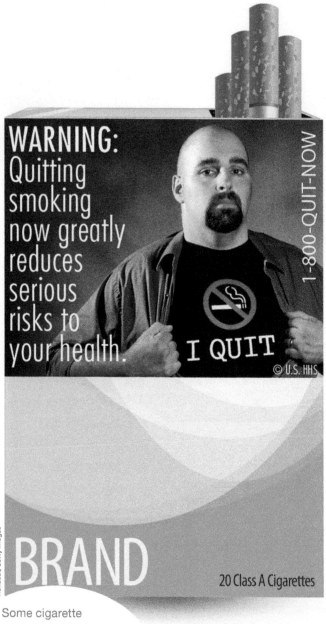

Some cigarette labels warn of the dangers of smoking; others emphasize the benefits of quitting.

tobacco use disorder A problematic pattern of tobacco use leading to clinically significant impairment or distress.

Genetics Researchers speculate that genes may account for about 50 percent of smoking behavior, with environment playing an equally important role. Studies have shown that identical twins, who have the same genes, are more likely than fraternal twins to have matching smoking profiles. If one identical twin is a heavy smoker, the other is also likely to be; if one smokes only occasionally, so does the other.

Weight Control Concern about weight is a significant risk factor for smoking among young women. Daily smokers are two to four times more likely to fast, use diet pills, and purge to control their weight than nonsmokers. Although black girls smoke at substantially lower rates than white girls, the common factor in predicting daily smoking among all girls, regardless of race, is concern with weight.

Mental Disorders About 38 percent of those with a mental illness or substance abuse disorder smoke.[8] People with mental illness account for nearly one-half of the tobacco market in the Unites States. Heavy smoking also is linked with an elevated risk of anxiety disorders in early adulthood.

Tobacco Use Disorder

In its *DSM-5*, the American Psychiatric Association defines a **tobacco use disorder** as "a problematic pattern of tobacco use leading to clinically significant impairment or distress," characterized by at least two of the following signs and symptoms within a 12-month period:

- Use of tobacco in larger amounts or over a longer period than was intended
- Persistent desire or unsuccessful efforts to cut down or control tobacco use
- A great deal of time spent in activities necessary to obtain or use tobacco
- Craving, or a strong desire or urge to use tobacco
- Interference with obligations at work, school, or home because of continued tobacco use
- Persistent or recurrent social or interpersonal problems, such as arguments about smoking, caused or exacerbated by tobacco
- Giving up or cutting back on important social, occupational, or recreational activities
- Recurrent tobacco use in physically hazardous situations, such as smoking in bed
- Continued tobacco use despite a persistent or recurrent physical or psychological problem caused or exacerbated by tobacco
- Tolerance, as indicated by a need for markedly increased amounts of tobacco to achieve the desired effect or a markedly diminished effect with continued use of the same amount of tobacco
- Withdrawal, as indicated by symptoms such as irritability, frustration, anger, anxiety, difficulty concentrating, increased appetite, restlessness, depressed mood, and insomnia, or use of tobacco or closely related substances to avoid such symptoms[9]

Cigarettes		Actual Use			Perceived Use		
Percent (%)		Male	Female	Total	Male	Female	Total
Never used		66.7	73.9	71.4	11.2	7.5	8.9
Used, but not in the last 30 days		18.1	15.5	16.4	15.9	13.5	14.3
Used 1–9 days		8.6	6.0	6.9	41.7	39.1	39.9
Used 10–29 days		2.6	1.5	1.9	17.0	19.7	18.8
Used all 30 days		3.9	3.0	3.4	14.2	20.1	18.2
Any use within the last 30 days		15.2	10.5	12.2	72.9	79.0	76.9

Source: American College Health Association. *American College Health Association-National College Health Assessment II: Reference Group Executive Summary Spring 2014.* Hanover, MD: American College Health Association, 2014.

✓**check-in** Have you experienced any of these symptoms?

Tobacco Use on Campus

About 12 percent of students report smoking in the previous 30 days. More than 7 in 10 have never smoked. (See Snapshot: On Campus Now.) Here is what we know about student smokers:

- Eight in 10 college smokers started smoking before age 18. They report smoking on twice as many days and smoke nearly four times as many cigarettes as those who began smoking at an older age.

- White students have the highest smoking rates, followed by Hispanic, Asian, and African American students. Although black students are least likely to smoke, more are doing so than in the past. Smoking rates remain lower at predominantly black colleges and universities, however.

- About equal percentages of college men and women smoke, although women are somewhat more likely than men to report smoking daily.

- Many college students say they smoke as a way of managing depression or stress. Studies consistently link smoking with depression and low life satisfaction. Smokers are significantly more likely to have higher levels of perceived stress than nonsmokers. The more depressed students, particularly women, are, the more likely they are to use nicotine as a form of self-medication.

- Male students who smoke are more likely than other men to say that smoking makes them feel more masculine and less anxious.

- More than half of female smokers feel that smoking helps them control their weight, although only 3 percent say it is their primary reason for smoking. Overweight female students are more likely to smoke to lose weight and to see weight gain as a barrier to quitting.

- Students can and do change their smoking behavior. As psychologists have noted, often those who quit smoking between ages 18 and 26 become less impulsive and negative over time, so they may "mature out" of this unhealthy behavior.

✓**check-in** How widespread is smoking on your campus?

Social Smoking

Some college students who smoke say they are "social smokers" who average less than one cigarette a day and smoke mainly in the company of others. On the positive side, social smokers smoke less often and less intensely than other smokers and are less dependent on tobacco.

However, they are still jeopardizing their health. The more they smoke, the greater the health risks they face. Even smokers who don't inhale or non-smokers who breathe in secondhand smoke are at increased risk for negative health effects. Here are some examples:

- Smoking less than a pack of cigarettes a week has been shown to damage the lining of blood vessels and to increase the risk of heart disease as well as of cancer.

- In women taking birth control pills, even a few cigarettes a week can increase the likelihood of heart disease, blood clots, stroke, liver cancer, and gallbladder disease.

- Pregnant women who smoke only occasionally still run an increased risk of giving birth to unhealthy babies.

- Social smokers are less motivated than smokers with tobacco use disorder to quit and make fewer attempts to do so. Many end up smoking more cigarettes for many more years than they intended.

✓**check-in** If you smoke, do you consider yourself a social smoker?

College Tobacco-Control Policies

The American College Health Association has recommended that all forms of tobacco be banned on college campuses, both indoors and outdoors. More than 1,300 schools have 100 percent smoke- or tobacco-free policies; others prohibit smoking everywhere but in designated areas.[10]

Universities that have banned smoking from designated residence halls report decreased damage to the buildings, increased retention of students, and improved enforcement of marijuana policies.

Enforcement of campus tobacco bans varies, and student smokers often ignore or disregard their schools' policies. Schools are experimenting with various ways to increase compliance, including passing out informational cards and training undergraduates as "ambassadors" to be advocates for no-tobacco policies.[11]

✓**check-in** Does your school ban tobacco entirely or in certain areas? Would you like to see more or fewer restrictions? Would you ask students smoking in a restricted area to put out their cigarettes?

Smoking, Gender, and Race

Almost 1 billion men in the world smoke—about 35 percent of men in developed countries and 50 percent of men in developing countries. Male smoking rates are slowly declining, but tobacco still kills about 5 million men every year. Men also face specific risks because smoking:

- Increases the risk of aggressive prostate cancer

- May affect male hormones, including testosterone

- Can reduce blood flow to the penis, impairing a man's sexual performance and increasing the likelihood of erectile dysfunction

About 20 million women and girls in the United States smoke. Women are as likely as men to die from smoking-related diseases. Their relative risk of dying from coronary heart disease is now higher than it is for men. Here are some other risks women face:

- More than 170,000 American women die of diseases caused by smoking every year.[12]

- Lung cancer now claims more women's lives than breast cancer. As discussed later in this chapter, both active and passive smoking increase a woman's risk of breast cancer.

- If she smokes, a woman's annual risk of dying more than doubles after age 45 compared with a woman who has never smoked.

- Teenage girls who smoke may be at increased risk of osteoporosis because girls who smoke build up less bone during this critical growth period in their lives.[13]

- Women who smoke are less fertile and experience menopause one or two years earlier than women who don't smoke. Smoking also greatly increases the possible risks associated with taking oral contraceptives.

- Women who smoke during pregnancy increase their risk of miscarriage and pregnancy complications, including bleeding, premature delivery, and birth defects such as cleft lip or palate. Smoking narrows the blood vessels and reduces blood flow to the fetus, resulting in lower birth weight, shorter length, smaller head circumference, and possibly lower IQ. Smoking may double or even triple the risk of stillbirth.[14]

- Youngsters whose mothers smoked during pregnancy tend to have problems with hyperactivity, inattention, and impulsivity. Some of these behavior problems persist through the teenage years into adulthood.

- Cigarette smoking is a major cause of disease and death in racial and ethnic minority groups. Among adults, Native Americans and Alaska Natives have the highest rates of tobacco use. African American and Southeast Asian men also have a high smoking rate. Asian American and Hispanic women have the lowest rates of smoking.

- Tobacco use is significantly higher among white college students than among Hispanic, African American, and Asian American students.

Tobacco's Immediate Effects

Tobacco, an herb that can be smoked or chewed, directly affects the brain. While its primary active ingredient is nicotine, tobacco smoke contains some 7,000 other compounds and chemicals, including gases, liquids, particles, tar, carbon monoxide, cadmium, pyridine, nitrogen dioxide, ammonia, benzene, phenol, acrolein, hydrogen cyanide, formaldehyde, and hydrogen sulfide.[15]

How Nicotine Works

A colorless, oily compound, **nicotine** is poisonous in concentrated amounts. If you inhale while smoking, 90 percent of the nicotine in the smoke is absorbed into your body. Even if you draw smoke only into your mouth and not into your lungs, you still absorb 25 to 30 percent of the nicotine. The FDA has concluded that nicotine is a dangerous, addictive drug that should be regulated. Yet in recent years tobacco companies have increased the levels of addictive nicotine.

Faster than an injection, smoking speeds nicotine to the brain in seconds (Figure 14.1). Nicotine affects the brain in much the same way as cocaine, opiates, and amphetamines, triggering the release of dopamine, a neurotransmitter associated with pleasure and addiction, as well as other messenger chemicals. Because nicotine acts on some of the same brain regions stimulated by interactions with loved ones, smokers subconsciously come to regard cigarettes as a friend that they turn to when they're stressed, sad, or mad.

Nicotine may enhance smokers' performance on some tasks but leaves other mental skills unchanged. Nicotine also acts as a sedative. How often you smoke and how you smoke determine nicotine's effect on you. If you're a regular smoker, nicotine will generally stimulate you at

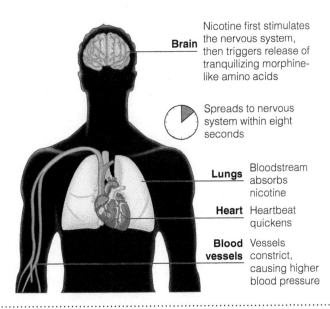

Brain Nicotine first stimulates the nervous system, then triggers release of tranquilizing morphine-like amino acids

Spreads to nervous system within eight seconds

Lungs Bloodstream absorbs nicotine

Heart Heartbeat quickens

Blood vessels Vessels constrict, causing higher blood pressure

FIGURE 14.1 The Immediate Effects of Nicotine on the Body

The primary active ingredient in tobacco is nicotine, a fast-acting and potent drug.

Sources: American Cancer Society, National Cancer Institute.

nicotine The addictive substance in tobacco; one of the most toxic of all poisons.

first and then tranquilize you. Shallow puffs tend to increase alertness because low doses of nicotine facilitate the release of the neurotransmitter *acetylcholine*, which makes the smoker feel alert. Deep drags, on the other hand, relax the smoker because high doses of nicotine block the flow of acetylcholine.

Nicotine stimulates the adrenal glands to produce adrenaline, a hormone that increases blood pressure, speeds up the heart rate by 15 to 20 beats a minute, and constricts blood vessels (especially in the skin). Nicotine also inhibits the formation of urine, dampens hunger, irritates the membranes in the mouth and throat, and dulls the taste buds so foods don't taste as good as they would otherwise.

Nicotine withdrawal usually begins within hours. Symptoms include craving, irritability, anxiety, restlessness, and increased appetite.

Tar and Carbon Monoxide

As it burns, tobacco produces **tar**, a thick, sticky dark fluid made up of several hundred different chemicals—many of them poisonous, some of them *carcinogenic* (enhancing the growth of cancerous cells). As you inhale tobacco smoke, tar and other particles settle in the forks of the branchlike bronchial tubes in your lungs, where precancerous changes are apt to occur. In addition, tar and smoke damage the mucus and the cilia in the bronchial tubes, which normally remove irritating foreign materials from your lungs.

Smoke from cigarettes, cigars, and pipes also contains **carbon monoxide**, the deadly gas that comes out of the exhaust pipes of cars, in levels 400 times those considered safe in industry. Carbon monoxide interferes with the ability of the hemoglobin in the blood to carry oxygen, impairs normal functioning of the nervous system, and is at least partly responsible for the increased risk of heart attacks and strokes in smokers.

tar A thick, sticky dark fluid produced by the burning of tobacco, made up of several hundred different chemicals, many of them poisonous, some of them carcinogenic.

carbon monoxide A colorless, odorless gas produced by the burning of gasoline or tobacco; it displaces oxygen in the hemoglobin molecules of red blood cells.

Health Effects of Cigarette Smoking

As many as 98 percent of tobacco-related deaths, including many due to secondhand smoke, are attributable to "combustible," or smokable, products.[56] Figure 14.2 shows a summary of the physiological effects of tobacco and the other chemicals in tobacco smoke. If you're a smoker who inhales deeply and started smoking before age 15, you're trading a minute of future life for every minute you now spend smoking.

Health Effects on Students

An estimated 6.4 million young people will eventually suffer premature death or diminished quality of life, or both, as a result of smoking-related diseases:

- Although little research has focused specifically on college students, young people who smoke are less physically fit and suffer diminished lung function and growth.

- Young smokers frequently report symptoms such as wheezing, shortness of breath, coughing, and increased phlegm. They also are more susceptible to respiratory diseases.

- Young adults who smoke are three times more likely to have consulted a doctor or mental health professional because of an emotional or psychological problem and almost twice as likely to develop symptoms of depression.

- Frequent smoking has been linked to panic attacks and panic disorder in young people.

- Long-term health consequences of smoking in young adulthood include dental problems, lung disorders (including asthma, chronic bronchitis, and emphysema), heart disease, and cancer.

- Young women who smoke may develop menstrual problems, including irregular periods and painful cramps. If they use oral contraceptives, they are at increased risk of heart disease or stroke.

- Male smokers suffer a more rapid decline in brain function as they age so that early-dementia-like symptoms may appear as early as age 45.

√**check-in** If you smoke, have you experienced any effects on your health?

Premature Death

Smoking kills, robbing smokers of a decade of life. Mortality among current smokers is two to three times as high as that of people who never smoked. Research has tied the higher death rates to 21 diseases proven to be caused by smoking. However, a long-term analysis has found that smoking also may increase the risk of dying by contributing to other diseases, including kidney failure, infections, various respiratory disorders, breast cancer, and prostate cancer.[16]

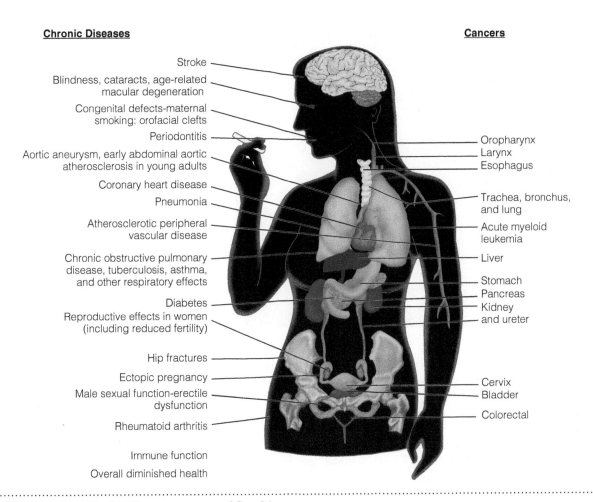

Stroke

Blindness, cataracts, age-related
macular degeneration

Congenital defects-maternal
smoking: orofacial clefts

Periodontitis

Aortic aneurysm, early abdominal aortic
atherosclerosis in young adults

Coronary heart disease

Pneumonia

Atherosclerotic peripheral
vascular disease

Chronic obstructive pulmonary
disease, tuberculosis, asthma,
and other respiratory effects

Diabetes

Reproductive effects in women
(including reduced fertility)

Hip fractures

Ectopic pregnancy

Male sexual function-erectile
dysfunction

Rheumatoid arthritis

Immune function

Overall diminished health

Oropharynx
Larynx
Esophagus

Trachea, bronchus,
and lung

Acute myeloid
leukemia

Liver

Stomach
Pancreas
Kidney
and ureter

Cervix
Bladder

Colorectal

FIGURE 14.2 The Health Consequences of Smoking

Source: The Health Consequences of Smoking—50 Years of Progress: A Report of the Surgeon General. Atlanta, GA: U.S. Department of Health and Human Services, Centers for Disease Control and Prevention, National Center for Chronic Disease Prevention and Health Promotion, Office on Smoking and Health, 2014

Smoking's effect on your chance of dying is similar to adding five to ten years to your age. A 55-year-old man or woman who smokes has about the same risk of dying in the next decade as a 65-year-old who never smoked. Smoking is responsible for 64 percent of deaths in current smokers and 28 percent in past smokers.

A cigarette smoker is

- 10 times more likely to develop lung cancer than a nonsmoker,

- 20 times more likely to have a heart attack,

- if female, more likely to develop breast cancer,

- more likely to have suicidal thoughts or attempt suicide.

Heart Disease and Stroke

Although a great deal of publicity has been given to the link between cigarettes and lung cancer, heart attack is actually the leading cause of death

for smokers. The federal Office of the Surgeon General blames cigarettes for 1 in every 10 deaths attributable to heart disease.

Smoking is more dangerous than the two most notorious risk factors for heart disease: high blood pressure and high cholesterol. If smoking is combined with one of these, the chances of heart attack are four times greater. Women who smoke and use oral contraceptives have a 10 times greater risk of suffering heart attacks than women who do neither. In addition to contributing to heart attacks, cigarette smoking increases the risk of stroke two to three times in men and women, even after other risk factors are taken into account.

The toxic chemicals in tobacco signal the heart to beat faster and harder. Blood vessels constrict, forcing blood to travel through a narrower space. Here are some of the consequences:

- Blood pressure increases—temporarily at first. Over time, smokers develop chronic high blood pressure.

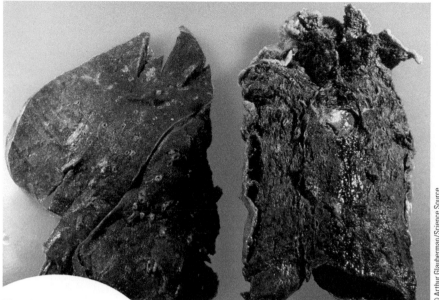

Healthy nonsmoker's lung (left) and smoker's lung (right). Healthy lungs are pink, with a smooth but porous texture. A smoker's lungs show obvious signs of impairment. Bronchial tubes are inflamed, air passages are constricted, and tar coats the bronchial tubes.

© Arthur Glauberman/Science Source

- Smoking increases harmful cholesterol (LDL); lowers beneficial cholesterol (HDL); promotes the buildup of plaque, or fatty deposits, within the arteries; and increases the risk of blood clots.

- Both current and former smokers have an increased risk for an abnormal heart rhythm.

- Smoking doubles the risk of heart disease and increases the risk of sudden death two to four times. The effect of smoking on risk of heart attack is greater in younger smokers. The number of cigarettes smoked daily may have a greater impact on the cardiovascular system than total years of smoking.

- Smokers who suffer heart attacks have only a 50 percent chance of recovering.

- Smokers have a 70 percent higher death rate from heart disease than nonsmokers, and those who smoke heavily have a 200 percent higher death rate.

Even people who have smoked for decades can reduce their risk of heart attack if they quit smoking. However, studies indicate some irreversible damage to blood vessels. Progression of atherosclerosis (hardening of the arteries) among former smokers continues at a faster pace than among those who never smoked.

Cancer

Smoking is linked to at least 10 different cancers and accounts for 30 percent of all deaths from cancer:

- Smoking is the cause of more than 80 percent of all cases of lung cancer. The more people

smoke, the longer they smoke, and the earlier they start smoking, the more likely they are to develop lung cancer. At highest risk are those who have accumulated 30 "pack-years" of smoking—for example, by smoking 20 cigarettes a day for 30 years.[17]

- Smoking causes about 130,000 lung cancer deaths each year. Smokers of two or more packs a day have lung cancer mortality rates 15 to 25 times greater than nonsmokers. If smokers stop smoking before cancer has started, their lung tissue tends to repair itself, even if there were already precancerous changes. However, their risk is never as low as that of individuals who never smoked.

- Cigarette smoking is associated with stomach and duodenal ulcers and with mouth, throat, and other types of cancer, including deadly bladder cancers.[18]

- Based on recent studies, liver cancer and colorectal cancer have been added to the long list of cancers caused by smoking.[19]

- The risk of breast cancer increases among women who smoke, especially among those who start smoking early.

Respiratory Diseases

Smoking quickly impairs the respiratory system, including the cough reflex, a vital protective response. Cigarette smokers are up to 18 times more likely than nonsmokers to die of noncancerous diseases of the lungs. Even some teenage smokers show signs of respiratory difficulty—breathlessness, chronic cough, excess phlegm production—compared with nonsmokers of the same age.

Cigarette smokers tend to miss work one-third more often than nonsmokers, primarily because of respiratory illnesses. The link between smoking and asthma has proven stronger than suspected, and individuals with asthma are much more likely to have a history of nicotine dependence.

Cigarette smoking is the major cause of chronic obstructive pulmonary disease (COPD), which includes emphysema and chronic bronchitis:

- COPD is characterized by progressive limitation of the flow of air into and out of the lungs.

- In emphysema, the limitation of air flow is the result of disease changes in the lung tissue, affecting the bronchioles (the smallest air passages) and the walls of the alveoli (the tiny air sacs of the lung). Eventually, many of the air sacs are destroyed, and the lungs become much less able to bring in oxygen and remove carbon dioxide. As a result, the heart has to work harder to deliver oxygen to all organs of the body.

- In chronic bronchitis, the bronchial tubes in the lungs become inflamed, thickening the walls of the bronchi, and the production of mucus increases. The result is a narrowing of the air passages.

....
√**check-in** Do you know anyone who has developed smoking-related illnesses?
....

Other Smoking-Related Problems

Smoking, which affects almost every organ system in the body, has other harmful effects. It:

- Can cause diabetes mellitus and rheumatoid arthritis[20]

- Contributes to gum disease and the loss of teeth and teeth-supporting bone, even in individuals with good oral hygiene

- Worsens the symptoms or complications of allergies, hypertension, cirrhosis of the liver, peptic ulcers, and disorders of the lungs or blood vessels

- Is an independent risk factor for high-frequency hearing loss and adds to the danger of hearing loss for those exposed to noise

- May increase the likelihood of anxiety, panic attacks, and social phobias

- May cause fires that claim thousands of lives

Emerging Tobacco Products

Cigarettes remain the most widely used form of tobacco, but more college students are trying new or "emerging" tobacco products, such as electronic cigarettes and hookahs (water pipes).[21] Some use multiple products, including cigarettes, bidis, clove cigarettes, smokeless tobacco, and snus.[22] "Polytobacco use" is more likely than any single form of tobacco to lead to nicotine addiction as well as additional health risks.[23]

Electronic Cigarettes

E-cigarettes are battery-powered devices that deliver aerosolized nicotine and additives flavored with chocolate, mint, candy, and other sweetness.

Designed to mimic the look and feel of smoking, they are marketed as a relatively benign alternative to cigarettes, without tar, carbon monoxide, and other harmful ingredients. "Vaping," the term for using e-cigarettes, comes from the cloud of vapor released by electronic cigarettes.[24] More than 100 brands are available, and sales have soared into the billions of dollars.

In a recent survey of students at four colleges/universities, more than 9 in 10 were aware of e-cigarettes; 30 percent had tried them at some point, and 15 percent were current users. While e-cigarettes were not usually the first tobacco product students tried, those who tried them were more likely to use cigarettes, other forms of tobacco, alcohol, and marijuana.[25]

Cigarette smokers report being attracted to e-cigarettes for several reasons, including lower cost, perceived lesser danger, freedom to use them in some places where cigarettes are banned, and enjoyment of the "smoking experience."

Researchers have found that puffing on e-cigarettes produces airway constriction and inflammation, which might lead to serious lung diseases such as emphysema. Other potential risks include headache, cough, dizziness, sore throat, nose bleeds, chest pain or other cardiovascular problems, and allergic reactions such as itchiness and swelling of the lips.

E-cigarettes also might have harmful effects on the developing brain as well as on the respiratory system and overall health of young users.[26] According to a recent review, "e-cigarettes may provide a less harmful source of nicotine than traditional cigarettes, but evidence of decreased harm with long-term use is not available."[27] (See Consumer Alert.)

Water Pipes (Hookahs)

A water pipe (known by different terms, such as hookah, narghile, arghile, and hubble-bubble, in different parts of the world) allows smoke to pass through water prior to inhalation. Although also used to smoke other substances, including marijuana and hashish, water pipes are most often used with flavored tobacco, made by mixing shredded tobacco with honey or molasses and dried fruit. This mix is most commonly called *shisha* in the United States. New forms of electronic hookah smoking include steam stones and hookah pens.

Water-pipe smoking usually occurs in a group setting. Commercial water-pipe venues, offering ready-to-smoke water pipes, have proliferated in many college towns.

In various surveys, 10 to 16 percent of Americans report ever having smoked a water pipe tobacco.[28] An estimated 15 to 41 percent of college

E-cigarettes

Electronic cigarettes first emerged as a form of nicotine substitution to help cigarette smokers break their habit. The first generation of "cigalikes," designed to look like conventional cigarettes, restricted the number of puffs and offered limited flavors. More sophisticated devices, perceived as more stylish and equipped with lithium batteries, deliver nicotine more efficiently. Vaping has gained popularity not just among smokers but also among adolescents and young adults, including many who have never smoked cigarettes.[29]

Facts to Know

- The sale, use, and advertising of e-cigarettes are permitted in the United States, but some individual states have imposed restrictions.

- There is not yet enough research to show whether e-cigarettes are any more or less toxic than traditional ones.

- E-cigarette smokers report mouth and throat irritation and dry cough with continuing use, and physiological tests reveal changes in respiratory function similar to those caused by cigarette smoking.

- Other potential risks include headache, cough, dizziness, sore throat, nosebleeds, chest pain or other cardiovascular problems, and allergic reaction such as itchiness and swelling of the lips.

- E-cigarette refill cartridges may contain toxic amounts of nicotine, which can remain on surfaces for weeks to months. This "environmental electronic smoke" may create the same dangers associated with secondhand and thirdhand smoke[30] (see page 435).

Steps to Take

- If you are not a smoker, don't try electronic cigarettes as a "healthier" alternative. There is no safe form of tobacco use.

- If you are trying to quit smoking, e-cigarettes may lessen symptoms such as irritability, but it is not yet known whether they help with long-term abstinence.

- Advertisements for e-cigarettes or depictions of vaping serve as visual cues that can trigger nicotine cravings in smokers and former smokers.[31]

- If you try e-cigarettes, use caution. There have been reports of the devices overheating, igniting, or exploding.

students have used a hookah.[32] (See Table 14.1.) Characteristics of users include the following:

- Male
- 18 to 24 years old
- White and, in some studies, Hispanic/Latino[33]
- Some college education
- Belonging to a sexual minority[34]
- Also using cigarettes, cigars, and other tobacco products

Many hookah smokers believe that water pipes pose less risk of tobacco-related disease than cigarettes. However, hookah smoke contains many of the same harmful toxins as cigarette smoke, including tar, carcinogens, hydrocarbons, and heavy metals. They can lead to dependence, heart disease, lung cancer, respiratory illness, low birth weight, and periodontal disease.[35]

The health effects of hookah use include these:

Short-term

- Increased heart rate
- Increased blood pressure
- Impaired lung function
- Carbon monoxide intoxication

Long-term

- Chronic bronchitis
- Emphysema
- Coronary artery disease
- Periodontal (gum) disease
- Osteoporosis
- Increased risk of lung, stomach, and esophageal cancer.[36]

Here are some of the facts you need to know about hookah use:

- The charcoal used to heat tobacco in the hookah produces smoke that contains high levels of carbon monoxide, metals, and cancer-causing chemicals.

- A hookah smoking session may expose the smoker to more smoke over a longer period of time than occurs when smoking a cigarette. The volume of smoke inhaled during a typical hookah session is about 90,000 milliliters, compared with 500 to 600 milliliters inhaled when smoking a cigarette.

- A typical one-hour-long hookah smoking session involves 200 puffs; smoking a cigarette, 20 puffs. Hookah smokers may absorb higher concentrations of the same toxins found in cigarettes.

TABLE 14.1 Tobacco from a Water Pipe (Hookah)

Percent (%)	Actual Use			Perceived Use		
	Male	Female	Average	Male	Female	Average
Never used	63.2	69.3	67.2	14.9	10.5	12.1
Used, but not in the last 30 days	26.4	23.1	24.2	20.7	18.1	19.0
Used 1–9 days	9.0	6.8	7.6	48.9	50.5	49.9
Used 10–29 days	1.0	0.6	0.7	10.9	15.2	13.7
Used all 30 days	0.4	0.1	0.3	4.6	5.6	5.3
Any use within the last 30 days	10.4	7.6	8.6	64.4	71.4	68.9

Source: American College Health Association. *American College Health Association-National College Health Assessment II: Reference Group Executive Summary Spring 2014.* Hanover, MD: American College Health Association, 2014).

Maksim Shmeljov/Shutterstock.com

- In a recent meta-analysis, water-pipe smoking was significantly associated with lung cancer, respiratory illnesses, low birth weight, and periodontal disease.
- In a six-month follow-up among college students, hookah users reported smoking more cigarettes more often over time.[37] When those who smoke both hookah and cigarettes try to quit, they have lower success rates than cigarette smokers.[38]

Other Forms of Tobacco

Two percent of Americans smoke cigars; 2 percent use smokeless tobacco. Ingesting tobacco may be less deadly than smoking cigarettes, but it is dangerous. Smoking cigars, clove cigarettes, and pipes and chewing or sucking on smokeless tobacco all put the user at risk of cancer of the lip, tongue, mouth, and throat, as well as other diseases and ailments. Despite claims of lower risk, "safer" cigarettes still jeopardize smokers' health.

Cigars

Cigar use has declined in the past few years. However, after cigarettes, cigars are the tobacco product most widely used by college students:

- About 16 percent of college men (and 4 percent of women) smoke cigars.
- White and African American students are more likely to smoke cigars than Hispanic or Asian American students.
- About 4 in 10 cigar smokers—particularly those who are female, younger, and less wealthy—report using flavored cigars.[39]

Even though cigar smokers may not inhale, a byproduct of nicotine called cotinine builds up. Cigars can cause cancer of the lung and the digestive tract. The risk of death related to cigars approaches that of cigarettes, depending on the number of cigars smoked and the amount of cigar smoke inhaled.

✓**check-in** Do you think that pipes or cigars are "healthier" alternatives to cigarettes?

Pipes

Many cigarette smokers switch to pipes to reduce their risk of health problems. But former cigarette smokers may continue to inhale, even though pipe smoke is more irritating to the respiratory system than cigarette smoke. People who have smoked only pipes and who do not inhale are less likely to develop lung and heart disease than cigarette smokers. However, they are likely to suffer respiratory problems and to develop—and die of—cancer of the mouth, larynx, throat, and esophagus.

Bidis

Skinny, sweet-flavored cigarettes called **bidis** (pronounced "beedees") have become a smoking fad among teens and young adults. For centuries, bidis were popular in India, where they are known as the poor man's cigarette and sell for less than five cents a pack. They look strikingly like clove cigarettes or marijuana joints and are available in flavors like grape, strawberry, and mandarin orange. Bidis are legal for adults and even minors in some states and are sold on the Internet as well as in stores.

Although bidis contain less tobacco than regular cigarettes, their unprocessed tobacco is more potent. Smoke from bidis has about three times as much nicotine and carbon monoxide and five times as much tar as smoke from regular filtered cigarettes. Because bidis are wrapped in nonporous brownish leaves, they don't burn as easily as cigarettes, and smokers have to inhale harder and more often to keep them lit. In one study, smoking a single bidi required 28 puffs, compared to 9 puffs for a cigarette.

Clove Cigarettes (Kreteks)

Sweeteners have long been mixed with tobacco, and clove, a spice, is an ingredient commonly added to the recipe for cigarettes. Clove cigarettes typically contain two-thirds tobacco and one-third clove. Consumers of these cigarettes are primarily teenagers and young adults.

Many users believe that clove cigarettes are safer because they contain less tobacco, but this isn't necessarily the case. The CDC reports that people who smoke clove cigarettes may be at risk of serious lung injury. Regular kretek smokers have 13 to 20 times the risk for abnormal lung function as nonsmokers.[40]

Clove cigarettes deliver twice as much nicotine, tar, and carbon monoxide as moderate-tar American brands. Eugenol, the active ingredient in cloves (which dentists have used as an anesthetic for years), deadens sensation in the throat, allowing smokers to inhale more deeply and hold smoke in their lungs for a longer time. Chemical relatives of eugenol can produce the kind of damage to cells that may lead to cancer.

bidis Skinny, sweet-flavored cigarettes.

Smokeless Tobacco

An estimated 3 percent of adults in the United States use smokeless tobacco products (sometimes called "spit"). Use of chewing tobacco by teenage boys, particularly in rural areas, has surged 30 percent in the past decade. About 9 percent of college men (and 0.4 percent of women) use smokeless tobacco. These substances include snuff, finely ground tobacco that can be sniffed or placed inside the cheek and sucked; and chewing tobacco, tobacco leaves mixed with flavoring agents such as molasses. With both, nicotine is absorbed through the mucous membranes of the nose or mouth.

Smokeless tobacco causes a user's heart rate, blood pressure, and epinephrine (adrenaline) levels to jump. In addition, it can cause cancer and noncancerous oral conditions and lead to nicotine addiction and dependence. People who use smokeless tobacco, or "snuff," become just as hooked on nicotine as cigarette smokers—if not more. Those who both smoke and use snuff may be especially nicotine dependent.

Powerful carcinogens in smokeless tobacco include nitrosamines, polycyclic aromatic hydrocarbons, and radiation-emitting polonium. Its use can lead to the development of white patches on the mucous membranes of the mouth, particularly on the site where the tobacco is placed. Most lesions of the mouth lining that result from the use of smokeless tobacco dissipate six weeks after the use of the tobacco product is stopped. However, when first found, about 5 percent of these lesions are cancerous or exhibit changes that progress to cancer within 10 years if not properly treated. Cancers of the lip, pharynx, larynx, and esophagus have all been linked to smokeless tobacco. Nicotine replacement with gum or patches decreases cravings for smokeless tobacco and helps with short-term abstinence. However, it does not improve long-term abstinence. Behavioral approaches are more effective for long-term quitting.

Snus

Snus (rhymes with "loose") is a smokeless tobacco product similar to snuff and chewing tobacco. It was originally developed in Sweden and banned elsewhere in Europe, but tobacco companies have introduced snus in the United States in recent years.

Users, generally white males between the ages of 18 and 24, pack snus under their upper lip and then swallow the byproduct rather than spit it out. Snus may pose less of a cancer risk than other forms of tobacco, but this does not mean that it is risk-free.[41]

Quitting Tobacco Use

The U.S. Public Health Service's most recent guidelines for treating tobacco use and dependence recognize tobacco dependence as "a chronic disease that often requires repeated intervention and multiple attempts to quit." Once a former smoker takes a single puff, the odds of a relapse are 80 to 85 percent. Smokers are most likely to quit in the third, fourth, or fifth attempt. Numbers show the difficulty of quitting, but there are effective treatments:

- More than half of all smokers attempt to quit each year, but only about 7 percent achieve long-term abstinence.[42]

- About half of whites who have smoked eventually were able to kick the habit, compared with 45 percent of Asian Americans, 43 percent of Hispanics, and 37 percent of African Americans. About 8 in 10 African Americans choose menthol cigarettes, compared with just one-quarter of adults of other races, which may make quitting harder.

- Smokers who work with a counselor specially trained to help them quit and who also use medications or nicotine patches or gum are three times more likely to kick the habit than smokers who try to quit without any help, according to a large recent study.[43]

Physical Benefits of Quitting

Young adults who quit smoking see improvements in coughing and other respiratory symptoms within a few weeks, according to a recent study of college students ages 18 to 24. Quitting eliminates the excess risk of dying from heart disease fairly quickly. After 15 smoke-free years, the risk of smoking-related cancers drops to that of someone who never smoked. (See Table 14.2 for a more complete list of reasons to quit smoking.)

Psychological Benefits of Quitting

Quitting may be as good for your mental health as it is for your physical health, according to analysis

Snus A smokeless tobacco product similar to snuff and chewing tobacco.

of three years of data on 4,800 daily smokers in the United States. Significantly fewer of those who quit were less likely to report alcohol or drug problems or anxiety or depression than those who continued to smoke.[44]

Quitting on Your Own

More than 90 percent of former smokers quit on their own—by throwing away all their cigarettes, by gradually cutting down, or by first switching to a less potent brand. One characteristic of successful quitters is that they see themselves as active participants in health maintenance and take personal responsibility for their own health.

Physically active smokers have greater success quitting, possibly because participating in one healthy behavior, such as exercise, leads to adoption of other positive behaviors. Often they experiment with a variety of strategies, such as learning relaxation techniques. In women, exercise has proved especially effective for quitting and avoiding weight gain. Making a home a smoke-free zone also increases a smoker's likelihood of successfully quitting.

Virtual Support

Electronic communications via cell phones, e-mails, text messages, blogs, and social networking sites may be particularly effective in helping young smokers quit. In the few research studies that have been done, these approaches generally resulted in higher quitting rates—but only if continued over time. Short text messages can help individuals track their smoking urges and provide encouragement in resisting them. Other options include apps for smart phones and online support groups.

Stop-Smoking Groups

Joining a support group doubles your chances of quitting for good. Options include the American Cancer Society's Freshstart program, the American Lung Association's Freedom from Smoking program, stop-smoking classes (available through student health services on many college campuses as well as through community public health departments), and commercial smoking-cessation programs.

Some smoking-cessation programs rely primarily on **aversion therapy**, which provides a negative experience every time a smoker has a cigarette. This may involve taking drugs that make tobacco smoke taste unpleasant, undergoing electric shocks, having smoke blown at you, or rapid smoking (inhaling smoke every six seconds until you're dizzy or nauseated).

TABLE 14.2 Why Quit?

Quitting is the smartest choice a smoker can make—and keeps paying off far into the future. Consider these facts:
• **20 minutes after quitting:** Your heart rate and blood pressure drop.
• **12 hours after quitting:** The carbon monoxide level in your blood drops to normal.
• **2 weeks to 3 months after quitting:** Your circulation improves and your lung function increases.
• **1 to 9 months after quitting:** Coughing and shortness of breath decrease; cilia (tiny hairlike structures that move mucus out of the lungs) regain normal function, increasing the ability to handle mucus, clean the lungs, and reduce the risk of infection.
• **1 year after quitting:** Your excess risk of coronary heart disease is half that of a smoker's.
• **5 years after quitting:** Your stroke risk is reduced to that of a nonsmoker.
• **10 years after quitting:** The lung cancer death rate is about half that of a continuing smoker's. Your risks of cancers of the mouth, throat, esophagus, bladder, cervix, and pancreas also decrease.
• **15 to 20 years after quitting:** Your risk of coronary heart disease is that of a nonsmoker's.

Source: American Cancer Society.

Nicotine Anonymous, a nonprofit organization based on the 12 Steps to recovery developed by Alcoholics Anonymous, acknowledges the power of nicotine and provides support to help smokers, chewers, and dippers live free of nicotine.

Nicotine Replacement Therapy (NRT)

NRT uses a variety of products that supply low doses of nicotine in a way that allows smokers to taper off gradually over a period of months. Nicotine replacement therapies include nonprescription products (nicotine gum, lozenges, nicotine-free cigarettes, and nicotine patches) and prescription products (nicotine nasal spray, nicotine inhalers, and e-cigarettes).

The nasal spray, dispensed from a pump bottle, delivers nicotine to the nasal membranes and reaches the bloodstream faster than any other nicotine replacement therapy product. The inhaler delivers nicotine into the mouth and enters the bloodstream much more slowly than the nicotine in cigarettes. Electronic cigarettes, or e-cigarettes, mimic the experience of smoking, right down to the glowing tip and smokelike vapor.

The FDA has approved the use of nicotine replacement gums, lozenges, and skin patches for a longer period of time.[45] None of these smoking cessation therapies appear to raise the risk of serious cardiovascular disease events.[46] Although not without some risks, these products are substantially less dangerous than cigarettes and other combustible forms of tobacco.

aversion therapy A treatment that attempts to help a person overcome a dependence or bad habit by making the person feel disgusted or repulsed by that habit.

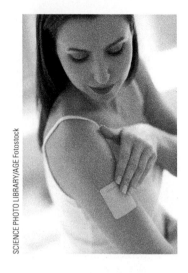

SCIENCE PHOTO LIBRARY/AGE Fotostock

A nicotine patch releases nicotine through the skin in measured amounts, which are gradually decreased over time.

environmental tobacco smoke Secondhand cigarette smoke; the third-leading preventable cause of death.

mainstream smoke The smoke inhaled directly by smoking a cigarette.

sidestream smoke The smoke emitted by a burning cigarette and breathed by everyone in a closed room, including the smoker; contains more tar and nicotine than mainstream smoke.

Although NRT is touted as an aid to permanent cessation of smoking, recent studies have found equivalent rates of relapse among smokers, regardless of whether they used nicotine replacement therapy, with or without professional counseling. Pregnant women and individuals with heart disease shouldn't use nicotine replacements.

The most effective approaches combine medication—nicotine patches or Zyban, for instance—with psychological intervention. Each doubles a person's chance of quitting successfully. Nicotine replacement therapy has proved more beneficial for men than for women—particularly with higher doses of nicotine.

Nicotine Gum   Nicotine gum (available as less expensive generic forms as well) contains a nicotine resin that's gradually released as the gum is chewed. Absorbed through the mucous membrane of the mouth, the nicotine doesn't produce the same rush as a deeply inhaled drag on a cigarette. However, the gum maintains enough nicotine in the blood to diminish withdrawal symptoms.

Although this gum is lightly spiced to mask nicotine's bitterness, many users say that it takes several days to become accustomed to its unusual taste. Its side effects include mild indigestion, sore jaws, nausea, heartburn, and stomachache. Also, because nicotine gum is heavier than regular chewing gum, it may loosen fillings or cause problems with dentures. Drinking coffee or other beverages may block absorption of the nicotine in the gum; individuals trying to quit smoking shouldn't ingest any substance immediately before or while chewing nicotine gum.

Most people use nicotine gum as a temporary crutch and gradually taper off until they can stop chewing it relatively painlessly. However, 5 to 10 percent of users transfer their dependence from cigarettes to the gum. When they stop using nicotine gum, they experience withdrawal symptoms, although the symptoms tend to be milder than those prompted by quitting cigarettes. Intensive counseling to teach smokers coping methods can greatly increase success rates.

Nicotine Patches   Nicotine transdermal delivery system products, or patches, provide nicotine, their only active ingredient, via a patch attached to the skin by an adhesive. Like nicotine gum, the nicotine patch minimizes withdrawal symptoms, such as intense craving for cigarettes. Nicotine patches help nearly 20 percent of smokers quit entirely after six weeks, compared with 7 percent on a placebo patch. Some insurance programs pay for patch therapy. Nicotine patches, which cost between $3.25 and $4 each, are replaced daily during therapy programs that run between 6 and 16 weeks. Extended use for 24 weeks provides added benefit.

Some patches deliver nicotine around the clock and others for just 16 hours (during waking hours). Those most likely to benefit from nicotine patch therapy are people who smoke more than a pack a day, are highly motivated to quit, and participate in counseling programs. While using the patch, 37 to 77 percent of people are able to abstain from smoking. When combined with counseling, the patch can be about twice as effective as a placebo, enabling 26 percent of smokers to abstain for six months. Occasional side effects include redness, itching, or swelling at the site of the patch application; insomnia; dry mouth; and nervousness.

Nicotine Inhaler   Available only by prescription, a nicotine inhaler consists of a mouthpiece and a cartridge containing a nicotine-impregnated plug. The smoker inhales through the mouthpiece, using either shallow or deep puffs. The inhaled air becomes saturated with nicotine, which is absorbed mainly through the tissues of the mouth. The inhaler releases less nicotine per puff than a cigarette and does not contain a cigarette's harmful tars, carbon monoxide, and smoke. Treatment is recommended for 3 months, with a gradual reduction over the next 6 to 12 weeks. Total treatment should not exceed 6 months.

Medications

Another alternative to the patch is *bupropion*, a drug initially developed to treat depression, that is marketed in a slow-release form for nicotine addiction as Zyban. In studies that have combined Zyban with nicotine replacement and counseling, 40 to 60 percent of those treated have remained smoke-free for at least a year after completing the program. This success rate is much higher than the 10 to 26 percent reported among smokers who try to quit by using nicotine replacement alone. For women, combining medication with behavioral therapy to address weight issues has proven effective. The combination of Zyban and nicotine replacement also prevented the initial weight gain that often accompanies quitting.

Another medication used to treat nicotine addiction is varenicline (Chantix), which may be more effective if taken for several weeks prior to quitting. It may be most effective combined with bupropion (Zyban or Wellbutrin) because the two drugs act in different ways.

Other Ways to Quit

Hypnosis may help some people quit smoking. Hypnotherapists use their techniques to create an atmosphere of strict attention and give smokers

- Because of its toxic effects on the heart and blood vessels, it may increase the risk of heart disease by an estimated 25 to 30 percent and cause about 46,000 heart disease deaths a year.

- Secondhand smoke may increase the risk of developing Alzheimer's disease or other dementias.

- Children are particularly vulnerable to secondhand smoke, beginning before birth. Prenatal exposure to tobacco can affect a child's growth, cognitive development, and behavior both before and after birth. Birth weight decreases in direct proportion to the number of cigarettes a mother smoked. As they grow, children of smokers tend to be shorter and weigh less than those of non-smokers. They also are at greater risk of heart disease as adults.[48]

✓**check-in** How would you describe your lifetime exposure to secondhand smoke?

Thirdhand Smoke

Thirdhand smoke is the nicotine residue that is left behind on furniture, walls, and carpet after a cigarette has been smoked in a room. According to scientists, particulates made up of ozone and nicotine can become airborne a second time and, because they are so small, easily penetrate into the deepest parts of the lung.

Thirdhand smoke remains in houses, apartments, and hotel rooms even after smokers move out.[49] The toxins it contains can enter the body by breathing, ingestion, or skin absorption.[50] Among the effects on nonsmokers is an increased risk of breathing problems and cancer.[51] The danger may be greatest to infants, children, pregnant women, and the elderly.

The Fight for Clean Air

Nonsmokers, realizing that their health is being jeopardized by environmental tobacco smoke, have increasingly turned to legislative and administrative measures to clear the air and protect their rights (Figure 14.4). Most states now have some restrictions on smoking in bars, restaurants, and workplaces. Nationally, the airlines have banned smoking on domestic flights. Many institutions, including medical centers and some universities, no longer allow smoking on their premises. States that have launched comprehensive antismoking programs, including higher cigarette taxes and a media campaign, have lowered smoking prevalence and secondhand smoke levels.

Community smoking policies can affect smoking by college students. In a recent study, undergraduates smoked less, and less often, after a city-wide ban on indoor smoking in restaurants, bars, and music clubs.[52]

✓**check-in** If you smoke, how do no-tobacco laws affect how much and how often you smoke? If you are not a smoker, do you think such restrictions are effective in reducing others' smoking?

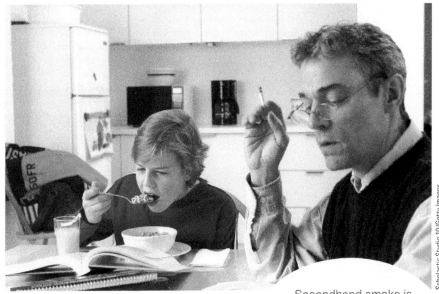

Secondhand smoke is the most common and hazardous form of indoor air pollution.

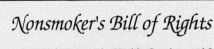

Nonsmoker's Bill of Rights

Nonsmokers Help Protect the Health, Comfort, and Safety of Everyone by Insisting on the Following Rights:

The Right to Breathe Clean Air

Nonsmokers have the right to breathe clean air, free from harmful and irritating tobacco smoke. This right supersedes the right to smoke when the two conflict.

The Right to Speak Out

Nonsmokers have the right to express — firmly but politely — their discomfort and adverse reactions to tobacco smoke. They have the right to voice their objections when smokers light up without asking permission.

The Right to Act

Nonsmokers have the right to take action through legislative means — as individuals or in groups — to prevent or discourage smokers from polluting the atmosphere and to seek the restriction of smoking in public places.

FIGURE 14.4 Nonsmoker's Bill of Rights

- Why do people smoke even when they're aware of the risks?
- What are the short- and long-term effects of tobacco on health?
- Are "emerging tobacco products" like electronic cigarettes and hookahs safe to use?
- Why are second- and third-hand smoke a danger to nonsmokers' health?

THE POWER OF NOW!
Becoming Smoke-Free

If you smoke—even just a few cigarettes a few times a week—you are at risk of nicotine addiction. Check the steps you will take to get back into control:

____ Delaying tactics. Have your first cigarette of the day 15 minutes later than usual, then 15 minutes later than that the next day, and so on.

____ Distracting yourself. When you feel a craving for a cigarette, talk to someone, drink a glass of water, or get up and move around.

____ Establishing nonsmoking hours. Instead of lighting up at the end of a meal, for instance, get up immediately, brush your teeth, wash your hands, or take a walk.

____ Never smoking two packs of the same brand in a row. Buy cigarettes only by the pack, not by the carton.

____ Making it harder to get to your cigarettes. Lock them in a drawer, wrap them in paper, or leave them in your coat or car.

____ Changing the way you smoke. Smoke with the hand you don't usually use. Smoke only half of each cigarette.

____ Stopping completely for just one day at a time. Promise yourself 24 hours of freedom from cigarettes; when the day's over, make the same commitment for one more day. At the end of any 24-hour period, you can go back to smoking and not feel guilty.

____ Spending more time in places where you can't smoke. Take up bike riding or swimming. Shower often. Go to movies or other places where smoking isn't allowed.

____ Going cold turkey. If you're a heavily addicted smoker, try a decisive and complete break. Smokers who quit completely are less likely to light up again than those who gradually decrease their daily cigarette consumption, switch to low-tar and low-nicotine brands, or use special filters and holders.

If these tactics don't work, talk to your doctor about nicotine replacement options or prescription medications.

What's Online

CENGAGE
brain.com

Visit www.cengagebrain.com to access course materials for this text, including the Behavior Change Planner, interactive quizzes, and more.

self survey

Are You Addicted to Nicotine?

	Yes	No
1. Do you smoke every day?	_____	_____
2. Do you smoke because of shyness and to build up self-confidence?	_____	_____
3. Do you smoke to escape from boredom and worries or while under pressure?	_____	_____

4. Have you ever burned a hole in your clothes, carpet, furniture, or car with a cigarette? _____ _____

5. Have you ever had to go to the store late at night or at another inconvenient time because you were out of cigarettes? _____ _____

6. Do you feel defensive or angry when people tell you that your smoke is bothering them? _____ _____

7. Has a doctor or dentist ever suggested that you stop smoking? _____ _____

8. Have you ever promised someone that you would stop smoking, then broken your promise? _____ _____

9. Have you ever felt physical or emotional discomfort when trying to quit? _____ _____

10. Have you ever successfully stopped smoking for a period of time, only to start again? _____ _____

11. Do you buy extra supplies of tobacco to make sure you won't run out? _____ _____

12. Do you find it difficult to imagine life without smoking? _____ _____

13. Do you choose only those activities and entertainments during which you can smoke? _____ _____

14. Do you prefer, seek out, or feel more comfortable in the company of smokers? _____ _____

15. Do you inwardly despise or feel ashamed of yourself because of your smoking? _____ _____

16. Do you ever find yourself lighting up without having consciously decided to? _____ _____

17. Has your smoking ever caused trouble at home or in a relationship? _____ _____

18. Do you ever tell yourself that you can stop smoking whenever you want to? _____ _____

19. Have you ever felt that your life would be better if you didn't smoke? _____ _____

20. Do you continue to smoke even though you are aware of the health hazards posed by smoking? _____ _____

If you answered yes to one or two of these questions, there's a chance that you are addicted or are becoming addicted to nicotine. If you answered yes to three or more of these questions, you are probably already addicted to nicotine.

Source: Nicotine Anonymous World Services, San Francisco.

MAKING THIS CHAPTER WORK FOR YOU

Review Questions

(LO 14.1) 1. Which of the following statements is true about tobacco consumption in the United States?
a. Smoking rates are lowest among the poor.
b. Asian and Hispanic women have the lowest smoking rates.
c. More than half of current smokers do not smoke daily.
d. Tobacco dependence is more prevalent among individuals aged 65 and older.

(LO 14.1) 2. Which of the following statements is true about factors associated with smoking behavior and tobacco addiction?
a. Smoking behavior is not influenced by genes.
b. Individuals with mental illnesses are unlikely to smoke.
c. Heavy smoking is linked with anxiety disorders in early adulthood.
d. A link between substance abuse disorder and smoking has not been found.

(LO 14.2) 3. Tobacco use on college campuses
a. is higher among black students.
b. continues to increase despite no-smoking policies by all schools.
c. is less than that of same-age peers who aren't in school.
d. is most often in the form of smokeless tobacco.

(LO 14.2) 4. Social smokers
a. have no negative health effects so long as they do not inhale.
b. have a higher risk of cancer than nonsmokers, even if they use less than a pack of cigarettes per week.
c. sometimes smoke more frequently and intensely than regular smokers and are more dependent on tobacco.
d. are more motivated to quit and make more committed attempts to do so.

(LO 14.3) 5. Women smokers
a. are more likely to die from breast cancer than lung cancer.
b. are less fertile than nonsmokers.
c. are less likely to develop osteoporosis.
d. bear children with fewer birth defects.

(LO 14.3) 6. Which of the following is among the differences in smoking behaviors for various racial and ethnic groups?
a. Asian American and Hispanic women have the highest rates of smoking.
b. Smoking rates among Hispanic youth have declined considerably in the past 10 years.
c. Among adults, Native Americans and Alaska Natives have the lowest rates of tobacco use.
d. Tobacco use is significantly higher among white college students than among other students.

(LO 14.4) 7. Nicotine
a. prevents the release of dopamine in the brain.
b. takes a long time to reach the brain.
c. stimulates the adrenal glands to produce adrenaline.
d. increases hunger.

(LO 14.4) 8. Among the thousands of chemicals produced in addition to nicotine as cigarettes burn is carbon monoxide, the side effects of which include _____.
a. increased ability of the blood to carry oxygen
b. impairment of normal functioning of the nervous system
c. increased risk of heart attacks and strokes in smokers
d. damaged mucus and cilia in the bronchial tubes

(LO 14.5) 9. The health effects of cigarette smoking include
a. a greater risk of heart attack in older smokers.
b. a higher incidence of panic attacks and panic disorder among young people who smoke than among nonsmokers.
c. a more rapid decline in brain function as they age among female smokers compared to males.
d. a smaller number of deaths than with other forms of substance abuse.

(LO 14.5) 10. The toxic chemicals in tobacco constrict blood vessels, leading to _____.
a. reduced blood pressure
b. increased beneficial cholesterol
c. increased risk of blood clots
d. reduced risk of heart attack

(LO 14.6) 11. Research conducted so far indicates that e-cigarettes
a. might have harmful effects on the developing brains of young users.
b. are less harmful to lung function than conventional cigarettes.
c. cause no allergic reactions in users.
d. are a relatively benign alternative to cigarettes.

(LO 14.6) 12. Health effects of hookah use include
a. decreased heart rate.
b. increased blood pressure.
c. little to no damage to lung function.
d. no carbon monoxide ingestion.

(LO 14.7) 13. Which of the following statements is *false*?
a. Using chewing tobacco can lead to lesions on the mucous membranes of the mouth.
b. Bidis come in several flavors.
c. The active ingredient in cloves lowers sensation in the throat, so clove-cigarette smokers inhale more deeply.
d. Smoking cigars is safe if you don't inhale.

(LO 14.7) 14. Which of the following statements is true about forms of tobacco other than cigarettes?
a. Ingesting tobacco can be more deadly than smoking cigarettes.
b. Water-pipe smoking has considerably fewer health risks than cigarette smoking.
c. The tobacco in bidis is unprocessed and more potent than the tobacco in cigarettes.
d. Clove cigarettes have not been found to cause any lung injuries.

(LO 14.8) 15. Quitting smoking
a. usually results in minor withdrawal symptoms.
b. will do little to reverse the damage to the lungs and other parts of the body.
c. can be aided by using nicotine replacement products.
d. is best done by cutting down on the number of cigarettes you smoke over a period of months.

(LO 14.8) 16. Ways to help yourself quit include all of the following *except*
a. join a support group.
b. make your home a smoke-free zone.
c. try acupuncture.
d. switch to bidis.

(LO 14.9) 17. Secondhand tobacco smoke is
a. the smoke inhaled by a smoker.
b. more hazardous than outdoor pollution as a cancer-causing agent.
c. less hazardous than mainstream smoke.
d. less likely to cause serious health problems in children than in adults.

(LO 14.9) 18. Sidestream smoke is
a. dirtier than mainstream smoke.
b. free of the tar particles and carbon monoxide found in mainstream smoke.
c. not a cause of serious health problems in small amounts.
d. not harmful in a well-ventilated room.

Answers to these questions can be found on page 623.

Critical Thinking Questions

1. Do many of your friends or family members smoke? Do any? What types of social activities continue to be associated with smoking?
2. How would you motivate someone you care about to stop smoking? What reasons would you give for them to stop? Discuss your strategy.
3. Have you ever been around people who have been intoxicated when you have been sober? What did you think of their behavior? Were they fun to be around? Was the experience difficult in any ways?
4. Have you ever been intoxicated? How do you behave when you are drunk? Do you find the experience enjoyable? What do the people around you think of your actions when you are drunk?

Additional Online Resources

www.cdc.gov/tobacco
This comprehensive feature on the Centers for Disease Control and Prevention (CDC) website provides educational information, research, a report from the U.S. Surgeon General, tips on how to quit, and much more.

www.joechemo.org
Based on the character Joe Chemo, an antismoking parody of Joe Camel, this site is highly interactive and allows visitors to test their "Tobacco IQ," get a personalized "Smoke-o-Scope," and send free Joe Chemo e-cards. There is also extensive information for teachers, antismoking activists, health-care providers, journalists, and smokers who wish to quit.

www.tobaccofacts.org
This excellent site provides access to many facts and resources regarding tobacco use.

http://tobacco.neu.edu
This site provides current information on tobacco-related litigation and legislation.

http://women.smokefree.gov/
This website provides information that is often important to women to support both their immediate and long-term needs as they become, and remain, nonsmokers.

www.ucanquit2.org
This Department of Defense-sponsored website provides the opportunity to develop a personalized plan for quitting, create a personal or public blog, and get live online help around the clock. It also offers the Train2Quit program to help track progress.

http://teen.smokefree.gov
This site sponsored by the National Cancer Institute educates teenagers so they can make their own informed decisions.

http://espanol.smokefree.gov
This National Cancer Institute site reaches out to Spanish-speaking people interested in quitting smoking.

Key Terms

The terms listed are used on the page indicated. Definitions of the terms are in the glossary at the end of the book.

aversion therapy 433

bidis 431

carbon monoxide 426

environmental tobacco smoke 434

mainstream smoke 434

nicotine 425

sidestream smoke 434

snus 432

tar 426

tobacco use disorder 422

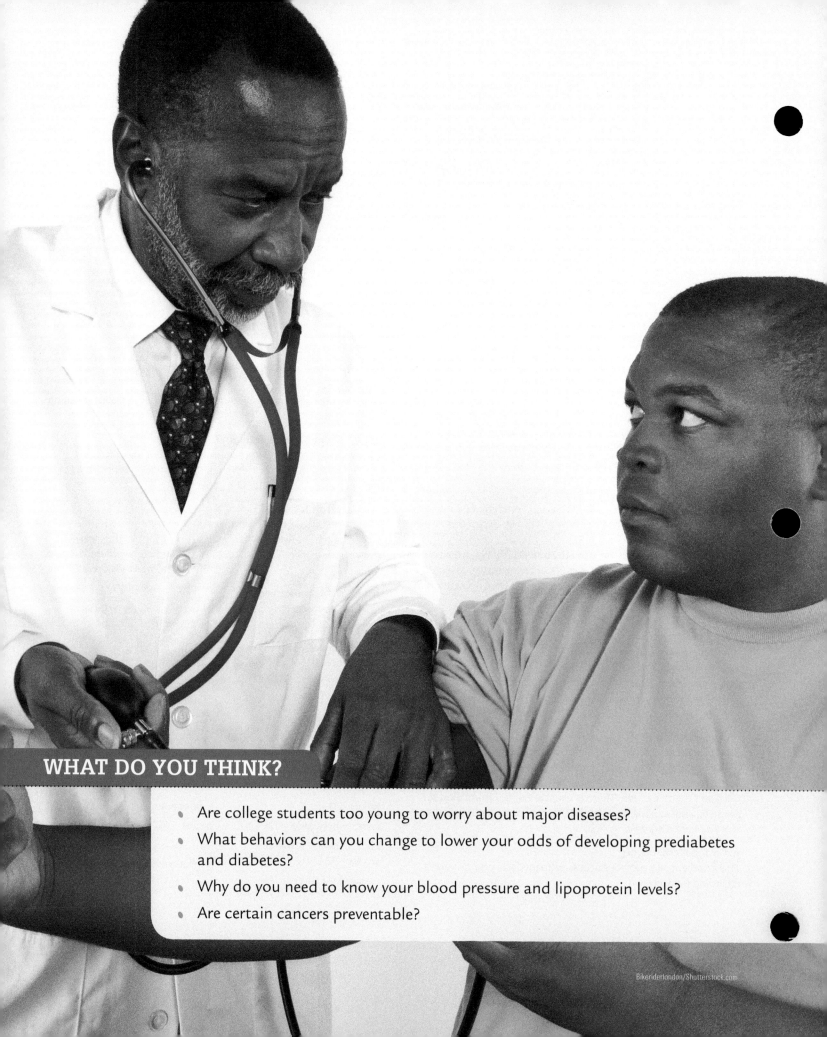

WHAT DO YOU THINK?

- Are college students too young to worry about major diseases?
- What behaviors can you change to lower your odds of developing prediabetes and diabetes?
- Why do you need to know your blood pressure and lipoprotein levels?
- Are certain cancers preventable?

15

Major Diseases

"What did your great-great-grandparents die of?"

Like many of the other students in her Personal Health class, Serena didn't know the answer to her teacher's question.

"Probably an infectious disease," she guessed—with good reason. At the turn of the twentieth century, the major killers of Americans were two deadly infections: tuberculosis and pneumonia.

By 1925, diseases of the heart had become the number-one cause of death in the United States, followed by pneumonia and influenza. By the 1940s, cancer had edged out pneumonia for the dubious distinction of being the nation's second-most-lethal disease. According to the most recent federal statistics, heart disease and cancer now account for nearly half of all deaths in the United States.[1]

Serena's family followed this pattern. Heart disease killed her great-grandfather; a series of strokes led to her great-grandmother's death. Her grandparents are still alive, but Serena worries about their health. Her grandfather has undergone bypass surgery for blocked arteries in his heart. Her grandmother is a breast cancer survivor.

Although she hates even to think about anything happening to her own parents, Serena knows that her father, who put on weight after a back injury, takes medication for high blood pressure and high cholesterol. Her mother has had several breast cancer scares, and Serena wonders if she too might be at risk. She's also come to realize that disease has an impact on life's quality as well as quantity.◄

After reading this chapter, you should be able to:

15.1 List the risk factors for cardiometabolic diseases.

15.2 Summarize the risks and signs of metabolic syndrome.

15.3 Explain the impact and treatment of diabetes.

15.4 Discuss the risk factors and management of hypertension.

15.5 Specify the effects and management of blood cholesterol levels.

15.6 Outline the risk factors and types of cardiovascular diseases.

15.7 Discuss treatment options for cardiovascular diseases.

15.8 Identify the risk factors and common causes of strokes.

15.9 Review the causes, risk factors, and types of cancer.

Modern medicine has won many victories against major threats such as cardiovascular disease and cancer, as well as life-threatening infectious illnesses. However, the number of healthy years you can expect to live depends largely on you. As this chapter demonstrates, by making healthier choices, boosting your defenses, and realizing when to seek treatment, you can add more years to your life and more life to your years.

Like the majority of college students, you are probably young—but not too young to think about serious health problems. Regardless of whether you're a teen, a twentysomething, or thirty-plus, the choices you make and the habits you develop now can put you at risk for a major disease that could sabotage your health and even shorten your life. The earlier in life that body fat, blood pressure, blood sugar, and cholesterol rise above optimal levels the greater the threat to well-being and longevity.

Fortunately, you can take steps to protect your health and prevent disease—and the sooner, you start the better.

✓ **check-in** Which of the American Heart Association's "simple seven" steps are you taking to safeguard your well-being?

___ Get moving. As new research confirms, being sedentary may be twice as deadly as being obese.[2] The good news: Increased physical activity, especially vigorous exercise, reduces cardiometabolic risks in the young, starting in adolescence.[3] (See Chapter 8.)

___ Eat healthfully. Diets lower in saturated and trans fats, sugar-sweetened drinks, and red or processed meats and higher in real fiber, nuts, coffee, and polyunsaturated fats (all discussed in Chapter 6) significantly reduce the risk of type 2 diabetes as well as heart disease and stroke.[4]

___ Maintain a healthy weight. General obesity increases the risk of cardiovascular disease and diabetes, while abdominal obesity increases the danger of dying of all causes, including cardiovascular illness and cancer.[5]

___ Control blood sugar. As long-term follow-up studies have shown, diabetics who intensively control their blood glucose early in their disease live longer than those who do not.[6]

___ Manage blood pressure. High systolic blood pressure—the top number in a reading—in young adults predicts a greatly increased risk of dying from heart disease over time.[7]

___ Control cholesterol. The sooner that blood fat levels rise and the longer they remain elevated, the greater the danger to your health.[8]

___ Stop smoking. Death rates among current smokers are two to three times as high as those of people who never smoked. (See Chapter 14.)

Men and women who adopt these healthy habits early in life enjoy longer lives, higher quality of life, and greater mobility and functioning as they age.[9]

Your Cardiometabolic Health

In recent years medical science has focused on the complex connections between various risk factors, symptoms, and diseases. Physical inactivity, for instance, increases the likelihood of obesity, which in turn leads to greater risk of many diseases. This awareness has led to a focus on **cardiometabolic** health. "Cardio" refers to the heart and blood vessels of the cardiovascular system; "metabolic" refers to the biochemical processes involved in the body's functioning.

Overall, America's cardiometabolic health is far from ideal. Every day more than 2,200 Americans die of cardiovascular diseases—an average of one death every 39 seconds. Cardiovascular diseases (all diseases of the heart and blood vessels) account for one of every three deaths, including an increasing number among younger adults ages 35 to 54. Medical scientists fear that the obesity epidemic and the rise in metabolic disorders may be responsible.

Only about half of young Americans get passing grades for heart-healthy behaviors. Although

cardiometabolic Referring to the heart and to the biochemical processes involved in the body's functioning.

many smoked, fewer than 1 percent eat "ideal" diets; about one-third have high-body mass indexes (BMIs) (discussed in Chapter 7), and one-third have unfavorable cholesterol readings.[10] Unhealthy habits in youth not only increase the odds of disease in old age but also lower the likelihood of surviving to age 55.[11]

The opposite is also true: For individuals who reached age 55 with low blood pressure and cholesterol levels, were not smoking, and were not diabetic, the risk for heart disease or a heart attack is significantly lower than for those with two or more risk factors.

Cardiometabolic Risk Factors

Specific risk factors determine your cardiometabolic health. Once you understand your risk, you can start making changes to lower your odds of developing metabolic syndrome, diabetes, and heart disease. (See Health on a Budget.)

✓**check-in** Are you "metabolically unhealthy"?

You are if you have two or more of the following risk factors:

___High cholesterol

___High blood pressure

___High blood sugar levels

___Elevated triglycerides

___Insulin resistance

___High C-reactive protein

Risk Factors You Can Control The choices you make and the habits you follow can have a significant impact on whether you remain healthy. For the sake of your cardiometabolic health, avoid the following potential risks.

Overweight/Obesity Excess weight, an increasingly common and dangerous cardiometabolic risk factor in both men and women, undermines good health:

- The higher your BMI during adolescence, according to a recent study, the greater your risk of type 2 diabetes and heart disease in the future. Even teens with a BMI in the high "normal" range face an increased likelihood of health problems.

- Overweight and obese individuals are more likely to have additional risk factors for cardiovascular disease, including physical

⦿ HEALTH ON A BUDGET

Lowering Your Cardiometabolic Risks

Yes, advances in treatment can help if you eventually develop a cardiometabolic condition. But changes in lifestyle can do even more. To make healthy changes, consider these behavioral modifications that require little or no expense.

Changes You Can Make Today

- Eat a good breakfast: whole-grain cereal, juice, yogurt, and so forth.
- Take a walk after lunch.
- Skip dessert at dinner.
- Eat one more serving of vegetables.
- Eat one more piece of fruit.
- Drink one more glass of water.
- Take the stairs for one or two flights rather than ride the elevator in your dorm or classroom building.
- Get seven to eight hours of sleep tonight.
- Don't smoke.

Changes You Can Make This Term

- **Block out time for exercise on your calendar.** Try for at least 30 minutes of physical activity most days.
- **If you haven't had your lipoproteins checked within the past year, schedule a test.**
- **If you don't know your blood pressure, find out what it is.**
- **Make a list of stress-reducing activities, such as meditation or listening to music.** Select two or three to try every week.
- **Learn your family history.** If you've inherited a predisposition to high blood pressure, diabetes, or heart disease, you need extra preventive care.
- **Develop and use a support system of friends and family members.** Identify individuals you can talk to, work out with, or call.

inactivity, hypertension, high cholesterol, and diabetes mellitus.

- Overweight teens who lose weight and keep their BMI within a healthy range as adults can eliminate the danger of diabetes, but being obese at any age endangers cardiovascular health.

✓**check-in** Is your weight increasing your risk of cardiometabolic disorders?

Body Fat Apple-shaped people who carry most of their excess weight around their waists are at greater risk of cardiometabolic conditions than are pear-shaped individuals who carry most of their excess weight below their waist. The more visceral (abdominal) fat that you have, the more resistant your body's cells become to the effects of your own insulin. However, as recent research suggests, fat alone, regardless of where it is stored, boosts the likelihood of heart attack or stroke. Subcutaneous fat (located under the skin) as well as visceral fat can pose dangers to cardiometabolic health.[12]

✓**check-in** Does your body shape or excess body fat put you at risk?

Waist Circumference A measurement of more than 40 inches in men and more than 35 inches in women indicates increased health risks. A "pot belly" raises risk even when a person's weight is normal. Rather than waist circumference alone, the ratio of waist to height may be a more precise indicator of risk. (See Chapter 7.)

✓**check-in** Do you know your waist measurement? Does it indicate increased risk?

Physical Inactivity As discussed in Chapter 8, about one-quarter of U.S. adults are sedentary and another third are not active enough to reach a healthy level of fitness. The risk for cardiometabolic conditions is higher for people who are inactive than for those who engage in regular physical activity.

Fitness may be more important than overweight or obesity for women's cardiometabolic risk. A minimum of 30 minutes a day of moderate activity at least five days a week can lift a woman from the "low-fitness category" and lessen her cardiometabolic risk.

The greater the exercise "dose," the more benefits it yields. In studies that compared individuals of different fitness levels, the least fit were at much greater risk of dying. In men, more rigorous exercise, such as jogging, produces greater protection against heart disease and boosts longevity.

✓**check-in** Did you know that the World Health Organization estimates that 3.2 million people around the globe die each year because they are not active enough?

Prolonged Sitting—defined as being seated from eight to twelve hours a day—significantly increases the odds of heart disease, diabetes, cancer, and dying, according to an analysis of about four dozen studies of the impact of inactivity.[13]

Healthy Diet A recent ten-year study has confirmed that closely following the Mediterranean diet—high in fresh fruits and vegetables, whole grains, beans, nuts, fish, and olive oil—can reduce the risk of heart disease by almost half. Additional benefits include weight loss, lower blood pressure and cholesterol levels, and a lower risk of diabetes.[14]

Tobacco Use Smoking's harmful effects include the following:

- Each year smoking causes more than 250,000 deaths from cardiovascular disease—far more than it causes from cancer and lung disease.

- Smokers who have heart attacks are more likely to die from them than are nonsmokers.

- Smoking is the major risk factor for peripheral arterial disease, in which the vessels that carry blood to the leg and arm muscles become hardened and clogged.

- Both active and passive smoking accelerate the process by which arteries become clogged and increase the risk of heart attacks and strokes.

✓**check-in** Is active or passive smoking putting you at risk?

High Blood Glucose As discussed in greater detail on page 450, your stomach and digestive system break down the food you eat into glucose, a type of sugar. The hormone insulin acts like a key, letting glucose into cells and providing energy. "Insulin-resistant" cells no longer respond well to insulin, and so glucose, unable to enter the cells, builds up in the bloodstream.

Frequent thirst, blurry vision, weakness, unexplained weight loss, and unusual hunger can be signs of high blood glucose. A simple blood test will tell you if your glucose levels are too high. Here is what the readings mean:

Healthy blood glucose	Under 100
Prediabetes	100–125
Diabetes	More than 125

✓**check-in** Have you ever had your blood glucose level tested? If so, what was it?

High Blood Pressure (Hypertension) Blood pressure is a result of the contractions of the heart muscle, which pumps blood through your body, and the resistance of the walls of the vessels through which the blood flows. Each time your heart beats, your blood pressure goes up and down within a certain range:

- It is highest when the heart contracts; this is called **systolic blood pressure**.

- It is lowest between contractions; this is called **diastolic blood pressure**.

- A blood pressure reading consists of the systolic measurement "over" the diastolic measurement, recorded in millimeters of mercury (mm Hg).

- High blood pressure, or **hypertension**, occurs when the artery walls become constricted so that the force exerted as the blood flows through them is greater than it should be. Physicians see blood pressure as a continuum: The higher the reading, the greater the risk of stroke and heart disease.

As a result of increased effort in pumping blood, the heart muscle of a person with hypertension can become stiffer. This stiffness increases resistance to filling up with blood between beats, which can cause the following:

- Shortness of breath with exertion

- Damage to the arteries in the kidneys, which can lead to kidney failure

- Accelerated development of plaque buildup in the arteries

✓**check-in** What's your blood pressure reading?

Lipoprotein Levels Cholesterol is a fatty substance found in certain foods and also manufactured by the body. Figure 15.1 shows food sources of cholesterol. The measurement of cholesterol in the blood is one of the most reliable indicators of the formation of plaque, the sludge-like substance that builds up on the inner walls of arteries. You can lower blood cholesterol levels by cutting back on high-fat foods and exercising more, thereby reducing the risk of a heart attack.

Lipoproteins are compounds in the blood that are made up of proteins and fat. The different types are classified by their size or density. The heaviest

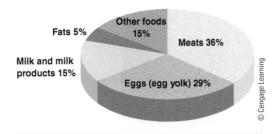

FIGURE 15.1 Cholesterol in Our Food
Food sources of cholesterol in the U.S. diet. Percentages indicate the proportion of cholesterol each type of food contributes to the diet.

are *high-density lipoproteins*, or HDLs, which have the highest proportion of protein. These "good guys," as some cardiologists refer to them, pick up excess cholesterol in the blood and carry it back to the liver for removal from the body. An HDL level of 40 mg/dL or lower substantially increases the risk of heart disease. (Cholesterol levels are measured in milligrams of cholesterol per deciliter of blood—mg/dL.) The average HDL for men is about 45 mg/dL; for women, it is about 55 mg/dL.

Low-density lipoproteins, or LDLs, and very low-density lipoproteins (VLDLs) carry more cholesterol than HDLs and deposit it on the walls of arteries—they're the "bad guys." The higher your LDL cholesterol, the greater your risk for heart disease. If you are at high risk of heart disease, any level of LDL higher than 100 mg/dL may increase your danger.

Triglycerides are fats that flow through the blood after meals and have been linked to increased risk of coronary artery disease, especially in women. Triglyceride levels tend to be highest in those whose diets are high in calories, sugar, alcohol, and refined starches. High levels of these fats may increase the risk of obesity, and cutting back on these foods can reduce high triglyceride levels.

✓**check-in** Have you ever had your lipoproteins measured?

Risk Factors You Can't Control

Family History Certain cardiometabolic risk factors, such as abnormally high blood levels of lipids, can be passed down from generation to generation. Individuals with an inherited vulnerability can lower the danger by changing the risk factors within their control, such as body weight and fat.

Race and Ethnicity Cardiometabolic risk factors occur at increased rates among ethnic minority populations such as African Americans, Hispanic

systolic blood pressure Highest blood pressure, which occurs when the heart contracts.

diastolic blood pressure Lowest blood pressure, which occurs between contractions of the heart.

hypertension High blood pressure that occurs when the blood exerts excessive pressure against the arterial walls.

cholesterol An organic substance found in animal fats; it is linked to cardiovascular disease, particularly atherosclerosis.

lipoproteins Compounds in blood that are made up of proteins and fat; high-density lipoproteins (HDL) pick up excess cholesterol in the blood; low-density lipoproteins (LDL) carry more cholesterol and deposit it on the walls of arteries.

triglycerides Fats that flow through the blood after meals and are linked to increased risk of coronary artery disease.

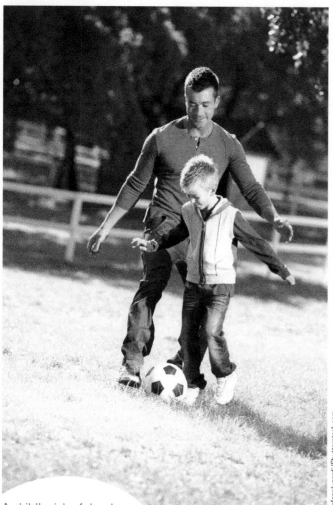

A child's risk of developing heart disease later in life depends on many factors, including family history, diet, and physical activity.

metabolic syndrome A cluster of disorders of the body's metabolism that make diabetes, heart disease, or stroke more likely.

Americans, and Native Americans. For reasons that aren't entirely clear, people of some races are more likely to develop diabetes:

- Blacks and Hispanics have double the rate of whites.

- Mexican-Americans are likely to have heart-damaging risk factors such as high blood pressure and high blood sugar levels, even if they are not obese.[15]

- The incidence of diabetes is even higher among American Indians. Among the Pima Indians of Arizona, half of all adults have type 2 diabetes, one of the highest rates of diabetes in the world.

- Nearly 4 in every 10 black adults have cardiovascular disease.

- Among Hispanic Americans, nearly 3 in 10 have cardiovascular disease.

- African Americans are twice as likely to develop high blood pressure as whites and suffer strokes at an earlier age and of greater severity.

- Black women are twice as likely as white women to suffer heart attacks and to die from heart disease. They are also less likely to receive common medications, such as cholesterol-lowering drugs, to lower their risk.

Poverty may be an unrecognized risk factor for minority groups, who are less likely to receive medical treatments or undergo corrective surgery. Family history, lifestyle, diet, and stress may also play a role, starting early in life.

Age Cardiometabolic risk factors increase as people get older, especially past age 45. This may be because many individuals tend to exercise less, lose muscle mass, and gain weight as they age.

Height Shorter men are more likely to develop cardiovascular disease, regardless of their smoking status, blood pressure, body mass index, blood fats, alcohol consumption, education level, or occupation. According to a recent data analysis, a man who is five feet tall has a 30 percent greater chance of developing heart disease than someone who is five feet six. Every extra 2.5 inches of height brings a 13.5 percent reduction in heart disease risk. Researchers theorize that the same gene variations that determine height may also affect the likelihood of atherosclerosis (page 465).[16]

✓**check-in** Do any of these factors put you at increased cardiometabolic risk?

Metabolic Syndrome

Metabolic syndrome, once called Syndrome X, or insulin-resistant syndrome, is not a disease but a cluster of disorders of the body's metabolism—including high blood pressure, high insulin levels, abdominal obesity, and abnormal cholesterol levels—that make a person more likely to develop diabetes, heart disease, or stroke. Each of these conditions is by itself a risk factor for other diseases. In combination, they dramatically boost the chances of potentially life-threatening illnesses.

Who Is at Risk?

Although the national prevalence of metabolic syndrome has fallen in the last decade, mainly because of a decrease in hypertension and high triglycerides, a significant number of Americans, especially black and Hispanic men and women, remain at risk:

- At a historically black college, about one-third of students had at least one criterion for metabolic disorder; one-fifth had two.[17]

- Young adults with metabolic syndrome are more likely than others their age to have thicker neck arteries, an indicator of atherosclerosis, the buildup of fatty plaques in arteries.

- Because retired professional football players have increased rates of metabolic syndrome and atherosclerosis, health professionals have called for regular screening of athletes, beginning in high school and college.

An all-too-common culprit for young people is consumption of sugary soft drinks, which, according to the American Heart Association, contributes to 130,000 new cases of diabetes and 14,000 new cases of heart disease every year.[18] Diet soft drinks also have been linked to the development of metabolic syndrome and type 2 diabetes.

What Are the Signs?

Three or more of the following characteristics indicate metabolic syndrome:

- **A larger-than-normal waist measurement:** 40 inches or more in men and 35 inches or more in women (for Asians and individuals with a genetic predisposition to diabetes, 37 to 39 inches in men and 31 to 35 inches in women).

- **A higher-than-normal triglyceride level:** 150 mg/dL or more.

- **A lower-than-normal high-density lipoprotein (HDL) level:** Less than 40 mg/dL in men or 50 mg/dL in women.

- **A higher-than-normal blood pressure:** 130 mm Hg systole over 85 mm Hg diastole (130/85), or higher.

- **A higher-than-normal fasting blood sugar:** 110 mg/dL or higher.

Compared with people with no factors of metabolic syndrome, those with three factors are nearly twice as likely to have a heart attack or stroke and more than 3 times more likely to develop heart disease. Men with four or five characteristics of the syndrome have nearly 4 times the risk of heart attack or stroke and more than 24 times the risk of diabetes.

√check-in Do you have any risk factors for metabolic syndrome?

College-age men and women who maintain their weights as they get older are much less likely to develop metabolic syndrome. Among those who are obese, losing 7 to 10 percent of their body weight may reverse the symptoms of metabolic syndrome.

Diabetes

Glucose is the primary form of sugar that body cells use for energy. When a person without diabetes eats a meal, the level of glucose in the blood rises, triggering the production and release of insulin by special cell clusters in the pancreas. Insulin enhances the movement of glucose into various body cells, bringing down the level of glucose in the blood.

In those who have diabetes, however, insulin secretion is either nonexistent or deficient. Without sufficient insulin, the glucose in the blood is unable to enter most body cells, so the energy needs of the cells aren't met. The levels of glucose in the blood rise higher and higher after each meal. This unused glucose eventually passes through the kidneys, which are unable to process the excessive glucose, and out of the body in urine.

Deprived of the fuel it needs, the body begins to break down stored fat as a source of energy. This process produces weak acids, called ketones. A buildup of ketones leads to ketoacidosis, an upheaval in the body's chemical balance that brings on nausea, vomiting, abdominal pain, lethargy, and drowsiness. Severe ketoacidosis can lead to coma and, eventually, death. (See Figure 15.2.)

An estimated 29 million Americans have diabetes. The Centers for Disease Control and Prevention (CDC) projects that up to one-third of Americans could have diabetes by 2050 if they continue to gain weight and avoid exercise.

The rate of diabetes is much higher in 15 states, mostly in the South. People living in this so-called diabetes belt are more likely to be obese, sedentary, and less educated than in the country as a whole. Certain racial and ethnic minorities—American Indians/Alaska Natives, African; Americans, and Hispanics—around the country also have higher rates of diabetes.

Before the development of insulin injections, diabetes was a fatal illness. Today diabetics can have normal life spans. However, diabetes still can lead to devastating complications. Uncontrolled glucose levels slowly damage blood vessels throughout the body; thus, individuals who become diabetic early in life may face major

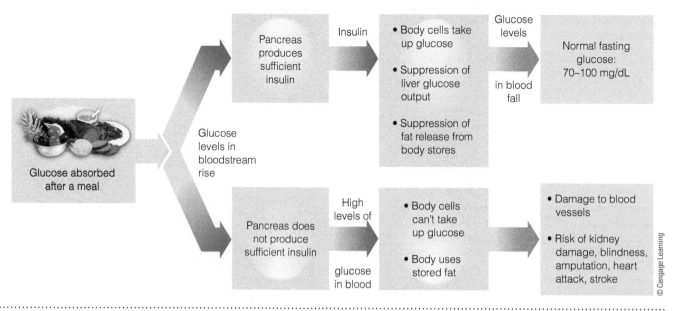

FIGURE 15.2 How Diabetes Affects the Body

Diabetes affects almost every organ system of the body in complex and often subtle ways.

complications even before they reach middle age. Diabetes is the number one cause of blindness, nontraumatic amputations, and kidney failure, and diabetes increases by two or three times the risk of heart attack or stroke.

Insulin Resistance

In a healthy body, the digestive system breaks down food into glucose, which then travels in the bloodstream to cells throughout the body. As blood glucose rises after a meal, the pancreas releases insulin to help cells take in the glucose. As noted earlier, **insulin resistance** is a condition in which the body produces insulin but does not use it properly.

When muscle, fat, and liver cells do not respond properly to insulin, the pancreas tries to keep up with the increased demand for insulin by producing more, but eventually it cannot. Excess glucose builds up in the bloodstream, setting the stage for diabetes. Many people with insulin resistance have high levels of both glucose and insulin circulating in their blood at the same time. Excess weight, particularly in men, and lack of physical activity, along with genetic factors, contribute to insulin resistance.[19]

Prediabetes

Sometimes called impaired fasting glucose or impaired glucose tolerance, **prediabetes** is a condition in which blood glucose levels are higher than normal but not high enough for a diagnosis of diabetes. According to the most

recent estimates from the CDC, more than one-third of adults in the United States—an estimated 79 million men and women—have prediabetes, although more than 90 percent are not aware of it. Among Americans age 65 and older, half may have prediabetes. All have an increased risk of cardiovascular events, such as heart attack and stroke.

One way to reduce this risk is by walking, as demonstrated in a study of more than 9,300 adults with prediabetes in 40 countries. For every 2,000 steps more per day participants took at the start of the study, they had a 10 percent lower risk for heart disease in subsequent years.[20] Following the Mediterranean diet, discussed in Chapter 6, also can lower the risk of diabetes, even in those at risk for heart disease.[13]

✓**check-in** Have you ever had your blood glucose tested?

Diabetes Mellitus

In those with **diabetes mellitus**, the pancreas, which produces insulin (the hormone that regulates carbohydrate and fat metabolism), doesn't function as it should. When the pancreas either stops producing insulin or doesn't produce sufficient insulin to meet the body's needs, almost every body system can be damaged. (See Figure 15.2.)

✓**check-in** Does anyone in your family have diabetes?

insulin resistance A condition in which the body produces insulin but does not use it properly.

prediabetes A condition in which blood glucose levels are higher than normal but not high enough for a diagnosis of diabetes.

diabetes mellitus A disease in which the inadequate production of insulin leads to failure of the body tissues to break down carbohydrates at a normal rate.

Diabetes mellitus, the seventh-leading cause of death in the United States, can shorten life expectancy by a decade or more.[21] The risk of premature death among people with diabetes is about twice that of people without the disease. Obesity, diabetes, and heart disease also can work together to speed dementia and other brain disorders, such as cognitive impairment.

Who is at Risk?

Several factors—some of which you can control—increase your risk for prediabetes and diabetes.

- Overweight or obese.

- Age 60 or older.

- Physically inactive.

- Parent or sibling with diabetes.

- Family background that is African American, Alaska Native, American Indian, Asian American, Hispanic/Latino, or Pacific Islander.

- Asian Americans start developing diabetes at lower weights. The reason may be that Asian Americans tend to deposit "visceral" fat around their internal organs (see page 446), which increases the risk of insulin resistance, a precursor to type 2 diabetes. The American Diabetes Association recommends that Asian Americans with a body mass index (BMI) of 23 or higher, rather than the 25 used for other races, undergo screening for type 2 diabetes.[22]

- Sitting—the more time that individuals spend on a chair or sofa, the greater their odds of developing high blood sugar.[15]

- Exercising fewer than three times a week.

- Giving birth to a baby weighing more than nine pounds or being diagnosed with diabetes during pregnancy.

- High blood pressure—140/90 or above—or being treated for high blood pressure.

- HDL, or "good," cholesterol level below 35 mg/dL or a triglyceride level above 250 mg/dL.

- Impaired fasting glucose (IFG) or impaired glucose tolerance (IGT) on previous testing.

- Other conditions associated with insulin resistance, such as severe obesity.

- History of cardiovascular disease.

- Sugary drinks—even a single can of sugary soda a day can increase the risk of prediabetes and diabetes by more then a fifth.[16]

- Certain common medications, including antibiotics such as penicillin[23] and cholesterol-lowering statin drugs,[24] may increase the risk of type 2 diabetes.

- Low levels of vitamin D may increase the risk for type 2 diabetes even in individuals who aren't overweight or obese.[25]

Types of Diabetes

Diabetes includes several conditions in which the body has difficulty controlling levels of glucose in the bloodstream. After an overnight fast, most people have blood glucose levels between 70 and 100 milligrams of glucose per deciliter of blood (mg/dL). This is considered normal. If your fasting blood glucose level is between 101 and 125 mg/dL, you have prediabetes. If your fasting blood glucose is consistently 126 mg/dL or higher, you have diabetes. There are three types of diabetes:

- **Type 1 diabetes:** In this form of diabetes (once called juvenile-onset or insulin-dependent diabetes), the body's immune system attacks the insulin-producing beta cells in the pancreas and destroys them. The pancreas then produces little or no insulin, and therefore blood glucose cannot enter the cells to be used for energy.

  Type 1 diabetes develops most often in young people but can appear in adults. About 15,000 children and 15,000 adults in the United States are diagnosed with type 1 diabetes every year.[26]

  People with type 1 diabetes lose an average of 11 years for men and 13 years for women to the chronic disease, compared to those without diabetes. The largest single cause of lost years is diabetes' impact on the heart. However, type 1 diabetics under age 50 also die because of conditions related to management of their disease, such as a diabetic coma triggered by low blood sugar.[27] Women with type 1 diabetes have a nearly 40 percent greater risk of dying from any cause and more than double the risk of dying from heart disease than men with type 1 diabetes. The reason may be that high levels of blood sugar may cause more damage to women's blood vessels than to men's.[28]

  Individuals with type 1 diabetes require insulin therapy because their own bodies no longer supply this vital hormone. As long-term follow-up studies have shown, people with type 1 diabetes who intensively control their blood glucose early in their disease are likely to live longer than those who do not.[29]

- **Type 2 diabetes:** In type 2 diabetes (once called adult-onset or non-insulin-dependent diabetes), either the pancreas does not make

YOUR STRATEGIES FOR PREVENTION

How to Lower Your Risk of Type 2 Diabetes

- Exercise 30 minutes on at least five days of the week.
- If you're overweight or obese, lose weight. Aim to lose 5 to 7 percent of your initial weight.
- Eat a diet rich in complex carbohydrates and high-fiber foods and low in sodium and fat. Among the eating patterns that lessen the risk of diabetes and cardiovascular complications are low-fat, low-glucose-index (see Chapter 6), Mediterranean, and high-protein diets.[30]
- Eat fruits and vegetables that are rich in antioxidants, substances that prevent oxygen damage to cells.
- If your doctor advises, take medications, such as metformin (Glucophage), to help lower your blood sugar.

enough insulin or the body is unable to use insulin correctly. Type 2 diabetes, which affects 90 to 95 percent of diabetics, is becoming more common in children and teenagers because of the increase in obesity in the young.[15]

Although type 1 and type 2 diabetes have different causes, two factors are important in both: an inherited predisposition to the disease and something in the environment that triggers diabetes. Genes alone are not enough. In most cases of type 1 diabetes, people need to inherit risk factors from both parents and to experience some environmental trigger, which might involve prenatal nutrition, a virus, or an unknown agent.

In type 2 diabetes, family history is one of the strongest risk factors for getting the disease, but only in Westernized countries. African Americans, Mexican Americans, and Native Americans have the highest rates, but people who live in less developed nations tend not to get type 2 diabetes, no matter how high their genetic risk.

Excess weight, especially around the waistline, is the major and most controllable risk factor for type 2 diabetes. Obese men are more likely than obese women to develop type 2 diabetes, perhaps because male muscles contain a protein that interferes with intake of glucose.[31] Losing weight greatly reduces this risk and, in individuals with the disease, can help get blood sugar under control.

- **Gestational diabetes:** Women who get diabetes while they are pregnant are more likely to have a family history of diabetes, especially on their mothers' side; they are at increased risk of developing diabetes later in life.

- Obese women who develop diabetes during pregnancy and then gain 11 or more pounds after giving birth have more than a 40 times higher risk of developing type 2 diabetes. Excess weight is a risk factor for both gestational and type 2 diabetes.[32]

- Children of mothers who develop gestational diabetes early in pregnancy may be at increased risk for autism spectrum disorders (discussed in Chapter 3). Early screening and good control of glucose levels during pregnancy may reduce this risk.[33]

Detecting Diabetes

To identify individuals with this disease as early as possible, the American Diabetes Association now recommends screening every three years for all men and women beginning at age 45. The American College of Endocrinology recommends screening at age 30 for individuals at risk, including those who are overweight, are sedentary, have a family history of diabetes, or have high blood pressure or heart disease.

Tests that can detect diabetes include these:

- **Random blood sugar test.** Because you don't necessarily fast for this test, your blood glucose may be high because you've just eaten. Even so, it shouldn't be higher than 200 mg/dL.

- **Fasting blood glucose test.** In general, glucose is lowest after an overnight fast. That's why the preferred way to test your blood sugar is after you've fasted overnight or for at least eight hours.

- **Glucose challenge test.** Often used to screen pregnant women for gestational diabetes, this test measures glucose before drinking eight ounces of an extremely sweet liquid after fasting for six hours, then every hour for a three-hour period. If your blood sugar rises more than expected and doesn't return to normal by the third hour, you likely have diabetes.

Diabetes Signs and Symptoms

About one-third of individuals with type 2 diabetes do not realize they have the illness. If you have risk factors for the disease, watch for the following warning signs:

- **Increased thirst and frequent urination:** Excess glucose circulating in your body draws water from your tissues, making you feel dehydrated. Drinking water and other beverages to quench thirst leads to more frequent urination.

- **Flu-like symptoms:** Type 2 diabetes can sometimes feel like a viral illness, with such symptoms as extreme fatigue and weakness. When glucose, your body's main fuel, doesn't reach cells, you may feel tired and weak.

- **Weight loss or weight gain:** Because your body is trying to compensate for lost fluids and glucose, you may eat more than usual and gain weight, or the opposite may occur. Although eating more than normal, you may lose weight because your muscle tissues don't get enough glucose to generate growth and energy.

- **Blurred vision:** High levels of blood glucose pull fluid from body tissues, including the lenses of the eyes, which affects ability to focus. Vision should improve with treatment of diabetes.

- **Slow-healing sores or frequent infections:** Diabetes affects the body's ability to heal and fight infection. Bladder and vaginal infections can be a particular problem for women.

- **Nerve damage (neuropathy):** Excess blood glucose can damage the small blood vessels to your nerves, leading to symptoms such as tingling and loss of sensation in hands and feet.

- **Red, swollen, tender gums:** Diabetes increases the risk of infection in your gums and in the bones that hold your teeth in place.

Diabetes Management

Before the development of insulin injections, diabetes was a fatal illness. Today diabetics can have normal lifespans. However, uncontrolled glucose levels slowly damage blood vessels throughout the body. Diabetes is the number-one cause of blindness, nontraumatic amputations, and kidney failure, and diabetes increases by two or three times the risk of heart attack or stroke.

Unlike many other medical conditions, patients must take charge of their diabetes and monitor their blood glucose regularly to prevent or delay the serious complications of the disease. Diabetes educators teach patients a new set of ABCs:

- **A** is for the *A1c test*. This test measures the amount of glucose attached to hemoglobin molecules, the iron-rich molecules in red blood cells that deliver oxygen to the body. The higher your blood glucose levels, the more hemoglobin molecules you will have with glucose attached—and the greater the risk of damage to eyes, kidneys, and feet. In general, the life cycle of a red blood cell is 75

to 90 days, which is why the A1c test shows average blood glucose levels for the past two to three months. The American Diabetes Association recommends a goal for A1c of less than 7 percent. The American College of Endocrinology recommends a goal of 6.5 percent. (Normal A1c levels are below 6.) Individuals with diabetes should have their A1c levels checked at least twice a year.

- **B** is for *blood pressure*. High blood pressure can cause heart attack, stroke, and kidney disease.

- **C** is for *cholesterol*. The LDL goal for most people is less than 160 mg/dL (see Table 15.2 on page 459). Bad cholesterol, or LDL, can build up and clog your blood vessels.

✓**check-in** If you have been diagnosed with diabetes, how vigilant are you in controlling your blood sugar levels?

Treatment

The goal for diabetics is to keep blood sugar levels as stable as possible to prevent complications, such as kidney damage. Home glucose monitoring, including new continuous glucose monitors, allows diabetics to check their blood sugar levels as many times a day as necessary and to adjust their diet or insulin doses as appropriate.

Types of insulin differ in how long they take to start working after injection (onset), when they work hardest (peak), and how long they last in the body (duration). Individuals with diabetes may use different types in various combinations, depending on time of day and timing of meals. New insulin inhalers offer an alternative to injections for those with type 2 diabetes.

Those with type 1 diabetes require daily doses of insulin via injections, an insulin infusion pump, or oral medication. Those with type 2 diabetes often can control their disease through a well-balanced diet, exercise, and weight management. However, insulin therapy may be needed to keep blood glucose levels normal or near normal, thereby reducing the risk of damage to the eyes, nerves, and kidneys. New medications help control weight and lower blood pressure and cholesterol.

One in every five diabetics between ages 18 and 39 lacks good medical care and has not seen a physician in the past six months. Younger diabetics also are less likely to monitor their cholesterol and blood pressure.[34]

Can Diabetes Be Cured?

In most cases, diabetes requires lifelong management and treatment. However, a cure for some patients no longer seems impossible. About 400 to 500 pancreas transplants are performed in the United States every year; when successful they normalize glucose levels, thereby curing diabetes. However, only about half of these transplants continue to function for ten years.

Gastric bypass surgery (which limits the amount of food a person can ingest) for extremely obese individuals has led to lasting remission of diabetes, sometimes even before a patient loses weight. (See Chapter 7.) Scientists believe that bypass surgery "cures" diabetes by changing the hormones and amino acids produced during digestion.[35] Some surgeons are advocating this approach for all diabetics with body mass indexes (BMIs) over 50; others, as an option for those with BMIs over 35.

Among other promising approaches are the use of stem cells to "rejuvenate" the pancreas, antibodies to block the autoimmune response of type 1 diabetes, and a more sophisticated artificial pancreas to monitor and manage glucose levels.

✓ **check-in** Could the future be pinch-free for diabetics?

On the horizon are several high-tech alternatives to the dreaded fingerstick, including cell phone apps, a contact lens to monitor blood sugar in tears, a breathalyzer, a saliva test, and a tattoo that would refract infrared light back through the skin to a monitor that could translate those readings into blood sugar levels.

Hypertension

Blood pressure refers to the force of blood against the walls of arteries. When blood pressure remains elevated over time—a condition called hypertension—the heart must pump harder than is healthy. Because the heart must force blood into arteries that are offering increased resistance to blood flow, the left side of the heart becomes enlarged. If untreated, high blood pressure can cause a variety of cardiovascular complications, including heart attack and stroke—as well as kidney failure and blindness (see Figure 15.3).

About a third of adults over age 20—some 80 million Americans—have hypertension.

The "silent killer" continues to live up to its nickname. Since 2000, the overall death rate from hypertension has increased 23 percent for both men and women, with the greatest spike in those ages 45 to 64.[35] People living in low-income states are more likely to have high blood pressure than the residents of more affluent states.[36]

Regulating blood pressure for all Americans could prevent 56,000 heart attacks and strokes and 13,000 deaths each year. However, 44 percent of adults with elevated blood pressure do not have it under control.[37] Globally, treating half of people with uncontrolled high blood pressure could prevent 10 million heart attacks and strokes over ten years.[38]

✓ **check-in** Are you too young to worry about blood pressure? Read the following section, and think again.

Hypertension in the Young

In a young person, even mild hypertension can cause organs such as the heart, brain, and kidneys to start to deteriorate. In an analysis of studies on more than 750,000 people, mild prehypertension—a blood pressure reading of 120–139/80–89 mm Hg.—increases the risk of stroke.[39]

High blood pressure can damage the structure of the brain in people as young as 40. In individuals at genetic risk, high blood pressure may spur development of the brain plaques characteristic of Alzheimer's disease.

Especially when combined with obesity, smoking, high cholesterol levels, or diabetes, hypertension greatly increases the risks of cardiovascular problems. Young adults in their 20s with even mildly elevated blood pressure may face an increased risk of clogged arteries by middle age, according to a 25-year-study of nearly 4,700 people.[40]

For young adults, high systolic blood pressure—the top number in a reading—may herald increased risk for heart disease. In a 30-year study of more than 27,000 young Americans (ages 18 to 49), a systolic reading of 140 mmHG or higher signaled a significantly greater likelihood of dying from heart disease over time: a 55 percent higher risk for women and a 23 percent higher one for men. The number of young adults with high systolic pressure has more than doubled as obesity has risen in recent years.[41] The take-home message: What you do as a young adult matters.

✓ **check-in** Do you know your systolic blood pressure?

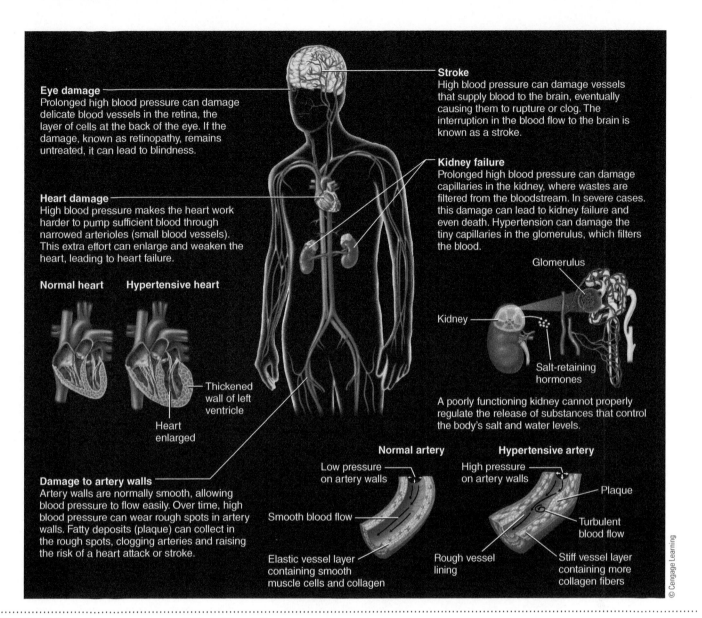

Eye damage
Prolonged high blood pressure can damage delicate blood vessels in the retina, the layer of cells at the back of the eye. If the damage, known as retinopathy, remains untreated, it can lead to blindness.

Stroke
High blood pressure can damage vessels that supply blood to the brain, eventually causing them to rupture or clog. The interruption in the blood flow to the brain is known as a stroke.

Heart damage
High blood pressure makes the heart work harder to pump sufficient blood through narrowed arterioles (small blood vessels). This extra effort can enlarge and weaken the heart, leading to heart failure.

Kidney failure
Prolonged high blood pressure can damage capillaries in the kidney, where wastes are filtered from the bloodstream. In severe cases. this damage can lead to kidney failure and even death. Hypertension can damage the tiny capillaries in the glomerulus, which filters the blood.

Normal heart   **Hypertensive heart**

Glomerulus

Kidney

Salt-retaining hormones

Thickened wall of left ventricle

Heart enlarged

A poorly functioning kidney cannot properly regulate the release of substances that control the body's salt and water levels.

Damage to artery walls
Artery walls are normally smooth, allowing blood pressure to flow easily. Over time, high blood pressure can wear rough spots in artery walls. Fatty deposits (plaque) can collect in the rough spots, clogging arteries and raising the risk of a heart attack or stroke.

Normal artery   **Hypertensive artery**

Low pressure on artery walls

High pressure on artery walls

Plaque

Smooth blood flow

Turbulent blood flow

Elastic vessel layer containing smooth muscle cells and collagen

Rough vessel lining

Stiff vessel layer containing more collagen fibers

© Cengage Learning

FIGURE 15.3 Consequences of High Blood Pressure
If left untreated, elevated blood pressure can damage blood vessels in several areas of the body and lead to serious health problems.

What You Need to Know Know your blood pressure numbers and, if needed, change your lifestyle to get them in normal range.[42] Why? Consider the following:

• Hypertension causes one in every eight deaths globally, making it the third-leading killer in the world.

• In the United States, high blood pressure is responsible for about one-third of cardiovascular problems, including heart attack and stroke, and for roughly one in six deaths among adults every year.

• For individuals who smoke, are overweight, don't exercise, or have high cholesterol levels, hypertension multiplies the risk of heart disease and stroke.

• Overweight people with high blood pressure are twice as likely to die of a heart attack or stroke as those with normal blood pressure. At ultrahigh risk are people with diabetes or kidney disease.

Who Is at Risk?

About 3 in 10 adults age 18 and older in the United States—some 65 million men and women—have high blood pressure.[43]

• Blood pressure has increased among children and adolescents as well as adults, with the highest rates among African American and Mexican American children. The primary culprit is the increase in obesity in the young.

- In some populations, such as residents of southern states, the odds of undiagnosed and uncontrolled hypertension are twice as high among blacks as whites.[44]

- An African American with the same elevated blood pressure reading as a Caucasian faces a greater likelihood of hospitalization and risk of stroke, heart disease, and kidney problems.[45]

- Family history increases the risk. "If you study healthy college students with normal blood pressures, those who have one parent with hypertension will have blood pressure that's a little higher than average," notes Rose Marie Robertson, MD, of the American Heart Association. "If two parents have high blood pressure, their levels will be a little higher, and they're destined to go higher still. If your parents have high blood pressure, have yours checked regularly."[46]

✓**check-in** Do you know if your parents have high blood pressure?

prehypertension A condition of slightly elevated blood pressure, which is likely to worsen in time.

- Men and women are equally likely to develop hypertension. Women who develop high blood pressure during pregnancy may face an increased risk of heart and kidney disease. Blood pressure also tends to rise around the time of menopause.

- People with chronic insomnia who take longer than 14 minutes to fall asleep may have a 300 percent higher risk of high blood pressure. The longer before sleep onset, the greater their risk.[47]

What Is a Healthy Blood Pressure?

Current guidelines (see Table 15.1) categorize a reading of 120–139/80–89 as **prehypertension**, a condition that is likely to worsen in time. A healthy reading is 115/75 mm Hg. Once blood pressure rises above this threshold, the risk of cardiovascular disease may increase.

In healthy adults, blood pressure screening should begin at age 21, with repeat evaluations at least every two years, or more often, depending on a person's current health, medical history, and risk factors for cardiovascular disease. According to the National College Health Assessment survey, about 9 in 10 students have done so.

✓**check-in** When was the last time you had your blood pressure checked?

To get an accurate blood pressure reading, you should visit the doctor's office at least twice and have your blood pressure taken two or more times while you're seated. The average of those measurements determines how your blood pressure is classified.

The current guidelines classify hypertension into two categories:

- **Stage 1:** This consists of a systolic pressure ranging from 140 to 159 or a diastolic pressure ranging from 90 to 99.

- **Stage 2:** The most severe form of hypertension occurs with a systolic pressure of 160 or higher or a diastolic reading of 100 or higher.

The most recent guidelines for treating blood pressure call for a target blood pressure of 140/90 mmHg for those at risk of heart attack and stroke and a goal of 130/80 mmHg for those with heart disease who already have had a heart attack, stroke, or ministroke or who show signs of arterial narrowing.[48]

Lowering High Blood Pressure

Lifestyle changes are a first-line weapon in the fight against high blood pressure. Rather than

TABLE 15.1 What Your Blood Pressure Reading Means

Normal Results

In adults, the systolic pressure should be less than 120 mm Hg and the diastolic pressure should be less than 80 mm Hg.

What Abnormal Results Mean

Prehypertension

The top number is consistently 120 to 139 or the bottom number reads 80 to 89.

Stage 1: Mild hypertension

The top number is consistently 140 to 159 or the bottom number reads 90 to 99.

Stage 2: Moderate to severe hypertension

The top number is consistently 160 or over or the bottom number reads 100 or over.

Low blood pressure (hypotension)

The top number reads lower than 90 mm Hg, or pressure 25 mm Hg lower than usual.

Blood pressure readings may be affected by many different conditions, including cardiovascular disorders; neurological conditions; kidney and urological disorders; psychological factors such as stress, anger, or fear; various medications; and "white coat hypertension," which may occur if the medical visit itself produces extreme anxiety.

Source: National Institute of Medicine National Institutes of Health.

Rob Marmion/Shutterstock.com

make a single change, a combination of behavioral changes, including losing weight, eating heart-healthy foods, reducing sodium, and exercising more, yields the best results.

Reducing Sodium
Reducing sodium consumption from the typical 3600 mg per day to about 2200 mg could save 280,000 to 500,000 lives over 10 years.

Too much sodium and too little potassium boost blood pressure in people who are sensitive to salt. For a healthful diet, aim for less than 1.5 grams of sodium a day and at least 4.7 grams of potassium. The lower the amount of sodium in the diet, the lower the blood pressure for both those with and those without hypertension and for both genders and all racial and ethnic groups. However, reducing dietary sodium has an even greater effect on blood pressure in blacks than in whites and in women than in men.

✓check-in Do you monitor your salt intake?

The DASH Eating Pattern
The National Heart, Lung, and Blood Institute (NHLBI) has developed the DASH eating pattern (for Dietary Approaches to Stop Hypertension), which has proved as effective as drug therapy in lowering blood pressure. An additional benefit: DASH also lowers harmful blood fats, including cholesterol and low-density lipoprotein, and the amino acid homocysteine (one of the new suspects in heart disease risk).

Exercise
Regular exercise, both aerobic workouts and resistance training, can lower blood pressure. Walking has proven as beneficial as running in lowering blood pressure and other cardiovascular risk factors. Alternative therapies, such as exercise, biofeedback, and transcendental meditation, may help lower blood pressure.[32] See Your Strategies for Change for ways to lower your blood pressure.

Medications
Making healthy lifestyle modifications can help reduce Stage 1 hypertension, but most people also require a medication. Drugs for lowering blood pressure come in a range of regimens (once a day to several times a day) with a range of effects on other conditions, interactions with other drugs, and potential side effects. They have been shown to lower the risk of stroke and add years to life expectancy.

Prompt and intense treatment at the first signs of rising blood pressure are essential for preventing heart attacks, strokes, and early death. Patients with a systolic blood pressure higher than 150 mmHG face an increased risk if they

YOUR STRATEGIES FOR CHANGE

How to Lower Your Blood Pressure

• **Get moving.** Regular exercise can lower blood pressure by 10 points, prevent the onset of high blood pressure, or enable you to reduce your dosage of blood pressure medications.

• **Eat your way to better blood pressure.** Choose more fruits, vegetables, low-fat dairy products, whole grains, poultry, fish, and nuts. Cut down on red meat, sweets, sugar-containing beverages, and saturated fat and cholesterol.

• **Lose 10.** Shedding 10 percent of your current weight—or even 10 pounds—can make a big difference.

• **Don't smoke.** A single cigarette can cause a 20-point spike in systolic blood pressure. Don't light up. See Chapter 13 for tips on quitting.

• **Hold the salt.** If you're salt sensitive, you may be spiking your blood pressure as you spice your food.

• **Stick with your medications.** If your doctor has prescribed medication to lower your blood pressure, take it conscientiously. Your future health may depend on it.

• **Avoid caffeinated energy drinks,** which can increase blood pressure and disrupt your heart rhythm.[a]

[a]"Energy Drinks May Increase Blood Pressure, Disturb Heart Rhythm." American Heart Association Meeting Report, March 21, 2013.

do not begin aggressive drug treatment within a month and a half of diagnosis or if they do not get a follow-up within about three months to see how well a medication is performing.[49]

Some of the medicines used to treat high blood pressure are

• Alpha blockers
• Angiotensin-converting enzyme (ACE) inhibitors
• Angiotension receptor blockers (ARBs)
• Beta-blockers
• Calcium channel blockers
• Central alpha agonists
• Diuretics
• Renin inhibitors, including aliskiren (Tekturna)
• Vasodilators

If your blood pressure is very high, you may need additional medications. Those with Stage 2 hypertension typically need at least two types of high blood pressure medications (antihypertensives) to reduce blood pressure to a safer level. The goal for most people with hypertension is to reduce blood pressure to below 140/90 mm Hg.

About 20 to 30 percent of people with high blood pressure have "resistant hypertension," which means that their blood pressure remains elevated despite taking three medications to lower it. In addition to medical conditions and certain medications, lifestyle factors, including excess weight, salt intake, and alcohol consumption, can contribute to this problem. New guidelines from the American Heart Association recommend weight loss, reduced salt, and decreased alcohol.

✓ **check-in** Did you know that only one-third of people with hypertension have it effectively controlled? Reducing blood pressure to healthy levels (140/9mmHG) could prevent one death in every 11 people treated for hypertension.

Your Lipoprotein Profile

Medical science has changed the way it views and targets the blood fats that endanger a healthy heart. In the past, the focus was primarily on total cholesterol in the blood. The higher this number was, the greater the risk of heart disease. The NHLBI's National Cholesterol Education Program has recommended more comprehensive testing, called a *lipoprotein profile*, for all individuals age 20 or older.

❗ CONSUMER ALERT

How to Get an Accurate Lipoprotein Profile

- Go to your primary health-care provider to get a lipoprotein profile. Although cholesterol tests at shopping malls or health fairs can help identify people at risk, the analyzers are often not certified technicians, and the readings may be inaccurate.

- Ask about accuracy. Find out if the lab is using the National Institutes of Health standards, and ask about the lab's margin for error (which should be less than 5 percent).

- Fast beforehand. Cholesterol tests are most accurate after a 9- to 14-hour fast. Women may not want to get tested at the end of their menstrual cycles, when minor elevations in cholesterol

levels occur because of lower estrogen levels. Cholesterol levels can also rise 5 to 10 percent during periods of stress. Reschedule the test if you come down with an intestinal flu because the viral infection could interfere with the absorption of food and thus with cholesterol levels. Let your doctor know if you're taking any drugs. Common medications, including birth control pills and hypertension drugs, can affect cholesterol levels.

- Sit down before allowing blood to be drawn or your finger to be pricked. Don't let a technician squeeze blood from your finger, which forces fluid from cells, diluting the blood sample and possibly leading to a falsely low reading.

This blood test, which should be performed after a 9- to 12-hour fast and repeated at least once every five years, provides readings of

- **Total cholesterol**
- **LDL (bad) cholesterol,** the main culprit in the buildup of plaque within the arteries
- **HDL (good** or **healthy) cholesterol,** which helps prevent cholesterol buildup
- **Triglycerides,** the blood fats released into the bloodstream after a meal

✓ **check-in** Are you too young to have to pay attention to how much fatty food you eat? Even if you are still in your teens, the answer is "no."

Long-term exposure to higher cholesterol levels can damage a person's future heart health. Individuals who live for more than a decade with high cholesterol have four times the risk of heart disease than those with shorter exposure. The longer your cholesterol remains high, the more likely you are to develop heart problems.[50]

What Is a Healthy Cholesterol Reading?

Total cholesterol is the sum of all the cholesterol in your blood. Less than 200 mg/dL total cholesterol is ideal, and 200–239 mg/dL is borderline high. Total cholesterol above 240 mg/dL is high and doubles your risk of heart disease. However, total cholesterol is not the only crucial number you should know. Because LDL increases your risk for heart disease, you always should find out your LDL level. Even if your total cholesterol is higher than 200, you may not be at high risk for a heart attack. Some people—such as women before menopause and young, active men who have no other risk factors—may have high HDL cholesterol and desirable LDL levels. Ask your doctor to interpret your results so you both know your numbers and understand what they mean. (See Table 15.2.)

HDL, good cholesterol, is important in everyone but particularly women. Federal guidelines define an HDL reading of less than 40 mg/dL as a major risk factor for developing heart disease. HDL levels of 60 mg/dL or more are protective and lower the risk of heart disease.

Triglycerides, the free-floating molecules that transport fats in the bloodstream, ideally should be below 150 mg/dL. Individuals with readings of 150 to 199 mg/dL, considered borderline, as well as those with higher readings, may benefit from weight control, physical activity, and, if necessary, medication.

TABLE 15.2 How to Interpret Your Lipoprotein Profile

Total Cholesterol Level	Category
Less than 200 mg/dL	Desirable level that puts you at lower risk for coronary heart disease. A cholesterol level of 200 mg/dL or higher raises your risk.
200 to 239 mg/dL	Borderline high
240 mg/dL and above	High blood cholesterol. A person with this level has more than twice the risk of coronary heart disease as someone whose cholesterol is below 200 mg/dL.

HDL Cholesterol Level	Category
Less than 40 mg/dL (for men)	Low HDL cholesterol. A major risk factor for heart disease.
Less than 50 mg/dL (for women)	
60 mg/dL and above	High HDL cholesterol. An HDL of 60 mg/dL and above is considered protective against heart disease.

LDL Cholesterol Level	Category
Less than 100 mg/dL	Optimal
100 to 129 mg/dL	Near or above optimal
130 to 159 mg/dL	Borderline high
160 to 189 mg/dL	High
190 mg/dL and above	Very high

Your LDL cholesterol goal depends on how many other risk factors you have.

- If you don't have coronary heart disease or diabetes and have one or no risk factors, your LDL goal is less than 160 mg/dL.

- If you don't have coronary heart disease or diabetes and have two or more risk factors, your LDL goal is less than 130 mg/dL.

- If you do have coronary heart disease or diabetes, your LDL goal is less than 100 mg/dL.

Triglyceride Level	Category
Less than 150 mg/dL	Normal
150–199 mg/dL	Borderline high
200–499 mg/dL	High
500 mg/dL or above	Very high

Source: National Cholesterol Education Program (NCEP) and American Heart Association. Adapted from http://www.americanheart.org/presenter.jhtml?identifier54500.

Lowering Cholesterol

According to federal guidelines, about one in five Americans may require treatment to lower his or her cholesterol level. However, nearly half of people who need cholesterol treatment, which can reduce the risk of heart disease by 30 percent over five years, don't get it. Depending on your lipoprotein profile and an assessment of other risk factors, your physician may recommend that you take steps to lower your LDL cholesterol.

Lifestyle Changes   Some individuals with elevated cholesterol can improve their lipoprotein profile with lifestyle changes:

- **Dietary changes:** In the past, dietary changes produced relatively modest improvements compared to the effects of medications, which can cut cholesterol by as much as 35 percent. However, a diet consisting of cholesterol-lowering foods, including nuts, soy, oats, and plant sterols (in margarine and green leafy vegetables), reduced LDL cholesterol by about 30 percent. Researchers are recommending this diet as an effective first treatment for individuals with high cholesterol levels, particularly coupled with exercise and weight loss.

- **Weight management:** For individuals who are overweight, losing weight can help lower LDL. This is especially true for those with high triglyceride levels and/or low HDL levels and those who have a large waist measurement (more than 40 inches for a man and more than 35 inches for a woman).

- **Physical activity:** Regular activity can help lower LDL, lower blood pressure, reduce triglycerides, and, particularly important, raise HDL. Again, these benefits are especially important for those with high triglyceride levels or large waist measurements.

√**check-in** Which lifestyle changes would you make to improve your cholesterol profile?

Lifestyle changes can lower harmful LDL levels by 5 to 10 percent. Alternative therapies, such as garlic, may have some limited benefit but remain unproven. A greater reduction of 30 to 40 percent requires either intensive lifestyle changes, including an extremely low-fat diet or the addition of cholesterol-lowering medication.

Medications   Drugs called statins—best known by brand names such as Lipitor, Mevacor, Pravachol, and Zocor—can cut the risk of dying of a heart attack by as much as 40 percent. Initially tested in men, statins have proved equally beneficial for women, including those whose cholesterol levels rise after menopause.

Statins work in the liver to block production of cholesterol. When the liver can't make cholesterol, it draws LDL cholesterol from the blood to use as raw material. This means that less LDL is available to trigger or promote the artery-clogging process known as atherosclerosis. Statins also appear to stabilize cholesterol-filled deposits in artery walls and to cool down inflammation. The combination of statins with moderate exercise, such as 30 minutes a day of brisk walking, has the most dramatic effect on cholesterol levels and reduced risk of dying.

Statins also protect patients who have not had a heart attack but are at high risk for developing cardiovascular disease because of high cholesterol or other risk factors. Large-scale studies indicate that statins protect against heart attacks and strokes even in older adults without known cardiovascular disease or diabetes and with low cholesterol—if these patients also have high levels of CRP or C-reactive protein (discussed on page 464).

Cardiovascular (Heart) Disease

Coronary heart disease causes about one of every seven deaths in the United States, killing about 375,000 Americans annually. Each year an estimated 635,000 Americans have their first heart attack; about 300,000 have a recurrence.[51]

√**check-in** Fewer than 20 percent of adults meet at least five of the following American Heart Association criteria for ideal heart health. Do you?

- Never smoked or quit more than a year ago
- Body mass index (BMI) less than 25
- Physical exercise—at least 150 minutes of moderate intensity or 75 minutes of vigorous intensity a week
- At least four components of a healthful diet, such as fewer calories and more fruits and vegetables (see Chapter 6)
- Total cholesterol lower than 200
- Blood pressure below 120/80
- Fasting blood sugar below 100

How the Heart Works

The heart is a hollow, muscular organ with four chambers that serve as two pumps (see Figure 15.4). Its key characteristics include the following:

- A human heart is about the size of a clenched fist.
- Each pump consists of a pair of chambers formed of muscles. The upper two—each called an **atrium**—receive blood, which then flows through valves into the lower two chambers, the **ventricles**, which contract to pump blood out into the arteries through a second set of valves.
- A thick wall divides the right side of the heart from the left side; even though the two sides are separated, they contract at almost the same time. Contraction of the ventricles is called **systole**; the period of relaxation between contractions is called **diastole**.
- The heart valves, located at the entrance and exit of the ventricular chambers, have flaps that open and close to allow blood to flow through the chambers of the heart.
- The *myocardium* (heart muscle) consists of branching fibers that enable the heart to contract, or beat, between 60 and 80 times per minute, or about 100,000 times a day. With each beat, the heart pumps about 2 ounces of blood. This may not sound like much, but it adds up to nearly 5 quarts of blood pumped by the heart in one minute, or about 75 gallons per hour.

atrium Either of the two upper chambers of the heart, which receive blood from the veins.

ventricles The two lower chambers of the heart, which pump blood out of the heart and into the arteries.

systole The contraction phase of the cardiac cycle.

diastole The period between contractions in the cardiac cycle, during which the heart relaxes and dilates as it fills with blood.

- The heart is surrounded by the *pericardium*, which consists of two layers of a tough membrane. The space between the two contains a lubricating fluid that allows the heart muscle to move freely. The *endocardium* is a smooth membrane lining the inside the heart and its valves.

- Blood circulates through the body by means of the pumping action of the heart, as shown in Figure 15.5. The right ventricle (on your own right side) pumps blood, via the *pulmonary arteries*, to the lungs, where it picks up oxygen (a gas essential to the body's cells) and gives off carbon dioxide (a waste product of metabolism). The blood returns from the lungs via the *pulmonary veins* to the left side of the heart, which pumps it, via the **aorta**, to the arteries in the rest of the body.

- The arteries divide into smaller and smaller branches and finally into **capillaries**, the smallest blood vessels of all (only slightly larger in diameter than a single red blood cell). The blood within the capillaries supplies oxygen and nutrients to the cells of the tissues and takes up various waste products.

- Blood returns to the heart via the veins: The blood from the upper body (except the lungs) drains into the heart through the *superior vena cava*, while blood from the lower body returns via the *inferior vena cava*.

The workings of this remarkable pump affect your entire body. If the flow of blood to or through the heart or to the rest of the body is reduced, or if a disturbance occurs in the small bundle of highly specialized cells in the heart that generate electrical impulses to control heartbeats, the result may at first be too subtle to notice. However, without diagnosis and treatment, these changes could develop into a life-threatening problem.

Heart Risks on Campus

Many people, including college students and other young adults, are unaware of habits and conditions that put their hearts at risk. Many undergraduates view heart disease as mainly a problem for white men and underestimate the risks for women and ethnic groups. Students rate their own knowledge of heart disease as lower than that of sexually transmitted infections and psychological disorders.

✓**check-in** How would you rate your knowledge of heart disease?

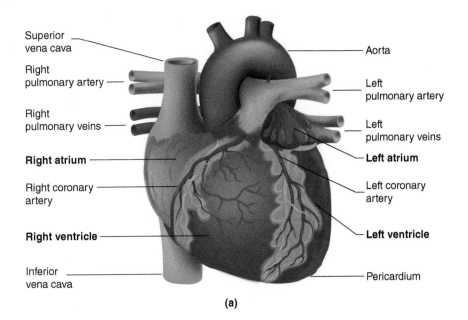

(a)

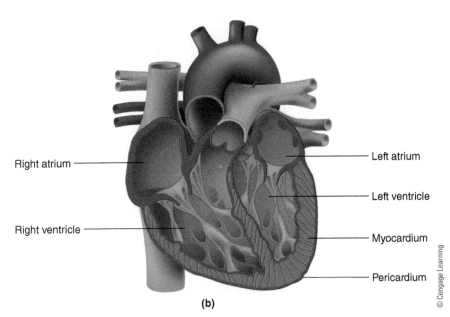

(b)

© Cengage Learning

FIGURE 15.4 The Healthy Heart

(a) The heart muscle is nourished by blood from the coronary arteries, which arise from the aorta. (b) The cross section shows the four chambers and the myocardium, the muscle that does the heart's work. The pericardium is the outer covering of the heart.

Here are some crucial facts:

- Heart disease is the third-leading cause of death among adults ages 25 to 44. Diabetes, family history, and other risk factors increase the likelihood of heart disease.

- It's never too soon to start protecting your heart. High aerobic fitness in the college-age years has been linked with a lower risk of heart attacks later in life.

aorta The main artery of the body, arising from the left ventricle of the heart.

capillaries Minute blood vessels that connect arteries to veins.

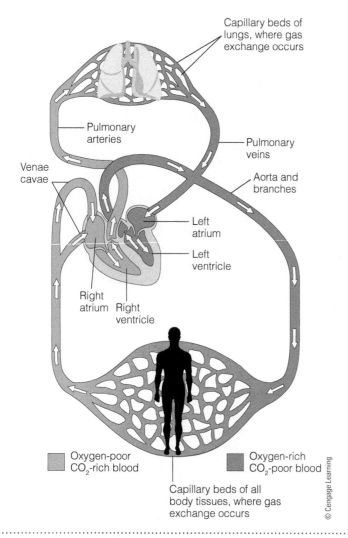

Capillary beds of lungs, where gas exchange occurs

Pulmonary arteries

Pulmonary veins

Venae cavae

Aorta and branches

Left atrium

Left ventricle

Right atrium Right ventricle

Oxygen-poor CO$_2$-rich blood

Oxygen-rich CO$_2$-poor blood

Capillary beds of all body tissues, where gas exchange occurs

© Cengage Learning

FIGURE 15.5 The Path of Blood Flow

Blood is pumped from the right ventricle into the pulmonary arteries, which lead to the lungs, where gas exchange (oxygen for carbon dioxide) occurs. Oxygenated blood returning from the lungs drains into the left atrium and is then pumped into the left ventricle, which sends the blood into the aorta and its branches. The oxygenated blood flows through the arteries, which extend to all parts of the body. Again, gas exchange occurs in the body tissues; this time oxygen is "dropped off" and carbon dioxide "picked up."

- Certain behaviors also put students' hearts at risk. According to a recent study, binge drinking may hinder the function of the blood vessels and increase the risk of stroke, sudden cardiac death, and heart attack.

- Young athletes face special risks. Each year, seemingly healthy teens or young adults die suddenly on playing fields and courts. The culprit in one of every three cases of sudden cardiac death in young athletes is a silent condition called hypertrophic cardiomyopathy (HCM), an excessive thickness of the heart muscle. Because of HCM, the heart is more prone to dangerous heart irregularities.

In research studies, cardiac screening with an electrocardiogram has revealed abnormalities in 21 to 37 percent of student athletes. Most were mild, but approximately 1 percent of the students had significant electrical problems in the heart that would have been missed without electrocardiography. Some medical groups have recommended routine electrocardiograms to reduce risk of sudden cardiac death in competitive collegiate sports; others believe that a simpler physical exam–based screening is sufficient.

The Power of Positive Emotions

Our psychological and social health affects not just our minds but our bodies, including the heart. While problems such as depression and stress may increase cardiovascular risk, happiness may help keep our hearts healthy. In a study that followed men and women for 10 years, those who showed more "positive" emotions—such as enthusiasm, joy, and contentment—were less likely to develop heart disease than less happy individuals. The happier people were, the lower their risk of heart disease became.

An optimistic outlook may also boost heart health. In a large study that adjusted for socioeconomic factors such as education and income, optimistic people were more likely to be in ideal cardiovascular health, with lower blood sugar, cholesterol, blood pressure, and BMIs, compared with the least optimistic.[52]

A sense of purpose affects your heart as well as your mind-set. Individuals who feel motivated by a sense of meaning and direction in life and view life as worth living are at lower risk of cardiovascular disease, stroke, and death from any cause.[53]

Psychological Risk Factors

Researchers classify psychological risk factors for heart disease into three categories:

- **Chronic factors**, such as job strain or lack of social support, play an important role in the buildup of artery-clogging plaque and may increase blood pressure. Even feeling that life has treated you unfairly boosts your chance of having a heart attack.

- **Episodic factors**, such as depression, can last from several weeks to two years and may lead to the creation of "unstable" plaque, which is more likely to break off and block a blood vessel within the heart.

- **Short-term, or acute, factors**, such as an angry outburst, can directly trigger a heart attack in people with underlying heart disease.

These factors may act alone or combine and exert different effects at different ages and stages of life. They may influence behaviors such as smoking, diet, alcohol consumption, and physical activity, as well as directly cause changes in physiology.

Stress   Stress itself can be acute, episodic, or chronic—and all three forms may affect heart health. Women tend to have higher chronic stress than men for many reasons, including other medical problems (such as diabetes or depression), family conflict, or the burden of caring for someone with a serious illness. Both women and younger adults with high stress prior to a heart attack have poorer prognosis for recovery afterward.[54]

One particularly stressful event, divorce, increases the lifetime risk of a heart attack. Divorced husbands and wives are both more likely to have a heart attack than continuously married spouses. If men remarry, their hearts are no longer in jeopardy, but that is not the case for women. Multiple divorces are as hazardous to women's hearts as risk factors like smoking and hypertension.[55]

Even stressed teenagers may be at risk. In a longitudinal analysis of data on almost 238,000 middle-aged men, those who had trouble coping with stress in adolescence encountered more future heart troubles, regardless of whether they exercised. In the study the teens with the "lowest stress resilience" had the highest risk for heart disease and for dying of heart disease.[56]

How you respond to everyday sources of stress can affect your heart as well as your overall health. While you may not be able to control the sources of stress, you can change how you habitually respond to it.

√check-in Do you think the way you respond to stress increases or decreases your cardiovascular risk?

Depression   Depression and heart disease often occur together. People with heart disease are more likely than others to be depressed, and some seemingly healthy people with depression are at greater risk of heart problems. Depressed women younger than age 60 are more likely to suffer a heart attack than those who do not suffer from depression.

The combination of stress, depression, and heart disease can be so deadline that researchers have dubbed the combination a "psychosocial perfect storm" that increases the risk of heart attack or death among men and women with heart disease.[57]

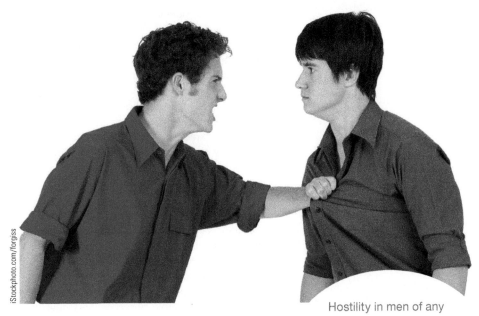

iStockphoto.com/forgiss

Hostility in men of any age can increase their risk of heart attacks and heart disease.

An additional benefit of treating depression with antidepressants is a lower risk of heart disease, stroke, and dying over a three-year period. The reason may be that, as symptoms of depression ease, people may be more inclined to exercise, practice good health habits, and comply with medical advice.[58]

Anger and Hostility   Anger and hostility have both short- and long-term consequences for the heart, particularly for men. In general, the angriest men are three times more likely to develop heart disease than the most placid ones. Hostility more than doubles the risk of recurrent heart attacks in men (but not women). Research has linked hostility to increased cardiac risk factors, to decreased survival in men with coronary artery disease below the age of 61, to an increased risk of heart attack in men with metabolic syndrome, and to an increased risk of abnormal heart rhythms. The risk of a heart attack or other cardiovascular "event" is highest in the two hours following an angry outburst. The more frequent the outbursts, the greater the danger to heart health.[40]

Angry young men may be putting their future heart health in jeopardy. In longitudinal studies the angriest young men were more likely to suffer heart attacks by age 55 and significantly to develop any form of cardiovascular disease.

√check-in If you are male, do you think anger may be putting your heart health at risk?

How does hostility harm the heart? Anger triggers a surge in stress hormones that can provoke abnormal and potentially lethal heart rhythms and activates platelets, the tiny blood cells that trigger blood clotting. High levels of anger can also trigger a spasm in a coronary artery, which results in the additional narrowing of a partially blocked blood vessel.

In women, anger and hostility do not always lead to heart troubles. However, women who outwardly express anger may be at increased risk if they also have other risk factors for heart disease, such as diabetes or unhealthy levels of lipoproteins.

Personality Types In addition to stress, anger, and depression, other psychological traits can increase the risk of heart disease. Based on more than a decade of research, Dutch scientists have identified a "Type D" (for distressed) personality type. Type D people tend to be anxious, self-conscious, irritable, insecure, and negative, and they go to great lengths not to say or do anything that others might not like. In the Dutch study, almost four times as many Type D individuals as others in cardiac rehabilitation programs died within an eight-year period.

In the past, other personality types were linked to disease; for example, hard-charging, hostile Type A's were associated with heart disease, and conflict-avoiding, emotion-suppressing Type C's with cancer. However, these traits have not proved to be significant risk factors for these illnesses.

Other Risk Factors

Researchers have identified other potential threats to heart health.

Inflammation and C-Reactive Protein

Inflammation—the process by which the body responds to fever, injury, or infection—plays an essential role in healing and recovering from infection. However, chronic low-grade inflammation may contribute to atherosclerosis and set the stage for heart attacks, strokes, and other forms of cardiovascular disease. The most common triggers of inflammation are smoking, lack of exercise, high-fat and high-calorie meals, and highly processed foods.

C-reactive protein (CRP), produced in the liver, rises whenever the body responds to inflammation. Individuals with the highest CRP levels are more likely to develop heart disease than those with the lowest levels. High concentrations of CRP also may predict greater risk of sudden death.

Homocysteine

Homocysteine High levels of *homocysteine*—an amino acid in the blood—have been linked to a greater risk of heart disease and stroke. Homocysteine may have an effect on atherosclerosis by damaging the inner lining of arteries and promoting blood clots. Several clinical trials are under way to test whether lowering homocysteine will reduce the risk of heart disease.

Illegal Drugs Illegal drugs pose many dangers —one of the most serious is their potentially deadly impact on the cardiovascular system. Ecstasy, amphetamines, and cocaine can cause a sudden rise in blood pressure, heart rate, and contractions of the left ventricle (the pumping chamber) of the heart, which can increase the risk of a heart attack.

The hallucinogens lysergic acid diethylamide (LSD) and psilocybin (psychoactive mushrooms) also have the potential for triggering irregular heartbeats and heart attacks, although less serious cardiac complications, such as a temporary rise in blood pressure, are more common. Morphine and heroin, which account for almost half of drug-related deaths, can lower blood pressure and affect the heart rate. Inhalants can produce fatal heartbeat irregularities. Marijuana, the most widely used illegal drug among young adults, can affect blood pressure and heart rate, but it is not known whether it can trigger a heart attack.

Bacterial Infection Certain bacteria may indeed put the heart at risk. *Streptococcus sanguis*, the bacterium found in dental plaque, has been implicated in the buildup of atherosclerotic plaque. Individuals with periodontal disease are at increased risk of heart disease and stroke. Regular brushing, flossing, and dental visits can reduce this danger.

Another common bacterium, *Chlamydia pneumoniae*, long linked to respiratory infections, also may threaten the heart. Individuals with high levels of antibodies to this bacteria are more likely to suffer a heart-related problem. Researchers have reported that antibiotics, taken to treat common infections, may protect against first-time heart attacks. A national clinical trial to determine whether antibiotics can reduce the risk of heart attack and stroke is under way.

Aspirin and the Heart

Daily low-dose aspirin has been recommended as a preventive step for men at high risk of cardiovascular disease because it reduces the stickiness of platelets (cells that cause blood clotting). This lowers the risk of blood clots, which can block a blood vessel and trigger a heart attack or stroke. Several research studies have demonstrated an association between aspirin use and reductions in heart attacks in men. However, while aspirin lowers the likelihood of heart attack, it may slightly increase stroke risk.

According to the U.S. Preventive Services Task Force, people should consider various factors including age, gender, diabetes, blood pressure, cholesterol levels, and smoking before deciding to use aspirin. The more risk factors they have, the more likely they are to benefit from aspirin.

The task force recommends against aspirin use in men under age 45 or women under age 55 because heart attacks and strokes are less likely in these age groups.

The Heart of a Woman

Many people still think of heart disease as a "guy problem." Men do have a higher incidence of cardiovascular problems than women before age 45, but women's hearts are also vulnerable:

- Every year 35,000 women under age 65 experience a heart attack.[59]

- More than 15,000 women younger than age 55 die from heart disease in the United States each year.[60]

- Younger women who suffer heart attacks tend to have more physical symptoms and a poorer quality of life.[61]

- Women between the ages of 30 and 55 often ignore early warning signs of a heart attack such as pain and dizziness, which may explain why they have higher rates of death from heart attack than men in their age group.[62]

Women need to know the early signs and symptoms of female heart disease:

- Tiredness, even after getting adequate sleep
- Trouble breathing
- Trouble sleeping
- Feeling sick to the stomach
- Feeling scared or nervous
- New or worse headaches
- An ache in the chest
- Feeling "heavy" or "tight" in the chest
- A burning feeling in the chest
- Pain in the back, between the shoulders
- Pain or tightness in the chest that spreads to the jaw, neck, shoulders, ear, or the inside of the arms
- Pain in the belly, above the belly button

Unhealthy lifestyles may be responsible for almost 75 percent of heart disease cases in young and middle-aged women.[63] Healthful habits can reduce the danger. Even a few bouts of moderate exercise each week can cut a middle-aged woman's odds for heart disease, blood clots, and stroke. More frequent exercises, at least in this study of more than 1.1 million middle-aged women with no history of heart disease, did not yield more benefits than walking, gardening, cycling, or engaging in other activities that caused sweating or increased heart rate two or three days a week.[64]

A study of almost 90,000 nurses followed for 20 years linked the six behaviors below with a significant decrease in the risk of heart disease.[65]

✓ **check-in** Would you like to cut your odds of heart disease by 90 percent over the next 20 years?

Here are six behaviors proven to do so:

___ Not smoking

___ Exercising at least 2.5 hours a week

___ Maintaining a healthy weight

___ Watching fewer than 7 hours of television a week

___ Following a healthy diet

___ Drinking no more than one glass of alcohol a day

Crises of the Heart

Coronary Artery Disease

The general term for any impairment of blood flow through the blood vessels, often referred to as "hardening of the arteries," is **arteriosclerosis**. The most common form is **atherosclerosis**, a disease of the lining of the arteries in which **plaque**—deposits of fat, fibrin (a clotting material), cholesterol, other cell parts, and calcium—narrows the artery channels. Inflammation also plays a crucial role.

Atherosclerosis This process begins when LDL cholesterol penetrates the wall of an artery. Ideally, HDL cholesterol carries the cholesterol out of the artery wall to the liver for disposal. However, if LDL accumulates, the artery responds by releasing chemical messengers called cytokines, which trigger active inflammation in the artery wall.

T-lymphocytes and macrophages, specialized white blood cells that are part of the body's defensive immune system, move from the bloodstream into the artery and engulf the LDL. As

arteriosclerosis Any of a number of chronic diseases characterized by degeneration of the arteries and hardening and thickening of arterial walls.

atherosclerosis A form of arteriosclerosis in which fatty substances (plaque) are deposited on the inner walls of arteries.

plaque A sludgelike substance that builds up on the inner walls of arteries.

they ingest the LDL, the macrophages enlarge and become foam cells, which rupture, releasing cholesterol into the artery wall, where the cycle of damage begins again. In response, the smooth muscle cells in the artery wall create a fibrous cap over the inflamed area (Figure 15.6).

These hard-capped plaques are dangerous: They narrow arteries, reduce the flow of blood, and produce **angina** (chest pain). However, the usual culprits in heart attacks are smaller, softer plaques that can rupture. As the body responds with clotting factors, platelets, and blood cells, a blood clot, or thrombus, forms on the disrupted plaque's surface. The clot ultimately blocks the artery and kills heart muscle cells. Similar clots can block blood flow to the brain and lead to other complications, including kidney failure and circulation problems in the legs and feet.

Unclogging the Arteries Reversing the buildup of plaque inside the arteries is possible with cholesterol-lowering drugs and a low-fat diet. A strict program of dietary and lifestyle change without any medication, developed by Dean Ornish, M.D., of the University of California, San Francisco, also has proved effective in reversing coronary artery disease. The following are the key elements of this approach:

- **A very low-fat, vegetarian diet,** including nonfat dairy products and egg whites, keeping fat intake to below 8 percent of total calories consumed. Ornish's recommended diet allows no meat, poultry, fish, butter, cheese, ice cream, or any form of oil.

- **Moderate exercise,** consisting of an hour of aerobic activity three times a week. Walking is recommended because more rigorous exercise might be dangerous for heart patients, who may develop increased risk of blood clots, irregular heartbeats, or coronary artery spasms during exertion.

- **Stress counseling.** Ornish's patients learn how the body's stress response can cause a rapid heartbeat and narrowing of the arteries, and how stress reduction can reduce cholesterol levels.

- **An hour a day of yoga, meditation, breathing, and progressive relaxation.** Some patients use visualization, for instance, imagining their arteries being cleared by a tunneling machine.

Angina Pectoris A temporary drop in the supply of oxygen to the heart tissue causes feelings of pain or discomfort in the chest known as **angina pectoris**. Some people suffer angina only when the demands on their hearts increase, such as during exercise or when under stress. Many people have angina for years and yet never suffer a heart attack; in some, the angina even disappears. However, angina should be considered a warning of danger if it becomes more severe or more frequent, occurs with less activity or exertion, begins to waken a person from a sound sleep at night, persists for more than 10 to 15 minutes, or causes unusual perspiration.

√**check-in** Did you know that on average someone in the United States has a coronary event every 34 seconds and someone dies of a coronary event approximately every 84 seconds?

angina Chest pain.

angina pectoris A severe, suffocating chest pain caused by a brief lack of oxygen to the heart.

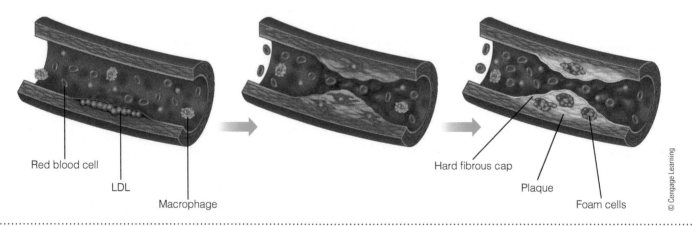

Red blood cell
LDL
Macrophage
Hard fibrous cap
Plaque
Foam cells

© Cengage Learning

FIGURE 15.6 How Atherosclerosis Happens

LDL cholesterol penetrates an artery wall, and the accumulation of LDL cholesterol triggers an inflammation. Macrophages engulf the LDL and become foam cells. The artery wall creates a fibrous cap over this plaque, and the artery is narrowed. If the plaque ruptures, blood clots can block blood flow to the heart or to the brain.

Heart Attack (Myocardial Infarction)

The medical name for a heart attack, or coronary, is **myocardial infarction (MI)**. The *myocardium* is the cardiac muscle layer of the wall of the heart. It receives its blood supply, and thus its oxygen and other nutrients, from the coronary arteries. If an artery is blocked by a clot or plaque, or by a spasm, the myocardial cells do not get sufficient oxygen, and the portion of the myocardium deprived of its blood supply begins to die.

Although such an attack may seem sudden, usually it has been building up for years, particularly if the person has ignored risk factors and early warning signs. According to research, 80 to 90 percent of those who develop heart disease and 95 percent of those who suffer a fatal heart attack have at least one major risk factor.

Is It a Heart Attack?

If they experience the following symptoms, individuals should seek immediate medical care and take an aspirin (325 milligrams) to keep the blood clot in a coronary artery from getting any bigger:

- A tight ache, heavy, squeezing pain, or discomfort in the center of the chest, which may last for 30 minutes or more and is not relieved by rest
- Chest pain that radiates to the shoulder, arm, neck, back, or jaw
- Anxiety
- Sweating or cold, clammy skin
- Nausea and vomiting
- Shortness of breath
- Dizziness, fainting, or loss of consciousness

Women often experience heart attacks differently than men. In the month before an attack, many report unusual fatigue and disturbed sleep. Far fewer women than men experience chest pain. More common symptoms are shortness of breath, weakness and fatigue, a clammy sweat, dizziness, and nausea.

✓**check-in** Would you recognize the symptoms of a heart attack?

Many everyday activities—eating, drinking coffee, having sex, even breathing—can spur a heart attack. Air pollution from traffic poses the greatest risk. Other triggers include coffee, alcohol, physical exertion, eating a heavy meal, and sex.

If you're with someone who's exhibiting the classic signs of heart attack, and if those signs last for two minutes or more, act at once. Expect the person to deny the possibility of anything as serious as a heart attack but insist on taking prompt action.

Time is of the essence when a heart attack occurs. Call 911 immediately. The sooner emergency personnel get to a heart attack victim and administer cardiac life support, the greater the odds of survival. Yet according to the American Heart Association, most patients wait three hours after the initial symptoms begin before seeking help. By that time, half of the affected heart muscle may already be lost.

Cardiac Arrest Cardiac arrest occurs when the heart stops beating. If circulation isn't restored within four or five minutes, the brain shuts down completely, and the person dies.

Cardiopulmonary resuscitation (CPR) is an emergency procedure for a person whose heart has stopped or who is no longer breathing. CPR can maintain circulation and breathing until emergency medical help arrives.

The combination of mouth-to-mouth "rescue" breathing and chest compressions performed by individuals trained in CPR is the most effective method. However, according to the most recent research, chest compressions or "hands-only" CPR, which does not require extensive training, also can keep blood circulating until emergency help arrives.

Automated external defibrillators (AEDs), portable computerized devices, can actually restart a heart with a lethal rhythm (ventricular fibrillation) or that is not beating at all. The machines, widely available on airplanes and in public places like stadiums and terminals, also can be purchased by individuals. Written and voice instructions allow laypeople as well as trained professionals to use them in case of emergency. A combination of CPR and defibrillation boosts the survival rate much higher than from CPR alone.

Saving Hearts

State-of-the-art treatments for heart attacks include clot-dissolving drugs, early administration of medications to thin the blood, intravenous nitroglycerin, and in some cases, a beta-blocker (which blocks many of the effects of adrenaline in the body, particularly its stimulating impact on the heart).

Percutaneous transluminal coronary angioplasty (PTCA), also called balloon angioplasty, is the most often performed heart operation. Less costly and less risky than bypass surgery, PTCA opens blood vessels in the heart that are

myocardial infarction (MI) A condition characterized by the dying of tissue areas in the myocardium, caused by interruption of the blood supply to those areas; the medical name for a heart attack.

cardiopulmonary resuscitation (CPR) Emergency treatment to maintain circulation in a person whose heart has stopped or who is no longer breathing.

How to Recognize a Stroke

Researchers have found that the following steps can identify facial weakness, arm weakness, and speech problems, all signs of stroke:

- **Ask the individual to smile.**

- **Ask him or her to raise both arms.**

- **Ask the person to speak a simple sentence, such as "It is sunny out today."**

If he or she has trouble with any of these tasks, call 911 immediately and describe the symptoms to the dispatcher.

later.[67] (See Your Strategies for Prevention for what to do if you think someone you know has had a stroke.)

As many as 80 percent of strokes are preventable, primarily through lifestyle modification. The most important steps are

- Treating hypertension

- Not smoking

- Managing diabetes

- Lowering cholesterol

- If you're a woman, taking aspirin (which reduces stroke risk in women but not in men)

√ **check-in** Which of these steps are you taking?

Quick treatment with a clot-busting drug at a hospital can reduce the chance of disability after a stroke, but few people recognize the signs of a stroke and seek medical care within three hours of the first symptoms.

Risk Factors

Risk factors for stroke, like those for heart disease, include some that can't be changed (such as gender, race, and age) and some that can be controlled:

- **Gender:** Up to age 85, men have a greater risk of stroke than women. However, women are at increased risk at times of marked hormonal changes, particularly pregnancy and childbirth. Although older oral contraceptives had been linked with stroke, particularly in women over age 35 who smoke, the newer low-dose oral contraceptives have not shown an increased stroke risk among women ages 18 to 44. Early menopause (before age 42) may double a woman's stroke risk.

- **Race:** The incidence of strokes is two to three times greater in blacks than whites in the same communities. Hispanics also are more likely to develop hemorrhagic strokes than whites.

- **Age:** A person's risk of stroke more than doubles every decade after age 55.

- **Obesity:** The more overweight individuals are, the more likely they are to have a stroke. Obesity may increase stroke risk by contributing to high blood pressure and diabetes.

- **Hypertension:** Detection and treatment of high blood pressure are the best means of stroke prevention.

- **High red blood cell count:** A moderate to marked increase in the number of a person's red blood cells increases the risk of stroke.

narrowed but not completely blocked. PTCA involves a precise, time-consuming technique called *cardiac catheterization*—the threading of a narrow tube or catheter through an artery to the heart.

A *coronary bypass* is a procedure in which an artery from the patient's leg or chest wall is grafted onto a coronary artery to detour blood around the blocked area. Each year hundreds of thousands of coronary bypasses are performed in the United States; about 1 to 5 percent of these patients die as a result of surgical complications.

Stroke

When the blood supply to a portion of the brain is blocked, a cerebrovascular accident, or **stroke**, occurs. The proportion of strokes among young adults between ages 20 and 45 has been rising, probably as a consequence of the higher incidence of obesity, hypertension, and diabetes. Young adults who suffer strokes are at higher risk of diabetes and further "vascular events."[66]

√ **check-in** Did you know that 10 percent of strokes occur in 18- to 50-year-olds?

Although the number and mortality rate have declined, strokes rank third, after heart disease and cancer, as a cause of death in this country.

Worldwide, stroke is second only to heart disease as a cause of death. An estimated 20 percent of stroke victims die within three months; 50 to 60 percent are disabled.

Among those who survive a stroke before age 50, one-third are unable to live independently or require assistance with daily activities 10 years

stroke A cerebrovascular event in which the blood supply to a portion of the brain is blocked.

- **Heart disease:** Heart problems can interfere with the flow of blood to the brain; clots that form in the heart can travel to the brain, where they may clog an artery.
- **Blood fats:** Although the standard advice from cardiologists is to lower harmful LDL levels, what may be more important to lower stroke risk is an increase in the levels of protective HDL.
- **Diabetes mellitus:** Diabetics have a higher incidence of stroke than nondiabetics.
- **Estrogen therapy:** In the Women's Health Initiative—a series of clinical trials of hormone therapy for postmenopausal women—estrogen-only therapy significantly increased the risk of stroke.
- **A diet high in fat and sodium:** Individuals consuming the largest amounts of fatty foods and sodium are at much greater risk than those eating low-fat, low-salt diets.
- **Marijuana:** According to recent research, smoking marijuana (discussed in Chapter 12) may double the risk of stroke in young adults.

√**check-in** Do you have any risk factors for stroke?

Causes of Stroke

There are two types of stroke:

- **Ischemic stroke** results from a blockage that disrupts blood flow to the brain. One of the most common causes is the blockage of a brain artery by a thrombus, or blood clot—a *cerebral thrombosis*. Clots generally form around deposits sticking out from the arterial wall. Sometimes a wandering blood clot (embolus), carried in the bloodstream, becomes wedged in one of the cerebral arteries. This is called a *cerebral embolism*, and it can completely plug up a cerebral artery.
- **Hemorrhagic stroke** occurs when a diseased artery in the brain floods the surrounding tissue with blood. The cells nourished by the artery are deprived of blood and can't function, and the blood from the artery forms a clot that may interfere with brain function. This is most likely to occur if the patient suffers from a combination of hypertension and atherosclerosis. Hemorrhage (bleeding) may also be caused by a head injury or by the bursting of an aneurysm, a blood-filled pouch that balloons out from a weak spot in the wall of an artery.

Brain tissue, like heart muscle, begins to die if deprived of oxygen, which may then cause difficulty speaking and walking, as well as loss of memory. (See Figure 15.7.) These effects may be slight or severe, temporary or permanent, depending on how widespread the damage and whether other areas of the brain can take over the function of the damaged area.

Silent Strokes

As many as one in ten middle-aged adults may suffer a "silent" stroke, known as a "silent cerebral infarct," that does not produce clear symptoms but causes damage within the brain. According to new research, silent strokes may be at least five times more common than full-blown strokes in people under age 65 and are not uncommon in those younger than 50. The parts of the brain affected by the stroke may not involve motion or speech, but silent strokes can affect mood or memory.

Doctors note that mild strokes are not really silent but "whisper," causing very subtle symptoms that people might ignore. However, on tests of mental and physical functioning, individuals who've had very mild strokes suffer clear impairments. Even if they do not cause.

Transient Ischemic Attacks (TIAs)

Sometimes a person will suffer **transient ischemic attacks (TIAs)**, "little strokes" that cause minimal damage but serve as warning signs of a potentially more severe stroke. A TIA doubles the risk for a heart attack. One of three people who suffer TIAs will have a stroke during the following five years if he or she doesn't get treatment. The two major types of TIAs are

- **Transient monocular blindness.** Blurring, a blackout or whiteout of vision, a sense of a shade coming down, or another visual disturbance in one eye.
- **Transient hemispheral attack.** Diminished blood flow to one side of the brain, causing numbness or weakness of one arm, leg, or side of the face, or problems speaking or thinking.

Many TIAs are caused by a narrowing of blood vessels in the neck (carotid arteries) because of a buildup of plaque. Specialists can diagnose this problem by feeling and listening to the arteries, by ultrasound, by measuring the pressure or circulation rate from the carotid arteries to the eyes, or by arterial angiography (injection of a

transient ischemic attacks (TIAs) Cerebrovascular events in which the blood supply to a portion of the brain is blocked temporarily; repeated attacks are predictors of more severe strokes.

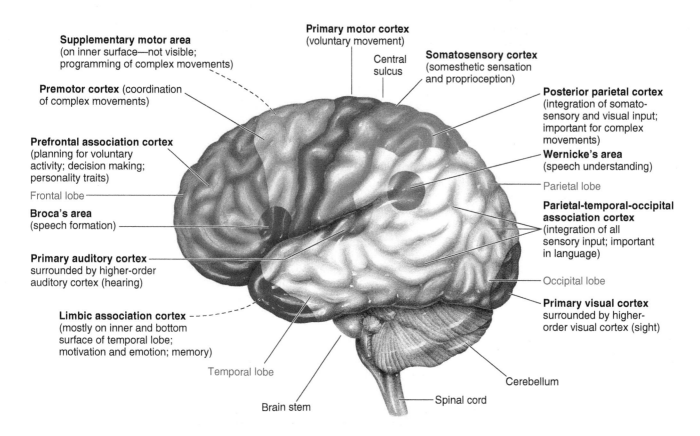

Supplementary motor area
(on inner surface—not visible;
programming of complex movements)

Primary motor cortex
(voluntary movement)

Central
sulcus

Somatosensory cortex
(somesthetic sensation
and proprioception)

Premotor cortex (coordination
of complex movements)

Posterior parietal cortex
(integration of somato-
sensory and visual input;
important for complex
movements)

Prefrontal association cortex
(planning for voluntary
activity; decision making;
personality traits)

Wernicke's area
(speech understanding)

Frontal lobe

Parietal lobe

Broca's area
(speech formation)

Parietal-temporal-occipital
association cortex
(integration of all
sensory input; important
in language)

Primary auditory cortex
surrounded by higher-order
auditory cortex (hearing)

Occipital lobe

Limbic association cortex
(mostly on inner and bottom
surface of temporal lobe;
motivation and emotion; memory)

Primary visual cortex
surrounded by higher-
order visual cortex (sight)

Temporal lobe

Cerebellum

Brain stem

Spinal cord

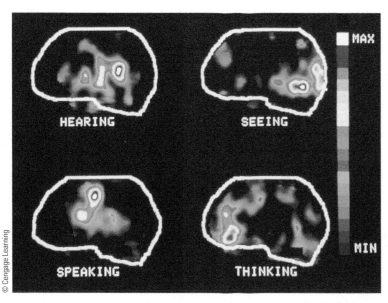

FIGURE 15.7 The Effects of Stroke on the Brain

dye into the arteries as X-rays are taken), a procedure that can be either dangerous, even deadly, or lifesaving.

✓**check-in** Did you know that on average someone in the United States has a stroke every 40 seconds and someone dies of a stroke approximately every 4 minutes?

Treatments for Strokes

Extremely rapid beating of the heart's upper chambers causes blood clots to form; they may enter the bloodstream and travel to the brain, where they can get stuck and choke off the blood supply. In the past, the only way to prevent such strokes was regular use of a medication called warfarin, which inhibits blood clotting and therefore increases the risk of severe bleeding. However, aspirin proved as effective as warfarin—without that dangerous side effect. Daily low-dose aspirin can cut in half the risk of strokes caused by abnormal heartbeats, which strike 75,000 Americans each year.

For patients who suffer a thrombotic stroke, thrombolytic drugs such as tissue-type plasminogen activator (tPa) can restore brain blood flow and save blood cells. Other medications called heparinoids can reduce the blood's tendency to clot. For thrombolytic drugs to be effective, they must be administered within three hours after the stroke; heparinoids must be given within 24 hours. People who get to a hospital within an hour of having the first symptoms of a stroke are twice as likely to receive tPa. However, more than one-third of people having a stroke do not call 911, and an equally large percentage live more than an hour away from a stroke center.[68]

Cancer

Cancer refers to a group of diseases characterized by "the uncontrolled growth and spread of abnormal cells." Second only to heart disease as a cause of death in the United States, cancer accounts for nearly one of every four deaths.[69]

Here are some basic facts about cancer in America:

- About 1,658,370 new cancers are diagnosed every year.

- About 589,430 Americans die of cancer every year.

- About 1,620 people die of cancer every day.

- The five-year survival rate for those diagnosed with cancer is 68 percent, up from about 50 percent four decades ago.[70]

Many cancers are preventable, including those caused by the following:

- Tobacco smoking

- Heavy alcohol consumption

- Overweight and obesity

- Physical inactivity

- Poor nutrition

- Excessive sun exposure and indoor tanning

- Infections that could be avoided by behavioral changes on vaccination[71]

Healthier lifestyles could prevent some 340,000 cancers a year. A third of cancers are related to smoking; another third, to obesity, poor diet, and lack of exercise.

A combination of healthy lifestyle behaviors has proven more effective than any one specific change in lowering the cancer risk.[72]

✓ **check-in** Which of the following preventive steps are you taking to reduce your risk of cancer?

____ Higher fruit and vegetable intake

____ Lower red meat intake

____ Lower fat intake

____ Lower BMI

____ Higher physical activity

Prevention, early detection, and improved treatment have lowered the death rates for cancers of the lungs, colon, breast, and prostate. Overall, cancer death rates have been falling an average of 1.5 percent per year.[73] For some cancers, such as breast and ovarian, survival rates are lower for blacks than whites, but survival rates for prostate cancer improved more among blacks than whites.[74]

Understanding Cancer

The uncontrolled growth and spread of abnormal cells causes cancer. Normal cells follow the code of instructions embedded in DNA (the body's genetic material); cancer cells do not. Think of the DNA within the nucleus of a cell as a computer program that controls the cell's functioning, including its ability to grow and reproduce itself. If this program or its operation is altered, the cell goes out of control. The nucleus no longer regulates growth. The abnormal cell divides to create other abnormal cells, which again divide, eventually forming *neoplasms* (new formations), or tumors.

External causes of cancer include

- Tobacco

- Infectious organisms

- Unhealthy diet

- Carcinogens in the environment

Often ten years or more may pass between exposure to external factors and cancer detection.

Internal causes of cancer include

- Genetic mutations

📷 Cancer Preventive Strategies

Percentage of students who	%
Used sunscreen regularly when outdoors	52
If male, performed a testicular self-exam in the past 30 days	33.4
If female, performed a breast self-exam in the past 30 days	35.2
If female, had a gynecological exam in the past 12 months	44.3

Simple steps can help you stay as healthy as possible as long as possible. Are you conscientious about these protective practices? Are you better at some than others? If not, why not? Are you too busy? Do you have other priorities? Is money an issue? Think through these issues and develop a personalized health maintenance plan. Write it down in your online journal.

Source: American College Health Association. *American College Health Association–National College Health Assessment II: Reference Group Executive Summary, Spring 2014.* Hanover, MD: American College Health Association, 2014.

• Hormones

• Immune conditions

Tumors can be either benign (slightly abnormal, not considered life-threatening) or malignant (cancerous). The only way to determine whether a tumor is benign is by microscopic examination of its cells. Cancer cells have larger nuclei than the cells in benign tumors; they vary more in shape and size; and they divide more often. In general, one billion cancer cells need to have formed before a cancer can be detected. This is the number of cells in a tumor that measures one centimeter (about a third of an inch.)

Cancer Staging

When cancer is detected, specialists focus on "staging" (describing the extent or spread of cancer at the time of diagnosis). A cancer's stage depends on the size and extent of the primary tumor and whether it has spread to nearby lymph nodes or other areas of the body. If cancer cells are present only in the layer of cells where they developed and have not spread, the stage is "in situ."

If cancer cells have penetrated beyond the original layer of tissue, the cancer has become invasive and is categorized as "local," "regional," or "distant," depending on the extent of the spread.

Oncologists (physicians who specialize in treating cancer) uses a different staging system called TNM:

• T for the extent of the primary tumor

• N for the absence or presence of regional lymph node involvement

• M for the absence or presence of distant metastases.

Once these categories are identified, a stage of 0, I, II, III, or IV is assigned, with stage 0 being in situ, stage I, early; and stage IV, the most advanced disease.

✓**check-in** Do you know your lifetime risk of developing cancer?

If you're male: slightly less than 1 in 2

If you're female: a little more than 1 in 3

Without treatment, cancer cells continue to grow, crowding out and replacing healthy cells. This process is called **infiltration**, or invasion. Cancer cells may also **metastasize**, or spread to other parts of the body via the bloodstream or lymphatic system (Figure 15.8). For many cancers, as many as 60 percent of patients may have metastases (which may be too small to be felt or seen without a microscope) at the time of diagnosis. Early detection and treatment result in the highest rate of cure.

Who Is at Risk?

Cancer strikes individuals at all social, economic, and educational levels. (See Table 15.3.)

Heredity An estimated 13 to 14 million Americans may be at risk of a hereditary cancer. In hereditary cancers, such as retinoblastoma (an eye cancer that strikes young children) or certain colon cancers, a specific cancer-causing gene is

infiltration A gradual penetration or invasion.

metastasize To spread to other parts of the body via the bloodstream or lymphatic system.

passed down from generation to generation. The odds of any child with one affected parent inheriting this gene and developing the cancer are 50–50.

Other people are born with genes that make them susceptible to having certain cells grow and divide uncontrollably, which may contribute to cancer development. The most well-known are mutations of the BRCA gene, linked with increased risk of breast, colon, and ovarian cancer.

Genetic tests can identify some individuals who are born with an increased susceptibility to cancer. Spotting a mutated gene in an individual may alert doctors to increase screening and possibly detect cancer years earlier than they otherwise would have. The most likely sites for inherited cancers to develop are the breast, brain, blood, muscles, bones, and adrenal glands.

✓**check-in** If you had a family history of cancer, would you undergo genetic tests to find out if you are at risk? Why or why not?

Racial and Ethnic Groups
Although cancer death rates have fallen in the United States, they vary in different racial and ethnic groups:

- Biological racial and ethnic differences can affect whether a cancer is aggressive and will spread beyond its initial site. In breast cancer, for instance, black women had a higher risk of dying compared with white women, even when both were diagnosed with small tumors.[75]

- African Americans have the highest rates of fatal cancers. Black women have the highest incidence of colorectal and lung cancers of any ethnic group, while black men have the highest rates of prostate, colorectal, and lung cancers. African Americans also have higher rates of incidence and deaths from other cancers, including those of the mouth, throat, esophagus, stomach, pancreas, and larynx. Cancer death rates have been declining annually since the 1990s for black men and women.

- Hispanics have a six times lower risk of developing melanoma than Caucasians yet tend to have a worse prognosis than Caucasians when they do develop this skin cancer.

- The incidence of female breast cancer is highest among white women and lowest among Native American women.

- Cervical cancer is most common in Hispanic women.

- Vietnamese men have much higher rates of liver cancer than whites, while Korean men and women are much more likely to develop stomach cancer.

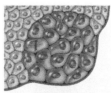 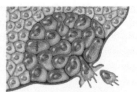

1 Benign neoplasms grow slowly and stay in their home tissue.

2 Cells of a malignant neoplasm can break away from their home tissue.

3 Malignant cells can become attached to the wall of a blood vessel or lymph vessel. They release enzymes that create an opening in the wall, then enter the vessel.

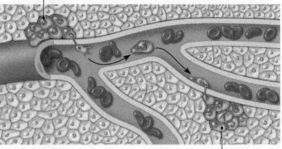

4 The cells creep or tumble along in blood vessels, then leave the bloodstream the same way they got in. They may start growing in other tissues, a process called metastasis.

© Cengage Learning

FIGURE 15.8 Metastasis, or Spread of Cancer

Cancer cells can travel through the blood vessels to spread to other organs or through the lymphatic system to form secondary tumors.

From Starr/Evers/Starr, Biology Today and Tomorrow without Physiology, 4E. © 2013 Cengage Learning

- Compared with other Asian Americans, Chinese and Vietnamese women have higher rates of lung cancer.

- Asian Americans who have lived in the United States the longest are likely to develop the cancers that are most common here, such as breast and colon cancer, although at lower rates than whites.

Obesity
Long recognized as threats to cardiovascular health, overweight and obesity may play a role in an estimated 90,000 cancer deaths each year.

The higher an individual's BMI, the greater the likelihood of dying of cancer. An unhealthy body weight increases the risk of many types of cancer, including non-Hodgkin's lymphoma, multiple myeloma, and cancers of the following:

- Breast (in postmenopausal women)

- Colon and rectum

- Kidney

- Cervix

- Ovary

TABLE 15.3 Leading New Cancer Cases and Deaths, 2015 Estimates

Cancer (Males)	Estimated New Cases*		Estimated Deaths		Cancer (Females)	Estimated New Cases*		Estimated Deaths	
Colon & Rectum	69,090	8%	26,100	8%	Brain & Other Nervous System			6,380	2%
Esophagus			12,600	4%	Breast	231,840	29%	40,290	15%
Kidney & Renal Pelvis	38,270	5%	9,070	3%	Colon & Rectum	63,610	8%	23,600	9%
Leukemia	30,900	4%	14,210	5%	Kidney & Renal Pelvis	23,290	3%		
Liver & Intrahepatic Bile Duct	25,510	3%	17,030	5%	Leukemia	23,370	3%	10,240	4%
Lung & Bronchus	115,610	14%	86,380	28%	Liver & Intrahepatic Bile Duct			7,520	3%
Melanoma of the skin	42,670	5%			Lung & Bronchus	105,590	13%	71,660	26%
Non-Hodgkin Lymphoma	39,850	5%	11,480	4%	Melanoma of the skin	31,200	4%		
Oral Cavity & Pharynx	32,670	4%			Non-Hodgkin Lymphoma	32,000	4%	8,310	3%
Pancreas			20,710	7%	Ovary			14,180	5%
Prostate	220,800	26%	27,540	9%	Pancreas	24,120	3%	19,850	4%
Urinary bladder	56,320	7%	11,510	4%	Thyroid	47,230	6%		
					Uterine corpus	54,870	7%	10,170	4%
All Sites	**848,200**	**100%**	**312,150**	**100%**	**All Sites**	**312,150**	**100%**	**277,280**	**100%**

*Excludes basal cell and squamous cell skin cancers and in situ carcinoma except urinary bladder

*Excludes basal cell and squamous cell skin cancers and in situ carcinoma except urinary bladder

© 2015, American Cancer Society, Inc., Surveillance Research

- Uterus
- Esophagus
- Gallbladder
- Stomach (in men)
- Liver
- Pancreas
- Prostate

The degree to which extra pounds affect cancer risk varies by the site of the cancer. Obesity elevates the risk of esophageal cancer fivefold; increases the risk of breast or uterine cancer by two to four times; and boosts the risk for colon cancer by 35 percent to twofold.

Infectious Agents Worldwide, an estimated 17 percent of cancers can be attributed to infection. In economically developing countries, infections cause or contribute to 26 percent of cancers. In developed countries, they play a role in 7 percent of new cases of cancer.

Among the cancers that have been linked with infectious agents are

- Human papillomavirus (HPV) with cancer of the cervix, mouth and throat, vulva, and anus.[76] (See Chapter 11 for details on human papillomavirus.)

- *Helicobacter pylori* with stomach cancer.

- Viruses with certain leukemias (cancers of the blood system) and lymphomas (cancers of the lymphatic system), cancers of the nose and pharynx, and liver cancer.

- Human immunodeficiency virus (HIV) with certain lymphomas and leukemias and a type of cancer called Kaposi's sarcoma.

Generally, the presence of a bacterium or a virus per se is not enough to cause cancer. A predisposing environment and other cofactors—most still unknown—are needed for cancer development and growth.

Common Types of Cancer

Cancer refers to a group of more than a hundred diseases characterized by abnormal cell growth. Although all cancers have similar characteristics, each is distinct. Some cancers are relatively simple to cure, whereas others are more threatening and mysterious. The earlier any cancer is found, the easier it is to treat and the better the patient's chances of survival.

Cancers are classified according to the type of cell and the organ in which they originate, such as the following:

- **Carcinoma,** the most common kind, which starts in the epithelium, the layers of cells that cover the body's surface or line internal organs and glands
- **Sarcoma,** which forms in the supporting, or connective, tissues of the body: bones, muscles, blood vessels
- **Leukemia,** which begins in the blood-forming tissues: bone marrow, lymph nodes, and the spleen
- **Lymphoma,** which arises in the cells of the lymph system, the network that filters out impurities

Skin Cancer   One of every five Americans can expect to develop skin cancer in his or her lifetime. Once scientists thought exposure to the B range of ultraviolet light (UVB), the wavelength of light responsible for sunburn, posed the greatest danger. However, longer-wavelength UVA, which penetrates deeper into the skin, also plays a major role in skin cancers. UV light can damage DNA in melanocytes, cells in the skin that make the substance called melanin, which gives skin its color. Damage to melanocytes can continue long after UV exposure, even in the dark.[77]

Exposure to tanning salons and sunlamps also increase the risk of skin cancer because they produce ultraviolet radiation. A half-hour dose of radiation from a sunlamp can be equivalent to the amount you'd get from an entire day in the sun. Often skin damage is invisible to the naked eye but shows up under special diagnostic lights.

According to a recent analysis of data on more than 400,000 people, more than one-third of all Americans—and nearly 6 out of 10 U.S. university students—have used indoor tanning.[78] Even when they perceive the seriousness of skin cancer, college students—particularly women—describe

suntanned skin as attractive, healthy, and athletic looking and view the benefits of getting a suntan as outweighing the risks of skin cancer or premature aging. (See Consumer Alert.) However, a CDC report concluded that indoor tanning is "simply not safe" and causes sunburn, infection, eye damage, and increased risk of skin cancer.

✓**check-in** Have you ever gone to indoor tanning salons? If so, how often?

The most common skin cancers are *basal cell* (involving the base of the epidermis, the top level of the skin) and *squamous cell* (involving cells in the epidermis). Their incidence is increasing among men and women under age 40. Long-term exposure to the sun is the biggest risk factor for these cancers.

Young men and women who use tanning beds are significantly more likely than nonusers to develop early-onset basal cell skin cancers before age 40. The more extensive their use, the greater their risk of skin cancers, particularly on the extremities and the torso. Researchers estimate that avoiding tanning beds could cut the percentages of early-onset skin cancer by 27 percent overall and by 43 percent among women.

Every year more than 5 million Americans develop skin lesions known as actinic keratoses (AKs), rough red or brown scaly patches that develop in the upper layer of the skin, usually on the face, lower lip, bald scalp, neck, back of the hands, and forearms. Forty percent of squamous cell carcinomas, the second-leading cause of skin cancer deaths, begin as AKs. Treatments include surgical removal, cryosurgery (freezing the skin), electrodesiccation (heat generated by an electric current), topical chemotherapy, and removal with lasers, chemical peels, or dermabrasion.

Malignant *melanoma*, the deadliest type of skin cancer, causes 1 to 2 percent of all cancer deaths. Melanoma rates have tripled since 1975 to about 23 cases per 100,000 people.[80] Melanoma has become the most common cancer among young adults between ages 25 and 29 and the second-most-common cancer among 15- to 24-year-olds. During the 1930s, the lifetime risk of melanoma was about 1 in 1,500. Today it is 1 in 75. This increase in risk is due mostly to overexposure to UV radiation. The use of a tanning bed 10 times or more a year doubles the risk for individuals over age 30.

Melanoma Both the amount and the intensity of lifetime sun exposure play key roles in determining risk for melanoma. People living in areas where the sun's ultraviolet rays reach Earth with extra intensity, such as tropical or high-altitude regions, are at increased risk. Although melanoma occurs more often among people over 40, it is increasing in younger people, particularly those who had severe sunburns in childhood.

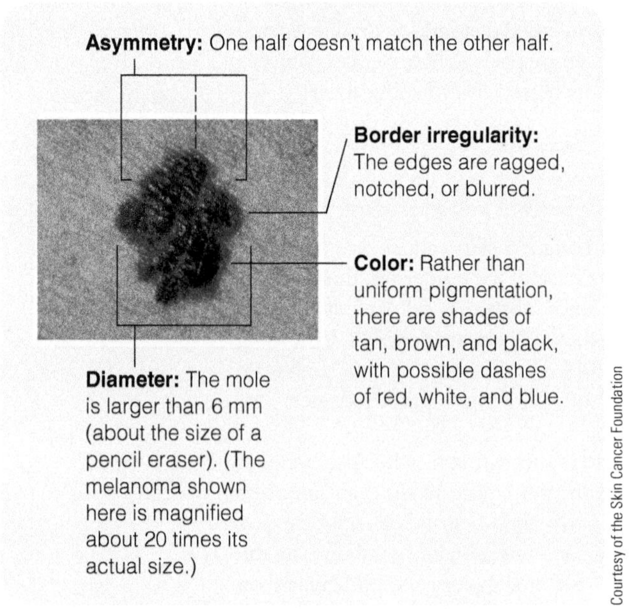

Asymmetry: One half doesn't match the other half.

Border irregularity: The edges are ragged, notched, or blurred.

Color: Rather than uniform pigmentation, there are shades of tan, brown, and black, with possible dashes of red, white, and blue.

Diameter: The mole is larger than 6 mm (about the size of a pencil eraser). (The melanoma shown here is magnified about 20 times its actual size.)

Courtesy of the Skin Cancer Foundation

FIGURE 15.9 ABCD: The Warning Signs of Melanoma

An estimated 95 percent of cases of melanoma arise from an existing mole. A normal mole is usually round or oval, less than 6 millimeters (about ¼ inch) in diameter, and evenly colored (black, brown, or tan). Seek prompt evaluation of any moles that change in ways shown in the photo.

Source: American Academy of Dermatology. All rights reserved.

Individuals with any of the following characteristics are at increased risk:

- Fair skin, light eyes, or fair hair
- A tendency to develop freckles and to burn instead of tan
- A history of childhood sunburn or intermittent, intense sun exposure
- A personal or family history of melanoma
- A large number of nevi, or moles (200 or more, or 50 or more if under age 20), or dysplastic (atypical) moles

Detection The most common predictor for melanoma is a change in an existing mole or development of a new and changing pigmented mole. The most important early indicators are change in color, an increase in diameter, and changes in the borders of a mole (Figure 15.9). An increase in height signals a corresponding growth in depth under the skin. Itching in a new or long-standing mole also should not be ignored.

In 2014, an estimated 15,780 new cases of cancer will be diagnosed, and 1,960 deaths from cancer will occur among children and adolescents aged birth to 19 years. The annual incidence rate of cancer in children and adolescents is 186.6 per 1 million children aged birth to 19 years. Approximately 1 in 285 children will be diagnosed with cancer before age 20 years, and approximately 1 in 530 young adults between the ages of 20 and 39 years is a childhood cancer survivor.

Treatment If caught early, melanoma is highly curable, usually with surgery alone. Once it has spread, chemotherapy with a single drug or a combination can temporarily shrink tumors in some people. However, the five-year survival rate for metastatic melanoma is only 14 percent. (See Your Strategies for Prevention.)

Breast Cancer Every 3 minutes, a woman in the United States learns that she has breast cancer. Every 12 minutes, a woman dies of breast cancer. Many women misjudge their own likelihood of developing breast cancer, either overestimating or underestimating their susceptibility. In a national poll, 1 in every 10 surveyed considered herself at no risk at all. This is never the case. Every woman is at risk for breast cancer simply because she's female. (See Table 15.3.)

✓**check-in** If you're a woman, do you examine your breasts regularly?

TABLE 15.4 A Woman's Risk of Developing Breast Cancer

By age 25	1 in 19,608
By age 30	1 in 2,525
By age 35	1 in 622
By age 40	1 in 217
By age 45	1 in 93
By age 50	1 in 50
By age 55	1 in 33
By age 60	1 in 24
By age 65	1 in 17
By age 70	1 in 14
By age 75	1 in 11
By age 80	1 in 10
By age 85	1 in 9
Ever	1 in 8

Source: Surveillance Program, National Cancer Institute.

The most common risk factors include the following:

- **Age:** As shown in Table 15.4, at 25, a woman's chance of developing breast cancer is 1 in 19,608; by age 45, it has increased to 1 in 93; by 65, it is 1 in 17. The mean age at which women are diagnosed is 63. However, more young women are being diagnosed with advanced metastatic breast cancer.[81]

- **Family history:** The overwhelming majority of breast cancers—90 to 95 percent—are not due to strong genetic factors. However, having a first-degree relative—mother, sister, or daughter—with breast cancer does increase risk, and if the relative developed breast cancer before menopause, the cancer is more likely to be hereditary.

- **Long menstrual history:** Women who had their first period before age 12 are at greater risk than women who began menstruating later. The reason is that the more menstrual cycles a woman has, the longer her exposure to estrogen, a hormone known to increase breast cancer danger. For similar reasons, childless women, who menstruate continuously for several decades, are also at greater risk. Neither miscarriage nor induced abortion increases the risk of breast cancer.

- **Age at birth of first child:** An early pregnancy—in a woman's teens or 20s—changes the actual maturation of breast cells and decreases risk. But if a woman has her first child in her 40s, precancerous cells may actually flourish with the high hormone levels of the pregnancy.

- **Breast biopsies:** Even if laboratory analysis finds no precancerous abnormalities, women who require such tests are more likely to develop breast cancer. Fibrocystic breast disease, a term often used for "lumpy" breasts, is not a risk factor.

- **Race and ethnicity:** Breast cancer rates are lower in Hispanic and Asian American populations than in whites and in African American women. Caucasian women over 40 have the highest incidence rate for breast cancer in this country, but African American women at every age have a greater likelihood of dying from breast cancer.[82] One reason may be that minority women wait longer for treatment, whether surgery or chemotherapy. Hispanic women, particularly those of Mexican descent, are more likely

YOUR STRATEGIES FOR PREVENTION

Save Your Skin

- **Once a month, stand in front of a full-length mirror to examine your front and back, as well as your left and right sides with your arms raised.** Check the backs of your legs, the tops and soles of your feet, and the surfaces between your toes. Use a hand mirror to check the back of your neck, behind your ears, and your scalp.

- **Watch for changes in the size, color, number, and thickness of moles.** Suspicious moles are likely to be asymmetrical (one half doesn't match the other), with ragged, notched, or blurred edges. Also look for any signs of darkly pigmented growth, oozing, scaliness, bleeding, or a change in sensation, itchiness, tenderness, or pain.

- **Don't put too much faith in sunscreens.** Wearing sunscreen (with a sun protection factor, or SPF, of at least 15) is good, but protective clothing is better—and staying in the shade is best. Check your shadow. One simple guideline for reducing the risk of skin cancer is avoiding the sun anytime your shadow is shorter than you are. According to the National Cancer Institute (NCI), this shadow method—based on the principle that the closer the sun comes to being directly overhead, the stronger its ultraviolet rays—works for any location and at any time of year.

- **Check for photosensitivity.** If you are taking any drugs, ask your doctor or pharmacist to see if the medication could make you more sensitive to sun damage. Be especially cautious about sun exposure if you have been using a synthetic preparation derived from vitamin A (Retin A) as an acne or anti-wrinkle treatment; it can increase your susceptibility.

- **Use extra caution near water, snow, and sand since they reflect the damaging rays of the sun and increase the risk of sunburn.** Wear protective clothing, such as a wide-brimmed cap or hat, whenever possible.

than white or black women to have hereditary forms of cancer.

- **Occupation:** Based on two decades of following more than a million women, Swedish researchers have developed a list of jobs linked with a high risk of breast cancer. These include pharmacists, certain types of teachers, schoolmasters, systems analysts and programmers, telephone operators, telegraph and radio operators, metal platers and coaters, and salon workers. Shift work, particularly at night, may be associated with an increased risk of breast cancer.

- **Alcohol:** Women's risk of breast cancer increases with the amount of alcohol they drink. Those who have two or more drinks per day are 40 percent more likely to develop breast cancer than women who don't drink at all. For a nondrinking woman, the lifetime risk of breast cancer by age 80 is 1 in 11. For heavy drinkers it's about 1 in 7, regardless of race, education, family history, use of hormone therapy, or other risk factors.

- **Smoking:** Cigarette smoking, with or without alcohol use, increases the risk of breast cancer, especially when women start smoking early in life.

- **Hormone therapy (HT):** Several studies confirm an increased risk with a combination of estrogen and progestin, particularly in women who use combination HT for five years or longer. With the decreasing use of hormone therapy, breast cancer rates declined.

- **Obesity:** Excess weight, particularly after menopause, increases the risk of getting breast cancer. Overweight women, both pre- and postmenopausal, with breast cancer are more likely to die of their disease.

- **Sedentary lifestyle:** According to the World Health Organization, regular physical activity may cut the risk of developing breast cancer by 20 to 40 percent, regardless of a woman's menopausal status or the type or intensity of the activity. The reason may be that exercise lowers levels of circulating ovarian hormones.

✓**check-in** Do you know which factors may lower a woman's risk of breast cancer?

*Breastfeeding for at least one year

*Regular moderate or vigorous exercise

*Maintaining a healthy body weight

*Taking one of two medications—tamoxifen and raloxifene—that have been approved

to reduce the likelihood of breast cancer in high-risk women

Screening for Breast Cancer Health providers vary in their recommendations for screening for breast cancer. Although it is a common practice, teaching breast self-examination has not been proven to reduce deaths from breast cancer. Some organizations encourage all women age 20 and older to monitor the normal appearance and feel of their breasts and promptly report any changes to their physicians.

In studies of clinical breast exams, the combination of an exam with **mammography** had the greatest sensitivity—but also the highest rate of false-positives.[83] Screening mammography has been shown to reduce breast cancer mortality, particularly among women 50 to 74 years of age. According to recent research, women in this age range who underwent mammography screening every two years were diagnosed at the same stage of disease as those screened annually.[84]

The U.S. Preventive Services Task Force initially recommended against routine biannual screening for women younger than 40, primarily because of the high rate of false-positives and the risks of overdiagnosis and overtreatment. The task force has since updated its recommendations to advise mammography on an individualized basis.

The primary downside or more frequent mammograms is a false-positive diagnosis—when breast cancer is first suspected but then ruled out with further testing—which can be extremely upsetting.

✓**check-in** If you are a woman, have you ever had a mammogram or breast biopsy?

Treatment Treatment options depend on the size of the tumor and the extent of spread, but may involve the following:

- Breast-conserving surgery (surgical removal of the tumor and surrounding tissue)

- **Mastectomy** (surgical removal of the breast)

As numerous studies have shown, women treated with breast-conserving surgery plus radiation and those who undergo mastectomy have similar long-term survival rates. Surgeons usually remove underarm lymph nodes to determine if a tumor has spread beyond the breast.

Breast cancer treatment also may involve the following:

- Radiation.

- Chemotherapy (before or after surgery).

mammography A diagnostic X-ray exam used to detect breast cancer.

mastectomy The surgical removal of an entire breast.

- Hormone therapy (with agents such as estrogen receptor modifiers or aromatase inhibitors). Women with early-stage breast cancer who test positive for hormone receptors benefit from at least five years of hormone therapy. Several targeted therapies are available for women whose cancer overexpresses a growth-promoting hormone called HER2.[85]

Survival About six in ten diagnosed breast cancers are localized and have not spread to lymph nodes or other locations outside the breast. The five-year survival rate for women with these cancers is 99 percent. If the cancer has spread to tissues or lymph nodes under the arm, the survival rate is 85 percent. If the cancer has spread to lymph nodes around the collarbone or more distant nodes or an organ, the survival rate falls to 25 percent. Survival rates are lower for black women, who may be diagnosed and seek treatment later. Breast cancer survivors who are more physically active, particularly after diagnosis, are less likely to die of breast cancer or other causes than those who are inactive.

Cervical Cancer Cervical cancer, the second-most-common cancer in women worldwide, claims 250,000 lives every year. An estimated 11,000 cases of invasive cervical cancer are diagnosed in the United States every year. The highest incidence rate occurs among Vietnamese, Alaska Native, Korean, and Hispanic women.

Human papillomavirus (HPV) infection is the primary risk factor for cervical cancer. (See Chapter 11.) Women are at higher risk for cervical cancer if they

- Engaged in sexual activity before age 16
- Have had multiple sexual partners (more than five in a lifetime)
- Have genital herpes
- Smoke
- Have been exposed to secondhand smoke

Screening Two types of tests are used for cervical cancer screening:

- The Pap test, which can find early cell changes and cancerous growths and treat them (see Table 15.5).
- The HPV test, which detects infections that can lead to cell changes and cancer. The HPV test may be used along with a Pap test or to help doctors decide how to treat women with an abnormal Pap test.

TABLE 15.5 What Pap Test Results Mean

A Pap test may come back as "normal," "unclear," or "abnormal."

Normal	A normal (or "negative") result means that no cell changes were found on the cervix.
Unclear	It is common for test results to come back unclear. Doctors may use other words to describe this result, such as inconclusive, or ASC-US. These mean the same thing: that some cervical cells could be abnormal, perhaps because of an infection. An HPV test will indicate whether the changes are related to HPV.
Abnormal	An abnormal result means that cell changes were found on the cervix. This usually does not indicate cervical cancer.
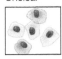	

© Cengage Learning

Abnormal changes on your cervix are likely caused by HPV. The changes may be minor (low-grade) or serious (high-grade). Most of the time, minor changes go back to normal on their own. But more serious changes can turn into cancer if the cells are not removed. The more serious changes are often called "pre-cancer" because they are not yet cancer but could turn into cancer over time.

The American Cancer Society's latest screening recommendations are as follows:

- All women should begin cervical cancer screening at age 21.
- Women between the ages of 21 and 29 should have a Pap test every three years but should not be tested for HPV unless they have an abnormal Pap test result.
- Women between the ages of 30 and 65 should have both a Pap test and an HPV test every five years. This is the preferred approach; a Pap test alone every three years also is acceptable.
- Women over age 65 who have had regular screenings with normal results should not be screened for cervical cancer. Women who have been diagnosed with cervical precancer should continue to be screened.
- Women who have had their uterus and cervix removed in a hysterectomy and have no history of cervical cancer or precancer should not be screened.
- Women who have had the HPV vaccine should still follow the screening recommendations for their age group.
- Women who are at high risk for cervical cancer—for example, those with HIV infection, organ transplant, or exposure to the drug DES—should talk with their doctor or nurse about more frequent screening.

Doctors no longer recommend annual Pap tests because it generally takes 10 to 20 years for cervical cancer to develop and overly frequent screening could lead to unneeded medical and surgical procedures.

✓ **check-in** If you're a woman, have you had any screening test for cervical cancer?

Ovarian Cancer

Ovarian cancer is the leading cause of death from gynecological cancers. Risk factors include

- A family history of ovarian cancer.
- Smoking
- Testing positive for inherited mutations in BRCA1 and BRCA2 genes. (Preventive surgery to remove the ovaries and fallopian tubes decreases the risk of these women.)

Among the factors that may reduce the risk of ovarian cancer are

- Pregnancy
- Long-term use of oral contraceptives
- Tubal ligation
- Hysterectomy (removal of the uterus)
- Salpingectomy (removal of the fallopian tubes)
- Personal history of breast cancer.
- Obesity.
- Infertility (because the abnormality that interferes with conception may also play a role in cancer development).
- Low levels of transferase, an enzyme involved in the metabolism of dairy foods.

Ovarian cancer may be diagnosed through pelvic examination, ultrasound, MRI, computed tomography, or PET (positron emission tomography) scan. Women with ovarian cancer are more likely to report abdominal pain, feeling full quickly after eating, and urinary urgency, but these symptoms are so common that they are often overlooked or dismissed.

Treatment involves surgery and usually chemotherapy. Survival rates depend on whether the cancer has spread to distant sites.

Testicular Cancer

In the past 20 years the incidence of testicular cancer has risen by about 50 percent in the United States, to 5.44 per 100,000. It is not clear why testicular cancer is on the rise, although researchers speculate that changing environmental or socioeconomic risk factors could have a role. Chronic use of marijuana increases the risk of an especially aggressive form of testicular cancer. Testicular cancer occurs mostly among young men between the ages of 18 and 35, who are not normally at risk of cancer.

Risk factors for testicular cancer include:

- An undescended testicle
- Family history of testicular cancer
- HIV infection
- Cancer in the other testicle
- Caucasian race (white men have a 4 to 5 times greater risk than black or Asian American men)

To detect possibly cancerous growths, men should perform monthly testicular self-exams.

✓ **check-in** If you're a man, do you examine your testicles regularly?

Often the first sign of this cancer is a slight enlargement of one testicle. There also may be a change in the way it feels when touched. Sometimes men with testicular cancer report a dull ache in the lower abdomen or groin, along with a sense of heaviness or sluggishness. Lumps on the testicles also may indicate cancer.

A man who notices any abnormality should consult a physician. If a lump is indeed present, a surgical biopsy is necessary to find out if it is cancerous. If the biopsy is positive, a series of tests generally is needed to determine whether the disease has spread.

Treatment for testicular cancer generally involves surgical removal of the diseased testis, sometimes along with radiation therapy, chemotherapy, and the removal of nearby lymph nodes. The remaining testicle is capable of maintaining a man's sexual potency and fertility. Only in rare cases is removal of both testicles necessary. Testosterone injections following such surgery can maintain potency. The chance for a cure is very high if testicular cancer is spotted early.

Colon and Rectal Cancer

Colon and rectal, or colorectal, cancer is the third most common cancer and accounts for 10 percent of cancer deaths. Most cases occur after age 50. Both age and gender influence the risk of colon cancer. Older individuals and men are more likely to develop polyps (nonmalignant growths that may turn cancerous at some point) and tumors in the colon than young people and women. Men who are physically fit in middle age are less likely to develop colon cancer later in life.[86]

Some factors may lower your odds of developing colon cancer. A healthy vegetarian diet that features fruits, vegetables, whole grains, beans, and nuts may cut the risk by as much as 20 percent.[87] Regular use of the nonprescription painkillers known as nonsteroidal anti-inflammatory drugs (NSAIDs), such as aspirin, naproxen (Aleve), and ibuprofen (Motrin, Advil), is associated with an overall lower risk of colon cancer but may only benefit those with certain genetic variations.[88]

Risk factors include

- Age (over 50)
- Personal or family history of colon and rectal cancer
- Polyps in the colon or rectum
- Ulcerative colitis
- Smoking
- Alcohol consumption
- Prolonged high consumption of red and processed meat
- High-fat or low-fiber diet
- Inadequate intake of fruits and vegetables
- Low calcium intake
- Obesity
- Physical inactivity

✓**check-in** Do you have any risk factors for color cancer? If so, are they modifiable?

Long-term constipation does not raise the risk of colorectal cancer.[89] Low doses of aspirin or other nonsteroidal anti-inflammatory drugs appear to reduce the risk of precancerous polyps that can lead to colon and rectal cancer. Smokers have a worse prognosis than nonsmokers.[90]

Current guidelines recommend that clinicians screen for colorectal cancer in average-risk adults starting at age 50 and in high-risk adults starting at age 40 or 10 years younger than the age at which the youngest affected relative was diagnosed with colorectal cancer. The screening options include a stool-based test, flexible sigmoidoscopy, and optical colonoscopy in patients who are at average risk.[71] The initial screening is crucial because it detects the largest, most dangerous polyps, which can then be removed. Removing polyps found during colonoscopies has proven to reduce deaths from colon and rectal cancer by 70 percent. If 80 percent of older adults underwent colon cancer screening, 21,000 fewer Americans would die of the cancer every year.[91]

Early signs of colorectal cancer are bleeding from the rectum, blood in the stool, and a change in bowel habits. Treatment may involve surgery, radiation therapy, and/or chemotherapy.

Prostate Cancer After skin cancer, prostate cancer is the most common form of cancer in American men. The risk of prostate cancer is 1 in 6; the risk of death due to metastatic prostate cancer is 1 in 30. More than one-quarter of men diagnosed with cancer have prostate cancer. The disease strikes African American men more often than white; Asian and American Indian men are affected less often.

The risk of prostate cancer increases with age, family history, exposure to the heavy metal cadmium, high number of sexual partners, and history of frequent sexually transmitted infections. A diet high in saturated fat may be a risk factor. An inherited predisposition may account for 5 to 10 percent of cases. A purported link between vasectomy and prostate cancer has been disproved. Statin drugs, commonly prescribed to lower cholesterol, also may lower the risk of prostate cancer.

Annual screening with a test that measures levels of a protein called prostate-specific antigen (PSA) in the blood is no longer recommended. Annual prostate cancer screening does not reduce deaths from the disease, regardless of the man's age or overall health.[92]

Some prostate cancers never progress. Since treatments, such as a radiation or surgery to remove the prostate, can cause significant side effects, more cancer specialists are recommending a conservative, wait-and-watch approach. However, most men opt for treatment, usually radiation, regardless of the severity of the disease.[93]

Other Major Illnesses

Other noninfectious diseases have a debilitating effect on many people. But most of the diseases discussed in this section can be controlled, if not cured.

Epilepsy and Seizure Disorders

About 10 percent of all Americans will have at least one seizure at some time. Between 0.5 and 1 percent of all Americans have recurrent seizures. Derived from the Greek word for seizure, **epilepsy** is the term used to refer to a variety of neurological disorders characterized by sudden attacks (seizures) of violent muscle contractions and unconsciousness. Epilepsy is rarely fatal; the primary danger to life is to suffer an attack while driving or swimming.

epilepsy A variety of neurological disorders characterized by sudden attacks (seizures) of violent muscle contractions and unconsciousness.

Seizures can be major, referred to as *grand mal*; minor, referred to as *petit mal*; or psychomotor. In a grand-mal seizure, the person loses consciousness, falls to the ground, and experiences convulsive body movements. Petit-mal seizures are brief, characterized by a loss of consciousness for 10 to 30 seconds, by eye or muscle flutterings, and occasionally by a loss of muscle tone. About 90 percent of all epileptics have grand-mal seizures; 40 percent suffer both petit-mal and grand-mal seizures. The frequency of attacks defines the severity of the epilepsy. Diagnosis is based on a history of recurring attacks and a study of the brain's electrical activity, called an electroencephalogram (EEG).

About half of all cases of epilepsy have no known cause and are therefore classified as *idiopathic*. Others stem from conditions that affect the brain, such as trauma, tumors, congenital malformations, or inflammation of the membranes covering the brain. Idiopathic epilepsy usually begins between the ages of 2 and 14. Seizures before age 2 are usually related to developmental defects, birth injuries, or a metabolic disease affecting the brain. (Fever-induced convulsions are not related to epilepsy.) Seizures after age 14 are generally symptoms of brain disease or injury.

Seizure disorders don't reflect or affect intellectual or psychological soundness; people who suffer from them have normal intelligence. Therapy with anticonvulsant drugs can control seizures in most people, and once seizures are under control, epileptics can live full, normal lives by continuing to take their medications.

If you're with a person who suffers a grand-mal seizure, make sure he or she isn't injured during the attack. Don't try to restrain the person or interfere with his or her movements, and don't try to force anything into the person's mouth.

Asthma

Asthma is a disease characterized by constriction of the breathing passages. As with allergy, asthma rates have skyrocketed in the last two decades. Approximately 26 million Americans have asthma. Asthma-related problems account for more than half a million hospital stays each year and 14 deaths each day in the United States, according to the Asthma and Allergy Foundation of America.

Asthma is more common among inner-city residents and blacks. The disease disproportionately affects African Americans. A black man in New York City is 11 times more likely to die from asthma than other men in the city.

While asthma is not always linked to allergy, the two are related. Among people with asthma, 90 percent of the children, 70 percent of young adults, and 50 percent of older adults also have allergies. According to epidemiologic research, 23 percent of youngsters diagnosed with allergies by age 1 develop asthma by age 6. Exposure to moisture or mold damage very early in life may increase the risk of developing asthma.[94] Symptoms include wheezing, coughing, shortness of breath, and chest tightness. If the symptoms are untreated or undertreated, they can worsen and damage the lungs. Oral contraceptives increase the risk in some women.

The number of people with asthma continues to increase into adulthood. However, as shown by a study that followed college students for 23 years, most report that their symptoms improve or disappear.

Over the last decade advances in asthma medications and tools have significantly improved management of this disease. Inhaled corticosteroids, long-acting bronchodilators (such as Advair), and leukotriene receptor antagonists (such as Singulair) have proven particularly helpful in controlling symptoms and preventing serious attacks that would require treatment with oral steroids.

If you have asthma, here are some steps you should take:

- **Get away from the asthma trigger** (cigarette smoke, cat, pollen, etc.).

- **Assess the severity of the attack.** The most precise way to do so is with a peak flow meter. If your peak flow is less than half your best value, the attack is severe.

- **Use a quick reliever.** The fastest way to relieve an asthma attack is to use a quick-acting bronchodilator such as albuterol.

- **Suppress inflammation.** Quick-relief bronchodilators treat only the constricted muscles surrounding the bronchial tubes. Treating the overproduction of mucus requires an anti-inflammatory medication, typically a corticosteroid, such as prednisone.

- **Know when to call for help.** Severe asthma attacks can be dangerous. If you don't feel improvement, get help immediately from your doctor or an urgent care or emergency health care center, or call 911.

Ulcers

Open sores, often more than an inch wide, that develop in the lining of the stomach or the duodenum (the first part of the small intestine) are called **ulcers**. They are caused by excessive acidic digestive juices. The major symptom is a burning pain felt throughout the upper abdomen. The pain may come and go, lasting up to three

asthma A disease or allergic response characterized by bronchial spasms and difficult breathing.

ulcers Lesions in, or erosion of, the mucous membrane of an organ.

hours. It may begin either right after eating or several hours later.

One in five men and one in ten women get ulcers of the stomach or duodenum, but the number of ulcers is declining. Risk factors include heavy use of cigarettes, alcohol, or caffeine; the ingestion of large amounts of painkillers that contain aspirin or ibuprofen; and advanced age. Bleeding is not common but may be dangerous, even life-threatening. An untreated stomach ulcer can lead to serious weight loss and anemia.

Researchers have identified a bacterium, *Helicobacter pylori*, that may infect the digestive system and set the stage for ulcers. According to various studies, most ulcer patients carry this organism. One theory is that infection leads to an inflammation of the stomach lining called gastritis, which increases vulnerability to other stressors, such as smoking, alcohol, or anxiety. Treatment with antibiotics leads to improvement in most patients.

Conventional therapy for ulcers includes self-help measures, such as avoiding aspirin; eating small, frequent meals; taking antacids; and not smoking or drinking alcohol or caffeine. Drugs such as cimetidine, ranitidine, and sucralfate can reduce the amount of acid produced by the stomach and relieve ulcer symptoms.

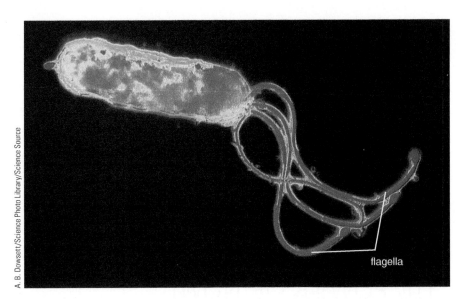

A. B. Dowsett/Science Photo Library/Science Source

flagella

The bacterium *Helicobacter pylori* has flagella that enable it to tunnel beneath the protective layer coating the stomach lining.

- Are college students too young to worry about major diseases?
- What behaviors can you change to lower your odds of developing prediabetes and diabetes?
- Why do you need to know your blood pressure and lipoprotein levels?
- Are certain cancers preventable?

THE POWER OF NOW!

Preventing Serious Illness

You may not be able to control every risk factor in your life or environment, but you can protect yourself from the obvious ones.

____ Not smoking. There's no bigger favor you can do for your heart or your lungs—your entire body.

____ Cutting down on saturated fats and cholesterol. This can help prevent high blood cholesterol levels, obesity, and heart disease.

____ Watching your weight. Even relatively modest gains can have a big effect on your risk of heart disease. Overweight and obesity are associated with increased risks for cancers at several sites: breast (among postmenopausal women), colon, endometrium, esophagus (adenocarcinoma), and kidney.

____ Moving more. Regular exercise can help lower your blood pressure, lower LDL, and reduce triglycerides.

____ Lowering your stress levels. If too much stress is a problem in your life, try the relaxation techniques described in Chapter 4.

____ Getting your blood pressure checked regularly. Knowing your numbers can alert you to a potential problem long before you develop any symptoms.

____ Avoiding excessive exposure to ultraviolet light. If you spend a lot of time outside, protect your skin by using sunscreen and wearing long-sleeve shirts and a hat. Also, wear sunglasses to protect your eyes. Don't purposely put yourself at risk by binge-sunbathing or by using sunlamps.

____ Controlling your alcohol intake. The risk of cancers of the mouth, pharynx, larynx, esophagus, liver, and breast increases substantially with intake of more than two drinks per day for men or one drink for women.

____ Being alert to changes in your body. You know your body's rhythms and appearance better than anyone else, and only you will know if certain things aren't right. Changes in bowel habits, skin changes, unusual lumps or discharges—anything out of the ordinary—may be clues that require further medical investigation.

What's Online

Visit www.cengagebrain.com to access course materials for this text, including the Behavior Change Planner, interactive quizzes, and more.

self survey

Diabetes Risk Test

Height	Weight (lbs.)		
4′ 10″	119–142	143–190	191+
4′ 11″	124–147	148–197	198+
5′ 0″	128–152	153–203	204+
5′ 1″	132–157	158–210	211+
5′ 2″	136–163	164–217	218+
5′ 3″	141–168	169–224	225+
5′ 4″	145–173	174–231	232+
5′ 5″	150–179	180–239	240+
5′ 6″	155–185	186–246	247+
5′ 7″	159–190	191–254	255+
5′ 8″	164–196	197–261	262+
5′ 9″	169–202	203–269	270+
5′ 10″	174–208	209–277	278+
5′ 11″	179–214	215–285	286+
6′ 0″	184–220	221–293	294+
6′ 1″	189–226	227–301	302+
6′ 2″	194–232	233–310	311+
6′ 3″	200–239	240–318	319+
6′ 4″	205–245	246–327	328+
	(1 Point)	(2 Points)	(3 Points)
	You weigh less than the amount in the left column (0 points)		

Adapted from Bang et al., Ann Intern Med 151:775-783,2009. Original algorithm was validated without gestational diabetes as part of the model.

1. How old are you?
   Less than 40 years (0 points)
   40–49 years (1 point)
   50–59 years (2 points)
   60 years or older (3 points)

2. Are you a man or a woman?
   Man (1 point)   Woman (0 points)

3. If you are a woman, have you ever been diagnosed with gestational diabetes?
   Yes (1 point)   No (0 points)

4. Do you have a mother, father, sister, or brother with diabetes?
   Yes (1 point)   No (0 points)

5. Have you ever been diagnosed with high blood pressure?
   Yes (1 point)   No (0 points)

6. Are you physically active?
   Yes (0 points)   No (1 point)

7. What is your weight status?
   (see chart at *left*)

Write your score in the box.

If you scored 5 or higher:
You are at increased risk for having type 2 diabetes. However, only your doctor can tell for sure if you do have type 2 diabetes or prediabetes (a condition that precedes type 2 diabetes in which blood glucose levels are higher than normal). Talk to your doctor to see if additional testing is needed.

Add up your score

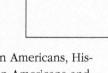

Type 2 diabetes is more common in African Americans, Hispanics/Latinos, American Indians, and Asian Americans and Pacific Islanders.

Higher body weights increase diabetes risk for everyone. Asian Americans are at increased diabetes risk at lower body weights than the rest of the general public (about 15 pounds lower).

For more information, visit us at diabetes.org/alert or call 1-800-DIABETES (1-800-342-2383)

MAKING THIS CHAPTER WORK FOR YOU

Review Questions

(LO 15.1) 1. _____ occurs when the artery walls become constricted so that the force exerted as the blood flows through them is greater than it should be.
a. Hypertension
b. Diabetes mellitus
c. Infiltration
d. Myocardial infarction

(LO 15.1) 2. Which of the following statements is true of high-density lipoproteins?
a. They cause the formation of plaque on arterial walls, leading to atherosclerosis and high blood pressure.
b. They pick up excess cholesterol in the body and carry it back to the liver for removal from the body.
c. They control the level of glucose in the blood.
d. They reduce the levels of low-density lipoproteins in the blood by blocking the production of cholesterol in the liver.

(LO 15.2) 3. _____ is a cluster of disorders, including high blood pressure, high insulin levels, abdominal obesity, and abnormal cholesterol levels, that make a person more likely to develop diabetes, heart disease, or stroke.
a. Down syndrome
b. Metabolic syndrome
c. Acute aortic syndrome
d. Chronic fatigue syndrome

(LO 15.2) 4. Which of the following characteristics is a sign of metabolic syndrome?
a. A higher-than-normal triglyceride level
b. A higher-than-normal high-density lipoprotein level
c. A lower-than-normal blood pressure
d. A lower-than-normal fasting blood sugar

(LO 15.3) 5. For people suffering from _____, the pancreas, which produces insulin, doesn't function as it should.
a. hepatitis
b. hypertension
c. meningitis
d. diabetes mellitus

(LO 15.3) 6. In _____, the body's immune system attacks the insulin-producing beta cells in the pancreas and destroys them.
a. adult-onset diabetes
b. type 2 diabetes
c. gestational diabetes
d. type 1 diabetes

(LO 15.4) 7. _____ occurs when blood pressure remains elevated over time and forces the heart to pump harder than is healthy.
a. Atherosclerosis
b. Arteriosclerosis
c. Hypertension
d. Myocardial infarction

(LO 15.4) 8. Which of the following statements is true about hypertension?
a. Men and women are equally likely to develop hypertension.
b. Low amounts of sodium in the diet lead to increased blood pressure in people with hypertension.
c. Lack of blood supply to the myocardium is the primary cause of hypertension.
d. Stage 1 hypertension is the most severe form of hypertension.

(LO 15.5) 9. _____ are the blood fats released into the bloodstream after a meal.
a. Monoglycerides
b. Diglycerides
c. Phospholipids
d. Triglycerides

(LO 15.5) 10. Drugs called _____ work in the liver to block production of cholesterol.
a. heparinoids
b. antibiotics
c. statins
d. beta-blockers

(LO 15.6) 11. The _____ is a smooth membrane that lines the inside of the heart and its valves.
a. pericardium
b. myocardium
c. endocardium
d. endothelium

(LO 15.6) 12. Pessimistic people tend to have poorer cardiovascular health than optimists, including _____.
a. higher blood sugar
b. lower cholesterol
c. lower BMIs
d. lower blood pressure

(LO 15.7) 13. _____ refers to a disease of the lining of the arteries in which plaque narrows the artery channels.
a. Atherosclerosis
b. Infiltration
c. Epilepsy
d. Metastasis

(LO 15.7) 14. Symptoms of a heart attack may include _____.
   a. headache
   b. feeling of being too warm
   c. extreme sleepiness
   d. anxiety

(LO 15.8) 15. _____ occurs when the blood supply to a portion of the brain is blocked.
   a. Melanoma
   b. Stroke
   c. Myocardial infarction
   d. Epilepsy

(LO 15.8) 16. _____ occurs when a diseased artery in the brain floods the surrounding tissue with blood.
   a. Cerebral thrombosis
   b. Ischemic stroke
   c. Hemorrhagic stroke
   d. Cerebral embolism

(LO 15.9) 17. _____ is a type of cancer that forms in the supporting, or connective, tissues of the body such as bones, muscles, and blood vessels.
   a. Lymphoma
   b. Carcinoma
   c. Leukemia
   d. Sarcoma

(LO 15.9) 18. A(n) _____ is a surgical treatment for breast cancer that removes only the cancerous tissue and a surrounding margin of normal tissue.
   a. lumpectomy
   b. mastectomy
   c. thrombectomy
   d. embolectomy

(LO 15.9) 19. Which of the following statements about epilepsy is true?
   a. People who have seizures have either *grand mal* or *petit mal* seizures, but never both.
   b. Epileptic seizures can be caused by allergies.
   c. About half of all cases have no known cause.
   d. Epilepsy usually accompanies a developmental disorder.

(LO 15.9) 20. Ulcers _____.
   a. cause heavy bleeding in the stomach
   b. may be triggered by a bacterium
   c. are not affected by the person taking aspirin
   d. are more common in women than in men

Answers to these questions can be found on page 623.

Critical Thinking Questions

1. Has anyone you know been diagnosed with diabetes? What were their early symptoms? Did they disregard the warning signs? What steps would you adopt to control your blood sugar levels?

2. Have you ever met a cancer survivor? When was his or her cancer diagnosed? What did you learn about the person's treatment procedures and coping strategies? Discuss your strategies for prevention and early diagnosis of cancer.

3. Think about the role of obesity in cardiovascular health. Discuss how weight increases the risk of the various health concerns discussed in this chapter. How does an active lifestyle reduce your risk of developing diseases?

4. A friend of yours, Karen, discovered a small lump in her breast during a routine self-examination. When she mentions it, you ask if she has seen a doctor. She tells you that she hasn't had time to schedule an appointment; besides, she says, she's not sure it's really the kind of lump one has to worry about. It's clear to you that Karen is in denial and procrastinating about seeing a doctor. What advice would you give her?

Additional Online Resources

www.diabetes.org

Here you will find the latest information on both type 1 and type 2 diabetes mellitus, including suggestions regarding diet and exercise. The online bookstore features meal planning guides, cookbooks, and self-care guides. Type in your zip code to find community resources.

www.heart.org/HEARTORG/

This comprehensive site features a searchable database of all major cardiovascular diseases, plus information on healthy lifestyles, current research, CPR, cardiac warning signs, risk awareness, low-cholesterol diets, and family health. The interactive Heart Profiles® provide personalized information about treatment options for common cardiovascular conditions such as hypertension, heart failure, and cholesterol.

www.fi.edu/learn/heart/index.html

This interesting site, developed by the Franklin Institute, provides an interactive multimedia tour of the heart, as well as statistics, resources, links, and information on how to monitor your heart's health by becoming aware of your vital signs.

www.cdc.gov/cancer

This site, sponsored by the Centers for Disease Control and Prevention (CDC), features current information on cancer of the breast, cervix, prostate, skin, and colon. The site also provides monthly spotlights on specific cancers, as well as links to the National Comprehensive Cancer Control Program and the National Program of Cancer Registries.

Key Terms

The terms listed are used on the pages indicated. Definitions of the terms are in the glossary at the end of the book.

angina 466

angina pectoris 466

aorta 461

arteriosclerosis 465

asthma 482

atherosclerosis 465

atrium 460

capillaries 461

cardiometabolic 444

cardiopulmonary resuscitation (CPR) 467

cholesterol 447

diabetes mellitus 450

diastole 460

diastolic blood pressure 447

epilepsy 481

hypertension 447

infiltration 472

insulin resistance 450

lipoproteins 447

mammography 478

mastectomy 478

metabolic syndrome 448

metastasize 472

myocardial infarction (MI) 467

plaque 465

prediabetes 450

prehypertension 456

stroke 468

systole 460

systolic blood pressure 447

transient ischemic attacks (TIAs) 469

triglycerides 447

ulcers 482

ventricles 460

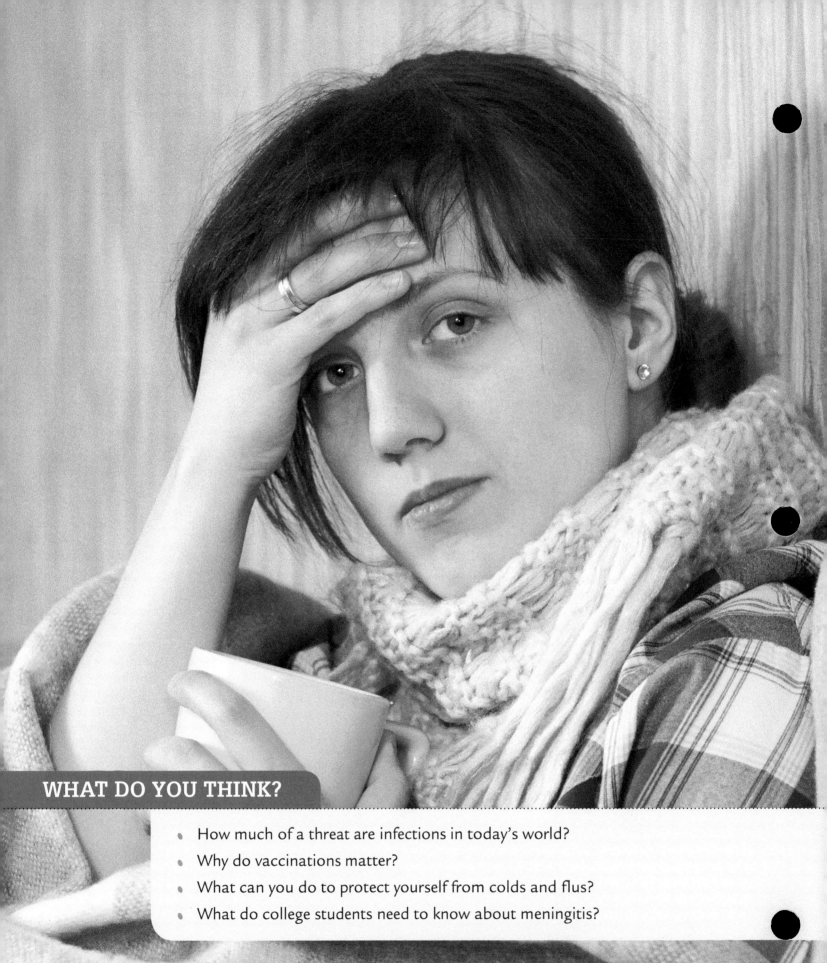

WHAT DO YOU THINK?

- How much of a threat are infections in today's world?
- Why do vaccinations matter?
- What can you do to protect yourself from colds and flus?
- What do college students need to know about meningitis?

16

Infectious Illnesses

Zach shrugged off the headache and sore throat he woke up with and rushed to class. During the lecture he started shivering. When he got up to leave, his legs felt shaky, and it hurt to walk. His entire body seemed stiff. Back in his dorm, Zach collapsed onto his bed. He felt feverish. His head throbbed. He started vomiting. Dark blotches broke out on his forehead, arms, and legs.

That evening his resident adviser drove Zach to the emergency room. The pain in his legs was excruciating, but his blood pressure was so low that the doctors couldn't give him pain medication. A spinal tap revealed that Zach had bacterial meningitis, a potentially deadly infection that causes swelling in the brain and spinal cord. Intensive treatment saved Zach's life, although he suffered hearing loss and severe nerve damage that required months of rehabilitation. Zach considers himself lucky. Bacterial meningitis can strike so unexpectedly and worsen so quickly that it can kill a healthy young person within days.

Throughout history, infectious diseases have claimed more lives than any military conflict or natural disaster. Although modern medicine has won many victories against the agents of infection, we remain vulnerable to a host of infectious illnesses. Drug-resistant strains of tuberculosis and *Staphylococcus* bacteria challenge current therapies. New

After reading this chapter, you should be able to:

16.1 Identify agents and vectors involved in the spread of infectious diseases.

16.2 Describe the role of the body's immune system.

16.3 List and describe immune disorders.

16.4 Evaluate the current recommendations regarding immunizations for adults and children.

16.5 Discuss prevention and treatments for upper respiratory infections.

16.6 Describe ways of preventing and recognizing meningitis.

16.7 Identify the types of hepatitis.

16.8 Name and describe other infectious illnesses.

16.9 Analyze the threat posed by emerging infectious diseases.

16.10 Identify and describe insect- and animal-borne infections.

16.11 Describe the symptoms and treatments of reproductive and urinary infections.

infectious diseases such as H1N1 flu are emerging and traveling around the world. Agents of infection also can be used as weapons of war and terrorism.

This chapter is a lesson in self-defense against all forms of infection. The information it provides can help you boost your defenses, recognize and avoid enemies, shield yourself from infections, and realize when to seek help. <

Understanding Infection

We live in a sea of microbes. Most of them don't threaten our health or survival; some, such as the bacteria that inhabit our intestines, are actually beneficial. Yet in the course of history, disease-causing microorganisms have claimed millions of lives. The twentieth century brought the conquest of infectious killers such as cholera and scarlet fever. Although modern science has won many victories against the agents of infection, infectious illnesses remain a serious health threat.

Infection is a complex process, triggered by various **pathogens** (disease-causing organisms) and countered by the body's own defenders. Physicians explain infection in terms of a **host** (either a person or a population) that contacts one or more agents in an environment. A **vector**—a biological or physical vehicle that carries the agent to the host—provides the means of transmission.

Agents of Infection

The types of microbes that can cause infection are viruses, bacteria, fungi, protozoa, and helminths (parasitic worms). (See Figure 16.1.)

Viruses   The tiniest pathogens—**viruses**—are also the toughest; they consist of a bit of nucleic acid (DNA or RNA, but never both) within a protein coat. Unable to reproduce on its own, a virus takes over a body cell's reproductive machinery and instructs it to produce new viral particles, which are then released to enter other cells. The common cold, the flu, herpes, hepatitis, and AIDS are viral diseases.

The most common viruses are these types:

- **Rhinoviruses and adenoviruses,** which get into the mucous membranes and cause upper respiratory tract infections and colds.

- **Coronaviruses,** named for their corona, or halo-like appearance, are second only to rhinoviruses in causing the common cold and other respiratory infections. A coronavirus is the cause of severe acute respiratory syndrome (SARS). A deadly new strain was identified in the Middle East and Great Britain in 2013.[1]

- **Influenza viruses,** which can change their outer protein coats so dramatically that individuals resistant to one strain cannot fight off a new one.

- **Herpes viruses,** which take up permanent residence in the cells and periodically flare up.

- **Papillomaviruses,** which cause few symptoms in women and almost none in men but may be responsible, at least in part, for a rise in the incidence of cervical cancer among younger women.

- **Hepatitis viruses,** which cause several forms of liver infection, ranging from mild to life-threatening.

- **Slow viruses,** which give no early indication of their presence but can produce fatal illnesses within a few years.

- **Retroviruses,** which are named for their backward (retro) sequence of genetic replication compared to other viruses. One retrovirus, human immunodeficiency virus (HIV), causes acquired immune deficiency syndrome (AIDS) (discussed in Chapter 11).

- **Filoviruses,** which resemble threads and are extremely lethal.

The problem in fighting viruses is that it's difficult to find drugs that harm the virus and not the cell it has commandeered. **Antibiotics** (drugs that inhibit or kill bacteria) have no effect on viruses. **Antiviral drugs** don't completely eradicate a viral infection, although they can decrease its severity and duration. Because viruses multiply very quickly, antiviral drugs are most effective when taken before an infection develops or in its early stages.

Bacteria   Simple one-celled organisms, **bacteria** are the most plentiful microorganisms as well as the most pathogenic. Most kinds of bacteria don't cause disease; some, like certain strains of *Escherichia coli* that aid in digestion, play important roles within our bodies. Even friendly bacteria, however, can get out of hand and cause acne, urinary tract infections, vaginal infections, and other problems.

pathogens Microorganisms that produce disease.

host A person or population that contracts one or more pathogenic agents in an environment.

vector A biological or physical vehicle that carries the agent of infection to the host.

viruses Submicroscopic infectious agents; the most primitive forms of life.

antibiotics Substances produced by microorganisms, or synthetic agents, that are toxic to bacteria.

antiviral drugs Substance that decrease the severity and duration of a viral infection if taken prior to or soon after onset of infection.

bacteria (singular, bacterium) One-celled microscopic organisms; they are the most plentiful pathogens.

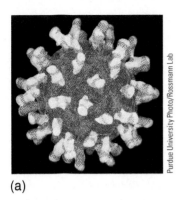
(a)

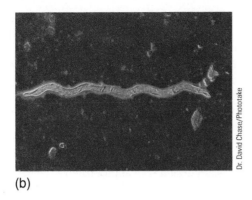
(b)

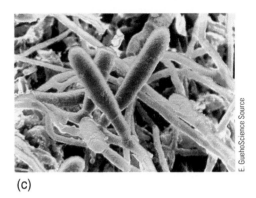
(c)

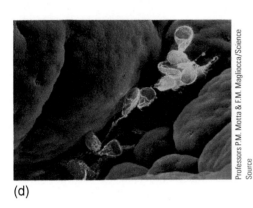
(d)

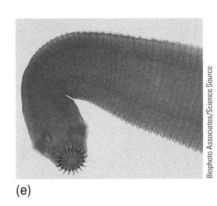
(e)

FIGURE 16.1 Examples of Major Categories of Organisms That Cause Disease in Humans.

Except for the helminths (parasitic worms), pathogens are microorganisms that can be seen only with the aid of a microscope. (a) Viruses: common cold, (b) Bacteria: syphilis, (c) Fungi: athlete's foot fungus, (d) Protozoa: *Giardia lamblia*, (e) Helminths: tapeworm.

Bacteria harm the body by releasing either enzymes that digest body cells or toxins that produce the specific effects of diseases such as diphtheria or toxic shock syndrome. In self-defense, the body produces specific proteins (called *antibodies*) that attack and inactivate the invaders. Tuberculosis, tetanus, gonorrhea, scarlet fever, and diphtheria are examples of bacterial diseases.

Because bacteria are sufficiently different from the cells that make up our bodies, antibiotics can kill them without harming our cells. Antibiotics work only against specific types of bacteria. If your doctor thinks you have a bacterial infection, tests of your blood, pus, sputum, urine, or stool can identify the particular bacterial strain.

Fungi Single-celled or multicelled organisms, **fungi** consist of threadlike fibers and reproductive spores. Fungi lack chlorophyll and must obtain their food from organic material, which may include human tissue. Fungi release enzymes that digest cells and are most likely to attack hair-covered areas of the body, including the scalp, beard, groin, and external ear canals. They also cause athlete's foot. Treatment consists of antifungal drugs.

Protozoa These single-celled, microscopic animals release enzymes and toxins that destroy cells or interfere with their function. Diseases caused by **protozoa** are not a major health problem in this country, primarily because of public health measures. Around the world, however, some 2.24 billion people (more than 40 percent of the world's population) are at risk for acquiring malaria—a protozoan-caused disease. Up to 3 million die from this disease annually. Many more come down with amoebic dysentery. Treatment for protozoa-caused diseases consists of general medical care to relieve the symptoms, replacement of lost blood or fluids, and drugs that kill the specific protozoan.

The most common disease caused by protozoa in the United States is *giardiasis,* an intestinal infection caused by microorganisms in human and animal feces. It has become a threat at day-care centers, as well as among campers and hikers who drink contaminated water. Symptoms include nausea, lack of appetite, gas, diarrhea, fatigue, abdominal cramps, and bloating. Many people recover in a month or two without treatment. However, in some cases the microbe causes recurring attacks over many years. Giardiasis can be life-threatening in small children and the elderly, who are especially prone to severe dehydration from diarrhea. Treatment usually consists of antibiotics.

fungi (singular, fungus) Organisms that reproduce by means of spores.

protozoa Microscopic animals made up of one cell or a group of similar cells.

Helminths (Parasitic Worms) Small parasitic worms that attack specific tissues or organs and compete with the host for nutrients are called **helminths**. One major worldwide health problem is *schistosomiasis*, a disease caused by a parasitic worm, the fluke, that burrows through the skin and enters the circulatory system. Infection with another helminth, the tapeworm, may be contracted from eating undercooked beef, pork, or fish containing larval forms of the tapeworm. Helminthic diseases are treated with appropriate medications.

✓**check-in** Which of the above agents do you see as the greatest threat to your health?

How Infections Spread

The major *vectors*, or means of transmission, for infectious disease are animals and insects, people, food, and water.

Animals and Insects
Disease can be transmitted by house pets, livestock, birds, and wild animals. Insects also spread a variety of diseases. The housefly may spread dysentery, diarrhea, typhoid fever, or trachoma (an eye disease rare in the United States but common in other parts of the world). Other insects, including mosquitoes, ticks, mites, fleas, and lice, can transmit such diseases as malaria, yellow fever, encephalitis, dengue fever (a growing threat in Mexico), and Lyme disease. West Nile virus (WNV) can be spread to humans by mosquitoes that bite infected birds; monkeypox virus is carried by various animals, including prairie dogs. Concern has grown about avian influenza, or bird flu, which has spread to wild and domestic birds around the world.[2]

The CDC has identified a new tick-borne pathogen: the "Bourbon virus," named for the Kansas county in which it was first discovered. An otherwise healthy man died of a related illness within two weeks of being bitten by ticks. The newly found virus belongs to a family of germs called Thogotoviruses, which have been linked to transmission by ticks and mosquitoes in parts of Europe, Asia, and Africa. Another tick-borne virus, the Heartland virus, was identified in Missouri in recent years.[3]

People
The people you're closest to can transmit pathogens through the air, through touch, or through sexual contact. To avoid infection, stay out of range of anyone who's coughing, sniffling, or sneezing, and don't share food or dishes. Carefully wash your dishes, utensils, and hands, and abstain from sex or make self-protective decisions about sexual partners.

✓**check-in** What precautions do you take to avoid being infected by others?

Food
Every year foodborne illnesses strike millions of Americans, sometimes with fatal consequences. Bacteria account for two-thirds of foodborne infections, and thousands of suspected cases of infection with *Escherichia coli* bacteria in undercooked or inadequately washed food have been reported.

Every year as many as 4 million Americans have a bout with *Salmonella* bacteria, which have been found in about one-third of all poultry sold in the United States. These infections can be serious enough to require hospitalization and can lead to arthritis, neurological problems, and even death. Consumers can greatly reduce the number of salmonella infections through proper handling, cooking, and refrigeration of poultry (see Chapter 6).

Water
Waterborne diseases, such as typhoid fever and cholera, are still widespread in less developed areas of the world. They have been rare in the United States, although outbreaks caused by inadequate water purification have occurred.

The Process of Infection

If someone infected with the flu sits next to you on a bus and coughs or sneezes, tiny viral particles may travel into your nose and mouth. Immediately, the virus finds or creates an opening in the wall of a cell, and the process of infection begins. During the **incubation period**, the time between invasion and the first symptom, you're unaware of the pathogen multiplying inside you. In some diseases, incubation may go on for months or even years; for most, it lasts several days or weeks.

The early stage of the battle between your body and the invaders is called the *prodromal period*. As infected cells die, they release chemicals that help block the invasion. Other chemicals, such as *histamines*, cause blood vessels to dilate, thus allowing more blood to reach the battleground. During all this, you feel mild, generalized symptoms, such as headache, irritability, and discomfort. You're also highly contagious. At the height of the battle—the typical illness period—you cough, sneeze, sniffle, ache, feel feverish, and lose your appetite.

Recovery begins when the body's forces gain the advantage. With time, the body destroys the last of the invaders and heals itself. However, the body is not able to develop long-lasting

helminths Parasitic roundworms or flatworms.

incubation period The time between a pathogen's entrance into the body and the first symptom.

immunity to certain viruses, such as colds, flu, or HIV.

Who Develops Infections?

Among the most vulnerable populations are the following groups:

- **Children and their families:** Youngsters get up to a dozen colds annually; adults average two a year. When a flu epidemic hits a community, about 40 percent of school-age boys and girls get sick, compared with only 5 to 10 percent of adults. Parents of young children get up to six times as many colds as other adults.

- **The elderly:** Statistically, fewer older men and women are likely to catch a cold or flu, but when they do, they face greater danger than the rest of the population. People over 65 who get the flu have a 1 in 10 chance of being hospitalized for pneumonia or other respiratory problems and a 1 in 50 chance of dying from the disease.

- **The chronically ill:** Lifelong diseases, such as diabetes, kidney disease, or sickle-cell anemia, decrease an individual's ability to fend off infections. Individuals taking medications that suppress the immune system, such as steroids, are more vulnerable to infections, as are those with medical conditions that impair immunity, such as infection with HIV.

- **Smokers and those with respiratory problems:** Smokers are a high-risk group for respiratory infections and serious complications, such as pneumonia. Chronic breathing disorders, such as asthma and emphysema, also greatly increase the risk of respiratory infections.

- **Those who live or work in close contact with someone sick:** Health-care workers who treat high-risk patients, nursing home residents, and others living in close quarters—such as students in dormitories—face greater risk of catching others' colds and flus.

- **Residents or workers in poorly ventilated buildings:** Building technology has helped spread certain airborne illnesses, such as tuberculosis, via recirculated air. Indoor air quality can be closely linked with disease transmission in winter, when people spend a great deal of time in tightly sealed rooms.

✓**check-in** How would you rate your risk?

How Your Body Protects Itself

Various parts of your body safeguard you against infectious diseases by providing **immunity**, or protection, from these health threats. Your skin, when unbroken, keeps out most potential invaders. Your tears, sweat, skin oils, saliva, and mucus contain chemicals that can kill bacteria. Cilia, the tiny hairs lining your respiratory passages, move mucus, which traps inhaled bacteria, viruses, dust, and foreign matter, to the back of the throat, where it is swallowed; the digestive system then destroys the invaders.

When these protective mechanisms can't keep you infection-free, your body's immune system, which is on constant alert for foreign substances that might threaten the body, swings into action. (See Health Now!)

The immune system includes structures of the lymphatic system—the spleen, thymus gland, lymph nodes, and lymph vessels—that help filter impurities from the body (Figure 16.2). The **lymph nodes**, or glands, are small tissue masses in which some protective cells are stored. If pathogens invade your body, many of them are carried to the lymph nodes to be destroyed. This is why your lymph nodes often feel swollen when you have a cold or the flu.

More than a dozen different types of white blood cells (lymphocytes) are concentrated in the organs of the lymphatic system or patrol the entire body by way of the blood and lymph vessels. Some of these white blood cells are generalists and some are specialists. The generalists include *macrophages*, which are large scavenger cells with insatiable appetites for foreign cells, diseased and run-down red blood cells, and other biological debris (Figure 16.3). The specialists are the *B cells* and *T cells*, which respond to specific invaders.

An *antigen* is any substance that the white blood cells recognize as foreign. B cells create antibodies, which are proteins that bind to antigens and mark them for destruction by other white blood cells. Antigens are specific to the pathogen, and the antibody to a particular antigen binds only to that antigen (see Figure 16.3). Once the human body produces antibodies against a specific antigen—the mumps virus, for instance—you're protected against that antigen for life. If you're again exposed to mumps, the antibodies previously produced prevent another episode of the disease.

But you don't have to suffer through an illness to acquire immunity. Inoculation with a vaccine

immunity Protection from infectious diseases.

lymph nodes Small tissue masses in which some immune cells are stored.

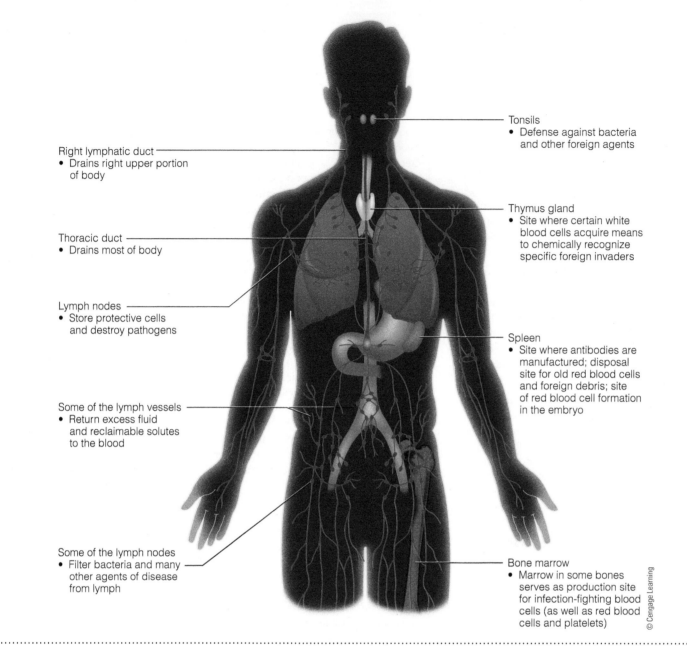

Right lymphatic duct
• Drains right upper portion of body

Thoracic duct
• Drains most of body

Lymph nodes
• Store protective cells and destroy pathogens

Some of the lymph vessels
• Return excess fluid and reclaimable solutes to the blood

Some of the lymph nodes
• Filter bacteria and many other agents of disease from lymph

Tonsils
• Defense against bacteria and other foreign agents

Thymus gland
• Site where certain white blood cells acquire means to chemically recognize specific foreign invaders

Spleen
• Site where antibodies are manufactured; disposal site for old red blood cells and foreign debris; site of red blood cell formation in the embryo

Bone marrow
• Marrow in some bones serves as production site for infection-fighting blood cells (as well as red blood cells and platelets)

© Cengage Learning

FIGURE 16.2 The Human Lymphatic System and Its Functions
The lymphatic system helps filter impurities from the body.

containing synthetic or weakened antigens can give you the same protection. The type of long-lasting immunity in which the body makes its own antibodies to a pathogen is called *active immunity*. Immunity produced by the injection of **gamma globulin**, the antibody-containing part of the blood from another person or animal that has developed antibodies to a disease, is called *passive immunity*.

Immune Response

Attacked by pathogens, the body musters its forces and fights. Sometimes the invasion is handled like a minor border skirmish; other times a full-scale battle is waged throughout the body. Together, the immune cells work like an internal police force:

• When an antigen enters the body, the T cells aided by macrophages engage in combat with the invader. Certain T cells (cytotoxic T cells) can destroy infected body cells or tumor cells by "touch-killing."

• Meanwhile, the B cells churn out antibodies, which rush to the scene and join in the fray.

gamma globulin The antibody-containing portion of the blood fluid (plasma).

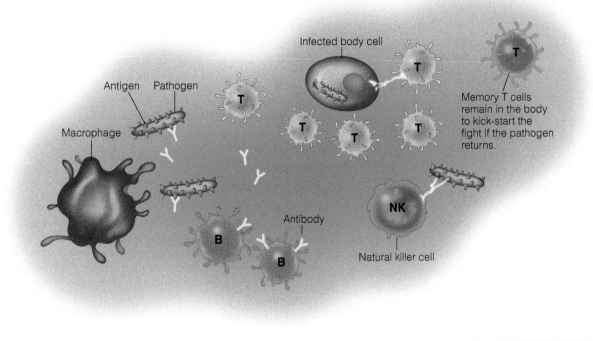

FIGURE 16.3 The Immune Response

Some T cells can kill infected body cells. B cells churn out antibodies to tag pathogens for destruction by macrophages and other white blood cells.

- Also busy at surveillance are natural killer cells that, like the elite forces of a SWAT team, seek out and destroy viruses and cancer cells (see Figure 16.3).

If the microbes establish a foothold, the blood supply to the area increases, bringing oxygen and nutrients to the fighting cells. Tissue fluids, as well as antibacterial and antitoxic proteins, accumulate. You may develop redness, swelling, local warmth, and pain—the signs of **inflammation**.

Chronic low-grade inflammation increases by twofold to fourfold the levels of cytokines, substances secreted by certain immune cells, in the bloodstream. These elevated levels serve as inflammatory markers that have emerged as major players in the development of several major diseases, including atherosclerosis, hypertension and other cardiovascular disorders, insulin resistance, metabolic syndrome, type 2 diabetes, and cancer.

As more tissue is destroyed, a cavity, or *abscess,* forms and fills with fluid, battling cells, and dead white blood cells (pus). If the invaders aren't killed or inactivated, the pathogens are able to spread into the bloodstream and cause **systemic disease**.

Some people have an **immune deficiency**—either inborn or acquired. A very few children are born without an effective immune system; their lives can be endangered by any infection. Although still experimental, therapy to implant a missing or healthy gene may offer new hope for a normal life.

Immunity and Stress

Whenever we confront a crisis, large or small, our bodies produce powerful hormones that provide extra energy. However, this stress response dampens immunity, reducing the number of some key immune cells and the responsiveness of others.

Stress affects the body's immune system in different ways, depending on two factors: the controllability or uncontrollability of the stressor and the mental effort required to cope with the stress. An uncontrollable stressor that lasts longer than 15 minutes may interfere with cytokine interleukin-6, which plays an essential role in activating the immune defenses.

Uncontrollable stressors also produce high levels of the hormone cortisol, which suppresses immune system functioning. The mental efforts required to cope with high-level stressors produce only brief immune changes that appear to have little consequence for health. However, stress has been shown to slow pro-inflammatory cytokine production, which is essential for healing.

inflammation A localized body response to tissue injury, characterized by swelling and dilation of the blood vessels.

systemic disease A pathologic condition that spreads throughout the body.

immune deficiency Partial or complete inability of the immune system to respond to pathogens.

Immunity and Gender

When the flu hits a household, the last one left standing is likely to be Mom. The female immune system responds more vigorously to common infections, offering extra protection against viruses, bacteria, and parasites.

The genders also differ in their vulnerability to allergies and autoimmune disorders. Although both men and women frequently develop allergies, allergic women are twice as likely to experience potentially fatal anaphylactic shock. A woman's robust immune system also is more likely to over-react and turn on her own organs and tissues. On average, three of four people with autoimmune disorders, such as multiple sclerosis, Hashimoto's thyroiditis, and scleroderma, are women.

Why are there such large gender differences in susceptibility? Scientists believe that the sex hormones have a great impact on immunity. Through a woman's childbearing years, estrogen, which protects heart, bone, brain, and blood vessels, also bolsters the immune system's response to certain infectious agents. Women produce greater numbers of antibodies when exposed to an antigen.

In contrast, testosterone may suppress this response—possibly to prevent attacks on sperm cells, which might otherwise be mistaken as alien invaders. When the testes are removed from mice and guinea pigs, their immune systems become more active.

Immune Disorders

Sometimes our immune system overreacts to certain substances, mistakes the body's own tissues for enemies, or doesn't react adequately. The results are immune disorders such as allergies and autoimmune disorders.

Allergic Rhinitis

Allergic rhinitis, the fifth most common chronic disease in the United States, affects nearly one in every six Americans. As defined by the American Academy of Otolaryngology, allergic rhinitis is an "inflammatory response of the nasal mucous membranes after exposure to inhaled allergens."[4] Allergic rhinitis can be seasonal or chronic, with intermittent or persistent symptoms.

....
✓**check-in** Do you have any allergies?
....

Allergies consistently rate as one of the top health problems among college students. In the ACHA survey, 21.5 percent of undergraduates reported a problem with allergies in the previous year.[5]

Among the substances that trigger allergic reactions are

- Pollen
- Dust mites
- Mold spores
- Pet dander
- Food (discussed in Chapter 6)
- Insect stings
- Medicine

In an allergic reaction, the immune system reacts as if it were defending the body against germs such as bacteria and viruses. When an allergic person first comes into contact with an allergen, the immune system generates large amounts of a type of antibody called immunoglobulin E or IgE. Each IgE antibody is specific for one particular substance, such as a particular pollen. The next time the allergen encounters its specific IgE, it attaches to it like a key fitting into a lock. This signals the cell to produce or release powerful chemicals like histamine that cause inflammation and the symptoms of allergy. The most common are these:

- Runny or clogged nose
- Sneezing
- Coughing
- Itching eyes, nose, and throat
- Eye irritation

Given the wide variety of tests and treatments used for managing allergic rhinitis, the American Academy of Otolaryngology has issued new guidelines:

- For someone with a stuffy nose, nasal passage discoloration, and/or red and watery eyes, allergy testing with exposure of skin or blood samples to possible allergen triggers is preferable to sinus imaging.

- Use "environmental controls" to eliminate problematic triggers, such as chemical agents to kill dust mites, air filter systems, and bedding with allergen barriers.

- Treat with nasal steroid sprays taken alone or in combination with newer antihistamines, which are less likely to cause drowsiness than earlier versions.

- If other treatments fail, drugs such as zafirlukast (Accolate) and montelukast (Singulair)—known as oral leukotriene receptor antagonists—may help.

allergic rhinitis An inflammatory response of the nasal mucous membranes after exposure to inhaled allergens.

allergies Hypersensitivities to particular substances in one's environment or diet.

- Immunotherapy—either desensitization shots or under-the-tongue pills—is an option when medication and environmental controls don't work well.

- Acupuncture, although not proven effective, can be an alternative for patients who want to avoid medications.[5]

Autoimmune Disorders

Sometimes the body's defenses go awry, and the immune system declares war on the cells, tissues, or organs it normally protects. **Autoimmune disorders** rank among the top ten killers and disablers of American adults, particularly women. They strike about three times as many women as men, possibly because of the effects of female hormones on the immune system. Women are most vulnerable in the prime of life, during their reproductive years.

Some autoimmune disorders directly damage a single organ, as happens with Addison's disease, which targets the adrenal glands, or Crohn's disease, which affects the gastrointestinal tract. Other autoimmune disorders attack multiple organs. Systemic lupus erythematosus, for instance, can affect the skin, joints, kidneys, heart, brain, and red blood cells.

For many people with autoimmune disorders, the biggest challenge is finding out what's wrong. Early symptoms, such as low-grade fever or achiness, often wax and wane and are dismissed or misdiagnosed by doctors. New blood tests for lupus and multiple sclerosis are promising faster, more accurate diagnoses, but for many autoimmune disorders, there are no conclusive laboratory tests.

Patients should keep a detailed record of when symptoms start, recur, flare, or subside, and seek a specialist—a rheumatologist, dermatologist, immunologist, or gastroenterologist, depending on symptoms—who has expertise in autoimmune disorders. New methods are revolutionizing treatments for many autoimmune disorders, including rheumatoid arthritis.

Immunization

One of the great success stories of modern medicine has been the development of vaccines that provide protection against many infectious diseases. Immunization has reduced cases of measles, mumps, tetanus, whooping cough, and other life-threatening illnesses by more than 95 percent.

Childhood Vaccinations

A small but growing number of parents, often clustered in specific areas,[6] have chosen not to have their children vaccinated, due largely to fears about childhood vaccines or the mistaken belief that the vaccine is not effective. Continuing concerns about vaccine safety date back to a fraudulent 1998 paper, later retracted, that falsely suggested a link between the measles-mumps-rubella (MMR) vaccine and autism. The lead author of that paper lost his medical license for having falsified his data. Several dozen studies and a report from the Institute of Medicine have found no link between any vaccines and the prevalence, severity, or age of onset of autism spectrum disorder (ASD) (discussed in Chapter 3).[7] Even siblings of autistic children, who are considered at higher risk, were no more likely than unvaccinated youngsters to develop ASD if given the MMR vaccine.[8]

The American Academy of Pediatrics, the U.S. Centers for Disease Control and Prevention, and the American Academy of Family Physicians all recommend that children receive the MMR vaccine at age 12 to 15 months and again at 4 to 6 years. The highly contagious measles virus can linger in an area up to two hours after an infected person leaves. Approximately 90 percent of people without immunity will become sick if exposed to the virus. Serious complications from measles include pneumonia and encephalitis, which can lead to long-term deafness or brain damage. An estimated one in 5,000 cases results in death.[9]

Although measles was declared eliminated in the United States in 2000, there have been recent outbreaks traced to residents of countries where measles is widespread or Americans who traveled abroad and brought the virus back home.[10] Public health officials blame the outbreaks on delayed or missed childhood vaccinations. At highest risk are infants too young to be vaccinated and children who are especially vulnerable due to certain illnesses or medications.[11]

√**check-in** Do you think that vaccination of children against common infectious diseases should be mandatory? Critics contend that no vaccine is safe. Advocates argue that unvaccinated children pose a threat to others. Summarize your view in a brief entry in your journal.

Adult Vaccinations

Although many people associate vaccination with children's health, the vast majority of

autoimmune disorders
Diseases caused by an attack on body tissue by an immune system that fails to recognize the tissue as self.

TABLE 16.1 Vaccines Recommended for College Students

Tetanus-diphtheria-pertussis (Tdap) vaccine*
Meningococcal vaccine
HPV vaccine series
Hepatitis A vaccine series
Hepatitis B vaccine series
Polio vaccine series
Measles-mumps-rubella (MMR) vaccine series
Varicella (chicken pox) vaccine series
Influenza vaccine
Pneumococcal polysaccharide (PPV) vaccine

*Recommended for previously unvaccinated college freshmen living in dormitories. © Cengage Learning

© Capifrutta/ShutterStock.com

vaccine-preventable deaths occur among adults. An estimated 40,000 to 50,000 American adults die every year from diseases that vaccines could have prevented.[12] Only slightly more than one-third of adults get an annual flu shot; many seniors have not gotten a pneumonia vaccination, a one-time shot recommended for everyone over age 65. Table 16.1 lists the vaccines recommended for college students, and Figure 16.4 shows the recommended adult immunization schedule.[13] (See Snapshot: On Campus Now.)

✓ **check-in** Have you received all the recommended vaccinations?

Upper Respiratory Infections

Every year, about 25 million cold sufferers in the United States visit their family doctors with uncomplicated upper respiratory infections. The common cold results in about 20 million days of absence from work and 22 million days of absence from school.

College and university students are at high risk for colds and influenza-like illnesses. In one study that followed more than 3,000 students from fall to spring, 9 in 10 had at least one cold or flu-like illness.

Common Cold

There are more than 200 distinct cold viruses. Although in a single season you may develop a temporary immunity to one or two, you may then be hit by a third. Americans come down with 1 billion colds annually.

Colds can strike in any season, but different cold viruses are more common at different times of year:

- Rhinoviruses cause most spring, summer, and early fall colds and tend to cause more symptoms above the neck (stuffy nose, headache, runny eyes)

- Adenoviruses, para-influenza viruses, coronaviruses, influenza viruses, and others that strike in the winter are more likely to get into the trachea and bronchi (the breathing passages) and cause more fever and bronchitis.

Cold viruses spread by coughs, sneezes, and touch. Cold sufferers who sneeze and then touch a doorknob or countertop leave a trail of highly contagious viruses behind them. A lack of sleep can increase your odds of getting a cold. People who get less than seven hours of sleep a night are three times more likely to catch a cold. Those who sleep poorly are five times more susceptible.

High levels of stress increase the risk of becoming infected by respiratory viruses and developing cold symptoms. People who feel unable to deal with everyday stresses have an exaggerated immune reaction that may intensify cold or flu symptoms once they've contracted a virus. Those with a positive emotional outlook are less vulnerable.

✓ **check-in** When was the last time you had a cold? Do you feel that stress made you more susceptible?

Preventing Colds According to a recent review of 30 published studies, taking vitamin C every day does not ward off the common cold or shorten its length or severity. Tests of high-dose vitamin C after the onset of cold symptoms showed no consistent effect on either the length of a cold or the severity of its symptoms. (See Health on a Budget.)

The findings on *Echinacea* are also mixed. In previous studies, the herbal supplement cut the chances of catching a cold by more than half and shortened the duration of a cold by an average of 1.4 days. However, a more recent report found no significant impact on the length or severity of a cold.[14]

According to a meta-analysis of research data, high-dose zinc acetate lozenges can substantially shorten the duration of various common cold symptoms. However, many zinc lozenges on the U.S. market either have too low a dose of zinc or contain ingredients that limit their effectiveness.[15]

SNAPSHOT: ON CAMPUS NOW

📷 Vaccinations

Vaccinated against	Percentage of students	Vaccinated against	Percentage of students
Hepatitis B	68	Varicella (chicken pox)	56
Measles-mumps-rubella	70.6	Influenza (within past 12 months)	45.1
Meningococcal meningitis	60.8		

Vaccinations are your first line of defense against potentially serious infectious diseases. Do you know your vaccination history? Do you keep track of recommendations for new or booster shots? Do you get a flu vaccination every year? Jot down what you see as the pros and cons of up-to-date vaccinations in your online journal.

Source: American College Health Association. *American College Health Association–National College Health Assessment II: Reference Group Executive Summary, Spring 2014.* Hanover, MD: American College Health Association. 2014.

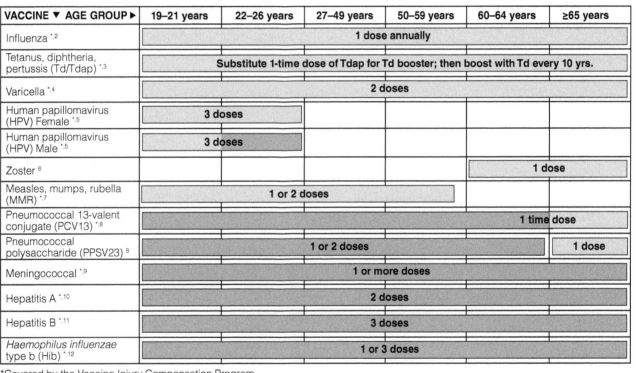

VACCINE ▼ AGE GROUP ▶	19–21 years	22–26 years	27–49 years	50–59 years	60–64 years	≥65 years
Influenza [*,2]	1 dose annually					
Tetanus, diphtheria, pertussis (Td/Tdap) [*,3]	Substitute 1-time dose of Tdap for Td booster; then boost with Td every 10 yrs.					
Varicella [*,4]	2 doses					
Human papillomavirus (HPV) Female [*,5]	3 doses					
Human papillomavirus (HPV) Male [*,5]	3 doses					
Zoster [6]					1 dose	
Measles, mumps, rubella (MMR) [*,7]	1 or 2 doses					
Pneumococcal 13-valent conjugate (PCV13) [*,8]	1 time dose					
Pneumococcal polysaccharide (PPSV23) [8]	1 or 2 doses					1 dose
Meningococcal [*,9]	1 or more doses					
Hepatitis A [*,10]	2 doses					
Hepatitis B [*,11]	3 doses					
Haemophilus influenzae type b (Hib) [*,12]	1 or 3 doses					

*Covered by the Vaccine Injury Compensation Program

▢ For all persons in this category who meet the age requirements and who lack documentation of vaccination or have no evidence of previous infection; zoster vaccine recommended regardless of prior episode of zoster

▢ Recommended if some other risk factor is present (e.g., on the basis of medical, occupational, lifestyle, or other indication)

▢ No recommendation

FIGURE 16.4 Recommended Adult Immunization Schedule, by Vaccine and Age Group—United States, 2014

Centers for Disease Control and Prevention, www.cdc.gov/vaccines/schedules/downloads/adult/adult-schedule.pdf

Caring for Your Cold

Fortunately, the most effective treatments for a cold are inexpensive—or even free:

- **Drink plenty of fluids, particularly warm ones.** Warmth is important because the aptly named "cold" viruses replicate at lower temperatures. Hot soups and drinks (particularly those with a touch of something pungent, like lemon or ginger) raise body temperature and help clear the nose. Tea may enhance the immune system.

- **Get plenty of rest.** Taking it easy reduces demands on the body, which helps speed recovery.

- **Do not take antibiotics.** They are ineffective against colds and flu.

- **Do not take aspirin or acetaminophen (Tylenol), which may suppress the antibodies the body produces to fight cold viruses and increase symptoms such as stuffiness.** Children, teenagers, and young adults should never take aspirin for a cold or flu because of the danger of Reye's syndrome, a potentially deadly disorder that can cause convulsions, coma, swelling of the brain, and kidney damage. A better alternative for achiness is ibuprofen (brand names include Motrin, Advil, and Nuprin), which doesn't seem to affect immune response.

- **Choose the right medicines for your symptoms.**

If you want to:	Choose medicine with:
Unclog a stuffy nose	Nasal decongestant
Quiet a cough	Cough suppressant
Loosen mucus so that you can cough it up	Expectorant
Stop runny nose and sneezing	Antihistamine
Ease fever, headaches, minor aches and pains	Pain reliever (analgesic)

- **Know when to call your doctor.** You usually do not have to call a doctor right away if you have signs of a cold or flu. But be sure to call in these situations:

  - Your symptoms get worse.

  - Your symptoms last a long time.

  - After feeling a little better, you show signs of a more serious problem. Some of these signs are a sick-to-your-stomach feeling, vomiting, high fever, shaking, chills, chest pain, or coughing with thick, yellow-green mucus.

✓**check-in** Which of the following steps do you take to prevent colds?

_____ Frequent hand washing

_____ Replacing toothbrushes often

_____ Exercising regularly

_____ Avoiding stress overload

Antibiotics Although colds and sore throats—a frequent cold symptom—are caused by viruses, many people seek treatment with antibiotics, which are effective only against bacteria. Unless you're coughing up green or foul yellow mucus (signs of a secondary bacterial infection), antibiotics won't help.[16] They also may make your body more resistant to such medications when you develop a bacterial infection in the future. For effective treatments, see Health on a Budget.

Excessive prescribing for antibiotics, more common in the South and West of the United States, accounts for more than half of all prescriptions.[17] In addition to their costs, antibiotics may increase risks to users and their contacts. Antibiotics can foster the growth of one or more strains of antibiotic-resistant bacteria for at least two to six months inside the person taking the pills—who can pass on this drug-resistant bug to family, roommates, and others.

influenza Any type of fairly common, highly contagious viral diseases.

The overuse of antibiotics to treat travelers' diarrhea may contribute to the spread of drug-resistant superbugs, according to new research.[18] Risk factors for catching antibiotic-resistant gut bacteria include taking antibiotics for travelers' diarrhea while abroad.

Influenza

Although similar to a cold, **influenza**—or the flu—causes more severe symptoms that last longer. Every year, 10 to 20 percent of Americans develop seasonal influenza, more than 200,000 are hospitalized, and 36,000 die from flu.

Flu viruses, transmitted by coughs, sneezes, laughs, and even normal conversation, are extraordinarily contagious, particularly in the first three days of the disease. The usual incubation period is two days, but symptoms can hit hard and fast. Two varieties of viruses—influenza A and influenza B—cause most flus.

The CDC recommends an annual flu shot for everyone over the age of 6 months, except for those with certain medical conditions. Vaccination with the live, nasal-spray flu vaccine (FluMist®) is an option for healthy people ages 5 to 49 years who are not pregnant. The spray provides a particular advantage for children since more than 30 percent of youngsters get the flu but most don't receive a flu shot.

√check-in Do you get a flu shot every year? If not, why not?

For those who don't get vaccinated, antiviral drugs, which must be taken within 36 to 48 hours of the first flu symptom, have provided the next-best line of defense. Two of the oldest of these medications, amantadine and rimantadine, which work only against the type A flu virus, are no longer effective, possibly because the flu virus has mutated and become resistant. According to a review of clinical trials, Tamiflu (oseltamivir) shortens the length of flu symptoms by about a day and reduces the risk of flu-related complications such as pneumonia. However, it is linked with more nausea and vomiting.[19] (See Your Strategies for Prevention for ways to protect yourself and others from influenza.)

Although regular exercise bolsters immunity, people with flu symptoms, such as fever, fatigue, muscle aches, and swollen lymph glands, should avoid exercise while sick and for two weeks after recovery, according to the American Council on Exercise.[20]

H1N1 Influenza (Swine Flu) The H1N1 virus is an influenza type A virus that was detected in people in the United States in April 2009, following infections in Mexico and other countries. It was originally referred to as "swine flu" because many of its genes were similar to influenza viruses that normally occur in pigs in North America. However, further study has shown that H1N1 is distinctive, with two genes from flu viruses that normally circulate in pigs in Europe and Asia plus avian genes and human genes. Scientists call this a "quadruple reassortant" virus. Annual flu shots now provide protection against both seasonal and H1N1 flu.

The symptoms of H1N1 flu are similar to the symptoms of regular flu: fever, cough, sore throat, body aches, headache, chills, and fatigue. A significant number of people infected with H1N1 also have reported diarrhea and vomiting. As with seasonal flu, severe illness and death have occurred as a result of infection with this virus.

The Threat of a Pandemic

Public health officials differentiate between an outbreak, an epidemic, and a pandemic:

- An outbreak is a sudden rise in the incidence of a disease.

- An epidemic affects an atypically large number of individuals within a population, community, or region at the same time.

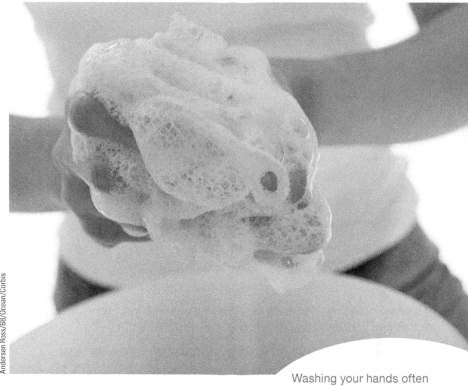

Andersen Ross/68/Ocean/Corbis

- A pandemic occurs over a wide geographic area and affects an exceptionally high proportion of the population. Influenza pandemics tend to occur when disease-causing organisms that typically affect only animals adapt and infect humans, then further adapt so they can pass easily from human to human. The flu pandemic of 1918–1919 claimed half a million lives.

Among the challenges health professionals face in a pandemic are inadequate supplies of vaccines or antiviral drugs; a shortage of medical supplies and facilities; and difficult decisions as to who should receive antiviral drugs and vaccines. A pandemic also has a significant economic and social impact as communities cancel events, businesses and schools close, and travel is restricted.

Meningitis

Meningitis, or invasive meningococcal disease, attacks the membranes around the brain and spinal cord and can result in hearing loss, kidney failure, and permanent brain damage. One of the most common types is caused by the bacterium *Neisseria meningitis*. Viral meningitis is typically less severe.

Washing your hands often with soap and hot water for 15 to 20 seconds will help protect you from germs. When soap and water are not available, you can use alcohol-based disposable hand wipes or gel sanitizers. If using gel, rub your hands until the gel is dry; the alcohol in the gel kills the germs.

meningitis An extremely serious, potentially fatal illness that attacks the membranes around the brain and spinal cord; caused by the bacterium *Neisseria meningitis*.

YOUR STRATEGIES FOR PREVENTION

How to Protect Yourself and Others from Influenza

If You Are Well

- **Get vaccinated.**

- **Do not share cups, glasses, bottles, dishes, or silverware.**

- **Frequently wash your hands with soap and water, especially after close contact with other people (on buses, in stores, at the gym, etc.).** Alcohol-based hand sanitizers are also effective.

- **Avoid touching your eyes, nose, or mouth.**

- **Try to avoid close contact with sick people.**

- **Reduce the time you spend in crowded settings.**

- **Stay in good general health: get plenty of sleep, be physically active, manage daily stress, drink plenty of fluids, and eat nutritious food.**

- **Follow public health advice regarding school closures, avoiding crowds, and other social distancing measures.**

- **Improve airflow in your living space by opening windows as much as possible.**

- **Know the facts about wearing a face mask.** There is no evidence that wearing a face mask in open areas (as opposed to enclosed spaces while in close contact with a person with flu-like symptoms) reduces the risk. If you do choose to wear one, place it carefully so it covers the mouth and nose, with minimal gaps between the face and mask. Once it's on, avoid touching the mask. Wash your hands immediately after removing it. Replace a mask with a new clean, dry one as soon as it becomes damp. Do not reuse single-use masks.

If You Have Symptoms

- **Cover your nose and mouth with a tissue when you cough or sneeze.** Throw the tissue in the trash after you use it.

- **Wash your hands often with soap and water, especially after you cough or sneeze.**

- **Be prepared to stay home, in your room, or in a designated quarantined area for a week or until you have been fever-free for at least a day.** Get a supply of over-the-counter medicines, alcohol-based hand rubs, tissues, and other related items to avoid the need to go out in public while you are sick and contagious.

- **To prevent the spread of influenza virus among family members or roommates, keep surfaces (especially bedside tables, bathroom sinks, and kitchen counters) clean by wiping them down with a household disinfectant.** Wash linens, eating utensils, and dishes before sharing them.

Most common in the first year of life, the incidence of bacterial meningitis rises in young people between ages 15 and 24. Adolescents and young adults account for nearly 30 percent of all cases of meningitis in the United States.

If not treated early, meningitis can lead to death or permanent disabilities. One in five of those who survive suffers from long-term side effects, such as brain damage, hearing loss, seizures, or limb amputation. Fatality rates are five times higher among 15- to 24-year-olds.

Each year 100 to 125 cases of meningitis occur on college campuses. An estimated 5 to 15 students die as a result. One in 5 survivors suffers long-term side effects.

Meningitis spreads through the exchange of respiratory droplets, which can come from sharing a drink, cigarette, or silverware; kissing; coughing; or sneezing. Even inhaling secondhand smoke can infect you with the disease.[21]

Preventing Meningitis

Vaccination is recommended for all American adolescents, with initial immunization at age 11 or 12 and a booster at age 16.[22] Vaccination protects against four of the five most common types of meningococcal bacteria. These four strains cause more than 80 percent of cases in adolescents and young adults. As with other immunizations, minor reactions may occur. These include pain and swelling at the injection site, headache, fatigue, or a vague sense of discomfort. The incidence of life-threatening meningitis has declined substantially since the vaccine was developed.

The CDC and other major health organizations, such as the American College Health Association, recommend routine vaccination with a new type of meningococcal vaccine, which provides longer-lasting protection than the previous type, and booster shots at age 16 for those previously vaccinated.[23]

√**check-in** Have you been vaccinated against meningitis? If not, why not?

Recognizing Meningitis

The early symptoms of meningitis may be mild and resemble symptoms of flu or other less severe infections. Bacterial meningitis symptoms may develop within hours; viral meningitis symptoms may develop quickly or over several days. Fever, headache, and neck stiffness are the hallmark symptoms of meningitis. Not all symptoms may appear, but they can progress very quickly, killing an otherwise healthy person in 48 hours or less, so it is critical to seek medical attention quickly.

The most common symptoms of meningitis are

- Sudden high fever

- Severe, persistent headache

- Neck stiffness and pain that makes it difficult to touch the chin to the chest

- Nausea and vomiting, sometimes along with diarrhea
- Confusion and disorientation (acting "goofy")
- Drowsiness or sluggishness
- Eye pain or sensitivity to bright light
- Pain or weakness in the muscles or joints

   Other possible signs and symptoms include

- Abnormal skin color
- Stomach cramps
- Ice-cold hands and feet
- Dizziness
- Reddish or brownish skin rash or purple spots
- Numbness and tingling
- Seizures

When to Seek Medical Care

If two or more of the symptoms of meningitis appear at the same time or if the symptoms are very severe or appear suddenly, seek medical care right away. If a red rash appears along with fever, see if the rash disappears when a glass is pressed against it. If it does not, this could be a sign of blood infection, which is a medical emergency. Call 911 without delay. Other symptoms that might require emergency treatment include loss of consciousness, seizures, muscle weakness, or sudden severe dementia.

A new rapid test can determine the presence of viral meningitis in just 2.5 hours. Because it can help quickly distinguish between viral and bacterial meningitis, the test could help reduce the unnecessary use of antibiotics. About 1 in 10 people who get meningitis dies from it. Of those who survive, another 11 to 19 percent lose fingers, arms, or legs; become deaf; have problems with their nervous systems; or suffer seizures, strokes, or brain damage. Thus it is critical to seek medical care for this infection. A new concern is the emergence of the first U.S. cases of bacterial meningitis resistant to a widely used antibiotic.

Hepatitis

An estimated 500,000 Americans contract hepatitis each year, and the number of hepatitis-related deaths has been rising in the past decade. At least five different viruses, referred to as **hepatitis** A,

B, C, Delta, and E, can cause this inflammation of the liver. Newly identified viruses also may be responsible for some cases of what is called "non-A, non-B" hepatitis.

Thanks largely to effective vaccines, rates of hepatitis A and hepatitis B infections have declined to their lowest rates in decades. Although there is no vaccine for hepatitis C, its incidence also has declined significantly. Nonetheless, hepatitis has surpassed HIV as a cause of death in the United States.

All forms of hepatitis target the liver, the body's largest internal organ. Symptoms include headaches, fever, fatigue, stiff or aching joints, nausea, vomiting, and diarrhea. The liver becomes enlarged and tender to the touch; sometimes the yellowish tinge of jaundice develops. Treatment consists of rest, a high-protein diet, and the avoidance of alcohol and drugs that may stress the liver. Alpha interferon, a protein that boosts immunity and prevents viruses from replicating, may be used for some forms.

Most people begin to feel better after two or three weeks of rest, although fatigue and other symptoms can linger. As many as 10 percent of those infected with hepatitis B and up to two-thirds of those with hepatitis C become carriers of the virus for several years or even life. Some have persistent inflammation of the liver, which may cause mild or severe symptoms and increase the risk of liver cancer.

Hepatitis A

Hepatitis A, a less serious form, is generally transmitted by poor sanitation, primarily fecal contamination of food or water, and is less common in industrialized nations than in developing countries. As many as 30 percent of individuals in the United States show evidence of past infection with the virus. Among those at highest risk in the United States are children and staff at day-care centers, residents of institutions for the mentally handicapped, sanitation workers, and workers who handle primates such as monkeys.

Gamma globulin can provide short-term immunity; vaccines against hepatitis A have been approved by the FDA. The CDC recommends routine immunization against hepatitis A in states with high rates, as well as for travelers to countries where hepatitis A is common, men who have sex with men, and persons who use illegal drugs.

Hepatitis B

Hepatitis B, a potentially fatal disease transmitted through the blood and other bodily fluids, infects an estimated 300 million people around the world. Once spread mainly by contaminated tattoo needles, needles shared by drug users, or

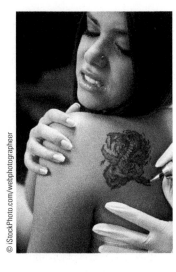

Getting a tattoo or a piercing can pose health risks, including bacterial infection and hepatitis.

hepatitis An inflammation and/or infection of the liver caused by a virus, often accompanied by jaundice.

transfusions of contaminated blood, hepatitis B is now transmitted mostly through sexual contact. Many cases resolve on their own, but hepatitis B can cause chronic liver infection, cirrhosis, and liver cancer. Medications for hepatitis B often must be taken long term, or the disease comes back even stronger.

Who Develops Hepatitis B?

At highest risk are the following:

- Young people. Seventy-five percent of new cases are diagnosed in those between ages 15 and 39. They usually contract hepatitis B through high-risk behaviors such as multiple sex partners and use of injected drugs.

- Athletes in contact sports, such as wrestling and football, who may transmit the hepatitis B virus in sweat. With the discovery that HBV is more common in athletes than had been suspected, health experts are calling for mandatory HBV testing and vaccination against hepatitis B for all athletes.

- Male homosexuals.

- Heterosexuals with multiple sex partners.

- Health-care workers with frequent contact with blood.

- Injection drug users.

- Infants born to infected mothers.

Vaccination can prevent hepatitis B and is recommended for all newborns and, if not already vaccinated, for travelers to certain regions, health-care workers, dialysis patients, and anyone engaging in unprotected sexual activity (homosexual or heterosexual).

Individuals who have tattoos or body piercing may also be at risk of various infections, including hepatitis B and C, being transmitted by unsterile tattooing or piercing practices.[24] (See Consumer Alert.)

If you choose to have a body piercing, avoid piercing guns and make certain that the piercing equipment has been sterilized. Tattoos from non-professionals pose two to four times greater risk than those done by professionals.

✓**check-in** Do have a tattoo or piercing?

Hepatitis C

About 3.2 million people in the U.S. are infected with hepatitis C virus (HCV), but most do not realize it because the virus causes so few symptoms. The most common are jaundice (a condition that causes yellow eyes and skin as well as dark urine), stomach pain, loss of appetite, nausea, and fatigue.

Hepatitis C virus is not spread by casual contact, such as hugging, kissing, or sharing food utensils. There is controversy about whether HCV can be transmitted sexually.

✓**check-in** Should you have a blood test for hepatitis C?

The CDC recommends one if any of the following are true:

- You received blood from a donor who later was found to have the disease.
- You have ever injected drugs.
- You got a blood transfusion or an organ transplant before July 1992.
- You received a blood product used to treat clotting problems before 1987.
- You were born between 1945 and 1965.
- You've had long-term kidney dialysis.
- You have HIV.
- You were born to a mother with hepatitis C.[25]

The treatments for HCV have changed in recent years. The latest is a once-daily pill called Harvoni, which combines two drugs—ledipasvir and sofosbuvir (Sovaldi)—and cures the disease in most people in eight to twelve weeks. This medication is very expensive; its most common side effects are fatigue and headache. Your doctor may also recommend a combination of other medications, including the traditional treatments: interferon (taken by injection) and/or ribavirin (available as a liquid, tablet, or capsule).[26]

About three-quarters of those infected with HCV develop chronic or long-term hepatitis. About one-quarter develop progressive, irreversible liver damage, with scar tissue (cirrhosis) gradually replacing healthy liver tissue. Hepatitis C also increases the risk of a rare form of liver cancer. If the liver no longer functions adequately, a patient may require liver transplantation.

Other Infectious Illnesses

Epstein-Barr Virus and Infectious Mononucleosis

Epstein-Barr virus (EBV), a member of the herpes virus family, infects most people at some time in their lives. As many as 95 percent of American adults between ages 35 and 45 have been infected. When infected in childhood, boys and girls usually show no or very mild symptoms. However, when infection with EBV occurs during adolescence or young adulthood, it causes infectious mononucleosis 35 to 50 percent of the time.

You can get **mononucleosis** through kissing—or any other form of close contact. "Mono" is a viral disease that targets people 15 to 24 years old. Its symptoms include a sore throat, headache, fever, nausea, and prolonged weakness. The spleen is swollen and the lymph nodes are enlarged. You may also develop jaundice or a skin rash similar to rubella (German measles).

The major symptoms usually disappear within two to three weeks, but weakness, fatigue, and often depression may linger for at least two more weeks. The greatest danger is from physical activity that might rupture the spleen, resulting in internal bleeding. The liver may also become inflamed. A blood test can determine whether you have mono. However, there's no specific treatment other than rest.

Myalgic Encephalomyelitis/ Chronic Fatigue Syndrome (ME/CFS)

The disorder once known as Chronic Fatigue Syndrome or **Myalgic Encephalomyelitis/ Chronic Fatigue Syndrome (ME/CFS)** has gained scientific recognition as a legitimate, serious, debilitating illness that affects 836,000 to 2.5 million Americans. (Since most people with this disorder have not yet been diagnosed, its exact prevalence is unknown). In a recent report, the Institute of Medicine has suggested a new name: Systemic Exertion Intolerance Disease (SEID).[27]

More likely to affect women than men, ME/CFS has five principal symptoms:

- Reduction or impairment in ability to carry out normal daily activities, accompanied by profound fatigue
- Post-exertional malaise (worsening of symptoms after physical, cognitive, or emotional effort)
- Unrefreshing sleep
- Cognitive impairment
- Worsening of symptoms when a person stands upright and improvement upon lying down

Also common are pain, failure to recover from a prior infection, and abnormal immune function. The average age of onset is 33, although ME/CFS has been reported in patients younger than age 10 and older than age 70. Symptoms can persist for years, and most patients never regain their predisease level of health. The cause of ME/CFS remains unknown, although recent research points toward a malfunctioning immune system. Rather than shutting down or reducing its response to an infection that has passed, the immune system continues to pump out large amounts of cytokines—chemical messengers that coordinate the response of the immune system's many cell types.[28]

There is no known cure for ME/CFS and little research on the efficacy of treatments used to manage its symptoms.

Herpes Gladiatorum (Mat Herpes, Wrestler's Herpes, Mat Pox)

Herpes gladiatorum is a skin infection caused by the herpes simplex type 1 virus and spread by direct skin-to-skin contact. It most commonly occurs among wrestlers, judo players, roller-derby skaters, or other athletes who have very close skin contact with each other.[29]

Within a few days of infection, some people develop a sore throat, swollen lymph nodes, fever, or tingling on the skin. *Herpes gladiatorum* lesions appear as a cluster of blisters on the face, extremities, or trunk. Generally, lesions appear within eight days after exposure to an infected person, but they may take longer to emerge. All wrestlers with skin sores or lesions should see a

mononucleosis An infectious viral disease characterized by an excess of white blood cells in the blood, fever, bodily discomfort, a sore throat, and kidney and liver complications.

myalgic encephalomyelitis/ chronic fatigue syndrome (ME/CFS) A cluster of symptoms whose cause is not yet known; a primary symptom is debilitating fatigue.

physician for evaluation and should not participate in practice or competition until their lesions have healed (usually four to five days).

Herpes gladiatorum infections can recur. The virus can "hide out" in the nerves and reactivate later, causing another infection. Generally, recurrent infections are less severe and don't last as long. However, a recurring infection is just as contagious as the original infection, so the same precautions are needed to prevent infecting others.

Tuberculosis

A bacterial infection of the lungs that was once the nation's leading killer, **tuberculosis (TB)** still claims the lives of more people than any acute infectious disease other than pneumonia. About 30 percent of the world's population is infected with the TB organism, although not all develop active disease. In the United States, rates are declining, but at a slower rate than in the past.[30] Immigration from countries where TB is common, poverty, homelessness, alcoholism and drug abuse, the HIV/AIDS epidemic, and the emergence of resistant strains of TB account for most new cases.

Although TB is most prevalent among high-risk groups, the overall danger increases as more people develop active disease because TB is highly contagious. TB outbreaks have occurred throughout the country in hospitals, nursing homes, prisons, and office buildings, where inadequate ventilation increases the risk of infection.

The "Superbug" Threat: MRSA

For decades most strains of the bacterium *Staphylococcus aureus* responded to treatment with penicillin. When the bacterium became resistant to penicillin, physicians switched to a newer antibiotic, methicillin. Within a year the first case of methicillin-resistant *S. aureus* (MRSA) was detected. This "superbug," which fights off traditional antibiotics, has become a major health threat.

One in three healthy people carry *S. aureus* bacteria on their skin. Of these as many as 1 in 100 may be carrying MRSA. In medical terms, these individuals are "colonized" but not infected. For infection to occur, MRSA must enter the body through an accidental injury such as a scrape or burn or via a deliberate break in the skin such as a surgical incision.

The rate of MRSA infections is highest in hospitals and health-care facilities, but MRSA also can develop among sports teams, child-care attendees, and prison inmates.

MRSA spreads by touch. In health-care settings, it can spread from patient to patient through contact with doctors and nurses with unwashed hands or contaminated gloves or contact with unsterile medical equipment.

Preventing MRSA Health advocates are calling for increased screening of patients for MRSA, isolating and treating MRSA carriers, more conscientious hand washing, and more diligent use of gowns, gloves, and masks to prevent transmission of MRSA.

Outside hospitals, community-associated MRSA (CA-MRSA) can occur in people without any established risks, including college students, who often live in close quarters and participate in contact sports such as football, wrestling, and fencing. According to a recent study, the risk of infection in a community gym is low, and commonsense health precautions can lower your risk.

According to CDC estimates, some 94,000 American get serious MRSA infections each year, and nearly 19,000 die. The number of these infections has decreased significantly in hospital intensive care units. Among the simple steps responsible for this decline are closer monitoring of hand washing, better means of disinfecting rooms, and improved tracking of patients as they transfer from one hospital or room to another. Another dangerous "superbug," carbapenem-resistant Enterobacteriaceae (CRE), is gaining a foothold in U.S. health-care facilities, particularly long-term health-care facilities.[31]

Who Is at Highest Risk? People at high risk of becoming infected with MRSA are those in close contact with carriers, as hospital patients are. MRSA poses the greatest danger to individuals who have the following:

• A weakened immune system

• A preexisting infection

tuberculosis (TB) A highly infectious bacterial disease that primarily affects the lungs and is often fatal.

YOUR STRATEGIES FOR PREVENTION

How to Avoid MRSA

• **Wash hands thoroughly and frequently.**

• **Ask health-care professionals if they've washed their hands before examining or treating you.**

• **Keep cuts and scrapes clean.** Cover them with a Band-Aid.

• **Avoid touching other people's cuts, incisions, or dressings.**

• **Don't share personal items such as towels or razors.**

• **If you go to a gym, wipe the equipment before working out.** Use a clean towel to prevent your skin from coming into direct contact with the machines. Shower after each workout.

- Open wounds, cuts, or burns
- Other types of wounds, such as skin breaks from an intravenous drug line
- Undergone surgery
- Taken antibiotics recently or for a long period

Also at great risk are

- Athletes in contact sports
- Elderly individuals
- Premature or newborn babies

Infections with the bacterium *Clostridium difficile* (*C. difficile*) also have become increasingly common in health-care facilities as well the community. The bacterium, which causes inflammation of the colon and potentially deadly diarrhea, is often linked to the use of antibiotics, which can destroy the natural bacterial balance in the colon and allow *C. difficile* to take over. These infections can be prevented by limiting antibiotics and effective infection-control procedures in health-care facilities treating patients infected with *C. difficile*. Although anyone can get *C. difficile*, women, whites, and those over age 65 are especially vulnerable.[32]

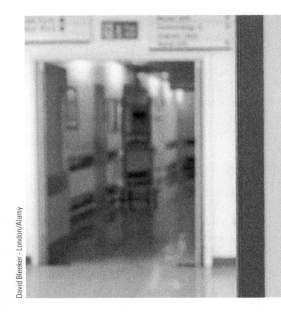

David Bleeker - London/Alamy

Insect- and Animal-Borne Infections

Common insects and animals, including ticks and mosquitoes, can transmit dangerous infections, among them Lyme disease and West Nile virus. Of all emerging infections, 75 percent originate in animals; of these, 61 percent can be transmitted to humans.

Lyme Disease

Lyme disease, the most commonly reported vector-borne infectious disease in the United States, affects about 20,000 to 30,000 Americans a year. This bacterial infection is spread by ixodid ticks that carry a particular bacterium—the spirochete *Borrelia burgdorferi*. Babesiosis, another tick-borne disease, is becoming a growing concern in the Northeast and upper Midwest.[33]

Here is what you need to know:

- Symptoms include joint inflammation, heart arrhythmias, blinding headaches, and memory

lapses. The disease can also cause miscarriages and birth defects.

- You are not likely to get Lyme disease if a tick is attached to your skin for less than 48 hours.
- About 70 to 80 percent of infected individuals develop a red rash at the site of the tick bite. Over a period of days to weeks, the rash grows larger. A ring of skin just beyond the bite site may fade, creating a ring or "bull's-eye" appearance. Rarely, the rash may burn or itch.
- Once diagnosed, Lyme disease is treated with antibiotics. Nonsteroidal anti-inflammatory drugs, such as aspirin or ibuprofen, can relieve fever and pain.

West Nile Virus

West Nile Virus (WNV), transmitted by a mosquito that feeds on an infected bird and then bites a human, flares up in the summer. WNV can also be spread through blood transfusions, organ transplants, and breast-feeding, as well as from mother to fetus during pregnancy. Things to remember about WNV include the following:

- WNV interferes with normal central nervous system functioning and causes inflammation of brain tissue.
- The risk of catching WNV is low. Relatively few mosquitoes carry WNV, and fewer than 1 percent of people who are bitten by mosquitoes experience any symptoms.

Hospitals can be dangerous places. MRSA spreads from patient to patient when hand washing is inadequate or when gloves or equipment are contaminated.

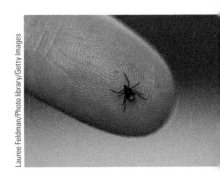

Lauree Feldman/Photo library/Getty Images

Ticks are responsible for the spread of Lyme disease. If you spot a tick, remove it as soon as possible with tweezers or small forceps. Put it in a plastic bag or sealed bottle and save it. If you develop a rash or other symptoms, take it with you to the doctor.

Lyme disease A disease caused by a bacterium carried by a tick; it may cause heart arrhythmias, neurological problems, and arthritis symptoms.

- Repellents that contain an EPA-registered insect repellent can protect against these mosquitoes.[34]

- There is no specific treatment for WNV infection. People with more severe cases usually require hospitalization and supportive treatment, including intravenous fluids and help with breathing.

Avian Influenza

Avian influenza, or bird flu, is caused by viruses that occur naturally among wild birds and usually does not infect humans. However, influenza viruses jumped from birds to humans three times in the twentieth century. In each case, a mutation in the genes of the virus allowed it to infect humans. Then a further change allowed the virus to pass easily from one human to another, and it spread rapidly around the world.

Emerging Infectious Diseases

The twenty-first century has ushered in new agents of infection and new apprehension about the lack of treatment protocols for them.

SARS

Severe acute respiratory syndrome (SARS) became a new global health threat in 2003 and 2004, with major outbreaks in several Asian countries, including China and Hong Kong, and in Toronto.

The average incubation period for SARS is six to ten days. Symptoms include high fever, coughing, headache, chills, muscle aches, and shortness of breath. Most of those infected develop pneumonia. There are no specific treatments for SARS. Patients receive supportive care, such as fluids to prevent dehydration and ventilators to aid breathing.

Ebola

The largest known outbreak of the Ebola virus disease occurred in several West African countries in 2014, with fatality rates as high as 60 percent. Americans who contracted the disease in Africa and health-care workers who cared for them were among those who became ill.[35] In an early-stage clinical trial, an experimental Ebola vaccine proved safe and effective in eliciting a "robust" immune response. The most common side effects were injection site pain and a temporary fever.[36]

Smallpox

Smallpox is a serious, contagious, and sometimes fatal infectious disease. Smallpox was eradicated decades ago after a successful worldwide vaccination program. The last case of smallpox in the United States was in 1949. The last naturally occurring case in the world was in Somalia in 1977. There is no treatment, and up to 30 percent of those infected with smallpox die.

Because of fear that terrorists might use smallpox as a biological weapon, the U.S. government has stockpiled enough vaccine to inoculate everyone in the event of an emergency. Most individuals vaccinated before 1972, when mandated smallpox immunization ended in the United States, retain some immunity for many years, some for up to 75 years. However, half of all Americans have never received the smallpox vaccine, and many scientists believe protection wanes over time for those who did. Those vaccinated in the past can safely be revaccinated for optimum protection. An Institute of Medicine committee has recommended against vaccinating the entire population at this time.

Reproductive and Urinary Tract Infections

Reproductive and urinary tract infections are very common. Many are not spread exclusively by sexual contact, so they are not classified as sexually transmitted diseases.

Vaginal Infections

Vaginal complaints account for approximately 10 million medical office visits a year. The most common are trichomoniasis, candidiasis, and bacterial vaginosis (Table 16.2).

Protozoa (*Trichomonas vaginalis*) that live in the vagina can multiply rapidly, causing itching, burning, and discharge—all symptoms of **trichomoniasis**. Male carriers usually have no symptoms, although some may develop urethritis or an inflammation of the prostate and seminal vesicles. Anyone with this infection should be screened for syphilis, gonorrhea, chlamydia, and HIV. Sexual partners must be treated with oral medication (metronidazole, trade name Flagyl), even if they have no symptoms, to prevent reinfection.

Populations of a yeast called *Candida albicans*—normal inhabitants of the mouth, digestive tract,

trichomoniasis An infection of the protozoan *Trichomonas vaginalis*; females experience vaginal burning, itching, and discharge, but male carriers may be asymptomatic.

TABLE 16.2 Common Reproductive Tract Infections

Infection	Transmission	Symptoms	Treatment
Bacterial vaginosis	Most common causative agent, *Gardnerella vaginalis* bacterium, sometimes transmitted through coitus	Women: Fishy- or musty-smelling thin discharge, like flour paste in consistency and usually gray Men: Mostly asymptomatic	Metronidazole (Flagyl) by mouth or intravaginal applications of topical metronidazole gel or clindamycin cream
Candidiasis (yeast infection)	*Candida albicans* fungus may accelerate growth when the chemical balance of the vagina is disturbed; also transmitted through sexual interaction	Women: White, "cheesy" discharge; irritation of vaginal and vulval tissues	Vaginal suppositories or topical cream, such as clotrimazol (GyneLotrimin) and miconazole (Monistat), or oral fluconazole
Trichomoniasis	Protozoan parasite *Trichomonas vaginalis*, usually passed through genital sexual contact	Women: White or yellow vaginal discharge with an unpleasant odor; sore and irritated vulva Men: No symptoms	Metronidazole (Flagyl) for both women and men

© Cengage Learning

and vagina—are usually held in check. Under certain conditions, however (such as poor nutrition, stress, or antibiotic use), the microbes multiply, causing burning, itching, and a whitish discharge, and producing what is commonly known as a yeast infection. Common sites for **candidiasis**, which is also called *moniliasis*, are the vagina, vulva, penis, and mouth.

The women most likely to test positive for candidiasis have never been pregnant, use condoms for birth control, have sexual intercourse more than four times a month, and have taken antibiotics in the previous 15 to 30 days. Vaginal medications, such as GyneLotrimin and Monistat, are nonprescription drugs that provide effective treatment. Women should keep the genital area dry and wear cotton underwear.

Male sexual partners may be advised to wear condoms during outbreaks of candidiasis.

Bacterial vaginosis is characterized by alterations in the microorganisms that live in the vagina, including depletion of certain bacteria and overgrowth of others. It typically causes a white or gray vaginal discharge with a distinctive fishy odor similar to that of trichomoniasis. Its underlying cause is unknown, although it occurs most frequently in women with multiple sex partners. Long-term dangers include pelvic inflammatory disease and pregnancy complications. Metronidazole, either in the form of a pill or a vaginal gel, is the primary treatment. According to CDC guidelines, treatment for male sex partners appears to be of little benefit, but some health practitioners recommend treatment for both partners in cases of recurrent infections. Antibiotic therapy may help prevent an infected woman from acquiring an STI.

Urinary Tract Infections

A urinary tract infection (UTI) can be present in any of the three parts of the urinary tract: the urethra, the bladder, or the kidneys. An infection involving the urethra is known as **urethritis**. If the bladder is also infected, it's called **cystitis**. If it reaches the kidneys, it's called *pyelonephritis*.

An estimated 40 percent of women report having had a UTI at some point in their lives. Three times as many women as men develop UTIs, probably for anatomical reasons. A woman's urethra is only 1.5 inches long; a man's is 6 inches. Therefore, bacteria, the major cause of UTIs, have a shorter distance to travel to infect a woman's bladder and kidneys. About one-fourth to one-third of all women between ages 20 and 40 develop UTIs, and 80 percent of those who experience one infection develop recurrences.

Conditions that can set the stage for UTIs include irritation and swelling of the urethra or bladder as a result of pregnancy, bike riding, irritants (such as bubble bath, douches, or a diaphragm), urinary stones, enlargement of the prostate gland in men, vaginitis, and stress. Early diagnosis is critical because infection can spread to the kidneys and, if unchecked, result in kidney failure. Symptoms include frequent, burning, or painful urination; chills; fever; fatigue; and blood in the urine.

Recurrent UTIs, a frequent problem among young women, have been linked with a genetic predisposition, sexual intercourse, and the use of diaphragms.

candidiasis An infection of the yeast *Candida albicans*, commonly occurring in the vagina, vulva, penis, and mouth and causing burning, itching, and a whitish discharge.

bacterial vaginosis A vaginal infection caused by overgrowth and depletion of various microorganisms living in the vagina, resulting in a malodorous white or gray vaginal discharge.

urethritis Infection of the urethra.

cystitis Infection of the urinary bladder.

- How much of a threat are infections in today's world?
- Why do vaccinations matter?
- What can you do to protect yourself from colds and flus?
- What do college students need to know about meningitis?

THE POWER OF NOW!
Protecting Yourself

As with other aspects of your well-being, your choices and behaviors affect your risk of acquiring infectious diseases. Which of the following steps have you taken?

____ Getting your "shots." Keep track of the vaccinations you've received and the dates you received them. Check with your doctor about any booster shots you may require. Get a tetanus booster every five years (an easy way not to forget: get one every time you celebrate a birthday ending in a 5 or 0, such as 25 and 30). Get your flu shot or spray. If you're a woman and have not been vaccinated against human papillomavirus (HPV), talk to your doctor about the potential benefits for you.

____ Washing your hands after you use the restroom or work out with weights and other exercise equipment and before you eat.

____ Washing/sanitizing your hands frequently during the cold and flu season.

____ Wiping down exercise equipment handles before using it.

____ Avoiding people who are sneezing or coughing.

____ Applying an insect spray containing an EPA-registered repellent when outdoors.

____ Wearing long-sleeved clothing and long pants when hiking.

____ Checking yourself for ticks after a walk or hike.

What's Online

 Visit www.cengagebrain.com to access course materials for this text, including the Behavior Change Planner, interactive quizzes, and more.

What's Your Infection IQ?

Check the items that apply to you.

____ I wash my hands with soap and water after I use the restroom.

____ I wash my hands with soap and water before I eat.

____ Before and after using exercise equipment, I wipe the handles.

____ I wash my hands with soap and water after working out with weights or exercise equipment at a gym.

____ I avoid contact with people who are coughing and sneezing.

____ I wash my hands with soap and water more often during the cold and flu season.

____ All of my vaccinations are current.

____ I eat at least 3 balanced meals a day.

____ I get 6 to 8 hours of sleep at night.

____ I use relaxation techniques to lower my stress level.

____ I do not smoke.

____ I do not drink or I keep alcohol consumption to a minimum.

____ I do not use drugs of any kind, including steroids.

____ I throw leftovers out after 3 days.

____ I wash fruits and vegetables before eating.

____ I check expiration dates on food items.

____ I apply insect spray (containing an EPA-registered repellent) when I am outdoors.

____ I wear long-sleeved clothing and long pants when hiking.

____ I check myself for ticks after a hike.

Scoring

Add up your checkmarks, and look for patterns in your protective behaviors. Are you conscientious about exercise and sleep, but careless about washing your hands or wiping down gym equipment? Do you protect yourself against food infections (discussed in Chapter 6) but not against sexually transmitted infections (discussed in Chapter 11)? Identify the aspects of infection protection that need the most work, and start practicing the defensive behaviors that will lower your risk.

MAKING THIS CHAPTER WORK FOR YOU

Review Questions

(LO 16.1) 1. When speaking of the infection process, a vector is:
   a. the area in which the infection occurred
   b. the biological or physical vehicle that carries the agent to the host
   c. the organism that causes the infection
   d. the person infected

(LO 16.1) 2. The time between the entry of a pathogen into your body and the first symptom is known as_____ .
   a. the incubation period
   b. the prodromal period
   c. the attack period
   d. dormancy

(LO 16.2) 3. Which of the following statements about the immune system is true?
   a. The immune system has two types of white blood cells: B cells, which produce antibodies that fight bacteria, and viruses.
   b. Immune system structures include the spleen, tonsils, lungs, thymus gland, and lymph nodes.
   c. Inoculation with a vaccine confers active immunity.
   d. The effect of stress on the human immune system is to increase its effectiveness.

(LO 16.2) 4. As part of the body's immune response, macrophages _____.
   a. act as specialist cells that respond to specific invaders
   b. are part of the bone marrow
   c. filter bacteria and many other agents of disease
   d. are scavenger cells that consume foreign cells as well as diseased red blood cells

(LO 16.3) 5. Allergic rhinitis is _____.
   a. a food allergy
   b. an allergic reaction to bee stings
   c. an inflammatory response of the nasal membranes to an allergen
   d. an infection of the ears that occurs after a person encounters an allergen

(LO 16.3) 6. _____ is considered to be an autoimmune disorder.
   a. Crohn's disease
   b. West Nile virus
   c. type 2 diabetes
   d. pancreatic cancer

(LO 16.4) 7. College students should have all of the following immunizations, except _____.
   a. hepatitis A
   b. pertussis
   c. measles
   d. zoster

(LO 16.4) 8. _____ is a highly infectious disease that was thought to be eliminated in the United States until outbreaks in 2014 and 2015.
   a. Polio
   b. Smallpox
   c. Measles
   d. Chicken pox

(LO 16.5) 9. Which of the following statements about the common cold and influenza is *true*?
   a. Influenza is just a more severe form of the common cold.
   b. Aspirin should be avoided by children and young adults who have a cold or influenza.
   c. The flu vaccine is also effective against most of the viruses that cause the common cold.
   d. Antibiotics are appropriate treatments for colds but not for influenza.

(LO 16.5) 10. The flu virus can be spread by all of the following except _____.
   a. sneezing
   b. laughing
   c. coughing
   d. texting

(LO 16.6) 11. The meningitis vaccination _____.
   a. is no longer recommended for all college freshmen
   b. protects against four of the five most common types of meningococcal bacteria
   c. also protects against gonorrhea
   d. may cause minor reactions such as fever or hives

(LO 16.6) 12. Viral meningitis _____.
   a. is usually less severe than bacterial meningitis
   b. can cause blindness
   c. is most common in people over age 65
   d. has slowly increased in frequency of occurrence over the last 10 years

(LO 16.7) 13. Hepatitis B _____.
   a. is spread mainly through contaminated needles
   b. infects mostly middle-aged people
   c. does not have a preventive vaccine
   d. can be spread in the sweat of athletes

(LO 16.7) 14. Hepatitis C can be contracted by _____.
   a. casual contact, such as kissing
   b. being a blood donor
   c. being born to a parent who has HCV
   d. having HIV

(LO 16.8) 15. Which statement about methicillin-resistant *Staphylococcus aureus* (MRSA) is *true*?
   a. MRSA can be spread by nurses rarely by doctors in a hospital.
   b. MRSA can be spread in community gyms.
   c. MRSA is carried on the skin of as many as one in three people.
   d. MRSA can develop among sports teams.

(LO 16.8) 16. Along with feelings of fatigue and unrefreshing sleep, symptoms of Myalgic Encephalomyelitis/Chronic Fatigue Syndrome include _____.
   a. slow recovery from infections
   b. migraine headaches
   c. severe allergic reaction to antibiotics
   d. nausea

(LO 16.9) 17. Lyme disease can be transmitted to humans by _____.
   a. bite from an infected tick
   b. a bite from an infected mosquito
   c. contact with an infected bird
   d. a kiss from someone who is infected with the disease

(LO 16.9) 18. West Nile virus _____.
   a. is highly contagious
   b. is easily treated with antiviral drugs
   c. affects at least 30% of the population
   d. interferes with normal central nervous system function

(LO 16.10) 19. Among the diseases that health experts say are eradicated is _____.
- a. polio
- b. smallpox
- c. mumps
- d. tuberculosis

(LO 16.10) 20. Which of the following about two emerging diseases, SARS and Ebola, is *true?*
- a. They are highly contagious.
- b. They cause blindness, among other serious symptoms.
- c. They are now treatable with a vaccine.
- d. They affect only people in Asian and African countries.

(LO 16.11) 21. Which statement about reproductive and urinary tract infections is *false?*
- a. Yeast infections can be treated with nonprescription drugs.
- b. Symptoms of UTIs include burning urination, chills, fever, and blood in the urine.
- c. Three times as many women as men develop UTIs.
- d. Bacterial vaginosis usually causes a vaginal discharge with a rotten-egg odor.

(LO 16.11) 22. If a urinary tract infection involves the bladder as well as the urethra, it is called _____.
- a. urethritis
- b. pyelonephritis
- c. cystitis
- d. blastosporosis

(LO 16.11) 23. Public health officials define a pandemic as
- a. sudden rise in the incidence of a particular disease.
- b. an atypically large number of people in a region suffering from the same disease.
- c. a high proportion of the population over a wide geographic area suffering from the same disease.
- d. more than 25 percent of the world's population suffering from the same disease.

Answers to these questions can be found on page 623.

Critical Thinking

1. Prior to reading this chapter, describe what you did to avoid contracting infectious disease. Now that you have read the chapter, will you be making any changes in your practices? Briefly explain the convenience, advantages, and disadvantages of each practice that you use and/or will be using to prevent infection.
2. At the pharmacy, the shelves are full of medications for cold and flu. How do you sort through them? Do you get recommendations from family and friends? Do you study the labels? Do you keep track of what works for you?
3. Did you get vaccinated for meningitis? Why or why not? Where did you get your information on the disease and the vaccine, and how did you make your decision?

Additional Online Resources

www.immunize.org
This site features comprehensive vaccination information for children, adolescents, and adults.

www.niaid.nih.gov
The National Institute of Allergy and Infectious Diseases is part of the National Institutes of Health. Its website provides information about current research and includes fact sheets about all manner of topics related to allergies and infectious diseases.

www.cdc.gov/ncezid
This comprehensive site, sponsored by the Centers for Disease Control and Prevention (CDC), features, news on emerging and zoonotic (spread from animals to humans) infectious diseases.

Key Terms

The terms listed are used on the page indicated. Definitions of the terms are in the glossary at the end of the book.

allergic rhinitis 498
allergies 498
antibiotics 492
antiviral drugs 492
autoimmune disorders 499
bacteria 492
bacterial vaginosis 511
candidiasis 511
cystitis 511
fungi 493
gamma globulin 496
helminth 493
hepatitis 505
host 492
immune deficiency 497
immunity 495
incubation period 493
inflammation 497

influenza 502
Lyme disease 509
lymph nodes 495
meningitis 503
mononucleosis 507
myalgic encephalomyelitis/chronic fatigue syndrome (ME/CFS) 507
pathogens 492
protozoa 493
systemic disease 497
trichomoniasis 510
tuberculosis (TB) 508
urethritis 511
vector 492
virus 492

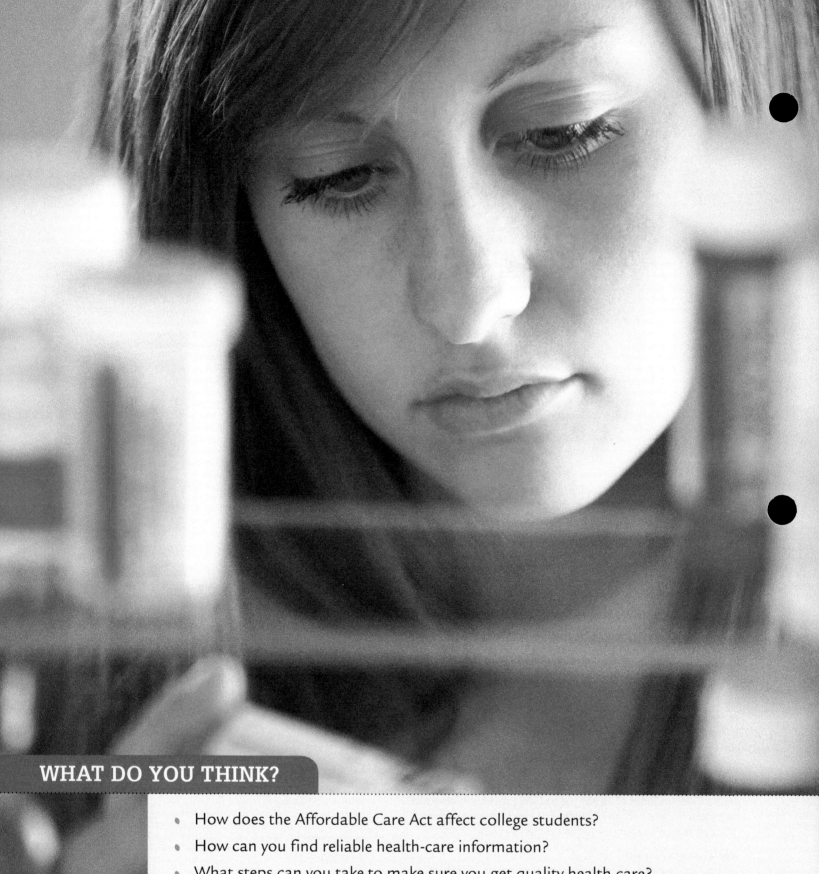

WHAT DO YOU THINK?

- How does the Affordable Care Act affect college students?
- How can you find reliable health-care information?
- What steps can you take to make sure you get quality health care?
- What do you need to know about complementary and alternative medicine?

SW Productions/Getty Images

17

Consumer Health

It sounded too good to be true: an herbal supplement that turned off appetite, burned up calories, melted away pounds. Of course, it was safe, her roommate reassured her. Doctors had been using it for severely obese patients for years. Yet anyone could get it online without a prescription. Lots of kids on campus had tried it. And just think: Karli could shed the weight she'd put on during her freshman year just in time for bikini season.

Karli rarely took any medications, even over-the-counter ones. She didn't smoke, drink alcohol, or experiment with drugs. And she definitely didn't consider herself a risk taker. But a quick, easy way to lose weight didn't strike her as risky. When her heart started beating rapidly, Karli blamed anxiety. She felt increasingly restless. Her head ached. She couldn't sleep. Her mouth felt dry, with an unpleasant taste that she couldn't gargle away.

One day Karli got so dizzy that a classmate insisted on taking her to the campus health center.

When the doctor inquired about drug use, she immediately said she didn't do drugs. But when asked about prescription medications, she mentioned the diet pills—and where they came from.

It had never occurred to her that they might be the culprit or that she might have been taking counterfeit pills with unknown ingredients. "Never again!" Karli swears. She isn't going to take any more chances with her health—and she's going to make better health-care choices. <

After reading this chapter, you should be able to:

17.1 Describe the impact of the Affordable Care Act on access to health care.

17.2 Discuss the concept of consumer-driven health care.

17.3 Explain the significance of personalized health care.

17.4 Describe what it means to be a savvy health-care consumer.

17.5 Outline your rights as a health-care consumer.

17.6 Discuss the pros and cons of elective treatments to enhance health or appearance.

17.7 Identify ways to recognize health hoaxes and medical quackery.

17.8 Assess the benefits and potential risks of complementary and alternative medicine (CAM).

17.9 Review the components of the health-care system, including types of practitioners and health-care facilities.

Although you may not realize it, every day you, too, make crucial decisions that affect your health. You choose what you eat, whether you exercise, whether you smoke or drink, and when to fasten your seat belt. You determine when to see a doctor, what kind of doctor, and with what sense of urgency. You decide what to tell the physician and whether to follow his or her advice, take a prescribed medication as directed, or seek further help or a second opinion. The entire process of maintaining or restoring health depends on your decisions. It cannot start or continue without them.

This chapter will help you take greater responsibility for your personal well-being. Whether you are monitoring your blood pressure, taking medication, or deciding whether to try an alternative therapy, you need to gather information, ask questions, weigh advantages and disadvantages, and take charge of your health. The reason: No one cares more about your health than you do, and no one will do more to protect your well-being.

✓ **check-in** Do you take good care of yourself? If you say yes, how? If you say no, what do you think you should be doing?

TABLE 17.1 Free Preventive Services under the ACA

- Alcohol misuse screening and counseling
- Aspirin to prevent cardiovascular disease for men and women of certain ages
- Blood pressure screening for all adults
- Cholesterol screening for adults of certain ages or at higher risk
- Colorectal cancer screening for adults over 50
- Depression screening for adults
- Diabetes (type 2) screening for adults with high blood pressure
- Diet counseling for adults at higher risk for chronic disease
- HIV screening for everyone ages 15 to 65
- Immunization vaccines for adults—doses, recommended ages, and recommended populations vary
- Obesity screening and counseling for all adults
- Sexually transmitted infection (STI) prevention counseling for adults at higher risk
- Syphilis screening for all adults at higher risk
- Tobacco use screening for all adults and cessation interventions for tobacco users

© 2017 Cengage Learning

The Affordable Care Act (ACA)

The Affordable Care Act (ACA), initially referred to as Obamacare and signed into law in 2010, has ushered in a new era in consumer health. Among the key reforms it has put in place are the following[1]:

- Health insurance exchanges, or marketplaces, for individuals, families, and small businesses to purchase guaranteed health insurance plans with affordable premiums.

- Subsidies for low-income purchasers to make buying health insurance more affordable.

- A tax penalty for those who do not purchase coverage.

- Insurance companies no longer allowed to refuse coverage or charge higher premiums to people with a preexisting condition.

- Elimination of annual and lifetime caps on how much an insurance company will pay a policyholder.

- No copayments, deductibles, or coinsurance for basic preventive care services. (See Table 17.1.)

Although the ACA continues to generate legal and political controversy, its impact has been profound. According to the Commonwealth Fund Biennial Health Insurance Survey, since the ACA's enactment, Americans have had significantly less trouble getting and paying for needed medical care:

- The number of uninsured working-age adults fell from a high of 22 percent in 2010 to 16 percent by mid-2014, with the greatest gains among blacks and Hispanics. [2]

- The number of adults who did not get needed health care because of cost declined from about 80 million (43 percent of the population) to 66 million (36 percent).[3]

- Fewer adults report that concern about cost has kept them from going to a doctor when sick; filling a prescription; having a recommended test, treatment, or follow-up visit; or seeking needed care from a specialist. However, even insured adults report delaying or avoiding needed care because of high deductibles or cost-sharing provisions in their health coverage.[4]

- Young adults realized the greatest gains in coverage of any age group. Among adults ages 19 to 25, the percentage who were uninsured decreased from 26.5 percent in 2013 to 20.4 percent in the first 9 months of 2014.[5]

✓ **check-in** Do you have health insurance? If so, what type of coverage?

What You Need to Know

College students have several choices for health coverage:

• If you are enrolled in your school's student health plan, check to see if it qualifies as coverage under the health law.

• If you are under age 26, you may be covered under a parent's health insurance plan. You can join or remain on a parent's plan even if you are married, attending school full or part time, not living at home, not financially dependent on your parents, or eligible to enroll in your employer's plan.

• Even if you have access to a student health plan, you can choose to buy a health plan at www .healthcare.gov. Based on your income, you may be able to obtain coverage at a lower cost.

• If you're under 30, you can buy a catastrophic health plan, which usually has lower monthly premiums but high deductibles. This means you pay for most of your care yourself, up to a certain amount. After that, the insurance company pays its share for covered services. Catastrophic plans are an affordable way to protect yourself from the high costs of worst-case scenarios, like an accident or a serious illness. They also cover three primary care visits per year before you meet your deductible, as well as certain preventive care benefits.

• If you do not obtain coverage, you will pay a penalty of either 1 percent of your income or $95 per adult ($47.50 per child), whichever is higher. This penalty will be charged on your income taxes.

Once you have a plan, make sure you know what it covers, including the following:

• **Prescriptions:** To find out which prescriptions are covered through a plan, visit your insurer's website to review a list of medications covered. Check the Summary of Benefits and Coverage that you received. You also can call your insurer. The number is on your insurance card and the insurer's website.

• **Doctor visits:** Most health plans give you the best deal on services when you see a doctor who has a contract with your health plan. While you may be able to see physicians who do not contract with your plan, visiting an "in-network" provider usually means you will have lower out-of-pocket costs. To find out if your current doctors and other health-care providers are covered through a new plan or to find a covered provider if you don't have one yet, visit your health plan's website and check the provider directory, which lists the doctors, hospitals, and other health-care providers that your plan contracts with to provide care.

• **Emergency care:** In an emergency, you should get care from the closest hospital that can help you. Your insurance company cannot require you to get prior approval before getting emergency services from a provider or hospital outside your plan's network or charge you more for such care.

✓ **check-in** Do you know what your health insurance plan covers?

Consumer-Driven Health Care

Increasingly Americans may approach "purchases" of health care the same way as other major investments, like buying a car. More than

YOUR STRATEGIES FOR PREVENTION
How to Boost Health Understanding

Always ask these three questions of your doctor, nurse, or pharmacist:

• **What is my main problem?**

• **What do I need to do?**

• **Why is it important for me to do this?**

• **If you don't understand, say,** "This is new to me. Can you explain it one more time?"

• **If you don't know the meaning of a medical term, don't hesitate to ask what it means.** Health professionals sometimes forget they're using technical terms, such as "myocardial infarction" for heart attack.

• **Write down a list of your health concerns,** and bring it with you whenever you seek health care.

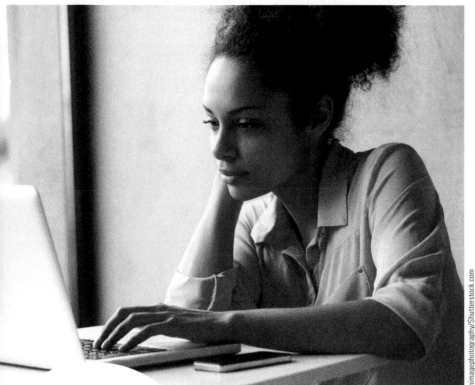

Millions of Americans go online to learn about medical problems and treatments and to chat with others who have similar conditions.

monitor cholesterol levels or blood sugar, manage a chronic disease, find health providers and services, or fill out necessary forms. According to research studies, people with limited health literacy are more likely to report poor health, to skip important preventive measures such as regular Pap smears, to have chronic conditions such as diabetes or asthma, to stop taking needed medications, and to have higher rates of preventable hospitalizations.[7]

Regardless of their literacy skills, college students often do not seek out information on health concerns. In one study that tracked college students' communications for a two-week period, they sought health-related advice and information in a little more than one-fourth of their communications about health. When they did seek help, they were most likely to turn to family members and friends. About half of students also turn to health educators for information, and most rank them and health center medical staff as trustworthy. Although students regularly get information from flyers, pamphlets, magazines, and television, they are less likely to consider these as authoritative, believable sources.

✓ **check-in** Where do you turn for health information? Which sources do you consider the most reliable?

ever, consumers will need clear, concise, and accurate information, not just on specific health conditions but also on factors such as out-of-pocket expenses and the effectiveness of a particular treatment.

The demand for this information coincides with the growth of personalized medicine, in which individuals' genetic profiles will help determine which drugs or cancer therapies to prescribe, as well as help predict the risk of future disease.[6]

This means that you will have to be a savvier, more sophisticated health-care consumer. By learning how to maintain your health, evaluate medical information, and spot early signs of a problem, you're more likely to get the best possible care.

✓ **check-in** How well informed a health-care consumer do you think you are?

Improving Your Health Literacy

According to federal estimates, about one-third of the population in the United States has limited ability to understand health information and to use that information to make good decisions about health and medical care. Because of poor **health literacy**, more than 90 million Americans may not understand how to take medication,

Finding Good Advice Online

More than one-third of Americans turn to the Internet to diagnose health problems. More than half of Internet users use the web to research health problems they have discussed with their doctors. Two-thirds go online to find health information.[8]

If you go to websites for medical information, here are some guidelines for evaluating them:

• **Check the creator.** Websites are produced by health agencies, health support groups, school health programs, health-product advertisers, health educators, and health-education organizations. Read site headers and footers carefully to distinguish biased commercial advertisements from unbiased sites created by scientists and health agencies.

• **If you are looking for the most recent research,** check the date the page was created and last updated, as well as the links. Several nonworking links signal that the site isn't carefully maintained or updated.

• **Check the references.** As with other health-education materials, web documents should provide the reader with references. Unreferenced suggestions may be scientifically unsound and possibly unsafe.

health literacy Ability to understand health information and use it to make good decisions about health and medical care.

mimagephotography/Shutterstock.com

- **Consider the author.** Is he or she recognized in the field of health education or otherwise qualified to publish a health information web document? Does the author list his or her occupation, experience, and education?

- **Look for possible bias.** Websites may attempt to provide health information to consumers, but they also may attempt to sell a product. Many sites are merely disguised advertisements. (See Table 17.2 for some doctor-endorsed websites.)

✓**check-in** Which websites have you used to find health information? Which ones do you trust? Which ones don't you trust?

Getting Medical Facts Straight

Cure! Breakthrough! Medical miracle! (See Consumer Alert above.) These words make headlines. Remember that although medical breakthroughs and cures do occur, most scientific progress is made one small step at a time. Rather than put your faith in the most recent report or the hottest trend, try to gather as much background information and as many opinions as you can.

When reading a newspaper or magazine story or listening to a radio or television report about a medical advance, look for answers to the following questions:

- **Who are the researchers?** Are they recognized, legitimate health professionals? What are their credentials? Are they affiliated with respected medical or scientific institutions? Be wary of individuals whose degrees or affiliations are from institutions you've never heard of, and be sure that the person's educational background is in a discipline related to the area of research reported.

- **Where did the researchers report their findings?** The best research is published in peer-reviewed professional journals, such as the *New England Journal of Medicine*. Research developments also may be reported at meetings of professional societies.

- **Is the information based on personal observations?** Does the report include testimonials from cured patients or satisfied customers? If the answer to either question is yes, be wary.

- **Does the article, report, or advertisement include words like *amazing*, *secret*, or *quick*?** Does it claim to be something the public has never seen or been offered before? Such sensationalized language is often a tip-off that the treatment is dubious.

TABLE 17.2 Doctor-Recommended Websites

National Library of Medicine: MedlinePlus	www.nlm.nih.gov/medlineplus/

MedlinePlus contains links to information on hundreds of health conditions and issues. The site also includes a medical dictionary, an encyclopedia with pictures and diagrams, and links to physician directories.

FDA Center for Drug Evaluation and Research	www.fda.gov

Click on Drugs@FDA for information on approved prescription drugs and some over-the-counter medications.

WebMD	www.webmd.com

WebMD is full of information to help you manage your health. The site's quizzes and calculators are a fun way to test your medical knowledge. Get diet tips, find information on drugs and herbs, and check out special sections on men's and women's health.

Mayo Clinic	www.mayoclinic.com

The renowned Mayo Clinic offers a one-stop health resource website. Use the site's Health Decision Guides to make decisions about prevention and treatment. Learn more about complementary and alternative medicine, sports medicine, and senior health in the Healthy Living Centers.

Centers for Disease Control and Prevention	www.cdc.gov

Stay up-to-date on the latest public health news and get the CDC's recommendations on travelers' health, vaccines and immunizations, and protecting your health in case of a disaster.

Medscape	www.medscape.com

Medscape delivers news and research specifically tailored to your medical interests. The site requires (free) registration.

© Cengage Learning

- **Is someone trying to sell you something?** Manufacturers that cite studies to sell a product have been known to embellish the truth.

- **Does the information defy all common sense?** Be skeptical. If something sounds too good to be true, it probably is.

Evidence-Based Medicine

Large randomized, controlled trials and large prospective studies provide the best evidence, or scientific proof, that a particular treatment is effective. **Evidence-based medicine** is a way of improving and evaluating patient care by combining the best research evidence with the patient's personal values.

Reviewing all available medical studies pertaining to an individual patient or group of patients helps doctors diagnose illnesses more precisely, choose the best tests, and select the best treatments or methods of disease prevention. By using evidence-based medical techniques for large groups of patients with the same illness, doctors can develop **practice guidelines** for evaluating and treating particular illnesses.

evidence-based medicine The choice of a medical treatment on the basis of large randomized, controlled research trials and large prospective studies.

practice guidelines Recommendations for diagnosis and treatment of various health problems, based on evidence from scientific research.

Too Good to Be True?

Almost every week you're likely to see an ad for a new health product that promises better sleep, more energy, clearer skin, firmer muscles, lower weight, brighter moods, longer life—or all of these combined. But you can't believe every promise you read or hear. Keep these general guidelines in mind the next time you come across a health claim.

Facts to Know

● **Do your own research.** Check with your doctor or with the student health center. Go to the library or do some online research to gather as much information as you can.

● **Check credentials.** Anyone can claim to be a scientist or a health expert. Find out if advocates of any type of therapy have legitimate degrees from recognized institutions and are fully licensed in their fields.

Steps to Take

● **Look for objective evaluations.** If you're watching an infomercial for a treatment or technique, you can be sure that the enthusiastic endorsements have been skillfully scripted and rehearsed. Even ads that claim to be presenting the science behind a new breakthrough are really sales pitches in disguise.

● **Consider the sources.** Research findings from carefully controlled scientific studies are reviewed by leading experts in the field and published in scholarly journals. Just because someone has conducted a study doesn't mean it was a valid scientific investigation.

● **If it sounds too good to be true, it probably is.** If a magic pill could really trim off excess pounds or banish wrinkles, the world would be filled with thin people with unlined skin. Look around, and you'll realize that's not the case.

Outcomes Research

Evidence-based medicine pays particular attention to **outcomes**—that is, the impact that a specific medication or treatment has on a patient's condition, overall health, and quality of life.

Outcomes research is designed to answer questions such as these: Is treatment better or worse than no treatment? Is one treatment better than another? If a treatment is effective, is a little just as good as a lot? Does quality of life change because of treatment? Are the benefits of treatment worth the cost or the risks to the patient?

Studies of outcomes look at how patients fared with or without a specific treatment, the costs involved, and the impact of undergoing or not undergoing treatment in terms of the patients' quality of life. Outcomes research can help determine which of several therapies or approaches provides the best results at the most reasonable costs.

outcomes The ultimate impacts of particular treatments or absence of treatment.

medical history Health-related information that a health-care professional collects while interviewing a patient.

✓**check-in** When you are diagnosed with a health problem, do you ask your doctor if the suggested treatment is based on the latest evidence and clinical guidelines? The National Guideline Clearinghouse provides a comprehensive database of evidence-based clinical practice guidelines for many common health problems, available at www.guideline.gov.

Personalizing Your Health Care

Thanks to advances in genomics (the study of the entire set of human genes), physicians are tailoring tests and treatments to individual patients. "Personalized" medicine can alert your doctor to potential threats that might be prevented, delayed, or detected at an earlier, more treatable stage and, if you do develop a disease, pinpoint the medications that will do the most good and cause the least harm.

But "personalizing" health care is also a personal responsibility. You can take charge of your own health by compiling a family health history and informing yourself about risks related to your gender, race, and ethnicity.

Your Family Health History

Someday a DNA scan from a single drop of blood may tell you the diseases you're most likely to develop. A family history can do the same—now.

Mapping your family **medical history** can help identify health risks you may face in the future. One way of charting your health history is to draw a medical family "tree" that includes your parents and siblings (who share your genes), as well as grandparents, uncles, aunts, and cousins. Depending on how much information you're able to obtain for each relative, your medical family tree can include health issues each family member has faced, including illnesses with a hereditary component, such as high blood pressure, diabetes, some cancers, and certain psychiatric disorders.

Although having a relative with a certain disease may mean you face increased risk for the condition, this likelihood also depends on your health habits, such as diet and exercise. Realizing that you have a relative with, say, colon cancer could mean that you should start screening tests 10 years before others because you're at risk of developing a tumor at an earlier age.

✓**check-in** Do you know your family's health history? For guidance on creating one, check this website from the office of the Surgeon General: https://familyhistory.hhs.gov/FHH/html/index.html

Gender Differences

The genders differ significantly in the way they use health-care services in the United States. Women see doctors more often than men, take more prescription drugs, are hospitalized more, and control the spending of three of every four health-care dollars.

Many experts believe that the need for birth control and reproductive health services gets women into the habit of making regular visits to health-care professionals, primarily gynecologists. There are no comparable specialists for men, who tend to visit urologists, specialists in male reproductive organs, only when they develop problems. In addition, men are conditioned to take a stoic, tough-it-out attitude to early symptoms of a disease. The length of time they wait to go for treatment may be one reason men die earlier than women.

In a survey of nearly 2 million patients who had recently been hospitalized, men tended to be more positive about their overall experiences. Women were less satisfied with staff responsiveness, discussions with nurses, communication about medications and discharge plans, and the general conditions of the hospital.

The genders also differ in the symptoms and syndromes they develop. For instance, men are more prone to back problems, muscle sprains and strains, allergies, insomnia, and digestive problems. Men develop heart disease about a decade earlier in life than women. More men develop ulcers and hernias; women are more likely to get migraines, gallbladder disease, and irritable bowel syndrome. Yet women and men spend similar proportions of their lifetimes—about 80 percent—free of disability.

Personal Health Apps and Monitors

Do you want to individualize your workout? Check your vital signs? Chart your menstrual cycles? Soothe your spirit? Put yourself to sleep? There's an app for that—tens of thousands, in fact, offering advice, encouragement, self-tests, and a host of home remedies. Although it cannot replace a doctor, a smartphone, watch, or wearable monitor can make you more aware of daily habits (healthful or not), provide access to useful information when and where you need it, remind you to take medications on time, and provide a minute-by-minute record of your daily calories and activity.

Can digital devices make you healthier? Medical scientists don't have definitive answers yet because the technology is relatively new and lacks any rigorous scientific evidence demonstrating possible benefits. Advocates cite many potential benefits for patients, including the following:

- Reminders to take medication at the prescribed times

- Instruction in correct use of devices such as asthma inhalers

- Monitoring of blood pressure or blood sugar

- More effective support for selecting healthful foods and losing weight

- Motivation, through apps or trackers like Fitbit and Jawbone, to be more physically active[9]

The FDA regulates only apps that turn smartphones into medical devices or accessories for measuring blood sugar, blood pressure, heart rate, and other vital signs. On the horizon are apps that may be able to detect antibodies against HIV and syphilis from a fingerprick of blood in just minutes.[10]

Skeptics argue that digital self-monitoring may create uncertainty and anxiety and transform healthy men and women into "young, asymptomatic, middle-class neurotics continuously monitoring their vital signs." As one physician recently argued, "Humanity is wasting its time on monitoring life rather than getting on and living it.[11]" Health apps that make deceptive claims—such as the capability to analyze skin moles to assess the risk of melanoma—could also lead to false positive or negative diagnoses and a failure to get needed treatment.

Health professionals do agree on the utility of some apps, including the following:

- **FitStar Personal Trainer.** By asking a simple set of questions, this app tailors workouts directly for you and your fitness goals, whether you're a beginner or an amateur athlete.

- **GoodRx:** This app compares prescription drug prices at virtually every pharmacy in the United States.

- **iTriage:** Created by two ER doctors, iTriage helps you evaluate any troubling symptoms and get suggestions for the best, nearest health-care facilities.

- **Cook It Allergy Free:** This app offers recipes free of gluten, dairy, nuts, and eggs.

✓**check-in** Do you use any health-monitoring apps or devices? If so, what do you like/dislike about them? Have they had an impact on your behavior?

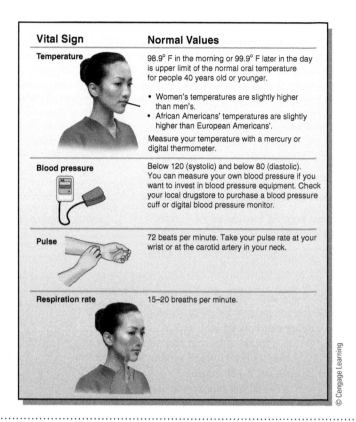

Vital Sign	Normal Values
Temperature	98.9° F in the morning or 99.9° F later in the day is upper limit of the normal oral temperature for people 40 years old or younger. • Women's temperatures are slightly higher than men's. • African Americans' temperatures are slightly higher than European Americans'. Measure your temperature with a mercury or digital thermometer.
Blood pressure	Below 120 (systolic) and below 80 (diastolic). You can measure your own blood pressure if you want to invest in blood pressure equipment. Check your local drugstore to purchase a blood pressure cuff or digital blood pressure monitor.
Pulse	72 beats per minute. Take your pulse rate at your wrist or at the carotid artery in your neck.
Respiration rate	15–20 breaths per minute.

© Cengage Learning

FIGURE 17.1 Do you know your vital signs?

TABLE 17.3 Home Health Tests: A Consumer's Guide

Type of Test	What It Does
Pregnancy	Determines whether a woman is pregnant by detecting the presence of human chorionic gonadotropin in urine. Considered 99% accurate.
Fertility	Measures levels of luteinizing hormone (LH), which rise 24 to 36 hours before a woman ovulates. Can help women increase their odds of conceiving.
Blood pressure	Measures blood pressure by means of an automatically inflating armband or a cuff for the finger or wrist; helps people taking hypertension medication or suffering from high blood pressure to monitor their condition.
Cholesterol	Checks cholesterol in blood from a finger prick; good for anyone concerned about cholesterol.
Colon cancer	Screening test to detect hidden blood in stool; recommended for anyone over 40 or concerned about colorectal disease.
Urinary tract infection	Diagnoses infection by screening for certain white blood cells in urine; advised for women who get frequent UTIs and whose doctors will prescribe antibiotics without a visit.
HIV infection	Detects antibodies to HIV in a blood sample sent anonymously to a lab. Controversial because no face-to-face counseling is available for those who test positive.

© Cengage Learning

Self-Care

Self-care means head-to-toe maintenance, including good oral care, appropriate screening tests, knowing your medical rights, and understanding the health-care system.

Most people do treat themselves. You probably prescribe aspirin for a headache, chicken soup or orange juice for a cold, or a weekend trip to unwind from stress. At the very least, you should know what your **vital signs** are and how they compare against normal readings (Figure 17.1).

At one time, a thermometer was the only self-testing equipment found in most American homes. Now hundreds of home tests are available to help consumers monitor everything from fertility to blood pressure to cholesterol levels (Table 17.3). More convenient and less expensive than a visit to a clinic or doctor's office, the new tests are generally as accurate as those administered by a professional.

Self-care can also mean getting involved in the self-help movement, which has grown into a major national trend. An estimated 20 million people participate in self-help support groups. Millions of others join virtual support communities online.

✓**check-in** When do you practice self-care?

Oral Health

Oral health involves more than healthy teeth; it refers to the entire mouth, including all the structures that allow us to talk, bite, chew, taste, swallow, smile, scream, and scowl. Oral health is a critical part of overall health. Research has revealed links between chronic oral infection and heart and lung diseases, stroke, low birth weight, premature births, and diabetes.

Poor oral health can lead to a variety of health problems. People with gum disease are at increased risk for developing heart disease, stroke, uncontrolled diabetes, preterm births, and respiratory disease. One recent study found an increased risk of pancreatic cancer in individuals who had experienced tooth loss.

Thanks to fluoridated water, toothpaste, and improved dental care, Americans' oral health is better today than in the past. However, without good self-care, you probably will lose some teeth to decay and gum disease. The best way to prevent such problems is through proper and regular brushing and flossing.

Gum disease, or periodontal disease, attacks the gum and bone that hold your teeth in place. The culprit is **plaque**, a sticky film of bacteria that forms on teeth. More than 300 species of bacteria live under the gum line, and about half a dozen have been linked to serious gum problems. The early stage of gum disease is called **gingivitis**. If untreated, it develops into a more serious form known as **periodontitis**, in which plaque moves down the tooth to the roots, which then become infected. In advanced periodontitis, the infection destroys the bone and fibers that hold teeth in place.

Taking care of your mouth isn't important only for dental health: It may affect how long you live. Gingivitis and periodontitis trigger an inflammatory response that causes the arteries to swell, which leads to a constriction of blood flow that can increase the incidence of cardiovascular disease. Periodontal disease also leads to a higher white blood cell count, an indicator that the immune system is under increased stress. The good news: You can prevent these problems by flossing daily and brushing your teeth and your tongue (to get rid of bacteria that can cause gum disease and bad breath).

✓**check-in** How would you rate your oral health care?

Becoming a Savvy Health-Care Consumer

Because physicians today have less time and less autonomy than they once had, patients today must do more. Your first step should be learning more about your body, any medical conditions or problems you develop, and your options for treatment. You can find a great deal of information online, via patient advocacy and support organizations, and from libraries.

Making the Most of a Medical Visit

Your visit to a health-care professional is an opportunity to learn, to share information, to get needed help, and to improve your health now and in the future. Here is how to ensure you get the greatest value from your health-care providers:

Scheduling the Appointment   When you schedule the appointment, you need to both get and give information:

____ Always check to see if a health-care provider accepts your insurance plan.

____ When you make your appointment, explain why you need to see the health-care provider.

YOUR STRATEGIES FOR PREVENTION
How to Take Care of Your Mouth

- **Brush your teeth every morning and every night.** Oral bacteria reach their highest count during sleep because fluids in the mouth accumulate. Nighttime cleaning reduces the bacterial population; morning cleaning reduces the buildup.

- **Use a toothpaste that has the American Dental Association (ADA) seal of acceptance and a toothbrush with soft, rounded bristles.** Replace your toothbrush after an illness or every three months.

- **Hold the brush at a 45-degree angle from your gums.** Pay particular attention to the space between your teeth and gums, especially on the inside, toward your tongue. Brush for two to five minutes. Don't brush too vigorously. If you scrub as hard as you can, you may damage your teeth and gums. Abrasion—a problem for more than half of American adults—erodes tooth surfaces, weakens teeth, and increases sensitivity to hot and cold foods. There is some evidence that powered toothbrushes are better at removing plaque and reducing the risk of gum disease than are ordinary manual toothbrushes.

- **Because brushing can't reach plaque and food trapped between teeth, daily flossing is essential.** Using waxed or unwaxed floss, start behind the upper and lower molars at one side of your mouth and work toward the other side.

- **See your dentist twice a year for routine cleaning and examination.** Your dentist should take a complete medical history from you and update it every six months, examine your mouth for signs of cancer, and thoroughly outline all treatment options.

- **Make sure that everyone who works on the inside of your mouth wears a mask and rubber gloves.** Such measures reduce the risk of disease transmission (that is, bacterial and viral infections, such as hepatitis, herpes, and HIV).

____ Are you scheduling a checkup?

____ Have you developed a new problem?

____ Is it urgent? Do you need to see a health-care provider right away?

____ If you want to see a specialist, find out if you need to a referral from your primary care provider.

____ If you prefer a female provider for religious or cultural reasons, make this clear.

Before Your Appointment   To get the most out of your appointment, you need to do some homework ahead of time:

____ Write down your questions, organize them in a logical fashion, and select the top ten queries you want answered. Start with your main problem so you can bring it up right away. Then list other concerns that you want to discuss. Make a copy of all your questions to review and leave with your doctor.

self-care Head-to-toe maintenance, including good oral care, appropriate screening tests, knowing your medical rights, and understanding the health-care system.

vital signs Measurements of physiological functioning—specifically temperature, blood pressure, pulse rate, and respiration rate.

gum disease Infection of the gums and bones that hold teeth in place.

plaque A sticky film of bacteria that forms on teeth.

gingivitis Inflammation of the gums.

periodontitis Severe gum disease in which the tooth root becomes infected.

_____ Make a list of all medications you take, including over-the-counter drugs, vitamins, and herbal supplements.

_____ Write down any symptoms or pain you are experiencing.

_____ If you are visiting a new health-care provider, download and bring any past medical records, or test results you have. You will need the names and contact information of your past health-care providers.

_____ Sum up your medical and surgical history. You can give it to the health-care provider or use it to fill out a standardized form.

_____ Provide the names and contact information of other doctors you've seen recently.

_____ Be sure you can describe what your symptoms feel like, when they started, and what makes them better.

_____ Think about bringing a support person who can act as your advocate. Choose someone who knows you and who has your best interests in mind.

_____ If English is not your first language or if you are hearing impaired, you may need an interpreter. Ask the office staff whether they can find one who is experienced in medical terms.

_____ Be sure to bring your health insurance card.

At Your Appointment

- Provide a complete health history, including

  _____ Illnesses and injuries

  _____ Hospitalizations

  _____ Surgical procedures

  _____ Drugs (ones you take now or have taken in the past)

  _____ Allergies, including bad reactions to drugs and foods

  _____ Immunizations

- Personal information, including

  _____ Exercise habits, diet, and alcohol use.

  _____ Relevant factors such as stress at work or, getting married, or moving

  _____ Harmful health behaviors such as smoking and drug use.

  _____ Family history of disease (include aunts, uncles, cousins, and grandparents as well as parents, brothers and sisters, and children).

_____ When a staff member checks your height, weight, blood pressure, and pulse, ask for the readings.

_____ Remember that you have a right to ask questions of anyone who is involved in your health care.

The Physical Examination Typically, your doctor will begin an exam by inspecting your body for any unusual marks or growths. Next, he or she may palpate your abdomen and other parts of your body to assess the consistency, location, size, tenderness, and texture of individual organs. Your doctor will use a stethoscope to listen to your heart and lungs as you take deep breaths. By using a technique known as _percussion_—tapping around the body as if it were a drum—your doctor checks for fluid in areas where it should not be, as well as locates the borders, consistency, and size of organs. Here are some other important points about a physical examination:

- Your health-care provider should make your physical examination as comfortable as possible. Speak up if something bothers or frightens you. Be clear about your modesty needs.

- A health-care professional (such as a nurse or nursing assistant) may remain throughout the exam. Let your doctor know if you want a friend or family member in the room.

- If you do not see your health-care providers wash their hands, you might ask, "Have you washed your hands?" Hand washing is the most important way your health-care provider can prevent the spread of infections.

Talking with Your Health-Care Provider

With the clues obtained during the _history_ and _physical examination_, a health-care provider can formulate a differential diagnosis—that is, a list of potential causes of the symptoms. Specific diagnostic tests generally confirm the cause or reveal other, previously unsuspected causes. When you are talking with your health-care provider, keep these points in mind:

- **If you have questions, ask them.** If the health-care provider asks you questions, answer them as best you can. Be honest.

- **Make sure you understand everything your health-care provider says.** Ask for simple, clear explanations. Take careful notes. If you have a friend or relative with you, ask that person to take notes so that you can listen more closely to what the health-care provider says.

- **If you are given a diagnosis and need further care, ask about the different treatments that are available.** You may want to ask the following questions:

  ____ What might have caused this condition?

  ____ What are the treatment choices?

  ____ What are the benefits and risks of each treatment?

  ____ How might the treatment affect my life?

  ____ Why is it important that I follow a certain treatment plan?

  ____ What might happen if I do not get treated?

- If you need a test, procedure, or surgery, the following are good questions to ask:

  ____ Why do I need it?

  ____ What does it involve? What do I need to do to get ready?

  ____ What should I expect? What are the side effects?

  ____ How will I find out the results?

  ____ How long will it take to recover?

- **If a medication is prescribed, make sure you find out the following:**

  ____ The brand and generic (common) names.

  ____ Instructions for taking the drug.

  ____ When you should take it and whether you should take it with food or on an empty stomach.

  ____ Whether you should avoid alcohol.

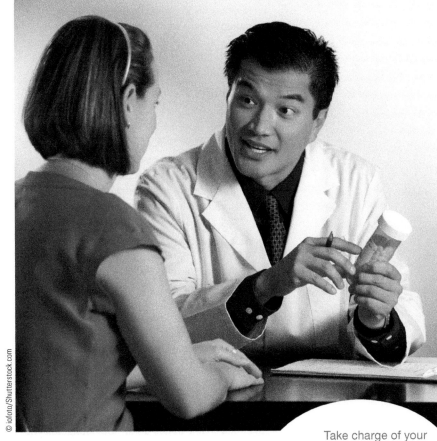

© iofoto/Shutterstock.com

____ How much you should take.

____ For how long you should take it.

____ Any side effects that may occur and what you should do about them. (See Health on a Budget.)

Take charge of your health by educating yourself and asking your doctor questions about your health and treatments.

HEALTH ON A BUDGET

Getting Your Money's Worth from the Health-Care System

The value of medical care depends not just on health-care professionals but also on you:

- **If you receive a diagnosis,** make sure you understand what may be wrong with you, as well as what medications you must take and why.

- **When your doctor writes a prescription for you,** make sure you can read it and know why and how you are to take the medication.

- **If your doctor recommends a screening test, ask**

  - **Am I at higher risk than the average person, and if so, why?**

- **How often does the test give false alarms?** How often does it provide falsely reassuring results?

- **Are any other tests just as good?**

- **If the test results are positive, are treatments available? What impact will they have on my life?**

- **If you must undergo surgery** and you can choose a hospital, select one at which many patients have had the procedure or surgery you need.

- **Ask about a "question hour."** Many health facilities aside a specific time of day for patients with call-in questions. Find out if your college health center offers this service. Does a nurse or physician's assistant field all calls? Can you get specific advice?

- **Go online.** Many medical offices answer queries by e-mail. Ask your doctor or physician's assistant if you can e-mail follow-up questions or progress reports on how you're feeling.

- **Interrupt the interrupter.** If you're having difficulty explaining what's wrong, say so. If your doctor tries to put words in your mouth, say, "Please just listen so I can tell you the whole story without getting sidetracked."

- **Ask for access to your medical record.** With the advent of electronic records, more health-care institutions are using secure Internet portals to offer patients online access to test results, medication lists, and other parts of their records. Primary care providers report some reservations, but patients express considerable enthusiasm and few fears.

At the end of your appointment, repeat what you have learned to the health-care provider. This recap will give your health-care provider a chance to correct any misunderstandings. If you need more time to talk about something, tell your health-care provider or see if you can schedule another appointment to continue your talk.

After Your Visit

At college health centers, clinics, and some health-care organizations, consumers may be assigned to a primary physician or restricted to certain doctors. Even if your choices are limited, don't suspend your critical judgment. If your assigned physician does not listen to your concerns or is not providing adequate care, you can—and should—request another physician. Your rapport with your primary physician and the feelings of mutual trust and respect that develop between you can have as much of an impact on your well-being as your doctor's technical expertise.

One key to making the health-care system work for you lies in choosing a good physician. After seeing your primary care physician, ask yourself the following questions to evaluate the quality of care you are getting.

- Did your physician take a comprehensive history? Was the physical examination thorough?

- Did your physician explain what he or she was doing during the exam?

- Did he or she spend enough time with you?

- Did you feel free to ask questions? Did your physician give you straight answers? Did he or she reassure you when you were worried?

- Does your physician seem willing to admit that he or she doesn't know the answers to some questions?

- Does your physician hesitate to refer you to a specialist even when you have a complex problem that warrants such care?

Look back at your answers. If they make you feel uneasy, have a talk with your physician. Or find a physician or a health plan that provides better service.

- If you question the diagnosis or recommended treatment, seek a second opinion about your problem and its treatment from another health-care provider.

✓ **check-in** Do you have a good, ongoing relationship with a primary care physician?

Diagnostic Tests If you are a woman, your physician will provide counseling on birth control and, if indicated, preconception care. Your doctor should also screen for intimate partner violence (discussed in Chapter 14) and, if you are at risk, for sexually transmitted infections.[12]

Besides the diagnostic tests just listed, the physician may order some laboratory and other tests, including the following:

- **Chest X-ray:** A chest X-ray can reveal abnormalities of the heart and lungs; if you're a smoker, the physician may insist on one.

- **Urinalysis:** Your urine may be analyzed by a medical laboratory. If sugar (glucose) is found in your urine, your physician may order a separate blood test to check for diabetes. The presence of blood cells may indicate infection of the bladder or kidneys. Abnormal amounts of albumin (protein) in the urine may also suggest kidney disease.

- **Blood tests:** A baseline blood test, an important part of your health record, may include analyses of your lipids, or blood fats, including cholesterol and triglycerides; glucose; kidney and liver function; and minerals such as potassium and calcium. An excess of white blood cells most often indicates an infection; a deficiency of red blood cells may indicate anemia. High levels of glucose can indicate diabetes, and high levels of uric acid may point to gout or kidney stones.

Screening Tests In recent years, the medical profession has changed its recommendations for many tests used to screen for or detect disease at early stages.

Here are the current recommendations for some of the most common screening tests:

- **Low back pain:** No imaging for low back pain within the first six weeks, unless there may be serious underlying conditions. Imaging of the lower spine before six weeks does not improve outcomes but does increase costs.

- **Osteoporosis screening:** No dual-energy X-ray absorptiometry (DEXA) screening for osteoporosis in women younger than 65 or men younger than 70 if they have no risk factors. DEXA is not cost-effective in younger, low-risk patients but is cost effective in older patients.[13]

- **Cardiac screening:** No annual electrocardiograms (EKGs), echocardiograms, or any other cardiac screening for low-risk patients without symptoms. False-positive tests are likely to lead to harm through unnecessary invasive procedures, overtreatment, and misdiagnosis.[14]

- **Mammography:** Breast cancer screening with mammography may be considered in women 40 to 49 years of age, based on patients' values and on potential benefits and harms. Mammography is recommended biennially in women 50 to 74 years of age.

- **Pap testing:** Pap smears are not recommended for women younger than 21. In teenage girls, most abnormalities regress (clear up) spontaneously; therefore, Pap smears for this age group can lead to unnecessary anxiety, additional testing, and cost. The American College of Obstetricians and Gynecologists recommends Pap testing every three years for women 21 to 65 years of age, with the option of co-testing for human papillomavirus (HPV) every five years for women ages 30 to 65.[15]

- **Pelvic exams:** Although pelvic exams have traditionally been performed to screen for sexually transmitted infections (STIs) and gynecologic cancers and to evaluate women before prescribing hormonal contraceptives, there is no scientific justification for such testing on a routine basis.[16] Some physicians continue to perform routine pelvic examinations for several reasons, including standard medical practice, patient reassurance, and identification of uterine and ovarian conditions.[17]

During a pelvic examination, a woman lies on her back, with her heels in stirrups at the end of the examining table and her legs spread out to the sides. The physician inspects the labia, clitoris, and vaginal opening. Using two gloved, lubricated fingers, the physician will check for abnormalities in the vagina, uterus, fallopian tubes, and ovaries. Many physicians will also perform a rectal or rectovaginal (one finger in the rectum and one in the vagina) examination. A nurse or other health-care worker should be present throughout the exam.

The *speculum* is a medical instrument that spreads the walls of the vagina so that the inside can be seen. As discussed in Chapter 11, doctors are using HPV tests as well as the conventional **Pap smear** to screen for cervical cancer.

✓**check-in** Which screening or diagnostic tests have you had?

Preventing Medical Errors

More people die from medical errors than from motor vehicle accidents, breast cancer, or AIDS. Medical errors occur when a planned part of medical care doesn't work properly or when the wrong plan was used in the first place. These errors can happen anywhere in the health-care system, from doctors' offices to pharmacies to hospitals to patients' homes. They may involve medications, diagnoses, tests, lab equipment, surgery, or infection. They are most likely to occur when doctors and patients have problems communicating.

Your best defense against medical errors is information. Your questions about your treatments can keep you safe and ensure that you get high-quality health care.

Avoiding Medication Mistakes

Whenever you get a prescription, be sure to learn as much as possible about it:

- Know the name of the drug, what it is supposed to do, and how and when to take it and for how long.

- Are there foods, drinks, other medications, or activities you should avoid while taking the medication?

- Ask if the drug causes any side effects and what you should do if any occur.

- Inform your doctor if you take popular herbal supplements such as gingko biloba and common over-the-counter drugs such as aspirin, which can interact with many prescription drugs to cause serious problems, such as excessive bleeding.

- If possible, always go to the same pharmacy, which can keep track of your prescriptions

Pap smear A test in which cells removed from the cervix are examined under a microscope for signs of cancer; also called a Pap test.

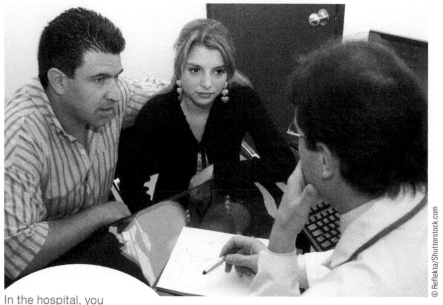
In the hospital, you can discuss patients' rights and other individual concerns with a patient advocate.

and identify any potentially harmful interactions.

- Don't use a kitchen spoon to dispense liquid medications. Household teaspoons can hold between 3 and 7 milliliters; a prescription "teaspoon" means 5 milliliters. Either measure the dose in the cup or dropper that came with the medicine or ask the pharmacist for a measuring device.

- Don't crush or chew a medicine without checking with your doctor or pharmacist first. Some medications are designed for gradual release rather than all at once and could be harmful if absorbed too quickly.

- Keep a record of all your medications, listing both their brand and generic (chemical) names and the reason you are taking them. Update the list regularly.

- Always turn on the lights when you take your medication. Familiarize yourself with the size, and shape of the imprint on each tablet or capsule so you can recognize each pill. If a refill looks different, check with your pharmacist or doctor before taking it.

- Never take someone else's medications. They could interact with your medications, or the dose may be different.

- Always check labels for warnings on interactions with alcohol and instructions on whether to take before, with, or after meals.

- Don't take medicine with grapefruit juice, which can interact with more than 200 medications, including cholesterol-lowering statins, sleeping pills, and antianxiety agents.

informed consent Permission (to undergo or receive a medical procedure or treatment) given voluntarily, with full knowledge and understanding of the procedure or treatment and its possible consequences.

- Don't leave medicines in a car for prolonged periods. Temperature extremes, along with moisture, light, and oxygen, can affect the potency of many medications.

√**check-in** Do you take any prescription medications on a regular basis? If so, what precautions are you using to avoid any mistakes or complications?

Your Medical Rights

As a consumer, you have basic rights that help ensure that you know about any potential dangers, receive competent diagnosis and treatment, and retain control and dignity in your interactions with health-care professionals. Many hospitals publish a Patient's Bill of Rights, including your rights to know whether a procedure is experimental; to refuse to undergo a specific treatment; to designate someone else to make decisions about your care if and when you cannot; and to leave the hospital, even against your physician's advice.

Your Right to Be Treated with Respect and Dignity

Make clear how you would like health-care providers to address you—for example, as "Mr." or "Ms." or by your first name or whatever you wish. If you feel that health-care professionals are being condescending or inconsiderate, say so—in the same tone and manner that you would like others to use with you. If you're hospitalized, find out if there's a patient advocate or representative at your hospital. These individuals can help you communicate with physicians, make any special arrangements, and get answers to questions or complaints.

Your Right to Information

By law, a patient must give consent for hospitalization, surgery, and other major treatments. **Informed consent** is a right, not a privilege. Use this right to its fullest. Ask questions. Seek other opinions. Make sure that your expectations are realistic and that you understand the potential risks, as well as the possible benefits, of a prospective treatment.

Your Right to Privacy and Access to Medical Records

Your medical records are your property. You have the right to see them whenever you choose and to limit who else can see them. Federal standards protecting the privacy of patients' medical information guarantee patients access to their medical records, give them more control over how personal health information is disclosed, and limit the ways that health plans, pharmacies, and hospitals can use personal medical information.

Key provisions include these:

- **Access to medical records:** As a patient, you should be able to see and obtain copies of your medical records and request corrections if there are errors. Health-care providers must provide these within 30 days; they may charge for the cost of copying and mailing records.

- **Notice of privacy practices:** Your providers must inform you of how they use personal medical information. Doctors, nurses, and other providers may not disclose information for purposes not related to your health care.

- **Prohibition on marketing:** Pharmacies, health plans, and others must obtain specific authorization before disclosing patient information for marketing.

- **Confidentiality:** Patients can request that doctors take reasonable steps to ensure confidential communications, such as calling a cell phone rather than home or office number.

A growing concern involves data breaches of protected health information. Since 2010, breaches involving more than 29 million health records have been reported, most accessed through laptops, portable devices, e-mail, and electronic health records.[18] Health professionals worry that patients concerned about their information being stolen or leaked may withhold certain details from their providers, which could "seriously undermine efforts to improve health.[19]"

✓**check-in** Think back on your health-care experiences. Were your rights as a patient respected? If not, what might you do differently in the future to ensure that they are?

Your Right to Quality Health Care

The essence of a *malpractice* suit is the claim that the physician failed to meet the standard of quality care required of a reasonably skilled and careful medical doctor. Although physicians don't have to guarantee good results to their patients and aren't held liable for unavoidable errors, they are required to use the same care as other physicians in the same specialty would use under similar circumstances. To protect themselves financially, physicians, particularly those in surgical specialties who are most likely to be sued, pay tens of thousands of dollars a year in malpractice insurance premiums. Some of this cost is passed on to patients.

Most lawsuits are based on negligence and assert that a physician failed to render diagnosis and treatment with appropriate professional knowledge and skill. Other cases are brought for failure to provide information, obtain consent, or respect a patient's confidentiality. However, analysis of malpractice cases has shown that, in 70 to 80 percent of cases, a doctor's attitude and inability to communicate effectively—by devaluing patients' views, delivering information poorly, failing to understand patients' perspectives, or displaying an air of superiority—also played a role.

Elective Treatments

As medical technology has developed new options, millions of Americans are trying elective procedures and products that are not medically necessary but that promise to enhance health or appearance. Some are new alternatives for correcting common problems, such as poor vision, while others offer the promise of looking younger or more attractive. In some cases, the procedures are scams or hoaxes.

Vision Surgery

Millions of people in the United States have undergone laser surgery to correct their vision. In LASIK (laser-assisted in situ keratomileusis), the most common technique, a surgeon uses a razorlike instrument to lift a flap of the cornea—the clear, stiff outer layer over the colored iris—and then reshapes the exposed area using a laser. The surgery alters the way the eye focuses light, correcting nearsightedness, farsightedness, and some astigmatism.

Laser surgery cannot make an aging eye's lens flexible again to improve close-up vision in middle-aged adults. Numbing eye drops make the treatment painless, although burning and scratchiness are normal for a couple hours afterward. An estimated 10 to 30 percent of patients require additional surgery, or "enhancements," to sharpen their vision. Other complications include glare, sensitivity to bright lights, and poor night vision.

Prices for LASIK have fallen, but ophthalmologists have warned consumers that some laser surgery centers have cut corners to cut prices, such as hiring inexperienced surgeons or using optometrists or technicians rather than MDs for pre- and postoperative checkups. A qualified eye surgeon should have a record of 100 or more LASIK procedures and at least 25 enhancements—but no more than 20 percent of his or her patients should require enhancements. Ideally, the surgeon should also be the one doing your pre- and postprocedure checks.

When Is LASIK Not for You?
You are probably NOT a good candidate for refractive surgery if

- **You are not a risk taker.** Certain complications are unavoidable in a percentage of patients, and there are no long-term data available for current procedures.

- **Cost is an issue.** Most medical insurance will not pay for refractive surgery. Although the cost is coming down, it is still significant.

- **You required a change in your contact lens or glasses prescription in the past year.** This is called refractive instability. Patients who are in their early 20s or younger, whose hormones are fluctuating due to disease such as diabetes, who are pregnant or breast-feeding, or who are taking medications that may cause fluctuations in vision are more likely to have refractive instability and should discuss the possible additional risks with their doctor.

- **You have a disease or are on medications that may affect wound healing.** Certain conditions, such as autoimmune diseases and diabetes, and some medications may prevent proper healing after a refractive procedure.

- **You actively participate in contact sports.** If you participate in boxing, wrestling, martial arts, or other activities in which blows to the face and eyes are a normal occurrence, LASIK is probably not right for you.

- **You are under 18.** Currently, no lasers are approved for LASIK on persons under the age of 18.

- **It will jeopardize your career.** Some jobs, including certain military assignments, prohibit refractive procedures.

Cosmetic Surgery

More than 15.6 million cosmetic treatments are performed every year.[20] About one-quarter of those undergoing plastic surgery are between the ages of 18 and 29.

✓**check-in** Have you undergone an elective procedure? If so, how did you make the decision to do it?

These are the most common cosmetic procedures:

- Injections of synthetic soft tissue fillers and botulinum toxin (Botox®), chemical peels, and laser hair removal account for more than 90 percent of cosmetic procedures. Health insurance rarely covers cosmetic procedures, which can run into the tens of thousands of dollars.

- Liposuction, the removal of fatty tissue by means of a vacuum device, can be performed on many areas of the body, from sagging jowls to midsection "love handles" or "muffin tops." The doctor first flushes the target area with a solution of lidocaine (a local anesthetic with a numbing effect), saline, and epinephrine (a drug that reduces bleeding by constricting blood vessels). Inserting a hollow, wandlike cannula under the skin, the doctor breaks up fatty deposits and suctions them, along with other body fluids, with a vacuum device.

  Risks and complications include infection, numbness, bleeding, discoloration, lumpiness, and, if too much tissue is removed without proper caution, potentially fatal complications. The American Society of Plastic Surgeons estimates that the mortality rate is 1 in 5,000 liposuction patients.

- Breast augmentation includes various approaches to increase the size or change the shape and texture of a woman's breasts. The Institute of Medicine, after reviewing all available evidence, has reported that there appears to be no link between breast implants and autoimmune disease, connective tissue disorders, or cancer. Patients still face possible complications, including rupture, scarring, infection, and leaking or hardening of their implants.[21] Women with implants also may run the risk of being diagnosed with more advanced breast cancer and of dying of the disease because implants can make early diagnosis more difficult.[22]

Buttock augmentation with fat grafting, implants, and lifts is becoming increasingly popular. The number of men having plastic surgery continues to rise. The top male-focused procedures are pectoral (chest) implants and male breast reduction.[23]

Body Art Perils

As discussed in Chapter 16, "body art" such as piercings and tattoos presents unique dangers, including adverse reactions to tattoo inks and bacterial and viral infections.[24] About one in five American adults has a tattoo; 14 percent say they regret having gotten tattoos. Dermatologists report about 100,000 tattoo removals a year; removal is a painful and painstaking process that typically requires 6 to 10 treatments, with a few weeks of healing required between each.[25]

Temporary tattoos that use henna and other dyes, meant to last several days to several weeks, also present risks. According to the FDA adverse-effects watch list, recipients of henna tattoos have reported redness, blistering, raised red weeping lesions, loss of pigmentation, increased sun sensitivity, and permanent scarring. Dyes using so-called black henna present greater risks because many contain a coal-tar hair dye called p-phenylenediamine (PPD), which is banned by law from cosmetics intended to be applied to the skin. Reactions to this compound may be severe enough to require emergency treatment.[26]

✓**check-in** Do you have a tattoo or piercing? If so, what precautions were taken to prevent complications? Did you experience any adverse effects?

Health Hoaxes and Medical Quackery

Every year millions of Americans search for medical miracles that never happen. In all, they spend more than $10 billion on medical **quackery**, unproven health products and services. Those who lose only money are the lucky ones. Many also waste precious time, during which their conditions worsen. Some suffer needless pain, along with crushed expectations.

Promoters of fraudulent health products often make claims and use particular practices to trick consumers into buying their products. Be suspicious when you see the following:

- Claims that a product is a "scientific break-through," "miraculous cure," "secret ingredient," or "ancient remedy."
- Claims that the product is an effective cure for a wide range of ailments. No product can cure multiple conditions or diseases.
- Claims that use impressive-sounding medical terms. They're often covering up a lack of good science.
- Personalized genetic cancer tests, which have not proven useful in guiding cancer treatment.
- Undocumented case histories of people who've had amazing results. It's too easy to make them up. And even if true, they can't be generalized to the entire population. Anecdotes are not a substitute for valid science.
- Claims that the product is available from only one source and payment is required in advance.
- Claims of a "money-back" guarantee.
- Websites that fail to list the company's name, physical address, phone number, or other contact information.

To keep from risking your life on false hope, follow these guidelines:

- Arm yourself with up-to-date information about your condition or disease from appropriate organizations, such as the American Cancer Society or the Arthritis Foundation, which keep track of unproven and ineffective methods of treatment.
- Ask for a written explanation of what a treatment does and why it works, evidence supporting all claims (not just testimonials), and published reports of the studies, including specifics on numbers treated, doses, and side effects. Be skeptical of self-styled "holistic practitioners," treatments supported by crusading groups, and endorsements from self-proclaimed experts or authorities.
- Don't part with your money quickly. Insurance companies won't reimburse for unproven therapies.
- Don't discontinue your current treatment without your physician's approval. Many physicians encourage supportive therapies—such as relaxation exercises, meditation, or visualization—as a supplement to standard treatments.

✓**check-in** Have you ever been taken in by a health "con"? Do you know anyone who has?

Nontraditional Health Care

Complementary and alternative medicine (CAM) refers to various medical and health-care systems, practices, and products that are not

quackery Medical fakery; unproven practices claiming to cure diseases or solve health problems.

complementary and alternative medicine (CAM) A term applied to all health-care approaches, practices, and treatments not widely taught in medical schools, not generally used in hospitals, and not usually reimbursed by medical insurance companies.

considered part of conventional medicine because there is not yet sufficient proof of their safety and effectiveness. CAM's varied healing philosophies, approaches, and therapies include preventive techniques designed to delay or prevent serious health problems before they start and **holistic** methods that focus on the whole person and the physical, mental, emotional, and spiritual aspects of well-being. Some approaches are based on the same physiological principles as traditional Western methods; others, such as acupuncture, are based on different healing systems.

Many medical schools now include training in CAM in their curricula. **Integrative medicine**, which combines selected elements of both conventional and alternative medicine in a comprehensive approach to diagnosis and treatment, has gained greater acceptance within the medical community.

✓ **check-in** Have you ever used any CAM treatments? If so, which ones?

According to a recent review of CAM trends since 2002, about a third of Americans age 18 and older report using a complementary health approach in the previous year, usually to complement conventional care rather than as a replacement. (See Table 17.4 for the most popular approaches.)

Here is a profile of what we know about CAM users (see Student Snapshot):

• Women use CAM more often than men.

holistic An approach to medicine that takes into account body, mind, emotions, and spirit.

integrative medicine An approach that combines traditional medicine with alternative/complementary therapies.

acupuncture A Chinese medical practice of puncturing the body with needles inserted at specific points to relieve pain or cure disease.

Ayurveda A traditional Indian medical treatment involving meditation, exercise, herbal medications, and nutrition.

TABLE 17.4 The Most Popular CAM Approaches

- Nonvitamin, nonmineral dietary supplements, used by about 18 percent of adults
- Deep-breathing exercises, either independently or as part of other approaches, used by 11 percent of adults
- Yoga, t'ai chi, and qui gong, used by 10 percent of adults
- Chiropractic and osteopathic manipulation, used by 8 percent of adults
- Meditation, also used by 8 percent of adults

Smaller percentages of Americans report the use of

- Homeopathic treatment
- Acupuncture
- Naturopathy
- Ayurveda
- Biofeedback
- Guide imagery hypnosis
- Energy healing

Source: Clarke T. C., et al. *Trends in the Use of Complementary Health Approaches among Adults.* National Health Statistics Report, Number 79 (February 10, 2015).

• Young adults ages 18 to 44 are more likely to use CAM than older Americans.

• White adults use CAM more often than Hispanic or black men and women.

• Adults with a college degree or higher use CAM more often than those with less education.[27]

Types of CAM

The National Center for Complementary and Alternative Medicine (NCCAM) has classified CAM therapies into five categories (Figure 17.2):

• Alternative medical systems
• Mind–body medicine
• Biologically based therapies
• Manipulative and body-based methods
• Energy therapies

Alternative Medical Systems Systems of theory and practice other than traditional Western medicine are included in this group. They include acupuncture, Eastern medicine, t'ai chi, external and internal qi, Ayurvedic medicine, naturopathy, and unconventional Western systems, such as homeopathy and orthomolecular medicine. (See Health Now.)

Acupuncture is an ancient Chinese form of medicine, based on the philosophy that a cycle of energy circulating through the body controls health. Pain and disease are the result of a disturbance in the energy flow, which can be corrected by inserting long, thin needles at specific points along longitudinal lines, or *meridians*, throughout the body. Each point controls a different corresponding part of the body. Once inserted, the needles are rotated gently back and forth or charged with a small electric current for a short time. Western scientists aren't sure exactly how acupuncture works but some believe that the needles alter the functioning of the nervous system.

Since the 1990s, studies have looked at acupuncture's effect on specific health conditions and how it affects the brain and nervous system, the neurological properties of meridians and acupuncture points, and methods for improving the quality of acupuncture research.

High-quality, randomized, controlled trials have shown that various forms of acupuncture, including so-called sham acupuncture during which no needles actually penetrate the skin, are equally effective for low-back pain—and more beneficial than standard care. However, even sham acupuncture can produce adverse effects, including infection and trauma.

Recent studies have found that acupuncture

• Helps alleviate nausea in cancer patients undergoing chemotherapy

	2002%	2007%	2012%
All forms	32.3	35.5	33.2
Whites	34.4	40.2	37.9
Blacks	22.9	22.9	19.3
Hispanics	26.4	21.6	22
Ages 18–44	33	34.2	32.2
Ages 45–64	36.5	40.1	36.8
65 and over	22.7	31.1	29.4

Source: Clarke T. C., et al. *Trends in the Use of Complementary Health Approaches among Adults.* National Health Statistics Report, Number 79 (February 10, 2015).

- Relieves pain and improves function for some people with osteoarthritis of the knee
- Helps in treating chronic lower back pain
- May or may not be of value for many other conditions, including irritable bowel syndrome and some neurologic disorders

Considered alternative in this country, **Ayurveda** is a traditional form of medical treatment in India, where it has evolved over thousands of years. Its basic premise is that illness stems from incorrect mental attitudes, diet, and posture. Practitioners use a discipline of exercise, meditation, herbal medication, and proper nutrition to cope with such stress-induced conditions as hypertension, the desire to smoke, and obesity.

Homeopathy is based on three fundamental principles: like cures like; treatment must always be individualized; and less is more—the idea that increasing dilution (and lowering the dosage) can increase efficacy. By administering doses of animal, vegetable, or mineral substances to a large number of healthy people to see if they all develop the same symptoms, homeopaths determine which substances may be given, in small quantities, to alleviate the symptoms. Some of these substances are the same as those used in conventional medicine: nitroglycerin for certain heart conditions, for example, although the dose is minuscule.

Naturopathy emphasizes natural remedies, such as sun, water, heat, and air, as the best treatments for disease. Therapies might include dietary changes (such as more vegetables and no salt or stimulants), steam baths, and exercise. Some naturopathic physicians (who are not MDs) work closely with medical doctors in helping patients.

Mind–Body Medicine Mind–body medicine uses techniques designed to enhance the mind's capacity to affect bodily function and symptoms. Some techniques that were considered alternative in the past have become mainstream (for example, patient support groups and cognitive-behavioral therapy). Other mind–body approaches are still considered CAM, including meditation, prayer (see Chapter 4), yoga, t'ai chi, visual imagery, mental healing, and therapies that use creative outlets such as art, music, or dance. About 30 percent of Americans report using relaxation techniques and imagery, biofeedback, and hypnosis; 50 percent use prayer.

homeopathy A system of medical practice that treats a disease by administering dosages of substances that would in healthy persons produce symptoms similar to those of the disease.

naturopathy An alternative system of treatment of disease that emphasizes the use of natural remedies such as sun, water, heat, and air. Therapies may include dietary changes, steam baths, and exercise.

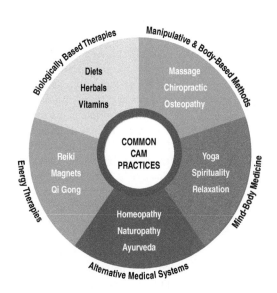

FIGURE 17.2 The Five Categories of CAM

Source: NCCAM, http://nccam.nih.gov.

HEALTH NOW!

Is a CAM Therapy Right for You?

You should never decide on any treatment—traditional or CAM—without fully evaluating it. Here are some key questions to ask:

- **Is it safe?** Be particularly wary of unregulated products.

- **Is it effective?** Check the website of the National Center for CAM: http://nccam.nih.gov.

- **Will it interact with other medicines or conventional treatments?** Many widely used alternative remedies can interact with prescription medications in dangerous ways.

- **Is the practitioner qualified?** Find out if your state licenses practitioners who provide acupuncture, chiropractic services, naturopathy, herbal medicine, homeopathy, and other treatments.

- **What has been the experience of others?** Talk to people who have used CAM for a similar problem, both recently and in the past.

- **Can you talk openly and easily with the practitioner?** You should feel comfortable asking questions and confident in the answers you receive. And the practitioner's office should put you at ease.

- **What are the costs?** Many CAM services are not covered by HMOs or health insurers.

Answer these questions in your online journal.

herbal medicine An ancient form of medical treatment using substances derived from trees, flowers, ferns, seaweeds, and lichens to treat disease.

chiropractic A method of treating disease, primarily through manipulating the bones and joints to restore normal nerve function.

The physical and emotional risks of using mind–body interventions are minimal. Although we need much more research on how these approaches work and when to apply them most effectively, there is considerable evidence that mind–body interventions have positive effects on psychological functioning and quality of life and may be particularly helpful for patients coping with chronic illnesses.

Mind–body approaches definitely have won some acceptance in modern medical care. Techniques such as hypnosis have proved helpful in reducing discomfort and complications during and after various surgical procedures and in relieving hot flashes in breast cancer survivors. With *biofeedback*, people can learn to control usually involuntary functions, such as circulation to the hands and feet, tension in the jaws, and heartbeat rates. Biofeedback has been used to treat dozens of ailments, including asthma, epilepsy, pain, and Raynaud's disease (a condition in which the fingers become painful and white when exposed to cold) and has produced small reductions in blood pressure.[28] Biofeedback has become accepted as a mainstream therapy, and many health insurers now cover biofeedback treatments.

Creative visualization (also discussed in Chapter 4) helps patients heal, including some diagnosed as terminally ill with cancer. Other patients use visualization to create a clear idea of what they want to achieve, whether the goal is weight loss or relaxation.

Biologically Based Therapies

Biologically based CAM therapies use substances such as herbs, foods, and vitamins. They include **herbal medicine** (botanical medicine or phytotherapy), the use of individual herbs or combinations; special diet therapies, such as macrobiotics, Ornish, Atkins, and high fiber; orthomolecular medicine (use of nutritional and food supplements for preventive or therapeutic purposes); and use of other products (such as shark cartilage) and procedures applied in an unconventional manner.

Dietary supplements include vitamins, minerals, herbs, botanicals, amino acids, and enzymes and are sold as tablets, capsules, softgels, or gelcaps. The most popular is fish oil (discussed in Chapter 6). More people are using probiotics and melatonin, while fewer are taking echinacea, glucosamine, chondroitin, garlic, ginseng, ginkgo biloba, and saw palmetto than in the past.[29]

Unlike drugs, supplements are not intended to treat, diagnose, prevent, or cure diseases. Many contain active ingredients that have strong and potentially unsafe biological effects in the body. This makes them particularly dangerous when used with medications (whether prescription or over-the-counter) or taken in high doses.

Liver injury related to herbal and dietary supplements has more than doubled in the past 10 years.[30]

Echinacea may cause liver damage if taken in combination with anabolic steroids. Several widely used herbs, including ginger, garlic, and ginkgo biloba, are dangerous if taken prior to surgery.

Canadian health authorities have pulled products containing a chemical called BMPEA off store shelves and warned that this amphetamine-like compound can increase blood pressure, heart rate, and body temperature; lead to serious cardiovascular complications (including stroke) at high doses; suppress sleep and appetite; and be addictive. A group of state attorneys have accused major retailers of selling contaminated herbal supplements and called on Congress to provide the FDA with more power to regulate supplements.

Manipulative and Body-Based Methods

CAM therapies based on manipulation and/or movement of the body are divided into three subcategories:

- **Chiropractic medicine:** This treatment method is based on the theory that many human diseases are caused by misalignment of the spine (subluxation). Chiropractors are licensed in all 50 states, but some consider **chiropractic** a mainstream therapy while others view it as a form of CAM. Significant research in the past 10 years has demonstrated its efficacy for acute lower-back pain. NIH is funding research on other potential benefits, including headaches, asthma, middle ear inflammation, menstrual cramps, and arthritis.

  Chiropractors, who emphasize wellness and healing without drugs or surgery, may use X-rays and magnetic resonance imaging (MRI) as well as orthopedic, neurological, and manual examinations in making diagnoses. However, chiropractic treatment consists solely of the manipulation of misaligned discs that may be putting pressure on nerve tissue and affecting other parts of the body. Many HMOs offer chiropractic services, which are the most widely used alternative treatment among managed care patients.

- **Massage therapy and body work:** This category includes osteopathic manipulation, Swedish massage, Alexander technique, reflexology, Pilates, acupressure, and rolfing.

- **Unconventional physical therapies:** This category includes colonics, hydrotherapy, and light and color therapies.

Energy Therapies   Various approaches focus on energy fields believed to exist in and around the body. Some use external energy sources, such as electromagnetic fields. Magnets are marketed to relieve pain, but there is little scientific evidence of their efficacy. Others, such as therapeutic touch, use a therapist's healing energy to repair imbalances in an individual's biofield.

The Health-Care System

As a college student, you may turn to the student health service if one is available on campus. There, a nurse, nurse practitioner, physician's assistant, or medical doctor may evaluate your symptoms and provide basic care. However, you may rely on a primary care physician in your hometown to perform regular checkups or manage a chronic condition such as asthma. If you're injured in an accident, you probably will be treated at the nearest emergency room. If you become seriously ill and require highly specialized care, you may have to go to a university-affiliated medical center to receive state-of-the-art treatment.

Under the Affordable Care Act (ACA) (discussed below), students can usually continue their health-care coverage under their parents' policy until age 26. However, if your parent belongs to an HMO with a local network of providers, you may not be covered for anything outside the plan's service area except for emergency care. A more open plan, like a preferred provider organization, may allow students to see doctors near school, but the costs may be high.

Most colleges offer some type of health insurance plan, with the student health center acting as the primary care provider. Many schools require participation if the student is not covered under any other plan. Check the plan carefully to see what is and is not covered.

✓check-in Does your school offer a health-care plan? If so, have you chosen to enroll in it?

Health-Care Practitioners

Fewer than 10 percent of health-care practitioners are physicians; other types of health professionals are assuming more important roles in delivering primary, or basic, health services. As a consumer, you should be aware of the range

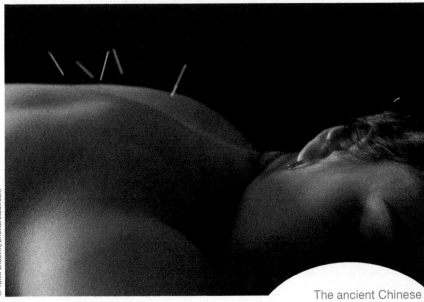

and special skills of the most common types of health-care providers.

Physicians   A medical doctor (MD) trained in American medical schools usually takes at least three years of premedical college courses (with an emphasis on biology, chemistry, and physics) and then completes four (but sometimes three or five) years of medical school. The first two years of medical school are devoted to the study of human anatomy, embryology, pharmacology, and similar basic subjects. During the last two years, students work directly with physicians in hospitals. Medical students who pass a series of national board examinations then enter a one-year internship in a hospital, followed by another two to five years of residency (depending on their specialty), which leads to certification in a particular field, or specialty.

The Health-Care Team   More than 60 types of health practitioners work together in providing medical services. Physician assistants provide a broad range of health-care services under the direction of medical doctors. They may conduct physical exams, diagnose and treat illnesses, order and interpret tests, prescribe medications, advise on preventive health care, and assist in surgery.

Registered nurses (RNs), who may have bachelor's or associate degrees from accredited schools of nursing, may specialize in certain areas, such as intensive care or nurse-midwifery. Nurse practitioners, RNs with advanced training and experience, may run community clinics or provide screening and preventive care at group medical practices.

Physician assistants, also known as PAs, serve on a health-care team under the supervision of

The ancient Chinese practice of acupuncture produces healing through the insertion and manipulation of needles at specific points, or meridians, throughout the body.

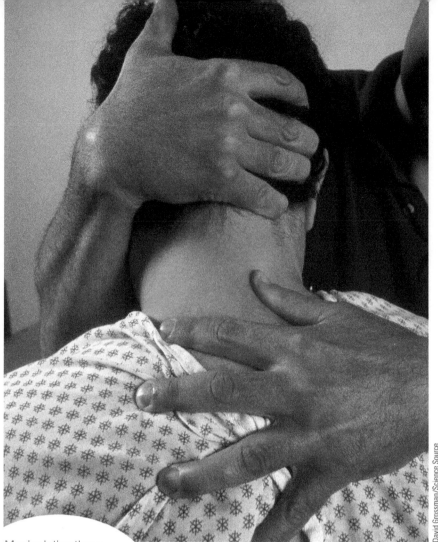

Manipulative therapies are among the most widespread forms of complementary and alternative medicine.

trained, licensed health-care professionals who specialize in problems of the feet.

Dentists Most dental students earn a bachelor's degree and then complete two more years of training in the basic sciences and two years of clinical work before graduating with a degree of DDS or DMD (Doctor of Dental Surgery or Doctor of Medical Dentistry) and taking licensing exams. Dentists may work in general practice or choose a specialty, such as orthodontics (straightening teeth).

Chiropractors Chiropractors hold the degree of Doctor of Chiropractic (DC), which signifies that they have had two years of college-level training, plus four years in a health-care school specializing in chiropractic, described earlier in this chapter.

Health-Care Facilities

As a prospective patient, you can choose from various options: a physician's office, a clinic, an emergency room, or a hospital. Most **primary care**—also referred to as ambulatory or outpatient care—is provided by a physician in an office, an emergency room, or a clinic. *Secondary care* usually is provided by specialists or subspecialists in either an outpatient or inpatient (hospital) setting. *Tertiary care*, available at university-affiliated hospitals and regional referral centers, includes special procedures such as kidney dialysis, open-heart surgery, and organ transplants.

College Health Centers The American College Health Association estimates that 1,500 institutions of higher learning provide direct health services. Student health centers, initially developed by departments of physical education and hygiene, range in size from small dispensaries staffed by nurses to large-scale, multispecialty clinics that provide both inpatient and outpatient care and are fully accredited by The Joint Commission. Some serve only students; others provide services for faculty, staff, and family members.

On some campuses, health educators work with student health centers to provide counseling on such topics as nutrition; tobacco, drug, and alcohol abuse; exercise and fitness; sexuality; and contraception. Some college health centers provide psychological counseling, as well as dental, pharmacy, and optometric services and sports-medicine services for student athletes. Services are paid for by various combinations of prepaid health fees, general university funds, fee-for-service charges, and health-insurance reimbursements.

physicians and surgeons. Formally educated to examine patients, diagnose injuries and illnesses, and provide treatment, they typically need a master's degree from an accredited educational program and a state license.

Licensed practical nurses (LPNs), also called licensed vocational nurses, are graduates of state-approved schools of practical nursing, who work under the supervision of RNs or physicians. Certified nursing assistants (CNAs), nursing aides, and orderlies assist in providing services directly related to the comfort and well-being of hospitalized patients.

Allied health professionals may specialize in a variety of fields. *Clinical psychologists* have graduate degrees and provide a wide range of mental health services but don't prescribe medications—as do *psychiatrists. Optometrists*, trained in special schools of optometry, diagnose visual abnormalities and prescribe lenses or visual aids; however, they don't prescribe drugs, diagnose or treat eye diseases, or perform surgery—functions performed by *ophthalmologists. Podiatrists* are specially

primary care Ambulatory or outpatient care provided by a physician in an office, an emergency room, or a clinic.

David Grossman/Science Source

Outpatient Treatment Centers Increasingly, procedures that once required hospitalization, such as simple surgery, are being performed at outpatient centers, which may be freestanding or affiliated with a medical center. Patients have any necessary tests performed beforehand, undergo surgery or receive treatment, and return home after a few hours to recuperate. Outpatient centers can handle many common surgical procedures, including cataract removal, tonsillectomy, breast biopsy, dilation and curettage (D and C), vasectomy, and cosmetic procedures, such as liposuction.

Freestanding emergency or urgent-care centers (those that are not part of a hospital) claim that they deliver high-quality medical treatment with maximum convenience in minimal time. Rather than go to a crowded hospital emergency room when they slice a finger in the kitchen, patients can go to a freestanding emergency center and receive prompt attention.

Hospitals and Medical Centers Different types of hospitals offer different types of care:

- The most common type of hospital is the *private*, or *community*, *hospital*, which may be run on a profit or a nonprofit basis, generally contains 50 to 400 beds, and provides more personalized care than public hospitals do. The quality of care individual patients receive depends mostly on the physicians themselves.

- *Public hospitals* include city, county, public health service, military, and Veterans Administration hospitals. The quality of patient care depends on the overall quality of the institution.

- Of the more than 6,500 hospitals nationwide, about 300 are major *academic medical centers* or *teaching hospitals*. Affiliated with medical schools, they generally provide the most up-to-date and experienced care because staff physicians must stay current in order to teach their students. These centers, with the best equipment, researchers, and resources, offer high-technology care—at a price. At major teaching hospitals with large graduate training programs for physicians and other health providers, the costs are as much as 45 percent higher than those at nonteaching hospitals.

The Joint Commission reviews all hospitals every three years. Eighty percent of hospitals qualify for Joint Commission accreditation, an important indicator of quality assurance.

Emergency Services Hospital emergency rooms should be used only in a true emergency. Most are overwhelmed, understaffed, and underfinanced—particularly in big cities. Patients usually see a different physician each time; he or she deals with a patient's main complaints but doesn't have time for a full examination. Arranging extensive tests and procedures in an emergency room is difficult, and patients who don't have truly urgent problems may have to wait a long time. Emergency-room fees are higher than those for standard office visits and are not always covered by medical insurance.

Inpatient Care Inpatient hospital care remains the most expensive form of health care. Health-insurance companies and health-care plans (described below) often demand a second opinion or make their own evaluation before approving coverage of an elective, or non-emergency, hospital admission.

Because hospital stays are shorter today than in the past, patients often leave "quicker and sicker"—after a shorter stay and not as far along in their recovery. Nevertheless, the benefits of shorter hospital stays, including reduced risk of infection (discussed in chapter 16) and more rapid resumption of normal life activities, may outweigh the slightly increased risks associated with early discharge.

Home Health Care With hospitals discharging patients sooner, **home health care**—the provision of equipment and services to patients in the home to restore or maintain comfort, function, and health—has become a major industry. Advances in technology have made it possible for treatments once administered only in hospitals—such as kidney dialysis, chemotherapy, and traction—to be performed at home at 10 to 40 percent of the cost of providing these treatments in a hospital.

home health care Provision of medical services and equipment to patients in the home to restore or maintain comfort, function, and health.

- How does the Affordable Care Act affect college students?
- How can you find reliable health-care information?
- What steps can you take to make sure you get quality health care?
- What do you need to know about complementary and alternative medicine?

THE POWER OF NOW!
Taking Charge of Your Health

You can do more to safeguard and enhance your well-being than any health-care provider. Here are some recommendations to keep in mind. Check the ones you have used or plan to use in the future.

_____ Trust your instincts. You know your body better than anyone else. If something is bothering you, it deserves medical attention. Don't let your health-care provider—or your health plan administrator—dismiss it without a thorough evaluation.

_____ Do your homework. Go to the library or online and find authoritative articles that describe what you're experiencing. The more you know about possible causes of your symptoms, the more likely you are to be taken seriously.

_____ Find a good primary care physician who listens carefully and responds to your concerns. Look for a family doctor or general internist who takes a careful history, performs a thorough exam, and listens and responds to your concerns.

_____ See your doctor regularly. If you're in your 20s or 30s, you may not need an annual exam, but it's important to get checkups at least every two or three years so you and your doctor can get to know each other and develop a trusting, mutually respectful relationship.

_____ Get a second opinion. If you are uncertain of whether to undergo treatment or which therapy is best, see another physician and listen carefully for any doubts or hesitation about what you're considering.

_____ Seek support. Patient support and advocacy groups can offer emotional support, information on many common problems, and referral to knowledgeable physicians.

_____ If your doctor cannot or will not respond to your concerns, get another one. Regardless of your health coverage, you have the right to replace a physician who is not meeting your health-care needs.

_____ Speak up. If you don't understand, ask. If you feel that you're not being taken seriously or being treated with respect, say so. Sometimes the only difference between being a patient or becoming a victim is making sure your needs and rights are not forgotten or overlooked.

_____ Bring your own advocate. If you become intimidated or anxious talking to physicians, ask a friend to accompany you, to ask questions on your behalf, and to take notes.

What's Online

Are You a Savvy Health-Care Consumer?

1. You want a second opinion, but your doctor dismisses your request for other physicians' names as unnecessary. What do you do?
   a. Assume that he or she is right and you would merely be wasting time.
   b. Suspect that your physician has something to hide and immediately switch doctors.
   c. Contact your health plan and request a second opinion.

2. As soon as you enter your doctor's office, you get tongue-tied. When you try to find the words to describe what's wrong, your physician keeps interrupting. When giving advice, your doctor uses such technical language that you can't understand what it means. What do you do?
   a. Prepare better for your next appointment.
   b. Pretend that you understand what your doctor is talking about.
   c. Decide you'd be better off with someone who specializes in complementary/alternative therapies and seems less intimidating.

3. You feel like you're running on empty, tired all the time, worn to the bone. A friend suggests some herbal supplements that promise to boost energy and restore vitality. What do you do?
   a. Immediately start taking them.
   b. Say that you think herbs are for cooking.
   c. Find out as much as you can about the herbal compounds and ask your doctor if they're safe and effective.

4. Your hometown physician's office won't give you a copy of your medical records to take with you to college. What do you do?
   a. Hope you won't need them and head off without your records.
   b. Threaten to sue.
   c. Politely ask the office administrator to tell you the particular law or statute that bars you from your records.

5. Your doctor has been treating you for an infection for three weeks, and you don't seem to be getting any better. What do you do?
   a. Talk to your doctor, by phone or in person, and say, "This doesn't seem to be working. Is there anything else we can try?"
   b. Stop taking the antibiotic.
   c. Try an herbal remedy that your roommate recommends.

6. Your doctor suggests a cutting-edge treatment for your condition, but your health plan or HMO refuses to pay for it. What do you do?
   a. Try to get a loan to cover the costs.
   b. Settle for whatever treatment options are covered.
   c. Challenge your health plan.

7. You call for an appointment with your doctor and are told nothing is available for four months. What do you do?
   a. Take whatever time you can get whenever you can get it.
   b. Explain your condition to the nurse or receptionist, detailing any symptoms and pain you're experiencing.
   c. Give up and decide you don't need to see a doctor at all.

8. Even though you've been doing sit-ups faithfully, your waist still looks flabby. When you see an ad for waist-whittling liposuction, what do you do?
   a. Call for an appointment.
   b. Talk to a health-care professional about a total fitness program that may help you lose excess pounds.
   c. Carefully research the risks and costs of the procedure.

9. You have a condition that you do not want anyone to know about, including your health insurer and any potential employer. What do you do?
   a. Use a false name.
   b. Give your physician a written request for confidentiality about this condition.
   c. Seek help outside the health-care system.

10. Your doctor suggests a biopsy of a funny-looking mole that's sprouted on your nose. Rather than using a laboratory that specializes in skin analysis, your HMO requires that all samples be sent to a general lab, where results may not be as precise. What do you do?
    a. Ask your doctor to request that a specialty pathologist at the general lab perform the analysis.
    b. Hope that in your case, the general lab will do a good-enough job.
    c. Threaten to change HMOs.

MAKING THIS CHAPTER WORK FOR YOU

Review Questions

(LO 17.1) 1. Which of the following is a change implemented under the Affordable Care Act?
   a. Fewer individuals will receive health care under Medicaid.
   b. Preventive services are no longer free.
   c. Insurance companies cannot deny coverage on the basis of preexisting medical conditions.
   d. Insurance companies can terminate coverage if a policyholder becomes ill.

(LO 17.1) 2. Which of the following statements is true of the Affordable Care Act?
   a. You cannot remain on your parent's health insurance plan if you are married.
   b. You can be covered under a parent's health insurance plan till you are 30.
   c. You can buy a catastrophic health plan if you are over 30.
   d. You will have to pay a penalty if you don't obtain coverage.

(LO 17.2) 3. Which of the following is true of health literacy in the United States?
   a. According to research studies, people with limited health literacy are less likely to report poor health.
   b. Most college students do not consider magazine and television as authoritative, believable sources for health literacy.
   c. College students are known to seek out information on health concerns.
   d. According to research studies, people with limited health literacy are more likely to have lower rates of preventable hospitalizations.

(LO 17.2) 4. When looking for medical information online, you should _____.
   a. look for sites that both provide advice and offer products for sale
   b. look for information that was recently published in a newspaper
   c. read testimonials about the product
   d. check the creator of the website to make sure it is a health or medical agency

(LO 17.3) 5. Which of the following statements is true of oral health?
   a. Oral health refers only to the health of teeth.
   b. Gingivitis and periodontitis can increase the incidence of cardiovascular disease.
   c. Periodontal disease leads to a lower white blood cell count.
   d. The early stage of gum disease is called periodontitis.

(LO 17.3) 6. The FDA monitors personal health apps that _____.
   a. monitor blood pressure
   b. provide reminders about when to take medication
   c. give instructions for the correct use of asthma inhalers
   d. track food intake and give tips for making healthier food choices

(LO 17.4) 7. Before an appointment with a health-care professional, you should _____.
   a. dress to look good
   b. expect the clinic to locate a copy of your medical history
   c. make a list of all medications you take except vitamins and herbal supplements
   d. keep track of everything you have eaten and drunk for the last week

(LO 17.4) 8. To avoid a mistake with a medication, make sure to _____.
   a. check with a friend to see if he or she has ever taken the drug
   b. count the number of pills in the bottle
   c. familiarize yourself with the color and shape of the pill
   d. always take the pill with grapefruit or orange juice

(LO 17.5) 9. As a health-care consumer, you have the right to _____.
   a. know about your doctor's record as a practitioner
   b. obtain your medical records at no cost
   c. leave the hospital against your physician's advice
   d. know if your physician is paying a malpractice insurance premium

(LO 17.5) 10. Most medical malpractice suits are filed because _____.
   a. the doctor acted with flagrant negligence
   b. the result was not what the doctor claimed
   c. the doctor made an unavoidable error
   d. the doctor communicated ineffectively with his or her patient

(LO 17.6) 11. Which of the following statements is true of LASIK?
   a. It can improve close-up vision in middle-aged adults.
   b. It does not require additional surgery.
   c. It may result in poor night vision.
   d. It cannot correct astigmatism.

(LO 17.6) 12. Getting a breast implant can lead to _____.
  a. connective tissue disorders
  b. rupture and scarring
  c. autoimmune diseases
  d. thinning blood vessels

(LO 17.7) 13. How can you protect yourself against medical hoaxes?
  a. Ask for a money-back guarantee.
  b. Choose products that cure a wide range of ailments.
  c. Choose products that are sold exclusively at one source.
  d. Ask for published reports of the studies.

(LO 17.7) 14. Which of the following is true of health hoaxes and medical quackery?
  a. Case histories of people who have had amazing results are a sign of effectiveness.
  b. Insurance companies reimburse for all kinds of treatments.
  c. A money-back guarantee is a sign of effective health services.
  d. There are organizations that keep track of unproven methods of treatment.

(LO 17.8) 15. _____ refers to various medical and health-care systems, practices, and products that are not considered a part of conventional medicine.
  a. Holistic medicine
  b. Personalized medicine
  c. Complementary and alternative medicine
  d. Preventive medicine

(LO 17.8) 16. Which of the following statements is true of complementary and alternative medicine (CAM)?
  a. CAM is only used by people with existing health conditions.
  b. CAM is not widely used in European countries.
  c. No health insurance provides coverage for CAM.
  d. Back pain is the most frequent reason Americans use CAM.

(LO 17.9) 17. Which of the following statements is true of health-care practitioners?
  a. Optometrists can perform eye surgery.
  b. Nurse practitioners can run community clinics.
  c. Clinical psychologists can prescribe medication.
  d. Podiatrists are licensed health-care professionals who specialize in problems of the stomach.

(LO 17.9) 18. In the current health care system, which of the following is true?
  a. Primary care is usually provided by specialists in a hospital.
  b. Nurses can perform simple surgical procedures if they are board-certified.
  c. Most hospitals in the U.S. are teaching hospitals affiliated with medical schools.
  d. Hospitals stays are generally shorter today than they were 10 years ago.

Answers to these questions can be found on page 623.

Critical Thinking Question

1. Think about an experience you've had with a traditional medical practitioner. How did you feel during the physical examination? Did you trust the practitioner? Were you comfortable with the level of communication? Assess your experience and share your opinion on the quality and value of the checkup.

Additional Online Resources

www.health.gov/nhic/
This excellent site, sponsored by the National Health Information Center (NHIC) of the U.S. Office of Disease Prevention and Health Promotion, is a health information referral service providing health professionals and consumers with a database of various health organizations. The site provides a searchable database, publications, and a list of toll-free numbers for health information.

http://nccam.nih.gov
This National Institutes of Health site features a variety of fact sheets on alternative therapies and dietary supplements, research, current news, and databases for the public as well as for practitioners.

www.medicinenet.com
This comprehensive site is written for the consumer by board-certified physicians and contains medical news, a directory of procedures, a medical dictionary, a pharmacy, and first aid information. You can use the information at MedicineNet .com to prepare for a doctor visit, learn about a diagnosis, or understand a prescribed treatment or procedure.

www.fda.gov
In addition to providing information on regulation and legislation relating to food and drugs, the FDA website offers information on strategies for evaluating health products and services.

http://ods.od.nih.gov/HealthInformation/
Health information on dietary supplements, including vitamins and minerals.

Key Terms

The terms listed are used on the page indicated. Definitions of the terms are in the glossary at the end of the book.

acupuncture 534

Ayurveda 534

chiropractic 536

complementary and alternative medicine (CAM) 533

evidence-based medicine 521

gingivitis 525

gum disease 525

health literacy 520

herbal medicine 536

holistic 534

home health care 539

homeopathy 534

informed consent 530

integrative medicine 534

medical history 522

naturopathy 534

outcomes 522

Pap smear 529

periodontitis 525

plaque 525

practice guidelines 521

primary care 538

quackery 533

self-care 525

vital signs 525

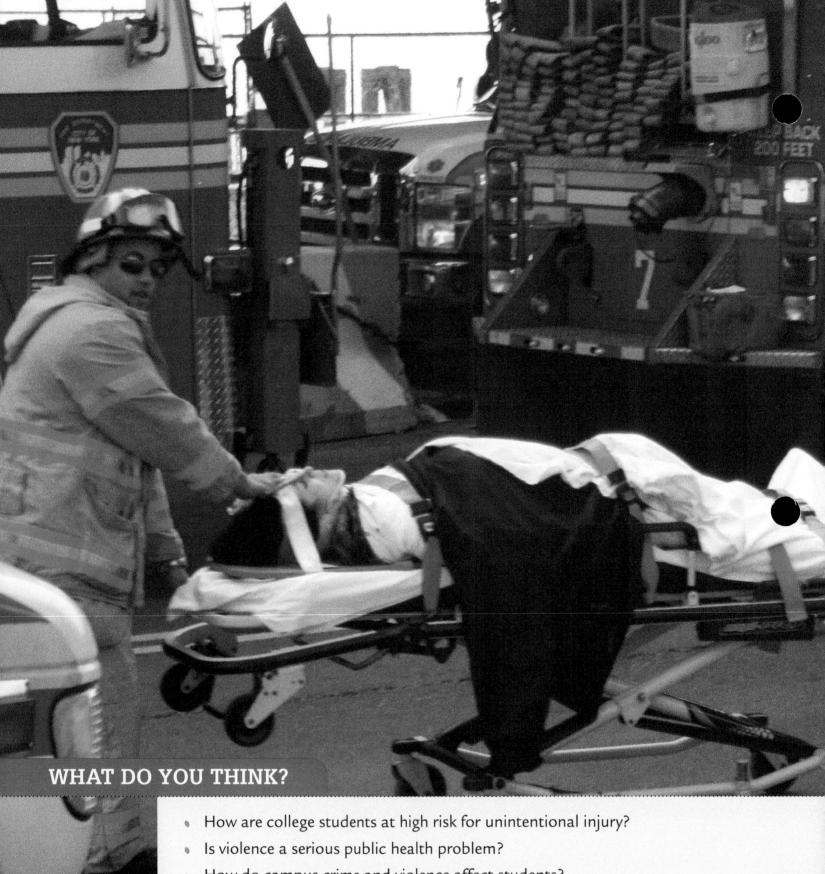

WHAT DO YOU THINK?

- How are college students at high risk for unintentional injury?
- Is violence a serious public health problem?
- How do campus crime and violence affect students?
- What is the impact of sexual victimization and violence?

18

Personal Safety

Jian just wanted to send his friends a quick text to let them know that he would be a few minutes late. When he glanced back at the road, all he could see were the headlights of an oncoming car. Then he heard the sickening sound of metal hitting metal and felt a terrible crushing pain shoot up through his legs.

Accidents, injuries, assaults, crimes—all seem like things that happen only to other people, only in other places. But no one, regardless of how young, healthy, or strong, is immune from danger. The risks to college students include alcohol-associated injuries and illnesses, traffic accidents, and physical and sexual assaults.

Recognizing the threat of intentional and unintentional injury is the first step to ensuring your personal safety. You may think that the risk of something bad happening is simply a matter of chance, of being in the wrong place at the wrong time. That's

not the case. Certain behaviors, such as using alcohol or drugs or not buckling your seat belt, greatly increase the risk of harm.

Ultimately, you have more control over your safety than anyone or anything else in your life. This chapter is a primer in self-protection that could help safeguard—perhaps even save—your life. Included are recommendations for common-sense safety on the road, at home, and at work. This chapter also explores other serious threats to personal safety in our society: violence and sexual victimization. **<**

After reading this chapter, you should be able to:

18.1 Identify the threats posed by unintentional injuries.

18.2 Outline the best practices for road safety.

18.3 Summarize safety precautions to implement at work and at home.

18.4 Comment on gender differences in vulnerability to injury.

18.5 Specify reasons why violence is a significant public health problem in America.

18.6 Discuss types of campus violence and their consequences for students.

18.7 Assess the impact of sexual victimization and violence.

18.8 Describe some approaches that can help rape victims.

Unintentional Injury

The major threat to the lives of college students isn't illness but injury. Almost 75 percent of deaths among Americans 15 to 24 years old are caused by "unintentional injuries" (a term public health officials prefer), suicides, and homicides. Accidents, especially motor vehicle crashes, kill more college-age men and women than all other causes combined; the greatest number of lives lost to accidents is among those 25 years of age.[1]

Accidents injure as well as kill. In a study of almost 20,000 university students from 26 low-, middle-, and high-income countries, about a quarter reported a nonfatal accidental injury. Students were most likely to be injured during sports activities and to suffer a broken bone/dislocated joint or a cut, puncture, or stab wound.[2]

YOUR STRATEGIES FOR PREVENTION

What to Do in an Emergency

Life-threatening situations rarely happen more than once or twice in any person's life. When they do, you must think and act quickly to prevent disastrous consequences.

- **Stop, look, and listen.** Your immediate response to an emergency may be overwhelming fear and anxiety. Take several deep breaths. Start by assessing the circumstances. Look for any possible dangers to you or the victim, such as a live electrical wire or a fire. Listen for sounds, such as a cry for help or a siren. Don't attempt rescue techniques, such as cardiopulmonary resuscitation (CPR), unless you're trained.

- **Don't wait for symptoms to go away or get worse.** If you suspect that someone is having a heart attack or stroke, or has ingested something poisonous, *phone for help immediately*. A delay could jeopardize the person's life.

- **Don't move a victim.** The person may have a broken neck or back, and attempting to move him or her could cause extensive damage or even death.

- **Don't drive.** Even if the hospital is just ten minutes away, you're better off waiting for a well-equipped ambulance with trained paramedics who can deliver emergency care on the spot.

- **Don't do too much.** Often well-intentioned good Samaritans make injuries worse by trying to tie tourniquets, wash cuts, or splint broken limbs. Also, don't give an injured person anything to eat or drink.

- **At home, keep a supply of basic first-aid items in a convenient place.** Beyond the emergency number 911, make sure that telephone numbers for your doctor and neighbors are handy.

The factors that increase the risk of unintentional injury in young adults include the following:

- Lower economic status
- Male gender
- Smoking
- Binge drinking
- Drunk driving
- Illicit drug use
- Short sleep duration
- Inadequate sleep
- Psychological distress (depression, anxiety)
- Danger or risk seeking
- Type-A behavior pattern (irritable, easily angered)
- Low social support[3]

Life can never be risk-free, but you can do more than anyone else to avoid unnecessary hazards and to maximize your ability to cope with potentially dangerous situations. According to research on survivors of various types of disasters, those who respond well in a crisis tend to have three underlying psychological attributes:

- They believe that they can influence events. (Refer to the discussion of self-efficacy in Chapter 1.)
- They are able to find meaningful purpose in turmoil and trauma. (See the discussion on spirituality in Chapter 2.)
- They know that they can learn from both positive and negative experiences.

Why Accidents Happen

Some of the many factors that influence an individual's risk of accident or injury are these:

- **Age.** Injury is the leading cause of death during the first four decades of life in the United States. Every day more than 2,000 children and teenagers die from an injury that could have been prevented. The five most common causes of unintentional injury are road traffic injuries, drowning, burns, falls, and poisoning. Most victims of fatal accidents are males. Feeling full of life and energy, they may take dangerous risks because they think they're invulnerable.

- **Alcohol.** An estimated 40 percent of Americans are involved in an alcohol-related accident sometime during their lives. Alcohol plays a role in about a quarter of fatal motor vehicle accidents and half of fatal motorcycle crashes.

- **Stress.** When we're tense and anxious, we all pay less attention to what we're doing. One common result is an increase in accidents. If you find yourself having a series of small mishaps or near-misses, do something to lower your stress level rather than wait for something more harmful to happen (see Chapter 4). When facing danger, take deep, controlled, regular breaths—a technique first-responders learn in their training.

- **Situational Factors.** Some situations—such as driving on a curvy, wet road in a car with worn tires—are so inherently dangerous that they greatly increase the odds of an accident. But even when there's greater risk, you can lower the danger: for instance, you can make sure your tires and brakes are in good condition.

- **Thrill Seeking.** To some people, activities that others might find terrifying—such as skydiving or parachute jumping—are stimulating. These thrill seekers may have lower-than-normal levels of the brain chemicals that regulate excitement. Because the stress of potentially hazardous sports may increase the levels of these chemicals, they feel pleasantly aroused rather than scared.

Accidents can happen to anyone at any time, so it's important that you be prepared.

✓**check-in** Do you think of yourself as accident-prone? Why or why not?

Safety on the Road

An average of 117 people die every day in motor vehicle crashes—approximately 1 every 12 minutes. Alcohol use is a factor in about 40 percent of these crashes; speeding, in about one-third. Rollovers caused by drivers losing control of their vehicles kill about 25 people daily.

The annual number of traffic fatalities has fallen in recent years. This decline, according to the National Highway Traffic Safety Administration (NHTSA), is due to several factors, including increased vehicle safety and rigorous campaigns to curtail drunk driving and encourage seat belt use. Yet drivers feel less safe on the road than they did five years ago. In a recent national study by the AAA Foundation for Traffic Safety, these wary drivers blamed distractions as the biggest reason for their insecurity.[4]

Teenage drivers and their passengers are at highest risks. According to a government analysis, teens and young adults are more likely than older victims to be so severely injured that they need to be taken to an emergency department following a motor vehicle accident.[4] Most accidents involving young drivers are due to three all-too-common errors:

- Failing to scan the environment by looking ahead and to the left and the right while driving

- Going too fast for road conditions (even if under the speed limit)

- Being distracted by something inside or outside the vehicle

College students aren't necessarily safer drivers than others their age. According to national data, full-time college students drink and drive more often than part-time students and other young adults, but they also are more likely to wear seat belts while driving and riding in cars. Young women who drink and drive have closed the gender gap and are at increasing risk of being in fatal accidents.[5]

✓**check-in** Have you ever had a car accident? What happened?

Avoid Distracted Driving

Distracted driving refers to any nondriving activity a person engages in that has the potential to distract him or her from the primary task of driving: eating, drinking, reaching for the phone, texting, talking to a passenger, etc. According to a study using video technology and in-vehicle sensors, drivers take their eyes off the road about 10 percent of the time they are behind the wheel.[6]

Nearly nine people die each day in the United States in crashes that involve distracted driving; another 1,060 are injured.[7] Distracted driving may be responsible for 20 percent of injury crashes, an estimated 5,474 deaths, and almost 450,000 injuries.[8] The number of pedestrians and bicyclists killed by distracted drivers has increased 50 percent in recent years.[9]

There are different types of distractions:

- **Visual.** Taking your eyes off the road—to read a text, check a navigation device, watch a video, look in the mirror, glance at something off to the side, etc.

- **Manual.** Taking your hands off the wheel to change a station or playlist, text, make a call, eat or drink something, etc.

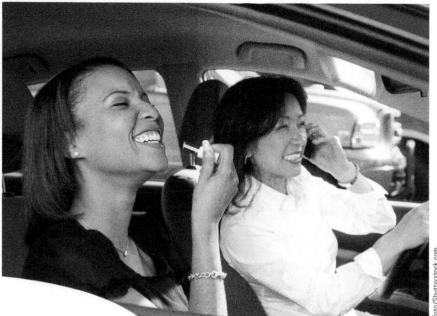

Chatting with friends while driving—whether on the phone or in person—can put you and others at risk.

An estimated 26 percent of all motor vehicle accidents are caused by drivers using a cell phone. Driving while dialing a cell phone makes the risk of a crash or near-crash three times more likely than if a driver were not distracted; texting increases the risk twentyfold.[11]

✓ **check-in** Did you know that nearly 50 percent of 18- to 24-year-old drivers report texting while driving?

In one study that simulated driving while texting, two-thirds of participants committed "lane excursions" and crossed into another lane with oncoming traffic or onto a shoulder.[12]

What makes talking or texting while driving so dangerous?

- These activities distract the brain as well as the eyes—much more so than talking to another person in the vehicle. Conversations between drivers and passengers tend to slow down or stop as driving conditions change.

- Conversation on any type of phone leads to what researchers call "inattention blindness"----, the inability to recognize objects encountered in the driver's visual field. This form of cognitive impairment may distract drivers for up to two minutes after a phone conversation has ended.

- Cell phone use delays a driver's reactions as much as having a blood-alcohol concentration at the legal limit of .08 percent.[13]

Many states have passed laws banning use of a cell phone to text or talk while driving. You can check the laws in your state at www.distraction.gov/content/get-the-facts/state-laws.html.

✓ **check-in** Have you ever texted while driving? Would you take a pledge never to text and drive?

- **Cognitive.** Taking your mind off what you're doing—to listen to lyrics, chat with a friend, place a call, pay attention to a podcast, think about what you have to do that day, etc.

- **Social.** Driving with passengers can be distracting—and dangerous. Young male drivers, at greater risk of automobile accidents than female and older drivers, drive faster when they have a friend in the car, particularly if in a happy mood.[10]

The U.S. Department of Transportation offers these safety precautions:

- Never text or talk on your cell phone while you're behind the wheel.

- Turn off the ringer on your phone and set the phone out of reach while you're driving.

- Never eat, drink, primp, focus on a GPS device, read, or surf through radio stations or playlists while you drive.

- If you happen to call someone who is driving, suggest that the driver call you back when he or she is done driving.

✓ **check-in** What is most likely to distract you while driving?

Don't Text or Talk

Although all distractions can endanger drivers' safety, texting is the most perilous because it involves three types of distractions. Even if your cell phone is a hands-free model, using it while driving is as dangerous as driving drunk.

Stay Sober and Alert

The number of fatalities caused by drunk driving, particularly among young people, has dropped. The NHTSA attributes this decline to several factors:

- Increases in the drinking age.

- Educational programs aimed at reducing nighttime driving by teens.

- The formation of Students Against Destructive Decisions (SADD, originally called Students Against Drunk Driving) and similar groups.

- Changes in state laws to lower the legal blood-alcohol concentration (BAC) level for young drivers. (Some states have zero tolerance blood-alcohol level for drivers under 21.)

Psychoactive drugs also impair driving, and the combination of two widely used mind-altering substances—alcohol and marijuana—has a much more severe impact than either one used alone.[14]

Falling asleep at the wheel is second only to alcohol as a cause of serious motor vehicle accidents. About half of drivers in the United States drive while drowsy. Nearly 14 million have fallen asleep at the wheel in the past year, according to the National Sleep Foundation. Men and young adults between the ages of 18 and 29 are at the highest risk for driving while drowsy or falling asleep at the wheel. Even after a night's sleep, the use of sleeping pills can impair driving ability, particularly in women and those who take extended-release formulations.[15]

√ **check-in** Have you ever driven while drowsy?

Buckle Up

Seat belts save an estimated 9,500 lives in the United States each year, and their use has reached an all-time high, with three in four Americans buckling up. States with seat belt laws have even higher rates of use: 80 percent. However, young people, especially men between ages 19 and 29, are less likely than others to use seat belts.

Here's what you need to know about buckling up:

- By official estimates, two-thirds of 15- to 20-year-olds killed in motor vehicle accidents were not wearing seat belts. (See Table 18.1.)

- When lap-shoulder belts are used properly, they reduce the risk of fatal injury to front-seat passengers by 45 percent and the risk of moderate to critical injury by 50 percent.

- Because an unrestrained passenger can injure others during a crash, the risk of death is lowest when all occupants wear seat belts, according to federal analysts. Seat belt use by everyone in a car may prevent about one in six deaths that might otherwise occur in a crash.

√ **check-in** Do you always buckle up when driving? Do you do the same as a passenger?

TABLE 18.1 Student Safety Strategies

	Percent (%)		
	Never	Rarely or sometimes	Mostly or always
Wear a seatbelt when you ride in a car	0.4	3.6	96.0
Wear a helmet when you ride a bicycle	38.2	24.9	36.9
Wear a helmet when you ride a motorcycle	7.7	7.2	85.2
Wear a helmet when you are inline skating	54.2	14.7	31.2

Source: American College Health Association. *American College Health Association–National College Health Assessment II: Reference Group Executive Summary, Spring 2014.* Hanover, MD: American College Health Association, 2014.

© arek_malang/Shutterstock.com

Check for Air Bags

An air bag, either with or without a seat belt, has proved the most effective means of preventing adult death, somewhat more so for women than for men. The combination of airbags and seat belts affords the best protection against spine fractures; an airbag alone decreases this risk but to a lesser extent.

Because there is controversy over the potential hazard air bags pose to children, the American Academy of Pediatrics recommends that children sit in the backseat, whether or not the car is equipped with a passenger air bag.

Rein in Road Rage

Emotional outbursts known as road rage are a factor in half of all fatal and nonfatal accidents, according to the NHTSA. The primary triggers are drivers' cutting in or weaving, speeding, and exhibiting hostile behaviors.[16]

Some strategies for reducing road rage include the following:

- **Lower the stress in your life.** Take a few moments to breathe deeply and relax your shoulders before putting the key in the ignition.

- **Consciously decide not to let other drivers get to you.** Tell yourself that whatever happens, it's not going to make your blood pressure go up.

- **Slow down.** If you're going 5 or 10 miles over the speed limit, you won't have the time you need to react to anything that happens.

- **Modify bad driving habits one at a time.** If you tend to tailgate slow drivers, spend a week driving at twice your usual following distance. If you're a habitual horn honker, silence yourself.

Bicycle Helmet Heads-Up

When will you fall off your bike? According to the Bicycle Helmet Safety Institute, the average careful bike rider can expect to crash about every 4,500 miles.

Facts to Know

- Bike helmets can prevent 85 percent of cyclists' head injuries, which cause 75 percent of bicycle-related deaths.
- Even a low-speed fall on a bicycle path can result in a head injury.
- Laws in 22 states and at least 192 localities require helmets.

Steps to Take

- Always look inside a helmet for a Consumer Product Safety Commission (CPSC) sticker before purchasing.

- Check the fit. A helmet should sit level on your head, touching all around, comfortably snug but not tight. The helmet should not move more than about an inch in either direction, regardless of how hard you tug at it.
- Pick a bright color for visibility. Avoid dark colors, thin straps, or a rigid visor that could snag in a fall.
- Look for a smooth plastic outer shell, not one with alternating strips of plastic and foam.
- Watch out for excessive vents, which put less protective foam in contact with your head in a crash.

- **Be courteous—even if other drivers aren't.** Don't dawdle in the passing lane. Never tailgate or switch lanes without signaling. Don't use your horn or high beams unless absolutely necessary.

- **Never retaliate.** Whatever another driver does, keep your cool. Count to 10. Take a deep breath. If you yell or gesture at someone who's upset with you, the conflict may escalate.

- **If you do something stupid, show that you're sorry.** On its website, the AAA Foundation for Traffic Safety solicited suggestions for automotive apologies. The most popular: slapping yourself on your forehead or the top of your head to indicate that you know you goofed. Such gestures can soothe a miffed motorist—and make the roads a slightly safer place for all of us.

Cycle Safely

Per vehicle mile, motorcyclists are 35 times more likely to die in a crash than passenger car occupants.

The most common motorcycle injury is head trauma, which can lead to physical disability, including paralysis and general weakness, as well as problems reading and thinking. It can also cause personality changes and psychiatric problems, such as depression, anxiety,

uncontrollable mood swings, and anger. Complete recovery from head trauma can take four to six years, and the costs can be staggering. Head injury can also result in permanent disability, coma, and death.

After years of steady increases, motorcycle deaths have begun to fall. Much of the credit goes to helmets, which are required in most states and dramatically reduce the risk not just of death but of head injury and spinal trauma that could otherwise lead to paralysis.

More than 80 million people ride bicycles, about half for basic transportation rather than recreation. Each year, bicycle crashes kill about 700 of these individuals and send 450,000 to 587,000 to emergency rooms. The number of bicyclist fatalities in the United States has increased dramatically in recent years as more Americans commute to school or work by bike. Two-thirds of the deaths occurred in riders who were not wearing helmets; eight in ten of the victims were adults, most of them men.[17]

Only about half of cyclists wear helmets. On college campuses, even fewer students—12 to 25 percent—opt for helmets. Yet in a study of students requiring emergency care for a bicycle-related head injury, only 4 percent were wearing helmets. Among the reasons college students give for not wearing helmets are the following:

- physical discomfort
- cost
- biking only a short distance
- inconvenience
- vanity
- concerns about ridicule
- impaired vision when wearing a helmet

✓**check-in** Do you always wear a helmet when on a motorcycle or bicycle?

Safety at Work and at Home

The workplace is second only to the home as the most frequent site of accidents. The industries with the highest fatality rates are mining; transportation, communication, and public utilities; construction; and agriculture, forestry, and fishing. Whatever your job, find out about potential hazards and learn the proper safety regulations. (Chapter 19 discusses some potential environmental hazards at work, including noise and toxic substances.)

According to a report by the National Research Council and Institute of Medicine, annually about one million workers suffer musculoskeletal disorders of the lower back and upper extremities as a result of their "particular jobs and working conditions—including heavy lifting, repetitive and forceful motions, and stressful working conditions." Many can be prevented.

Computers and Your Health

As computers have become part of daily life for everyone from preschoolers to seniors, health professionals have learned a great deal about potential health problems, including repetitive motion injuries and vision-related difficulties.

Repetitive Motion Injuries **Repetitive motion injuries (RMIs)** have surpassed back and neck injuries as the number one claim for workers' compensation injuries. Repeating motions—such as the hand and arm movements made while using a computer keyboard—all day, every day can result in muscle and tendon strain and inflammation. About 20 percent of people with pain, tingling, or numbness in the hands may have carpal tunnel syndrome, an overuse injury caused by repetitive motions in the hands and wrists. Symptoms include pain, swelling, and numbness and weakness in the hands or the arms. If these problems are identified early, permanent damage can generally be avoided by altering the work environment and allowing for more breaks during the day.

The slope and height of a computer keyboard can affect the likelihood of repetitive motion injuries. If you work at a computer, good posture and correct positioning of the computer screen and keyboard can help prevent repetitive motion injuries, eyestrain, and back strain (Figure 18.1). Here are some additional tips:

- Place the keyboard so that your elbows are bent at a 90-degree angle and you don't have to bend your wrists to type.

- Use a chair that provides ample back support. Keep your thighs parallel to the floor and your feet on the floor. If your feet don't reach the floor, use a footrest.

- If you experience neck strain, place a document holder next to your screen so that you can view the materials more easily.

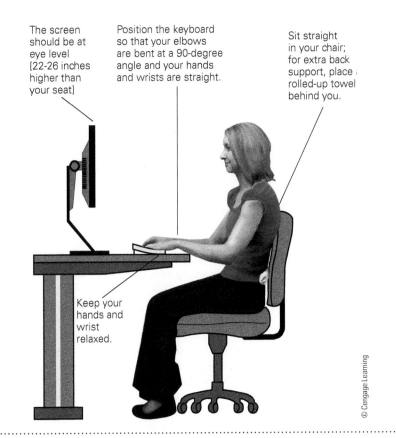

The screen should be at eye level [22-26 inches higher than your seat]

Position the keyboard so that your elbows are bent at a 90-degree angle and your hands and wrists are straight.

Sit straight in your chair; for extra back support, place a rolled-up towel behind you.

Keep your hands and wrist relaxed.

© Cengage Learning

FIGURE 18.1 Safe Computing

By paying attention to your posture and your computer's position, you can help protect yourself from repetitive motion injury, back strain, and eyestrain.

- Every 15 minutes take a 30-second break, stretch your arms, and walk around the office. Take a 15-minute break at least once every two hours.

Vision Problems **Computer vision syndrome** is a condition marked by tired and sore eyes; blurred vision; headaches; and neck, shoulder, and back pain. The American Optometric Association estimates that it afflicts nearly 90 percent of workers who use computers and also is common among children and students of all ages. The symptoms result from repeatedly stressing some aspect of the visual system, but they often disappear as soon as the person stops working at the computer.

The eye focuses on a computer image differently from the way it focuses on a printed one. The pixels that appear on a computer screen, unlike printed characters, are bright in the center and gradually fade away into the background color. This makes it difficult for the eye to sustain focus. Optometrists have developed a specific method, called a PRIO examination, that simulates how the eye responds to pixels on a computer screen. It can determine the need and proper prescription for computer-only eyeglasses.

repetitive motion injuries (RMIs) Inflammation of or damage to parts of the body due to repetition of the same movements.

computer vision syndrome A condition caused by computer use marked by tired and sore eyes; blurred vision; headaches; and neck, shoulder, and back pain.

At Home

Every year home accidents cause nearly 25 million injuries. Over 30 percent of fatal injuries to adolescents occur in the home. According to a recent study of home safety, households tend to be safe in some ways but not in others. For instance, some homes have smoke detectors but also have exposed electrical cords. Poison poses the greatest threat, causing about 30,000 deaths every year; 93 percent are the result of drug overdose, mostly from opioid pain medications. Half a million children swallow poisonous materials each year. Adults may also be poisoned by mistakenly taking someone else's prescription drugs or taking medicines in the dark and swallowing the wrong one. In case of poisoning, call 911 or 1-800-222-1222 for help 24 hours every day.

Falls of all kinds are the second leading cause of death from unintentional injury in the United States. High heels or worn footgear, poor lighting, slippery or uneven walkways, broken stairs and handrails, loose or worn rugs, and objects left where people walk all increase the likelihood of a slip.

You can prevent fires by making sure that the three ingredients of fire—fuel, a heat source, and oxygen—don't get a chance to mix. Almost anything can act as fuel for fire, including paper, wood, and flammable liquids such as oils, gasoline, and some paints. A heat source can be a spark from a lighted match, a pilot light, or an electrical wire. Oxygen is necessary for the chemical reaction between the fuel and heat source that causes combustion.

If a fire starts and it's small, you may be able to put it out with a portable fire extinguisher before it spreads. However, if the fire does get out of control, you might have only two to five minutes to get out of the house or building alive. A fire-escape plan can save time and lives. Sketch a plan of your house, apartment building, dormitory, or fraternity or sorority house. Identify two ways out of each room or apartment. Make sure everyone is familiar with these escape routes. Designate an area outside where all family members or dorm residents should meet after escaping from a fire.

In a national survey, the majority of colleges had at least one dorm without a sprinkler system. If a fire breaks out in your dorm room, get out as quickly as possible, but don't run. Before opening a room door, place your hand on it. If it's hot, don't open it. If the door feels cool, open it slightly to check for smoke; if there's none, leave by your planned escape route. If you're on an upper floor and your escape routes are blocked, open a window (top and bottom, if possible) and wait or signal from the window for help. Never try to use an elevator in a fire.

Which Gender Is at Greater Risk?

Just like illness, injury doesn't discriminate against either gender. Both men and women can find themselves in harm's way—but for different reasons. Here are some gender differences in vulnerability:

- Men are ten times more likely to die of an occupational injury than women.

- Males are most often the victims and the perpetrators of homicides in the United States. In about 68 percent of cases reported by the Bureau of Justice Statistics, both the offender and the victim were male.

- Overall, men are 3.6 times more likely than women to be murdered and 9 times more likely to commit murder. Both men and women are more likely to kill or attempt to kill male victims than female victims.

- Men are more likely than women to be assaulted as adults.

- The genders also differ in their fear of crime. In a recent study, women—but not men—tended to become less apprehensive and to feel less vulnerable as they became older. Increased income correlated with higher levels of fear for men but lower levels for women.[18]

Violence in America

The World Health Organization (WHO) defines violence as "the intentional use of physical force or power, threatened or actual, against oneself, another person, or a group or community, that either results in, or has a high likelihood of resulting in injury, death, psychological harm, maldevelopment, or deprivation." A simpler way of putting it is that "violence is anything you wouldn't want someone to do to you." Although anyone is capable of violent crime, being aware of certain behaviors in a person may keep you safer. (See Table 18.2, Warning Signs of Violence.)

Violence, a significant public health problem in this country, kills 55,000 people in the United States every year. Every day 13 young people between the ages of 10 and 24 die as a result of violence, making homicide the third leading cause of death for this age group.[19] The rate of violent injuries and deaths in the United States far exceeds that in any other high-income "peer" nation.

There are ethnic and racial differences in patterns of violence. African Americans are at greater risk of victimization by violent crime than whites or persons of other racial groupings. Hispanics are at greater risk of violent victimization than non-Hispanics. There is little difference between white women and nonwhite women in rape, physical assault, or stalking. Native American and Alaska Native women are significantly more likely than white women or African American women to report being raped. Mixed-race women also have a significantly higher incidence of rape than white women. Native American and Alaska Native men report significantly more physical assaults than Asian and Pacific Islander men.

There is no simple answer to explain why a person becomes violent and punches, kicks, stabs, or fires a gun at someone else.[20] Among the motives identified by psychologists are as follows:

- **Expression.** Some people use violence to release feelings of anger or frustration.

- **Manipulation.** For some, violence is a way of controlling others or getting something they want.

- **Retaliation.** Individuals may use violence to get back at those who have hurt them or their loved ones.[21]

Gun Violence

Gun violence causes an estimated 74,000 injuries and 32,000 deaths every year.[22] The most common form of fatal gun violence is suicide, which accounts for almost two-thirds of such deaths. Beginning in adolescence, suicide risk is highest in white males, while black males are at highest risk of fatal shootings.[23]

Only car accidents kill more Americans. In a recent survey, one in five Americans reported knowing a victim of gun violence—a family member, a friend, or even themselves. Young people between the ages of 18 and 20 were among those most likely to know a gun violence victim.[24] Those between the ages of 15- and 24 are most likely to be targets of gun violence. (see Table 18.3.)

√**check-in** Do you or does anyone in your family own a gun?

TABLE 18.2 Warning Signs of Violence

Some signs of potential for violence may be historical or static (unchangeable) factors, such as the following:

- A history of violent or aggressive behavior
- Young age at first violent incident
- Having been a victim of bullying
- A history of discipline problems or frequent conflicts with authority
- Early childhood abuse or neglect
- Having witnessed violence at home
- Family or parent condones use of violence
- A history of cruelty to animals
- Having a major mental illness
- Being callous or lacking empathy for others
- A history of vandalism or property damage

Other signs of potential violence may escalate or contribute to the risk of violence given a certain event or activity:

- Serious drug or alcohol use
- Gang membership or strong desire to be in a gang
- Access to or fascination with weapons, especially guns
- Trouble controlling feelings like anger
- Withdrawal from friends and usual activities
- Regularly feeling rejected or alone
- Feeling constantly disrespected

Some signs of potential violence may be new or active:

- Increased loss of temper
- Frequent physical fighting
- Increased use of alcohol or drugs
- Increased risk-taking behavior
- Declining school performance
- Acute episode of major mental illness
- Planning how to commit acts of violence
- Announcing threats or plans for hurting others
- Obtaining or carrying a weapon

Adapted from materials developed by the American Psychological Association, www.apa.org.

TABLE 18.3 Incidences of firearms use

Firearms are involved in

- 68% of homicides
- 52% of suicides
- 43% of robberies
- 21% of aggravated assaults
- 85% of fatal suicide attempts

Source: Federal Bureau of Investigation

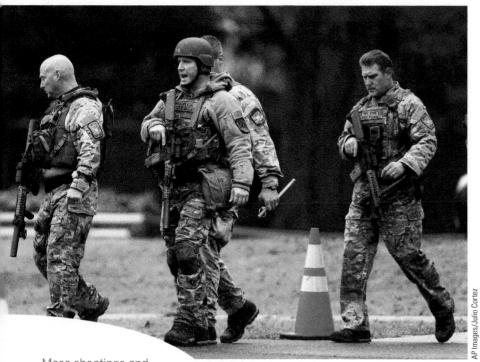

Mass shootings and terrorist threats have brought armed first responders to some college campuses.

Compared with other industrialized nations, the United States has low rates of violent assaults but uniquely high mortality rates from gun homicide and suicide.[25]

Mass Shootings

Mass murder—the killing of four or more people at a single location—has emerged as a national concern, with far too many tragic shootings occurring at schools, college campuses, movie theaters, and public events in recent years. Although there have been few studies, researchers have identified underlying psychosocial issues in mass shooters, including the following:

- Social alienation
- Problems with self-esteem
- A persecutory/paranoid outlook
- Narcissism
- Depression
- Suicidality
- Family dysfunction

Mass shootings often reinforce common misconceptions, including the assumptions that mental illness causes gun violence, that psychiatrists can predict gun crime, that shootings represent the deranged acts of mentally ill loners, and that gun control won't prevent other mass shootings. Yet surprisingly little research-based evidence supports these notions. As mental health professionals note,

- Less than 3 to 5 percent of crimes involve people with mental illness, and the percentage for gun-related crimes committed by those with mental illness is lower than the national average for persons not diagnosed with mental illness.
- Fewer than 5 percent of the 120,000 gun-related killings in the United States are perpetrated by people diagnosed with mental illness.
- Mass shootings represent distortions of, rather than depictions of, the actions of mentally ill people as a whole.
- The vast majority of people diagnosed with psychiatric disorders do not commit violent acts. Only about 4 percent of violence in the United States can be attributed to people diagnosed with mental illness.[26]

✓**check-in** Has your life ever been touched by violence? In what way?

A Public Health Approach

Gun control remains one of the most controversial political issues, with intense disagreement about Second Amendment interpretations of the right to bear arms. However, medical groups are focusing on violence as a public health challenge involving sociocultural, educational, behavioral, and product safety issues rather than solely gun ownership.[27] As they point out, this sort of multidimensional approach has led to great success in reducing smoking rates by more than half since 1966 and in saving thousands of lives by making cars and roads safer.[28]

In order to prevent gun violence, many public health initiatives have been proposed, including the following:

- Prohibiting the purchase and possession of firearms by people with multiple criminal convictions related to alcohol abuse
- Prohibiting firearm purchase by people convicted of violent misdemeanor crimes, such as assault and battery
- Requiring background checks on recipients to help prevent prohibited people from acquiring firearms anonymously and illegally from private parties, including via the Internet[29]

✓**check-in** Which public policy changes do you think might help lessen the toll of gun violence in the United States?

SNAPSHOT: ON CAMPUS NOW

How Safe Do Students Feel?

Percentage Feeling "Very Safe"

	Male	Female	Average
On their campus (daytime)	90.1	87.9	88.4
On their campus (nighttime)	57.6	30.4	39.7
In the community surrounding their school (daytime)	65.3	55.8	58.9
In the community surrounding their school (nighttime)	34.6	16	22.5

Do you give much thought to your day-to-day safety? What do you think is the greatest threat to your well-being?

Source: American College Health Association. *American College Health Association–National College Health Assessment II: Reference Group Executive Summary, Spring 2014.* Hanover, MD: American College Health Association, 2014.

Violence and Crime on Campus

Most college students feel safe on campus, especially during the daytime, but less so at night and in the community surrounding their school. (See Snapshot: On Campus Now.) According to the Bureau of Justice Statistics, college students are victims of almost half a million violent crimes a year, including assault, robbery, sexual assault, and rape. (See Table 18.4.)

Although this number may seem high, the overall violent crime rate has dropped from 88 to 41 victimizations per 1,000 students in the past decade. You can take steps to lower your risk—at little or no financial cost.

College students ages 18 to 24 are less likely to be victims of violent crime, including robbery and assault, than nonstudents of the same age. More than half (58 percent) of crimes against students are committed by strangers. More than nine in ten occur off campus, most often in an open area or street, on public transportation, in a place of business, or at a private home. In about two-thirds of the crimes, no weapon is involved. Most off-campus crimes occur at night, while on-campus crimes are more frequent in the day.

✓**check-in** Do you feel safe on your campus? Why or why not?

Male college students are twice as likely as female students to be victims of violence overall. White undergraduates have higher rates of violent victimization than students of other races.

TABLE 18.4 Violence, Abusive Relationships, and Personal Safety

Within the last 12 months, college students reported experiencing the following:

	Percent (%)		
	Male	Female	Total
A physical fight	9.5	2.8	5.2
A physical assault (not sexual assault)	4.3	3.0	3.5
A verbal threat	22.7	14.3	17.3
Sexual touching without their consent	3.3	8.9	7.0
Sexual penetration attempt without their consent	0.9	3.9	2.9
Sexual penetration without their consent	0.7	2.5	1.9
Stalking	2.8	6.3	5.1
An emotionally abusive intimate relationship	6.3	10.5	9.1
A physically abusive intimate relationship	1.7	2.0	2.0
A sexually abusive intimate relationship	1.0	2.1	1.7

Source: American College Health Association. *American College Health Association–National College Health Assessment II: Reference Group Executive Summary, Spring 2014.* Hanover, MD: American College Health Association, 2014.

Simple assault accounts for two-thirds of violent crimes against students; sexual assault or rape accounts for around 6 percent.

Substance use increases the risk of sexual and physical victimization of college students. College women are more likely to report sexual violence associated with most forms of substance use, while college men are more likely to be victims of physical violence.

About three in four campus crimes are never reported to the police. The main reasons students give for not reporting crimes are that they are too minor or private or they are not certain that the action was a crime. Individuals also may be ashamed or too emotionally overwhelmed to contact authorities.

According to researchers, only 2 percent of victimized college women report crimes to the police. The most frequent reason for not reporting sexual and physical incidents is that they didn't seem serious enough. However, women who were sexually victimized also felt ashamed, feared that they would be held responsible, or didn't want anyone to know what happened. Nonwhite women were significantly more likely than white women to say that they did not report an incident to the police because they thought they would be blamed or because they did not want the police involved.

According to surveys of undergraduates, LGBT individuals and male undergraduates are less likely to report a sexual assault or seek help.[30]

The Jeanne Clery Disclosure of Campus Security Policy and Campus Crime Statistics Act, originally known as the Student Right-to-Know and Campus Security Act, requires colleges to publish annual crime statistics for their campuses. However, the act excludes certain offenses, such as theft, threats, harassment, and vandalism, so the picture it presents may not be complete. The most recent crime statistics for the nation's colleges, universities, and career schools are posted on the Internet at http://ope.ed.gov/security.

hazing Any activity that humiliates, degrades, or poses a risk of emotional or physical harm for the sake of joining a group or maintaining full status in that group.

√**check-in** How safe is your school? (See Table 18.4 to compare your school's numbers with ACHA statistics.)

Campuses have implemented dozens of programs to halt violence, and many have proven effective. Some use posters to raise awareness of dating violence. Others have designed sexual violence prevention programs for members of fraternities, sororities, and intercollegiate athletic teams. Many have established codes of conduct barring the use of alcohol and drugs, fighting, and sexual harassment and have instituted policies requiring suspension or expulsion for students who violate the codes. Some schools are experimenting with social media messages and training bystanders to intervene to prevent problems such as violence against women.[31]

Hazing

Hazing refers to any activity that humiliates, degrades, or poses a risk of emotional or physical harm for the sake of joining a group or maintaining full status in that group. This behavior may occur in fraternities and sororities, athletic teams, or other campus organizations. Its forms include verbal ridicule and abuse, forced consumption of alcohol or ingestion of vile substances, sexual violation, sleep deprivation, paddling, beating, burning, and branding.

HEALTH ON A BUDGET

A Do-It-Yourself Security Program

These simple, no-cost steps can provide greater protection than an elaborate alarm system. The key is to employ them every day and never let your guard down.

- **Avoid walking alone in the evening or night.** Take advantage of campus shuttle or escort services. If none is available, stick to well-lit routes.

- **Train yourself to be aware of your surroundings and the people around you.** Visualize potential exit routes in case of an emergency.

- **Always carry your cell phone and enough money so that you can take a taxi home if you find yourself in a dicey situation.**

- **Program the campus security number into your cell phone's speed dial numbers so you can access it with a single key stroke.**

- **Always lock your doors and any first- and second-floor windows at night.** Don't compromise your safety for a roommate or friend who asks you to leave the door unlocked.

- **Never leave your ID, wallet, checkbook, jewelry, cameras, and other valuables in open view.**

- **Be careful what information and which photographs you post online on social networking sites.** You never know who will see them.

- **Never drive when you're drowsy or under the influence of alcohol or drugs.** Always wear a seat belt. Never give a ride to hitchhikers or anyone you don't know.

Hate or Bias Crimes

The term *hate crime* generally refers to a criminal offense committed against a person or property that is motivated, in whole or in part, by bias or prejudice against race, national or ethnic origin, religion, sexual orientation, or disability.

More than half of hate or bias crimes on campus are motivated by race. Twenty percent of students, faculty, and staff surveyed fear for their physical safety because of their sexual orientation or gender identity. These crimes can take the form of graffiti; verbal slurs; bombings; threatening notes, e-mails, or phone calls; and physical attacks. They often generate fear and intimidation in large groups of students, undermining health, academic work, and the basic security of a campus.

Victims of anti-gay hate crime report significant levels of fear of revictimization and frequently make changes in their behavior to avoid future harassment or violence, including changing the way they dress, attempting to act "straight," and staying away from situations and areas known to be associated with lesbians and gay men. These strategies may increase susceptibility to mental health problems.

Beyond the immediate victims, hate crimes affect the psychological and emotional well-being of entire groups, with individuals of similar backgrounds or orientations reporting depression, anxiety, pain, and anger that, for some, result in feelings of inadequacy and low self-worth.[32]

✓**check-in** Do you know of hate or bias crimes on your campus? Have they ever been directed at you or your friends?

Shootings, Murders, and Assaults

Shootings of students and faculty members have occurred at several campuses in recent years. However, like murder and manslaughter, they remain uncommon. There are about 3,000 aggravated assaults—an attack with a weapon or one that causes serious injury—each year. Weapons are involved in about one-third of violent college crimes. Firearms have been used in 9 percent of all violent crimes and 8 percent of assaults. Most state colleges ban guns on campus, but some schools have allowed concealed weapons. This policy does not seem to have made a noticeable difference in life on campus.[33]

Campus shootings have a psychological impact on students on other campuses as well. In a study of students at a school in the same geographical

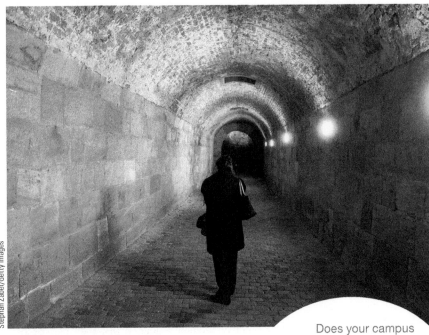

Stephan Zabel/Getty Images

area, the most common reaction was greater caution in social settings.

The American College Health Association has recommended various strategies to keep campuses safe, including these:

- Enforcing codes of conduct

- Imposing tougher sanctions, including expulsion, for serious misconduct

- Implementing zero-tolerance policies for campus violence

- Building a sense of community

- Screening out students who pose a real threat

- Warning students about criminal activity at orientation, through the campus newspaper, in residence halls, and through campus Internet communications devices

✓**check-in** What is your school doing to keep students, faculty, and staff safe?

Consequences of Campus Violence

Crime and violence take a great toll at colleges and universities. Violence can seriously injure people as well as claim lives. Moreover, victims of violent crime often suffer lasting psychological and emotional effects. Some victims take a leave of absence or transfer to another school. Those who remain in school may have problems concentrating, studying, and attending classes, and they may avoid academic and social activities. Some develop clinical symptoms that affect their mental and physical health. (See Chapter 4, on stress.)

Does your campus have regular security patrols, surveillance cameras, or late-night escorts? Have you taken advantage of these services?

Sexual Victimization and Violence

Sexual victimization refers to any situation in which a person is deprived of free choice and forced to comply with sexual acts. This is not only a woman's issue; men also are victimized. In recent years, researchers have come to view acts of sexual victimization along a continuum, ranging from street hassling, stalking, and obscene telephone calls to rape, battering, and incest.

In a recent survey of almost 2,000 students, 38 percent (29 percent of men and 43 percent of women) reported sexual violence victimization. Almost 6 percent (15 percent of men and 4 percent of women) admitted that they had perpetrated sexual violence.[34]

Sexual violence often has its roots in social attitudes and beliefs that demean a particular gender and condone aggression. According to international research, much sexual violence takes place within families, marriage, and dating relationships. In many settings, rape is a culturally approved strategy to control and discipline women. In these places, laws and policies to improve women's status are critical to ending sexual coercion.

Cyberbullying and Sexting

The Internet, which brings friends and fans together to share common interests, also has given rise to new forms of victimization. (See Chapter 5 for more on social networking.) One is **cyberbullying**, defined as an aggressive, intentional act carried out by a group or individual using electronic forms of contact repeatedly and over time against a victim who cannot easily defend him- or herself. Here is what we have learned about this behavior:

- As many as 20 percent of adolescents and young adults have reported being cyber-victims or cyberbullies; some describe themselves as both.

- Both cyberbullies and their victims are likely to experience psychiatric and psychosomatic problems. One in four of those who had been victimized reported fearing for his or her safety.

- Male and female undergraduates agreed that cyberbullying is easier than face-to-face bullying because it is less personal and more indirect. Many students minimized it as a problem

and argued that simply using technology—signing up for Facebook, for instance—qualifies as consent.

Sexting is defined as "the sharing of images or videos of sexually explicit content."[35] In the United States, about seven in ten of adolescents (ages 12 to 18) reported having received sexually oriented material, while two-thirds reported having sent it.[36]

A photo that may be sent as a joke or intended for only one person can quickly make its way to countless viewers. As discussed in Chapter 5, such violations of privacy can be emotionally devastating. In some states they also are illegal, and tough new laws are cracking down on cyberbullying and the transmission of sexual materials.

Sexual Harassment

All forms of **sexual harassment** or unwanted sexual attention—from the display of pornographic photos to the use of sexual obscenities to a demand for sex by anyone in a position of power or authority—are illegal. They nonetheless occur on college campuses and elsewhere:

- Nearly two-thirds of students experience sexual harassment at some point during college, including nearly one-third of first-year students.

- Nearly one-third of students say they have experienced physical harassment, such as being touched, grabbed, or pinched in a sexual way.

- Sexual comments and jokes are the most common form of harassment. More than half of female students and nearly half of male students say they have experienced this type of harassment.

- Lesbian, gay, bisexual, transgender, and questioning (LGBTQ) students, as well as those with physical disabilities such as deafness, are more likely than other students to be sexually harassed.

- Sexual harassment takes an especially heavy toll on female students, who often feel upset, self-conscious, embarrassed, or angry. Men are much less likely to admit to being very or somewhat upset. One-third of harassed college women say they have felt afraid; one-fifth say they have been disappointed in their college experience as a result of sexual harassment.

- About half of college men and one-third of women admit that they have sexually harassed someone on campus. Private college students are more likely than their public college peers to have ever done so. Students

---

cyberbullying Aggressive, intentional act carried out by a group or individual using electronic forms of contact repeatedly and over time against a victim who cannot easily defend him- or herself.

sexting The sharing of digital images or videos of sexually explicit content over the Interm.

sexual harassment Uninvited and unwanted sexual attention.

at large schools (population 10,000 or more) are more likely than students at small schools with fewer than 5,000 students to say they have experienced sexual harassment.

- The most common rationale for harassment is "I thought it was funny." Harassment occurs in dorms or student housing as well as outside on campus grounds and in classrooms or lecture halls.

··
√**check-in** Have you ever experienced or observed sexual harassment on campus?
··

If you encounter sexual harassment as a student, report it to the department chair or dean. If you don't receive an adequate response to your complaint, talk with the campus representatives who handle matters involving affirmative action or civil rights. Federal guidelines prevent any discrimination against you in terms of grades or the loss of a job or scholarship if you report harassment. Schools that do not take measures to remedy harassment could lose federal funds.

Stalking

Stalking, the willful, repeated, and malicious following, harassing, or threatening of another person, is common on college campuses—perhaps more so than in the general population.

An estimated 8 percent of women and 2 percent of men may meet the legal criteria for stalking.[37]

Stalking is not a benign behavior and can result in emotional or psychological distress, physical harm, or sexual assault. The most common consequence is psychological, with victims reporting emotional or psychological distress. Simply because they are young and still learning how to manage complex social relationships, some individuals may not recognize their behavior as stalking or even as disturbing.

College students may be targeted for several reasons:

- College students tend to live close to each other and to have flexible schedules and large amounts of unsupervised time.

- Most college women know their stalkers. About half are acquaintances; a high percentage of them are classmates, boyfriends, or ex-boyfriends.

- In one study, about half of the women stalked on campus said they had not sought help from anyone. Those who did seek assistance turned to friends, parents, residence hall advisers, or police.

Intimate Partner (Dating) Violence

Intimate partner violence can occur between heterosexual, homosexual, or bisexual partners and can take different forms:

- **Physical violence.** The threat of or the use of force on one's partner to cause harm or death.

- **Sexual violence.** The threat of or the use of force to engage a partner in sexual activity without consent, an attempted or completed sexual act without consent, or abusive sexual contact.

- **Psychological violence.** The use of threats, actions, or coercive tactics that cause trauma or emotional harm to a partner.

All forms of intimate partner violence can have devastating psychological, physical, interpersonal, and occupational effects on the victim, his or her friends and family, and society in general.

Young women ages 18 to 24, regardless of whether they are in college, are frequent targets of intimate partner violence.[38] Almost one in three undergraduate women at a college in the United States was assaulted by a male dating partner in the past year. At 31 different sites worldwide, 17 to 49 percent of college students reported perpetrating physical assault against a dating partner in the past year. The median rate was 29 percent.[39]

Violent intimate relationships are often characterized by mutual aggression, and partners may be both victims and perpetrators. They are often also victims or perpetrators of other forms of violence. College students may be at greater risk for several reasons, including alcohol use, drug use, and risky sexual behaviors. Perpetrators may engage in a host of behaviors that prevent victims from fully engaging in college. This may increase the risk of dropping classes, scholastic failure, and school withdrawal, which can impair their academic performance.[40]

Risk Factors for Intimate Partner Violence Factors that increase the likelihood of intimate partner violence include the following:

- **Gender.** Both men and women experience acts of violence and aggression by their partners, but the violence perpetrated against women by men is likely to be much more severe and potentially injurious.

- **Sexual minority.** Compared with heterosexual students, male and female sexual-minority undergraduates (defined as having had any

stalking The willful, repeated, and malicious following of another person.

same-sex sexual experience) report significantly higher rates of physical sexual violence, sexual assault, and unwanted pursuit. Sexual-minority women (but not men) reported significantly higher rates of physical dating violence than heterosexual students.[41]

- **Violence in the family of origin.** Childhood exposure to violence and abuse are risk factors for dating violence, especially for women.

- **Emotional states and mental health.** Negative emotions, particularly anger, anxiety, and depression, are associated with dating violence. Women who behave violently are more likely to be victims of partner violence and to have high levels of depression, anger, and hostility. Men who behave violently show more antisocial personality characteristics and have lower educational and economic status.[42]

- **Substance use and abuse.** Drugs and alcohol reduce the ability to resist unwanted physical or sexual advances and/or may prevent a victim from being able to interpret warning cues of a potential assault.[43]

- **Sexual risk taking.** Involvement with strangers and individuals who are close acquaintances may increase the risk for dating violence.[44]

Disclosure and Support Most victims of dating violence disclose what happened to at least one person, usually a friend, family member, classmate, coworker, or neighbor. They are more likely to do so if they

- Are female
- Are white
- Are younger
- Are of higher socioeconomic status
- Attach anger/jealousy motives to the violence
- Feel less shame or fear regarding the violence
- Experience psychological or stalking-related violence
- Experience greater severity and frequency of violence
- Have someone witness the violence

Victims report that the most helpful reaction following disclosure is emotional support; the least helpful reactions are expressing disbelief and blaming the victim. Disclosure and social support following disclosure are associated with better mental health and psychological recovery.[45]

Innovative programs, such as Friends Helping Friends, train young adults ages 18 to 22 in skills that could help them recognize and intervene in dating violence.[46]

Nonvolitional Sex and Sexual Coercion

Nonvolitional sex is sexual behavior that violates a person's right to choose when and with whom to have sex and what sexual behaviors to engage in. The more extreme forms of this behavior include sexual coercion or forced sex, rape, childhood sexual abuse, and violence against people with nonconventional sexual identities. Other forms, such as engaging in sex to keep one's partner or to pass as heterosexual, are so common that many think of them as normal.

Sexual coercion can take many forms, including exerting peer pressure, taking advantage of one's desire for popularity, threatening to end a relationship, getting someone intoxicated, stimulating a partner against his or her wishes, or insinuating an obligation based on the time or money one has expended. Men may feel that they need to live up to the sexual stereotype of taking advantage of every opportunity for sex. Women are far more likely than men to encounter physical force. Alcohol use increases a woman's risk.

Estimates of the prevalence of sexual coercion range from 29 to 33 percent. Intimate partners may use overwhelming psychological pressure to obtain sex, escalating to physical force if they do not get their way.[47]

About 20 percent of students say they have coerced a partner into sex in the previous 12 months, and 24 percent of students report having been victims of sexual coercion. Rates of sexual coercion—for example, making a partner have sex without a condom or insisting on sex when a partner does not want to—are higher for men than women. In a study of 387 college men, sexual arousal was significantly related to "overperception" of a woman's sexual interest and to sexually coercive behaviors.[48]

Researchers use the term **covictimization** to describe experiencing both physical and sexual forms of intimate partner violence. In one study of college women, 64 percent were covictimized since adolescence, although not necessarily by the same partner. These women, who report more psychological abuse, more intimidation, and more severe forms of physical and sexual violence, are at greater risk for anxiety, traumatic stress, and depression. Even after a breakup, their former partners are more likely to pursue, stalk, threaten, or assault them.[49]

Many schools are alerting incoming female students about what researchers call "the red zone," a period of time early in one's first undergraduate year when women are at particularly high risk

nonvolitional sex Sexual behavior that violates a person's right to choose when and with whom to have sex and what sexual behaviors to engage in.

sexual coercion Sexual activity forced upon a person by the exertion of psychological pressure by another person.

covictimization experiencing both physical and sexual forms of intimate partner violence.

for unwanted sexual experiences. One university defines the red zone more precisely as "the time period between freshman move-in and fall break wherein there is a particularly high risk of victimization." Unwanted touching and attempted intercourse are the most common behaviors reported, although researchers have also documented sexual assaults and rapes. Women who had a nonconsensual sexual experience while drinking prior to college are at increased risk.

In a recent survey of more than 1,000 undergraduates, nearly two-thirds reported knowing one or more women who have been victims of sexual assault, and over half (52.4%) reported knowing one or more men who have perpetrated sexual assault.[50]

√check-in Have you encountered any form of sexual coercion? Do you know any victims of sexual assault? Do you know any perpetrators?

Rape

Rape generally refers to sexual intercourse with an unconsenting partner under actual or threatened force. In 2012 the Justice Department updated the legal definition of rape as "the penetration, no matter how slight, of the vagina or anus with any body part or object, or oral penetration by a sex organ of another person, without the consent of the victim." Previously rape had been defined as "the carnal knowledge of a female forcibly and against her will."

Sexual intercourse between a male over the age of 16 and a female under the age of consent (which ranges from 12 to 21 in different states) is called *statutory rape*. In *acquaintance rape*, or *date rape*, the victim knows the rapist. In *marital* or *spousal rape*, the perpetrator is the victim's spouse. In *stranger rape*, the rapist is an unknown assailant. Both acquaintance and stranger rapes are serious crimes that can have a devastating impact on their victims.

All states now recognize as rape the assault of a victim who is incapable of giving consent because of alcohol or other substances. However, many women who experience a sexual encounter that meets this legal definition do not label it as a rape or even as sexual victimization. Compared with stranger rapes, these assaults are typically less violent and involve less force by the assailant, less resistance by the victim, and less injury to the victim. Yet women who do not acknowledge an unwanted sexual experience as rape nonetheless suffer psychological consequences, including distress and other trauma symptoms.

Over the course of five years (the national average for a college career), including summers and vacations, one of every four or five female students is raped. In a single academic year, 3 percent of coeds are raped—35 rapes for every 1,000 women. According to the U.S. Department of Justice, a campus with 6,000 coeds averages 1 rape a day every day for the entire school year.

In nine surveys of male university students, between 3 and 6 percent had been raped by other men; up to 25 percent had been sexually assaulted. Like female rape victims, male victims suffer long-term psychological problems and physical injuries and are at risk of contracting sexually transmitted infections.

For many years, the victims of rape were blamed for doing something to bring on the attack. However, researchers have shown that women are raped because they encounter sexually aggressive men, not because they look or act a certain way. Although no woman is immune to attack, many rape victims are children or adolescents.[51]

Women who successfully escape rape attempts do so by resisting verbally and physically, usually by yelling and fleeing. Women who use forceful verbal or physical resistance (screaming, hitting, kicking, biting, and running) are more likely to avoid rape than women who try pleading, crying, or offering no resistance.

Types of Rape   Although rape has long been viewed as an act of violence and domination, recent studies indicate that not all rapes follow a single pattern. Within the broad category of rape are specific, but not mutually exclusive, subcategories of the crime, including anger rape, power rape, sadistic rape, gang rape, and sexual gratification rape:

- *Marital rape*, the most common around the world, is a form of domestic abuse. Once ignored or condoned by the laws in many countries, it is now considered a crime in many nations.

- *Anger rape*, usually on a total stranger, is motivated by hatred and a desire for revenge for the rejection the rapist feels he's suffered from women. Anger rapists often harbor long-standing hostility toward women, use far more physical violence than is needed to get submission, and usually don't find the rape sexually gratifying.

- *Power rape* is generally a premeditated attack motivated by a desire to dominate and control another person. Power rapists, unable to deal with stress and their sense of failure, may rape to regain a sense of power. They use only as much force as needed to make their

rape Sexual penetration of a female or a male by means of intimidation, force, or fraud.

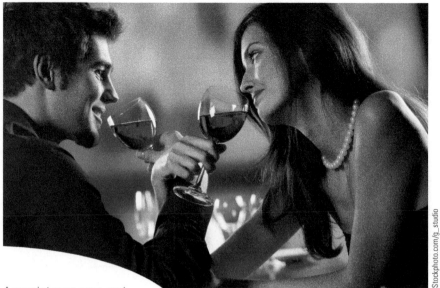

Acquaintance rape and alcohol use are very closely linked. Both men and women may find their judgment impaired or their communications unclear as a result of drinking.

victims submit and may find the rape sexually gratifying, even though that's not their primary motive.

- *Sadistic rape* is a premeditated assault that often involves bondage, torture, or sexual abuse. Sadistic rapists find power and anger sexually arousing and may subject victims to rituals of humiliation or torture. They're often preoccupied with violent pornography; their motives are more complex and difficult to understand than those of other types of rapists.

- *Gang rape* involves three or more rapists. Men in close groups that drink and party together—such as fraternities or athletic teams—are most likely to participate in such assaults. The reasons may go beyond aggression and sexual gratification to the excitement and camaraderie the men feel while sharing the experience.

- *Sexual gratification rape* is usually an impulsive attack by someone willing to use physical coercion for the sake of sex. These rapists generally use no more force than needed to get a partner to submit and may stop the attack if it becomes clear they'll have to use extreme violence to overcome resistance. Many acquaintance rapes fit into this category.

Acquaintance, or Date, Rape   According to data from the U.S. Bureau of Justice, 9 in 10 reported rapes and sexual assaults in the United States involve a single offender with whom the victim had a prior relationship.

Both women and men report having been forced into sexual activity by someone they know. Many college students are in the age group most likely to face this threat: women ages 16 to 25 and men under 25. Women are most vulnerable and men are most likely to commit assaults during their senior year of high school and their first year of college.

According to surveys of undergraduates, LGBT individuals and male undergraduates are less likely to report a sexual assault or to seek help afterward.[52]

The same factors that lead to other forms of sexual victimization can set the stage for date rape. Socialization into an aggressive role, acceptance of rape myths, and a view that force is justified in certain situations increase the likelihood of a man's committing date rape. (See Health Now! How to Avoid Date Rape.)

✓**check-in** What steps do you take to prevent acquaintance rape? Compare your response with that of a classmate of the other sex.

Other factors that play a role in sexual aggression are:

- **Personality and early sexual experiences.** These may include first sexual experience at a very young age, earlier and more frequent than usual childhood sexual experiences (both forced and voluntary), hostility toward women, irresponsibility, lack of social consciousness, and a need for dominance over sexual partners.

- **Situational variables (what happens during the date).** Men who initiate a date, pay all expenses, and provide transportation are more likely to be sexually aggressive, perhaps because they feel they can call all the shots.

- **Rape myths.** As several studies have confirmed, college men hold more rape-tolerant attitudes than do college women. For example, college men are significantly more likely than college women to agree with statements such as "Some women ask to be raped and may enjoy it" and "If a woman says 'no' to having sex, she means 'maybe' or even 'yes.'"

- **Social norms.** Some social groups, such as fraternities and athletic teams, may encourage the use of alcohol; reinforce stereotypes about masculinity; and emphasize violence, force, and competition. The group's shared values, including an acceptance of sexual coercion, may keep individuals from questioning their behavior. They also may keep bystanders from intervening to prevent a potential rape.

- **Drinking.** Alcohol use is one of the strongest predictors of acquaintance rape. Men who have been drinking may not react to subtle signals, may misinterpret a woman's behavior as a come-on, and may feel more sexually aroused. At the same time, drinking may impair a woman's ability to effectively communicate her wishes and to cope with a man's aggressiveness.

- **Date rape drugs.** Drugs such as Rohypnol (flunitrazepam) and GHB (gamma-hydroxybutyrate) have been implicated in cases of acquaintance, or date, rape. Since both drugs are odorless and tasteless, victims have no way of knowing their drink has been tampered with. The subsequent loss of memory leaves victims with no explanation for where they've been or what's happened. Rohypnol—which can cause impaired motor skills and judgment, lack of inhibitions, dizziness, confusion, lethargy, very low blood pressure, coma, and death—has been outlawed in the United States. Deaths also have been attributed to GHB overdoses.

   College women often aren't aware of the possibility that their drinks may be tampered with or that they may have been given a date-rape drug. As a result, many see no risk in leaving their drinks unattended. Even if they start feeling ill at a party, many do not suspect that a date-rape drug could be the cause. The victims of prior assaults tend to be slower at picking up on and responding to potentially dangerous dating situations, possibly because they feel that personal risks are unavoidable and beyond their control.

- **Gender differences in interpreting sexual cues.** In research comparing college men and women, the men typically overestimated the woman's sexual availability and interest, seeing friendliness, revealing clothing, and attractiveness as deliberately seductive. In one study of date rape, the men reported feeling "led on," in part because their female partners seemed to be dressed more suggestively than usual.

Stranger Rape Rape prevention consists primarily of making it as difficult as possible for a rapist to make you a victim:

- **Don't advertise that you're a woman living alone.** Use initials on your mailbox. Install and use secure locks on doors and windows; change door locks after losing keys or moving into a new residence.

- **Don't open your door to strangers.** If a repairperson or public official is at your door, ask him to identify himself and call his office to verify that he is a reputable person on legitimate business.

- **Lock your car when it is parked and drive with locked car doors.** If your car breaks down, attach a white cloth to the antenna and lock yourself in. If someone other than a uniformed officer stops to offer help, ask that person to call the police or a garage but do not open your locked car door.

- **Avoid dark and deserted areas** and be aware of your surroundings when you're walking. If a driver asks for directions when you're a pedestrian, avoid approaching his car. Instead, call out your reply from a safe distance.

- **Have house or car keys in hand as you approach the door.** Check the backseat before getting into your car.

- **Carry a device for making a loud noise,** like a whistle or, even better, a pint-sized compressed air horn available in many sporting goods and boat supply stores. Sound the noise alarm at the first sign of danger.

√**check-in** How would you rate your safety awareness and personal protection skills?

Male Nonconsensual Sex and Rape No one knows how common male rape is because men are even less likely to report such assaults than women. Researchers estimate that the victims in about 10 percent of acquaintance rape cases are men. These hidden victims often keep silent because of embarrassment, shame, or humiliation, as well as their own feelings and fears about homosexuality and conforming to conventional sex roles.

Although many people think men who rape other men are always homosexuals, most male rapists consider themselves to be heterosexual. Young boys aren't the only victims. The average age of male rape victims is 24. Rape is a serious problem in prison, where men may experience brutal assaults by men who usually resume sexual relations with women once they're released.

Impact of Rape Rape-related injuries include unexplained vaginal discharge, bleeding, infections, multiple bruises, and fractured ribs. Victims of sexual violence often develop chronic symptoms, such as headaches, backaches, high blood pressure, sleep disorders, pelvic pain, and sexual fertility problems. But sexual violence has both a physical and a psychological impact. The psychological scars of a sexual assault take a long time to heal. Therapists have linked sexual victimization with hopelessness, low self-esteem, high levels

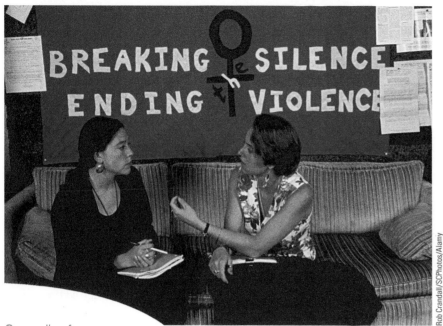

Counseling from a trained professional can help ease the trauma suffered by a rape victim.

and treatment for sexually transmitted infections and postintercourse conception.

Even an unsuccessful rape attempt should be reported because the information a woman may provide about the attack—the assaulter's physical characteristics, voice, clothes, and car, or even an unusual smell—may prevent another woman from being raped.

Helping the Victims of Violence

As their numbers have grown and their anguish has been recognized, the victims of violence have received greater attention. Hundreds of shelters for battered wives and their children have been set up across the country. They offer physical and psychological treatment and a haven where women can begin to rebuild their shattered self-esteem as well as their daily lives. Rape counseling and crisis centers on college campuses and in the community provide various forms of assistance to victims of rape. Educational programs that train bystanders to intervene to de-escalate conflict and prevent sexual violence on campus have proved to be effective on college campuses.[54] In many cities, the telephone directory lists hotlines and resources. More than 400 victims' advocacy groups have been set up across the country to advise those hurt by crime. Support organizations help many survivors deal with the emotional aftermath of their experiences.

Sometimes well-intentioned friends and relatives add to the stress felt by the victims of violence. Here's how to offer comfort without implying criticism:

- **Don't try to deny that it happened.** Although it may be hard to talk about—or even listen to—what happened, the reality of the event must not be ignored. Denial makes victims doubt their own experience and question themselves at a time when they crave reassurance.

- **Don't pressure the victim to talk—or not to talk.** Some individuals need to go over every detail of what happened, again and again, until they work out their feelings of outrage and become ready to get on with their lives. Others find going into details too humiliating. Let the victim set the tone and limits for disclosure. Don't pry or prod.

- **Don't blame the victim.** Even when no one doubts that the victim is completely innocent,

of self-criticism, and self-defeating relationships. An estimated 30 to 50 percent of women develop posttraumatic stress disorder (see Chapter 3) following a rape. Many do not seek counseling until a year or more after an attack, when their symptoms have intensified or become chronic.[53]

Acquaintance rape may cause fewer physical injuries but greater psychological torment. Often too ashamed to tell anyone what happened, victims may suffer alone, without skilled therapists or sympathetic friends to reassure them. Women raped by acquaintances blame themselves more, see themselves less positively, question their judgment, have greater difficulty trusting others, and have higher levels of psychological distress. Nightmares, anxiety, and flashbacks are common. The women may avoid others, become less capable of protecting themselves, and continue to be haunted by sexual violence for years. A therapist can help these victims begin the slow process of healing.

What to Do in Case of Rape Fewer than 5 percent of college rapes are reported. Women who are raped should call a friend or a rape crisis center. A rape victim should not bathe or change her clothes before calling. Semen, hair, and material under her fingernails or on her apparel all may be useful in identifying the man who raped her.

A rape victim who chooses to go to a doctor or hospital should remember that she may not necessarily have to talk to police. However, a doctor can collect the necessary evidence, which will then be available if she later decides to report the rape to police. All rape victims should talk with a doctor or health-care worker about testing

individuals may be plagued by regrets and self-accusation: Why didn't I lock the windows? Why did I park on that dark street? Any second-guessing or implied criticism adds to this burden of blame and shame.

- **Don't try to rush the victim to leave the past behind and get on with his or her life.**

Recovery from any traumatic event takes time, and only the victim knows the appropriate pace. If, however, months pass without any lessening of symptoms or improvement in day-to-day functioning, family members and friends shouldn't hesitate to recommend that their loved one see a mental health professional.

WHAT DID YOU DECIDE?

- How are college students at high risk for unintentional injury?
- Is violence a serious public health problem?
- How do campus crime and violence affect students?
- What is the impact of sexual victimization and violence?

THE POWER OF NOW!

Protecting Yourself

Like other aspects of your health, safety is your personal responsibility. Are you as safe as you can be? Answer the questions below by providing a numerical score from zero to ten to describe to what extent you usually behave this way:

____ I am alert to my surroundings.

____ I do not pursue relationships with people out of a feeling that I should rescue them.

____ I am careful to observe others long and well before allowing them into an intimate position in my life.

____ If someone behaves strangely, I move away and keep my distance.

____ I do not let people "guilt" or pressure me into situations that make me feel uncomfortable or unsafe.

____ I take appropriate precautions if alone in unfamiliar surroundings.

____ I do not lend money.

____ I buy only from reputable merchants.

____ I avoid Internet scams.

____ I keep a close eye on my credit and identification cards.

____ I get the sleep I need.

____ I wear a helmet when biking or skateboarding.

____ I wear a seat belt whenever I'm in a vehicle.

____ I avoid unnecessary risks when engaging in any sport.

____ I practice safe sex.

____ I lock the doors and windows to my car, room, apartment, or dormitory.

____ I do not let strangers enter my car or residence.

____ I know where fire alarms and fire extinguishers are located.

____ I carry my cell phone with me and know how to reach campus security.

____ I control my alcohol intake so I can keep my wits about me in any situation.

Review your responses. Which behaviors rate lowest? Think through ways in which you can consciously improve them. Make a to-do list of the changes you will implement today, in the coming week, and by the end of the term.

What's Online

CENGAGE
brain.com

Visit www.cengagebrain.com to access course materials for this text, including the Behavior Change Planner, interactive quizzes, tutorials, and more.

self survey

Rate Your Safety/Problem Prevention Skills

Put a check beside each of the following questions for which the answer is yes. And yes, these questions apply to both genders. Remember, more violent crimes are committed against college men than women.

On the road

_____ Do you always wear a safety belt?

_____ Do you never drive under the influence of alcohol or drugs?

_____ Do you never drive when you're drowsy?

_____ Do you slow down in bad weather conditions?

_____ Do you check your tires, brakes, and so on regularly?

_____ Do you always stay within five miles of the speed limit?

_____ Do you always wear a helmet when on a bike or motorcycle?

_____ Do you avoid isolated roads and shortcuts?

_____ Do you always keep your vehicle locked, even while driving?

_____ Do you always park in well-lit areas?

_____ Do you never pick up hitchhikers or give rides to people you don't know well?

_____ Do you always lock car doors and take the keys when you leave your car?

_____ Do you keep all valuables out of sight in the trunk?

At home

_____ Do you keep your doors locked when you are there and when away?

_____ Do you use peepholes to identify people before opening the door?

_____ Do you require identification from service providers?

_____ Do you not let anyone you don't know well inside your residence to use the phone or bathroom?

_____ Do you close the curtains and shades at night?

_____ Do you refrain from doing laundry in a deserted or poorly lit facility?

_____ Do you always have your key out for a quick entry into your home?

_____ Do you have a phone near your bed for quick use at night?

_____ Do you immediately report any stranger who looks "wrong" in your residence hall?

_____ Do you never lend your keys or ID card to anyone?

_____ Do you never prop open locked doors?

Out and about

_____ Do you avoid walking alone in the evening or at night?

_____ Do you stay in well-lit areas away from alleys or bushes?

_____ Do you walk confidently, directly, and at a steady pace?

_____ Do you walk on the side of the street facing traffic?

_____ Do you never accept rides from people you don't know well?

_____ Do you pay attention to your money and wallet?

_____ Do you count your change?

_____ Do you avoid using credit cards unless necessary?

_____ Do you pay off your credit balance every month?

_____ Do you know your checkbook balance?

_____ Do you not lend money?

On a date

_____ Do you communicate your limits clearly and verbally?

_____ Do your trust your instincts?

_____ If a situation doesn't feel right, do you leave?

_____ Do you avoid drugs and alcohol, or use them only moderately?

_____ Do you never leave a party, concert, or bar with someone you just met or don't know well?

_____ Do you always carry your cell phone and money so that you can call a taxi to get home?

_____ Have you taken a self-defense class?

_____ Do you abstain from sex until you know a potential partner well, including sexual history and health status?

_____ Do you always carry and use condoms?

Count the number of checks, and compare to the possible maximum of 40. Do you score high in vigilance on the road but low in taking precautionary steps at home? Do you see any patterns? Do you leave valuables in sight in your car? Lend your keys or ID to people you don't know well? Leave a party or bar with someone you don't know? Think through the implications of such choices. Identify three ways in which you could make yourself and your belongings safer. Put them into action—now.

MAKING THIS CHAPTER WORK FOR YOU

Review Questions

(LO 18.1) 1. Which of the following is a common cause of unintentional injury?
   a. Drowning
   b. Suicide
   c. Stabbing
   d. Homicide

(LO 18.1) 2. Which of the following underlying psychological attributes do individuals tend to exhibit while responding well in a crisis?
   a. They do not believe in learning from past experiences.
   b. They fail to recognize the threat of unintentional injuries.
   c. They assume risks to be a matter of chance.
   d. They believe that they can influence events.

(LO 18.2) 3. A majority of motor vehicle crashes are due to _____.
   a. speeding
   b. alcohol use
   c. distracted driving
   d. rollovers

(LO 18.2) 4. Which of the following strategies can reduce road rage?
   a. Resisting apologies
   b. Speeding
   c. Being courteous
   d. Retaliating

(LO 18.3) 5. _____ is the third-leading cause of death for people between the ages of 10 and 24 in the United States.
   a. Homicide
   b. Suicide
   c. Head trauma
   d. Drunk driving

(LO 18.3) 6. _____ is a primary psychological issue identified among mass shooters.
   a. Societal acceptance
   b. Self-efficacy
   c. Depression
   d. Self-acceptance

(LO 18.4) 7. Which of the following statements is true about violence on college campuses?
   a. Most crimes against students occur on campus.
   b. Men are more likely than women to be victims of physical violence.
   c. On-campus crimes are more frequent at night than during the day.
   d. Incidents of violence are always reported to higher authorities.

(LO 18.4) 8. _____ refers to any activity that humiliates, degrades, or poses a risk of emotional or physical harm for the sake of joining a group or maintaining full status in that group.
   a. Discrimination
   b. Bragging
   c. Hazing
   d. Hate

(LO 18.5) 9. The willful, repeated, and malicious following, harassing, or threatening of another person is called _____.
   a. dating
   b. stalking
   c. hazing
   d. bragging

(LO 18.5) 10. Which of the following is true about the occurrence of intimate partner violence?
   a. Sexual violence is more prevalent than other forms of violence.
   b. It can have psychological effect on a victim's family.
   c. Partners of a violent intimate relationship are always the victims and not the perpetrators.
   d. College campuses are free from intimate partner violence.

Answers to these questions can be found on page 623.

Critical Thinking

1. Can you name two risk factors in your daily life that might increase the likelihood of accidental injury? What actions have you taken to keep yourself safe? Are there other risk factors you could minimize or eliminate? What might you do about them?

2. A friend of yours, Eric, frequently makes crude or derogatory comments about women. When you finally call him on this, his response is, "I didn't say anything wrong. I like women." What might you say to him?

Additional Online Resources

www.rainn.org
This site provides great information from an organization fighting against rape, assault, and incest.

www.rapecrisis.com
This private nonprofit organization provides support to victims of sexual violence and their families, including a 24/7 crisis hotline and several advocacy programs.

www.nsc.org
The mission of the NSC is to educate and influence society to adopt safety, health, and environmental policies, practices, and procedures that prevent human suffering and economic losses arising from preventable causes.

www.safeyouth.gov
This is the website for Striving to Reduce Youth Violence (STRYVE), a national initiative led by the CDC that takes a public health approach to preventing youth violence before its starts.

Key Terms

The terms listed are used on the page indicated. Definitions of the terms are in the glossary at the end of the book.

computer vision syndrome   553

covictimization   562

cyberbullying   560

hazing   558

nonvolitional sex   562

rape   563

repetitive motion injuries (RMIs)   553

sexting   560

sexual coercion   562

sexual harassment   560

stalking   561

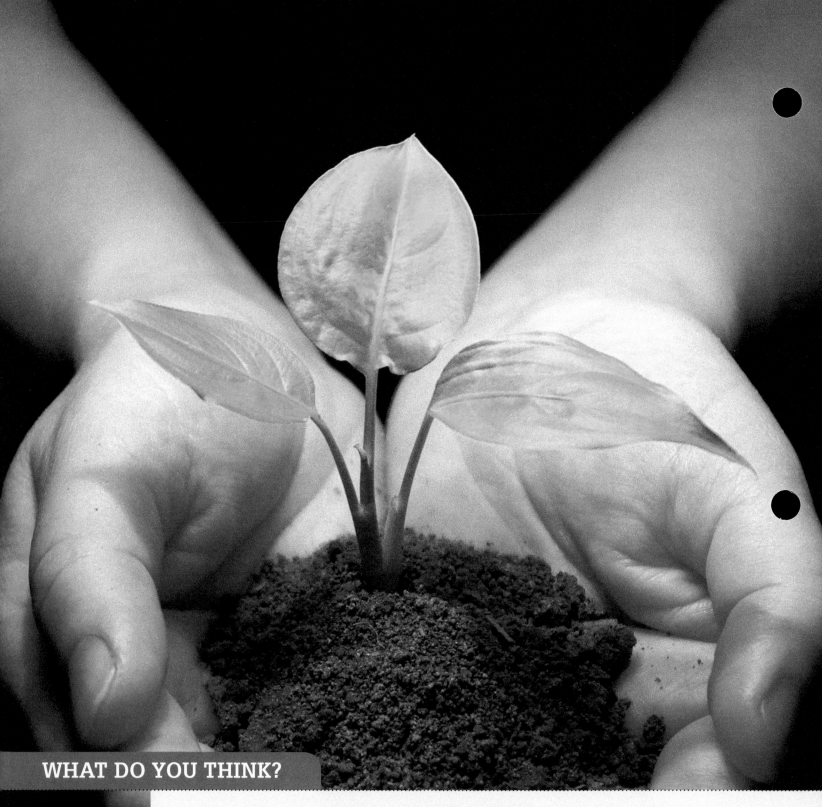

WHAT DO YOU THINK?

- Does climate change pose a risk to global health?
- Does the air you breathe affect your well-being?
- How can you reduce your exposure to indoor pollutants?
- Are you jeopardizing your hearing health?

© Pakhnyushcha/Shutterstock.com

19

A Healthier Environment

Until college Neri's commitment to the environment consisted of carrying the recyclables out to the curb every week. She opted to live in a "green" residence hall on campus because she liked the light, airy architecture, the plantings everywhere, and the opportunity to join a community of individuals committed to a shared cause. But as Neri learned more about energy sources and usage, living green became a way of life. She stopped

buying plastic bottles of water, relied on natural light whenever possible, and switched to energy-efficient lightbulbs. Like a growing number of students, she joined an environmental action group whose activities included planting trees, setting up recycling centers, and launching energy-conservation makeovers on campus. (See Snapshot: On Campus Now on page 574.)

Some describe the campaign to create a healthier environment and combat climate change as this generation's equivalent of the civil rights movement. Without doubt these issues cannot be ignored. Although

environmental concerns may seem so enormous that nothing any individual can do will have an effect, this is not the case. All of us, as citizens of the world, can help find solutions to the challenges confronting our planet. The first step is realizing that you have a personal responsibility for safeguarding the health of your environment and, thereby, your own well-being.

This chapter explores the complex interrelationships between your world and your well-being. It discusses major threats to the environment, including climate changes; atmospheric changes; air, water, and noise pollution; chemical risks; and radiation. <

After reading this chapter, you should be able to:

19.1 Discuss the relationship between human health and the environment.

19.2 Comment on the impact of pollution on health.

19.3 Describe the health threats posed by polluted air.

19.4 Summarize various paths to achieving sustainability.

19.5 Specify the importance of safe drinking water.

19.6 Explain the impact of indoor air pollution.

19.7 Identify harmful effects of exposure to toxic chemicals on humans.

19.8 Discuss health threats posed by radiation.

19.9 Outline the factors that lead to hearing loss.

🔲 Do Students Care about the Environment?

Incoming freshmen who consider it very important to	Percent
• become involved in programs to clean up the environment	26.4
• participate in a community action program	29.9
• adopt "green" practices to protect the environment	40.7

How would you describe your commitment to a healthier environment? Have you participated in any environmental cleanups? Have you adopted "green" practices in your life? Describe what you've done or what you are ready to commit to doing for the environment's sake in your online journal.

Source: Eagan, K.et al. *The American Freshman: National Norms Fall 2014.* (Los Angeles: Higher Education Research Institute, UCLA, 2014).

The Environment and Your Health

Ours is a planet in peril. Glaciers are melting. Sea levels are rising. Forests are being destroyed. Droughts have become more frequent and more intense. Heat waves have killed tens of thousands of people. Hurricanes and floods have ravaged cities. Millions have died from the effects of air pollution and contaminated water.

The planet Earth—once taken for granted as a ball of rock and water that existed for our use for all time—is a single, fragile **ecosystem** (a community of organisms that share a physical and chemical environment). Our environment is a closed ecosystem, powered by the sun. The materials needed for the survival of this planet must be recycled over and over again. Increasingly, we're realizing just how important the health of this ecosystem is to our own well-being and survival.

For good or for ill, we cannot separate our individual health from that of the environment in which we live. However, efforts to clean up the environment are paying off. According to the American Lung Association, air quality in many cities, particularly in the Northeast and Midwest, has improved in the last decade. In addition to air quality, the water we drink and the chemicals we use also have an impact on the quality of our lives. At the same time, the lifestyle choices we make, the products we use, and the efforts we undertake to clean up a beach or save wetlands affect the quality of our environment. (See Health Now! Protecting the Planet.)

✓ **check-in** What do you see as the greatest environment threat?

Climate Change

The Intergovernmental Panel on Climate Change of the United Nations, made up of leading scientists from around the world, has reported with absolute certainty that the world's climate is changing in significant ways and will continue to do so in the foreseeable future. These experts predict an increase in extreme weather events (such as hurricanes and heat waves), greater weather variability, and rising water temperatures. The American Association for the Advancement of Science (AAAS) and other prestigious institutions around the world have issued warnings on the growing dangers of global climate change.

Global Warming

Earth's average temperature increased about one to two degrees in the twentieth century to approximately 59 degrees, but the rate of warming in the last three decades has been three times the average rate since 1900. Seas have risen about six to eight feet globally over the last century and are rising at a higher rate.

Why is our planet getting warmer? Figure 19.1 shows the normal greenhouse effect: Certain gases in Earth's atmosphere trap energy from the sun

ecosystem A community of organisms sharing a physical and chemical environment and interacting with each other.

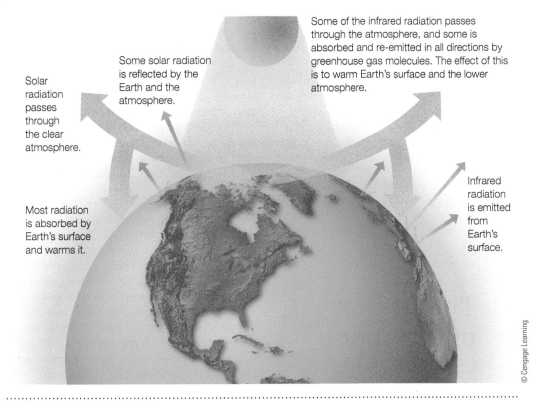

Some solar radiation is reflected by the Earth and the atmosphere.

Solar radiation passes through the clear atmosphere.

Some of the infrared radiation passes through the atmosphere, and some is absorbed and re-emitted in all directions by greenhouse gas molecules. The effect of this is to warm Earth's surface and the lower atmosphere.

Most radiation is absorbed by Earth's surface and warms it.

Infrared radiation is emitted from Earth's surface.

© Cengage Learning

FIGURE 19.1 The Greenhouse Effect

The normal greenhouse effect warms Earth to a hospitable temperature. An increase in greenhouse gases intensifies the greenhouse effect, trapping more heat and raising Earth's temperature.

and retain heat somewhat like the glass panels of a greenhouse. These greenhouse gases include carbon dioxide, methane, and nitrous oxide. Human activities, scientists now say with 90 percent certainty, have increased the greenhouse gases in our atmosphere. We burn fossil fuels (oil, natural gas, and coal) and wood products, which release carbon dioxide into the atmosphere. We produce coal, natural gas, and oil, which emit methane. Livestock and the decomposition of organic wastes also produce methane. Agricultural and industrial processes emit nitrous oxide. These emissions enhance the normal greenhouse effect, trapping more heat and raising the temperature of the atmosphere and Earth's surface.

After years of doubt and debate, most leading experts agree that the buildup of greenhouse gases is changing natural climate and weather patterns in new and potentially dangerous ways. Carbon dioxide levels are higher now than at any time in the past 800,000 years and, according to the AAAS, are "heading for levels not experienced for millions of years."

The Health Risks

Some scientists argue that climate change is "the greatest threat to global health."[1] Global warming

and related changes can imperil health indirectly through the following:

- More frequent and intense heat waves
- Flooding
- More extreme weather, such as hurricanes, tornadoes, cyclones, and tsunamis
- More severe droughts

All of these could jeopardize physical and psychological well-being, particularly among the most vulnerable members of society, such as children and the elderly.[2]

Global warming also affect health indirectly by changing the patterns of infectious diseases, supplies of fresh water, and food availability. For example, as the planet continues to warm, infectious diseases—particularly mosquito-borne illnesses such as malaria, dengue fever, yellow fever, and encephalitis—may spread to more regions. Already in the United States, mosquitoes and other insects that carry diseases such as West Nile virus, Rocky Mountain spotted fever, and Lyme disease are spreading to areas once considered too cold for these insects to survive. The rise in global temperatures has already led to a greater pollen load and more allergies among more people.

Climate change poses a serious risk to global health, a recent analysis concluded, but it is not any more catastrophic than other threats, such as poverty and lack of access to clean water and adequate nutrition. This is true in part because of the time lag between exposure to greenhouse emissions and their impact on the environment.[3] However, if steps are not taken to reduce global warming, Earth's inhabitants will face ever-increasing dangers in the future.

√**check-in** How concerned are you about climate change as a threat to your health? To others on the planet? To the next generation?

The Impact of Pollution

Any change in the air, water, or soil that could reduce its ability to support life is a form of **pollution**. Natural events, such as smoke from fires triggered by lightning, can cause pollution. However, most sources of pollution are man-made. There are now about ten times as many cars around the world as there were 50 years ago. The number of people living in cities has increased by more than a factor of four, and global energy consumption by nearly a factor of five.

The effects of pollution depend on the concentration (amount per unit of air, water, or soil) of the **pollutant**, how long it remains in the environment, and its chemical nature. An *acute effect* is a severe, immediate reaction, usually after a single, large exposure. For example, pesticide poisoning can cause nausea, dizziness, and even death. A *chronic effect* may take years to develop or may be a recurrent or continuous reaction, usually after repeated exposure. Years of exposure to traffic pollution, for instance, has been linked to an increase in blood pressure.

Environmental agents that trigger changes, or *mutations*, in the genetic material (the DNA) of living cells are called **mutagens**. The changes that result can lead to the development of cancer. A substance or agent that causes cancer is a **carcinogen**: All carcinogens are mutagens; most mutagens are carcinogens. Furthermore, when a mutagen affects an egg or a sperm cell, its effects can be passed on to future generations. Mutagens that can cross the placenta of a pregnant woman and cause a spontaneous abortion or birth defects in the fetus are called *teratogens*.

Pollution is a hazard to all who breathe. Deaths caused by air pollution exceed those from motor vehicle injuries. Those with respiratory illnesses and other chronic health problems are at greatest risk during days when smog or allergen counts are high. However, as a recent study showed, even healthy college students suffer impairments in their heart and circulatory systems as a result of urban air pollution. The effects of carbon monoxide are much worse in smokers, who already have higher levels of the gas in their blood.

Pollution can even pose a threat to unborn children. One recent study linked exposure in the womb to chemicals commonly found in plastics to lower IQs and poorer learning skills at age 7.[4] According to other reports, children born to mothers exposed to high levels of air pollution late in pregnancy may have an increased risk of developing autism spectrum disorder[5] and experiencing blood pressure abnormalities as newborns.[6]

As carbon dioxide levels in the air rise due to the greenhouse effect, air quality will worsen. Gases found in polluted air—such as ozone, sulfur dioxide, and nitrogen dioxide—contribute to heart disease and worsen the health of individuals who already have heart conditions. Poor air quality also contributes to breathing difficulties and may be responsible for the dramatic increase in asthma in

pollution Any change in the air, water, or soil that could reduce its ability to support life.

pollutant A substance or agent in the environment, usually the by-product of human industry or activity, that is injurious to human, animal, or plant life.

mutagens Agents that cause alterations in the genetic material of living cells.

carcinogen A substance or agent that causes cancer.

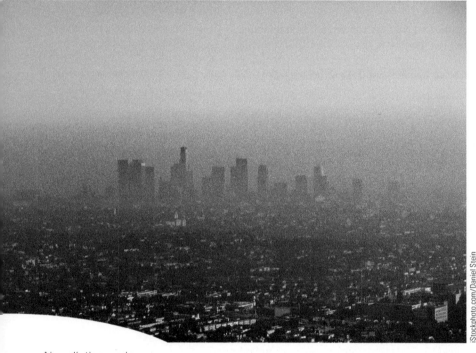

iStockphoto.com/Daniel Stein

Air pollution endangers the well-being of more than half of Americans, including many city dwellers.

recent decades. Elevated carbon dioxide levels can trigger asthma attacks and allergies by increasing ragweed pollen. Greater carbon dioxide in the air also stimulates the growth of poison ivy and other nuisance plants.

Toxic substances in polluted air can enter the human body in three ways: through the skin, through the digestive system, and through the lungs. The combined interaction of two or more hazards can produce an effect greater than that of either one alone. Pollutants can affect an organ or organ system directly or indirectly.

Among the health problems that have been linked with pollution are the following:

- Headaches and dizziness

- Decline in cognitive functioning[7]

- Eye irritation and impaired vision

- Nasal discharge

- Cough, shortness of breath, and sore throat

- Constricted airways

- Constriction of blood vessels and increased risk of heart disease

- Increased risk of stroke and of dying from a stroke

- Chest pains and aggravation of the symptoms of colds, pneumonia, bronchial asthma, emphysema, chronic bronchitis, lung cancer, and other respiratory problems

- Birth defects and reproductive problems including lower success with in-vitro fertilization

- Nausea, vomiting, and stomach cancer

- Allergies and asthma from diesel fumes in polluted air

The Air You Breathe

Remember the last time you stood at a busy intersection as a bus or truck spewed brownish fumes in your face? Maybe your eyes stung, or your throat burned. But breathing polluted air can do more than irritate: It can take months or even years off your life. Fortunately, as air pollution in the United States has declined, American life expectancy has improved.[8]

However, more than half the nation's population still live in areas with dangerous levels of air pollution. As pollutants destroy the hairlike cilia that remove irritants from the lungs, individuals may suffer chronic bronchitis,

characterized by excessive mucus flow and continuous coughing. Emphysema may develop or worsen, as pollutants constrict the bronchial tubes and destroy the air sacs in the lungs, making breathing more difficult. Long-term exposure to air pollution may speed up the process of atherosclerosis (discussed in Chapter 10).[9] Other health threats include stroke, heart failure, and lung troubles.[10]

Even healthy individuals can be affected, particularly if they exercise outdoors during high-pollution periods or spend long periods in dirty air. Breathing air pollution can increase the risk for heart attack by nearly 5 percent.[11] Some people are at increased risk, including those

- Who have had a heart attack or angioplasty

- Who have angina, heart failure, some types of heart rhythm problems, or diabetes

- Who have asthma

- With known risk factors for heart disease, such as smoking cigarettes

- With high blood pressure or high blood cholesterol

- With a family history of stroke or early heart disease (father or brother diagnosed before 55 years of age; mother or sister diagnosed before 65 years of age)

- Who are older than 65 years of age

Ozone

Ozone, the primary ingredient of smog air pollution, can impair the body's immune system and cause long-term lung damage. (Ozone in the upper atmosphere protects us by repelling harmful ultraviolet radiation from the sun, but ozone in the lower atmosphere is a harmful component of air pollution.) Automobiles also produce carbon monoxide, a colorless and odorless gas that diminishes the ability of red blood cells to carry oxygen. The resulting oxygen deficiency can affect breathing, hearing, and vision in humans and stunt the growth of plants and trees.

Several large investigations have confirmed that ozone at levels currently found in the United States can shorten lives. Even on days when ozone levels are below the national standard, the risk of premature death is greater in areas with higher levels. The individuals most vulnerable to the effects of ozone are children, senior citizens, people who work or exercise outdoors, those with a respiratory disease such as asthma, and "responders" who are otherwise healthy but respond intensely to ozone.

Ozone's other ill effects include shortness of breath, chest pain when inhaling deeply,

ozone A component of smog that can impair the body's immune system and cause long-term lung damage.

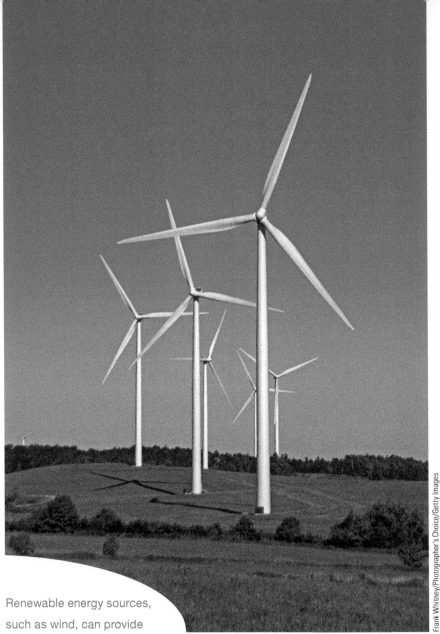

Renewable energy sources, such as wind, can provide more environmentally friendly alternatives. However, individual choices and behaviors also have an impact on the state of our world.

sustainability A method of using a resource so that the resource is not depleted or permanently damaged.

precycling The use of products that are packaged in recycled or recyclable material.

recycling The processing or reuse of manufactured materials to reduce consumption of raw materials.

or sneeze large particles out of our bodies, but they don't keep out smaller particles, which get trapped in the lungs. The smallest ones pass through the lungs into the bloodstream.

Particle pollution damages the body in ways similar to cigarette smoking. Even short-term exposure can be deadly because particle pollution increases the risk of heart attacks and strokes, especially among the elderly and those with heart conditions. It also diminishes lung function, causes inflammation of lung tissue in young, healthy adults, increases the number and severity of asthma attacks, and increases mortality in infants and young children.

Living near highways or spending time in heavy traffic, whether driving or taking public transportation, may be especially dangerous. Several studies have found an increased risk of premature death in those who live, work, drive, or ride in high-traffic areas.[12]

Particle pollution—considered the most dangerous because it can be an immediate as well as a long-term threat to life—has increased in the eastern part of the United States but decreased in the West. Cities that have reduced particle pollution—such as Pittsburgh, Buffalo, Los Angeles, Indianapolis, and St. Louis—have reported gains in life expectancy.

wheezing, coughing, and increased susceptibility to respiratory infections. Studies of college freshmen who were lifelong residents of Los Angeles or the San Francisco Bay Area found that long exposure to elevated ozone levels had reduced their "lung function," that is, their lungs' ability to work efficiently. Although ozone levels have declined, Los Angeles, Bakersfield, and Visalia, all in California, remain the most ozone-polluted cities in the United States.

Particle Pollution

Scientists refer to the mix of very tiny solid and liquid particles in the air as *particle pollution*. The particles themselves can range in size from microscopic to one-tenth the diameter of a strand of hair. Our natural defenses help us to cough

Working toward Sustainability

More universities are developing programs to achieve **sustainability**, the use of as little as possible of resources that cannot be renewed. Innovative programs include green dorms and campaigns to reduce energy waste. Not all undergraduates share this concern, but higher numbers express commitment to environmental action than in the past.

Three important paths to sustainability are precycling, recycling, and composting. **Precycling** refers to buying products packaged in recycled materials. According to the consumer group Earthworks, packaging makes up a third of what people in the United States throw away. When you precycle, you consider how you're going to dispose of a product and the packaging materials before purchasing it. For example, you might choose eggs in recyclable cardboard packages, rather than in foam cartons, and look for juice and milk in refillable bottles.

Recycling—collecting, reprocessing, marketing, and reusing materials once considered

Frank Whitney/Photographer's Choice/Getty Images

trash—serves several important functions, including the following:

- **Preserving natural resources.** Reprocessing used materials to make new products and packaging reduces the consumption of natural resources. Recycling steel saves iron ore, coal, and limestone. Recycling newsprint, office paper, and mixed paper saves trees.

- **Saving energy.** Recycling used aluminum cans, for instance, requires only about 5 percent of the energy needed to produce aluminum. Recycling just one can save enough electricity to light a 100-watt bulb for 3½ hours.

- **Reducing greenhouse gas emissions.** Recycling cuts these gases by decreasing the amount of energy used to produce and transport new products.

- **Decreasing the need for landfill storage or incineration.** Both are more costly and can contribute to air pollution.

Different communities take different approaches to recycling. Many provide regular curbside pickup of recyclables, and others have drop-off centers. Buyback centers pay for recyclables. In some places, reverse vending machines accept returned beverage containers and provide deposit refunds.

Discarded computers, other electronic devices, and printer cartridges also should be recycled, by donating them to schools or charitable organizations. "Tech trash" buried in landfills is creating a new hazard because trace amounts of potentially hazardous agents, such as lead and mercury, can leak into the ground and water. Find out if your campus has a program to recycle electronic devices.

With *composting*—which some people describe as nature's way of recycling—you can see the benefits as close as your backyard. Organic products, such as leftover food and vegetable peels, are mixed with straw or other dry material and kept damp. Bacteria eat the organic material and turn it into a rich soil. Some people keep a compost pile (which should be stirred every few days) in their backyards; others take their organic garbage (including mowed grass and dead leaves) to community gardens or municipal composting sites.

The Water You Drink

Fears about the public water supply have led many Americans to turn off their taps. About two-thirds take steps to drink purer water, either by using filtration and distillation methods or by drinking bottled water. However, Consumers Union, a nonprofit advocacy group, maintains that the United States has the safest water supply in the world. The Environmental Protection Agency has set standards for some 80 contaminants. These include many toxic chemicals and heavy metals—including lead, mercury, cadmium, and chromium—that can cause kidney and nervous system damage and birth defects.

Each year the CDC reports an average of 7,400 cases of illness related to the water people drink. The most common culprits include parasites, bacteria, viruses, chemicals, and lead. Traces of prescription drugs also have been found in the water of some communities. Home filters can block certain pathogens that can cause diarrhea and other gastrointestinal problems, but they do not seem to remove most chemical contaminants. If you

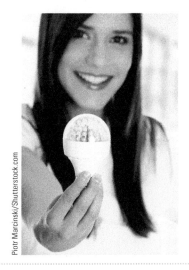

⚠ CONSUMER ALERT

What Difference Does a Lightbulb Make?

Facts to Know

- Not all lightbulbs are the same. Incandescent bulbs use electricity to heat a metal filament until it becomes white hot or incandescent. In a compact fluorescent bulb (CFL), an electric current flows between electrodes at each end of a tube containing gases, producing ultraviolet (UV) light that is transferred into visible light when it strikes a phosphor coating on the inside of the bulb. In LED (light emitting diode) products, an electrical current passes through semiconductor material, which illuminates the tiny diodes.

- A CFL bulb that qualifies for the government's Energy Star symbol lasts about ten times longer and saves about $30 or more in electricity over an incandescent bulb. Because of its even higher efficiency and lower power usage, an LED bulb is 80 percent cheaper to run than a conventional bulb.

- LEDs, which cost significantly more to purchase, are more environmentally friendly and economical in the long run. They last longer, don't produce heat and carbon dioxide emissions like incandescent bulbs do, and normally don't contain any toxic materials like the mercury vapor in CFLs.

Steps to Take

- When shopping for a lightbulb, look for the federal Energy Star label. This indicates that the bulb uses about 70 to 90 percent less energy than traditional incandescent bulbs, lasts 10 to 25 times longer, saves $30 to $80 in electricity costs over its lifetime, and produces about 70 to 90 percent less heat so it is safer to operate.

- If you buy CFL bulb be careful when removing them from their packaging and unscrewing them because they are made of glass and contain mercury. Screw and unscrew bulbs by their bases, not the glass. Never forcefully twist a CFL into a light socket.

- Some LED bulbs may look like familiar lightbulbs and some may not, but they can outperform traditional lightbulbs— if they carry an Energy Star label. A general-purpose LED bulb that does not qualify for the Energy Star label may not distribute light in all directions and therefore not work well in a table lamp.

decide to use a filter, clean it regularly to prevent a buildup of bacteria.

✓**check-in** Do you use a water filter? If so, clean or replace it regularly to prevent buildup of bacteria.

Is Bottled Better?

Consumers seem convinced that bottled water is purer than tap. The market for bottled water in the United States has been growing by 10 percent per year, making it second only to soft drinks as America's favorite beverage. On average we drink about 25 gallons of bottled water every year, compared to 51.5 gallons of soft drinks and 21 gallons of beer.

However, medical researchers have not found a scientific reason to recommend bottled water over tap water. Dentists report an increase in cavities among children and teenagers who drink bottled water rather than fluoridated tap water. Recent studies found a "negligible" risk of exposure to chemicals in plastic products for young children.[13] Despite images of mountain streams and glacier peaks on the labels, most bottled water comes from urban water supplies.

✓**check-in** Did you know that an estimated 25 to 30 percent of bottled water sold in this country is, in fact, tap water, sometimes further treated and sometimes not?

Portable Water Bottles

The simplest, safest, most ecofriendly water container is a glass. If you want to carry water with you, you have plenty of alternatives, but some portable drinking containers may pose risks to you or to the environment.

Most disposable water bottles are made with lightweight polyethylene terephthalate (PET). Reusing these bottles may pose some health dangers, although there is little scientific agreement on how serious these risks may be. Your mouth leaves a residue of bacteria when you drink from a bottle, and these bacteria may accumulate with repeated use. Disposable bottles also pose a risk to the environment. The manufacture of the estimated 30 billion PET water bottles sold annually in the United States requires about 17 million barrels of oil. About 86 percent of these bottles become waste.

✓**check-in** Did you know that it may take as long as 400 to 1,000 years for some disposable water bottles to degrade once dumped in a landfill?

Many consumers have switched to harder bottles made with polycarbonate plastic (known by brand names such as Camelbak and Nalgene). Portable metal containers are another option. Some bottles are aluminum with a nontoxic liner; others are simply made of stainless steel.

Indoor Pollutants: The Inside Story

You may think of pollution as primarily a threat when you're outdoors, but people in industrialized societies spend more than 90 percent of their time inside buildings. Think of how much time you spend in your dorm, apartment, or home and in classrooms, dining halls, movie theaters, offices, stores, and shops. The quality of the air you breathe inside these places can have an even greater impact on your well-being than outdoor pollution. (See Health on a Budget.)

Some sources—such as building materials and household products such as air fresheners—release pollutants more or less continuously. Other sources—such as tobacco smoke, solvents in cleaning products, and pesticides—can produce high levels of pollutants that remain in the air for long periods after their use.

Wood-burning fireplaces and stoves also pose a risk to both indoor and outdoor air quality because the smoke contains fine particles that, as discussed earlier in this chapter, can injure the lungs, blood vessels, and heart.[14]

Environmental Tobacco Smoke (ETS)

The mixture of smoke from the burning end of a cigarette, pipe, or cigar and a smoker's exhalations contains over 4,000 compounds, more than 40 of which are known to cause cancer in humans or animals. More than half of U.S. states have enacted smoking bans in private worksites, restaurants, bars, airports, schools, hospitals, and many other locations. However, some states, mainly in the South and parts of the West, have resisted comprehensive bans. As a result, about 88 million nonsmokers in the United States are still exposed to environmental tobacco smoke.

Secondhand Smoke At greatest risk for the dangers of "passive smoking" or "secondhand smoke" are infants and young children and youngsters with asthma or other respiratory problems. Children exposed to secondhand

No- and Low-Cost Ways to Green Your Space

Whether you live in a dorm, apartment, or house, you can take simple, inexpensive steps to create a greener personal environment. Here are some ways to get started. (See Figure 19.2 for more ideas.)

- **Buy furniture and household items secondhand, or recycle your parents' things.** If you can't find everything you need in the attic or basement, try a website such as **www.freecycle.com**, where you can barter your way to greener furnishings.

- **Choose recycled notebooks and printer paper and ecofriendly shampoos, conditioners, and lotions.**

- **Rather than relying on air-conditioning or central heat, use a space heater or fan, depending on the season, to regulate the temperature around you.**

- **Buy a stainless steel or coated aluminum water bottle instead of using disposable bottles.**

- **Use green cleaning products like vinegar and baking soda instead of expensive and potentially harmful chemicals.**

- **Tote books and groceries in canvas bags rather than paper or plastic ones.**

- **Chip in with roommates or friends so you can buy in bulk, which saves money and requires less packaging.**

- **Don't throw anything out before asking yourself if it can be recycled, donated, or simply used in another way.**

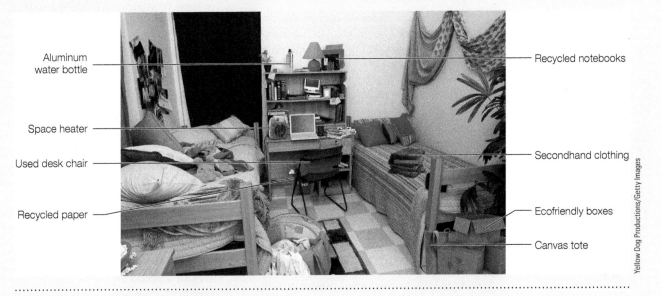

Aluminum water bottle

Space heater

Used desk chair

Recycled paper

Recycled notebooks

Secondhand clothing

Ecofriendly boxes

Canvas tote

Yellow Dog Productions/Getty Images

FIGURE 19.2 Greening Your Space

smoke face a much higher likelihood of high blood pressure and other risks for heart disease by age 13 than other children. (See Chapter 14 for a further discussion of the health risks of environmental tobacco smoke.)

Health effects of secondhand smoke include eye, nose, and throat irritation; headaches; and lung cancer. In children, the health effects include increased risk of lower respiratory tract infections, such as bronchitis and pneumonia, and ear infections; buildup of fluid in the middle ear; increased severity and frequency of asthma episodes; and decreased lung function. Pregnant women who live or work with smokers may be at higher risk of having a stillbirth. The greater your exposure to secondhand smoke, the more

likely you are to develop early signs of heart disease.[15]

Thirdhand Smoke   Tobacco smoke creates more than an odor in a room. According to a recent study, tobacco residue—dubbed "thirdhand smoke"—contains cancer-causing toxins that stick to a variety of surfaces, where they can get into the dust and be picked up on the fingers. Babies and young children are most likely to be exposed to these harmful chemicals.

Radon

Created by the breakdown of uranium in rocks, soil, and water, radon is the second-leading cause of lung cancer. Colorless and odorless, this radioactive gas enters homes through dirt floors, cracks in concrete walls and floors, floor drains, and sumps. When radon becomes trapped in buildings and concentrations build up indoors, exposure to the gas becomes a concern.

- **Sources:** Earth and rock beneath home; well water; building materials. Houses in the Northeast and Midwest tend to have higher radon levels than those elsewhere in the United States.

- **Health Effects:** No immediate symptoms. Exposure to high levels of radon increases the risk of lung cancer. Smokers are at higher risk of developing radon-induced lung cancer. Each year lung cancer caused by radon exposure kills about 21,000 Americans.[16]

- **Steps to Reduce Exposure:**

  - If you have any reason to suspect a radon problem in your home, you can buy inexpensive, do-it-yourself radon test kits online and in hardware stores. Look for ones that are state-certified or have met the requirements of a national radon proficiency program.

  - If testing reveals unsafe levels, contractors trained to fix radon problems can make changes to reduce the risk.

  - For more information on radon, contact your state radon office, or call 800-SOS-RADON.

Molds and Other Biological Contaminants

Bacteria, mildew, viruses, animal dander, cat saliva, house dust mites, cockroaches, and pollen can all pose a threat to health. One of the oldest and most widespread substances on Earth, mold—a type of fungus that decomposes organic matter and provides plants with nutrients—has emerged as a major health concern. Common molds include *Aspergillus, Penicillium,* and *Stachybotrys,* a slimy, dark green mold that has been blamed for infant deaths and various illnesses, from Alzheimer's disease to cancer, in adults that breathe in its spores. Faulty ventilation systems and airtight buildings have been implicated as contributing to the increased mold problem.

- **Sources:** Wet or moist walls, ceilings, carpets, and furniture; poorly maintained humidifiers, dehumidifiers, and air conditioners; bedding; household pets.

- **Health Effects:** Eye, nose, and throat irritation; shortness of breath; dizziness; lethargy; fever; digestive problems. Diseases like

humidifier fever are associated with exposure to toxins that can grow in ventilation systems of large buildings. However, these diseases can also be traced to microorganisms in home heating and cooling systems and humidifiers. Children, the elderly, and people with breathing problems, allergies, and lung diseases are particularly susceptible to disease-causing biological agents in the indoor air.

- **Steps to Reduce Exposure:**

  - Use fans vented to outdoors in kitchens and bathrooms.

  - Clean cool-mist and ultrasonic humidifiers in accordance with manufacturer's instructions and refill with clean water daily.

  - Empty water trays in air conditioners, dehumidifiers, and refrigerators frequently.

  - Keep your personal living space clean. No, your mother may not be checking on you, but regular cleaning reduces house dust mites, pollens, animal dander, and other allergy-causing agents.

Household Products

- **Sources:** The liquids, foams, gels, and other materials you use to clean, disinfect, degrease, polish, wax, and preserve contain powerful chemicals that can pollute indoor air during and for long periods after their use. Researchers have found levels of some 55 common organic pollutants in common products such as soaps, lotions, detergents, cleaners, sunscreens, air fresheners, kitty litters, shaving creams, vinyl shower curtains, cosmetics, and perfumes.

- **Health Effects:** Eye, nose, and throat irritation; headaches, loss of coordination, and nausea; damage to liver, kidney, and central nervous system. In women they also may lower estrogen and lead to earlier menopause. Exposure to bisphenol A (BPA), a controversial chemical commonly used to make plastics such as that used to hold packaged food and drinks, may increase a healthy person's risk of developing heart disease later in life.

- **Steps to Reduce Exposure:**

  - Follow instructions carefully. If the label says to use the product in a well-ventilated area, go outdoors or open windows to provide the maximum amount of outdoor air possible.

  - Use one household care product at a time. Mixing can create dangerous chemical reactions.

  - Throw away partially full containers of old or unneeded chemicals, which can leak gases even when closed. Do not simply toss them in the garbage can. Find out if your local government or any organization in your community sponsors special days for the collection of toxic household wastes. If no such collection days are available, think about organizing one.

- Buy limited quantities. Purchase only as much as you will use right away.

- Keep to a minimum any exposure to emissions from products containing methylene chloride, such as paint strippers, adhesive removers, and aerosol spray paints. Methylene chloride is converted to carbon monoxide in the body and can cause symptoms associated with exposure to carbon monoxide.

√**check-in** Have you ever had an adverse reaction to a cleaning product or a cosmetic?

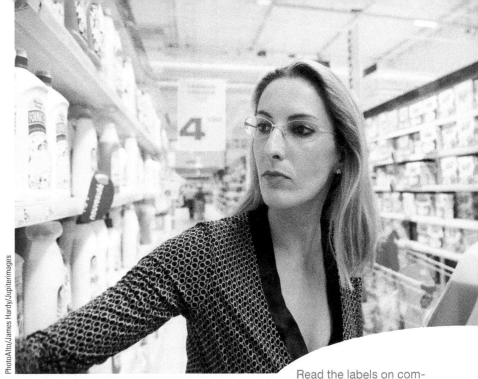

Read the labels on common cleaning products and follow instructions for use and storage to avoid possible health risks.

Formaldehyde

Some indoor pollutants come from the very materials that buildings are made of and from the appliances inside them. Formaldehyde is commonly used in building materials, carpet backing, furniture, foam insulation, plywood, and particle board. This chemical can cause nausea, dizziness, headaches, heart palpitations, stinging eyes, and burning lungs. Formaldehyde gas, which is colorless and odorless, has been shown to cause cancer in animals. Most manufacturers have voluntarily quit using it, but many homes already contain materials made with urea-formaldehyde, which can seep into the air.

The rate at which products like pressed wood or textiles release formaldehyde can change. Formaldehyde emissions will generally decrease as products age. When the products are new, high indoor temperatures or humidity can cause increased release of formaldehyde from these products.

- **Sources:** Pressed wood products (hardwood plywood wall paneling, particle board, fiberboard) and furniture made with these pressed wood products; urea-formaldehyde foam insulation (UFFI); combustion sources and environmental tobacco smoke; durable press drapes, other textiles, and glues.

- **Health Effects:** Watery eyes, burning sensations in the eyes and throat, nausea, and difficulty in breathing. High concentrations may trigger attacks in people with asthma. Has been shown to cause cancer in animals and may cause cancer in humans.

Pesticides

According to a recent survey, 75 percent of U.S. households used at least one pesticide product indoors during the past year. Products used most often are insecticides and disinfectants.

The EPA requires manufacturers to put information on the label about when and how to use a pesticide. Remember that the "-cide" in pesticides means "to kill." Pesticides are also made up of ingredients that are used to carry the active agent. These carrier agents are called "inerts" because they are not toxic to the targeted pest; nevertheless, some inerts are capable of causing health problems.

- **Sources:** Pesticides used in and around the home include products to control insects (insecticides), termites (termiticides), rodents (rodenticides), fungi (fungicides), and microbes (disinfectants). They are sold as sprays, liquids, sticks, powders, crystals, balls, and foggers.

- **Health Effects:** High levels of certain pesticides can produce various symptoms, including headaches, dizziness, muscle twitching, weakness, tingling sensations, and nausea. They also might cause long-term damage to the liver and the central nervous system, as well as an increased risk of cancer and of shorter pregnancies and smaller babies.

- **Steps to Reduce Exposure:**
  - Follow instructions. It is illegal to use any pesticide in any manner inconsistent with the directions on its label.

- Use only the pesticides approved for use by the general public and then only in recommended amounts; increasing the amount does not offer more protection. Ventilate the area well after pesticide use.

- If possible, take plants and pets outside when applying pesticides to them.

- Dispose of unwanted pesticides according to the directions on the label or on special household hazardous waste collection days.

- Use nonchemical methods of pest control where possible.

- Keep indoor spaces clean, dry, and well ventilated to avoid pest and odor problems.

- Minimize exposure to moth repellents, which contain paradichlorobenzene, a chemical known to cause cancer in animals. If using mothballs, place them and the items to be protected in trunks or other containers that can be stored in areas such as attics and detached garages. Do not buy air fresheners that contain paradichlorobenzene.

Asbestos

This mineral fiber has been used commonly in a variety of building construction materials for insulation and as a fire-retardant. The government has banned several asbestos products, and manufacturers have also voluntarily limited use of asbestos. Today asbestos is most commonly found in older homes, pipe and furnace insulation materials, asbestos shingles, millboard, textured paints, and floor tiles.

- **Sources:** Deteriorating, damaged, or disturbed insulation, fireproofing, acoustical materials, and floor tiles.

- **Health Effects:** Too small to be visible, the most dangerous asbestos fibers accumulate in the lungs and can cause lung cancer, mesothelioma (a cancer of the chest and abdominal linings), and asbestosis (irreversible lung scarring that can be fatal). Symptoms of these diseases do not show up until many years after exposure began. Smokers are at higher risk of developing asbestos-induced lung cancer.

- **Steps to Reduce Exposure:**

  - Leave undamaged asbestos material alone if it is not likely to be disturbed.

  - Use trained and qualified contractors for control measures that may disturb asbestos and for cleanup.

  - Follow proper procedures in replacing woodstove door gaskets that may contain asbestos.

Lead

People are exposed to lead, a long-recognized health threat, through air, drinking water, food, contaminated soil, deteriorating paint, and dust. Airborne lead enters the body when an individual breathes or swallows lead particles or dust. Before its risks were known, lead was used in paint, gasoline, water pipes, and many other products. Although lead exposure has declined, about 2.6 percent of children ages 1 to 5 still have dangerous levels of lead in their blood.[17] Boys are at greater risk than girls because female hormones may protect the brain against lead's harmful effects.[18]

- **Sources:** Lead-based paint; contaminated soil, dust, and drinking water.

- **Health Effects:** Lead affects practically all systems within the body. Lead at high levels can cause convulsions, coma, and even death. Lower levels of lead can cause adverse health effects on the central nervous system, kidney, and blood cells. In pregnant women, even small amounts can significantly increase blood pressure. Infants and children are more vulnerable to lead exposure than adults—lead is more easily absorbed into growing bodies, and the tissues of small children are more sensitive to the damaging effects of lead. Children may have higher exposures since they are more likely to get lead dust on their hands and then put their fingers or other lead-contaminated objects into their mouths.

- **Steps to Reduce Exposure:**

  - Keep areas where children play as dust-free and clean as possible.

  - Leave lead-based paint undisturbed if it is in good condition; do not sand or burn off paint that may contain lead.

  - Do not remove lead paint yourself.

  - Do not bring lead dust into the home.

  - If your work or hobby involves lead, change clothes and use doormats before entering your home.

  - Eat a balanced diet rich in calcium, iron, and vitamin C. High levels of ascorbic acid (vitamin C) have been associated with a lower rate of elevated blood lead levels.

Carbon Monoxide and Nitrogen Dioxide

Carbon monoxide (CO) gas—which is tasteless, odorless, colorless, and nonirritating—can be deadly. Produced by the incomplete combustion of fuel in space heaters, furnaces, water heaters, and engines, CO reduces the delivery of oxygen in the blood. Every year an estimated 10,000 Americans seek treatment for CO inhalation; at least 250 die because of this silent killer. Those most at risk are the chronically ill, the elderly, pregnant women, and infants.

- **Sources:** Unvented kerosene and gas space heaters; leaking chimneys and furnaces; back-drafting from furnaces, gas water heaters, woodstoves, and fireplaces; gas stoves; automobile exhaust from attached garages.

- **Health Effects:** At low concentrations, fatigue in healthy people and chest pain in people with heart disease. At higher concentrations, impaired vision and coordination; headaches; dizziness; confusion; nausea. Can cause flu-like symptoms that clear up after leaving home. Fatal at very high concentrations.

Another dangerous gas, nitrogen dioxide (NO_2), can reach very high levels if you use a natural gas or propane stove in a poorly ventilated kitchen. This gas may lead to respiratory illnesses. Pilot lights are a steady source of nitrogen dioxide; to reduce exposure, switch to spark ignition.

- **Sources:** Kerosene heaters, unvented gas stoves and heaters.

- **Health Effects:** Eye, nose, and throat irritation. May cause impaired lung function and increased respiratory infections in young children.

- **Steps to Reduce Exposure to Both CO and NO_2:**
  - Keep appliances properly adjusted.
  - Open flues when fireplaces are in use.
  - Do not idle a car inside the garage.

Chemical Risks

Various chemicals, including benzene, asbestos, and arsenic, have been shown to cause cancer in humans. Probable carcinogens include DDT and PCB. Risks can be greatly increased with simultaneous exposures to more than one carcinogen—for example, tobacco smoke and asbestos.

According to the CDC, the levels of potentially harmful chemicals, including pesticides and lead, in Americans' blood have declined. Still, an estimated 50,000 to 70,000 U.S. workers die each year of chronic diseases related to past exposure to toxic substances, including lung cancer, bladder cancer, leukemia, lymphoma, chronic bronchitis, and disorders of the nervous system. **Endocrine disruptors**, chemicals that act as or interfere with human hormones, particularly estrogen, may pose

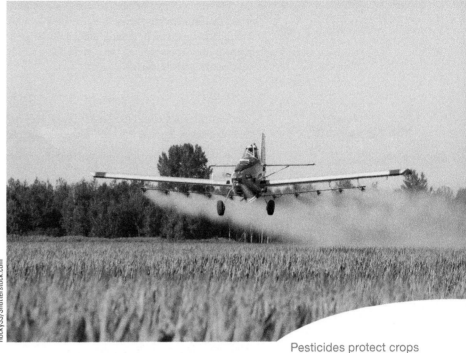

Pesticides protect crops from harmful insects, plants, and fungi but may endanger human health.

a different threat. Scientists are investigating their impact on fertility, falling sperm counts, and cancers of the reproductive organs. Exposure to toxic chemicals causes about 3 percent of developmental defects.

Agricultural Pesticides

High quantities of toxic chemical waste from unused or obsolete pesticides are posing a continuing and worsening threat to people and the environment in Eastern Europe, Africa, Asia, the Middle East, and Latin America. The world's most popular pesticide, Roundup, has been linked to a range of health problems, including cancer, Parkinson's, and infertility.[18] In the United States, the FDA estimates that 33 to 39 percent of our food supply contains residues of pesticides that may pose a long-term danger to our health. Scientists have detected traces of pesticides in groundwater in both urban and rural areas. Exposure to pesticides may pose a risk to pregnant women and their unborn children. Men whose jobs routinely expose them to pesticides may be at increased risk of prostate cancer. Parental exposure does not increase the likelihood of childhood brain cancer.

Chlorinated hydrocarbons include several high-risk substances—such as DDT, kepone, and chlordane—that have been restricted or banned because they may cause cancer, birth defects, neurological disorders, and damage to wildlife and the environment. They are extremely resistant to breakdown.

Organophosphates, including chemicals such as malathion, break down more rapidly than

endocrine disruptors Synthetic chemicals that interfere with the ways that hormones work in humans and wildlife.

chlorinated hydrocarbons Highly toxic pesticides, such as DDT and chlordane, that are extremely resistant to breakdown; may cause cancer, birth defects, neurological disorders, and damage to wildlife and the environment.

organophosphates Toxic pesticides that may cause cancer, birth defects, neurological disorders, and damage to wildlife and the environment.

the chlorinated hydrocarbons. Most are highly toxic, causing cramps, confusion, diarrhea, vomiting, headaches, and breathing difficulties. Higher levels in the blood can lead to convulsions, paralysis, coma, and death.

Chemical Weapons

Terrorist threats include the possibility of the use of chemical weapons. Possible bioterror agents include poison gases, herbicides, and other types of chemical substances that can kill, maim, or temporarily incapacitate. Chemical agents can be dispersed as liquids, vapors, gases, and aerosols that attack nerves, blood, skin, or lungs. In contrast to biological weapons, chemical weapons can kill rapidly, often within hours or minutes, and sometimes with just a small drop. Possible protection against chemical weapons includes gas masks, shelters, and sealed suits and vehicles. Treatment and antidotes can sometimes help after exposure. If contaminated, you need to flush your eyes and skin immediately for at least five to ten minutes while awaiting emergency help.

Multiple Chemical Sensitivity

The proliferation of chemicals in modern society has led to an entirely new disease, **multiple chemical sensitivity (MCS)**, also called environmentally triggered illness, universal allergy, or chemical AIDS. MCS was first described almost a half century ago when a Chicago allergist treated a number of patients who reported becoming ill after being exposed to various petrochemicals. Since that time, many more cases of MCS have been reported, yet there is no agreed-upon definition of the condition, no medical test that can diagnose it, and no proven treatment.

According to medical theory, people become chemically sensitive in a two-step process: First, they experience a major exposure to a chemical, such as a pesticide, a solvent, or a combustion product. The sensitized person then begins to react to low-level chemical exposures from ordinary substances, such as perfumes and tobacco smoke. Symptoms include a runny nose, breathing difficulties, memory problems, chest pain, depression, dizziness, fatigue, headache, inability to concentrate, nausea, aches and pains in muscles and joints, and heart palpitations.

Invisible Threats

Among the unseen threats to health are various forms of *radiation*, energy radiated in the form of waves or particles.

Electromagnetic Fields

Any electrically charged conductor generates two kinds of invisible fields: electric and magnetic. Together they're called **electromagnetic fields (EMFs)**. For years, these fields, produced by household appliances, home wiring, lighting fixtures, electric blankets, and overhead power lines, were considered harmless. However, epidemiological studies have revealed a link between exposure to high-voltage lines and cancer (especially leukemia, a blood cancer) in electrical workers and children.

Exposure to electromagnetic fields can break DNA chains, damage proteins, disturb sleep, cause fatigue, impair memory and concentration, and affect brain and hormonal development.[19]

Researchers have documented increases in breast cancer deaths in women who worked as electrical engineers, electricians, or in other high-exposure jobs, and a link between EMF exposure and increased risk of leukemia and possibly brain cancer.

The National Institute of Environmental Health Sciences concluded that the evidence of a risk of cancer and other human disease from the electric and magnetic fields around power lines is "weak." This finding applies to the extremely low-frequency electric and magnetic fields surrounding both the big power lines that distribute power and the smaller but closer electric lines in homes and appliances. However, the researchers also noted that EMF exposure "cannot be recognized as entirely safe."

Cell Phones

Since cellular phone service was introduced in the United States in 1984, mobile and handheld phones have become ubiquitous, and concern has grown about their possible health risks. The federal government sets upper exposure limits for exposure to electromagnetic energy from cell phones, known as the specific absorption rate (SAR). A phone emits the most radiation during a call, but it also emits small amounts periodically whenever it's turned on.

Researchers have found that a one-hour cell phone conversation stimulates the areas of the brain closest to the phone's antenna, but they do not know if these effects pose any long-term risk. More than 70 research papers on the potentially harmful effects of cell phone use have raised concerns about cancer, neurological disorders, sleep problems, or headaches; others have shown no association or have been inconclusive. A recent British study found no significant increase in the incidence of brain tumors in men and women in the decade after cell phones became widespread.

multiple chemical sensitivity (MCS) A sensitivity to low-level chemical exposures from ordinary substances, such as perfumes and tobacco smoke, that results in physiological responses such as chest pain, depression, dizziness, fatigue, and nausea. Also known as environmentally triggered illness.

electromagnetic fields (EMFs) The invisible electric and magnetic fields generated by an electrically charged conductor.

Other adverse effects of cell phone use include changes in brain activity, reaction times, and sleep patterns. Drivers using cell phones, whether handheld or hands-free, have a three- to four-times greater chance of an accident because of the distraction.[20]

The Food and Drug Administration (FDA) and Federal Communications Commission (FCC) have stated that "the available scientific evidence does not show that any health problems are associated with using wireless phones. There is no proof, however, that wireless phones are absolutely safe." Additional studies are under way.

✓ **check-in** How much time do you spend talking on your cell phone every day?

Microwaves

Microwaves (extremely high-frequency electromagnetic waves) increase the rate at which molecules vibrate; this vibration generates heat. There's no evidence that existing levels of microwave radiation encountered in the environment pose a health risk to people, and all home microwave ovens must meet safety standards for leakage.

A concern about the safety of microwave ovens stems from the chemicals in plastic wrapping and plastic containers used in microwave ovens. Chemicals may leak into food. In high concentrations, some of the chemicals (such as DEHA, which makes plastic more pliable) can cause cancer in mice. Consumers should be cautious about using clingy plastic wrap when reheating leftovers, and plastic-encased metal "heat susceptors" included in convenience foods such as popcorn and pizza. Although these materials seem safe when tested in conventional ovens at temperatures of 300° to 350° Fahrenheit, microwave ovens can boost temperatures to 500° Fahrenheit.

Ionizing Radiation

Radiation that possesses enough energy to separate electrons from their atoms, leaving charged ions, is called **ionizing radiation**. Its effects on health depend on many factors, including the amount, length of exposure, type, part of the body exposed, and the health and age of the individual.

We're surrounded by low-level ionizing radiation every day. Most comes from cosmic rays and radioactive minerals, which vary according to geography. (Denver has more than Atlanta, for instance, because of its altitude.) Man-made sources, including medical and dental X-rays, account for approximately 18 percent of the

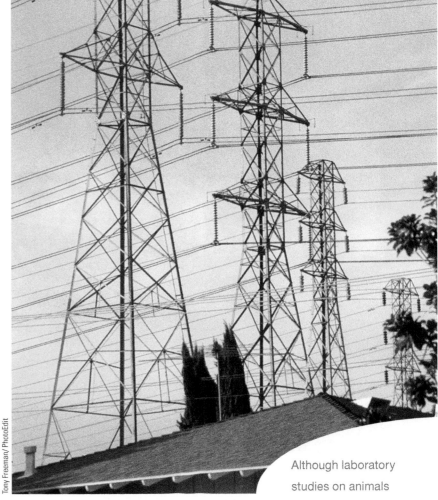

Tony Freeman/ PhotoEdit

average person's lifetime exposure. Exposure to some dental X-rays performed in the past, when radiation levels were higher, may increase the risk of meningioma, a common type of brain tumor.

Radiation exposure in humans is measured in units called rads and rems. A rad (radiation absorbed dose) is a measure of the energy deposited by ionizing radiation when it's absorbed by an object. A rem (roentgen equivalent man) is a measure of the biological effect of ionizing radiation. Different types of radiation cause different amounts of damage. The rem measurement takes this into account. For X-rays, rads and rems are equivalent. A quantity of 1 rad or 1 rem is a substantial dose of radiation. Smaller doses are measured in millirads (thousandths of a rad) or millirems (thousandths of a rem). The average annual radiation exposure for a person in the United States is about one-tenth of a rem.

Diagnostic X-Rays

The EPA estimates that 30 to 50 percent of the 700 million X-rays taken every year in the United States are unnecessary. However, doctors

Although laboratory studies on animals indicate that EMFs affect human cell membranes, research on humans has found only a weak connection between EMFs and disease.

microwaves Extremely high-frequency electromagnetic waves that increase the rate at which molecules vibrate, thereby generating heat.

ionizing radiation A form of energy emitted from atoms as they undergo internal change.

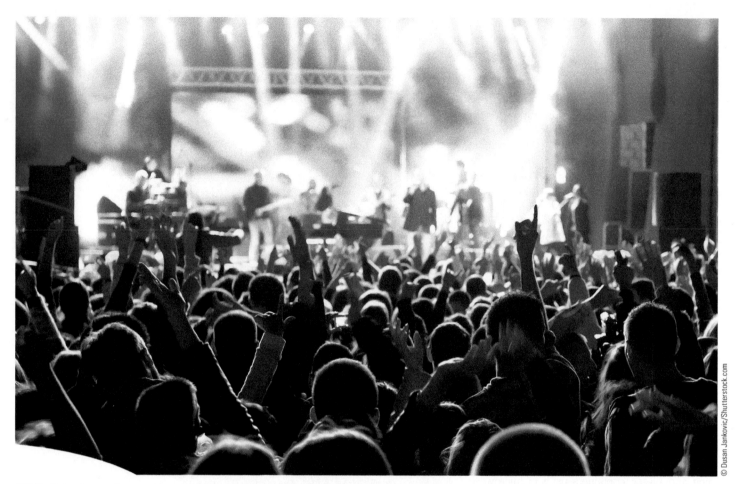

While listening to the music at your next concert, tune into the noise level and how your ears are feeling.

sometimes prescribe X-rays or newer imaging techniques involving radiation, such as CT scans, to protect themselves from malpractice suits, and hospitals benefit financially from the heavy use of X-ray equipment.

Dental X-rays involve little radiation, but many people receive so many so often that they're second only to chest examinations in frequency. New technology has significantly reduced radiation exposure.

Your Hearing Health

Hearing loss is the third-most-common chronic health problem, after high blood pressure and arthritis, among older Americans. Noise-induced hearing loss is the most frequent preventable disability. Nearly 22 million Americans between ages 20 and 69 have irreversibly damaged hearing because of excessive noise exposure. Regular use of over-the-counter painkillers also can lead to hearing loss, especially in younger men.

decibels (dB) Units for measuring the intensity of sounds.

How Loud Is That Noise?

Loudness, or the intensity of a sound, is measured in **decibels (dB)**. A whisper is 20 decibels; a conversation in a living room is about 50 decibels. On this scale, 50 isn't two and a half times louder than 20, but 1,000 times louder: Each 10-dB rise in the scale represents a tenfold increase in the intensity of the sound. Very loud but short bursts of sounds (such as gunshots and fireworks) and quieter but longer-lasting sounds (such as power tools) can induce hearing loss.

Sounds under 75 dB don't seem harmful. However, prolonged exposure to any sound over 85 dB (the equivalent of a power mower or food blender) or brief exposure to louder sounds can harm hearing. The noise level at rock concerts can reach 110 to 140 dB, about as loud as an air raid siren.

Effects of Noise

Noise-induced hearing loss is 100 percent preventable—and irreversible. Hearing aids are the only treatment, but they do not correct the problem; they just amplify sound to compensate for hearing loss.

The healthy human ear can hear sounds within a wide range of frequencies (measured in hertz), from the low-frequency rumble of thunder at 50 hertz to the high-frequency overtones of a piccolo at nearly 20,000 hertz. High-frequency noise damages the delicate hair cells that serve as sound receptors in the inner ear. Damage first begins as a diminished sensitivity to frequencies around 4,000 hertz, the highest notes of a piano.

Early symptoms of hearing loss include difficulty understanding speech and *tinnitus* (ringing in the ears). Brief, very loud sounds, such as an explosion or gunfire, can produce immediate, severe, and permanent hearing loss. Longer exposure to less intense but still hazardous sounds, such as those common at work or in public places, can gradually impair hearing, often without the individual's awareness.[21]

Are Earbuds Hazardous to Hearing?

Although there is limited research, audiologists (who specialize in hearing problems) report seeing greater noise-induced hearing loss in young people. One probable culprit is extended use of earbuds, tiny earphones used with portable music players that deliver sound extremely close to the eardrum. Hearing loss can be temporary or permanent.

√**check-in** How often do you use earbuds?

The dangers to your hearing depend on how loud the music is and how long you listen. Because personal music players have long-lasting rechargeable batteries, people—especially young ones—both listen for long periods and turn up the volume because they feel "low personal vulnerability" to hearing loss. As long as the sound level is within safety levels (see Figure 19.3), you can listen as long as you'd like. If you listen to music so loud that someone else can hear it two or three feet away, it's too loud.

For safe listening, limit listening to a portable music player with earphones or earbuds at 60 percent of its potential volume to one hour a day. At the very least, take a five-minute break after an hour of listening and keep the volume low.

Ask yourself the following questions to determine if you should have your hearing checked:

- Do you frequently have to ask people to repeat themselves?
- Do you have difficulty hearing when someone speaks in a whisper?
- Do people complain that you turn up the volume too much when watching television or listening to music?

- Do you have difficulty following conversation in a noisy environment?
- Do you avoid groups of people because of hearing difficulty?
- Have your friends or family suggested you might have hearing loss?

Hearing Loss

Hearing loss is not just for seniors. About one in five 6- to 19-year-olds has impaired hearing. In a recent study, as many as one-quarter of college students suffered mild hearing loss, including some who believed their hearing was normal. This loss could be the result of use of personal music devices such as MP3 players. Exposure to urban noise, such as the sounds of subways and ferries, also increases the risk of hearing problems.

Hearing loss generally increases with age, affecting a third of American ages 65 to 74 and almost half of those over 75.[22]

Consider getting your hearing tested if

- You frequently ask "What?" during conversations.
- You have to turn your TV or music player up high to hear.
- You need to read lips or strain to hear.
- You hear a ringing in your ears.

YOUR STRATEGIES FOR PREVENTION

How to Protect Your Ears

- **If you must live or work in a noisy area, wear hearing protectors to prevent exposure to blasts of very loud noise.** Don't think cotton or facial tissue stuck in your ears can protect you; foam or soft plastic earplugs are more effective. Wear them when operating lawn mowers, weed trimmers, or power tools.

- **Give your ears some quiet time.** Rather than turning up the volume on your personal music player to blot out noise, look for truly quiet environments, such as the library, where you can rest your ears and focus your mind.

- **Soundproof your home by using draperies, carpets, and bulky furniture.** Put rubber mats under washing machines, blenders, and other noisy appliances. Seal cracks around windows and doors.

- **Beware of large doses of aspirin.** Researchers have found that eight aspirin tablets a day can aggravate the damage caused by loud noise; twelve a day can cause ringing in the ears (tinnitus).

- **Don't drink in noisy environments.** Alcohol intensifies the impact of noise and increases the risk of lifelong hearing damage.

- **When you hear a sudden loud noise, press your fingers against your ears.** Limit your exposure to loud noise. Several brief periods of noise seem less damaging than one long exposure.

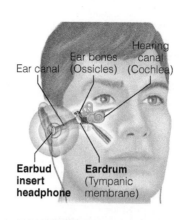

Ear canal
Ear bones (Ossicles)
Hearing canal (Cochlea)

Earbud insert headphone
Eardrum (Tympanic membrane)

Decibels	Example	Zone
0	The softest sound a typical ear can hear	Safe
10 dB	Just audible	
20 dB	Watch ticking; leaves rustling	
30 dB	Soft whisper at 16 feet	
40 dB	Quiet office; suburban street (no traffic)	
50 dB	Interior of typical urban home; rushing stream	1,000 times louder than 20 dB
60 dB	Normal conversation; busy office	
70 dB	Vacuum cleaner at 10 feet; hair dryer	
80 dB	Alarm clock at 2 feet; loud music; average daily traffic	1,000 times louder than 50 dB
90 dB*	Motorcycle at 25 feet; jet 4 miles after takeoff	Risk of injury
100 dB*	Video arcade; loud factory; subway train	
110 dB*	Car horn at 3 feet; symphony orchestra; chain saw	1,000 times louder than 80 dB
120 dB	Jackhammer at 3 feet; boom box; nearby thunderclap	Injury
130 dB	Rock concert; jet engine at 100 feet	
140 dB	Jet engine nearby; amplified car stereo; firearms	1,000 times louder than 110 dB

© Cengage Learning

FIGURE 19.3 Louder and Louder

The human ear perceives a 10-decibel increase as a doubling of loudness. Thus, the 100 decibels of a subway train sound much more than twice as loud as the 50 decibels of a rushing stream.

*Note: The maximum exposure allowed on the job by federal law, in hours per day: 90 decibels, 8 hours; 100 decibels, 2 hours; 110 decibels, ½ hour.

- Does climate change pose a risk to global health?
- Does the air you breathe affect your well-being?
- How can you reduce your exposure to indoor pollutants?
- Are you jeopardizing your hearing health?

THE POWER OF NOW!

Taking Care of Mother Earth

Environmental problems can seem so complex that you may think there's little you can do about them. That's not the case. This world can be made better instead of worse. The job isn't easy, and all of us have to do our part. Just as many diseases of the previous century have been eradicated, so in time we may be able to remove or reduce many environmental threats. Your future—and our planet's future—may depend on it.

____ Plant a tree. Even a single tree helps absorb carbon dioxide and produces cooling that can reduce the need for air conditioning.

____ Limit your driving. If you usually drive to campus, check out alternatives, such as carpooling and public or campus transportation.

____ Precycle. Surf the web for sites that sell products made from recycled materials. Click on www.ecomall.com/ for listings.

____ Save the juice. Plug your appliances and e-gadgets, which drain electricity even when turned off, into a power strip. Whenever you leave, flicking off the switch effectively unplugs them.

____ Integrate a new green habit into your life every week. Turn the thermostat down in winter and up in summer. Spend a little less time in the shower. Use both sides of printer paper. Once a week declare a "spare the air" day and don't drive.

____ Avoid disposables. Use a mug instead of a paper or foam cup, a sponge instead of a paper towel, a cloth napkin instead of a paper one.

____ Recycle. Buy products made from recycled materials. Shop for used furniture or clothing. Don't throw away anything someone else may be able to use.

____ Be water wise. Turn off the tap while you shave or brush your teeth. Install water-efficient faucets, toilets, and shower heads. Wash clothes in cold water. Drink tap rather than bottled water.

____ Spare the seas. If you live near the coast or are picnicking or hiking near the ocean, don't use plastic bags (which are often blown into the water) or plastic six-pack holders (which can get caught around the necks of sea birds).

What's Online

 Visit www.cengagebrain.com to access course materials for this text, including the Behavior Change Planner, interactive quizzes, tutorials, and more.

self survey

Are You Doing Your Part for the Planet?

You may think that there is little you can do, as an individual, to save Earth. But everyday acts can add up and make a difference in helping or harming the planet on which we live.

	Almost Never	Sometimes	Always
1. Do you walk, cycle, carpool, or use public transportation as much as possible to get around?	____	____	____
2. Do you recycle?	____	____	____
3. Do you reuse plastic and paper bags?	____	____	____
4. Do you try to conserve water by not running the tap as you shampoo or brush your teeth?	____	____	____
5. Do you use products made of recycled materials?	____	____	____
6. Do you drive a car that gets good fuel mileage and has up-to-date emission control equipment?	____	____	____
7. Do you turn off lights, televisions, and appliances when you're not using them?	____	____	____
8. Do you avoid buying products that are elaborately packaged?	____	____	____
9. Do you use glass jars and waxed paper rather than plastic wrap for storing food?	____	____	____
10. Do you take brief showers rather than baths?	____	____	____
11. Do you use cloth towels and napkins rather than paper products?	____	____	____
12. When listening to music, do you keep the volume low?	____	____	____
13. Do you try to avoid any potential carcinogens, such as asbestos, mercury, or benzene?	____	____	____
14. Are you careful to dispose of hazardous materials (such as automobile oil or antifreeze) at appropriate sites?	____	____	____
15. Do you follow environmental issues in your community and write your state or federal representatives to support green legislation?	____	____	____

Count the number of items you've checked in each column. If you've circled 10 or more in the "Always" column, you're definitely helping to make a difference. If you've mainly circled "Sometimes," you're moving in the right direction, but you need to be more consistent and more conscientious. If you've circled 10 or more in the "Never" column, carefully read this chapter and identify steps you can take to improve. Make a note in your journal and identify one or two things you could do differently.

MAKING THIS CHAPTER WORK FOR YOU

Review Questions

(LO 19.1) 1. The _____ is a direct health risk attributable to climatic changes.
a. availability of food
b. supply of fresh water
c. spread of mosquito-borne infectious diseases
d. incidence of domestic violence

(LO 19.1) 2. Which of the following greenhouse gases is released into the atmosphere when fossil fuels are burned?
a. Carbon dioxide
b. Methane
c. Nitrous oxide
d. Propane

(LO 19.2) 3. Which of the following is an example of a chronic effect caused by pollution?
a. Dizziness
b. Nausea
c. Increased blood pressure
d. Death

(LO 19.2) 4. Mutagens are environmental agents that trigger changes in the _____.
a. composition of pollutants
b. genetic material of living cells
c. average temperature of the atmosphere
d. impact of greenhouse gases

(LO 19.3) 5. _____ is a health risk caused by pollutants constricting the bronchial tubes.
a. High blood pressure
b. Heart failure
c. Stroke
d. Emphysema

(LO 19.3) 6. Air pollutants destroy the _____, exposing individuals to lung disorders.
a. air sacs
b. cilia
c. bronchial tubes
d. blood vessels

(LO 19.4) 7. Sustainability, with reference to the environment, means _____.
a. using resources as needed for the present
b. using resources in ways that do not deplete or permanently damage them
c. using materials that can be easily discarded
d. using materials that can be found easily in nature

(LO 19.4) 8. Precycling refers to _____.
a. discarding packaging at the store where you bought the product
b. buying only products that can be composted
c. choosing products that are packaged in recycled or recyclable materials
d. gathering up trash and disposing of it

(LO 19.5) 9. Water bottles made with lightweight polyethylene terephthalate _____.
a. cannot be disposed after use
b. are the simplest, safest, and most ecofriendly water containers
c. do not pose any threat to the environment
d. can lead to an accumulation of bacteria in the mouth

(LO 19.5) 10. Consumers in the United States prefer to use bottled water over tap water due to _____.
a. fears about public water supply
b. scientific recommendations of medical researchers
c. reports of decreased cavities among children drinking bottled water
d. decrease in the usage of reusable bottles

(LO 19.6) 11. Which of the following is a health effect of secondhand smoke in children?
a. Stillbirth
b. Pneumonia
c. Osteoporosis
d. Hypertension

(LO 19.6) 12. The inhalation of _____ reduces the delivery of oxygen in the blood, leading to fatal health effects.
a. lead
b. carbon dioxide
c. carbon monoxide
d. formaldehyde

(LO 19.7) 13. Which of the following can be used as bioterror agents?
a. Herbicides
b. Antidotes
c. Endocrine disruptors
d. Asbestos

(LO 19.7) 14. Which of the following is true about chemical risks?
a. Risks can decrease with simultaneous exposure to multiple carcinogens.
b. Exposure to chemicals can cause cancer in humans.
c. Human hormones are immune to chemical exposures.
d. Treatments and antidotes provide the least protection against chemical exposures.

(LO 19.8) 15. Which of the following are natural sources of low-level ionizing radiation?
a. Cosmic rays
b. Medical X-rays
c. Microwaves
d. Electromagnetic fields

(LO 19.8) 16. According to scientific researches, electromagnetic fields _____.
a. can be recognized as entirely safe
b. can be linked to cancer in children
c. are harmless irrespective of the level of exposure
d. are visible fields threatening to health

(LO 19.9) 17. _____ is the third-most-common chronic health problem among older Americans.
a. Osteoporosis
b. Arthritis
c. High blood pressure
d. Hearing loss

(LO 19.9) 18. Noise produced from a(n) _____ is the least harmful to the human ears.
a. whisper
b. rock concert
c. earbud
d. gunshot

Answers to these questions can be found on page 623.

Critical Thinking Questions

1. How do you contribute to environmental pollution? How might you change your habits to protect the environment?

2. An excerpt from a recent newspaper article stated, "Children living in a public housing project near a local refinery suffer from a high rate of asthma and allergies, and an environmental group says the plant may be to blame." The refinery has met all the local air quality standards, employs hundreds in the community, and pays substantial city taxes, which support police, fire, and social services. If you were a city council member, how would you balance health and environmental concerns with the need for industry in your community? What actions would you recommend in this particular situation?

3. In one Harris poll, 84 percent of Americans said that, given a choice between a high standard of living (but with hazardous air and water pollution and the depletion of natural resources) and a lower standard of living (but with clean air and drinking water), they would prefer clean air and drinking water and a lower standard of living. What about you? What exactly would you be willing to give up: air conditioning, convenience packaging and products, driving your own car rather than using public transportation? Do you think most people are willing to change their lifestyles to preserve the environment?

Key Terms

The terms listed are used on the page indicated. Definitions of the terms are in the glossary at the end of the book.

carcinogen 576	mutagens 576
chlorinated hydrocarbons 585	organophosphates 585
decibels (dB) 588	ozone 577
ecosystem 574	pollutant 576
electromagnetic fields (EMFs) 586	pollution 576
endocrine disruptors 585	precycling 578
ionizing radiation 587	recycling 578
microwaves 587	sustainability 578
multiple chemical sensitivity (MCS) 586	

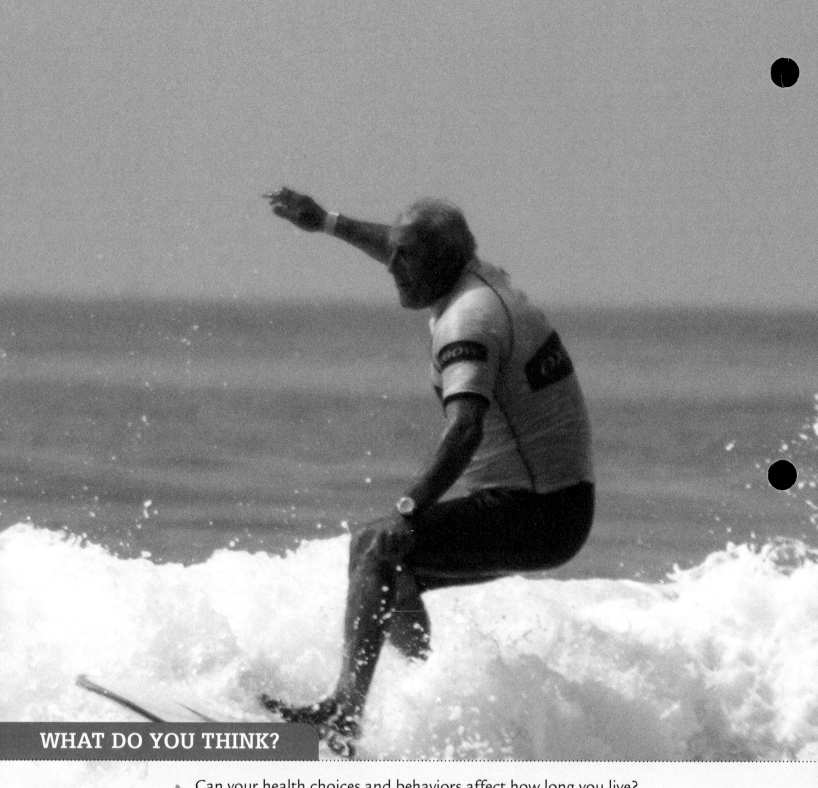

WHAT DO YOU THINK?

- Can your health choices and behaviors affect how long you live?
- What will be the greatest challenge you expect to face in old age?
- Are you prepared for medical crises that may affect you or your family?
- How do people respond to dying or the loss of a loved one?

Nik Taylor Sport/Alamy

20

A Lifetime of Health

Lauren decided to do something different for her term project for her Personal Health course. Unlike other students, who analyzed their diets or launched fitness programs, she assembled three generations of her family—some in person, some on phones or computers—on the annual National Healthcare Decisions Day to talk about a subject most people avoid: planning for illness, aging, and death. (See page 615.)

The oldest generation—Lauren's two surviving grandparents—had already completed advance directives that gave her mother a health-care power of attorney and spelled out the type of medical treatments they did or did not want at the end of life. Yet her parents, both in their 60s, had never disclosed their preferences. Laura and her husband, just turning 30, had never discussed their own wishes.

Talking about the inevitable challenges that aging brings wasn't easy, but it brought Lauren and her family closer and made them more appreciative of each other. It also served as a reality check. Lauren,

seeing some of the medical complications affecting her parents and grandparents, realized that the health choices she was making every day would affect not only how long she might live but also how she might feel and fare as she aged.

This chapter provides a preview of the changes age brings, the steps you can take to age healthfully, and the ways you can make the most of all the years of your life.

Invariably, though, no one gets out of this life alive. Death is the natural completion of things, as much a part of the real world as life itself. In time we

After reading this chapter, you should be able to:

20.1 Discuss life expectancy in the United States.

20.2 Examine the factors that influence successful aging and the characteristics of old age.

20.3 Explain the physiological changes involved in aging.

20.4 Assess different ways to prepare for medical crises and the end of life.

20.5 Discuss the emotional and psychological responses to dying.

20.6 Describe the process of dying.

20.7 Discuss the reasons why people commit suicide.

20.8 Outline some practicalities of death.

20.9 Summarize the effects of grief at the death of a loved one.

all lose people we cherish: grandparents, aunts and uncles, parents, friends, neighbors, coworkers, and siblings. With each loss, part of us may seem to die, yet each loss also reaffirms how precious life is.

This chapter explores the meaning of death, describes the process of dying, provides information on end-of-life issues, and offers advice on comforting the dying and helping their survivors. <

An Aging Nation

Within just 10 years, there will be 1 billion more older people around the globe.[1] By 2030 the number of Americans over age 65 will more than double to 70.3 million (20 percent of the total population).[2] The number of Americans age 85 and over, the fastest-growing cohort in the country, is projected to grow from 5.8 million today to 19 million in 2050. Of those who survive to age 85, women can expect to live an average of 6.8 more years; men, 5.7 years.[3]

Worldwide life expectancy by 2030 is expected to rise to 85.3 years for women and 78.1 for men.[4] Despite gains in life expectancy and survival rates, Americans live shorter lives and experience more injuries and illnesses than people in other high-income countries.

Seniors in the United States have more chronic health problems and take more medications than seniors in 10 other industrialized countries, according to a recent global survey. Almost nine in ten over age 65 suffer at least one chronic illness; the majority of these men and women have two or more ongoing health conditions.[5]

√**check-in** How old is the oldest person you know? Do you expect to live as long as that person? Why or why not?

Will You Live to 50?

If you're 20 to 25 years old—or even 30 to 35—the question may strike you as absurd. "Of course," you say. Life expectancies at birth have been rising steadily since the early 1900s, when they ranged from 40 to 50 years. The U.S. Census Bureau projects that by 2020 life expectancy at birth, now 78.8 years, will reach 79.5 years.[6] (See Figure 20.1.)

Yet according to a recent report, "U.S. Health in International Perspective: Shorter Lives, Poorer Health," by a panel convened by the prestigious Institute of Medicine and National Research

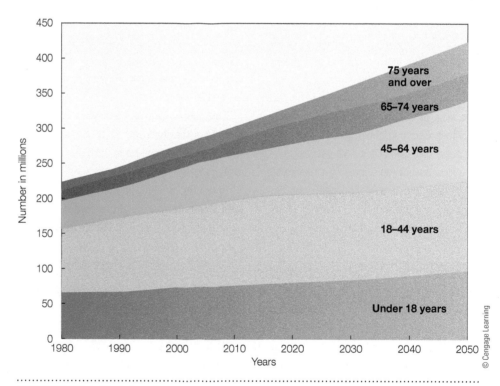

FIGURE 20.1 The Age Boom

The baby boomers (those born between 1946 and 1964) started turning 65 in 2011, and the number of older people will increase dramatically. The older population in 2030 is projected to be twice as large as in 2000.

Council, as an American you—regardless of your age, gender, race, ethnicity, education, and socioeconomic status—are less likely to hit the half-century mark than your peers in 16 other affluent countries: Australia, Austria, Canada, Denmark, Finland, France, Germany, Italy, Japan, Norway, Portugal, Spain, Sweden, Switzerland, the Netherlands, and the United Kingdom. If you do survive to celebrate your fiftieth birthday—and the odds are nonetheless good that you will—you're likely to be in much worse health than citizens of America's "peer" nations.[7]

"The tragedy is not that the United States is losing a contest with the other countries," the report states, "but that Americans are dying and suffering from illness and injury at rates that are demonstrably unnecessary."

Consider these findings:

- Since 1980 Americans have had the lowest or next-to-lowest probability of surviving to age 50 among all the nations studied.

- At age 50 Americans are in poorer health than their counterparts in other high-income countries and face greater sickness and mortality rates due to chronic illnesses, such as obesity and diabetes, established earlier in life.

- Men in the United States had the lowest life expectancies in the study, lagging 3.7 years behind the longest-living males—in Switzerland.

- Women in the United States ranked next to last in life expectancy, 5.2 years behind the longest-living females—in Japan.

- The United States had higher mortality rates than almost all the other nations, even when only high-income, non-Hispanic white men and women were considered.

- Major contributors to the excess years of life lost by Americans before age 50 include intentional injuries (murder and suicide) and motor vehicle accidents and injuries not related to transportation. For American men between ages 20 and 24, the risk of dying from violence is nearly seven times higher than in any other developed country.

As discussed in Chapter 1, there are many complex reasons for the growing health and longevity gap between the United States and similar nations.

Americans who smoke, have high blood pressure, have high blood sugar, and are overweight may be shortening their life expectancy by an average of four years. The patterns of smoking, high blood pressure, high blood glucose, and overweight/obesity account for almost 75 percent of differences in cardiovascular deaths and up to 50 percent of differences in cancer deaths in various areas of the United States.

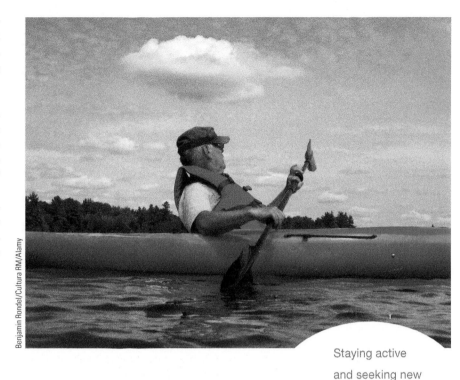

Benjamin Rondel/Cultura RM/Alamy

Staying active and seeking new adventures can add many vital years to your life.

Here is the difference in life expectancy each of these health hazards can make:

- **High blood pressure:** 1.5 years for men, 1.6 years for women.

- **Obesity:** 1.3 years for both men and women.

- **High blood sugar:** .5 years for men, .3 years for women.

- **Smoking:** 10 years for both men and women, but those who quit before age 35 can gain back these years.[8]

✓ **check-in** What do you think is the biggest threat to your reaching age 50? What can you do to overcome it?

Successful Aging

Are people as young as they feel? Recent research suggests that the old saying may be true. In an eight-year study that followed more than 6,000 men and women older than age 52, those who reported feeling three or more years younger than their actual age experienced a lower death rate than those who felt either their actual age or a little older. The reason might be optimism, which can be, as one scientist put it, "a self-fulfilling prophecy" when it comes to health.[9]

Although **aging**—the characteristic pattern of normal life changes that occur as humans, plants,

aging The characteristic pattern of normal life changes that occur as living things grow older.

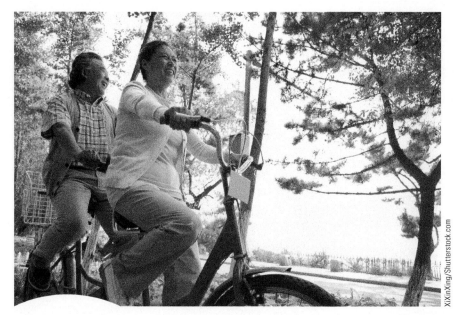

Keeping both brain and body active can enhance physical health, cognitive ability, and emotional well-being as we age.

and animals grow older—remains inevitable, you can do a great deal to influence the impact that the passage of time has on you. Whether you're in your teens, 20s, 30s, or older, now is the time to take the steps that will add healthy, active, productive years to your life.

According to research on "exceptional longevity" (survival to at least age 90), the key factors to living long and well are maintaining a healthy lifestyle (including regular exercise, weight management, and smoking avoidance) and avoiding or delaying chronic illnesses. Genetic factors contribute to healthy aging and exceptional longevity, but researchers have not been able to pinpoint specific "aging" genes.

One factor that predicts successful aging isn't physical but psychological: happiness. "Enjoyment of life contributes to healthier and more active old age," said the lead author of a study that tracked almost 3,200 British men and women ages 70 and older. Those reporting greater enjoyment were less likely to die over the next five to eight years than those with lower enjoyment of life.

However, it's important to be cautious about the conclusions. "All we can conclude is some kind of relation between physical health and happiness and life satisfaction," the researchers noted. "The findings do not tell us whether a great sense of well-being results in improved health or whether improved health results in a greater sense of well-being."[10]

✓ **check-in** How successfully do you think you will age? What do you think will help you most? What may get in your way?

Physical Activity: It's Never Too Late

Lack of physical activity, dangerous even for the young, becomes deadly among the old. Simply sitting for prolonged periods increases "all-cause mortality," the risk of dying for any reason, in both sexes and all age groups, regardless of general health, body mass index (BMI), and physical activity levels. Despite the potential benefits of being active, many seniors are sedentary. By age 75, about one in three men and one in two women engage in no physical activity.

Even some activity is better than none. Thirty minutes of physical activity a day can be as protective as 10-plus hours of sitting is harmful.[11] Gardening, dancing, and brisk walking, as well as more intense exercise, can delay chronic physical disability and cognitive decline. In fact, the effects of ongoing activity are so profound that gerontologists sometimes refer to exercise as "the closest thing to an anti-aging pill."

Exercise slows many changes associated with advancing age, such as loss of lean muscle tissue, increase in body fat, and decrease in work capacity. Consistent lifelong exercise preserves heart muscle in the elderly to levels that match or even exceed those of healthy young sedentary individuals.

Physical activity offers older Americans many other benefits, including the following:

- Greater ability to live independently.
- Increased stamina and strength.
- Enhanced mental well-being, reduced stress and anxiety, and increased self-esteem.
- Healthier bones, muscles, and joints.
- Reduced risk of falling and fracturing bones.
- Protection against many health problems, including cardiovascular disease; cancers of the colon, breast, lung, and prostate; type 2 diabetes; and muscular-skeletal disorders such as arthritis and osteoporosis.
- Reduced risk of dying from coronary heart disease and of developing high blood pressure, colon cancer, and diabetes.
- Reduced blood pressure in some people with hypertension.
- Fewer symptoms of anxiety and depression.
- Improvements in mood and feelings of well-being.
- Lower health-care costs. (See Health on a Budget.)

Reduce Your Future Health-Care Costs

Healthy seniors with no chronic conditions average $5,186 annually in health-care costs, compared to $25,132 for those with five or more chronic health problems. You may be able to reduce your expenses by following four basic steps:

- **Keep your arteries young.** If your arteries are clear and healthy, you're more likely to have a healthy heart and a sharper brain and less likely to develop high blood pressure, high cholesterol, kidney problems, and memory impairment. For your arteries' sake, exercise regularly, avoid high-fat foods, watch your weight, and find ways to manage daily stress (see Chapter 4).

- **Avoid illness.** Most individuals who live to celebrate their hundredth birthdays don't suffer from chronic diseases. Defend yourself by eating a healthy diet, not smoking, avoiding weight gain in middle age, recognizing and treating conditions like high blood pressure and elevated cholesterol, and keeping up with immunizations.

- **Stay strong.** As landmark studies with frail nursing home residents in their 80s and 90s have shown, strength training at any age builds muscle and bone, speeds up metabolic rate, improves sleep and mobility, boosts the spirit, and enhances self-confidence.

- **Maintain your zest for living.** Just as with muscles, the best advice to keep your brain strong is "use it or lose it." Keep challenging yourself, asking questions, and pursuing new passions. Individuals who are optimistic, sociable, and happy generally outlive their more pessimistic, grumpier peers.

No one is ever too old to get in shape. The American College of Sports Medicine (ACSM) encourages seniors to engage in a full range of physical activities, including aerobic conditioning. With regular conditioning, 60-year-olds can regain the fitness they had at age 40 to 45.

The ACSM recommends that older adults develop a fitness plan with a health professional to manage risks and take into account health conditions. Its basics should consist of

- Moderately intense aerobic exercise 30 minutes a day, five days a week

  or

- Vigorously intense aerobic exercise 20 minutes a day, three days a week

  and

- Eight to ten strength-training exercises, with 10 to 15 repetitions of each exercise, two or three times a week

  and

- Balance exercises

✓**check-in** Are you active enough to keep your body "young" as long as possible?

Nutrition and Obesity

The most common nutritional disorder in older people is obesity. Overweight men and women over age 65 face increased risk of diabetes, heart disease, stroke, and other health problems, including arthritis.

Although excess pounds can undermine the quality of seniors' lives, they don't necessarily cut them short. In a review of almost 100 studies involving 3 million people, being somewhat overweight correlated with a 6 percent lower risk of dying compared to people considered "normal weight." However, researchers caution that the so-called obesity paradox may be deceiving because being thin, especially in old age, is often a sign of serious illness.[12]

According to recent research, the Mediterranean diet (discussed in Chapter 6)—rich in whole grains, vegetables, legumes, nuts, fish, and olive oil—is associated with longer telomere length, an indicator of slower aging. Prior studies have linked the Mediterranean diet with better heart health as well as lower risk for chronic disease and premature death.[13]

✓**check-in** What effects do you think your weight may have on the way you age?

The Aging Brain

Scientists used to think that the aging brain, once worn out, could never be fixed. Now they know that the brain can and does repair itself. When neurons (nerve cells) in the brain die, the surrounding cells develop "fingers" to fill the gaps and establish new connections, or synapses, between surviving neurons. Although self-repair occurs more quickly in young brains, the process continues in older brains. Even victims of Alzheimer's disease, the most devastating form of dementia, have enough healthy cells in the diseased brain to regrow synapses. Scientists hope

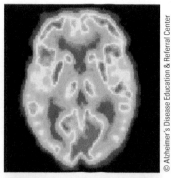

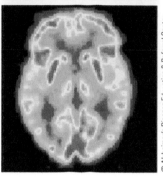

In these PET scans, the red and yellow show greater neuron activity in the young adult. The brain of the older person shows less activity and more dark areas, indicating that the fluid-filled ventricles have grown larger. Recent research shows, however, that older brains do repair themselves.

menopause The complete cessation of ovulation and menstruation for 12 consecutive months.

perimenopause The period from a woman's first irregular cycles to her last menstruation.

to develop drugs that someday may help the brain repair itself.

The brain, like the rest of the body, may begin to show signs of aging in middle age. Researchers have documented dips in memory, reasoning, and other cognitive functions beginning at age 45, although the declines are greater in older people. However, just as exercise can maintain physical health, mental workouts can benefit our brains. Individuals who engage in activities such as reading and playing mind-engaging games may lower a protein in the brain linked with Alzheimer's disease. The higher the level of cognitive stimulation in young and middle-aged adults, the lower the risk of Alzheimer's later in life. Among healthy seniors, a lifetime of speaking a second language has proven to keep the brain sharper and more efficient.[14]

Cognitive Aging Mental ability does not decline along with physical vigor. Older people who remain mentally healthy think just as quickly and sharply as college students. In cognitive tests administered to undergraduates, adults ages 60 to 74, and adults ages 75 to 90, the response time of the 60- and 70-year-olds was almost equal to that of the students. The accuracy of the answers was comparable across all age groups.

Wisdom increases because more mature minds can better see multiple points of view, search for compromise, and solve social conflicts. Older adults may find it more difficult to multitask and split their focus between two tasks. The ability to remember newly learned information also declines with age. The reason may be that structural changes in the brain interfere with sleep quality, which in turn impairs memory. Sleeping well earlier in life may lead to better mental functioning as people age. According to an analysis of fifty years of sleep studies, good sleep in midlife (defined as ages 30 to 60) predicts fewer changes in memory and thinking in later years.[15]

✓**check-in** Did you realize that people who live to age 85 may have slept nearly 250,000 hours—the equivalent of more than 10,000 full days?

Memory According to data from a National Institute on Aging survey, memory loss and cognitive problems are becoming less common among older Americans. The reasons may be that today's seniors have more formal education, higher economic status, and better health care for problems such as high blood pressure and high cholesterol that can jeopardize brain function.

Higher education does not prevent cognitive decline over time, but schooling does yield an advantage: Individuals with more education continue to have a higher level of cognitive functioning into old age, so they remain independent for a longer period.

There is growing evidence that using your brain as you age—by reading, playing games, solving crossword puzzles, and doing crafts such as pottery or quilting—greatly decreases the risk of memory loss. Even work helps—if it involves the mind as well as the body. Jobs requiring intellectually challenging tasks have proven to help preserve thinking skills and memory as workers age.[16]

✓**check-in** How do you exercise your brain to keep it healthy?

Women at Midlife

In the next two decades some 40 million, American women will end their reproductive years.

Medical specialists have identified several stages that characterize the aging of the female reproductive system:

- **Late reproductive stage**. Declines in fertility and changes in the menstrual cycle.

- **Early menopausal transition.** Increased variability in menstrual cycles.

- **Late menopausal transition.** Hormonal changes and amenorrhea, or lack of menstrual bleeding, for 60 days or longer.

- **Early postmenopause.** Five to eight years after the final menstrual period, when hormones fluctuate and then stabilize.

- **Late postmenopause.** Limited changes in reproductive hormones.

While the average age of **menopause**—defined as the complete cessation of menstrual periods for 12 consecutive months—is 51.5, a woman's reproductive system begins changing more than a decade earlier. Genes may determine the age at which women begins the transition to menopause.

For many women, **perimenopause**—the four to ten-year span before a woman's last period—is more baffling and bothersome than the years after. During this time the egg cells, or oocytes, in a woman's ovaries start to senesce, or die off, at a faster rate. Eventually, the number of egg cells drops to a tiny fraction of the estimated 2 million packed into her ovaries at birth. Trying to coax some of the remaining oocytes to ripen, the pituitary gland churns out extra follicle-stimulating hormone (FSH). This surge is the earliest harbinger of menopause, occurring six to ten years before a woman's final periods. Eventually, the other menstrual messenger, luteinizing hormone (LH), also increases, but at a slower rate.

These hormonal shifts can trigger an array of symptoms. The most common is night sweats (a *subdromal hot flash*, in medical terms), which can be intense enough to disrupt sleep. The drop in estrogen levels also may cause hot flashes (bursts of perspiration that last from a few seconds to 15 minutes).

A woman's habits and health history also have an impact. Women with a lifelong history of depression are more likely to experience early perimenopause. The fluctuating hormones of perimenopause may increase depressive symptoms even in women who have never had previous depressions. Smokers experience more symptoms at an earlier age than nonsmokers. Heavier women also have more severe symptoms.

✓**check-in** If you're a woman, do you know the age your mother entered perimenopause or went through menopause? Have you ever talked with her about her experience?

Menopause About 10 to 15 percent of women breeze through this transition with only trivial symptoms. Another 10 to 15 percent are virtually disabled. The majority fall somewhere in between these extremes. Women who undergo surgical or medical menopause (the result of removal of their ovaries or chemotherapy) often experience abrupt symptoms, including flushing, sweating, sleeplessness, early morning awakenings, involuntary urination, changes in libido, mood swings, perception of memory loss, and changes in cognitive function. An estimated 50 percent to 82 percent of women going through menopause have hot flashes and night sweats that can cause sleep problems and disrupt their daily lives for years.[17]

Race and ethnicity profoundly affect women's experience. African American women report more hot flashes and night sweats but have more positive attitudes toward menopause. Japanese and Chinese women experience more muscle stiffness and fewer hot flashes but view menopause more negatively. Hispanic women reach menopause a year or two earlier than Caucasian women; Asian women reach menopause a year or two later.

Dwindling levels of estrogen subtly affect many aspects of a woman's health, from her mouth (where dryness, unusual tastes, burning, and gum problems can develop) to her skin (which may become drier, itchier, and overly sensitive to touch). With less estrogen to block them, a woman's androgens, or male hormones, may have a greater impact, causing acne, hair loss, and, according to some anecdotal reports, surges in sexual appetite. (Other women, however, report a drop in sexual desire.)

At the same time, a woman's clitoris, vulva, and vaginal lining begin to shrivel, sometimes resulting in pain or bleeding during intercourse. Since the thinner genital tissues are less effective in keeping out bacteria and other pathogens, urinary tract infections may become more common. Some women develop breast or ovarian cysts, which usually go away on their own. Eventually, a woman's ovaries don't respond at all to her pituitary hormones. After the last ovulatory cycle, progesterone is no longer secreted, and estrogen levels decrease rapidly. A woman's testosterone level also falls.

In the United States, the average woman who reaches menopause has a life expectancy of about 30 more years. However, she faces risks of various diseases, including an increased risk of obesity, metabolic syndrome, heart disease, stroke, and breast cancer. Women can reduce these risks through exercise, good nutrition, and weight control both before and after menopause.

Hormone Replacement Therapy Medical thinking on **hormone therapy (HT)**, long believed to prevent heart disease and stroke and help women live longer, has changed, particularly related to the combination of estrogen and progestin. Based on the Women's Health Initiative (WHI)—a series of clinical trials begun in 1991 on postmenopausal women—HT now is recommended for fewer than five years as "a reasonable option" for the relief of moderate to severe symptoms such as hot flashes.[18] As various studies have confirmed, longer-term combination therapy increases the risk of breast cancer, heart disease, blood clots, stroke, and ovarian cancer.[19] In the latest analysis of the WHI data, the risks to women who took estrogen-only therapy faded after they stopped their treatment.

Middle-aged women who take hormone therapy are not at increased risk of heart attack, memory loss, or dementia years down the road, according to a new study. Earlier research had raised alarms that hormone therapy might increase the risk of these health problems. Many of the women in these studies were older than 65 and had started taking hormones 20 years past menopause. Younger women taking replacement hormones did face a slightly elevated risk of breast cancer.

hormone therapy (HT) The use of supplemental hormones during and after menopause.

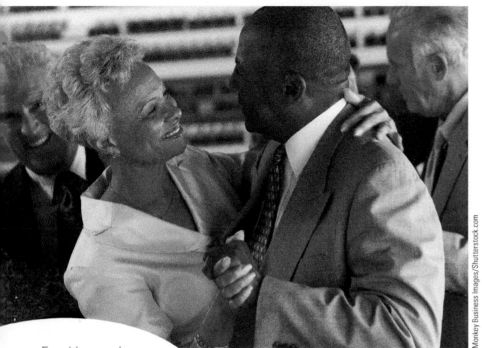

For older couples, sexual desire and pleasure can be enhanced by years of intimacy and affection.

In its most recent practice guidelines, the American College of Obstetricians and Gynecologists recommended the following options for relief of hot flashes and night sweats:

- Minimal doses of hormone therapy, with estrogen alone or estrogen plus progestin
- Low doses of certain antidepressants, such as Prozac or Paxil
- The anti-seizure drug gabapentin
- The blood pressure medication clonidine[20]

In a recent review of 16 studies involving 2,027 menopausal women, **black cohosh** didn't do any better than a placebo at relieving hot flashes and was far less effective than hormone therapy. Soy supplements and acupuncture have not been shown to improve a women's quality of life during menopause.

Men at Midlife

Although men don't experience the dramatic hormonal upheaval that women do, they do experience a decline by as much as 30 to 40 percent in their primary sex hormone, testosterone, between the ages of 48 and 70. This change, sometimes called *andropause*, may cause a range of symptoms, including decreased muscle mass, greater body fat, loss of bone density, flagging energy, lowered fertility, and impaired virility.

As they age, men who smoke may lose more Y chromosomes from their cells, a change that has been correlated with a shorter life span and an increased risk of dying from cancer.[21]

black cohosh A plant used as a traditional folk remedy for conditions such as menstrual cramps and hot flashes.

Low Testosterone As men age, they produce somewhat less testosterone, especially compared to the years of peak testosterone production during adolescence and early adulthood. Although the media have popularized the concepts of male menopause and "low T" (low testosterone), there is very little scientific evidence that normally decreasing testosterone levels are responsible for many changes that take place in older men. Yet increased numbers of men with normal or untested testosterone levels are using testosterone, often in gel form.[22]

As recent studies have shown, testosterone supplements pose serious risks to middle-aged and older men. In a study of more than 7,000 men ages 65 and older, testosterone supplements doubled the risk of cardiovascular disease. In another group of 48,000 middle-aged men with previous histories of heart disease, testosterone almost tripled the risk of heart attacks within 90 days of beginning treatment.[23]

✓ **check-in** You've probably seen television commercials aimed at men with "low T." If you are a man, would you ever consider taking supplemental testosterone? Why or why not?

Prostate Problems After age 40, the prostate gland, which surrounds the urethra at the base of the bladder, enlarges. This condition, called *benign prostatic hypertrophy*, occurs in every man. By age 50, half of all men have some enlargement of the gland; after 70, three-quarters do. As it expands, the prostate tends to pinch the urethra, decreasing urinary flow and creating a sense of urinary urgency, particularly at night. Other warning signs of prostate problems include difficult urination, blood in the urine, painful ejaculation, or constant lower-back pain.

Medical treatments for benign prostate hypertrophy include drugs that improve urine flow and reduce obstruction of the bladder outlet as well as medications that partially shrink the enlarged prostate by lowering the level of the major male hormone inside the prostate. In some cases, surgical treatment is necessary.

Sexuality and Aging

Health and sexuality interact in various ways as we age. When they are healthy and have a willing partner, a substantial number of older men remain sexually active. The fittest men and women report more frequent sexual activity. Better health translates into a better sex life. Healthy people are more likely to express an interest in sex, engage in sex, and enjoy sex.

On average, 55-year-old men can expect to remain sexually active for another 15 years, while women the same age can expect about 11 more sexually active years. Women with partners remain sexually active longer. Being in good health gains men an additional five to seven years of sexual life expectancy.[23]

Aging does cause some changes in sexual response: Women produce less vaginal lubrication. An older man needs more time to achieve an erection or orgasm and to attain another erection after ejaculating. Both men and women experience fewer contractions during orgasm. However, none of these changes reduces sexual pleasure or desire.

The Challenges of Age

No matter how well we eat, exercise, and take care of ourselves, some physical changes are inevitable as we age. Figure 20.2 shows some of these changes, but most of them are not debilitating, and people can remain active and vital into extreme old age. Aging brains and bodies do become vulnerable to diseases like Alzheimer's and osteoporosis. Other common life problems, such as depression, substance misuse, and safe driving, become more challenging as we age. Nearly 40

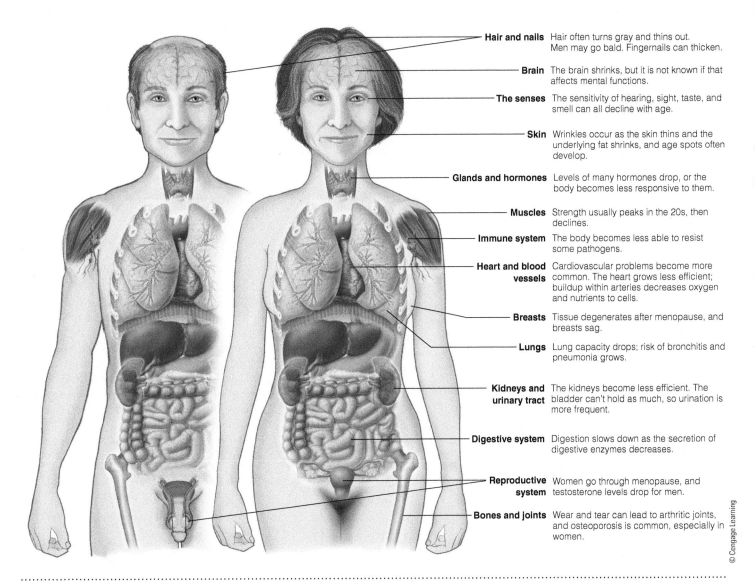

Hair and nails Hair often turns gray and thins out. Men may go bald. Fingernails can thicken.

Brain The brain shrinks, but it is not known if that affects mental functions.

The senses The sensitivity of hearing, sight, taste, and smell can all decline with age.

Skin Wrinkles occur as the skin thins and the underlying fat shrinks, and age spots often develop.

Glands and hormones Levels of many hormones drop, or the body becomes less responsive to them.

Muscles Strength usually peaks in the 20s, then declines.

Immune system The body becomes less able to resist some pathogens.

Heart and blood vessels Cardiovascular problems become more common. The heart grows less efficient; buildup within arteries decreases oxygen and nutrients to cells.

Breasts Tissue degenerates after menopause, and breasts sag.

Lungs Lung capacity drops; risk of bronchitis and pneumonia grows.

Kidneys and urinary tract The kidneys become less efficient. The bladder can't hold as much, so urination is more frequent.

Digestive system Digestion slows down as the secretion of digestive enzymes decreases.

Reproductive system Women go through menopause, and testosterone levels drop for men.

Bones and joints Wear and tear can lead to arthritic joints, and osteoporosis is common, especially in women.

FIGURE 20.2 The Effects of Aging on the Body

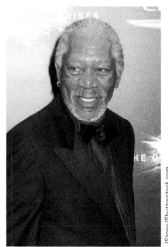

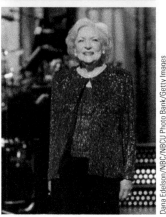

What life after 70 can look like.

mild cognitive impairment (MCI) A slight but noticeable and measurable decline in cognitive abilities, including memory and thinking skills.

dementia Deterioration of mental capability.

Alzheimer's disease A progressive deterioration of intellectual powers due to physiological changes within the brain; symptoms include diminishing ability to concentrate and reason, disorientation, depression, apathy, and paranoia.

percent of Americans over the age of 65 live with at least one disability that affects their hearing, sight, walking, thinking, self-care, or independent living, according to a government report. The most common—reported by two-thirds of seniors with a disability—is difficulty walking or climbing stairs.[24]

Mild Cognitive Impairment (MCI)

An estimated 10 to 20 percent of those ages 65 and older may suffer **mild cognitive impairment (MCI)** , which causes a slight but noticeable and measurable decline in cognitive abilities, including memory and thinking skills. The changes are not severe enough to interfere with independent living, but people with MCI have an increased risk of developing Alzheimer's disease or another type of dementia.

According to the American Psychiatric Association's *Diagnostic and Statistical Manual of Mental Disorders* (*DSM-5*), MCI can affect one or more cognitive abilities, including complex attention, executive functions, learning and memory, language, and perceptions, movement, or social cognition. There are no tests to diagnose MCI conclusively. Physicians evaluate patients on the basis of a medical history, neuropsychological testing, assessment of mental status, input from family, and laboratory tests.[25]

No medications are currently approved to treat mild cognitive impairment. Taking vitamin B_{12} or folic acid supplements, contrary to previous studies, does not have any effect on thinking and memory and does not reduce the risk of Alzheimer's disease as people age.[26] Drugs that treat symptoms of Alzheimer's disease have not shown any lasting benefit in delaying or preventing progression of MCI to dementia. However, the following coping strategies may help slow decline in thinking skills:

- Exercise to benefit blood vessels, including those that nourish the brain.

- Reduce cardiovascular risk factors (see Chapter 10) to protect the heart and the blood vessels that support brain function.

- Participate in mentally stimulating and socially engaging activities.

Alzheimer's Disease

About 15 percent of older Americans lose previous mental capabilities, a brain disorder called **dementia**. Sixty percent of these—an estimated 2.4 to 4.5 million—suffer from the type of dementia called **Alzheimer's disease**, a progressive deterioration of brain cells and mental capacity. The number of people with Alzheimer's disease in the United States will more than double by 2050, when one in five Americans will be age 65 or older.[27]

In addition to its physical and psychological benefits, physical activity may reduce the risk of dementia. In a study of sedentary adults between the ages of 57 and 75, three hours of aerobic exercise a week enhanced memory and brain function.[28]

Age is the top risk factor for Alzheimer's, but cognitive decline may begin up to six years before it is evident. Someone in America develops Alzheimer's every 72 seconds; by 2050 the rate will increase to every 33 seconds. The percentage of people with Alzheimer's doubles for every five-year age group beyond 65. By age 85, nearly half of men and women have Alzheimer's. A person with the disease typically lives eight years after the onset of symptoms, but some live as long as 20 years. Some 7.7 million older Americans will develop Alzheimer's by 2030. The greatest increase will be among people age 85 and older.

People whose parents have been diagnosed with Alzheimer's disease or dementia may be more likely to experience memory loss themselves in middle age. Scientists have identified multiple genes that make people more likely to develop Alzheimer's.[29]

Women are more likely to develop Alzheimer's than men, and women with Alzheimer's perform significantly worse than men in various visual, spatial, and memory tests. Black Americans are about two times more likely to develop Alzheimer's than whites; Hispanics face about 1.5 times the risk.

Various factors, such as regular exercise and weight management, may lower the likelihood of Alzheimer's. A healthful diet—rich in nuts, fish, tomatoes, poultry, and dark and green leafy vegetables and low in high-fat foods, red meat, and butter—may help protect the brain. Elderly people who report feeling lonely are more likely to develop dementia, regardless of other risk factors.

The early signs of dementia are usually subtle and insidious:

- Sleep problems
- Irritability
- Increased sensitivity to alcohol and other drugs
- Decreased energy
- Lower tolerance of frustration
- Depression[30]

Diagnosis requires a comprehensive assessment of an individual's medical history, physical health, and mental status, often involving brain scans and a variety of other tests.

Cholesterol-lowering statin drugs, discussed in Chapter 10, and low-dose daily aspirin may reduce the risk of Alzheimer's, regardless of a person's genetic risk for the disease. Vitamins C, D, and E, as well as calcium supplements, once touted as possible memory preservers, have not proven to lower the risk of dementia or Alzheimer's in older adults.[28]

Even though medical science cannot restore a brain that is in the process of being destroyed by an organic brain disease like Alzheimer's, medications can control difficult behavioral symptoms and enhance or partially restore cognitive ability. Often physicians find other medical or psychiatric problems, such as depression, in these patients; recognizing and treating these conditions can have a dramatic impact.

The FDA has approved several prescription drugs for people with mild to moderate dementia, including Aricept, Exelon, Reminyl, and Namenda. Although these medications do not cure Alzheimer's, they slow deterioration and improve cognitive and daily functioning.[29]

✓**check-in** Have any of your close relatives developed cognitive impairment or Alzheimer's? Would you be able to recognize the early signs?

Osteoporosis

Another age-related disease is *osteoporosis*, a condition in which losses in bone density become so severe that a bone will break with even slight trauma or injury. A chronic disease, osteoporosis is silent for years or decades before a fracture occurs. Each year more than one-third of Americans age 65 and older experience falls, and nearly 16,000 die as a result of their injuries. Even a low-trauma fracture increases the risk of dying during the subsequent five years, and a hip fracture heightens this risk for ten years.

Women, who have smaller skeletons, are more vulnerable to osteoporosis than men; in extreme cases, their spines may become so fragile that just bending causes severe pain. But although commonly seen as an illness of women, osteoporosis occurs frequently in men. One in every two women and one in four men over 50 will have an osteoporosis-related fracture in their lifetimes.

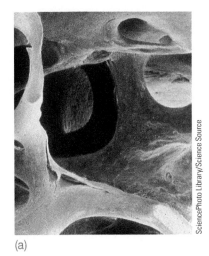

(a)   (b)

SciencePhoto Library/Science Source

Rome/SciencePhoto Library/Science Source

The effect of osteoporosis on bone density. (a) Normal bone tissue. (b) After the onset of osteoporosis, bones lose density and become hollow and brittle.

✓**check-in** Are you taking steps now to prevent future bone problems?

Preparing for Medical Crises and the End of Life

Throughout this book, we have stressed the ways in which you can determine how well and how long you live. You can also make decisions about the end of your life. When facing a serious, potentially life-threatening illness, people typically have practical, realistic goals, such as maintaining their quality of life, remaining independent, being comfortable, and providing for their families. (See Health Now!)

According to a recent study, most Americans—almost three-quarters in a sample of nearly 8,000 people—do not deal with end-of-life issues. Women, whites, married people, and those with a college degree or postgraduate training are more likely to prepare advance directives ("living wills"), while black and Hispanic respondents, regardless of education, are less likely to do so. The most common reason overall is lack of awareness.[31]

Various racial and ethnic groups have different preferences for their end-of-life wishes. Many Arab Americans prefer not to go to nursing homes as they near the end of their lives, while many African Americans are comfortable with nursing homes and hospitals. Hispanic individuals express strong concerns about dying with dignity. Many white people don't want their families to take care of them, although they—like members of most other racial and ethnic groups—want their families nearby as they live out their last days.

✓**check-in** Has your family discussed each member's preferences in case of a medical crisis? Have you thought through and communicated your own preferences?

Advance Directives

All states and the District of Columbia have laws authorizing the use of **advance directives** to specify the kind of medical treatment individuals want in case of a medical crisis. These documents are important because, without clear indications of a person's preferences, hospitals and other institutions often make decisions on an individual's behalf, particularly if family members are not available or disagree among themselves. Only about a quarter of American adults have prepared advance health directives, according to a nationally representative survey.[32]

The two most common advance directives are health-care proxies and living wills. Each state has different legal requirements for these forms. You can find state-specific forms at www.caringinfo .org. Once the forms are completed, make copies of your advance directives and give them to anyone who might have input into decisions on your behalf. Also give copies to your physician or health-care organization and ask that they be made part of your medical record.

Health-Care Proxies A *health-care proxy* is an advance directive that gives someone else the power to make health decisions on your behalf. This advance directive is also called medical power of attorney or health-care power of attorney. People typically name a relative or close friend as their agent. Let family members and friends know that you have completed a health-care proxy. You should tell your primary physician, but you should not designate your doctor as your agent. Many states prohibit this. Even when allowed, it is not a good idea because your doctor's primary responsibility is to administer care.

Living Wills Individuals can use a **living will** (also called health-care directive or physician's directive) to indicate whether they want or don't want all possible medical treatments and technology used to prolong their lives. Living wills are most effective when they focus on priorities and goals rather than on how to achieve them.

Most states recognize living wills as legally binding, and a growing number of health-care professionals and facilities offer patients help in drafting living wills.

The Five Wishes An innovative document called "Five Wishes" helps aged and seriously ill people, as well as their loved ones and caregivers, prepare for medical crises. Written with the help of the American Bar Association's Commission on the Legal Problems of the Elderly, the Five Wishes document has a health-care proxy, a health-care directive, and three other "wishes." People using this document can specify the following:

- Which person they want to make health-care decisions for them when they are no longer able to do so
- Which kinds of medical treatments they do or don't want
- How comfortable they want to be made
- How they want people to treat them
- What they want loved ones to know

The Five Wishes document (available at www. agingwithdignity.org) is legally valid in thirty-eight states. Churches, synagogues, hospices, hospitals, physicians, social service agencies, and employers also are distributing the document to help people plan for their own care or that of aging parents.

✓**check-in** Do you know what your grandparents', parents', or partner's five wishes would be? Do they know yours?

DNR Orders You can sign an advance directive specifying that you want to be allowed to die naturally—that you do not want to be resuscitated when your heart stops beating.

advance directives Documents that specify an individual's preferences regarding treatment in a medical crisis.

living will An advance directive that provides instructions for the use of life-sustaining procedures in the event of terminal illness or injury.

YOUR STRATEGIES FOR PREVENTION

Keep Your Bones Healthy

- **Get adequate calcium**. Increased calcium intake, particularly during childhood and the growth spurt of adolescence, can produce a heavier, denser skeleton and reduce the risk of the complications of bone loss later in life. College-age women also can strengthen their bones and reduce their risk of osteoporosis by increasing their calcium intake and physical activity.

- **Drink alcohol only moderately**. More than two or three alcoholic beverages a day impairs intestinal calcium absorption.

- **Don't smoke**. Smokers tend to be thin and enter menopause earlier.

- **Let the sunshine in (but don't forget your sunscreen)**. Vitamin D, a vitamin produced in the skin in reaction to sunlight, boosts calcium absorption.

- **Exercise regularly**. Both aerobic exercise and weight training can help preserve bone density.

Do-not-resuscitate (DNR) orders apply mainly to hospitalized, terminally ill patients and must be signed by a physician. However, in some states, it is possible to complete a *nonhospital DNR* form that specifies an individual's wish not to be resuscitated at home. Patients in the final stages of advanced cancer or AIDS may choose to use such forms to protect their rights in case paramedics are called to their homes.

Holographic Wills Perhaps you think that only wealthy or older people need to write wills. However, if you're married, have children, or own property, you should either hire a lawyer to draw up a will or at least write a **holographic will** yourself, specifying who should inherit your possessions. If you die *intestate* (without a will), the state will make these decisions for you. Even a modest estate can be tied up in court for a long period of time, depriving family members of money when they need it most.

A holographic will is a handwritten (not typed) statement that some states will recognize. You can

- **Name a family member or friend** as the executor, the person who sees that your wishes are carried out.

- **List the things you own** and to whom you want them to go; include addresses and telephone numbers, if possible.

- **Select a guardian for your children** (if any), presumably someone whose ideas about raising children are similar to your own. Be sure that any named guardians are willing and able to accept this responsibility before writing them into your will.

- **Specify any funeral arrangements.**

Be sure to keep the will in a safe place, where your executor, family members, or closest beneficiary can find it quickly and easily; tell them where it is.

Ethical Dilemmas

Modern medicine can do more to delay or defy death than was once thought possible. However, the ability to sustain life in patients with no hope of recovery has created wrenching medical and moral dilemmas. Increasingly, lawyers, ethicists, and consumer advocates are arguing that health-care providers must recognize a fundamental right of patients: the right to die.

Health economists, noting that more than half of U.S. health-care dollars are spent in the last year of life, have questioned "heroic" measures to prolong the life of chronically ill elderly patients or those with fatal diseases. Policies on such aggressive measures vary from hospital to hospital and state to state; often medical staff are not aware of patients' wishes.

Some health-care facilities require that staff members try to resuscitate any patient whose heart stops unless a do-not-resuscitate (DNR) order has been written, usually with the family's permission.

Families may demand aggressive medical care near the end of life on the basis of religious grounds, such as a conviction that every moment of life is a gift from God worth preserving at any cost. However, doctors are not obliged to provide a treatment they consider medically inappropriate or inhumane simply because of the family's religious beliefs. Ideally, doctors and family members, perhaps with the aid of a chaplain, work together to reach a consensus on the appropriate limits to life-sustaining treatment.

Another major ethical concern is the fate of an estimated 5,000 to 10,000 unconscious Americans who are being kept alive by artificial means. Some are in a **coma**, a state of total unconsciousness. They may have no sense of where they are, no memory, and no experience of pain. Others are in a **persistent vegetative state**, in which they're awake and yet unaware. They open their eyes; their brain waves show the characteristic patterns of waking and sleep. They can usually breathe on their own after a few weeks on artificial respiration; they can cough; the pupils of their eyes respond to light; but they do not respond to pain.

The Gift of Life

If you're at least 18 years old, you can fill out a donor card agreeing to designate, in the event of your death, any organs or tissues needed for transplantation (see Figure 20.3). Corneas may help a blind person see, for example. Kidneys, or even a heart, may be transplanted. The donation takes effect upon your death and is a generous way of

do-not-resuscitate (DNR) orders An advance directive that expresses an individual's preference that resuscitation efforts not be made during a medical crisis.

holographic will A will wholly in the handwriting of its author.

coma A state of total unconsciousness.

persistent vegetative state A state of being awake and capable of reacting to physical stimuli, such as light, while being unaware of pain or other environmental stimuli.

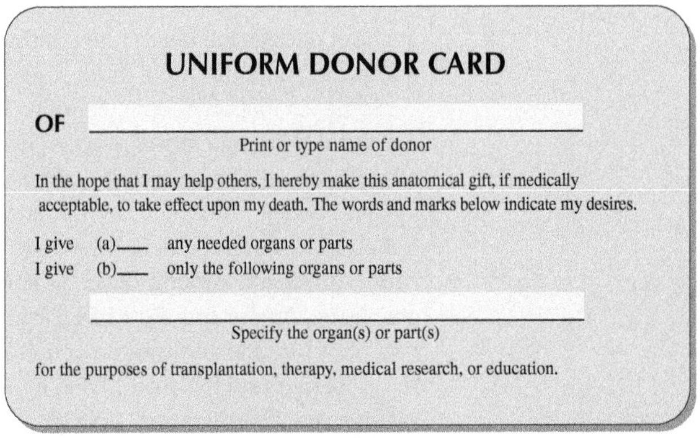

UNIFORM DONOR CARD

OF _____
Print or type name of donor

In the hope that I may help others, I hereby make this anatomical gift, if medically acceptable, to take effect upon my death. The words and marks below indicate my desires.

I give (a)____ any needed organs or parts
I give (b)____ only the following organs or parts

_____
Specify the organ(s) or part(s)

for the purposes of transplantation, therapy, medical research, or education.

© Cengage Learning

FIGURE 20.3 Example of a Uniform Donor Card

Dying Young: Leading Causes of Death

Men		Women	
Ages 20–24	**Ages 25–34**	**Ages 20–24**	**Ages 25–34**
Unintentional injuries	Unintentional injuries	Unintentional injuries	Unintentional injuries
Homicide	Suicide	Suicide	Cancer
Suicide	Homicide	Homicide	Heart disease
Cancer	Heart disease	Cancer	Suicide
Heart disease	Cancer	Heart disease	Homicide

Source: National Vital Statistics Report. Mortality Tables at www.cdc.gov/nchs/deaths.htm.

What have been the primary causes of death among young men and women in your community?

giving others the possibilities for life that you have had yourself. The card should be filled out and signed; some must be signed in the presence of two witnesses. Attach the donor card to the back of your driver's license or I.D. card. (Whole-body donations may require other arrangements.)

The reasons for becoming an organ donor or agreeing to donate a loved one's organs are complex. Older men and women generally have higher donation rates. Families often base their decision on a loved one's explicit desire either to donate organs or not. Concerns about disfigurement and feelings of emotional exhaustion also play a role.

✓**check-in** Have you signed up to be an organ donor? Why or why not?

Death and Dying

According to medical statisticians, your risk of death doubles every eight years after about age 20 or 30. Although previously thought to level off at about age 80, the death rate continues to rise at about the same rate until at least age 106.

Some 2.4 million people die in the United States each year. Although most are older, death occurs in all age groups. The causes of death vary with both age and gender. Among those under age 35, intentional and non-intentional injury are the primary causes of death. Among older Americans, cancer and heart disease are the top killers. In fact, cancer, heart disease, and stroke continue to claim the most lives around the world. Men typically die at a younger age than women. College-age individuals are most likely to die as a result of accidents, homicide, or suicide. (See Snapshot: On Campus Now.)

Death Education

Death used to be such a taboo subject that people for a long time avoided even mentioning it, let alone treating it as a subject worthy of study and discussion. This attitude is changing, as "death education," which consists of a variety of educational activities and experiences related to death, dying, and bereavement, becomes more widespread in colleges and schools for health professionals.

Formal death education may involve courses, independent research, and clinical experiences, offered at every educational level, from elementary to graduate school, or seminars or workshops for health professionals and the public. Informal death education can take place whenever and wherever a "teachable moment" occurs, whether it's the death of a family pet or media coverage of a mass shooting. The goal is to challenge individuals to acknowledge their personal mortality so they can create a more meaningful life.

According to research on college students' views, undergraduates generally accept death as another life experience. However, compared to college women, male students are significantly less concerned about death and its inevitability, fear death less although they do not welcome it, and consider themselves less frightened of death than others. College men also consistently put themselves at greater risk of death through behaviors such as driving after drinking, getting into physical fights, and not wearing seat belts.

✓**check-in** Do you think that learning about death can reduce fears of dying?

Defining Death

In our society, death isn't a part of everyday life, as it once was. Because machines can now keep alive people when they would have died in the past, the definition of death has become more complex. Death has been broken down into the following categories:

- **Functional death**. The end of all vital functions, such as heartbeat and respiration.

- **Cellular death.** The gradual death of body cells after the heart stops beating. If placed in a tissue culture or, as is the case with various organs, transplanted to another body, some cells can remain alive indefinitely.

- **Death.** The moment the heart stops beating.

- **Brain death.** The end of all brain activity, indicated by an absence of electrical activity (confirmed by an electroencephalogram [EEG]) and a lack of reflexes. The notion of brain death is bound up with what we consider to be the actual person, or self. The destruction of a person's brain means that his or her personality no longer exists; the lower brain centers controlling respiration and circulation no longer function.

- **Spiritual death.** The moment the soul, as defined by many religions, leaves the body.

When does a person actually die? The traditional legal definition of death is failure of the lungs or heart to function. However, because respiration and circulation can be maintained by artificial means, most states have declared that an individual is considered dead only when the brain, including the brain stem, completely stops functioning. Brain-death laws prohibit a medical staff from "pulling the plug" if there is any hope of sustaining life.

Denying Death

Most of us don't quite believe that we're going to die. A reasonable amount of denial helps us focus on the day-to-day realities of living. However, excessive denial can be life-threatening. Some drivers, for instance, refuse to buckle their seat belts because they refuse to acknowledge that a drunk driver might collide with them. Similarly, cigarette smokers deny that lung cancer will ever strike them, and people who eat high-fat meals deny that they'll ever suffer a heart attack.

One important factor in denial is the nature of the threat. It's easy to believe that death is at hand when someone's pointing a gun at you; it's much harder to think that cigarette smoking might cause your death 20 or 30 years down the road. The late Elisabeth Kübler-Ross, a psychiatrist who extensively studied the process of dying, described the downside of denying death in *Death: The Final Stage of Growth*:

> It is the denial of death that is partially responsible for people living empty, purposeless lives; for when you live as if you'll live forever, it becomes too easy to postpone the things you know that you must do. You live your life in preparation for tomorrow or in the remembrance of yesterday—and meanwhile, each today is lost. In contrast, when you fully understand that each day you awaken could be the last you have, you take the time that day to grow, to become more of who you really are, to reach out to other human beings.[33]

Emotional Responses to Dying

Kübler-Ross identified five typical stages of reaction that a person goes through when facing death (Figure 20.4).

1. **Denial ("No, not me").** At first knowledge that death is coming, a terminally ill patient rejects the news. The denial overcomes the initial shock and allows the person to begin to gather together his or her resources. Denial, at this point, is a healthy defense mechanism. It can become distressful, however, if it's reinforced by the relatives and friends of the dying patient.

YOUR STRATEGIES FOR CHANGE

Learning about Death

College students enrolled in death education classes have passed along some of the lessons they've learned from the experience:

- **If you have anyone you need to forgive, do it now.** If that person is you, write yourself a letter absolving yourself of blame for whatever wrong you feel that you did.

- **Write a letter to someone, dead or alive, to say thank you.** This could be a grandparent who cherished you as a child or a friend you lost touch with long ago. Reflect on your gratitude for their gifts to you.

- **Don't assume that it's ever too late for love.** Until their final breath, people find strength and solace in expressing their feelings, touching and being touched, and reaching out to others.

- **Accept the prospect of death but don't focus on it.** People of every age—from the very young to the extremely old—die every day. The point is to live life to the fullest no matter how much is left.

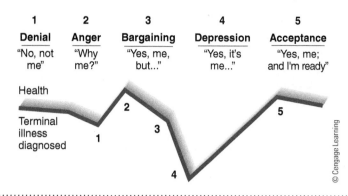

1	2	3	4	5
Denial	**Anger**	**Bargaining**	**Depression**	**Acceptance**
"No, not me"	"Why me?"	"Yes, me, but..."	"Yes, it's me..."	"Yes, me; and I'm ready"

© Cengage Learning

FIGURE 20.4 Kübler-Ross's Five Stages of Adjustment to Facing Death

2. **Anger ("Why me?").** In the second stage, the dying person begins to feel resentment and rage regarding imminent death. The anger may be directed at God or at the patient's family and caregivers, who can do little but try to endure any expressions of anger, provide comfort, and help the patient on to the next stage.

3. **Bargaining ("Yes, me, but . . .").** In this stage, a patient may try to bargain, usually with God, for a way to reverse or at least postpone dying. The patient may promise, in exchange for recovery, to do good works or to see family members more often. Alternatively, the patient may say, "Let me live long enough to see my grandchild born" or "to see the spring again."

4. **Depression ("Yes, it's me").** In the fourth stage, the patient gradually realizes the full consequences of his or her condition. This may begin as grieving for health that has been lost and then become anticipatory grieving for the loss that is to come of friends, loved ones, and life itself. This stage is perhaps the most difficult: The dying person should not be left alone during this period. Neither should loved ones try to cheer up the patient, who must be allowed to grieve.

5. **Acceptance ("Yes, me; and I'm ready").** In this last stage, the person has accepted the reality of death: The moment looms as neither frightening nor painful, neither sad nor happy—only inevitable. The person who waits for the end of life may ask to see fewer visitors, to separate from other people, or perhaps to turn to just one person for support.

Several stages may occur at the same time and some may happen out of sequence. Each stage may take days or only hours or minutes. Throughout, denial may come back to assert itself unexpectedly, and hope for a medical breakthrough or a miraculous recovery is forever present.

Some experts dispute Kübler-Ross's basic five-stage theory as too simplistic and argue that not all people go through such well-defined stages in the dying process. The way a person faces death is often a mirror of the way he or she has faced other major stresses in life: Those who have had the most trouble adjusting to other crises will have the most trouble adjusting to the news of their impending death.

An individual's will to live can postpone death for a while. In a study of elderly Chinese women, researchers found that their death rate decreased before and during a holiday during which the senior women in a household play a central role; it increased after the celebration. A similar temporary drop occurs among Jews at the time of Passover. However, different events may have different effects. The prospect of an upcoming birthday postpones death in women but hastens it in men. The will to live typically fluctuates in terminal patients, varying along with depression, anxiety, shortness of breath, and a sense of well-being.

The family of a dying person experiences a spectrum of often wrenching emotions. Family members, too, may deny the verdict of death, rage at the doctors and nurses who can't do more to save their loved one, bargain with God to give up their own health if necessary, sink into helplessness and depression, and finally accept the reality of their anticipated loss. Dying can be seen from different perspectives. The Renz model, for example, views it as a process of maturation consisting of pretransition, transition, and posttransition. The initial response is an upsurge of emotions, including anger, grief, feelings of personal emptiness, and despair. These may emerge again and again.

However, as patients confront reality, they eventually can "let go and let be." As one researcher observed, "There is happiness and well-being in the midst of illness. In the course of the dying process spiritual experiences of such intensity often happen more than just once. After a shorter or longer struggle, patients reach a new mental state, a gift of grace beyond human endeavor and power."

How We Die

Life can end in very different ways. Sudden death, by accident or assault, for instance, brings an abrupt end to life in individuals who may have been in optimal health. A terminal illness, such as an aggressive and fatal cancer, can lead to a steep drop in functioning prior to death. When organs such as the kidneys fail, a patient's well-being tends to plummet and then recover but in a downward pattern. The frailty of old age leads to a gradual decline to ever lower levels of functioning and eventual death.

Most people who have a fatal or **terminal illness** prefer to know the truth about their health and chances for recovery. Even when they're not officially informed by a doctor or relative, most fatally ill people know or strongly suspect that they're dying. Dying people usually make it clear whether they want to talk about death and to what extent. The most frequent concern is how much time is left. Usually physicians can give only a rough estimate, such as "several weeks or months."

A "Good" Death

Although Americans are living longer, an increasing number suffer pain, depression, and other distressing symptoms in their final year.[34]

Many health-care professionals as well as citizens and social organizations have begun to demand a better way of caring for those who are dying.

The Center to Improve Care of the Dying, in Washington, D.C., has set goals for reintegrating dying within living, thus enhancing the prospect for growth at the end of life. These experts talk of "dying well," "living while dying," and "physician-assisted living." They aim to change our way of thinking about dying so that we view the end of life as a time of love and reconciliation and a transcendence of suffering.

Various psychological factors can affect those at risk of dying. Elderly people who lack hope in the future are much more likely to die within the next few years. Researchers speculate that hopelessness may lead to biochemical and nervous system abnormalities or that hopeless individuals may not eat well, take medications as prescribed, or follow a doctor's recommendations.

Spirituality plays a major role. In various surveys, many patients say they want their doctors and nurses to address their spiritual concerns. In one survey, even 45 percent of nonreligious patients thought physicians should inquire politely about patients' spiritual needs. However, some worry that such queries may be inappropriate or detract from a doctor's primary mission.

Caregiving

When someone becomes terminally ill, a woman—usually the patient's wife, daughter, or sister—is most likely to provide day-to-day care, often for periods longer than a year. Caregiving takes a different toll on men and women. In one study of adult daughters and husbands caring for terminally ill breast cancer patients, the daughters experienced more symptoms of anxiety and depression and greater family strain.

The impact of caregiving continues even after the death of an ill spouse. In one study, the health of older caregivers who had experienced strain prior to a spouse's death did not deteriorate. They showed no increase in depressive symptoms or use of antidepressant drugs and did not lose weight. Those who had not been caregivers were more likely to experience depression and weight loss.

Hospice: Caring When Curing Isn't Possible

A **hospice** helps dying men and women live their final days to the fullest, as free as possible from disabling pain and mental anguish.

Race and ethnicity affect the use of hospice. In a study of patients over age 65 (and all covered by Medicare) with terminal cancer, Asian American and black patients were less likely to enroll in a hospice program than whites and Hispanics. They also were more likely to be hospitalized in an intensive care unit at least twice during their last month of life.

Hospice workers generally work in teams, usually consisting of a nurse, physician, social worker, chaplain, and trained volunteers. Other professionals, such as a physical therapist, may join the team when needed. These workers provide the comfort, support, and care dying patients need until they die.

Hospice programs offer a combination of medical and emotional care that involves not only the patient but also the family members or others concerned with caring for the patient. Most hospice patients have life expectancies of six months or less and are no longer receiving treatments aimed at curing their diseases. When someone is available to provide care, patients remain in their own homes. Hospice nurses regularly visit all home patients and are available around the clock.

For patients requiring care that the family cannot provide, round-the-clock care is available at a hospice facility. Unlike a traditional hospital, where the focus is on diagnosis, cure, and treatment, a hospice works to make what is left of life pain-free and comfortable. Visiting hours for relatives and friends are flexible, with no restrictions on visits by children and grandchildren. Hospice services are covered, in full or in part, by most private and government insurance.

terminal illness An illness in which death is inevitable.

hospice A homelike health-care facility or program committed to supportive care for terminally ill people.

Near-Death Experiences

Interest in near-death experiences has grown, thanks largely to popular books such as *Proof of Heaven* by neurosurgeon Eben Alexander. Most accounts are remarkably similar, whether they occur in children or adults, whether they're the result of accidents or illnesses, even whether the individuals actually are near death or only think they are. Some individuals who have survived a close brush with death report **autoscopy** (watching, from several feet in the air, resuscitation attempts on their own bodies) or **transcendence** (the sense of passing into a foreign region or dimension). Some see light, often at the end of a tunnel. Their vision seems clearer; their hearing, sharper. Some recall scenes from their lives or feel the presence of loved ones who have died. Many report profound feelings of joy, calm, and peace. Fewer than 1 percent of those who've reported near-death experiences described them as frightening or distressing, although a larger number recall transitory feelings of fear or confusion.

Many near-death experiences occur in individuals who've been sedated or given other medications; however, many others do not. Several studies have shown that individuals who received medication or anesthesia were actually less likely to remember near-death experiences than those who hadn't had any drugs. Some scientists have speculated that lack of oxygen, changes in blood gases, altered brain functioning, or the release of neurotransmitters (messenger chemicals in the brain) may play a role in near-death experiences. However, there's little solid evidence that physiological events are responsible. There's also no proof that wishful thinking, cultural conditioning, posttraumatic stress, or other psychological mechanisms may be at work. For now, the most that scientists can say for sure about this medical mystery is that it needs further study.

autoscopy The sensation of one's self being outside its body, often experienced by individuals in near-death medical crises.

transcendence The sense of passing into a foreign region or dimension, often experienced by a person near death.

euthanasia The painless killing of a patient with an incurable fatal disease or in an irreversible coma.

assisted suicide Providing the means to end life to a patient by a health professional.

Suicide

Suicide increases with age and is most common in persons age 65 and older. Elderly men, particularly non-Hispanic white men, have much higher suicide rates than women. For every completed suicide, there are 10 to 40 unsuccessful attempts.

As discussed in Chapter 3, an estimated one in ten college students seriously considers suicide, and nearly half suffer from significant depression. Other factors that may place a college student at risk for suicide include substance abuse, a family history of suicide, impulsive and aggressive behavior, and relationship difficulties. (Chapter 3 presents a detailed discussion of the risk factors and warning signs of suicide.)

One of the main factors leading to suicide is illness, especially terminal illness. Simply receiving a diagnosis of cancer increases the danger of suicide. A great deal of debate centers on quality of life, yet there is no reliable or consistent way to measure this. Patients who are dying may feel some quality of life, even when others do not recognize it, or their evaluations of the quality of their lives may fluctuate. Dying patients who say their lives are not worth living may be suffering from depression; hopelessness is one of its characteristic symptoms.

"Rational" Suicide

An elderly widow suffering from advanced cancer takes a lethal overdose of sleeping pills. A young man with several AIDS-related illnesses shoots himself. A woman in her 50s, diagnosed as having Alzheimer's disease, asks a doctor to help her end her life. Are these suicides "rational" because these individuals used logical reasoning in deciding to end their lives?

The question is intensely controversial. Advocates of the right to "self-deliverance" argue that individuals in great pain or faced with the prospect of a debilitating, hopeless battle against an incurable disease can and should be able to decide to end their lives. As legislatures and the legal system tackle the thorny questions of an individual's right to die, mental health professionals worry that, even in those with fatal diseases, suicidal wishes often stem from undiagnosed depression.

Because depression may indeed warp the ability to make a rational decision about suicide, mental health professionals urge physicians and family members to make sure individuals with chronic or fatal illnesses are evaluated for depression and given medication, psychotherapy, or both. It is also important for everyone to allow enough time—an average of three to eight weeks—to see if treatment for depression will make a difference in their desire to keep living.

Euthanasia and Assisted Suicide

Euthanasia, the administration of a lethal medication by a physician or another person, is illegal in the United States. **Assisted suicide**, in which a health professional gives a patient the means to end his or her life, has been legalized by the states of Oregon, Washington, Montana, Vermont, and New Mexico for patients of sound mind with a confirmed terminal illness.

If patients have a right to die, should doctors help them end their lives? Physicians could stop any extraordinary efforts to sustain life (for example, by withholding oxygen or ending intravenous feedings); such actions are referred to as passive *euthanasia*, or *dyathanasia*. Euthanasia, the active form of so-called mercy killing, has generally been viewed as illegal and unethical. Euthanasia is tolerated and legally pardoned in the Netherlands in cases of hopeless and unbearable suffering, but remains illegal in all European countries. The demand for physician-assisted death in the Netherlands has not risen, and patients and physicians have become more reluctant to ask for or offer this option over the past few years.

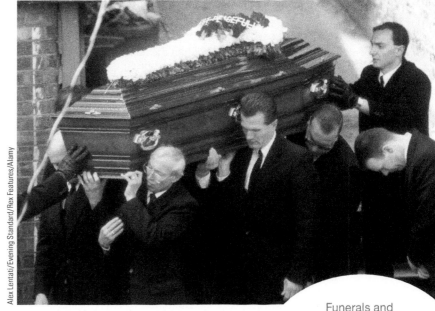

Alex Lentati/Evening Standard/Rex Features/Alamy

Funerals and memorial services help those in mourning to honor the deceased and to come to terms with their loss.

The Practicalities of Death

At a time of great emotional pain, grieving family members must cope with medical, legal, and practical concerns, including obtaining a medical certificate of the cause of death, registering the death, and making funeral arrangements. They also may want to arrange for organ donations and, in some circumstances, an autopsy.

Funeral Arrangements

A body can be either buried or cremated. Burial requires the purchase of a cemetery plot, which many families do decades before death. A burial is typically one of the most expensive investments of a lifetime. The average national costs range as high as $6,000, although they vary considerably. Memorial societies are voluntary groups that help people plan in advance for death. They obtain services at moderate cost, keep the arrangements simple and dignified, and—most important, perhaps—ease the emotional and financial burden on the rest of the family when death finally does come.

If the body is to be cremated, you must comply with some additional formalities, with which the funeral director can help you. After a *cremation*

(incineration of the remains), you can either collect the ashes to keep, bury, or scatter yourself, or ask the crematorium to dispose of them.

The tradition of a funeral may help survivors come to terms with the death, enabling them to mourn their loss and to celebrate the dead person's life. Funerals are usually held two to four days after the death. Many have two parts: a religious ceremony at a church or funeral home, and a burial ceremony at the grave site.

Alternatively, the body may be disposed of immediately, through burial, cremation, or bequeathal to a medical school, and a memorial service held later. In a memorial service, the body is not present, which may change the focus of the service from the person's death to his or her life.

Autopsies

An autopsy is a detailed examination of a body after death, also called a postmortem exam. There are two types:

- **Medicolegal.** This type of autopsy is performed to establish the cause of death and to gather information about the death for use as evidence in any legal proceedings. It is done to detect any crimes and to help identify the proper person for prosecution, to investigate possible industrial hazards or contagious diseases that may endanger the public health, or to establish the cause of death for insurance purposes.

- **Medical/educational.** This type of autopsy is performed, usually in the hospital where the person died, to increase medical knowledge and to determine a more exact cause of death. It may be requested by the attending physician or the family, but it cannot be performed without the family's permission.

Autopsies can be extremely valuable in establishing an accurate cause of death, revealing a different diagnosis that might have led to a change in therapy and prolonged survival in about 10 percent of cases. Thirty years ago about 50 percent of patients who died in hospitals were autopsied. However, the autopsy rate in the United States has been steadily declining, and today about 10 to 20 percent of deaths in teaching hospitals are autopsied.

Grief

An estimated 8 million Americans lose a member of their immediate family each year. Each death leaves an average of five people bereaved. Such loss may be the single most upsetting and feared event in a person's life. It produces a wide range of reactions, including anxiety, guilt, anger, and financial concern.

Many may see the death of an old person as less tragic than the death of a child or young person. A sudden death is more of a shock than one following a long illness. A suicide can be particularly devastating, because family members may wonder whether they could have done anything to prevent it.

The cause of death also can affect the reactions of friends and acquaintances. Some people express less sympathy and support when individuals are murdered or take their own lives.

According to the stage theory of grief, individuals respond to the loss of a loved one by progressing through several steps, just like people facing death. These consist of

- shock-numbness
- yearning-searching
- disorganization-despair
- reorganization

All these reactions can occur simultaneously, although most peak within six months. Acceptance continues to increase over time. The most common and one of the most painful experiences is the death of a parent. When both parents die, even adult individuals may feel like orphaned children. They mourn not just for the father and mother who are gone but also for their lost role of being someone's child.

Bereavement is not a rare occurrence on college campuses, but it is largely an ignored problem. Counselors have called upon universities to help students who have lost a loved one through initiatives such as training nonbereaved students to provide peer support and raising consciousness about bereavement.

✓**check-in** If you have suffered the loss of a loved one, how did you experience grief?

YOUR STRATEGIES FOR CHANGE

How to Cope with Grief

- **Accept your feelings—sorrow, fear, emptiness, whatever—as normal.** Don't try to deny emotions such as anger, guilt, despair, or relief.

- **Let others help you—by bringing you food, taking care of daily necessities, providing companionship and comfort.** (It will make them feel better, too.)

- **Face each day as it comes.** Let yourself live in the here-and-now until you're ready to face the future. Give yourself time—perhaps more than you ever imagined—for the pain to ebb, the scars to heal, and your life to move on.

- **Don't think there's a right or wrong way to grieve.** Mourning takes many forms, and there's no set timetable for working through the various stages of grief.

- **Seek professional counseling if your grief does not ease over time.** Therapy can help prevent potentially serious physical and psychological problems.

Grief's Effects on Health

Men and women who lose partners, parents, or children endure so much stress that they're at increased risk of serious physical and mental illness, and even of premature death. Studies of the health effects of grief have found the following:

- Grief produces changes in the respiratory, hormonal, and central nervous systems and may affect functions of the heart, blood, and immune systems.

- Grieving adults may experience mood swings between sadness and anger, guilt and anxiety.

- Grievers may feel physically sick, lose their appetites, sleep poorly, or fear that they're going crazy because they "see" the deceased person in different places.

- Friendships and remarriage offer the greatest protection against health problems.

- Some widows may have increased rates of depression, suicide, and death from cirrhosis of the liver. The greatest risk factors are poor previous mental and physical health and a lack of social support.
- Grieving parents, partners, and adult children are at increased risk of serious physical and mental illness, suicide, and premature death.

Sometimes grief progresses from an emotionally painful but normal experience to a more persistent problem, called *complicated grief*. Individuals who experience very long-lasting or severe symptoms, including inability to accept a loved one's death, persistent thoughts about the death, and preoccupation with the lost loved one, can benefit from professional treatment.

WHAT DID YOU DECIDE?

- Can your health choices and behaviors affect how long you live?
- What will be the greatest challenge you expect to face in old age?
- Are you prepared for medical crises that may affect you or your family?
- How do people respond to dying or the loss of a loved one?

THE POWER OF NOW!
Staying Alive and Well

"Every man desires to live long," wrote Jonathan Swift, "but no man would be old." We all wish for long lives, yet we want to avoid the disease and disability that can tarnish our golden years. Which of the following steps will you take to ensure a lifetime of health?

____ Exercise regularly. By improving blood flow, staving off depression, warding off heart disease, and enhancing well-being, regular workouts help keep mind and body in top form.

____ Don't smoke. This habit can take an estimated ten years off a lifespan. Even light smokers (one to nine cigarettes a day) are twice as likely to die as nonsmokers.[35]

____ Watch your weight and blood pressure. Increases in these vital statistics can increase your risk of hypertension, cardiovascular disease, stroke, and other health problems.

____ Eat more fruits and vegetables. These foods, rich in vitamins and protective antioxidants, can reduce your risk of cancer and damage from destructive free radicals.

____ Cut down on fat. Fatty foods can clog the arteries and contribute to various cancers.

____ Limit drinking. Alcohol can undermine physical health and sabotage mental acuity.

____ Cultivate stimulating interests. Elderly individuals with complex and interesting lifestyles are most likely to retain sharp minds and memories beyond age 70.

____ Don't worry; be happy. At any age, emotional turmoil can undermine well-being. Relaxation techniques, such as meditation, help by reducing stress.

____ Reach out. Try to keep in contact with other people of all ages and experiences. Make the effort to invite them to your home or go out with them. On a regular basis, do something to help another person.

____ Make the most of your time. Greet each day with a specific goal—to take a walk, write letters, visit a friend.

In your online journal, describe the life you envision for yourself at ages 50, 60, 75, and 100.

What's Online

 Visit www.cengagebrain.com to access course materials for this text, including the Behavior Change Planner, interactive quizzes, and more.

What Is Your Aging IQ?

Answer True or False.

1. **True** or **False**: Everyone becomes "senile" sooner or later, if he or she lives long enough.

2. **True** or **False**: American families have by and large abandoned their older members.

3. **True** or **False**: Depression is a serious problem for older people.

4. **True** or **False**: The numbers of older people are growing.

5. **True** or **False**: The vast majority of older people are self-sufficient.

6. **True** or **False**: Mental confusion is an inevitable, incurable consequence of old age.

7. **True** or **False**: Intelligence declines with age.

8. **True** or **False**: Sexual urges and activity normally cease around ages 55 to 60.

9. **True** or **False**: If a person has been smoking for 30 or 40 years, it does no good to quit.

10. **True** or **False**: Older people should stop exercising and rest.

11. **True** or **False**: As you grow older, you need more vitamins and minerals to stay healthy.

12. **True** or **False**: Only children need to be concerned about calcium for strong bones and teeth.

13. **True** or **False**: Extremes of heat and cold can be particularly dangerous to old people.

14. **True** or **False**: Many older people are hurt in accidents that could have been prevented.

15. **True** or **False**: More men than women survive to old age.

16. **True** or **False**: Deaths from stroke and heart disease are declining.

17. **True** or **False**: Older people on the average take more medications than younger people.

18. **True** or **False**: Snake oil salesmen are as common today as they were on the frontier.

19. **True** or **False**: Personality changes with age, just like hair color and skin texture.

20. **True** or **False**: Sight declines with age.

Scoring

1. **False.** Even among those who live to be 80 or older, only 20 to 25 percent develop Alzheimer's disease or some other incurable form of brain disease. "Senility" is a meaningless term that should be discarded.

2. **False.** The American family is still the number one caretaker of older Americans. Most older people live close to their children and see them often; many live with their spouses. In all, eight out of ten men and six out of ten women live in family settings.

3. **True.** Depression, loss of self-esteem, loneliness, and anxiety can become more common as older people face retirement, along with the deaths of relatives and friends, and other such crises—often at the same time. Fortunately, depression is treatable.

4. **True.** By the year 2030, one in four people will be over 65 years of age.

5. **True.** Only a small percentage of the older population live in nursing homes. The rest live independently or with relatives or caregivers.

6. **False.** Mental confusion and serious forgetfulness in old age can be caused by Alzheimer's disease or other conditions that cause incurable damage to the brain, but some 100 other problems can cause the same symptoms. A minor head injury, a high fever, poor nutrition, adverse drug reactions, and depression can all be treated and the confusion will be cured.

7. **False.** Intelligence per se does not decline without reason. Most people maintain their intellect or improve as they grow older.

8. **False.** Most older people can lead an active, satisfying sex life.

9. **False.** Stopping smoking at any age not only reduces the risk of cancer and heart disease but also leads to healthier lungs.

10. **False.** Many older people enjoy—and benefit from—exercises such as walking, swimming, and bicycle riding. Exercise at any age can help strengthen the heart and lungs, and lower blood pressure. See your physician before beginning a new exercise program.

11. **False.** Although certain requirements, such as that for "sunshine" vitamin D, may increase slightly with age, older people need the same amounts of most vitamins and minerals as younger people. Older people in particular should eat nutritious food and cut down on sweets, salty snack foods, high-calorie drinks, and alcohol.

12. **False.** Older people require fewer calories, but adequate intake of calcium for strong bones can become more important as you grow older. This is particularly true for women, whose risk of osteoporosis increases after menopause. Milk and cheese are rich in calcium, as are cooked dried beans, collards, and broccoli. Some people need calcium supplements as well.

13. **True.** The body's thermostat tends to function less efficiently with age, and the older person's body may be less able to adapt to heat or cold.

14. **True.** Falls are the most common cause of injuries among the elderly. Good safety habits, including proper lighting, nonskid carpets, and keeping living areas free of obstacles, can help prevent serious accidents.

15. **False.** Women tend to live 5 to 10 percent longer than men.

16. **True.** Fewer men and women are dying of stroke or heart disease.

17. **True.** The elderly consume 25 percent of all medications and, as a result, have many more problems with adverse drug reactions.

18. **True.** Medical quackery is a $10 billion business in the United States. People of all ages are commonly duped into "quick cures" for aging, arthritis, and cancer.

19. **False.** Personality doesn't change with age. Therefore, all old people can't be described as rigid and cantankerous. You are what you are for as long as you live. But you can change what you do to help yourself to good health.

20. **False.** Although changes in vision become more common with age, any change in vision, regardless of age, is related to a specific disease. If you are having problems with your vision, see your doctor.

In your online journal, identify at least one change or behavior that you can initiate now that may affect how long and how well you live. What is the first step you are willing to take? When and how will you begin?

Source: National Institute on Aging, http://www.counselingnotes.com/seniors/age/age_iq.htm.

MAKING THIS CHAPTER WORK FOR YOU

Review Questions

(LO 20.1) 1. In which of the following countries do women have the highest life expectancy?
   a. Japan
   b. The United States
   c. Canada
   d. Denmark

(LO 20.1) 2. In which of the following countries do men have the highest life expectancy?
   a. Austria
   b. Japan
   c. Switzerland
   d. Spain

(LO 20.2) 3. Compared to their peers who are not fit, physically fit people over age 60 _____.
   a. have a lower risk of dying from coronary heart disease
   b. can regain the fitness level of a 25-year-old
   c. show no difference in levels of anxiety and depression
   d. have higher health-care expenses

(LO 20.2) 4. Which of the following is true of men older than 40?
   a. Their prostate glands decrease in size.
   b. Their prostate glands enlarge.
   c. They produce greater amounts of testosterone.
   d. They experience more contractions during orgasm.

(LO 20.3) 5. Steps for protecting against bone loss include _____.
   a. having at least two drinks per day
   b. getting moderate exposure to sunlight
   c. avoiding heavy exercise
   d. having a diet low in calcium

(LO 20.3) 6. Which of the following is an early sign of dementia?
   a. Insomnia
   b. Insensitivity to alcohol
   c. Increased energy
   d. Craving for fatty foods

(LO 20.4) 7. A health-care proxy _____.
  a. indicates who should have your property in the event that you die
  b. gives someone else the power to make health decisions on your behalf
  c. can specify your desires related to the use of medical treatments and technology to prolong your life
  d. designates your doctor as your health agent by default

(LO 20.4) 8. What is the purpose of a DNR order?
  a. It designates, in the event of your death, any organs or tissues needed for transplantation.
  b. It gives someone else the power to make health decisions on your behalf.
  c. It specifies how comfortable you need to be made in case of a terminal illness.
  d. It specifies that you do not want to be resuscitated in case your heart stops beating.

(LO 20.5) 9. An absence of electrical activity and a lack of reflexes are indicators of _____.
  a. cellular death
  b. functional death
  c. brain death
  d. spiritual death

(LO 20.5) 10. The first stage a person goes through when facing death is:
  a. anger
  b. denial
  c. bargaining
  d. depression

(LO 20.6) 11. Having a "good" death involves _____.
  a. Dying soon after a diagnosis of terminal illness.
  b. Being sedated so that death is pain-free.
  c. Reintegrating dying within living so that it is a part of the life cycle.
  d. Taking antidepressants to alleviate depression about one's impending death.

(LO 20.6) 12. Some persons who have experienced near-death experiences report:
  a. Confusion
  b. Fear
  c. Overwhelming sense of loss
  d. Transcendence

(LO 20.7) 13. Which of the following statements is true of suicide?
  a. Suicide is most common in people ages 35 and younger.
  b. Elderly women have much higher suicide rates than men.
  c. A family history of suicide increases a person's risk for suicide.
  d. Being diagnosed with a terminal illness does not increase the danger of suicide.

(LO 20.7) 14. Which of the following factors can place a college student at risk for suicide?
  a. Rash driving
  b. Low alcohol intake
  c. Substance abuse
  d. A large number of friends

(LO 20.8) 15. An important purpose of a funeral or memorial service is to:
  a. Help survivors comes to terms with the death of the loved one
  b. Establish that the person is legally dead
  c. Give the family an occasion to see old friends
  d. Serve as a necessary prerequisite to burial.

(LO 20.8) 16. Autopsies performed to establish cause of death are termed:
  a. medical/educational
  b. medicolegal
  c. police procedural
  d. necessary by law

(LO 20.9) 17. Which of the following offers the greatest protection against health problems that result from grief?
  a. Medication
  b. Low alcohol intake
  c. Regular exercise
  d. Friendships and remarriage

(LO 20.9) 18. What is the first stage that individuals go through in the process of responding to the death of a loved one?
  a. Yearning-searching
  b. Shock-numbness
  c. Disorganization-despair
  d. Reorganization

Answers to these questions can be found on page 623.

Critical Thinking Question

1. Have your parents and grandparents written advance directives or a living will? Have you discussed with them their preferences regarding treatment in the event of a medical crisis? If you haven't had this discussion with your family, how can you begin the process of helping your parents or grandparents communicate their wishes?

Additional Online Resources

www.nia.nih.gov
This government site features a comprehensive array of resources on aging, including publications on a variety of geriatric health topics, current news events, and a resource directory for older people.

www.realage.com
This site features diet and exercise assessment tools—such as a BMI calculator, exercise estimator, and RealAge assessment quizzes on a variety of health topics—to help you determine your risk of disease and what you can do to reduce this risk. The main feature is an interactive, online personal lifestyle assessment that also gives you options for "growing younger."

Key Terms

The terms listed are used on the pages indicated. Definitions of the terms are in the glossary at the end of the book.

advance directives 608

aging 599

Alzheimer's disease 606

black cohosh 604

assisted suicide 614

autoscopy 614

coma 609

dementia 606

do-not-resuscitate (DNR) orders 609

euthanasia 614

holographic will 609

hormone therapy (HT) 603

hospice 613

living will 608

menopause 602

mild cognitive impairment (MCI) 606

perimenopause 602

persistent vegetative state 609

terminal illness 613

transcendence 614

Making This Chapter Work for You

Answers to Review Questions

Chapter 1
1. c; 2. b; 3. d; 4. b; 5. c; 6. a; 7. d; 8. c

Chapter 2
1. d; 2. b; 3. a; 4. c; 5. c; 6. d; 7. a; 8. d; 9. b; 10. d

Chapter 3
1. a; 2. d; 3. a; 4. c; 5. b; 6. c; 7. b; 8. c; 9. d; 10. b; 11. c; 12. a; 13. d; 14. b

Chapter 4
1. b; 2. b; 3. a; 4. c; 5. d; 6. d; 7. c; 8. b; 9. d; 10. d; 11. d; 12. a; 13. b; 14. c; 15. d; 16. a; 17. c; 18. c; 19. b

Chapter 5
1. d; 2. b; 3. a; 4. b; 5. c; 6. d; 7. a; 8. d; 9. c; 10. b; 11. a; 12. c; 13. b; 14. c; 15. d; 16. b; 17. d; 18. a

Chapter 6
1. c; 2. d; 3. c; 4. c; 5. a; 6. d; 7. a; 8. c; 9. a; 10. a; 11. b; 12. d; 13. c; 14. c

Chapter 7
1. a; 2. b; 3. a; 4. a; 5. d; 6. a; 7. d; 8. a; 9. c; 10. d; 11. b; 12. d; 13. b; 14. c; 15. a; 16. c; 17. b; 18. d

Chapter 8
1. a; 2. b; 3. c; 4. a; 5. d; 6. c; 7. b; 8. b; 9. c; 10. c; 11. b; 12. d; 13. b; 14. b; 15. a; 16. c; 17. d; 18. c; 19. a; 20. b; 21. d; 22. a

Chapter 9
1. a; 2. b; 3. d; 4. b; 5. d; 6. d; 7. a; 8. b; 9. a; 10. a; 11. c; 12. b; 13. d; 14. b; 15. c; 16. c

Chapter 10
1. b; 2. c; 3. b; 4. a; 5. d; 6. a; 7. d; 8. c; 9. b; 10. d; 11. c; 12. a; 13. b; 14. b

Chapter 11
1. c; 2. c; 3. a; 4. b; 5. a; 6. d; 7. a; 8. c

Chapter 12
1. c; 2. c; 3. b; 4. d; 5. a; 6. d; 7. c; 8. a; 9. c; 10. d; 11. c; 12. b; 13. c; 14. a; 15. d; 16. d; 17. c; 18. d

Chapter 13
1. d; 2. b; 3. a; 4. b; 5. a; 6. a; 7. b; 8. d; 9. c; 10. d; 11. a; 12. c; 13. c; 14. d

Chapter 14
1. b; 2. c; 3. c; 4. b; 5. b; 6. d; 7. c; 8. b; 9. b; 10. c; 11. a; 12. b; 13. d; 14. c; 15. c; 16. d; 17. b; 18. a

Chapter 15
1. a; 2. c; 3. b; 4. a; 5. d; 6. d; 7. c; 8. a; 9. d; 10. c; 11. c; 12. a; 13. a; 14. d; 15. b; 16. c; 17. d; 18. a; 19. c; 20. b

Chapter 16
1. b; 2. a; 3. c; 4. d; 5. c; 6. a; 7. d; 8. c; 9. b; 10. d; 11. b; 12. a; 13. d; 14. d; 15. d; 16. a; 17. a; 18. d; 19. b; 20. a; 21. d; 22. c

Chapter 17
1. c; 2. d; 3. b; 4. d; 5. b; 6. a; 7. c; 8. c; 9. c; 10. d; 11. c; 12. b; 13. d; 14. d; 15. c; 16. d; 17. b; 18. d

Chapter 18
1. a; 2. d; 3. b; 4. c; 5. a; 6. c; 7. b; 8. c; 9. b; 10. b

Chapter 19
1. c; 2. a; 3. c; 4. b; 5. d; 6. b; 7. b; 8. c; 9. d; 10. a; 11. b; 12. c; 13. c; 14. b; 15. a; 16. b; 17. a; 18. d

Chapter 20
1. a; 2. c; 3. a; 4. b; 5. b; 6. a; 7. b; 8. d; 9. b; 10. d; 11. c; 12. d; 13. c; 14. c; 15. a; 16. b; 17. d; 18. b

Glossary

absorption The passage of substances into or across membranes or tissues.

abstinence Voluntary refrainment from sexual intercourse.

acquired immune deficiency syndrome (AIDS) The final stages of HIV infection, characterized by a variety of severe illnesses and decreased levels of certain immune cells.

active stretching A technique that involves stretching a muscle by contracting the opposing muscle.

acupuncture A Chinese medical practice of puncturing the body with needles inserted at specific points to relieve pain or cure disease.

acute injuries Physical injuries, such as sprains, bruises, and pulled muscles, that result from sudden traumas, such as falls or collisions.

addiction A behavioral pattern characterized by compulsion, loss of control, and continued repetition of a behavior or activity in spite of adverse consequences.

additive Characterized by a combined effect that is equal to the sum of the individual effects.

adoption The legal process for becoming the parent to a child of other biological parents.

advance directives Documents that specify an individual's preferences regarding treatment in a medical crisis.

aerobic exercise Physical activity in which sufficient or excess oxygen is continually supplied to the body.

aging The characteristic pattern of normal life changes that occur as living things grow older.

alcoholism A chronic, progressive, potentially fatal disease characterized by impaired control of drinking; a preoccupation with alcohol; continued use of alcohol despite adverse consequences; and distorted thinking, most notably denial.

alcohol use disorder Problematic pattern of alcohol use leading to significant impairment or distress.

allergic rhinitis An inflammatory response of the nasal mucous membranes after exposure to inhaled allergens.

allergies Hypersensitivities to particular substances in one's environment or diet.

altruism Acts of helping or giving to others without thought of self-benefit.

Alzheimer's disease A progressive deterioration of intellectual powers due to physiological changes within the brain; symptoms include diminishing ability to concentrate and reason, disorientation, depression, apathy, and paranoia.

AmED (alcohol mixed with energy drinks) Any combination of alcohol with caffeine and other stimulants.

amenorrhea The absence or suppression of menstruation.

amino acids Organic compounds containing nitrogen, carbon, hydrogen, and oxygen; the essential building blocks of proteins.

amnion The innermost membrane of the sac enclosing the embryo or fetus.

amphetamines Any of a class of stimulants that trigger the release of epinephrine, which stimulates the central nervous system; users experience a state of hyperalertness and energy, followed by a crash as the drug wears off.

anabolic steroids Synthetic derivatives of the male hormone testosterone that promote the growth of skeletal muscle and increase lean body mass.

anaerobic exercise Physical activity in which the body develops an oxygen deficit.

androgyny The expression of both masculine and feminine traits.

angina Chest pain.

angina pectoris A severe, suffocating chest pain caused by a brief lack of oxygen to the heart.

anorexia nervosa A psychological disorder in which refusal to eat and/or an extreme loss of appetite leads to malnutrition, severe weight loss, and possibly death.

antagonistic Opposing or counteracting.

antibiotics Substances produced by microorganisms, or synthetic agents, that are toxic to bacteria.

antidepressants Drugs used primarily to treat symptoms of depression.

antioxidants Substances that prevent the damaging effects of oxidation in cells.

antiviral drugs Substances that decrease the severity and duration of a viral infection if taken prior to or soon after onset of infection.

anxiety disorders A group of psychological disorders involving episodes of apprehension, tension, or uneasiness, stemming from the anticipation of danger and sometimes accompanied by physical symptoms, which cause significant distress and impairment to an individual.

aorta The main artery of the body, arising from the left ventricle of the heart.

appetite A desire for food, stimulated by anticipated hunger, physiological changes within the brain and body, the availability of food, and other environmental and psychological factors.

arteriosclerosis Any of a number of chronic diseases characterized by degeneration of the arteries and hardening and thickening of arterial walls.

artificial insemination The introduction of viable sperm into the vagina by artificial means for the purpose of inducing conception.

assisted suicide Providing the means to end life to a patient by a health professional.

asthma A disease or allergic response characterized by bronchial spasms and difficult breathing.

atherosclerosis A form of arteriosclerosis in which fatty substances (plaque) are deposited on the inner walls of arteries.

atrium Either of the two upper chambers of the heart, which receive blood from the veins.

attention-deficit/hyperactivity disorder (ADHD) A spectrum of difficulties in controlling motion and sustaining attention, including hyperactivity, impulsivity, and distractibility.

autism spectrum disorder A neurodevelopmental disorder that causes social and communication impairments.

autoimmune disorders Diseases caused by an attack on body tissue by an immune system that fails to recognize the tissue as self.

autonomy The ability to draw on internal resources; independence from familial and societal influences.

autoscopy The sensation of one's self being outside its body, often experienced by individuals in near-death medical crises.

aversion therapy A treatment that attempts to help a person overcome a dependence or bad habit by making the person feel disgusted or repulsed by that habit.

axon The long fiber that conducts impulses from the neuron's nucleus to its dendrites.

axon terminal The ending of an axon, from which impulses are transmitted to a dendrite of another neuron.

Ayurveda A traditional Indian medical treatment involving meditation, exercise, herbal medications, and nutrition.

bacteria (singular, bacterium) One-celled microscopic organisms; the most plentiful pathogens.

bacterial vaginosis (BV) A vaginal infection caused by overgrowth and depletion of various microorganisms living in the vagina, resulting in a malodorous white or gray vaginal discharge.

ballistic stretching Rapid bouncing movements.

barbiturates Antianxiety drugs that depress the central nervous system, reduce activity, and induce relaxation, drowsiness, or sleep; often prescribed to relieve tension and treat epileptic seizures or as a general anesthetic.

barrier contraceptives Birth control devices that block the meeting of egg and sperm, either by physical barriers, such as condoms, diaphragms, or cervical caps, or by chemical barriers, such as spermicide, or both.

basal metabolic rate (BMR) The number of calories required to sustain the body at rest.

behavioral therapy A technique that emphasizes application of the principles of learning to substitute desirable responses and behavior patterns for undesirable ones.

benzodiazepine An antianxiety drug that depresses the central nervous system, reduces activity, and induces relaxation, drowsiness, or sleep; often prescribed to relieve tension, muscular strain, sleep problems, anxiety, and panic attacks; also used as an anesthetic and in the treatment of alcohol withdrawal.

bidis Skinny, sweet-flavored cigarettes.

binge For a man, having five or more alcoholic drinks at a single sitting; for a woman, having four drinks or more at a single sitting.

binge eating The rapid consumption of an abnormally large amount of food in a relatively short time.

binge-eating disorder A psychiatric disorder characterized by binge-eating once a week or more for at least a three-month period.

biofeedback A technique of becoming aware, with the aid of external monitoring devices, of internal physiological activities in order to develop the capability of altering them.

bipolar disorder Severe depression alternating with periods of manic activity and elation.

bisexuality Sexually oriented toward both sexes.

black cohosh A plant used as a traditional folk remedy for conditions such as menstrual cramps and hot flashes.

blastocyst In embryonic development, a ball of cells with a surface layer and an inner cell mass.

blended families Families formed when one or both of the partners bring children from a previous union to the new marriage.

blood-alcohol concentration (BAC) The amount of alcohol in the blood, expressed as a percentage.

body composition The relative amounts of fat and lean tissue (bone, muscle, organs, water) in the body.

body mass index (BMI) A mathematical formula that correlates with body fat; the ratio of weight to height squared.

bulimia nervosa Episodic binge eating, often followed by forced vomiting or laxative abuse, and accompanied by a persistent preoccupation with body shape and weight.

burnout A state of physical, emotional, and mental exhaustion resulting from constant or repeated emotional pressure.

caesarean delivery The surgical procedure in which an infant is delivered through an incision made in the abdominal wall and uterus.

calories The amount of energy required to raise the temperature of 1 gram of water by 1 degree Celsius. In everyday usage related to the energy content of foods and the energy expended in activities, a calorie is actually the equivalent of a thousand such calories, or a kilocalorie.

calorie balance The relationship between calories consumed from foods and beverages and calories expended in normal body functions and through physical activity. If the calories consumed equal calories expended, you have calorie balance.

candidiasis An infection of the yeast *Candida albicans*, commonly occurring in the vagina, vulva, penis, and mouth and causing burning, itching, and a whitish discharge.

cannabinoids A group of closely related compounds that include cannabinol and the active constituents of cannabis (marijuana).

capillaries Minute blood vessels that connect an artery to a vein.

carbohydrates Organic compounds, such as starches, sugars, and glycogen, that are composed of carbon, hydrogen, and oxygen and are sources of bodily energy.

carbon monoxide A colorless, odorless gas produced by the burning of gasoline or tobacco; it displaces oxygen in the hemoglobin molecules of red blood cells.

carcinogen A substance or agent that causes cancer.

cardiometabolic Referring to the heart and to the biochemical processes involved in the body's functioning.

cardiopulmonary resuscitation (CPR) Emergency treatment to maintain circulation in a person whose heart has stopped or who is no longer breathing.

cardiorespiratory fitness The ability of the heart and blood vessels to circulate blood through the body efficiently.

cathinone An amphetamine-like stimulant derived from the khat plant.

celibacy Abstention from sexual activity; can be partial or complete, permanent or temporary.

certified social workers or licensed clinical social workers (LCSWs) Persons who have completed a two-year graduate program in counseling people with mental problems.

cervical cap A thimble-size rubber or plastic cap that is inserted into the vagina to fit over the cervix and prevent the passage of sperm into the uterus during sexual intercourse; used with a spermicidal foam or jelly, it serves as both a chemical and a physical barrier to sperm.

cervix The narrow, lower end of the uterus that opens into the vagina.

chancroid A soft, painful sore or localized infection usually acquired through sexual contact.

chiropractic A method of treating disease, primarily through manipulating the bones and joints to restore normal nerve function.

chlamydia A sexually transmitted infection caused by the bacterium *Chlamydia trachomatis*, often asymptomatic in women, but sometimes characterized by urinary pain; if undetected and untreated, may result in pelvic inflammatory disease (PID).

chlorinated hydrocarbons Highly toxic pesticides, such as DDT and chlordane, that are extremely resistant to breakdown; may cause cancer, birth defects, neurological disorders, and damage to wildlife and the environment.

cholesterol An organic substance found in animal fats; linked to cardiovascular disease, particularly atherosclerosis.

circumcision The surgical removal of the foreskin of the penis.

clitoris A small erectile structure on the female, corresponding to the penis on the male.

club drugs A variety of drugs including MDMA, GHB, GBL, ketamine, fentanyl, Rohypnol, and nitrites that first became popular at nightclubs, bars, and raves.

cocaine A white crystalline powder extracted from the leaves of the coca plant that stimulates the central nervous system and produces a brief period of euphoria followed by a depression.

codependency An emotional and psychological behavioral pattern in which the spouses, partners, parents, children, and friends of individuals with addictive behaviors allow or enable their loved ones to continue their self-destructive habits.

cognitive therapy A technique used to identify an individual's beliefs and attitudes, recognize negative thought patterns, and educate in alternative ways of thinking.

cohabitation Two people living together as a couple, without official ties such as marriage.

coitus interruptus The removal of the penis from the vagina before ejaculation.

coma A state of total unconsciousness.

complementary and alternative medicine (CAM) A term applied to all health-care approaches, practices, and treatments not widely taught in medical schools, not generally used in hospitals, and not usually reimbursed by medical insurance companies.

complementary proteins Incomplete proteins that, when combined, provide all the amino acids essential for protein synthesis.

complete protein A protein that contains all the amino acids needed by the body for growth and maintenance.

complex carbohydrates Starches, including cereals, fruits, and vegetables.

computer vision syndrome A condition caused by computer use marked by tired and sore eyes; blurred vision; headaches; and neck, shoulder, and back pain.

conception The merging of a sperm and an ovum.

condoms Latex or polyurethane sheaths worn over the penis during sexual acts to prevent conception and/or the transmission of disease; the female condom lines the walls of the vagina.

contraception The prevention of conception; birth control.

corpus luteum A yellowish mass of tissue that is formed, immediately after ovulation, from the remaining cells of the follicle; it secretes estrogen and progesterone for the remainder of the menstrual cycle.

covictimization Experiencing both physical and sexual forms of intimate partner violence.

Cowper's glands Two small glands that discharge into the male urethra; also called bulbourethral glands.

culture The set of shared attitudes, values, goals, and practices of a group that are internalized by an individual within the group.

cunnilingus Sexual stimulation of a woman's genitals by means of oral manipulation.

cyberbullying Deliberate, repeated, and hostile actions that use information and communication technologies, including online web pages and text messages, with the intent of harming others by means of intimidation, control, manipulation, false accusations, or humiliation.

cyberstalking A form of cyberbullying that uses online sites, Twitter, e-mail messages, and social media to harass victims and try to damage their reputation or turn others against them.

cystitis Infection of the urinary bladder.

decibels (dB) Units for measuring the intensity of sounds.

defense mechanisms Psychological processes that alleviate anxiety and eliminate mental conflict; include denial, displacement, projection, rationalization, reaction formation, and repression.

delirium tremens (DTs) The delusions, hallucinations, and agitated behavior following withdrawal from long-term chronic alcohol abuse.

dementia Deterioration of mental capability.

dendrites Branching fibers of a neuron that receive impulses from axon terminals of other neurons and conduct these impulses toward the nucleus.

designer drugs Illegally manufactured psychoactive drugs that have dangerous physical and psychological effects.

detoxification The supervised removal of a poisonous or harmful substance (such as a drug) from the body; a therapy for alcoholics in which they are denied alcohol in a controlled environment.

diabetes mellitus A disease in which the inadequate production of insulin leads to failure of the body tissues to break down carbohydrates at a normal rate.

diaphragm A bowl-like rubber cup with a flexible rim that is inserted into the vagina to cover the cervix and prevent the passage of sperm into the uterus during sexual intercourse; used with a spermicidal foam or jelly, it serves as both a chemical and a physical barrier to sperm.

diastole The period between contractions in the cardiac cycle, during which the heart relaxes and dilates as it fills with blood.

diastolic blood pressure Lowest blood pressure, which occurs between contractions of the heart.

dietary fiber The nondigestible form of carbohydrates found in plant foods, such as leaves, stems, skins, seeds, and hulls.

distress A negative stress that may result in illness.

do-not-resuscitate (DNR) orders Advance directives expressing an individual's preference that resuscitation efforts not be made during a medical crisis.

dopamine A brain chemical associated with feelings of satisfaction and euphoria.

drug Any substance, other than food, that affects bodily functions and structures when taken into the body.

drug abuse The excessive use of a drug in a manner inconsistent with accepted medical practice.

drug dependence Continued substance use even when its use causes cognitive, behavioral, and physical symptoms.

drug diversion The transfer of a drug from the person for whom it was prescribed to another individual.

drug misuse The use of a drug for a purpose (or person) other than that for which it was medically intended.

dynamic flexibility The ability to move a joint quickly and fluidly through its entire range of motion with little resistance.

dynamic stretching Stretching that increases the range of motion around a joint or group of joints by using active muscular effort, momentum, and speed.

dysfunctional Characterized by negative and destructive patterns of behavior between partners or between parents and children.

dysmenorrhea Painful menstruation.

dyspareunia A sexual difficulty in which a woman experiences pain during sexual intercourse.

eating disorders Unusual, often dangerous patterns of food consumption, including anorexia nervosa and bulimia nervosa.

ecosystem A community of organisms sharing a physical and chemical environment and interacting with each other.

Ecstasy (MDMA) A synthetic compound, also known as methylenedioxymethamphetamine, that is similar in structure to methamphetamine and has both stimulant and hallucinogenic effects.

ectopic pregnancy A pregnancy in which the fertilized egg has implanted itself outside the uterine cavity, usually in the fallopian tube.

ejaculation The expulsion of semen from the penis.

ejaculatory ducts The canals connecting the seminal vesicles and vas deferens.

electromagnetic fields (EMFs) The invisible electric and magnetic fields generated by an electrically charged conductor.

embryo An organism in its early stage of development; in humans, the embryonic period lasts from the second to the eighth week of pregnancy.

emergency contraception (EC) Types of oral contraceptive pills, usually taken within 72 hours after intercourse, that can prevent pregnancy.

emotional health The ability to express and acknowledge one's feelings and moods and exhibit adaptability and compassion for others.

emotional intelligence The ability to monitor and use emotions to guide thinking and actions.

enabling Unwittingly contributing to a person's addictive or abusive behavior. Components of enabling include shielding or covering up for an abuser/addict; controlling him or her; taking over responsibilities; rationalizing addictive behavior; or cooperating with him or her.

enabling factors The skills, resources, and physical and mental capabilities that shape our behavior.

endocrine disruptors Synthetic chemicals that interfere with the ways that hormones work in humans and wildlife.

endocrine system The group of ductless glands that produce hormones and secrete them directly into the blood for transport to target organs.

endometrium The mucous membrane lining the uterus.

environmental tobacco smoke Secondhand cigarette smoke; the third-leading preventable cause of death.

epididymis That portion of the male duct system in which sperm mature.

epilepsy A variety of neurological disorders characterized by sudden attacks (seizures) of violent muscle contractions and unconsciousness.

erectile dysfunction (ED) The consistent inability to maintain a penile erection sufficient for adequate sexual relations.

erogenous Sexually sensitive.

essential nutrients Nutrients that the body cannot manufacture for itself and must obtain from food.

estrogen The female sex hormone that stimulates female secondary sex characteristics.

ethyl alcohol The intoxicating agent in alcoholic beverages; also called ethanol.

eustress Positive stress, which stimulates a person to function properly.

euthanasia The painless killing of a patient with an incurable fatal disease or in an irreversible coma.

evidence-based medicine The choice of a medical treatment on the basis of large randomized controlled research trials and large prospective studies.

exercise A type of physical activity that requires planned, structured, and repetitive bodily movement with the intent of improving one or more components of physical fitness.

failure rate The number of pregnancies that occur per year for every 100 women using a particular method of birth control.

fallopian tubes The pair of channels that transport ova from the ovaries to the uterus; the usual site of fertilization.

families Groups of people united by marriage, blood, or adoption—each residing in the same household; maintaining a common culture; and interacting with one another on the basis of their roles within the group.

fellatio Sexual stimulation of a man's genitals by means of oral manipulation.

fertilization The fusion of sperm and egg nucleus.

fetal alcohol effects (FAE) Milder forms of FAS, including low birth weight, irritability as newborns, and permanent mental impairment as a result of the mother's alcohol consumption during pregnancy.

fetal alcohol syndrome (FAS) A cluster of physical and mental defects in the newborn, including low birth weight, smaller-than-normal head circumference, intrauterine growth retardation, and permanent mental impairment caused by the mother's alcohol consumption during pregnancy.

fetus The human organism developing in the uterus from the ninth week until birth.

FITT A formula that describes the frequency, intensity, type, and length of time for physical activity.

flexibility The range of motion allowed by one's joints; determined by the length of muscles, tendons, and ligaments attached to the joints.

folic acid A form of folate used in vitamin supplements and fortified foods.

functional fiber Isolated, nondigestible carbohydrates that have beneficial effects in humans.

functional fitness The ability to perform real-life activities, such as lifting a heavy suitcase.

fungi (singular, fungus) Organisms that reproduce by means of spores.

gambling disorder Persistent and recurrent problematic gambling that leads to significant impairment or distress.

gamma globulin The antibody-containing portion of the blood fluid (plasma).

GBL (gamma butyrolactone) The main ingredient in gamma hydroxybutyrate (GHB); once ingested, GBL converts to GHB and can cause the ingestor to lose consciousness.

gender Maleness or femaleness, as determined by a combination of anatomical and physiological factors, psychological factors, and learned behaviors.

generalized anxiety disorder (GAD) An anxiety disorder characterized as chronic distress.

generic A consumer product with no brand name or registered trademark.

GHB (gamma hydroxybutyrate) A brain messenger chemical that stimulates the release of human growth hormone; commonly abused for its high and its alleged ability to trim fat and build muscles. Also known as "blue nitro" or the "date rape drug."

gingivitis Inflammation of the gums.

glia Support cells for neurons in the brain and spinal cord that separate the brain from the bloodstream, assist in the growth of neurons, speed transmission of nerve impulses, and eliminate damaged neurons.

gonadotropins Gonad-stimulating hormones produced by the pituitary gland.

gonorrhea A sexually transmitted infection caused by the bacterium *Neisseria gonorrhoeae*; symptoms include discharge from the penis; women are generally asymptomatic.

gum disease Infection of the gums and bones that hold teeth in place.

hallucinogens Drugs that cause hallucinations.

hashish A concentrated form of a drug derived from the cannabis plant, that contains the psychoactive ingredient THC, which causes a sense of euphoria when inhaled or eaten.

hazing Any activity that humiliates, degrades, or poses a risk of emotional or physical harm for the sake of joining a group or maintaining full status in that group.

health A state of complete well-being, including physical, psychological, spiritual, social, intellectual, and environmental dimensions.

health belief model (HBM) A model of behavioral change that focuses on the individual's attitudes and beliefs.

health literacy Ability to understand health information and use it to make good decisions about health and medical care.

health promotion Any planned combination of educational, political, regulatory, and organizational supports for actions and conditions of living conducive to the health of individuals, groups, or communities.

helminths Parasitic roundworms or flatworms.

hepatitis An inflammation and/or infection of the liver caused by a virus, often accompanied by jaundice.

herbal medicine An ancient form of medical treatment using substances derived from trees, flowers, ferns, seaweeds, and lichens to treat disease.

herpes simplex A condition caused by one of the herpes viruses and characterized by lesions of the skin or mucous membranes; herpes simplex virus 2 is sexually transmitted and causes genital blisters or sores.

heterosexual Primary sexual orientation toward members of the other sex.

holistic An approach to medicine that takes into account body, mind, emotions, and spirit.

holographic will A will wholly in the handwriting of its author.

home health care Provision of medical services and equipment to patients in the home to restore or maintain comfort, function, and health.

homeopathy A system of medical practice that treats a disease by administering dosages of substances that would in healthy persons produce symptoms similar to those of the disease.

homeostasis The body's natural state of balance or stability.

homosexuals Those with primary sexual orientation toward members of the same sex.

hooking up An experience in which partners engage in intimate behaviors without explicit expectation of future romantic commitment.

hookup Refers to a range of physically intimate behaviors—from kissing to intercourse—with no expectation of emotional intimacy or a romantic relationship.

hormones Substances released in the blood that regulate specific bodily functions.

hormone therapy (HT) The use of supplemental hormones during and after menopause.

hospice A homelike health-care facility or program committed to supportive care for terminally ill people.

host A person or population that contracts one or more pathogenic agents in an environment.

human immunodeficiency virus (HIV) A virus that causes a spectrum of health problems, ranging from a symptomless infection to changes in the immune system, to the development of life-threatening diseases because of impaired immunity.

human papillomavirus (HPV) A pathogen that causes genital warts and increases the risk of cervical cancer.

hunger The physiological drive to consume food.

hypertension High blood pressure that occurs when the blood exerts excessive pressure against the arterial walls.

hypothermia An abnormally low body temperature; if not treated appropriately, coma or death could result.

immune deficiency Partial or complete inability of the immune system to respond to pathogens.

immunity Protection from infectious diseases.

immunotherapy A series of injections of small but increasing doses of an allergen, used to treat allergies.

implantation The embedding of the fertilized ovum in the uterine lining.

incomplete protein Protein that lacks one or more of the amino acids essential for protein synthesis.

incubation period The time between a pathogen's entrance into the body and the first symptom.

infertility The inability to conceive a child.

infiltration A gradual penetration or invasion.

inflammation A localized body response to tissue injury, characterized by swelling and the dilation of the blood vessels.

influenza Any type of fairly common, highly contagious viral diseases.

informed consent Permission (to undergo or receive a medical procedure or treatment) given voluntarily, with full knowledge and understanding of the procedure or treatment and its possible consequences.

inhalants Substances that produce vapors having psychoactive effects when sniffed.

insulin resistance A condition in which the body produces insulin but does not use it properly.

integrative medicine An approach that combines traditional medicine with alternative/complementary therapies.

intercourse Sexual stimulation by means of entry of the penis into the vagina; coitus.

interpersonal therapy (IPT) A technique used to develop communication skills and relationships.

intimacy A state of closeness between two people, characterized by the desire and ability to share one's innermost thoughts and feelings with each other either verbally or nonverbally.

intoxication Maladaptive behavioral, psychological, and physiologic changes that occur as a result of substance abuse.

intramuscular Into or within a muscle.

intrauterine device (IUD) A device inserted into the uterus through the cervix to prevent pregnancy by interfering with implantation.

intravenous Into a vein.

ionizing radiation A form of energy emitted from atoms as they undergo internal change.

isokinetic Having the same force; exercise with specialized equipment that provides resistance equal to the force applied by the user throughout the entire range of motion.

isometric Of the same length; exercise in which muscles increase their tension without shortening in length, such as when pushing an immovable object.

isotonic Having the same tension or tone; exercise requiring the repetition of an action that creates tension, such as weight lifting or calisthenics.

labia majora The fleshy outer folds that border the female genital area.

labia minora The fleshy inner folds that border the female genital area.

labor The process leading up to birth: effacement and dilation of the cervix; the movement of the baby into and through the birth canal, accompanied by strong contractions; and contraction of the uterus and expulsion of the placenta after the birth.

laparoscopy A surgical sterilization procedure in which the fallopian tubes are observed with a laparoscope inserted through a small incision, and then cut or blocked.

lipoproteins Compounds in blood that are made up of proteins and fat; a high-density lipoprotein (HDL) picks up excess cholesterol in the blood; a low-density lipoprotein (LDL) carries more cholesterol and deposits it on the walls of arteries.

living will An advance directive that provides instructions for the use of life-sustaining procedures in the event of terminal illness or injury.

locus of control An individual's belief about the sources of power and influence over his or her life.

long-acting reversible contraceptives (LARCs) Contraceptive devices that provide protection from pregnancy for an extended period without any action by users. Examples include intrauterine devices, injections, and implants.

LSD (lysergic acid diethylamide) A synthetic psychoactive substance originally developed to explore mental illness.

Lyme disease A disease caused by a bacterium carried by a tick; it may cause heart arrhythmias, neurological problems, and arthritis symptoms.

lymph nodes Small tissue masses in which some immune cells are stored.

macronutrients Nutrients required by the human body in the greatest amounts, including water, carbohydrates, proteins, and fats.

mainstream smoke The smoke inhaled directly by smoking a cigarette.

major depressive disorder Sadness that does not end; ongoing feelings of utter helplessness.

mammography A diagnostic X-ray exam used to detect breast cancer.

marijuana The drug derived from the cannabis plant, containing the psychoactive ingredient THC, which causes a mild sense of euphoria when inhaled or eaten.

marriage and family therapists Psychiatrists, psychologists, or social workers who specialize in marriage and family counseling.

mastectomy The surgical removal of an entire breast.

masturbation Manual (or nonmanual) self-stimulation of the genitals, often resulting in orgasm.

medical abortion Method of ending a pregnancy within nine weeks of conception using hormonal medications that cause expulsion of the fertilized egg.

medical history Health-related information that a health-care professional collects while interviewing a patient.

meditation A group of approaches that use quiet sitting, breathing techniques, and/or chanting to relax, improve concentration, and become attuned to one's inner self.

menarche The onset of menstruation at puberty.

meningitis An extremely serious, potentially fatal illness that attacks the membranes around the brain and spinal cord; caused by the bacterium *Neisseria meningitis*.

menopause The complete cessation of ovulation and menstruation for 12 consecutive months.

menstruation Discharge of blood from the vagina as a result of the shedding of the uterine lining at the end of the menstrual cycle.

mental disorder A behavioral or psychological syndrome associated with distress or disability or with a significantly increased risk of suffering death, pain, disability, or loss of freedom.

mental health The ability to perceive reality as it is, respond to its challenges, and develop rational strategies for living.

metabolic fitness The reduction in risk for diabetes and cardiovascular disease, which can be achieved through a moderate-intensity exercise program.

metabolic syndrome A cluster of disorders of the body's metabolism that make diabetes, heart disease, or stroke more likely.

metastasize To spread to other parts of the body via the bloodstream or lymphatic system.

MET (metabolic equivalent of task) The amount of energy used at rest.

micronutrients Vitamins and minerals needed by the body in very small amounts.

microaggressions Subtle racial expressions.

microassaults Conscious and intentional actions and slurs.

microinsults Verbal and nonverbal communications that subtly convey rudeness and insensitivity.

microinvalidations Communications that subtly exclude, negate, or nullify the thoughts, feelings, or experiential reality of a person of color.

microwaves Extremely high-frequency electromagnetic waves that increase the rate at which molecules vibrate, thereby generating heat.

mild cognitive impairment (MCI) A slight but noticeable and measurable decline in cognitive abilities, including memory and thinking skills.

mindfulness A method of stress reduction that involves experiencing the physical and mental sensations of the present moment.

minerals Naturally occurring inorganic substances, small amounts of some being essential in metabolism and nutrition.

minipills, progestin-only pills Oral contraceptives containing a small amount of progestin and no estrogen, which prevents contraception by making the mucus in the cervix so thick that sperm cannot enter the uterus.

miscarriage A pregnancy that terminates before the twentieth week of gestation; also called spontaneous abortion.

mononucleosis An infectious viral disease characterized by an excess of white blood cells in the blood, fever, bodily discomfort, a sore throat, and kidney and liver complications.

monophasic pills Oral contraceptives that release synthetic estrogen and progestin at constant levels throughout the menstrual cycle.

mons pubis The rounded, fleshy area over the junction of the female pubic bones.

mood A sustained emotional state that colors one's view of the world for hours or days.

multiphasic pills Oral contraceptives that release different levels of estrogen and progestin to mimic the hormonal fluctuations of the natural menstrual cycle.

multiple chemical sensitivity (MCS) A sensitivity to low-level chemical exposures from ordinary substances, such as perfumes and tobacco smoke, that results in physiological responses such as chest pain, depression, dizziness, fatigue, and nausea. Also known as environmentally triggered illness.

muscular endurance The ability to withstand the stress of continued physical exertion.

muscular strength Physical power; the maximum weight one can lift, push, or press in one effort.

muscle dysmorphia A condition that affects mostly male bodybuilders in which they become obsessed with appearance and size of muscles.

mutagens Agents that cause alterations in the genetic material of living cells.

Myalgic Encephalomyelitis/Chronic Fatigue Syndrome (ME/CFS) A cluster of symptoms whose cause is not yet known; a primary symptom is debilitating fatigue.

myocardial infarction (MI) A condition characterized by the dying of tissue areas in the myocardium, caused by interruption of the blood supply to those areas; the medical name for a heart attack.

naturopathy An alternative system of treatment of disease that emphasizes the use of natural remedies such as sun, water, heat, and air. Therapies may include dietary changes, steam baths, and exercise.

NEAT (nonexercise activity thermogenesis) Nonvolitional movement that can be an effective way of burning calories.

neurons Nerve cells; the basic working units of the brain, which transmit information from the senses to the brain and from the brain to specific body parts; each neuron consists of a cell body, an axon terminal, and dendrites.

neuropsychiatry The study of the brain and mind.

neurotransmitters Chemicals released by neurons that stimulate or inhibit the action of other neurons.

nicotine The addictive substance in tobacco; one of the most toxic of all poisons.

nongonococcal urethritis (NGU) Inflammation of the urethra caused by organisms other than the *Gonococcus* bacterium.

nonvolitional sex Sexual behavior that violates a person's right to choose when and with whom to have sex and what sexual behaviors to engage in.

nucleus The central part of a cell, contained in the cell body of a neuron.

nutrition The science devoted to the study of dietary needs for food and the effects of food on organisms.

obesity The excessive accumulation of fat in the body; class 1 obesity is defined by a BMI between 30.0 and 34.9; class 2 obesity by a BMI between 35.0 and 39.9; class 3, or severe obesity, is a BMI of 40 or higher.

obsessive-compulsive disorder (OCD) An anxiety disorder characterized by obsessions and/or compulsions that impair one's ability to function and form relationships.

omega-3 and omega-6 Polyunsaturated fatty acids with recognized health benefits. Omega-3 fatty acids are found in fatty fish such as salmon and sardines, flaxseed, and walnuts. Omega-6 fatty acids are found in vegetable oils, nuts, seeds, meat, poultry, and eggs.

opioids Drugs that have sleep-inducing and pain-relieving properties, including opium and its derivatives and nonopioid, synthetic drugs.

optimism The tendency to seek out, remember, and expect pleasurable experiences.

oral contraceptives Preparations of synthetic hormones that inhibit ovulation; also referred to as *birth control pills* or simply *the pill*.

organic Term designating food produced with, or production based on the use of, fertilizers originating from plants or animals, without the use of pesticides or chemically formulated fertilizers.

organophosphates Toxic pesticides that may cause cancer, birth defects, neurological disorders, and damage to wildlife and the environment.

orgasm A series of contractions of the pelvic muscles occurring at the peak of sexual arousal.

osteoporosis A condition in which the bones become increasingly soft and porous, making them susceptible to injury.

outcomes The ultimate impacts of particular treatments or absence of treatment.

ovaries The female sex organs that produce egg cells, estrogen, and progesterone.

overloading A method of physical training that involves increasing the number of repetitions or the amount of resistance gradually to work the muscle to temporary fatigue.

overload principle The idea that for the body to get stronger, you must provide a greater stress or demand on the body than it is normally accustomed to handling.

over-the-counter (OTC) Medications that can be obtained legally without a prescription from a medical professional.

overtrain Working muscles too intensely or too frequently, resulting in persistent muscle soreness, injuries, unintended weight loss, nervousness, and an inability to relax.

overuse injuries Physical injuries to joints or muscles, such as strains, fractures, and tendinitis, which result from overdoing a repetitive activity.

overweight A condition of having a BMI between 25.0 and 29.9.

ovulation The release of a mature ovum from an ovary approximately 14 days prior to the onset of menstruation.

ovum (plural, ova) The female gamete (egg cell).

ozone A component of smog that can impair the body's immune system and cause long-term lung damage.

panic attacks Short episodes characterized by physical sensations of light-headedness, dizziness, hyperventilation, and numbness of extremities, accompanied by an inexplicable terror, usually of a physical disaster such as death.

panic disorder An anxiety disorder in which the apprehension or experience of recurring panic attacks is so intense that normal functioning is impaired.

Pap smear A test in which cells removed from the cervix are examined under a microscope for signs of cancer; also called a Pap test.

passive stretching A stretching technique in which an external force or resistance (your body, a partner, gravity, or a weight) helps the joints move through their range of motion.

pathogens Microorganisms that produce disease.

PCP (phencyclidine) A synthetic psychoactive substance that produces effects similar to other psychoactive drugs when swallowed, smoked, sniffed, or injected, but also may trigger unpredictable behavioral changes.

pelvic inflammatory disease (PID) An inflammation of the internal female genital tract, characterized by abdominal pain, fever, and tenderness of the cervix.

penis The male organ of sex and urination.

perimenopause The period from a woman's first irregular cycles to her last menstruation.

perineum The area between the anus and vagina in the female and between the anus and scrotum in the male.

periodontitis Severe gum disease in which the tooth root becomes infected.

persistent vegetative state A state of being awake and capable of reacting to physical stimuli, such as light, while being unaware of pain or other environmental stimuli.

phobias Anxiety disorders marked by an inordinate fear of an object, a class of objects, or a situation, resulting in extreme avoidance behaviors.

physical activity Any movement produced by the muscles that results in expenditure of energy.

physical dependence Physiological attachment to, and need for, a drug.

physical fitness The ability to respond to routine physical demands, with enough reserve energy to cope with a sudden challenge.

phytochemicals Chemicals such as indoles, coumarins, and capsaicin, which exist naturally in plants and have disease-fighting properties.

placenta An organ that develops after implantation and to which the embryo attaches, via the umbilical cord, for nourishment and waste removal.

plaque A sludgelike substance that builds up on the inner walls of arteries.

pollutant A substance or agent in the environment, usually the by-product of human industry or activity, that is injurious to human, animal, or plant life.

pollution Any change in the air, water, or soil that could reduce its ability to support life.

polyabuse The misuse or abuse of more than one drug.

posttraumatic stress disorder (PTSD) The repeated reliving of a trauma through nightmares or recollection.

potentiating Making more effective or powerful.

practice guidelines Recommendations for diagnosis and treatment of various health problems based on evidence from scientific research.

preconception care Health care to prepare for pregnancy.

precycling The use of products that are packaged in recycled or recyclable material.

prediabetes A condition in which blood glucose levels are higher than normal but not high enough for a diagnosis of diabetes.

predisposing factors The beliefs, values, attitudes, knowledge, and perceptions that influence our behavior.

predrinking Consuming alcoholic beverages, usually with friends, before going out to bars or parties; also called pregaming, preloading, or front-loading.

prehypertension A condition of slightly elevated blood pressure, which is likely to worsen in time.

premature ejaculation A sexual difficulty in which a man ejaculates so rapidly that his partner's satisfaction is impaired.

premature labor Labor that occurs after the twentieth week but before the thirty-seventh week of pregnancy.

premenstrual dysphoric disorder (PMDD) A disorder that causes symptoms of psychological depression during the last week of the menstrual cycle.

premenstrual syndrome (PMS) A disorder that causes physical discomfort and psychological distress prior to a woman's menstrual period.

prevention Information and support offered to help healthy people identify their health risks, reduce stressors, prevent potential medical problems, and enhance their well-being.

primary care Ambulatory or outpatient care provided by a physician in an office, an emergency room, or a clinic.

progesterone The female sex hormone that stimulates the uterus, preparing it for the arrival of a fertilized egg.

progressive overloading Gradually increasing physical challenges once the body adapts to the stress placed upon it to produce maximum benefits.

progressive relaxation A method of reducing muscle tension by contracting, then relaxing, certain areas of the body.

proof The alcoholic strength of a distilled spirit, expressed as twice the percentage of alcohol present.

prostate gland A structure surrounding the male urethra that produces a secretion that helps liquefy the semen from the testes.

protection Measures that an individual can take when participating in risky behavior to prevent injury or unwanted risks.

proteins Organic compounds composed of amino acids; one of the essential nutrients.

protozoa Microscopic animals made up of one cell or a group of similar cells.

psychiatric drugs Medications that regulate a person's mental, emotional, and physical functions to facilitate normal functioning.

psychiatric nurses Nurses with special training and experience in mental health care.

psychiatrists Licensed medical doctors with additional training in psychotherapy, psychopharmacology, and treatment of mental disorders.

psychoactive Mind-affecting.

psychodynamic Interpreting behaviors in terms of early experiences and unconscious influences.

psychological dependence Emotional or mental attachment to the use of a drug.

psychologists Mental health care professionals who have completed a doctoral or graduate program in psychology and are trained in psychotherapeutic techniques, but who are not medically trained and do not prescribe medications.

psychotherapy Treatment designed to produce a response by psychological rather than physical means, such as suggestion, persuasion, reassurance, and support.

quackery Medical fakery; unproven practices claiming to cure diseases or solve health problems.

range of motion The fullest extent of possible movement in a particular joint.

rape Sexual penetration of a female or a male by means of intimidation, force, or fraud.

Rating of Perceived Exertion (RPE) A self-assessment scale that rates symptoms of breathlessness and fatigue.

receptors Molecules on the surface of neurons on which neurotransmitters bind after their release from other neurons.

recycling The processing or reuse of manufactured materials to reduce consumption of raw materials.

refractory period The period of time following orgasm during which the male cannot experience another orgasm.

reinforcing factors Rewards, encouragement, and recognition that influence our behavior in the short run.

relapse prevention An alcohol recovery treatment method that focuses on social skills training to develop ways of preventing or minimizing a relapse.

repetitive motion injuries (RMIs) Inflammation of or damage to parts of the body due to repetition of the same movements.

reps (or repetitions) In weight training, multiple performances of a movement or exercise.

resting heart rate The number of heartbeats per minute during inactivity.

reuptake Reabsorption by the originating cell of neurotransmitters that have not connected with receptors and have been left in synapses.

reversibility principle The idea that the physical benefits of exercise are lost through disuse or inactivity.

rhythm method A birth control method in which sexual intercourse is avoided during those days of the menstrual cycle in which fertilization is most likely to occur.

rubella An infectious disease that may cause birth defects if contracted by a pregnant woman; also called German measles.

salvia An herb with hallucinogenic properties when smoked or inhaled.

same-sex marriage Governmentally, socially, or religiously recognized marriage in which two people of the same sex live together as a family.

satiety The sensation of feeling full after eating.

saturated fats A chemical term indicating that a fat molecule contains as many hydrogen atoms as its carbon skeleton can hold. These fats are normally solid at room temperature.

schizophrenia A general term for a group of mental disorders with characteristic psychotic symptoms, such as delusions, hallucinations, and disordered thought patterns during the active phase of the illness, and a duration of at least six months.

scrotum The external sac or pouch that holds the testes.

secondary sex characteristics Physical changes associated with maleness or femaleness, induced by the sex hormones.

self-actualization A state of wellness and fulfillment that can be achieved once certain human needs are satisfied; living to one's full potential.

self-care Head-to-toe maintenance, including good oral care, appropriate screening tests, knowing your medical rights, and understanding the health-care system.

self-compassion A healthy form of self-acceptance in the face of perceived inadequacy or failure.

self-disclosure Sharing personal information and experiences with another that he or she would not otherwise discover; self-disclosure involves risk and vulnerability.

self-efficacy Belief in one's ability to accomplish a goal or change a behavior.

self-esteem Confidence and satisfaction in oneself.

semen The viscous whitish fluid that is the complete male ejaculate; a combination of sperm and secretions from the prostate gland, seminal vesicles, and other glands.

seminal vesicles Glands in the male reproductive system that produce the major portion of the fluid of semen.

sets In weight training, multiples of repetitions of the same movement or exercise.

sex Maleness or femaleness, resulting from genetic, structural, and functional factors.

sexting The sharing of digital images or videos of sexually explicit content over the Internet.

sexual coercion Sexual activity forced upon a person by the exertion of psychological pressure by another person.

sexual dysfunction The inability to react emotionally and/or physically to sexual stimulation in a way expected of the average healthy person or according to one's own standards.

sexual harassment Uninvited and unwanted sexual attention.

sexual health The integration of the physical, emotional, intellectual, social, and spiritual aspects of sexual being in ways that are positively enriching and that enhance personality, communication, and love.

sexuality The behaviors, instincts, and attitudes associated with being sexual.

sexually transmitted disease (STD) A disease that is caused by a sexually transmitted infection that produces symptoms.

sexually transmitted infection (STI) The presence in the human body of an infectious agent that can be passed from one sexual partner to another.

sexual orientation The direction of an individual's sexual interest, either to members of the opposite sex or to members of the same sex.

sidestream smoke The smoke emitted by a burning cigarette and breathed by everyone in a closed room, including the smoker; contains more tar and nicotine than mainstream smoke.

simple carbohydrates Sugars; like all carbohydrates, they provide the body with glucose.

Snus A smokeless tobacco product similar to snuff and chewing tobacco.

social anxiety disorder A fear and avoidance of social situations.

social contagion The process by which friends, friends of friends, acquaintances, and others in our social circle influence our behavior and our health—both positively and negatively.

social norm A behavior or attitude that a particular group expects, values, and enforces.

specificity principle The idea that each part of the body adapts to a particular type and amount of stress placed upon it.

sperm The male gamete produced by the testes and transported outside the body through ejaculation.

spermatogenesis The process by which sperm cells are produced.

spiritual health The ability to identify one's basic purpose in life and to achieve one's full potential.

spiritual intelligence The capacity to sense, understand, and tap into ourselves, others, and the world around us.

spirituality A belief in someone or something that transcends the boundaries of self.

stalking The willful, repeated, and malicious following of another person.

static flexibility The ability to assume and maintain an extended position at one end point in a joint's range of motion.

static stretching A stretching technique in which a gradual stretch is held for a short time of 10 to 30 seconds.

sterilization A surgical procedure to end a person's reproductive capability.

stimulants Agents, such as drugs, that temporarily relieve drowsiness, help in the performance of repetitive tasks, and improve capacity for work.

stress The nonspecific response of the body to any demands made upon it; may be characterized by muscle tension and acute anxiety, or may be a positive force for action.

stress response The cascade of internal changes that mobilize the body's resources for action.

stressor A specific or nonspecific agent or situation that causes the stress response in a body.

stroke A cerebrovascular event in which the blood supply to a portion of the brain is blocked.

subcutaneous Under the skin.

suction curettage A procedure in which the contents of the uterus are removed by means of suction and scraping.

sustainability A method of using a resource so that the resource is not depleted or permanently damaged.

synapse A specialized site at which electrical impulses are transmitted from the axon terminal of one neuron to a dendrite of another.

synergistic Characterized by a combined effect that is greater than the sum of the individual effects.

syphilis A sexually transmitted infection caused by the bacterium *Treponema pallidum* and characterized by early sores, a latent period, and a final period of life-threatening symptoms, including brain damage and heart failure.

systemic disease A pathologic condition that spreads throughout the body.

systole The contraction phase of the cardiac cycle.

systolic blood pressure Highest blood pressure, which occurs when the heart contracts.

tar A thick, sticky dark fluid produced by the burning of tobacco, made up of several hundred different chemicals, many of them poisonous, some of them carcinogenic.

target heart rate Fifty to 85 percent of the maximum heart rate; the heart rate at which one derives maximum cardiovascular benefit from aerobic exercise.

tend and befriend A behavioral response to stress characterized by increased feelings of trust.

terminal illness An illness in which death is inevitable.

testes (singular, testis) The male sex organs that produce sperm and testosterone.

testosterone The male sex hormone that stimulates male secondary sex characteristics.

tobacco use disorder A problematic pattern of tobacco use leading to clinically significant impairment or distress.

tolerance A need for markedly increased amounts of alcohol or a drug to achieve the desired effect or a markedly diminished effect with continued use of a substance.

toxicity Poisonousness; the dosage level at which a drug becomes poisonous to the body, causing either temporary or permanent damage.

toxic shock syndrome (TSS) A disease characterized by fever, vomiting, diarrhea, and often shock, caused by a bacterium that releases toxic waste products into the bloodstream.

transcendence The sense of passing into a foreign region or dimension, often experienced by a person near death.

***trans* fat** Fat formed when liquid vegetable oils are processed to make table spreads or cooking fats; also found in dairy and beef products; considered to be especially dangerous dietary fats.

transgender Having a gender identity opposite one's biological sex.

transient ischemic attacks (TIAs) Cerebrovascular events in which the blood supply to a portion of the brain is blocked temporarily; repeated attacks are predictors of more severe strokes.

transtheoretical model A model of behavioral change that focuses on the individual's decision making; it states that an individual progresses through a sequence of six stages as he or she makes a change in behavior.

trichomoniasis An infection of the protozoan *Trichomonas vaginalis*; females experience vaginal burning, itching, and discharge, but male carriers may be asymptomatic.

triglycerides Fats that flow through the blood after meals and are linked to increased risk of coronary artery disease.

tubal ligation The suturing or tying shut of the fallopian tubes to prevent pregnancy.

tubal occlusion The blocking of the fallopian tubes to prevent pregnancy.

tuberculosis (TB) A highly infectious bacterial disease that primarily affects the lungs and is often fatal.

12 Step program Self-help group program based on the principles of Alcoholics Anonymous.

ulcer A lesion in, or an erosion of, the mucous membrane of an organ.

unsaturated fats A chemical term indicating that a fat molecule contains fewer hydrogen atoms than its carbon skeleton can hold. These fats are normally liquid at room temperature.

urethra The canal through which urine from the bladder leaves the body; in the male, also serves as the channel for seminal fluid.

urethral opening The outer opening of the thin tube that carries urine from the bladder.

urethritis Infection of the urethra.

uterus The female organ that houses the developing fetus until birth.

vagina The canal leading from the exterior opening in the female genital area to the uterus.

vaginal contraceptive film (VCF) A small dissolvable sheet saturated with spermicide that can be inserted into the vagina and placed over the cervix.

vaginal spermicide A substance that kills or neutralizes sperm, inserted into the vagina in the form of a foam, cream, jelly, suppository, or film.

vaginismus A sexual difficulty in which a woman experiences painful spasms of the vagina during sexual intercourse.

values The criteria by which one makes choices about one's thoughts, actions, goals, and ideals.

vas deferens Two tubes that carry sperm from the epididymis into the urethra.

vasectomy A surgical sterilization procedure in which each vas deferens is cut and tied shut to stop the passage of sperm to the urethra for ejaculation.

vector A biological or physical vehicle that carries the agent of infection to the host.

ventricles The two lower chambers of the heart, which pump blood out of the heart and into the arteries.

viruses Submicroscopic infectious agents; the most primitive forms of life.

visualization, or guided imagery An approach to stress control, self-healing, or motivating life changes by means of seeing oneself in the state of calmness, wellness, or change.

vital signs Measurements of physiological functioning—specifically temperature, blood pressure, pulse rate, and respiration rate.

vitamins Organic substances that the body needs in very small amounts and that carry out a variety of functions in metabolism and nutrition.

waist-to-hip-ratio (WHR) The proportion of one's waist circumference to one's hip circumference.

wellness A deliberate lifestyle choice characterized by personal responsibility and optimal enhancement of physical, mental, and spiritual health.

withdrawal Development of symptoms, such as sweating, rapid pulse, tremor, nausea, vomiting, temporary hallucinations, physical agitation, anxiety, or seizures, when substance use is stopped.

zygote A fertilized egg.

References

Chapter 1

1. Allen, N. B., et al. "Blood Pressure Trajectories in Early Adulthood and Subclinical Atherosclerosis in Middle Age." *Journal of the American Medical Association* vol. 311, no. 5 (February 5, 2014): pp. 490–497.

2. Barthold, D., et al. "Analyzing Whether Countries Are Equally Efficient at Improving Longevity for Men and Women." *American Journal of Public Health* (December 12, 2013).

3. Centers for Disease Control and Prevention. *National Vital Statistics Report* vol. 62, no. 7 (January 6, 2014) www.cdc.gov/nchs/data/nvsr/nvsr62/nvsr62_07.pdf

4. National Research Council and Institute of Medicine. *U.S. Health in International Perspective: Shorter Lives, Poorer Health*. Panel on Understansing Cross-National Health Differences among High-Income Countries, Steven. H. Woolf and Lauden Aron (eds.) Committee on Population, Division of Behavioral and Social Sciences and Education, and Board on Population Health and Public Health Practice, Institute of Medicine. Washington, DC: National Academics Press (2013).

5. National Health Survey. "Summary Health Statistics for U.S. Adults. National Health Survey, 2012. *Vital and Health Statistics* series 10, no. 260. Hyattsville, MD: Department of Health and Human Services (February 2014).

6. U.S. Burden of Disease Collaborators. "The State of U.S. Health, 1990–2010," *Journal of the American Medical Association* vol. 301, no. 6 (2013): pp. 591–608.

7. National Research Council. *U.S. Health in International Perspective.*

8. Ibid.

9. Grollman, E. A. "Multiple Disadvantaged Statuses and Health." *Journal of Health and Social Behavior* vol. 55, no. 1 (March 2014): pp. 3–19.

10. National Heart, Lung, and Blood Institute. *Hispanic Community Health Study/Study of Latinos (HCHS/SOL).* www.nhlbi.nih.gov/resources/obesity/pop-studies/hchs.htm

11. Whiteside, Y. O., et al. "Progress Along the Continuum of HIV—United States, 2010." *Morbidity and Mortality Weekly Report* (MWWR) vol. 63, no. 5 (February 7, 2014): pp. 86–89.

12. Brigham and Women's Hospital. "Charting the Course: A National Policy Summit on the Future of Women's Health (March 3, 2014) www.brighamandwomens.org/Departments_and_Services/womenshealth/ConnorsCenter/Policy/summithome.aspx

13. Ibid.

14. Ibid.

15. National Center for Education Statistics. nces.ed.gov.

16. Hartman, L. A. "Community college students' awareness and use of college information." *Dissertation Abstracts International Section A: Humanities and Social Sciences* vol. 75 (2015).

17. Kenzig, M. "Health status during college students' transition to adulthood: Health behaviors, negative experiences, and the mediating effects of personal development" *Dissertation Abstracts International: Section B: The Sciences and Engineering* vol. 75, (2015).

18. Deforche, B., et al. "Changes in weight, physical activity, sedentary behaviour and dietary intake during the transition to higher education: a prospective study." *I. Int J Behav Nutr Phys Act.* vol. 12, no. 1 (December 2015): p. 173.

19. Ibid.

20. Kenzig. "Health status during college students' transition to adulthood."

21. Ibid.

22. American College Health Association. *American College Health Association-National College Health Assessment II: Reference Group Executive Summary Spring 2014.* Hanover, Md.: American College Health Association (2014).

23. Simon, J. E. and C. L. Docherty. "Current Health-Related Quality of Life is Lower in Former Division 1 Collegiate Athletes Than in Non-collegiate Athletes," *American Journal of Sports and Medicine* vol. 42, no. 2 (February 2014): pp. 423–429.

24. Plotnikoff, R. C. "Effectiveness of interventions targeting physical activity, nutrition and healthy weight for university and college students: a systematic review and meta-analysis." *Int J Behav Nutr Phys Act.* vol. 12, no. 1 (April 1, 2015): p. 45. doi: 10.1186/s12966-015-0203-7.

25. Ibid.

26. Högström, G., et al. "High Aerobic Fitness in Late Adolescence Is Associated with a Reduced Risk of Myocardial Infarction Later in Life: A Nationwide Cohort Study in Men." *European Heart Journal* (January 7, 2014).

27. ACHA, 2014.

28. Ibid.

29. Holford, T. R., et al. "Tobacco Control and the Reduction in Smoking-Related Premature Deaths in the United States, 1964–2012," *Journal of the American Medical Association* vol. 311, no. 2 (January 8, 2014): pp. 164–171.

30. Montanaro, E. A., & Bryan, A. D. "Comparing theory-based condom interventions: Health belief model versus theory of planned behavior." *Health Psychology* vol. 33, no. 10 (2014): pp. 1251–1260.

31. Lodyga, M. G. "The relationship between health belief model constructs and factors influencing cancer self-examinations in college students." *Dissertation Abstracts International Section A: Humanities and Social Sciences* vol. 75 (2015).

32. McNamara, Robert S., et al. "Motivational Interviewing Intervention With College Student Tobacco Users: Providers' Beliefs and Behaviors." *Journal of American College Health* just-accepted (2015).

33. Epton, T., Harris, P. R., Kane, R., van Koningsbruggen, G. M., & Sheeran, P. "The impact of self-affirmation on health-behavior change: A meta-analysis." *Health Psychology* vol. 34, no. 3 (2015): pp. 187–196.

34. Falk, Emily B., et al. "Self-affirmation alters the brain's response to health messages and subsequent behavior change." *Proceedings of the National Academy of Sciences* vol. 112, no. 7 (2015): pp. 1977–1982.

35. Gillison, F., et al. "Processes of behavior change and weight loss in a theory-based weight loss intervention program: A test of the process model for lifestyle behavior change." *The International Journal of Behavioral Nutrition and Physical Activity* 12 (2015).

36. Turano, N. A., et al. "Perceived Control Reduces Mortality Risk at Low, Not High, Education Levels." *Health Day.* www.medlineplus.gov. (February 3, 2014).

Chapter 2

1. Jeste, D. V., and Palmer, B. W. "What Is Positive Psychiatry?" In *Positive Psychiatry*, edited by Dilip V. Jeste and Barton W. Palmer. Washington, D.C.: American Psychiatric Publishing (2015): pp. 1–18.

2. Seligman, M. E. "Foreword." In *Positive Psychiatry*, edited by Dilip V. Jeste and Barton W. Palmer. Washington, D.C.: American Psychiatric Publishing (2015): p. xvii.

3. Parks, A. C., et al. "Positive Psychotherapeutic and Behavioral Intervention." In *Positive Psychiatry*, edited by Dilip V. Jeste and Barton W. Palmer. Washington, D.C.: American Psychiatric Publishing (2015): pp. 261–284.

4. Moore, R. C., et al. "Biology of Positive Psychiatry." In *Positive Psychiatry*, edited by Dilip V. Jeste and Barton W. Palmer. Washington, D.C.: American Psychiatric Publishing (2015): pp. 261–284.

5. Zeller, M., et al. "Self-compassion in recovery following potentially traumatic stress: longitudinal study of at-risk youth." *J Abnorm Child Psychol* vol. 43, no. 4 (May 2015): pp. 645–53.

6. Simon-Thomas, E., and J. Breines. "Can an Online Course Boost Happiness?" Greater Good: The Science of a Meaningful Life http://greatergood.berkeley.edu/.

7. Lyubominsky, S. *The Myths of Happiness.* New York: Penguin (2013).

8. Stewart-Brown, S., et al. *Br J Psychiatry.* (March 19, 2015). pii: bjp.bp.114.147280.

9. Lyubominsky, S. *The Myths of Happiness.*

10. Nelson, S. K., et al. "In Defense of Parenthood: Children Are Associated with More Joy Than Misery." *Psychological Science* vol. 24, no. 1 (January 1, 2013): pp. 3–10.

11. Martin, A. S., et al. "Positive Psychological Traits." Socioeconomic gradients and mental health: implications for public health. *Positive Pscychiatry.* Washington, D.C.: American Psychiatric Publishing (2015): pp. 19–44.

12. Summers, R. F., and Lord, J. A. "Positivity in Supportive and Psychodynamic Therapy." In *Positive Psychiatry*, edited by Dilip V. Jeste and Barton W. Palmer. Washington, D.C.: American Psychiatric Publishing (2015): pp. 167–192.

13. Larsen, R. Personal interview.

14. Verburgh, L., et al. "Physical Exercise and Executive Functions in Preadolescent Children, Adolescents, and Young Adults: A Meta-Analysis." *British Journal of Sports Medicine* (March 6, 2013).

15. Martin, et al. "Positive Psychological Traits."

16. Brechting, Emily H., and Charles R. Carlson. "Religiousness and Alcohol Use in College Students: Examining Descriptive Drinking Norms as Mediators." *Journal of Child & Adolescent Substance Abuse* vol. 24, no. 1 (2015): pp. 1–11.

17. Phillips, L., et al. "Eating disorders and spirituality in college students." *J Psychosoc Nurs Ment Health Serv.* vol. 53, no. 1 (January 1, 2015): pp. 30–7.

18. Cohen, R. Presentation, American Heart Association meeting, Baltimore, MD (March 6, 2015).

19. Yu, L., et al. "Purpose in life and cerebral infarcts in community-dwelling older people." *Stroke* vol. 46, no. 4 (April 2015): pp. 1071–1076.

20. Edwards, P. Personal interview.

21. Olver, L. *Investigation Prayer: Impact on Health and Quality of Life*. New York: Springer (2013).

22. Mills, P. J., Redwine, L., & Chopra, D. "A grateful heart may be a healthier heart." *Spirituality in Clinical Practice* vol. 2, no. 1 (2015): pp. 23–24.

23. Boardman, S., and Doraiswamy, P. M. "Integrating Positive Psychiatry into Clinical Practice." In *Positive Psychiatry*, edited by Dilip V. Jeste and Barton W. Palmer. Washington, D.C.: American Psychiatric Publishing (2015): pp. 239–260

24. American College Health Association. American College Health Association-National College Health Assessment II: Reference Group Executive Summary Spring 2014. Hanover, Md.: American College Health Association (2014).

25. Mitchell, J. A., et al. "Sleep Duration and Adolescent Obesity." *Pediatrics* vol. 5, no. 131 (May 2013): pp. 1428–1434.

26. Benedict, C., et al. "Acute Sleep Deprivation Increases Serum Levels of Neuron-Specific Enolase (NSE) and S100 Calcium-Binding Protein B (S-100B) in Healthy Young Men." *Sleep* vol. 1, no. 37 (January 1, 2014): pp. 195–198.

27. Reite, M., and M. Weissberg. "Sleep–Wake Disorders." In *Textbook of Psychiatry* (6th ed.), edited by R. E. Hales, et al. Washington, DC: American Psychiatric Publishing (2014).

28. Kalmbach, D. A., et al. "The Impact of Sleep on Female Sexual Response and Behavior: A Pilot Study." *J Sex Med*. vol. 2, no. 1 (March 16, 2015).

29. Hysing, M., et al. "Sleep and use of electronic devices in adolescence: results from a large population-based study." *BMJ Open*. vol. 5, no. 1 (February 2, 2015): p. e006748

30. Ferret, B., et al. "Napping reverses the salivary interleukin-6 and urinary norepinephrine changes induced by sleep restriction." *J Clin Endocrinol Metab*. vol. 100, no. 3 (March 2015): pp. E416–26.

31. Ye, L., Johnson, S. H., Keane, K., Manasia, M., & Gregas, M. "Napping in college students and its relationship with nighttime sleep." *Journal of American College Health* vol. 63, no. 2 (2015): pp. 88–97.

32. Ibid.

33. Ibid.

34. Osorio, R. S., et al. "Sleep-disordered breathing advances cognitive decline in the elderly." *Neurology* vol. 84, no. 19 (May 12, 2015): pp. 1964–71.

35. Sharpless, B. A. "Exploding head syndrome is common in college students." *J Sleep Res*. (March 13, 2015).

Chapter 3

1. *Understanding Mental Disorders*. Washington, D.C.: American Psychiatric Association (2015).

2. Substance Abuse and Mental Health Services Administration (SAMHSA). *Results from the 2010 National Survey on Drug Use and Health: Mental Health Finding*. NSDUH Series H-42. HHS Publication No. (SMA) 11-4667. Rockville, MD: Substance Abuse and Mental Health Services Administration (2012).

3. *Understanding Mental Disorders*.

4. American Psychiatric Association. *Diagnostic and Statistical Manual of Mental Disorders*. 5th ed. (DSM-5). Arlington, VA: American Psychiatric Association (2013).

5. Walker E. R., et al. "Mortality in Mental Disorders and Global Disease Burden Implications: A Systematic Review and Meta-analysis." *JAMA Psychiatry* vol. 72, no. 4 (April 1, 2015): pp. 334–41.

6. Bunevicius, A., et al. "Decreased Physical Effort, Fatigue, and Mental Distress in Patients with Coronary Artery Disease: Importance of Personality-Related Differences." *International Journal of Behavioral Medicine* (February 28, 2013) (e-pub).

7. Brandy, J. M., et al. "Factors predictive of depression in first-year college students. *J Psychosoc Nurs Ment Health Serv*. vol. 53, no. 2 (February 1, 2015): pp. 38–44.

8. Beiter, R., et al. "The prevalence and correlates of depression, anxiety, and stress in a sample of college students." *Journal of Affective Disorders* vol. 173 (2015): pp. 90–96.

9. American College Health Association. American College Health Association-National College Health Assessment II: Reference Group Executive Summary Spring 2014. Hanover, Md.: American College Health Association (2014).

10. Beiter, et al. "The prevalence and correlates of depression, anxiety, and stress in a sample of college students."

11. Shatkin, J. P., and Diamond, U. "Psychiatry's Next Generation: Teaching College Students About Mental Health." *Acad Psychiatry* (March 6, 2015).

12. Martel, Adele L.; Sood, Aradhana Bela. In *The Virginia Tech massacre: Strategies and challenges for improving mental health policy on campus and beyond* edited by Aradhana Bela Sood and Robert Cohen. New York: Oxford University Press (2015).

13. Beiter, et al. "The prevalence and correlates of depression, anxiety, and stress in a sample of college students."

14. Ibid.

15. Ibid.

16. Cleveland, S. D., et al. "Mental Health Symptoms Among Student Service Members/Veterans and Civilian College Students." *J Am Coll Health* (November 14, 2014) (epub).

17. Walsemann, K. M., et al. "Sick of our loans: Student borrowing and the mental health of young adults in the United States." *Soc Sci Med*. vol. 124 (January 2015): pp. 85–93.

18. Hoggard, L. S., et al. "The lagged effects of racial discrimination on depressive symptomology and interactions with racial identity." *Journal of Counseling Psychology* vol. 62, no. 2 (April 2015): pp. 216–225.

19. Salami, T. K., & Walker, R. L. "Socioeconomic status and symptoms of depression and anxiety in African American college students: The mediating role of hopelessness." *Journal of Black Psychology* vol. 40, no. 3 (2014): pp. 275–290.

20. Linden-Carmichael, A. N., et al. "Protective behavioral strategies as a mediator between depressive symptom fluctuations and alcohol consumption: a longitudinal examination among college students." *J Stud Alcohol Drugs*. vol. 76, no. 1 (January 2015): pp. 80–8.

21. American College Health Association. Executive Summary (2014).

22. Copeland, William E., et al. "Increase in Untreated Cases of Psychiatric Disorders During the Transition to Adulthood." *Psychiatr Serv*. vol. 66, no. 4 (April 1, 2015): pp. 397–403.

23. Miranda, R., et al. "Mental Health Treatment Barriers Among Racial/Ethnic Minority Versus White Young Adults 6 Months After Intake at a College Counseling Center." *J Am Coll Health* (February 18, 2015): pp. 1–8.

24. Pompeo, A. "College students' perceived and personal mental health stigma: The influence on help-seeking attitudes and intentions." *Dissertation Abstracts International: Section B: The Sciences and Engineering* vol., I 7-B (2015).

25. Williams, Sha-Lai L. "Examining the Role of Predictive Factors in Mental Health Service Utilization Among African American College Students." Society for Social Work and Research 19th Annual Conference: The Social and Behavioral Importance of Increased Longevity. *SSWR* (2015).

26. Han, M., & Pong, H. "Mental health help-seeking behaviors among Asian American community college students: The effect of stigma, cultural barriers, and acculturation." *Journal of College Student Development* vol. 56, no. 1 (2015): pp. 1–14.

27. Copeland, et al. "Increase in Untreated Cases of Psychiatric Disorders."

28. Miranda, et al. "Mental Health Treatment Barriers."

29. Beiter, et al. "The prevalence and correlates of depression, anxiety, and stress in a sample of college students."

30. Brandy, et al. "Factors predictive of depression in first-year college students."

31. Weigand, S., et al. "Susceptibility for Depression in Current and Retired Student Athletes." *Sports Health: A Multidisciplinary Approach* (March 25, 2013) http://sph.sagepub.com/content/early/2013/03/20/1941738113480464.

32. McGuire, L. C. "Temporal changes in depression and neurocognitive performance in collegiate student-athletes: A repeated measures evaluation pre- and post-concussion injury." *Dissertation Abstracts International: Section B: The Sciences and Engineering* vol. 75, issue 9-B(E) (2015).

33. Weaver, A., et al. "Urban vs rural Residence and the Prevalence of Depression and Mood Disorder Among African American Women and Non-Hispanic White Women." *JAMA Psychiatry* (April 8, 2015).

34. Burt, V. K., et al. "Treatment of Women," in *Textbook of Psychiatry* (6th ed.), edited by R. E. Hales, et al. Washington, DC: American Psychiatric Publishing (2014).

35. McInnis, M. G., et al. "Depressive Disorders," in *Textbook of Psychiatry* (6th ed.), edited by R. E. Hales, et al. Washington, DC: American Psychiatric Publishing (2014).

36. American Psychiatric Association. *Diagnostic and Statistical Manual*.

37. McInnis, "Depressive Disorders."

38. Hill, R. M., et al. "Enhancing depression screening to identify college students at risk for persistent depressive symptoms." *J Affect Disord*. vol. 174 (March 15, 2015): pp. 1–6.

39. American Psychiatric Association. *Diagnostic and Statistical Manual*.

40. Sinyor, Mark, and Amy H. Cheung. "Antidepressants and risk of suicide." *BMJ* vol. 350 (2015): p. h783.

41. Cheung, Kiki, et al. "Antidepressant use and the risk of suicide: A population-based cohort study." *Journal of Affective Disorders* vol. 174 (2015): pp. 479–484.

42. Ibid.

43. Ketter, T. A., and K. D. Chang. "Bipolar and Related Disorders," in *Textbook of Psychiatry* (6th ed.), edited by Hales, R. E., et al. Washington, DC: American Psychiatric Publishing (2014).

44. Kessing, Lars Vedel, Eleni Vradi, and Per Kragh Andersen. "Life expectancy in bipolar disorder." *Bipolar Disorders* (2015).

45. Stein, M. B., et al. "Anxiety Disorders," in *Textbook of Psychiatry* (6th ed.), edited by Hales, R. E., et al. Washington, DC: American Psychiatric Publishing (2014).

46. Paul, I. M., et al. "Postpartum Anxiety and Maternal–Infant Health Outcomes." *Pediatrics* vol. 131, no. 4 (April 2013): pp. e1218–e1224.

47. Beiter, et al. "The prevalence and correlates of depression, anxiety, and stress in a sample of college students."

48. MacDonald, E. M., et al. "An examination of distress intolerance in undergraduate students high in symptoms of generalized anxiety disorder." *Cognitive Behaviour Therapy* vol. 44, no. 1 (2015): pp. 74–84.

49. Dougherty, D. D., et al. "Obsessive Compulsive and Related Disorders," in *Textbook of Psychiatry* (6th ed.), edited by Hales, R. E., et al. Washington, DC: American Psychiatric Publishing (2014).

50. Figee, M., et al. "Deep Brain Stimulation Restores Frontostriatal Network Activity in Obsessive-Compulsive Disorder." *Nature Neuroscience* vol. 16, no. 4 (April 2013): pp. 386–387.

51. Bruner, M. R., et al. "Attention-deficit/hyperactivity disorder symptom levels and romantic relationship quality in college students." *J Am Coll Health* vol. 63, no. 2 (2015): pp. 98–108.

52. Abbeduto, L., et al. "Neurodevelopmental Disorders," in *Textbook of Psychiatry* (6th ed.), edited by Hales, R. E., et al. Washington, DC: American Psychiatric Publishing (2014).

53. American Psychiatric Association. *Diagnostic and Statistical Manual*.

54. Chang, Z., et al. "Serious Transport Accidents in Adults with Attention-Deficit/Hyperactivity Disorder and the Effect of Medication: A Population-Based Study." *JAMA Psychiatry* vol. 71, no. 3 (2014): pp. 319–325.

55. Bruner, et al. "Attention-deficit/hyperactivity disorder symptom levels."

56. Prevatt, F., Dehili, V., Taylor, N., & Marshall, D. "Anxiety in college students with ADHD: Relationship to cognitive functioning." *Journal of Attention Disorders* vol. 19, no. 3 (2015): pp. 222–230.

57. Gray, Sarah A., et al. "Symptom Manifestation and Impairments in College Students With ADHD." *Journal of Learning Disabilities* (2015): 0022219415576523.

58. Bruner, et al. "Attention-deficit/hyperactivity disorder symptom levels."

59. Benson, Kari, et al. "Misuse of Stimulant Medication Among College Students: A Comprehensive Review and Meta-analysis." Clinical Child and Family Psychology Review (2015): pp. 1–27.

60. Baio, J. "Prevalence of Autism Spectrum Disorder Among Children Aged 8 Years." Autism and Developmental Disabilities Monitoring Network, 11 Sites, United States, 2010. *MMWR Surveillance Summaries* vol 2, no. 63 (March 28, 2014): pp. 1–21.

61. Lopes, A. M., et al. "Human Spermatogenic Failure Purges Deleterious Mutation Load from the Autosomes and Both Sex Chromosomes, Including the Gene DMRT1." *PLoS Genetics* vol. 9, no. 3 (March 2013): p. e1003349.

62. Ronemus, M., et al. "The Role of de Novo Mutations in the Genetics of Autism Spectrum Disorders." *Nature Reviews Genetics* vol. 15 (January 16, 2014): pp. 133–141.

63. Elison, J. T., et al. "White Matter Microstructure and Atypical Visual Orienting in 7-Month-Olds at Risk for Autism." *American Journal of Psychiatry* vol. 170, no. 8 (August 1, 2013): pp. 899–908.

64. Abbeduto, "Neurodevelopmental Disorders."

65. D'Onofrio, B. M., et al. "Paternal Age at Childbearing and Offspring Psychiatric and Academic Morbidity." *JAMA Psychiatry* vol. 71, no. 4 (April 2014): pp. 432–438.

66. Jain, A., et al. "Autism occurrence by MMR vaccine status among US children with older siblings with and without autism." *JAMA* vol. 313, no. 15 (April 21, 2015): pp. 1534–40.

67. Rollins, P. R., et al. "A community-based early intervention program for toddlers with autism spectrum disorders." *Autism* (April 23, 2015). pii: 1362361315577217.

68. Matthews, Nicole L., Agnes R. Ly, and Wendy A. Goldberg. "College Students' Perceptions of Peers with Autism Spectrum Disorder." *Journal of Autism and Developmental Disorders* vol. 45, no. 1 (2015): pp. 90–99.

69. Gillespie-Lynch, Kristen, et al. "Changing College Students' Conceptions of Autism: An Online Training to Increase Knowledge and Decrease Stigma." *Journal of Autism and Developmental Disorders* (2015): pp. 1–14.

70. Croen, Lisa A., et al. "The health status of adults on the autism spectrum." *Autism* (2015): 1362361315577517.

71. Stroup, T. S., et al. "Schizophrenia Spectrum and Other Psychotic Disorders," in *Textbook of Psychiatry* (6th ed.), edited by R. E. Hales, et al. Washington, DC: American Psychiatric Publishing (2014).

72. American Psychiatric Association. *Diagnostic and Statistical Manual*.

73. Kimhy, D., et al. "The Impact of Aerobic Exercise on Brain-Derived Neurotrophic Factor and Neurocognition in Individuals With Schizophrenia: A Single-Blind, Randomized Clinical Trial." *Schizophr Bull*. (March 23, 2015). pii: sbv022.

74. American Psychiatric Association. *Diagnostic and Statistical Manual*.

75. American College Health Association (2013).

76. Taliaferro, Lindsay A., and Jennifer J. Muehlenkamp. "Risk factors associated with self-injurious behavior among a national sample of undergraduate college students." *Journal of American College Health* vol. 63, no. 1 (2015): pp. 40–48.

77. Ibid.

78. Kaplan, A. "Panic Attacks and Suicide." *Psychiatric Times* vol. 30, no. 2 (February 2013): p. 1.

79. *Understanding Mental Disorders*.

80. Ploskonka, R. A., and Sevaty-Seib, H. L. "Belongingness and suicidal ideation in college students." *J Am Coll Health* vol. 63, no. 2 (2015): pp. 81–7.

81. Pease, James L., et al. "Military Service and Suicidal Thoughts and Behaviors in a National Sample of College Crisis" vol. 12 (January 2015): pp. 1–9.

82. Ploskonka. "Belongingness and suicidal ideation."

83. Farabaugh, Amy, et al. "Screening for Suicide Risk in the College Population." *Journal of Rational-Emotive & Cognitive-Behavior Therapy* (2015): pp. 1–17.

84. King, C. A., et al. "Online Suicide Risk Screening and Intervention With College Students: A Pilot Randomized Controlled Trial." *J Consult Clin Psychol*. (February 16, 2015).

85. American Psychiatric Association. *Diagnostic and Statistical Manual*.

86. Kaplan, "Panic Attacks."

87. Bower, P., et al. "Influence of Initial Severity of Depression on Effectiveness of Low Intensity Interventions: Meta-analysis of Individual Patient Data." *BMJ* vol. 346 (February 26, 2013): p. f540.

88. Hollis, C., et al. "Technological innovations in mental healthcare: harnessing the digital revolution." *Br J Psychiatry* vol. 206, no. 4 (April 2015): pp. 263–265.

89. Boardman, S., and Doraiswamy, P. M., "Integrating Positive Psychiatry into Clinical Practice." In *Positive Psychiatry*, edited by Dilip V. Jeste and Barton W. Palmer. Washington, D.C.: American Psychiatric Publishing (2015): pp. 239–260.

90. Horgan, A., et al. "An Evaluation of an Online Peer Support Forum for University Students with Depressive Symptoms." *Archives of Psychiatric Nursing* vol. 27, no. 2 (April 2013): pp. 84–89.

91. Ursano, R. J., and R. B. Carr. "Psychodynamic Psychotherapy," in *Textbook of Psychiatry* (6th ed.), edited by Hales, R. E., et al. Washington, DC: American Psychiatric Publishing (2014).

92. Wright, J. H., et al. "Cognitive-Behavior Therapy," in *Textbook of Psychiatry* (6th ed.), edited by Hales, R. E., et al. Washington, DC: American Psychiatric Publishing (2014).

93. "Is Telephone CBT as Effective as Face-to-Face CBT?" *American Family Physician* vol. 87, no. 1 (January 1, 2013): p. 56.

94. Olfson, Mark. "Surveillance of Adverse Psychiatric Medication Events." *JAMA* vol. 313, no. 12 (March 24/31, 2015).

Chapter 4

1. American College Health Association. American College Health Association-National College Health Assessment II: Reference Group Executive Summary Spring 2014. Hanover, Md.: American College Health Association (2014).

2. Wright, K. B., et al. "Functions of Social Support and Self-verification in Association with Loneliness, Depression, and Stress." *Journal of Health Communication* vol. 19, no. 1 (January 2014): pp. 82–99.

3. Lederer, A. M., et al. "The Impact of Work and Volunteer Hours on the Health of Undergraduate Students." *J Am Coll Health* (February 18, 2015).

4. Stress in America: Paying with Our Health. Washington, D.C.: American Psychological Association, 2015. http://apa.org/news/press/releases/stress/2014/stress-report.pdf.

5. Ibid.

6. American College Health Association (2014).

7. Ibid.

8. Hurst, C. S., et al. "College Student Stressors: A Review of the Qualitative Research." *Stress and Health* vol. 29, issue 3 (August 2013): pp. 275–285.

9. Hintz, S., et al. "Evaluating an online stress management intervention for college students." *J Couns Psychol*. vol. 62, no. 2 (April 2015): pp. 137–147.

10. Deatherage, S., et al. "Stress, Coping, and Internet Use of College Students." *Journal of American College Health* vol. 62, no. 1 (January 2014): pp. 40–46.

11. Hoggard, L. S., et al. "The lagged effects of racial discrimination on depressive symptomology and interactions with racial identity." *Journal of Counseling Psychology* vol. 62, no. 2 (April 2015): pp. 216–225.

12. Han, M., & Pong, H. "Mental health help-seeking behaviors among Asian American community college students: The effect of stigma, cultural barriers, and acculturation." *Journal of College Student Development* vol. 56, no. 1 (2015): pp. 1–14.

13. Sirin, S. R., et al. "Discrimination-Related Stress Effects on the Development of Internalizing Symptoms Among Latino Adolescents." *Child Dev*. (February 11, 2015).

14. Besser, A., et al. "Positive Personality Features and Stress among First-Year University Students: Implications for Psychological Distress, Functional Impairment, and Self-esteem." *Self and Identity* vol. 13, no. 1 (January 2014): pp. 24–44.

15. American College Health Association (2014).

16. "The American Freshman." *HERI Research Brief* (January 2013).

17. Lazzarino, A. I., et al. "The Combined Association of Psychological Distress and Socioeconomic Status with All-Cause Mortality: A National Cohort Study." *JAMA Internal Medicine* vol. 173, no. 1 (January 14, 2013): pp. 22–27.

18. Pelzer, B., et al. "Coping with Unemployment: The Impact of Unemployment on Mental Health, Personality, and Social Interaction Skills." *Work* (March 26, 2013) (e-pub).

19. Mewes, R., et al. "Job Insecurity versus Unemployment: Unequal in Socioeconomic Status but Comparable Detrimental Effects on Mental Health and Health Care Utilization." *Psychotherapie, Psychosomatik, Medizinische Psychologie* vol. 63, no. 3–4 (March 2013): pp. 138–144.

20. Strack, J., Lopes, P. N., & Esteves, F. "Will you thrive under pressure or burn out? Linking anxiety motivation and emotional exhaustion." *Cognition and Emotion* vol. 29, no. 4 (2015): pp. 578–591.

21. *Understanding Mental Disorders*. Washington, D.C.: American Psychiatric Association (2015).

22. Stoddard, F. J., et al. "Trauma- and Stressor-Related Disorders." In *Textbook of Psychiatry* (6th ed.), edited by Hales, R. E., et al. Washington, DC: American Psychiatric Publishing (2014).

23. Zeller, M., et al. "Self-compassion in recovery following potentially traumatic stress: longitudinal study of at-risk youth." *J Abnorm Child Psychol.* vol. 43, no. 4 (May 2015): pp. 645–53.

24. Stoddard, "Trauma- and Stressor-Related Disorders."

25. Hales, R. E., et al. (eds.). *Textbook of Psychiatry* (6th ed.). Washington, DC: American Psychiatric Publishing (2014).

26. Stoddard, "Trauma- and Stressor-Related Disorders."

27. Warner, L. M., Gutiérrez-Doña, B., Angulo, M. V., & Schwarzer, R. "Resource loss, self-efficacy, and family support predict posttraumatic stress symptoms: A 3-year study of earthquake survivors." *Anxiety, Stress & Coping: An International Journal* vol. 28, no. 3: pp. 239–253.

28. Kim, S. H., et al. "Mind–Body Practices for Posttraumatic Stress Disorder." *Journal of Investigative Medicine* vol. 61, no. 5 (June 2013): pp. 827–834.

29. Cardoso, D., et al. "Stress-Induced Negative Mood Moderates the Relation Between Oxytocin Administration and Trust: Evidence for the Tend-and-Befriend Response to Stress." *Psychoneuroendocrinology* vol. 38, no. 11 (November 2013): pp. 2800–2804.

30. Lazarus, R., and R. Launier. "Stress-Related Transactions between Person and Environment." In *Perspectives in Interactional Psychology*. New York: Plenum (1978).

31. Bergh, Cecilia, et al. "Stress Resilience and Physical Fitness in Adolescence and Risk of Coronary Heart Disease in Middle Age." *Heart* vol. 101, no. 8 (2015): pp. 623–629.

32. Bruno, L. "Brain–Gut Interactions in Inflammatory Bowel Disease." *Gastroenterology* vol. 144, no. 1 (January 2013): pp. 36–49.

33. McDonald, P. G., et al. "Psychoneuroimmunology and Cancer: A Decade of Discovery, Paradigm Shifts, and Methodological Innovations." *Brain, Behavior, and Immunity* vol. 30 (2013): pp. S1–S9.

34. Spiegel, D. "Minding the Body: Psychotherapy and Cancerno." British Journal of Health Psychology (2013) (epub).

35. Hintz, et al. "Evaluating an online stress management intervention for college students."

36. Ben-Zeev, D., Scherer, E. A., Wang, R., Xie, H., & Campbell, A. T. "Next-generation psychiatric assessment: Using smartphone sensors to monitor behavior and mental health." *Psychiatric Rehabilitation Journal.* doi: http://dx.doi.org/10.1037/prj0000130.

37. Marchand, W. R. "Mindfulness Meditation Practices as Adjunctive Treatments for Psychiatric Disorders." *Psychiatric Clinics of North America* vol. 36, no. 1 (March 2013): pp. 141–152.

38. Rogers, H. B. "Mindfulness Meditation for Increasing Resilience in College Students." *Psychiatric Annals* vol. 43, no. 12 (December 2013): pp. 545–548.

39. Ramler, T. R., Tennison, L. R., Lynch, J., & Murphy, P. "Mindfulness and the college transition: The efficacy of an adapted mindfulness-based stress reduction intervention in fostering adjustment among first-year students." Mindfulness, published online March 12, 2015.

40. Köhn, M., et al. "Medical Yoga for Patients with Stress-Related Symptoms and Diagnoses in Primary Health Care: A Randomized Controlled Trial." *Evidence-Based Complementary and Alternative Medicine* (February 26, 2013) (e-pub).

41. Akhtar, P., et al. "Effects of Yoga on Functional Capacity and Well Being." *International Journal of Yoga* vol. 6, no. 1 (January 2013): pp. 76–79.

Chapter 5

1. Wood, L., et al. "The Pet Factor–Companion Animals as a Conduit for Getting to Know People, Friendship Formation and Social Support." *PLoS One.* vol. 10, no. 4 (April 29, 2015): p. e0122085

2. American College Health Association. American College Health Association-National College Health Assessment II: Reference Group Executive Summary Spring 2014. Hanover, Md.: American College Health Association (2014).

3. Holt-Lunstad, J., et al. "Loneliness and social isolation as risk factors for mortality: a meta-analytic review." *Perspect Psychol Sci.* vol. 10, no. 2 (March 2015): pp. 227–237.

4. Jaremka, L. M., et al. "Loneliness Predicts Pain, Depression, and Fatigue: Understanding the Role of Immune Dysregulation." *Psychoneuroendocrinology* vol. 38, no. 8 (August 2013): pp. 1310–1317.

5. American Psychiatric Association. *Diagnostic and Statistical Manual of Mental Disorders* (5th ed.). Arlington, VA: American Psychiatric Association (2013).

6. Schreier, H. M., et al. "Effect of Volunteering on Risk Factors for Cardiovascular Disease in Adolescents: A Randomized Controlled Trial." *JAMA Pediatrics* vol. 167, no. 4 (April 1, 2013): pp. 327–332.

7. Aston-Lebold, Me. Online Socializing vs. In-Person Socializing: Psychological Sense of Community Is Equivalent. Ann Arbor, MI: ProQuest Information and Learning (2013).

8. Derbyshire, K. L., et al. "Problematic Internet Use and Associated Risks in a College Sample." *Comprehensive Psychiatry* vol. 54, no. 5 (July 2013): pp. 415–422.

9. Yang, C.-C., and B. B. Brown. "Motives for Using Facebook, Patterns of Facebook Activities, and Late Adolescents' Social Adjustment to College." *Journal of Youth and Adolescence* vol. 42, no. 3 (March 2013): pp. 403–416.

10. Egan, K. G., et al. "College Students' Responses to Mental Health Status Updates on Facebook." *Issues in Mental Health Nursing* vol. 34, no. 1 (January 2013): pp. 46–51.

11. Toma, C., and J. Hancock. "Self-Affirmation Underlies Facebook Use." *Personality and Social Psychology Bulletin* vol. 39, no. 3 (March 2013): pp. 321–331.

12. Lepp, Andrew, et al. "Exploring the relationships between college students' cell phone use, personality and leisure." *Computers in Human Behavior* 43 (2015): pp. 210–219.

13. Lepp, A., et al. "The Relationship between Cell Phone Use, Academic Performance, Anxiety, and Satisfaction with Life in College Students." *Computers in Human Behavior* vol. 31 (February 2014): pp. 343–350.

14. Lepp, A., et al. "The Relationship between Cell Phone Use, Physical and Sedentary Activity, and Cardiorespiratory Fitness in a Sample of U.S. College Students." *International Journal of Behavioral Nutrition and Physical Activity* vol. 10 (June 21, 2013): p. 79.

15. Panek, E. "Left to their own devices: College students' 'guilty pleasure' media use and time management." *Communication Research* vol. 41, no. 4 (2014): pp. 561–577.

16. Derbyshire et al., "Problematic Internet Use."

17. American College Health Association (2013).

18. Selkie, E. M., Kota, R., Chan, Y., & Moreno, M. "Cyberbullying, depression, and problem alcohol use in female college students: A multisite study." *Cyberpsychology, Behavior, and Social Networking* vol. 18, no. 2 (2015): pp. 79–86.

19. Crosslin, K., & Golman, M. "'Maybe you don't want to face it'"—College students' perspectives on cyberbullying." *Computers in Human Behavior,* vol. 41 (2014): pp. 14–20.

20. Selkie, et al. "Cyberbullying, depression, and problem alcohol use in female college students."

21. Dreßing, H., et al. "Cyberstalking in a large sample of social network users: prevalence, characteristics, and impact upon victims." *Cyberpsychol Behav Soc Netw.* vol. 17, no. 2 (February 2014): pp. 61–67.

22. Fournier, A., et al. "Alcohol and the Social Network: Online Social Networking Sites and College Students' Perceived Drinking Norms." *Psychology of Popular Media Culture* vol. 2, no. 2 (April 2013): pp. 86–95.

23. Liu, G., et al. "Trends and Patterns of Sexual Behavior among Adolescents and Adults Aged 14 to 59 Years, United States." *Sexually Transmitted Diseases* vol. 42, no. 1 (January 2015): pp. 20–27.

24. Bachtel, M. K. "Do Hookups Hurt? Exploring College Students' Experiences and Perceptions." *Journal of Midwifery and Women's Health* vol. 58, no. 1 (January–February 2013): pp. 41–48.

25. Monto, M. A., Carey, A. G. "A new standard of sexual behavior? Are claims associated with the 'hookup culture' supported by general social survey data?" *J Sex Res.* vol. 51, no. 6 (2014): pp. 605–615.

26. Robertson, P. N., et al. "Hooking up during the college years: is there a pattern?" *Cult Health Sex.* vol. 17, no. 5 (May 2015): pp. 576–591.

27. Braithwaite, Scott R., et al. "The influence of pornography on sexual scripts and hooking up among emerging adults in college." *Archives of Sexual Behavior* vol. 44, no. 1 (2015): pp. 111–123.

28. Fielder, R. L., et al. "Are Hookups Replacing Romantic Relationships? A Longitudinal Study of First-Year Female College Students." *Journal of Adolescent Health* vol. 52, no. 5 (May 2013): pp. 657–659.

29. Fielder, R. L., et al. "Sexual Hookups and Adverse Health Outcomes: A Longitudinal Study of First-Year College Women." *Journal of Sex Research* vol. 51, no. 2 (2014): pp. 131–144.

30. Kenney, Shannon R., et al. "Development and validation of the Hookup Motives Questionnaire (HMQ)." *Psychological Assessment* vol. 26, no. 4 (2014): p. 1127.

31. Vrangalova, Z. "Hooking Up and Psychological Well-Being in College Students: Short-Term Prospective Links Across Different Hookup Definitions." *J Sex Res.* (July 29, 2014): pp. 1–14.

32. Bersamin, M. M., et al. "Risky Business: Is there an association between casual sex and mental health in emerging adults?" *Journal of Sex Research* vol. 51, no. 1 (2014): pp. 43–51.

33. Fuller, et al. "Sexual Hookups and Adverse Health Outcome."

34. Vrangalova, Z. "Does Casual Sex Harm College Students' Well-Being? A Longitudinal Investigation of the Role of Motivation." *Archives of Sexual Behavior* (February 5, 2014) (e-pub).

35. Olmstead, S. B., et al. "Sex, Commitment, and Casual Sex Relationships among College Men: A Mixed-Methods Analysis." *Archives of Sexual Behavior* vol. 42, no. 4 (May 2013): pp. 561–571.

36. Cooper, J. C., et al. "The Role of the Posterior Temporal and Medial Prefrontal Cortices in Mediating Learning from Romantic Interest and Rejection." *Cerebral Cortex* (April 18, 2013) (e-pub).

37. Takahashi, K. "Imaging the passionate stage of romantic love by dopamine dynamics." *Front Hum Neurosci.* vol. 9 (April 9, 2015): p. 191. doi: 10.3389/fnhum.2015.00191. eCollection 2015.

38. Jaremka, L. M., et al. "Synergistic Relationships among Stress, Depression, and Troubled Relationships: Insights from Psychoneuroimmunology." *Depression and Anxiety* vol. 30, no. 4 (April 2013): pp. 288–296.

39. Johnson, W. I., et al. "Intimate Partner Violence and Depressive Symptoms during Adolescence and Young Adulthood." *Journal of Health and Social Behavior* vol. 55 (March 2014): pp. 39–55.

40. American College Health Association (2013).

41. Tsui, E. K., Santamaria, E. K. "Intimate Partner Violence Risk among Undergraduate Women from an Urban Commuter College: the Role of Navigating Off- and On-Campus Social Environments." *J Urban Health.* (February 3, 2015).

42. Sylaska, K. M., Edwards, K. M. "Disclosure experiences of sexual minority college student victims of intimate partner violence." *Am J Community Psychol.* vol. 55, no. 3-4 (June 2015): pp. 326–35.

43. Ibid.

44. French, M. T., et al. "Personal Traits, Cohabitation, and Marriage." *Social Science Research* vol. 45 (May 2014): pp. 184–199.

45. Uchino, B. N., et al. "Spousal Relationship Quality and Cardiovascular Risk: Dyadic Perceptions of Relationship Ambivalence Are Associated with Coronary-Artery Calcification." *Psychological Science* vol. 25, no. 4 (April 2014): pp. 1037–1042.

46. Haas, S. M., Whitton, S. W. "The Significance of Living Together and Importance of Marriage in Same-Sex Couples." *J Homosex.* (April 7, 2015).

47. Campion, E. W., et al. "In Support of Same-Sex Marriage." *N Engl J Med.* (April 22, 2015).

48. Wight, R. G., et al. "Same-Sex Legal Marriage and Psychological Well-Being: Findings from the California Health Interview Survey." *American Journal of Public Health* vol. 103, no. 2 (February 2013): pp. 339–346.

49. Doss, D. B., et al. "Marital Therapy, Retreats and Books: The Who, What, When, and Why of Relationship Help-Seeking." *Journal Marital and Family Therapy* vol. 35, no. 1, pp. 18–29.

50. Sbarra, D. A., et al. "Divorce and Health: Beyond Individual Differences." *Curr Dir Psychol Sci.* vol. 24, no. 2 (April 1, 2015): pp. 109–113.

51. Kennedy, S., and S. Ruggles. "Breaking Up Is Hard to Count: Divorce and Cohabitation Instability in the United States, 1980-2010." *Demography* vol. 51, no. 2 (April 2014) pp. 587–598.

52. Ibid.

53. Dupree, M. E., et al. "Association Between Divorce and Risks for Acute Myocardial Infarction." *Circulation* (April 2015) (online).

Chapter 6

1. Callejas, J. "Food insecurity on college campuses." *The Chronicle* (April 28, 2015). http://www.dukechronicle.com/.

2. Patton-López, M. M., et al. "Prevalence and Correlated of Food Insecurity among Students Attending a Midsize Rural University in Oregon." *Journal of Nutrition Education and Behavior* vol. 46, no. 3 (May–June 2014): pp. 209–214.

3. Executive Summary. Scientific Report of the 2015 Dietary Guidelines Advisory Committee. http://health.gov/dietaryguidelines/2015-scientific-report/02-executive-summary.asp

4. Del Gobbo, L. C., et al. "Assessing global dietary habits: a comparison of national estimates from the FAO and the Global Dietary Database." *Am J Clin Nutr.* vol. 101, no. 5 (May 2015): pp. 1038–46.

5. Rahavi, E., et al. "Updating the dietary guidelines for Americans: status and looking ahead." *J Acad Nutr Diet.* vol. 115, no. 2 (February 2015): pp. 180–182.

6. Executive Summary. Scientific Report of the 2015 Dietary Guidelines Advisory Committee.

7. Luu, Hung N., et al. "Prospective evaluation of the association of nut/peanut consumption with total and cause-specific mortality." *JAMA Intern Med* (2015).

8. Yang, Q., et al. "Added Sugar Intake and Cardiovascular Diseases Mortality among US Adults." *JAMA Internal Medicine* vol. 174, no. 4 (April 2014): pp. 516–524.

9. Erickson, J., Slavin, J. "Total, added, and free sugars: are restrictive guidelines science-based or achievable?" *Nutrients.* vol. 7, no. 4 (April 15, 2015): pp. 2866–2878.

10. Huang, T., et al. "Consumption of whole grains and cereal fiber and total and cause-specific mortality: prospective analysis of 367,442 individuals." *BMC Med.* vol. 13, no. 59 (March 24, 2015).

11. Chowdhury, R., et al. "Association of Dietary, Circulating, And Supplement Fatty Acids with Coronary Risk: A Systemic Review and Meta-analysis." *Annals of Internal Medicine* vol. 160, no. 6 (2014): pp. 398–406.

12. Grey, A., and M. Bolland. "Clinical Trial Evidence and Use of Fish Oil Supplements." *JAMA Internal Medicine* vol. 174, no. 3 (March 2014): pp. 460–462.

13. Writing Group for the AREDS2 Research Group. "Effect of long-chain ω-3 Fatty Acids and Lutein + Zeaxanthin Supplements on Cardiovascular Outcomes: Results of the Age-Related Eye Disease Study 2 (AREDS2) Randomized Clinical Trial." *JAMA Internal Medicine* vol. 174, no. 5 (May 1, 2014): pp. 763–771.

14. Rizos, E. C., and E. E. Ntzani. "ω-3 Fatty Acids and Lutein + Zeaxanthin Supplementation for the Prevention of Cardiovascular Disease." *JAMA Internal Medicine* vol. 174, no. 5 (May 1, 2014): pp. 771–772.

15. Suren, P., et al. "Association between Maternal Use of Folic Acid Supplements and Risk of Autism Spectrum Disorders in Children." *JAMA* vol. 309, no. 6 (February 13, 2013): pp. 570–577.

16. Vollset, S. E., et al. "Effects of Folic Acid Supplementation on Overall and Site-Specific Cancer Incidence during the Randomised Trials: Meta-analyses of Data on 50,000 Individuals." *The Lancent* vol. 381 (March 2013): pp. 1029–1036.

17. Chowdhury, R., et al. "Vitamin D and Risk of Cause Specific Death: Systemic Review and Meta-analysis of Observational Cohort and Randomised Intervention Studies." *British Medical Journal* vol. 348 (April 1, 2014): pp. g1903.

18. Ibid.

19. Theodoratou, E., et al. "Vitamin D and Multiple Health Outcomes: Umbrella Review and Systemic Reviews and Meta-analyses of Observational Studies and Randomised Trials." *British Medical Journal* vol. 348 (April 1, 2014): pp. g2035.

20. Reid, I. R., et al. "Effects of Vitamin D Supplements on Bone Mineral Density: A Systemic Review and Meta-analysis." *The Lancet* vol. 282, no. 9912 (January 11, 2014): pp. 146–155.

21. Beveridge, L. A., et al. "Effect of Vitamin D Supplementation on Blood Pressure: A Systematic Review and Meta-analysis Incorporating Individual Patient Data." *JAMA Intern Med.* (March 16, 2015).

22. Bolland, M. J., et al. "The Effect of Vitamin D Supplementation on Skeletal, Vascular, or Cancer Outcomes: A Trial Sequential Meta-analysis." *The Lancet Diabetes & Endocrinology* vol. 2, no. 4 (April 2014): pp. 207–320.

23. Cashman, K. D. "Vitamin D: dietary requirements and food fortification as a means of helping achieve adequate vitamin D status." *J Steroid Biochem Mol Biol.* vol. 148 (April 2015): pp. 19–26.

24. Farquhar, W. B., et al. "Dietary sodium and health: more than just blood pressure." *J Am Coll Cardiol.* vol. 65, no. 10 (March 17, 2015): pp. 1042–1050.

25. Gillespie, C., et al. "Sodium content in major brands of US packaged foods, 2009." *Am J Clin Nutr.* vol. 101, no. 2 (February 2015): pp. 344–353.

26. Oyebode, O., et al. "Fruit and Vegetable Consumption and All-cause, Cancer and CVD Mortality: Analysis of Health Survey for England Data." *Journal of Epidemiology Community Health* (March 31, 2014) (epub).

27. Clemens, R., et al. "Squeezing fact from fiction about 100% fruit juice." *Adv Nutr.* vol. 6, no. 2 (March 13, 2015): pp. 236S–243S.

28. Schwingshackl, L., et al. "Dietary supplements and risk of cause-specific death, cardiovascular disease, and cancer: a protocol for a systematic review and network meta-analysis of primary prevention trials." *Syst Rev.* vol. 4, no. 1 (March 26, 2015): p. 34.

29. Ibid.

30. Lieberman, H. R., et al. "Patterns of dietary supplement use among college students." *Clin Nutr.* (November 7, 2014). pii: S0261-5614(14)00262-3.

31. Panagiotakos, D. B., et al. "Adherence to Mediterranean diet offers an additive protection over the use of statin therapy: results from the ATTICA study (2002–2012)." *Curr Vasc Pharmacol.* (April 16, 2015).

32. Sala-Vila, A., et al. "Changes in Ultrasound-Assessed Carotid Intima-Media Thickness and Plaque with a Mediterranean Diet: A Substudy of the PREDIMED Trial." *Arteriosclerosis, Thrombosis, and Vascular Biology* vol. 34, no. 2 (February 2014): pp. 439–445.

33. Sherzai, A. Z., Elkind, M. S. "Advances in stroke prevention." *Ann N Y Acad Sci.* vol. 1338, no. 1 (March 2015): pp. 1–15.

34. Panagiotakos, et al. "Adherence to Mediterranean Diet."

35. "Veggie-Rich Diets May Mean Lower Heart Risks." MedlinePlus *HealthDay* (March 5, 2015). www.medlineplus.gov.

36. Yang, et al. "Added Sugar Intake and Cardiovascular Diseases Mortality among US Adults."

37. "Dropping One Sugary Soda a Day Could Cut Diabetes Risk," MedlinePlus *HealthDay* (May 1, 2015). www.medlineplus.gov.

38. Ibid.

39. Bleich, S. N., et al. "Diet-Beverage Consumption and Caloric Intake among US Adults, Overall and by Body Weight." *American Journal of Public Health* vol. 104, no. 3 (March 2014): pp. e72–e78.

40. Miller, L. M., et al. "Relationships among food label use, motivation, and dietary quality." *Nutrients.* vol. 7, no. 2 (February 5, 2015): pp. 1068–80.

41. Levings, J. L., et al. "Reported use and perceived understanding of sodium information on US nutrition labels." *Prev Chronic Dis.* vol. 12 (April 9, 2015): p. E48.

42. Anagnostou, K., et al. "The rapidly changing world of food allergy in children." *F1000Prime Rep.* vol. 7, no. 5 (March 3, 2015).

Chapter 7

1. Ogden, C. L., et al. "Prevalence of Childhood and Adult Severe Obesity in the United States, 2011–2012." *JAMA* vol. 311, no. 8 (February 26, 2014): pp. 806–814.

2. Skinner, A. C., and J. A. Skelton. "Prevalence and Trends in Obesity and Sever Obesity among Children in the United States, 1999–2012." *JAMA Pediatrics* vol. 168, no. 6 (June 1, 2014): pp. 561–566.

3. Ng, S. W., et al. "Turning Point for US Diets? Recessionary Effects or Behavioral Shifts in Foods Purchased and Consumed." *American Journal of Clinical Nutrition* vol. 99, no. 3 (March 2014): pp. 609–616.

4. Weight-Control Information Network. "Overweight and Obesity Statistics," http://win.niddk.nih.gov/statistics/.

5. Nanney, M. S., et al. "Weight and Weight-Related Behaviors Among 2-Year College Students." *J Am Coll Health*. (February 18, 2015): pp. 1–9.

6. American College Health Association. American College Health Association-National College Health Assessment II: Reference Group Executive Summary Spring 2014. Hanover, Md.: American College Health Association (2014).

7. Nanney, M. S., et al. "Weight and Weight-Related Behaviors."

8. Laska, Melissa N., et al. "Disparities in Weight and Weight Behaviors by Sexual Orientation in College Students." *American Journal of Public Health* vol. 105, no. 1 (2015): pp. 111–121.

9. Odlaug, B. L., et al. "Prevalence and correlates of being overweight or obese in college." *Psychiatry Res.* vol. 227, no. 1 (May 30, 2015): pp. 58–64.

10. Nanney, M. S., et al. "Weight and Weight-Related Behaviors."

11. Ladabaum, U., et al. "Obesity, abdominal obesity, physical activity, and caloric intake in US adults: 1988 to 2010." *Am J Med.* vol. 127, no. 8 (August 2014): pp. 717–727.e12.

12. Nanney, M. S., et al. "Weight and Weight-Related Behaviors."

13. Cerhan, J. R., et al. "A Pooled Analysis of Waist Circumference and Mortality in 650,000 Adults." *Mayo Clinic Proceedings* vol. 89, no. 3 (March 2014): pp. 335–345.

14. Crockett, A. C., et al. "Boredom proneness and emotion regulation predict emotional eating." *J Health Psychol.* vol. 20, no. 5 (May 2015): pp. 670–680.

15. Tobias, D., et al. "BMI and Mortality among Adults with Incident Type 2 Diabetes." *New England Journal of Medicine* vol. 370, no. 14 (April 3, 2014): pp. 1363–1364.

16. Barrington, W. E., et al. "Associations of obesity with prostate cancer risk differ between U.S. African-American and non-Hispanic white men: results from the selenium and vitamin e cancer prevention trial." *Cancer Epidemiol Biomarkers Prev.* vol. 24, no. 4 (April 2015): p. 765.

17. Zhang, X., et al. "Early life body fatness and risk of colorectal cancer in U.S. women and men—results from two large cohort studies." *Cancer Epidemiol Biomarkers Prev.* vol. 24, no. 4 (April 2015): pp. 690–697.

18. Esteghamati, A., et al. "Complementary and alternative medicine for the treatment of obesity: a critical review." *Int J Endocrinol Metab.* vol. 13, no. 2 (April 20, 2015): e19678.

19. Borell, L. N., and L. Samuel. "Body Mass Index Categories and Mortality Risk in US Adults: The Effect of Overweight and Obesity on Advancing Death." *American Journal of Public Health* vol. 104, no. 3 (March 2014): pp. 512–519.

20. Cao, S., et al. "J-shapedness: An Often Missed, Often Miscalculated Relation: *Journal of Epidemiology and Community Health* (March 2014).

21. Ma, Y., et al. "Single-component versus multicomponent dietary goals for the metabolic syndrome: a randomized trial." *Ann Intern Med.* vol. 162, no. 4 (February 17, 2015): pp. 248–57.

22. Leidy, H. J., et al. "The role of protein in weight loss and maintenance." *Am J Clin Nutr.* (April 29, 2015).

23. Gudzune, K. A., et al. "Efficacy of commercial weight-loss programs: an updated systematic review." *Ann Intern Med.* vol. 162, no. 7 (April 7, 2015): pp. 501–12.

24. Esteghamati, et al. "Complementary and alternative medicine."

25. Ibid.

26. Olson, K. L. and Emery, C. F. "Mindfulness and weight loss: a systematic review." *Psychosom Med.* vol. 77, no. 1 (January 2015): pp. 59–67.

27. Emery, C., et al. "Home environment and psychosocial predictors of obesity status among community-residing men and women." *International Journal of Obesity* (April 28, 2015).

28. Beamish, A. J., et al. "Bariatric surgery in adolescents: what do we know so far?" *Scand J Surg.* vol. 104, no. 1 (March 2015): pp. 24–32.

29. Kwok, C. S., et al. "Bariatric Surgery and Its Impact on Cardiovascular Disease and Mortality: A Systemic Review and Meta-analysis. *International Journal of Cardiology* vol. 173, no. 1 (April 15, 2015): pp. 20–28.

30. Johansson, K., et al. "Outcomes of pregnancy after bariatric surgery." *N Engl J Med.* vol. 372, no. 9 (February 26, 2015): pp. 814–24.

31. Risstad, H., et al. "Five-year outcomes after laparoscopic gastric bypass and laparoscopic duodenal switch in patients with body mass index of 50 to 60: a randomized clinical trial." *JAMA Surg.* vol. 150, no. 4 (April 1, 2015): pp. 352–61.

32. American Psychiatric Association. *Diagnostic and Statistical Manual of Mental Disorders,* 5th edition (DSM-5). Washington, DC: American Psychiatric Association (2013).

33. Cerhan, et al. "A Pooled Analysis."

34. "Eating Disorders." In *Understanding Mental Disorders,* 145–158. Washington, D.C.: American Psychiatric Association (2015).

35. Bakalar, J. L., et al. "Recent advances in developmental and risk factor research on eating disorders." *Curr Psychiatry Rep.* vol. 17, no. 6 (June 2015): p. 585.

36. Mabe, A. G., Forney, K. J., and Keel, P. K. "Do you 'like' my photo? Facebook use maintains eating disorder risk," *International Journal of Eating Disorders* vol. 47, issue 5 (July 2014): pp. 516–523.

37. "Eating Disorders."

38. Mitchell, J. F., and S. A. Wonderlich. "Feeding and Eating Disorders." In *Textbook of Psychiatry* (6th ed.), edited by R. E. Hales, et al.

39. Ibid.

40. "Eating Disorders."

Chapter 8

1. American College Health Association. American College Health Association-National College Health Assessment II: Reference Group Executive Summary Spring 2014. Hanover, MD.: American College Health Association (2014).

2. Young, D. R., et al. "Effects of Physical Activity and Sedentary Time on the Risk of Heart Failure." *Circulation: Heart Failure* vol. 7, no. 1 (January 2014): pp. 21–27.

3. Beddhu, S., et al. "Light-Intensity Physical Activities and Mortality in the United States General Population and CKD Subpopulation." *Clin J Am Soc Nephrol.* (April 30, 2015). pii: CJN.08410814.

4. Ibid.

5. American College of Sports Medicine. Exercise Is Medicine toolkit. www.exerciseismedicine.org.

6. Gebel, K., et al. "Effect of Moderate to Vigorous Physical Activity on All-Cause Mortality in Middle-aged and Older Australians." *JAMA Intern Med.* (April 6, 2015). doi: 10.1001/jamainternmed.2015.0541.

7. Boyle, T., et al. "Lifetime physical activity and the risk of non-Hodgkin lymphoma." *Cancer Epidemiol Biomarkers Prev.* vol. 24, no. 5 (May 2015): pp. 873–7.

8. Warden, S. J., "Physical Activity When Young Provides Lifelong Benefits to Cortical Bone Size and Strength in Men." *Proceedings of the National Academy of Science* vol. 111, no. 14 (April 8, 2014): pp. 5337–5342.

9. Iso-Markku, P., et al. "Physical activity and dementia: Long-term follow-up study of adult twins." *Ann Med.* vol. 47, no. 2 (March 2015): pp. 81–87.

10. Verburgh, L., et al. "Physical Exercise and Executive Functions in Preadolescents and Young Adults: A Meta-analysis." *British Journal of Sports and Medicine* vol. 48, no. 12 (June 2014): pp. 973–979.

11. Richards, J., et al. "Don't worry, be happy: cross-sectional associations between physical activity and happiness in 15 European countries." *BMC Public Health.* vol. 15, no. 53 (January 31, 2015).

12. Iso-Markku, et al. "Physical activity and dementia."

13. Fitzgerald, J. D., et al. "Association of objectively measured physical activity with cardiovascular risk in mobility-limited older adults." *J Am Heart Assoc.* vol. 4, no. 2 (February 18, 2015). pii: e001288.

14. Simon, R. M., et al. "The Association of Exercise with Both Erectile and Sexual Function in Black and White Men." *J Sex Med.* (March 20, 2015).

15. Gebel, K et al. Effect of moderate to vigorous physical activity on all-cause mortality in middle-aged and older Australians. *JAMA Internal Medicine* vol. 175, no. 6 (June 2015): pp. 970–977.

16. Ross, R., et al. "Effects of exercise amount and intensity on abdominal obesity and glucose tolerance in obese adults: a randomized trial." *Ann Intern Med.* vol. 162, no. 5 (March 3, 2015): pp. 325–34.

17. Arem H et al. Leisure time physical activity and mortality: a detailed pooled analysis of the dose-response relationship. *JAMA Internal Medicine* vol. 175, no. 6 (June 2015): pp. 959–967.

18. Pillay, J. D., et al. "Steps That Count: Physical Activity Recommendations, Brisk Walking and Steps per Minute—How Do They Relate?" *Journal of Physical Activity and Health* vol. 11, no. 3 (March 2014): pp. 502–508.

19. Kaplan, Y., et al. "Referent Body Weight Values in Over Ground Walking, Over Ground Jogging, Treadmill Jogging, and Elliptical Exercise." *Gait Posture* vol. 39, no. 1 (January 2014): pp. 558–562.

20. Srikanthan, P., and A. S. Karlamangla. "Muscle Mass Index as a Predictor of Longevity in Older-Adults." *American Journal of Medicine* vol. 127, no. 6 (June 2014): pp. 547–553.

21. Clarke, T., et al. "Trends in the Use of Complementary Health Approaches Among Adults." National Health Statistics Reports, no. 79 (February 10, 2015).

22. Kiccolt-Glaser, J. K. "Yoga's Impact on Inflammation, Mood, and Fatigue in Breast Cancer Survivors: A Randomized Controlled Trial." *Journal of Clinical Oncology* vol. 32, no. 10 (April 1, 2014): pp. 1040–1049.

23. Battle, C. L., et al. "Potential for prenatal yoga to serve as an intervention to treat depression during pregnancy." *Women's Health Issues.* vol. 25, no. 2 (March–April 2015): pp. 134–41.

24. Hoy, D., et al. "The Global Burden of Low Back Pain: Estimates from the Global Burden of Disease 2010 Study." *Annals of Rheumatic Diseases* (March 24, 2014) (e-pub).

25. Cheung, R. T., and Ngai, S. P. "Effects of footwear on running economy in distance runners: A meta-analytical review." *J Sci Med Sport.* (March 14, 2015). pii: S1440-2440(15)00057-2.

26. Earhart, E. L., et al. "Effects of oral sodium supplementation on indices of thermoregulation in trained, endurance athletes." *J Sports Sci Med.* vol. 14, no. 1 (March 1, 2015): pp. 172–178.

27. Richards, J., et al. "A Study of the Combined Effects of Physical Activity and Air Pollution on Mortality in Elderly Urban Residents: The Danish Diet, Cancer, and Health Cohort." *Environ Health Perspect.* (January 27, 2015).

Chapter 9

1. Hensel, D. J., and J. D. Fortenberry. "A Multidimensional Model of Sexual Health and Sexual and Prevention Behavior among Adolescent Women."

Journal of Adolescent Health vol. 52, no. 2 (February 2013): pp. 219–227.

2. Lechner, K. F., et al. "College Students' Sexual Health: Personal Responsibility or the Responsibility of the College?" *Journal of College Health* vol. 61, no. 1 (January 2013): pp. 28–35.

3. Ibid.

4. Riley, M., et al. "Health Maintenance in Women." *American Family Physicians* vol 87, no. 1 (January 1, 2013): pp. 30–38.

5. Nguyen, G. T., et al. "The Annual Pelvic Examination. Preventive Time Not Well Spent." *American Family Physician* vol. 87, no. 1 (January 1, 2013): pp. 8–9.

6. Chrisler, Joan C., et al. "Body appreciation and attitudes toward menstruation." *Body Image* vol. 12 (2015): pp. 78–81.

7. Zarei, Z., and S. Bazzazian. "The relationship between premenstrual syndrome disorder, stress and quality of life in female students." *Iranian Journal of Psychiatric Nursing* vol. 2, no. 4 (2015): pp. 49–58.

8. Matsumoto, T. et al. "Biopsychological Aspects of Premenstrual Syndrome and Premenstrual Dysphoric Disorder." *Gynocological Endocrinology* vol. 29, no. 1 (January 2013): pp. 67–73.

9. Santamaría, Miriam, and Irantzu Lago. "Premenstrual Experience Premenstrual Syndrome and Dysphoric Disorder." In *Psychopathology in Women* edited by Margarita Sáenz-Herrero. Springer International Publishing vol. 2, no. 4 (2015): pp. 423–449.

10. Veale, D. et al. Am I normal? A systematic review and construction of nomograms for flaccid and erect penis length and circumference in up to 15,521 men. BJU International. doi: 10.1111/bju.13010.

11. Ibid.

12. Nelson, Roxanne. "New CDC guidelines recommend circumcision to cut HIV risk." *The Lancet Infectious Diseases* vol. 15, no. 3 (2015): pp. 269–270.

13. Manago, Adriana M., L. Monique Ward, and Adriana Aldana. "The Sexual Experience of Latino Young Adults in College and Their Perceptions of Values About Sex Communicated by Their Parents and Friends." *Emerging Adulthood* vol. 3, no. 1 (2015): pp. 14–23.

14. Liu, G. et al. "Trends and Patterns of Sexual Behavior among Adolescents and Adults Aged 14 to 59 Years, United States" *Sexually Transmitted Diseases* vol. 42, no.1 (January 2015) pp. 20–27.

15. Ibid.

16. American College Health Association. *American College Health Association–National College Health Assessment II: Reference Group Executive Summary.* Hanover, MD: American College Health Association, Spring 2014).

17. Becasen, Jeffrey, et al. "138. Sexual and Healthcare Seeking Behaviors of Young Adults by College Enrollment." *Journal of Adolescent Health* vol. 56, no. 2 (2015): S72.

18. Kenney, Shannon R., et al. "Development and validation of the Hookup Motives Questionnaire (HMQ)." *Psychological Assessment* vol. 26, no. 4 (2014): p.1127.

19. Bachtel, M. "Do Hookups Hurt? Exploring College Students' Experiences and Perceptions." *Journal of Midwifery and Women's Health* vol. 58, no. 1 (January/February 2013): pp. 41–48.

20. Kenny, et al. "Development and validation of the Hookup Motives Questionnaire."

21. Braithwaite, Scott R., et al. "The influence of pornography on sexual scripts and hooking up among emerging adults in college." *Archives of Sexual Behavior* vol. 44, no. 1 (2015): pp. 111–123.

22. Kenny, et al. "Development and validation of the Hookup Motives Questionnaire."

23. Ibid.

24. Bersamin, M. M. et al. "Risky Business: Is there an association between casual sex and mental health in emerging adults?" *Journal of Sex Research* vol. 51, no. 1 (2014): pp. 43–51.

25. Olmstead, S. B., et al. "Sex, Commitment, and Casual Sex Relationships among College Men: A Mixed-Methods Analysis." *Archives of Sexual Behavior.* (January 8, 2013) (e-pub).

26. Dodge, B., et al. "Sexual Behaviors and Experiences among Behaviorally Bisexual Men in the Midwestern United States." *Archives of Sexual Behavior* vol. 42, no. 2 (February 2013): pp. 247–256.

27. Schrimshaw, E. W., et al. "Disclosure and Concealment of Sexual Orientation and the Mental Health of Non-Gay-Identified, Behaviorally Bisexual Men." *Journal of Consulting and Clinical Psychology* vol. 81, no. 1 (February 2013): pp. 141–153.

28. Harbaugh, Evan, and Eric W. Lindsey. "Attitudes Toward Homosexuality Among Young Adults: Connections to Gender Role Identity, Gender-Typed Activities, and Religiosity." *Journal of Homosexuality* just-accepted (2015).

29. Fields, Errol Lamont, et al. "I Always Felt I Had to Prove My Manhood": Homosexuality, Masculinity, Gender Role Strain, and HIV Risk Among Young Black Men Who Have Sex With Men." *American Journal of Public Health* vol. 105, no. 1 (2015): pp. 122–131.

30. American Academy of Pediatrics. "Four Stages of Coming Out," www.healthychildren.org/English/ages-stages/teen/dating-sex/Pages/Four-Stages-of-Coming-Out.aspx.

31. Brittain, D. R. and M. K. Dinger. "An examination of health inequities among college students by sexual orientation identity and sex." *Journal of Public Health Research* vol. 4, no. 1 (2015).

32. Richardson, Hannah B., et al. "Sexual Violence and Help-Seeking Among LGBQ and Heterosexual College Students." *Partner Abuse* vol. 6, no. 1 (2015): pp. 29–46.

33. Braithwaite. "The influence of pornography on sexual scripts."

34. Grubbs, Joshua B., et al. "Internet pornography use: Perceived addiction, psychological distress, and the validation of a brief measure." *Journal of Sex & Marital Therapy* vol. 41, no. 1 (2015): pp. 83–106.

35. Grubbs J. B. et al. "Transgression as addiction: religiosity and moral disapproval as predictors of perceived addiction to pornography." Arch Sex Behav. vol. 44, no. 1 (January 205): pp. 125–136.

36. Whipple, Beverly. "Ejaculation, female." *The International Encyclopedia of Human Sexuality* (2015).

37. Vlachopoulos, Charalambos. "Definition and Assessment of Erectile Dysfunction." *Erectile Dysfunction in Hypertension and Cardiovascular Disease,* edited by Margus Viigimaa, Charalambos Vlachopoulos, and Michael Doumas, 1–8. Springer International Publishing (2015).

38. Fang, Shona C., et al. "Changes in Erectile Dysfunction over Time in Relation to Framingham Cardiovascular Risk in the Boston Area Community Health (BACH) Survey." *The Journal of Sexual Medicine* vol. 12, no. 1 (2015): pp. 100–108.

39. Kingsberg, Sheryl A., and Terri Woodard. "Female Sexual Dysfunction: Focus on Low Desire." *Obstetrics & Gynecology* vol. 125, no. 2 (2015): pp. 477–486.

Chapter 10

1. Khurana, Atika, and Amy Bleakley. "Young adults' sources of contraceptive information: variations based on demographic characteristics and sexual risk behaviors." *Contraception* vol. 91, no. 2 (2015): pp. 157–163.

2. Johnson, Abigail Z., et al. "The Roles of Partner Communication and Relationship Status in Adolescent Contraceptive Use." *Journal of Pediatric Health Care* vol. 29, no. 1 (2015) pp. 61–69.

3. Goldstein, R. L., U. D., Upadhyay, and T. R. Raine. "With Pills, Patches, Rings, and Shots: Who Still Uses Condoms? A Longitudinal Cohort Study." *Journal of Adolescent Health* vol. 52, no. 1 (January 2013): pp. 77–82.

4. Li, Daniel, Allen J. Wilcox, and David B. Dunson. "Benchmark Pregnancy Rates and the Assessment of Post-coital Contraceptives: An Update." *Contraception* (2015).

5. Bellizzi, S., et al. "Underuse of modern methods of contraception: underlying causes and consequent undesired pregnancies in 35 low- and middle-income countries." Human Reproduction. (February 3, 2015).

6. Sitruk-Ware, R., A. Nath, and D. R. Mishell, Jr. "Contraception Technology: Past, Present and Future." *Contraception* vol. 87, no. 3 (March 2013): pp. 319–330.

7. Goldstein, et al. "With Pills."

8. Daniels, K., et al. Current contraceptive status among women aged 15-44: United States, 2011-2013. NCHS Data Brief. vol. 173 (December 2014): pp. 1–8.

9. Sutherland, M. A., Fantasia, H. C., and Fontenot, H. "Reproductive Coercion and Partner Violence among College Women." *Journal of Obstetric, Gynecologic, & Neonatal Nursing* (2015).

10. American College Health Association (ACHA). *American College Health Association–National College Health Assessment II: Reference Group Executive Summary.* Hanover, MD: American College Health Association (Spring 2014).

11. Herbenick, D., et al. "Characteristics of Condom and Lubricant Use among a Nationally Representative Probability Sample of Adults Ages 18–59 in the United States." *Journal of Sexual Medicine* vol. 10, no. 2 (February 2013): pp. 474–483.

12. Crosby, R. A., et al. "Understanding Problems with Condom Fit and Feel: An Important Opportunity for Improving Clinic-Based Safer Sex Programs." *Journal of Primary Prevention* vol. 34 (April 2013): pp. 109–115.

13. Habel, Melissa A., Jeffrey S. Becasen, and Patricia J. Dittus. "143. The State of Sexual Health Services at US Colleges & Universities." *Journal of Adolescent Health* vol. 56, no. 2 (2015): pp. S74–S75.

14. Wilson A. M., Ickes, M. J. "Purchasing condoms near a college campus: environmental barriers." Sex Health. (February 9, 2015).

15. American College Health Association.

16. Crosby, et al. "Understanding Problems."

17. Jin, J. "Oral Contraceptives." *Journal of the American Medical Association* vol. 311, no. 5. (January 15, 2014): p. 321.

18. Wallis, L. "Women's Access to Contraception." *American Journal of Nursing* vol. 113, no. 2 (February 2013): p. 18.

19. Brache, V., L. J. Payán, and A. Faundes. "Current Status of Contraceptive Vaginal Rings." *Contraception* vol. 87, no. 3 (March 2014): pp. 264–272.

20. Branum, Amy, et al. "Trends in Long-acting Reversible Contraception Use Among U.S. Women Aged 15-44." National Center for Health Statistics, U.S. Centers for Disease Control and Prevention (February 4, 2015).

21. Wildemeersch, D., Hasskamp, T., Goldstuck, N. "Intrauterine devices that do not fit well cause side effects, become embedded, or are expelled and can even perforate the uterine wall." *J Minim Invasive Gynecol.* vol. 22, no. 2 (February 2015) pp. 309–310.

22. American College Health Association.

23. Daniels, K., et al. "Use of Emergency Contraception among Women Aged 15–44: United States, 2006–2010. *NCHS Data Brief,* no. 112 (February 2013).

24. Papic, Melissa, et al. "Same-Day Intrauterine Device Placement is Rarely Complicated by Pelvic Infection." *Women's Health Issues* vol. 25, no. 1 (2015): pp. 22–27.

25. Mulligan, Karen. "Access to Emergency Contraception and its Impact on Fertility and Sexual Behavior." *Health economics* (2015).

26. Gemzell-Danielsson, K., C. Berger, and P. G. L. Lalnkumar. "Emergency Contraception: Mechanisms of Action." *Contraception* vol. 87, no. 3 (March 2013): pp. 300–308.

27. Schwarzer, J. U., and H. Steinfatt. "Current Status of Vasectomy Reversal." *Nature Reviews: Urology,* February 12, 2013 (e-pub).

28. www.cdc.gov

29. Upadhyay, Ushma D., et al. "Incidence of Emergency Department Visits and Complications After Abortion." *Obstetrics & Gynecology* vol. 125, no. 1 (2015): pp. 175–183.

30. Hall, M. et al. "Association between Intimate Partner Violence and Termination of Pregnancy: A Systematic Review and Meta-analysis." *PLoS Men.* vol. 11, no.1 (January 2014), e1001581.

31. Ibid.

32. Foster, D. G., et al. "A comparison of depression and anxiety symptom trajectories between women who had an abortion and women denied one." *Psychological Medicine* (2015): pp. 1–10.

33. Roberts, S. C., Fuentes, L., Kriz, R., Williams, V., Upadhyay, U. "Implications for women of Louisiana's law requiring abortion providers to have hospital admitting privileges." *Contraception* (February 9, 2015).

34. Martin, J. A., et al. "Births: Final Data for 2013" *National Vital Statistics Reports* vol. 64, no. 1 (January 15, 2015).

35. Sedgh, Gilda, et al. "Adolescent Pregnancy, Birth, and Abortion Rates Across Countries: Levels and Recent Trends." *Journal of Adolescent Health* vol. 56, no. 2 (2015): pp. 223–230.

36. Poston, L. "Healthy Eating in Pregnancy." *British Medical Journal* vol. 348 (March 2014): p. 1739.

37. Englund-Ogge, L., et al. "Maternal Dietary Patterns and Preterm Delivery: Results for a Large Prospective Cohort Study." *British Medical Journal* vol. 48 (March 4, 2014): p. 1446.

38. Dodd, J. M., et al. "Antenatal Lifestyle Advice for Women Who Are Overweight or Obese: LIMIT Randomised Trial." *British Medical Journal* vol. 348 (February 2014): p. 1285.

39. Gupta, R., et al. "To Eat or Not to Eat: What Foods Are Safe to Consume During Pregnancy?" *JAMA Pediatrics* vol. 168, no. 2 (February 1, 2014): pp. 109–110.

40. Barakat, Ruben, Alejandro Lucía, and Jonatan Ruiz. "Exercise and Pregnancy." *Handbook of Sports Medicine and Science: The Female Athlete* (2015): pp. 110–119.

41. Stroud, L. R., et al. "Prenatal Glucocorticoids and Maternal Smoking during Pregnancy Independently Program Adult Nicotine Dependence in Daughters: A 40-Year Prospective Study." *Biological Psychiatry* vol. 75, no. 1 (January 2014): pp. 47–55.

42. Hyland, A., et al. "Associations of Lifetime Active and Passive Smoking with Spontaneous Abortion, Stillbirth and Tubal Ectopic Pregnancy: A Cross-sectional Analysis of Historical Data from the Women's Health Initiative." *Tobacco Control* (February 26, 2014).

43. Nykjaer, C., et al. "Maternal Alcohol Intake prior to and during Pregnancy and Risk of Adverse Birth Outcomes: Evidence from a British Cohort." *Journal of Epidemiology and Community Health* vol. 68, no. 6 (June 1, 2014): pp. 543–599.

44. Liew, Z., et al. "Acetaminophen Use during Pregnancy, Behavioral Problems and Hyperkinetic Disorders." *JAMA Pediatrics* vol. 168, no. 4 (April 1, 2014): pp. 313–320.

45. Daniel, S., et al. "Fetal Exposure to Nonsteroidal Anti-inflammatory Drugs and Spontaneous Abortions." *Canadian Medical Association Journal* vol. 186, no. 16 (March 18, 2014): pp. 177–182.

46. Creanga, Andreea A., et al. "Pregnancy-related mortality in the United States, 2006–2010." *Obstetrics & Gynecology* vol. 125, no. 1 (2015): pp. 5–12.

47. D'Onotrio, B. M., et al. "Paternal Age at Childbearing and Offspring Psychiatric and Academic Morbidity." *JAMA Psychiatric* vol. 1, no. 4 (April 1, 2014): pp. 432–438.

48. Hamilton, B. E., et al, "Annual Summary of Vital Statistics," *Pediatrics* vol. 131, no. 3 (March 2013): pp. 548–558.

49. Dohle, G. R. "Male Factors in Couple's Infertility." In *Clinical Uro-Andrology* edited by Vincenzo Mirone, 197-201. Springer Berlin Heidelberg (2015).

Chapter 11

1. www.cdc.gov.

2. Smith, Haley. "Sexually transmitted infections." *Professional Nursing Today* vol. 18, no. 1 (2015): pp. 29–32.

3. Crosby, R., and L. A. Shrier. "A Partner-Related Risk Behavior Index to Identify People at Elevated Risk for Sexually Transmitted Infections." *Journal of Primary Prevention* (January 25, 2013) (e-pub).

4. Brown, Monique J., River Pugsley, and Steven A. Cohen. "Meeting Sex Partners Through the Internet, Risky Sexual Behavior, and HIV Testing Among Sexually Transmitted Infections Clinic Patients." *Archives of Sexual Behavior* (2015): pp. 1–11.

5. Herbenick, D., et al. "Characteristics of Condom and Lubricant Use among a Nationally Representative Probability Sample of Adults Ages 18–59 in the United States." *Journal of Sexual Medicine* vol. 10, no. 2 (February 2013): pp. 474–483.

6. Crosby, R. A., et al. "Understanding Problems with Condom Fit and Feel: An Important Opportunity for Improving Clinic-Based Safer Sex Programs." *Journal of Primary Prevention* (January 25, 2013) (e-pub).

7. American College Health Association. American College Health Association-National College Health Assessment II: Reference Group Executive Summary Spring 2014. Hanover, MD.: American College Health Association (2014).

8. Habel, Melissa A., Jeffrey S. Becasen, and Patricia J. Dittus. " The State of Sexual Health Services at US Colleges & Universities." *Journal of Adolescent Health* vol. 56, no. 2 (2015): pp. S74–S75.

9. Wang, X. "Negotiating Safer Sex: A Detailed Analysis of Attitude Functions, Anticipated Emotions, Relationship Status and Gender." *Psychol Healt* vol. 28, no. 7 (January 2013): pp. 800–817.

10. Lindley, L. L., et al. "Receipt of the Human Papillomavirus Vaccine among Female College Students in the United States, 2009." *Journal of American College Health* vol. 61, no. 1 (January 2013): pp. 18–27.

11. Jemal, A., et al. "Annual Report to the Nation on the Status of Cancer, 1975–2009. Featuring the Burden and Trends in Human Papillomavirus (HPV)-Associated Cancers and HPV Vaccination Coverage Levels." *Journal of the National Cancer Insitutute* vol. 105, no. 3 (February 6, 2013): pp. 175–201.

12. Lindley, "Receipt of the Human Papillomavirus Vaccine."

13. Brisson, M., et al. "Inequalities in Human Papillomavirus (HPV)-Associated Cancers: Implications for the Success of HPV Vaccination." *Journal of the National Cancer Institute* vol. 105, no. 3 (February 6, 2013): pp. 158–161.

14. Djajadiningrat, Rosa S., et al. "Human papillomavirus prevalence in invasive penile cancer and association with clinical outcome." *The Journal of Urology* vol. 193, no. 2 (2015): pp. 526–531.

15. Jemal et al., "Annual Report."

16. Bednarczyk, R. A. "How Do We Best Address Parent and Physician Concerns?" *JAMA Intern Med.* Published online February 9, 2015.

17. Mullins, Tanya L. Kowalczyk, et al. "HPV Vaccine Risk Perceptions and Subsequent Sexual Behaviors and Sexually Transmitted Infections Among Adolescent Girls." *Journal of Adolescent Health* vol. 56, no. 2 (2015): p. S14.

18. Jena, Anupam B., Dana P. Goldman, and Seth A. Seabury. "Incidence of Sexually Transmitted Infections After Human Papillomavirus Vaccination Among Adolescent Females." *JAMA Internal Medicine* (2015).

19. Baandrup, L., et al. "Significant Decrease in the Incidence of Genital Warts in Young Danish Women after Implementation of a National Human Papillomavirus Vaccination Program." *Sexually Transmitted Diseases*, vol. 40, no. 2 (February 2013): pp. 130–135.

20. Balder-Felskov, B., et al. "Early Impact of Human Papillomavirus Vaccination on Cervical Neoplasia—Nationwide Follow-up of Young Danish Women." *Journal of the National Cancer Institute* vol 106, no. 3 (March 1, 2014). Crowe, E. et al. "Effectiveness of Quadrivalent Human Papillomavirus Vaccine for the Prevention of Cervical Abnormalities: Case-Control Study Nested within a Population Based Screening Programme in Australia." *British Medical Journal* vol. 28 (2014) p. 1458.

21. Herweijer, E., et al. "Association of Varying Number of Doses of Quadrivalent Human Papillomavirus Vaccine with Incidence of Condyloma." *Journal of the American Medical Association,* vol. 311, no. 6 (February 12, 2014): pp. 597–603.

22. Skinner, S. Rachel, et al. "Efficacy, safety, and immunogenicity of the human papillomavirus 16/18 AS04-adjuvanted vaccine in women older than 25 years: 4-year interim follow-up of the phase 3, double-blind, randomised controlled VIVIANE study." *The Lancet* vol. 384, no. 9961 (2015): pp. 2213–2227.

23. Lindley et al., "Receipt of the Human Papillomavirus Vaccine."

24. Royer, H. R., et al. "Genital Herpes Beliefs: Implications for Sexual Health." *Journal of Pediatric and Adolescent Gynecology,* (January 18, 2013).

25. Leone, Peter. "Expert commentary: genital herpes transmission." *Herpes* vol. 11, no. 2 (2015): pp. 48–49.

26. Royer, H. R., et al. "Genital Herpes Beliefs."

27. Jackson, Jaleesa A., Tiffany S. McNair, and Jenell S. Coleman. "Over-screening for chlamydia and gonorrhea among urban women age ≥ 25 years." *American Journal of Obstetrics and Gynecology* vol. 212, no. 1 (2015): pp. 40–e1.

28. Simmons, Susan. "Understanding pelvic inflammatory disease." *Nursing2015* vol. 46, no. 2 (2015): pp. 65–66.

29. Kerani, Roxanne P., et al. "Gonorrhea Treatment Practices in the STD Surveillance Network, 2010–2012." *Sexually Transmitted Diseases* vol. 42, no. 1 (2015): pp. 6–12.

30. www.cdc.gov.

31. "The Global HIV/AIDS Epidemic." Fact Sheet, Kaiser Family Foundation (February 2013).

32. Hamilton, B. E., et al. "Annual Summary of Vital Statistics: 2010–2011." *Pediatrics* vol. 131, no. 13 (March 2013): pp. 548–558.

33. Zeglin, Robert J., and J. Paul Stein. "Social determinants of health predict state incidence of HIV and AIDS: a short report." *AIDS care* vol. 27, no. 2 (2015): pp. 255–259.

34. "Black Americans and HIV/AIDS." Fact Sheet, Kaiser Family Foundation (February 2013).

35. Whiteside, Y. O. "Progress along the Continuum of HIV Care among Blacks with Diagnosed HIV—United States, 2010." *Morbidity & Mortality Weekly Report,* vol. 63, no. 5 (February 7, 2014): pp. 85–89.

36. Chan, S. K., et al. "Likely Female-to-Female Sexual Transmission of HIV—Texas, 2012." *Morbidity & Mortality Weekly Report* vol. 63, no. 10 (March 14, 2014): pp. 209–212.

37. Feldblum, P. J., M. J. Welsh, and M. J. Steiner. "Don't overlook condoms for HIV prevention [editorial]." *Sexually Transmitted Infections* vol. 79 (2015): pp. 268–269.

38. Scott, H. M., Fuqua, V., and Raymond, H.F. "Utilization of HIV Prevention Services Across Racial/Ethnic Groups Among Men Who Have Sex with Men in San Francisco, California, 2008." *AIDS Behavior* vol. 18, supplement 3 (April 2014): pp. 316–323.

39. Buchbinder, S. P., et al. "HIV Pre-exposure Prophylaxis in Men Who Have Sex with Men and Transgender Women: A Secondary Analysis of a Phase 3 Randomised Controlled Efficacy Trial." *The Lancet Infect Diseases* (March 6, 2014) pii: S1473-3099(14)70025-8.

40. Agwu, A. L., et al. "CD4 Counts of Nonperinatally HIV-Infected Youth and Young Adults Presenting for HIV Care between 2002 and 2010." *JAMA Pediatrics* vol. 168, no. 4 (April 1, 2014): pp. 381–383.

41. Rosenberg, Nora E., et al. "How can we better identify early HIV infections?." *Current Opinion in HIV and AIDS* vol. 10, no. 1 (2015): pp. 61–68.

42. Ananworanich, Jintanat, and John W. Mellors. "A cure for HIV: what will it take?." *Current Opinion in HIV and AIDS* vol. 10, no. 1 (2015): pp. 1–3.

Chapter 12

1. Johnston, L. D., O'Malley, P. M., Miech, R. A., Bachman, J. G., & Schulenberg, J. E. "Monitoring the Future national survey results on drug use: 1975-2014: Overview, key findings on adolescent drug use." Ann Arbor: Institute for Social Research, The University of Michigan (2015).

2. Johnston, L. D., O'Malley, P. M., Bachman, J. G., Schulenberg, J. E. & Miech, R. A. "Monitoring the Future national survey results on drug use, 1975–2013: Volume 2, College students and adults ages 19–55." Ann Arbor: Institute for Social Research, The University of Michigan (2014).

3. American College Health Association. American College Health Association-National College Health Assessment II: Reference Group Executive Summary Spring 2014. Hanover, Md.: American College Health Association (2014).

4. Meshesha, L. Z. et al. "Polysubstance use is associated with deficits in substance-free reinforcement in college students." *J Stud Alcohol Drugs.* vol. 76, no. 1 (January 2015): pp. 106–16.

5. Ibid.

6. Yau, Y. H., Potenza, M. N. "Gambling disorder and other behavioral addictions: recognition and treatment." *Harv Rev Psychiatry.* vol. 23, no. 2 (March-April 2015): pp. 134–46.

7. Scholes-Balog, K. E., et al. "A Prospective Study of Adolescent Risk and Protective Factors for Problem Gambling Among Young Adults." *Journal of Adolescence* vol. 37, no. 2 (February 2014): pp. 215–224.

8. American Psychiatric Association. *Diagnostic and Statistical Manual of Mental Disorders*, 5th ed. Arlington, VA: American Psychiatric Association (2013).

9. Arria, A. M., et al. "Discontinuous College Enrollment: Associations with Substance Use and Mental Health." *Psychiatric Services* vol. 64, no. 2 (February 1, 2013): pp. 165–172.

10. Johnston, L. D. et al. (2015).

11. American College Health Association.

12. Brandt, S. A. et al. "A survey of nonmedical use of tranquilizers, stimulants, and pain relievers among college students: patterns of use among users and factors related to abstinence in non-users." *Drug Alcohol Depend.* vol. 143 (October 1, 2014): pp. 272–276.

13. Thompson, K. et al. "The Relationship of Higher Education to Substance Use Trajectories: Variations as a Function of Timing of Enrollment" *Am J Stud Alcohol Drugs.* vol. 76, no. 1 (January 2015): pp. 95–105.

14. Snipes, D.J. et al. "Religiosity in the non-medical use of prescription medication in college students." *Am J Drug Alcohol Abuse* vol. 41, no. 1 (January 2015): pp. 93–9.

15. American College Health Association.

16. Merrill, R. M. "Use of marijuana and changing risk perceptions." *Am J Health Behav.* (May 2015) vol. 39, no. 3: pp. 308–17.

17. Varner, M. W., et al. "Association Between Stillbirth and Illicit Drug Use and Smoking During Pregnancy." *Obstetrics & Gynecology* vol. 123, no. 1 (January 2014): pp. 113–125.

18. Hahn, K. A. et al. "Caffeine and caffeinated beverage consumption and risk of spontaneous abortion." *Hum Reprod.* (March 18, 2015) pii: dev063.

19. Borota, D., et al. "Post-Study Caffeine Administration Enhances Memory Consolidation in Humans." *Nature Neuroscience* vol. 17, no. 2 (February 2014): pp. 201–203.

20. Panza, F. I. et al. "Coffee, tea, and caffeine consumption and prevention of late-life cognitive decline and dementia: a systematic review." *J Nutr Health Aging.* vol. 19, no. 3 (2015): pp. 313–28.

21. Ahluwalia, N. and Herrick, K. "Caffeine intake from food and beverage sources and trends among children and adolescents in the United States: review of national quantitative studies from 1999 to 2011." *Adv Nutr.* vol. 6, no. 1 (January 15, 2015): pp. 102–11.

22. Ibrahim, N. K. and Iftikhar, R. "Energy drinks: Getting wings but at what health cost?" *Pak J Med Sci.* vol. 30, no. 6 (November-December 2014): pp. 1415–9.

23. Sorkin, B. C., Coates, P. M. "Caffeine-containing energy drinks: beginning to address the gaps in what we know." *Adv Nutr.* vol. 5, no. 5 (September 2014): pp. 541–3.

24. Breslow, R. A., et al. "Prevalence of alcohol-interactive prescription medication use among current drinkers: United States, 1999 to 2010." *Alcohol Clin Exp Res.* vol. 39, no. 2 (February 2015): pp. 371–379.

25. American Psychiatric Association. *Diagnostic and Statistical Manual of Mental Disorders*, 5th ed.

26. Ibid.

27. Hartz, S. M., et al. "Comorbidity of Severe Psychotic Disorders with Measures of Substance Use." *JAMA Psychiatry* vol. 71, no. 3 (March 2014): pp. 248–254.

28. Dart, R. C., et al. "Trends in opioid analgesic abuse and mortality in the United States." *N Engl J Med.* vol. 372, no. 3 (January 15, 2015): pp. 241–248.

29. Johnston, L. D., et al (2015).

30. Looby, A., et al. "Challenging Expectancies to Prevent Nonmedical Prescription Stimulant Use: A Randomized, Controlled Trial." *Drug and Alcohol Dependence* (April 6, 2013).

31. Cicero, T. J., et al. "Factors Influencing the Selection of Hydrocodone and Oxycodone as Primary Opioids in Substance Abusers Seeking Treatment in the United States." *Pain* vol. 154, no. 12 (December 2013): pp. 2639–2648.

32. Benson, K., et al. "Misuse of Stimulant Medication Among College Students: A Comprehensive Review and Meta-analysis." *Clin Child Fam Psychol Rev.* vol. 18, no. 1 (March 2015): pp. 50–76.

33. Ibid.

34. Ibid.

35. Reid, A. M., et al. "Frequent Nonprescription Stimulant Use and Risky Behaviors in College Students: The Role of Effortful Control." *Journal of American College Health* vol. 63, no. 1 (2015): pp. 23–30.

36. Benson, K., et al. "Misuse of Stimulant Medication Among College Students."

37. Johnston, L.D., et al. (2014).

38. Ibid.

39. Gilman, J. M., et al. "Cannabis use is quantitatively associated with nucleus accumbens and amygdala abnormalities in young adult recreational users." *J Neurosci.* vol. 34, no. 16 (April 16, 2014): pp. 5529–38.

40. Bagot, K. S., et al. "Adolescent Initiation of Cannabis Use and Early-Onset Psychosis." *Subst Abus.* (March 16, 2015).

41. American Stroke Association. "Smoking Marijuana Associated with Higher Stroke Risk in Young Adults." News release (February 6, 2013).

42. Smith, M. J., et al. "Cannabis-Related Working Memory Deficits and Associated Subcortical Morphological Differences in Healthy Individuals and Schizophrenia Subjects." *Schizophrenia Bulletin* vol. 40, no. 2 (March 2014): pp. 287–299.

43. Kramer, J. L. "Medical marijuana for cancer." *CA Cancer J Clin.* vol. 65, no. 2 (March 2015): pp. 109–122.

44. Ibid.

45. Ibid.

46. Hall, W., Weier, M. "Assessing the public health impacts of legalising recreational cannabis use in the USA." *Clin Pharmacol Ther.* (March 16, 2015).

47. McGeeney, B. E. "Cannabinoids and Hallucinogens for Headache." *Headache* vol. 53, no. 3 (March 2013): pp. 447–458.

48. Room, R. "Legalizing a Market for Cannabis for Pleasure: Colorado, Washington, Uruguay and Beyond." *Addiction* vol. 109, no. 3 (March 2014): pp. 345–351.

49. AAP Reaffirms Opposition to Legalizing Marijuana for Recreational or Medical Use http://www.healthychildren.org/English/news/Pages/ AAP-Reaffirms-Opposition-toLegalizing-Marijuana-for-Recreational-or-Medical-Use.aspx

50. Johnston, L. D., et al. (2014).

51. Woo, T. M., and J. R. Hanley. "How High Do They Look?" Identification and Treatment of Common Ingestions in Adolescents." *Journal of Pediatric Health Care* vol. 27, no. 2 (March–April 2013): pp. 135–144.

52. Johnston, L. D., et al. (2014).

53. "Synthetic Drugs." Office of National Drug Control Policy, www.whitehouse.gov/ondcp

54. Woo and Hanley, "'How High Do They Look?'"

55. Seely, K. A., et al. "Forensic Investigation of K2, Spice, and 'Bath Salt' Commercial Preparations: A Three-Year Study of New Designer Drug Products Containing Synthetic Cannabinoid, Stimulant, and Hallucinogenic Compounds." *Forensic Science International* vol. 233, no. 1–3 (December 2013): pp. 416–422.

56. Monte, A., et al. "An Outbreak of Exposure to a Novel Synthetic Cannabinoid." *New England Journal of Medicine* vol. 370 (January 2014): pp. 389–390.

57. "Acute Kidney Injury Associated with Synthetic Cannabinoid Use—Multiple States, 2012." Centers for Disease Control and Prevention. *Morbidity and Mortality Weekly Report* vol. 62, no. 6 (February 15, 2013): pp. 93–98.

58. Wood, K. E. "Exposure to Bath Salts and Synthetic Tetrahydrocannabinol from 2009 to 2012 in the United States." *Journal of Pediatrics* (February 4, 2013).

59. Woo and Hanley, "'How High Do They Look?'"

60. Artenie, A. A., et al. "Associations of substance use patterns with attempted suicide among persons who inject drugs: can distinct use patterns play a role?" *Drug Alcohol Depend.* vol. 147 (February 1, 2015): pp. 208–214.

61. Lyon, I. K., et al. "Predisposition to and effects of methamphetamine use on the adolescent brain." *Mol Psychiatry* (February 10, 2015).

62. Curtin, K., et al. "Methamphetamine/amphetamine abuse and risk of Parkinson's disease in Utah: a population-based assessment." *Drug Alcohol Depend.* vol. 146 (January 1, 2015): pp. 30–38.

63. Artenie, A. A., et al. "Association of substance abuse patterns."

64. "U.S. Officials Target Escalating Drug Overdoses." *HealthDay* (February 11, 2014)..www.medlineplus.gov.

65. "Heroin Overdose Deaths Quadrupled since 2000." *HealthDay,* Medline Plus (March 4, 2015).

66. Sahker, E., et al. "National analysis of differences among substance abuse treatment outcomes: college student and nonstudent emerging adults." *J Am Coll Health.* vol. 63, no. 2 (2015): pp. 118–24.

Chapter 13

1. National Institute on Alcohol Abuse and Alcoholism. www.niaaa.nih.gov.

2. Ibid.

3. Popovici, I., and M. T. French. "Does Unemployment Lead to Greater Alcohol Consumption?" *Industrial Relations* (Berkeley), vol. 52, no. 2 (April 2013): pp. 444–466.

4. Virtanen, M., et al. "Long working hours and alcohol use: systematic review and meta-analysis of published studies and unpublished individual participant data." *BMJ* 350 (January 13, 2015): p. g7772.

5. American College Health Association. *American College Health Association-National College Health Assessment II: Reference Group Executive Summary Spring 2014.* Hanover, MD: American College Health Association (2014).

6. College Drinking—Changing the Culture. www.collegedrinkingprevention.gov.

7. Www.niaaa.nih.gov.

8. Ibid.

9. American College Health Association.

10. American College Health Association.

11. Cacciola, E. E., Nevid, J.S. "Alcohol consumption in relation to residence status and ethnicity in college students." *Psychol Addict Behav* vol. 28, no. 4 (December 2014): pp. 1278–83. doi: 10.1037/a0038362. Epub December 1, 2014.

12. Neighbors, C., et al. "Reliance on God, Prayer, and Religion Reduces Influence of Perceived Norms on Drinking." *Journal of Studies on Alcohol and Drugs* vol. 74, no. 3 (May 2013): pp. 361–368.

13. Van Damme, J., et al. "Social Motives for Drinking in Students Should Not Be Neglected in Efforts to Decrease Problematic Drinking." *Health Education Research* (March 13, 2013) (e-pub).

14. Armeli, S., et al. "A Longitudinal Study of the Effects of Coping Motives, Negative Affect and Drinking Level on Drinking Problems among College Students." *Anxiety, Stress, & Coping* (February 20, 2014) (epub).

15. Pedersen, E. R., et al. "Demographic and Predeparture Factors Associated with Drinking and Alcohol-Related Consequences for College Students Completing Study Abroad Experiences." *Journal of American College Health* (February 5, 2014) (e-pub).

16. Henslee, A. M., et al. "The impact of campus traditions and event-specific drinking." *Addict Behav.* vol. 45C (February 2, 2015): pp. 180–183. doi: 10.1016/j.addbeh.2015.01.033. [Epub ahead of print].

17. Lee, C. M., et al. "Randomized Controlled Trial of a Spring Break Intervention to Reduce High-Risk Drinking." *Journal of Consulting and Clinical Psychology* (February 3, 2014) (e-pub).

18. Lewis, M. A., et al. "Sex on the Beach: The Influence of Social Norms and Trip Companion on Spring Break Sexual Behavior." *Prevention Science* (January 25, 2014).

19. Barry, A. E. et al. "Alcohol use among college athletes: do intercollegiate, club, or intramural student athletes drink differently?" *Subst Use Misuse* vol. 50, no. 3 (February 2015): pp. 302–307. doi: 10.3109/10826084.2014.977398. (epub).

20. LaBrie, J. W., et al. "Alcohol abstinence or harm-reduction? Parental messages for college-bound light drinkers." *Addict Behav.* vol. 46C (February 26, 2015): pp. 10–13. doi: 10.1016/j.addbeh.2015.02.019.

21. Selkie, E. M., et al. "Cyberbullying, depression, and problem alcohol use in female college students: a multisite study." *Cyberpsychol Behav Soc Netw.* vol. 18, no. 2 (February 2015): pp. 79–86. doi: 10.1089/cyber.2014.0371.

22. Turchik, J. A., and C. M. Hassija. "Female Sexual Victimization among College Students: Assault Severity, Health Risk Behaviors, and Sexual Functioning." *Journal of Interpersonal Violence* (February 5, 2014) (e-pub).

23. Clanky A. K., et al. "Child abuse exposure, emotion regulation, and drinking refusal self-efficacy: an analysis of problem drinking in college students." *Am J Drug Alcohol Abuse* vol. 41, no. 2 (March 2015): pp. 188–196.

24. Tripp, J. C., et al. "PTSD Symptoms, Emotion Dysregulation, and Alcohol-Related Consequences Among College Students with a Trauma History." *J Dual Diagn.* vol. 20 (March 2015).

25. O'Hara, R. E., et al. "Perceived racial discrimination and negative-mood-related drinking among African American college students." *J Stud Alcohol Drugs* vol. 76, no. 2 (March 2015): pp. 229–236.

26. Koordeman, R., et al. "Self-control and the effects of movie alcohol portrayals on immediate alcohol consumption in male college students." *Front Psychiatry* vol. 5 (February 3, 2015): p. 187. doi: 10.3389/fpsyt.2014.00187. eCollection 2014.

27. Bauer, L. O., and N. A. Ceballos. "Neural and Genetic Correlates of Binge Drinking among College Women." *Biological Psychology* (February 14, 2014) (e-pub).

28. Plunk, A. D., et al. "The Persistent Effects of Minimum Legal Drinking Age Laws on Drinking Patterns Later in Life." *Alcoholism: Clinical and Experimental Research* vol. 37, no. 3 (March 2013): pp. 463–469.

29. LaBrie, J. W., et al. "Are They All the Same? An Exploratory, Categorical Analysis of Drinking Game Types." *Addictive Behaviors* vol. 38, no. 5 (May 2013): pp. 2133–2139.

30. Martin, J. L., et al. "Disordered eating and alcohol use among college women: Associations with race and big five traits." *Eat Behav.*17C (February 23, 2015): pp. 149–152. doi: 10.1016/j.eatbeh.2015.02.002. [Epub ahead of print].

31. Napper, L. E., et al. "Gender as a moderator of the relationship between preparty motives and event-level consequences." *Addict Behav.* vol. 45C (February 21, 2015): pp. 263–268. doi: 10.1016/j.addbeh.2015.02.010. [Epub ahead of print].

32. www.niaaa.nih.gov.

33. Winickoff, J. P., M. Gottlieb, and M. M. Mello. "Tobacco 21—An Idea Whose Time Has Come." *New England Journal of Medicine* vol. 370, no. 4 (January 23, 2014): pp. 297–299.

34. McKetin R., Coen, A. "The effect of energy drinks on the urge to drink alcohol in young adults." *Alcohol Clin Exp Res.* vol. 38, no. 8 (August 2014): pp. 2279–2285.

35. Smoyak, S. A., et al. "High energy drinks, with and without alcohol: what do nurses know and do?" *J Psychosoc Nurs Ment Health Serv.* vol. 53, no. 1 (January 1, 2015): pp. 39–44.

36. Peacock, A., et al. "Patterns of Use and Motivations for Consuming Alcohol Mixed with Energy Drinks." *Psychology of Addictive Behaviors* vol. 27, no. 1 (March 2013): pp. 202–206.

37. Peacock, A., and R. Bruno. "'High' Motivation for Alcohol: What Are the Practical Effects of Energy Drinks on Alcohol Priming?" *Alcoholism: Clinical and Experimental Research* vol. 37, no. 2 (February 2013): pp. 185–187.

38. Howland, J., and D. J. Rohsenow. "Risks of Energy Drinks Mixed with Alcohol." *JAMA* vol. 309, no. 3 (January 16, 2013): pp. 245–246.

39. Snipes, D. J., and E. G. Benotsch. "High-Risk Cocktails and High-Risk Sex: Examining the Relation between Alcohol Mixed with Energy Drink Consumption, Sexual Behavior, and Drug Use in College Students." *Addictive Behaviors* vol. 38, no. 1 (January 2013): 1418–1423.

40. Mallett, K. A., et al. "Are All Alcohol and Energy Drink Users the Same? Examining Individual Variation in Relation to Alcohol Mixed with Energy Drink Use, Risky Drinking, and Consequences." *Psychology of Addictive Behaviors* (March 25, 2013) (e-pub).

41. American College Health Association.

42. Lewis, M. A., et al. "Sex on the Beach."

43. Scott-Sheldon, L. A., et al. "Efficacy of Alcohol Interventions for First-Year College Students: A Meta-Analytic Review of Randomized Controlled Trials." *Journal of Consulting and Clinical Psychology* (January 20, 2014).

44. Moreno, M. A. et al., "Emergence and Predictors of Alcohol Reference Displays on Facebook During the First Year of College." *Comput Human Behav* (January 30, 2014).

45. Shorey, R. C., et al. "The Temporal Relationship between Alcohol, Marijuana, Angry Affect, and Dating Violence Perpetration: A Daily Diary Study with Female College Students." *Psychology of Addictive Behaviors* (November 25, 2013).

46. Shorey, R. C., et al. "Acute Alcohol Use Temporally Increases the Odds of Male Perpetrated Dating Violence: A 90-Day Diary Analysis." *Addictive Behaviors* (2014).

47. American College Health Association.

48. Henson, J. M., et al. "Defining and characterizing differences in college alcohol intervention efficacy: A growth mixture modeling application." *J Consult Clin Psychol.* vol. 83, no. 2 (April 2015): pp. 370–381.

49. Borsari B et al. "In-session processes of brief motivational interventions in two trials with mandated college students." *Journal of Consulting and Clinical Psychology* vol. 83, no. 1 (February 2015): pp. 56–67.

50. Mermelstein, L. C., and Garske, J. P. "A Brief Mindfulness Intervention for College Student Binge Drinkers: A Pilot Study." *Psychol Addict Behav.* (November 17, 2014).

51. Black, N., Mullan, B. "An Intervention to Decrease Heavy Episodic Drinking in College Students: The Effect of Executive Function Training." *J Am Coll Health* (December 16, 2014).

52. Canale, N., et al. "The efficacy of computerized alcohol intervention tailored to drinking motives among college students: a quasi-experimental pilot study." *Am J Drug Alcohol Abuse* vol. 41, no. 2 (March 2015): pp. 183–187.

53. Woo, T. M., and J. R. Hanley. "'How High Do They Look?': Identification and Treatment of Common Ingestions in Adolescents." *Journal of Pediatric Health Care* vol. 27, no. 2, (March/April 2013): pp. 135–144.

54. Hultgren, B. A., et al. "How Estimation of Drinking Influences Alcohol-Related Consequences Across the First Year of College." *Alcoholism: Clinical and Experimental Research* (January 24, 2014).

55. Marczinski, C. A., and A. L. Stamates. "Artificial Sweeteners Versus Regular Mixers Increase Breath Alcohol Concentrations in Male and Female Social Drinkers." *Alcoholism: Clinical and Experimental Research* vol. 37, no. 4 (April 2013): pp. 696–702.

56. Ibid.

57. Gruenewald, P. J., and Mair, C. "Heterogeneous dose-response and college student drinking: examining problem risks related to low drinking levels." *Addiction* (February 16, 2015.)

58. Kanny, D., et al. "Vital signs: alcohol poisoning deaths – United States, 2010–2012." *MMWR Morb Mortal Wkly Rep.* vol. 63, no. 53 (January 9, 2015): pp. 1238–42.

59. Askgaard, G., et al. "Alcohol drinking pattern and risk of alcoholic liver cirrhosis: A prospective cohort study." *J Hepatol.* (January 20, 2015).

60. Nelson, D. E., et al. "Alcohol-Attributable Cancer Deaths and Years of Potential Life Lost in the United States." *American Journal of Public Health* vol. 103, no. 4 (April 2013): pp. 641–648.

61. Ebrahim, I. O., et al. "Alcohol and Sleep I: Effects on Normal Sleep." *Alcoholism: Clinical and Experimental Research* vol. 37, no. 4 (April 2013): pp. 539–549.

62. Popovici, I., and M. T. French. "Binge Drinking and Sleep Problems among Young Adults." *Drug and Alcohol Dependence* (March 2, 2013) (e-pub).

63. Fornier, C. B., et al. "Widespread effects of alcohol on white matter microstructure." *Alcoholism: Clinical & Experimental Research* (November 18, 2014) [Epub ahead of print]. PMID: 25406797.

64. Centers for Disease Control and Prevention (CDC). "Vital Signs: Binge Drinking in Young Women and Girls." *MMWR. Morbidity and Mortality Weekly Report* vol. 62, no. 1 (January 11, 2013): pp. 9–13.

65. Www.niaaa.nih.gov.

66. American Psychiatric Association. *Diagnostic and Statistical Manual of Mental Disorders*, 5th ed. Arlington, VA: American Psychiatric Association (2013).

67. Hales, R. E., et al. *American Psychiatric Publishing Textbook of Psychiatry*. Arlington, VA: American Psychiatric Association (2014).

68. Www.niaaa.nih.gov.

69. Soyka, M., Lieb, M. "Recent Developments in Pharmacotherapy of Alcoholism." *Pharmacopsychiatry* (March 11, 2015).

70. Kosten, T. R., et al. "Substance-Related and Addictive Disorders." In *American Psychiatric Publishing Textbook of Psychiatry*, 6th edition, edited by R. E. Hales, et al. Washington DC: American Psychiatric Publishing (2014).

71. Www.niaaa.nih.gov.

Chapter 14

1. Roberts, M. E., et al. "What predicts early smoking milestones?" *J Stud Alcohol Drugs* vol. 76, no. 2 (March 2015): pp. 256–266.

2. Johnston, L. D., O'Malley, P. M., Miech, R. A., Bachman, J. G., and Schulenberg, J. E. "Monitoring the Future national survey results on drug use: 1975–2014: Overview, key findings on adolescent drug use." Ann Arbor: Institute for Social Research, The University of Michigan (2015).

3. American College Health Association. *American College Health Association-National College Health Assessment II: Reference Group Executive Summary* Spring 2014. Hanover, Md.: American College Health Association (2014).

4. "Current Cigarette Smoking among Adults in the United States." Centers for Disease Control. http://www.cdc.gov/tobacco/data_statistics/fact_sheets/adult_data/cig_smoking/index.htm.

5. *The Health Consequences of Smoking—50 Years of Progress: A Report of the Surgeon General.* Atlanta, GA: U.S. Department of Health and Human Services, Centers for Disease Control and Prevention, National Center for Chronic Disease Prevention and Health Promotion, Office on Smoking and Health (2014).

6. "Current Cigarette Smoking among Adults in the United States."

7. Fiore, M. C., et al. "Smoke, the Chief Killer—Strategies for Targeting Combustible Tobacco Use." *New England Journal of Medicine* vol. 370, no. 4 (January 23, 2014): pp. 297–299.

8. Preidt, R. "People with Mental Illness Make Up Large Share of U.S. Smokers." *Healthday*, MedlinePlus. www.medlineplus.gov.

9. American Psychiatric Association. *Diagnostic and Statistical Manual.*

10. Butler, K. M., et al. "Polytobacco Use among College Students." *Nicotine Tob Res.* (March 13, 2015).

11. Kuntz M. et al. "Enforcing a tobacco-free campus through an ambassador-based program: a phenomenology." *J Am Coll Health* vol. 63, no. 3 (April 2015): pp. 195–202.

12. "Women and Smoking." Centers for Disease Control. http://www.cdc.gov/tobacco/data_statistics/sgr/50th-anniversary/pdfs/fs_women_smoking_508.pdf.

13. Dorn, L. D., et al. "Longitudinal Impact of Substance Use and Depressive Symptoms on Bone Accrual among Girls Aged 11–19 Years." *Journal of Adolescent Health* vol. 52, no. 4 (April 2013): pp. 393–399.

14. Ebbert, J. O., et al. "Combination Varenicline and Bupropion SR for Tobacco-Dependence Treatment in Cigarette Smokers: A Randomized Trial." *JAMA* vol. 311, no. 2 (January 8, 2014): pp. 155–163.

15. *The Health Consequences of Smoking.*

16. Carter, B. D., et al. "Smoking and mortality—beyond established causes." *N Engl J Med* vol. 372, no. 7 (February 12, 2015): pp. 631–640.

17. *The Health Consequences of Smoking.*

18. Mitra, A. P., et al. "Combination of Molecular Alterations and Smoking Intensity Predicts Bladder Cancer Outcome: A Report from the Los Angeles Cancer Surveillance Program." *Cancer* vol. 119, no. 4 (February 15, 2013): pp. 756–765.

19. *The Health Consequences of Smoking.*

20. Ibid.

21. Meier, E. M., et al. "Which nicotine products are gateways to regular use? First-tried tobacco and current use in college students." *Am J Prev Med.* vol. 48(1 Suppl 1) (January 2015): pp. S86–93.

22. Lee, Y. O., et al. "Youth tobacco product use in the United States." *Pediatrics* vol. 135, no. 3 (March 2015): pp. 409–15. doi: 10.1542/peds.2014-3202.

23. Butler, K. M., et al. "Polytobacco Use among College Students."

24. Fillon, M. "Electronic cigarettes may lead to nicotine addiction." *J Natl Cancer Inst.* vol. 107, no. 3 (March 5, 2015). pii: djv070.

25. Saddleson, M. L., et al. "Risky behaviors, e-cigarette use and susceptibility of use among college students." *Drug Alcohol Depend.* vol. 149 (April 1, 2015): pp. 25–30.

26. Fillon, M. "Electronic cigarettes may lead to nicotine addiction."

27. Callahan-Lyon, P. "Electronic cigarettes: human health effects." *Tob Control* vol. 23(Suppl 2) (May 2014): pp. ii36–40. doi: 10.1136/tobaccocontrol-2013-051470. Review.

28. Cavazos-Rehg, P. A., et al. "Risk Factors Associated With Hookah Use." *Nicotine Tob Res.* (February 2, 2015): pii: ntv029.

29. Meier, E. M., et al.

30. Protano, C., et al. "Electronic cigarette: a threat or an opportunity for public health? State of the art and future perspectives." *Clin Ter.* vol. 107, no. 3 (January–February 2015): pp. 32–37.

31. Maloney, E. K., Cappella, J. N. "Does Vaping in E-Cigarette Advertisements Affect Tobacco Smoking Urge, Intentions, and Perceptions in Daily, Intermittent, and Former Smokers?" *Health Commun.* (March 11, 2015): pp. 1–10.

32. Moreno, M. A. "JAMA Pediatrics Patient Page. Risks of hookah smoking." *JAMA Pediatr.* vol. 169, no. 2 (February 2015): p. 196.

33. Cavazos-Rehg, P. A., et al. "Risk Factors Associated With Hookah Use."

34. Salloum, R. G. et al. "Water pipe tobacco smoking in the United States: Findings from the National Adult Tobacco Survey." *Prev Med.* vol. 71 (February 2015): pp. 88–93.

35. Shihadeh, A., et al. "Toxicant content, physical properties and biological activity of waterpipe tobacco smoke and its tobacco-free alternatives." *Tob Control* 24(Suppl 1) (March 2015): pp. i22–i30. doi: 10.1136/tobaccocontrol-2014-051907. Epub February 9, 2015.

36. El-Zaatari, Z. M., et al. "Health effects associated with waterpipe smoking." *Tob Control* vol. 24(Suppl 1) (March 2015): pp. i31–i43.

37. Doran, N., et al. "Hookah Use Predicts Cigarette Smoking Progression Among College Smokers." *Nicotine Tob Res.* (January 12, 2015): pii: ntu343.

38. Thomas, J. L., et al. "Abstinence rates among college cigarette smokers enrolled in a randomized clinical trial evaluating Quit and Win contests: The impact of concurrent hookah use." *Prev Med.* (March 13, 2015).

39. King, B. A., et al. "Flavored Cigar Smoking among U.S. Adults: Findings from the 2009–2010 National Adult Tobacco Survey." *Nicotine and Tobacco Research* vol. 15, no. 2 (February 2013): pp. 608–614.

40. BeTobaccoFree.gov. "Smoked Tobacco Products." http://betobaccofree.hhs.gov/about-tobacco/Smoked-Tobacco-Products/

41. Goldberg, R. *Drugs across the Spectrum.* Belmont, CA: Wadsworth Cengage Learning (2014).

42. Caponnetto, P., et al. "Electronic cigarettes—from smoking cessation to smoking sensation and back." *Addiction* vol. 110, no. 4 (April 2015): pp. 678–679.

43. Kotz, D., Brown, J., West, R. "Real-World' Effectiveness of Smoking Cessation Treatments: A Population Study." *Addiction* vol. 109, no. 3 (March 2014): pp. 491–499.

44. Hartz, S. M. "Comorbidity of Severe Psychotic Disorders with Measures of Substance Use." *JAMA Psychiatry* vol. 109, no. 1 (January 1, 2014): pp. 35–43.

45. U.S. Food and Drug Administration. "FDA Gives Nod to Longer Use of Nicotine Patch, Gum." News release (April 1, 2013).

46. Mills, E. J., et al. "Cardiovascular Events Associated with Smoking Cessation Pharmacotherapies: A Network Meta-analysis." *Circulation* vol. 129, no. 1 (January 7, 2014): pp. 28–41.

47. Foulds J., et al. "Development of a questionnaire for assessing dependence on electronic cigarettes among a large sample of ex-smoking E-cigarette users." *Nicotine Tob Res.* vol. 17, no. 2 (February 2015): pp. 186–192.

48. Mendelson, M. M., de Ferranti, S. D. "Childhood Environmental Tobacco Smoke Exposure: A 'Smoking Gun' for Atherosclerosis in Adulthood." *Circulation* (March 23, 2015).

49. Sleiman, M., et al. "Inhalable constituents of thirdhand tobacco smoke: chemical characterization and health impact considerations." *Environ Sci Technol.* vol. 48, no. 22 (November 18, 2014): pp. 13093–101. doi: 10.1021/es5036333. Epub October 31, 2014.

50. Martins-Green, M., et al. "Cigarette smoke toxins deposited on surfaces: implications for human health." *PLoS One* vol. 9, no. 1 (January 29, 2014): p. e86391.

51. Ramírez, N., et al. "Exposure to nitrosamines in thirdhand tobacco smoke increases cancer risk in non-smokers." *Environ Int.* vol. 71 (October 2014): pp. 139–47. doi: 10.1016/j.envint.2014.06.012. Epub July 16, 2014.

52. Cance, J. D., et al. "The Impact of a City-Wide Indoor Smoking Ban on Smoking and Drinking Behaviors across Emerging Adulthood." *Nicotine Tob Res.* (March 5, 2015). pii: ntv050.

Chapter 15

1. Mozaffarian, Dariush, et al. "Heart Disease and Stroke Statistics—2015 Update A Report From the American Heart Association." *Circulation* vol. 131, no. 4 (2015): pp. e29–e322.

2. Ekelund, Ulf, et al. "Physical Activity and all-cause mortality across levels of general and abdominal adiposity: The European Prospective Investigation into Cancer and Nutrition Study (EPIC)." (2015).

3. Rendo-Urteaga, Tara, et al. "The combined effect of physical activity and sedentary behaviors on a clustered cardio-metabolic risk score: The Helena study." *International Journal of Cardiology* vol. 186 (2015): pp. 186–195.

4. Rhee, Jinnie J., et al. "Dietary Diabetes Risk Reduction Score, Race and Ethnicity, and Risk of Type 2 Diabetes in Women." *Diabetes Care* (2015): dc141986.

5. Cheong, Kee C., et al. "The discriminative ability of waist circumference, body mass index and waist-to-hip ratio in identifying metabolic syndrome: Variations by age, sex and race." *Diabetes & Metabolic Syndrome: Clinical Research & Reviews* (2015).

6. Orchard, Trevor J., et al. "Association between 7 Years of Intensive Treatment of Type 1 Diabetes and Long-term Mortality." *JAMA* vol. 313, no. 1 (2015): pp. 45–53.

7. Yano, Yuichiro, et al. "Isolated systolic hypertension in young and middle-aged adults and 31-year risk for cardiovascular mortality: the Chicago Heart Association Detection Project in Industry study." *Journal of the American College of Cardiology* vol. 65, no. 4 (2015): pp. 327–335.

8. Navar-Boggan, A. M., et al. "Hyperlipidemia in early adulthood increases long-term risk of coronary heart disease." *Circulation* vol. 131, no. 5 (February 3, 2015): pp. 451–458.

9. Dhamoon, M. S., et al. "Ideal cardiovascular health predicts functional status independently of vascular events: the Northern Manhattan Study." *J Am Heart Assoc.* vol. 4, no. 2 (February 12, 2015). pii: e001322.

10. Navar-Boggan. "Hyperlipidemia in early adulthood."

11. Saydah, S., et al. "Cardiometabolic Risk Factors among U.S. Adolescents and Young Adults and Risk of Early Mortality." *Pediatrics* vol. 131, no. 3 (March 2013) pp. e679–e686.

12. Cheong. "The discriminative ability of waist circumference."

13. Biswas, Aviroop, et al. "Sedentary Time and Its Association With Risk for Disease Incidence, Mortality, and Hospitalization in Adults: A Systematic Review and Meta-analysis." *Annals of Internal Medicine* vol. 162, no. 2 (2015): pp. 123–132.

14. Georgousopoulou, E. N., et al. "Adherence to Mediterranean is the most important protector against the development of fatal and non-fatal cardiovascular event: 10-year follow-up of the Attica Study." *Journal of the American College of Cardiology* vol. 65, no. 10_S (2015).

15. Laing, S. T., et al. "Subclinical atherosclerosis and obesity phenotypes among Mexican Americans." *J Am Heart Assoc.* vol. 4, no. 3 (March 18, 2015). pii: e001540.

16. Nelson, C. P., et al. "Genetically Determined Height and Coronary Artery Disease." *N Engl J Med.* (April 2015).

17. Topè, A. M., and P. F. Rogers. "Metabolic Syndrome among Students Attending a Historically Black College: Prevalence and Gender Differences." *Diabetology and Metabolic Syndrome* vol. 5, no. 1 (January 12, 2013): p. 2.

18. Romaguera, D., et al. "Consumption of Sweet Beverages and Type 2 Diabetes Incidence in European Adults: Results from EPIC-InterAct." *Diabetologia* (April 26, 2013) (e-pub).

19. Samaan, M. Constantine, et al. "Sex differences in skeletal muscle Phosphatase and tensin homolog deleted on chromosome 10 (PTEN) levels: A cross-sectional study." *Scientific Reports* vol. 5 (2015).

20. Yates T et al. "Association Between Change in Daily Ambulatory Activity and Cardiovascular Events in People with Impaired Glucose Tolerance (NAVIGATOR trial): A Cohort Analysis." *The Lancet* vol. 383, no. 9922 (March 22, 2014): pp. 1059–1066.

21. Huxley, Rachel R., et al. "Risk of all-cause mortality and vascular events in women versus men with type 1 diabetes: a systematic review and meta-analysis." *The Lancet Diabetes & Endocrinology* vol. 3, no. 3 (2015): pp. 198–206.

22. Romeo, Giulio R., and Martin J. Abrahamson. "The 2015 Standards for Diabetes Care: Maintaining a Patient-Centered Approach." *Annals of Internal Medicine* (2015).

23. Boursi, Ben, et al. "The effect of past antibiotic exposure on diabetes risk."*European Journal of Endocrinology* (2015): p. EJE-14.

24. Blackburn, David F., Jonathan Y. Chow, and Amy D. Smith. "Statin use and incident diabetes explained by bias rather than biology." *Canadian Journal of Cardiology* (2015).

25. Clemente-Postigo, Mercedes, et al. "Serum 25-Hydroxyvitamin D and Adipose Tissue Vitamin D Receptor Gene Expression: Relationship With Obesity and Type 2 Diabetes." *The Journal of Clinical Endocrinology & Metabolism* (2015).

26. Huxley. "Risk of all-cause mortality and vascular events in women versus men with type 1 diabetes."

27. Livingstone, Shona J., et al. "Estimated life expectancy in a Scottish cohort with type 1 diabetes, 2008–2010." *JAMA* vol. 313, no. 1 (2015): pp. 37–44.

28. Huxley. "Risk of all-cause mortality and vascular events in women versus men with type 1 diabetes."

29. Orchard. "Association between 7 Years of Intensive Treatment of Type 1 Diabetes."

30. Rhee. "Dietary Diabetes Risk Reduction Score."

31. Samaan. "Sex differences in skeletal muscle Phosphatase and tensin homologue."

32. Bao, Wei, et al. "Long-term risk of type 2 diabetes mellitus in relation to BMI and weight change among women with a history of gestational diabetes mellitus: a prospective cohort study." *Diabetologia* (2015): pp. 1–8.

33. Xiang, A. H., et al. "Association of Maternal Diabetes With Autism in Offspring." *JAMA* vol. 313, no. 14 (April 14, 2015): pp. 1425–1434.

34. Villarroel, Maria A., Anjel Vahratian, and Brian W. Ward. "Health Care Utilization Among US Adults With Diagnosed Diabetes, 2013." *NCHS Data Brief* vol. 183 (2015): pp. 1–8

35. Kung, Hsiang-Ching, et al. "Hypertension-Related Mortality in the United States." Washington D.C.: National Center for Health Statistics (2015).

36. Fan, Amy Z., et al. "Peer Reviewed: State Socioeconomic Indicators and Self-Reported Hypertension Among US Adults, 2011 Behavioral Risk Factor Surveillance System." *Preventing Chronic Disease* vol. 12 (2015).

37. Moran, A. E., et al. "Cost-effectiveness of hypertension therapy according to 2014 guidelines." *N Engl J Med.* vol. 372, no. 5 (January 29, 2015): pp. 447–455.

38. Angell, Sonia Y., Kevin M. De Cock, and Thomas R. Frieden. "A public health approach to global management of hypertension." *The Lancet* vol. 385, no. 9970 (2015): pp. 825–827.

39. Huang, Y., et al. "Prehypertension and the Risk of Stroke." *Neurology* vol. 82, no. 13 (April 2014): pp. 1153–61.

40. Allen, N. B., et al. "Blood Pressure Trajectories in Early Adulthood and Subclinical Atherosclerosis in Middle Age." *JAMA* vol. 311, no. 5 (February 5, 2014): pp. 490–497.

41. Yano. "Isolated systolic hypertension in young and middle-aged adults."

42. Sarafidis, P. A., and Bakris, G. L. "Early Patterns of Blood Pressure Change and Future Coronary Atherosclerosis." *JAMA* vol. 311, no. 5 (February 5, 2014): pp. 471–472.

43. www.cdc.gov.

44. Sampson, U. K., et al. "Factors Associated with the Prevalence of Hypertension in the Southeastern United States: Insights from 69 211 Blacks and Whites in the Southern Community Cohort Study." *Circulation: Cardiovascular and Quality Outcomes* vol. 7, no. 1 (January 1, 2014): pp. 33–54.

45. Centers for Disease Control and Prevention. "Tips for Minorities: Prevent High Blood Pressure." www.cdc.gov.

46. Robertson, R. M. Personal interview.

47. Fernandez-Mendoza, Julio, et al. "Abstract MP71: Short Sleep Duration Modifies the Relationship Between Hypertension and All-Cause Mortality."*Circulation* vol. 131 (Suppl 1) (2015): pp. AMP71–AMP71.

48. Rosendorff, C., et al. "Treatment of Hypertension in Patients With Coronary Artery Disease: A Scientific Statement From the American Heart Association, American College of Cardiology, and American Society of Hypertension." *Hypertension* (2015); published online before print March 31, 2015.

49. Xu, Wenxin, et al. "Optimal systolic blood pressure target, time to intensification, and time to follow-up in treatment of hypertension: population based retrospective cohort study." *BMJ* vol. 350 (2015): p. h158.

50. Navar-Boggan. "Hyperlipidemia in early adulthood."

51. http://www.cdc.gov/HeartDisease/facts.htm.

52. Hernandez, Rosalba, et al. "Optimism and Cardiovascular Health: Multi-Ethnic Study of Atherosclerosis (MESA)." *Health Behavior and Policy Review* vol. 2, no. 1 (2015): pp. 62–73.

53. "A Sense of Purpose May Help Your Heart." Medline Plus *HealthDay* (March 6, 2015).

54. Xu. "Optimal systolic blood pressure target."

55. Dupree, M. E., et al. "Association Between Divorce and Risks for Acute Myocardial Infarction" *Circulation* (April 2015) (online).

56. Bergh, Cecilia, et al. "Stress resilience and physical fitness in adolescence and risk of coronary heart disease in middle age." *Heart* (2015): heartjnl-2014.

57. Alcántara, Carmela, et al. "Perfect Storm Concurrent Stress and Depressive Symptoms Increase Risk of Myocardial Infarction or Death." *Circulation: Cardiovascular Quality and Outcomes* vol. 8, no. 2 (2015): pp. 146–154.

58. May, Heidi Thomas, et al. "The Association of Antidepressant and Statin Use to Future Death and Incident Cardiovascular Disease Varies by Depression Severity." *Journal of the American College of Cardiology* 65.10_S (2015).

59. Xu. "Optimal systolic blood pressure target."

60. Lichtman, Judith H., et al. "Symptom recognition and healthcare experiences of young women with acute myocardial infarction." *Circulation: Cardiovascular Quality and Outcomes* vol. 8, no. 2 (Suppl 1) (2015): pp. S31–S38.

61. Dreyer, Rachel P., et al. "Gender differences in pre-event health status of young patients with acute myocardial infarction: A VIRGO study analysis." *European Heart Journal: Acute Cardiovascular Care* (2015): 2048872615568967.

62. Lichtman. "Symptom recognition and healthcare experiences."

63. Chomistek, Andrea K., et al. "Relationship of sedentary behavior and physical activity to incident cardiovascular disease: results from the Women's Health Initiative." *Journal of the American College of Cardiology* vol. 61, no. 23 (2013): pp. 2346–2354.

64. Armstrong, Miranda E. G., et al. "Frequent physical activity may not reduce vascular disease risk as much as moderate activity: large prospective study of UK women." *Circulation* (2015): CIRCULATIONAHA-114.

65. Chromistek. "Relationship of sedentary behavior and physical activity to incident cardiovascular disease."

66. Rutten-Jacobs, L. C., et al. "High Incidence of Diabetes after Stroke in Young Adults and Risk of Recurrent Vascular Events: The FUTURE Study." *PLoS One* vol. 9, no. 1 (January 23, 2014): p. e87171.

67. Synhaeve, N. E., et al. "Poor Long-Term Functional Outcome after Stroke Among Adults Aged 18 to 50 Years: Follow-up of Transient Ischemic Attack and Stroke Patients and Unelucidated Risk Factor Evaluation (FUTURE) Study." *Stroke* vol. 45, no. 4 (April 2014): pp. 1157–1160.

68. Mullen, M. T., et al. "Optimization modeling to maximize population access to comprehensive stroke centers." *Neurology* 84(12) (March 24, 2015): pp. 1196–205.

69. Torre, L. A., et al. "Global cancer statistics, 2012." *CA Cancer J Clin.* vol. 65, no. 2 (March 2015): pp. 87–108.

70. Siegel, Rebecca L., Kimberly D. Miller, and Ahmedin Jemal. "Cancer statistics, 2015." *CA: A Cancer Journal for Clinicians* vol. 65, no. 1 (2015): pp. 5–29.

71. American Cancer Society. "Cancer Facts & Figures 2014."

72. Thomson, C. A., et al. "Nutrition and Physical Activity Cancer Prevention Guidelines, Cancer Risk, and Mortality in the Women's Health Initiative." *Cancer Prev Res (Phila)* vol. 7, no. 1 (January 2014): pp. 42–53.

73. Kohler, B. A., et al "Annual report to the nation on the status of cancer, 1975–2011, featuring incidence of breast cancer subtypes by race/ethnicity, poverty, and state." *J Natl Cancer Inst.* vol. 65, no. 1 (March 30, 2015). pii: djv048.

74. Zeng, Chenjie, et al. "Disparities by Race, Age, and Sex in the Improvement of Survival for Major Cancers: Results From the National Cancer Institute Surveillance, Epidemiology, and End Results (SEER) Program in the United States, 1990 to 2010." *JAMA Oncology* (2015).

75. Iqbal, Javaid, et al. "Differences in breast cancer stage at diagnosis and cancer-specific survival by race and ethnicity in the United States." *JAMA* vol. 313, no. 2 (2015): pp. 165–173.

76. Jemal, A., et al. "Annual Report to the Nation on the Status of Cancer, 1975–2009, Featuring the Burden and Trends in Human Papillomavirus (HPV)–Associated Cancers and HPV Vaccination Coverage Levels." *Journal of the National Cancer Institute*, January 7, 2013 (e-pub).

77. Premi, S., et al. "Photochemistry. Chemiexcitation of melanin derivatives induces DNA photoproducts long after UV exposure." *Science* vol. 347, no. 6224 (February 20, 2015): pp. 842–847.

78. Wehner, M. R., et al. "International Prevalence of Indoor Tanning: A Systematic Review and Metaanalysis." *JAMA Dermatology* vol. 150, no. 4 (April 2014): pp. 390–400.

79. Cartmel, B., et al. "Novel gene identified in an exome-wide association study of tanning dependence." *Exp Dermatol.* vol. 23, no. 10 (October 2014): pp. 757–759.

80. American Cancer Society.

81. Johnson, R. H., et al. "Incidence of Breast Cancer with Distant Involvement among Women in the United States, 1976 to 2009." *JAMA* vol. 309, no. 8 (February 27, 2013): pp. 800–805.

82. "Breast Cancer Disparities among U.S. Women." www.cdc.gov.

83. Tria Tirona, M. "Breast Cancer Screening Update." *American Family Physician* vol. 87, no. 4 (February 15, 2013): pp. 274–278.

84. Kerlikowske, K., et al. "Outcomes of Screening Mammography by Frequency, Breast Density, and Postmenopausal Hormone Therapy." *JAMA Internal Medicine* vol. 173, no. 9 (May 13, 2013): pp. 807–816.

85. American Cancer Society.

86. Lakoski, Susan G., et al. "Midlife Cardiorespiratory Fitness, Incident Cancer, and Survival After Cancer in Men: The Cooper Center Longitudinal Study." *JAMA Oncology* (2015).

87. Power, A. M., et al. "Association between Constipation and Colorectal Cancer: Systematic Review and Meta-Analysis of Observational Studies." *American Journal of Gastroenterology* (March 12, 2013) (e-pub).

88. Nan H, et al. "Association of aspirin and NSAID use with risk of colorectal cancer according to genetic variants." *JAMA* vol. 313, no. 11 (March 17, 2015): pp. 1133–1142.

89. Orlich, Michael J., et al. "Vegetarian dietary patterns and the risk of colorectal cancers." *JAMA Internal Medicine* (2015).

90. Phipps, A. I., et al. "Associations between Cigarette Smoking Status and Colon Cancer Prognosis among Participants in North Central Cancer Treatment Group Phase III Trial N0147." *Journal of Clinical Oncology* (April 1, 2013) (e-pub).

91. Meester, Reinier G. S., et al. "Public health impact of achieving 80% colorectal cancer screening rates in the United States by 2018." *Cancer* (2015).

92. Gulati, R., et al. "Comparative Effectiveness of Alternative Prostate-Specific Antigen–Based Prostate Cancer Screening Strategies: Model Estimates of Potential Benefits and Harms." *Annals of Internal Medicine* vol. 158, no. 3 (February 5, 2013): pp. 145–153.

93. Chamie, Karim, Stephen B. Williams, and Jim C. Hu. "Population-Based Assessment of Determining Treatments for Prostate Cancer." *JAMA Oncology* (2015).

94. Karvonen, Anne M., et al. "Moisture Damage and Asthma: A Birth Cohort Study." *Pediatrics* (2015): peds-2014.

Chapter 16

1. "U.S. Warns Health Officials to Be Alert for Deadly New Virus," medlineplus.gov (March 7, 2013).

2. Lam, T. T., et al. "Dissemination, divergence and establishment of H7N9 influenza viruses in China." *Nature* (March 11, 2015).

3. "Emerging Infectious Diseases" U.S. Centers for Disease Control and Prevention (February 20, 2015).

4. Seidman, M. D., et al. "Clinical practice guideline: allergic rhinitis executive summary." *Otolaryngol Head Neck Surg.* vol. 152, no. 2 (February 2015): pp. 197–206.

5. Ibid.

6. Lieu, T. A., et al. "Geographic clusters in underimmunization and vaccine refusal." *Pediatrics* vol. 135, no. 2 (February 2015): pp. 280–289.

7. King, B. H. "Promising Forecast for Autism Spectrum Disorders." *JAMA* vol. 313, no. 15 (April 21, 2015): pp. 1518–1519.

8. Jain, A., et al. "Autism Occurrence by MMR Vaccine Status Among US Children With Older Siblings With and Without Autism." *JAMA* vol. 313, no. 15 (April 21, 2015): pp. 1534–1540.

9. Zipprich, Jennifer, et al. "Measles outbreak—California, December 2014–February 2015." *MMWR Morb Mortal Wkly Rep* vol. 64, no. 6 (2015): 153–154.

10. Majumder, Maimuna S., et al. "Substandard Vaccination Compliance and the 2015 Measles Outbreak." *JAMA Pediatrics* (2015).

11. Hussey, H. H. "Immunity Against Contagious Diseases: Inadequacies." *JAMA* vol. 313, no. 15 (April 21, 2015): p. 1577

12. Kim, D. K., et al. "Advisory committee on immunization practices recommended immunization schedule for adults aged 19 years or older—United States, 2015." *MMWR Morb Mortal Wkly Rep.* vol. 64, no. 4 (February 6, 2015): pp. 91–92.

13. Centers for Disease Control and Prevention. "2013 Vaccine Recommendations: What They Mean for You." www.cdc.gov.

14. Karsch-Völk, Marlies, Bruce Barrett, and Klaus Linde. "Echinacea for Preventing and Treating the Common Cold." *JAMA* vol. 313, no. 6 (2015): p. 618–619.

15. Hemilä, Harri, and Elizabeth Chalker. "The effectiveness of high dose zinc acetate lozenges on various common cold symptoms: a meta-analysis." *BMC Family Practice* vol. 16, no. 1 (2015): p. 24.

16. Meropol, S. B., et al. "Risks and Benefits Associated with Antibiotic Use for Acute Respiratory Infections: A Cohort Study." *Annals of Family Medicine* vol. 11, no. 2, (March/April 2013): pp. 165–172.

17. Hicks, L. A., et al. "U.S. Outpatient Antibiotic Prescribing, 2010." *New England Journal of Medicine* Vol. 368, no. 15, (April 11, 2013): pp. 1461–1462.

18. Kantele., A. "As far as Travelers' Risk of Acquiring Resistant Intestinal Microbes is Considered, no Antibiotics (Absorbable or Nonabsorbable) are Safe." *Clin Infect Dis.* (March 3, 2015). pii: civ174.

19. Dobson, Joanna, et al. "Oseltamivir treatment for influenza in adults: a meta-analysis of randomised controlled trials." *The Lancet* (2015).

20. Dallas, M. E. "Got the Flu? Rest First, Exercise Later." *HealthDay*, medlineplus.gov (January 22, 2013).

21. Adriani, K. S., M. C. Brouwer, and D. van de Beek. "Risk factors for community-acquired bacterial meningitis in adults." *Neth J Med* 2 (2015): p. 53–60. http://www.cdc.gov/hepatitis/C/cFAQ.htm#overview

22. Centers for Disease Control and Prevention. "Meningococcal Disease: Help Prevent It." www.cdc.gov.

23. Centers for Disease Control and Prevention. "Meningococcal Vaccines: What You Need to Know." www.cdc.gov/meningitis/vaccine_info.html/

24. American Academy of Dermatology. "Dermatologist Warns Consumers about Complications Linked to Newer Tattoo Inks." (March 1, 2013).

25. Centers for Disease Control. www.cdc.gov.

26. Ibid.

27. Clayton, E. W., et al. "Beyond Myalgic Encepholamyelitis/Chronic Fatigue Syndrome." Washington, D.C.: Institute of Medicine (2015).

28. Hornig, M., et al. "Cytokine network analysis of cerebrospinal fluid in myalgic encephalomyelitis/chronic fatigue syndrome." *Science Advances.* (February 2015).

29. "Germs Fly in Roller-Derby Games, Study Finds." medlineplus.gov (March 12, 2013).

30. Scott, C., et al. "Tuberculosis trends—United States, 2014." *MMWR Morb Mortal Wkly Rep.* vol. 64, no. 10 (March 20, 2015): pp. 265–269.

31. Kuehn, Bridget. "'Nightmare' Bacteria on the Rise in U.S. Hospitals, Long-Term Care Facilities." *JAMA* vol 309, no. 1 (April 17, 2013): pp. 1573–1574.

32. Lessa, F. C., et al. "Burden of Clostridium difficile infection in the United States." *N Engl J Med.* vol. 372, no. 9 (February 26, 2015): pp. 825–834.

33. Kuehn, B. "Emerging Tick-Borne Diseases Expand beyond Range along with Rebounding Deer Populations." *JAMA* vol. 309, no. 2 (January 9, 2013): pp. 124–125.

34. Centers for Disease Control and Prevention. "West Nile Virus (WNV) Fact Sheet." www.cdc.gov.

35. Levin-Sparenberg, Elizabeth, et al. "Ebola: The Natural and Human History of a Deadly Virus By David Quammen." *American Journal of Epidemiology* vol. 181, no. 2 (2015).

36. Agnandji, S. T., et al. "Phase 1 Trials of rVSV Ebola Vaccine in Africa and Europe—Preliminary Report." *N Engl J Med.* (April 1, 2015).

Chapter 17

1. https://www.healthcare.gov/.

2. "Quality & Disparities Report: Access to Health Care Improving Among all Racial and Ethnic Groups Following Affordable Care Act; Additional Work Remains." April 2015. Agency for Healthcare Research and Quality, Rockville, MD.

3. Collins, S. R., et al. "The Rise in Health Care Coverage and Affordability since Health Reform Took Effect." Xx: Commonwealth Fund (January 2015.)

4. Ibid.

5. Martinez, M. E., and Cohen, R. A. "Health Insurance Coverage: Early Release of Estimates From the National Health Interview Survey, January–September 2014." Washington, D.C.: National Center for Health Statistics (2015).

6. Jaffe, S. "The Affordable Care Act's Insurance Programme Takes Effect." *The Lancet* vol. 383, no. 9912 (January 11-17, 2014): pp. 112–113.

7. Bauer, A. M., et al. "Health Literacy and Antidepressant Medication Adherence among Adults with Diabetes: The Diabetes Study of Northern California (DISTANCE)." *Journal of General Internal Medicine* (March 20, 2013) (e-pub).

8. Kuehn, B. "More Than One Third of U.S. Individuals Use the Internet to Self-Diagnose." *JAMA*, vol. 309, no. 8 (February 27, 2013): pp. 756–757.

9. Husain, I., et al. "Can healthy people benefit from health apps?" *British Medical Journal* vol. 350 (April 2015): p. h1887

10. Laksanasopin, T., et al. "A smartphone dongle for diagnosis of infectious diseases at the point of care." *Sci Transl Med.* vol. 7, no. 273 (February 4, 2015): p. 273re1.

11. Husain, et al. "Can healthy people benefit from health apps?"

12. Riley, M. "Health Maintenance in Women." *American Family Physician* vol. 87, no. 1 (January 1, 2013): pp. 30–37.

13. Ibid.

14. Chou, Roger. "Cardiac Screening With Electrocardiography, Stress Echocardiography, or Myocardial Perfusion Imaging: Advice for High-Value Care From the American College of Physicians." *Annals of Internal Medicine* vol. 162, no. 6 (2015): pp. 438–447.

15. Berkowitz, Z., et al. "Cervical Cancer Screening Intervals, 2006 to 2009: Moving Beyond Annual Testing." *JAMA Internal Medicine* (April 8, 2013) (e-pub), pp. 1–3.

16. Nguyen, G. T., and P. F. Cronholm. "The Annual Pelvic Examination: Preventive Time Not Well Spent." *American Family Physician* vol. 87, no. 1 (January 1, 2013): pp. 8–9.

17. Henderson, J. T., et al. "Routine Bimanual Pelvic Examinations: Practices and Beliefs of U.S. Obstetrician-Gynecologists." *American Journal of Obstetrics and Gynecology* vol. 208, no. 2 (February 2013): p. 109.

18. Liu, V., et al. "Data Breaches of Protected Health Information in the United States." *JAMA* vol. 313, no. 14 (April 14, 2015): pp. 1471–1473.

19. Blumenthal, David, and Deven McGraw. "Keeping Personal Health Information Safe: The Importance of Good Data Hygiene." *JAMA* vol. 313, no. 14 (April 14, 2015): p. 1424.

20. "American Society of Plastic Surgeons Reports Cosmetic Procedures Increased 3 Percent in 2014." American Society of Plastic Surgeons news release (February 16, 2015).

21. U.S. Food and Drug Administration. "5 Things to Know about Breast Implants." Consumer Updates, February 20, 2013, www.fda.gov/ForConsumers/ConsumerUpdates/ucm338144.htm.

22. Lavigne, E., et al. "Breast Cancer Detection and Survival among Women with Cosmetic Breast Implants: Systematic Review and Meta-analysis of Observational Studies." *BMJ* vol. 346 (April 29, 2013): p. f2399.

23. "American Society of Plastic Surgeons Reports."

24. American Academy of Dermatology. "Dermatologist Warns Consumers about Complications Linked to Newer Tattoo Inks." News release (March 1, 2013).

25. Dallas, M. "Want to Get Rid of That Old Tattoo? You're Not Alone." MedlinePlus (February 8, 2013), www.nlm.nih.gov/medlineplus/.

26. U.S. Food and Drug Administration. "Temporary Tattoos May Put You at Risk." *Consumer Updates* (March 25, 2013), www.fda.gov/ForConsumers/ConsumerUpdates/ucm343932.htm.

27. Clarke, T. C., et al. *Trends in the Use of Complementary Health Approaches among Adults.* National Health Statistics Report, no. 79 (February 10, 2015).

28. American Heart Association. "Alternative Therapies May Help Lower Blood Pressure." News release (April 22, 2013).

29. Clarke, et al. Trends in the Use of Complementary Health Approaches.

30. Navarro, V. J., et al. "Liver injury from herbals and dietary supplements in the U.S." *Drug-Induced Liver Injury Network Hepatology* vol. 60, issue 4 (October 2014): pp. 1399–1408.

Chapter 18

1. National Center for Health Statistics. www.cdc.gov/nchs.

2. Peltzer, Karl, and Supa Pengpid. "Factors Associated with Unintentional Injury among University Students in 26 Countries." *Public Health Nursing* (2015).

3. Ibid.

4. Albert, M. and L. F. McCaig "Emergency department visits for motor vehicle traffic injuries: United States, 2010–2011." *NCHS Data Brief.* vol. 185 (January 2015): pp. 1–8.

5. Vaca, F. E. et al. "Female drivers increasingly involved in impaired driving crashes: actions to ameliorate the risk." *Acad Emerg Med.* vol. 21, no. 12 (December 2014): pp. 1485–1492.

6. Simons-Morton, B. G., et al. "Experimental Effects of Injunctive Norms on Simulated Risky Driving Among Teenage Males." *Health Psychology* (January 27, 2014).

7. Centers for Disease Control and Prevention. "Distracted Driving." www.cdc.gov/Motorvehiclesafety/Distracted_Driving.

8. Project Yellow Light. www.distraction.gov

9. Stimpson, J. P., et al. "Fatalities of Pedestrians, Bicycle Riders, and Motorists Due to Distracted Driving: Motor Vehicle Crashes in the U.S., 2005–2010." *Public Health Reports* vol. 128, no. 6 (November–December 2013) pp. 436–442.

10. Rhodes, Nancy, Kelly Pivik, and Marnie Sutton. "Risky driving among young male drivers: The effects of mood and passengers." *Transportation Research Part F: Traffic Psychology and Behaviour* vol. 28 (2015): pp. 65–76.

11. Lawrence, Natalie Kerr. "Highlighting the injunctive norm to reduce phone-related distracted driving." *Social Influence* vol. 10, no. 2 (2015): pp. 109–118.

12. Rumschlag, Gordon, et al. "The effects of texting on driving performance in a driving simulator: the influence of driver age." *Accident Analysis & Prevention* vol. 74 (2015): pp. 145–149.

13. Preidt, R. "Phones, Texting May Be as Dangerous as Alcohol for Drivers." *MedlinePlus* (March 15, 2013). www.nlm.nih.gov/medlineplus/.

14. Dubois, Sacha, et al. "The combined effects of alcohol and cannabis on driving: Impact on crash risk." *Forensic Science International* vol. 248 (2015): pp. 94–100.

15. Kuehn, B. "FDA Warning: Driving May Be Impaired the Morning Following Sleeping Pill Use." *JAMA* vol. 309, no. 7 (February 20, 2013) pp. 645–646.

16. Wickens, C. M., et al. "Driver Anger on the Information Superhighway: A Content Analysis of Online Complaints of Offensive Driver Behaviour." *Accident Analysis and Prevention* vol. 51 (March 2013): pp. 84–92.

17. Williams, Allan. "Spotlight on Safety: Bicyclist Safety." Governors Highway Safety Association. http://www.ghsa.org/html/files/pubs/spotlights/bikes_2014.pdf

18. Franklin, C. A., and T. W. Franklin. "Predicting Fear of Crime: Considering Differences across Gender." *Feminist Criminology* vol. 4, no. 1: pp. 83–106.

19. Centers for Disease Control and Prevention (CDC). "Preventing Violent Deaths in America." www.cdc.gov.

20. Klein, Robert H., and Victor L. Schermer. "Toward understanding and treating violence in America: some contributions from group dynamic and group therapy perspectives: introduction to part i." *International Journal of Group Psychotherapy* vol. 65, no. 1 (2015): pp. iv–28.

21. Centers for Disease Control and Prevention. "Preventing Violent Deaths in America." www.cdc.gov/features/ViolentDeathsAmerica/.

22. Wintemute, Garen J. "The epidemiology of firearm violence in the twenty-first century United States." *Annual Review of Public Health* vol. 36 (2015): pp. 5–19.

23. Braga, Anthony A., and David L. Weisburd. "Focused deterrence and the prevention of violent gun injuries: practice, theoretical principles, and scientific evidence." *Annual Review of Public Health* vol. 36 (2015): pp. 55–68.

24. Preidt, R. "1 in 5 Americans Know a Victim of Gun Violence: Poll." MedlinePlus, (February 28, 2013), www.nlm.nih.gov/medlineplus/.

25. Braga and Weisburd. "Focused deterrence and the prevention of violent gun injuries."

26. Metzl J. M. and K. T. MacLeish. "Mental Illness, Mass Shootings, and the Politics of American Firearms." *American Journal of Public Health* vol. 105, no. 2 (February 2015): pp. 240–249.

27. Webster, Daniel W. "Commentary: evidence to guide gun violence prevention in America." *Annual Review of Public Health* vol. 36 (2015): pp. 1–4

28. Hemenway, D., and M. Miller. "Public Health Approach to the Prevention of Gun Violence." *New England Journal of Medicine* (April 12, 2013) (e-pub).

29. Butts, Jeffrey A., et al. "Cure violence: a public health model to reduce gun violence." *Annual review of public health* vol. 36 (2015): pp. 39–53.

30. Richardson, Hannah B., et al. "Sexual Violence and Help-Seeking Among LGBQ and Heterosexual College Students." *Partner Abuse* vol. 36 (2015): pp. 29–46.

31. Amar, Angela F., et al. "Friends Helping Friends: A Non-Randomized Control Trial of a Peer Based Response to Dating Violence." *Nursing Outlook* (2015).

32. Bell, James G., and Barbara Perry. "Outside looking in: the community impacts of anti-lesbian, gay, and bisexual hate crime." *Journal of Homosexuality* vol. 36 (2015): pp. 98–120.

33. Perez-Pena, R., and S. Saulny. "Colleges Become Major Front in Fight over Carrying Guns." *New York Times*, (February 16, 2013).

34. Sutherland, J. L. et al. "Victimization and perpetration of sexual violence in college-aged men and women." *J Forensic Nurs.* vol. 10, no. 3 (July-September 2014): pp. 153–159.

35. Davidson, Judith. *Sexting: Gender and Teens.* Springer (2015).

36. Pellai, L. A., et al. "Epidemiology of sexting." *Minerva pediatrica* vol. 67, no. 1 (2015): p. 1

37. Brooks-Russell, A. et al. "Dating Violence" *Handbook of Adolescent Behavioral Problems,* edited by Thomas P. Gullotta, et al. New York: Springer (2015): pp. 559–576.

38. Coker, Ann L., et al. "Are Interpersonal Violence Rates Higher Among Young Women in College Compared With Those Never Attending College?" *Journal of Interpersonal Violence* (2015).

39. Sutherland, et all. "Victimization and perpetration of sexual violence."

40. Kaukinen C. "Dating Violence among College Students: The Risk and Protective Factors." *Trauma, Violence, & Abuse* (February 14, 2014).

41. Edwards, Katie M., et al. "Physical Dating Violence, Sexual Violence, and Unwanted Pursuit Victimization A Comparison of Incidence Rates Among Sexual-Minority and Heterosexual College Students." *Journal of interpersonal violence* vol. 30, no. 4 (2015): pp. 580–600.

42. Dardis, C. M., et al. "An Examination of the Factors Related to Dating Violence Perpetration Among Young Men and Women and Associated Theoretical Explanations: A Review of the Literature." *Trauma, Violence, & Abuse* (January 13, 2014).

43. Littleton H. "Interpersonal Violence on College Campuses: Understanding Risk Factors and Working to Find Solutions." *Trauma, Violence, & Abuse* (January 30, 2014).

44. Kaukinen C. "Dating Violence among College Students."

45. Sabina, C., and L. Y. Ho. "Campus and College Victim Responses to Sexual Assault and Dating Violence: Disclosure, Service Utilization, and Service Provision." *Trauma, Violence, & Abuse* (February 2014).

46. Amar, et al. "Friends Helping Friends."

47. Katz, Jennifer, and Hillary Rich. "Partner Covictimization and Post-Breakup Stalking, Pursuit, and Violence: A Retrospective Study of College Women." *Journal of Family Violence* (2015): pp. 1–11.

48. Bouffard, J. A., and H. A. Miller. "The Role of Sexual Arousal and Overperception of Sexual Intent within the Decision to Engage in Sexual Coercion." *Journal of Interpersonal Violence* (January 8, 2014).

49. Katz and Rich. "Partner Covictimization and Post-Breakup Stalking."

50. Sorenson, S. B., M. Joshi, and E. Sivitz. "Knowing a Sexual Assault Victim or Perpetrator: A Stratified Random Sample of Undergraduates at One University." *Journal of Interpersonal Violence* vol. 29, no. 3 (February 2014): pp. 394–416.

51. Bourke, Joanna. *Rape: A History from 1860 to the Present.* Hachette UK (2015).

52. Brooks-Russell, et al. "Dating Violence."

53. Kohler, Rachel. "Campus sexual assault: Effects of trauma on student survivors and how campuses intervene." *7th Biennial National Conference on Health and Domestic Violence.* nchdv (2015).

54. Moynihan, Mary M., et al. "Encouraging Responses in Sexual and Relationship Violence Prevention: what Programs Remain Effective 1 Year Later?" *Journal of Interpersonal Violence* vol. 30, no. 1 (2015): pp. 110–132.

Chapter 19

1. Papworth, A. et al. "Is climate change the greatest threat to global health?" *The Geographical Journal,* published online (December 3, 2014). doi. 10.1111/geoj.12127.

2. Barrett, B. et al. "Climate change, human health, and epidemiological transition." *Prev Med* vol. 70C (January 2015): pp. 69–75.

3. Papworth, et al. "Is climate change the greatest threat?"

4. Factor-Litvak, P. et al. "Persistent Associations between Maternal Prenatal Exposure to Phthalates on Child IQ at Age 7 Years." *PLoS One.* vol. 9, no. 12 (December 2014): pp. e114003.

5. Raz, R. et al. "Autism Spectrum Disorder and Particulate Matter Air Pollution before, during, and after Pregnancy: A Nested Case-Control Analysis within the Nurses' Health Study II Cohort." *Environ Health Perspect.* (December 18, 2014).

6. Van Rossem, L. et al. "Prenatal Air Pollution Pressure and Newborn Blood Pressure." *Environmental Health Perspectives,* published online. doi.org/10.1289/ehp.1307419.

7. Weuve, J., et al. "Exposure to Particulate Air Pollution and Cognitive Decline in Older Women." *Archives of Internal Medicine* vol. 172, no. 3 (February 13, 2012) pp. 219–227.

8. Gold, D. R., and J. M. Samet. "Air Pollution, Climate, and Heart Disease." *Circulation* vol. 128, no. 21 (November 19, 2013): pp. e411–e414.

9. Adar, S. D., et al. "Fine Particulate Air Pollution and the Progression of Carotid Intima-Medial Thickness: A Prospective Cohort Study from the Multi-ethnic Study of Atherosclerosis and Air Pollution." *PLoS Medicine* 10, no. 4 (April 2013).

10. Gold and Samet, "Air Pollution, Climate, and Heart Disease."

11. Ensor, K. B., et al. "A Case-Crossover Analysis of Out-of-Hospital Cardiac Arrest and Air Pollution." *Circulation* 127, no. 11 (March 19, 2013). pp. 1192–1199.

12. Jakubiak-Lasocka, J. et al. "Impact of Traffic-Related Air Pollution on Health." *Adv. Exp. Medicine, Biology—Neuroscience and Respiration* vol. 3 (2015): pp. 21–29.

13. Zare-Jeddi, M. et al. "Concentration of phthalates in bottled water under common storage condition: Do they pose a health risk to children?" *Food Research International.* (March 2015): pp. 256–265.

14. Dallas, M. E. "Indoor Wood-burning Can Affect Air Quality." MedlinePlus *HealthDay* (January 2, 2015).

15. Yankelevitz, D. F., et al. "Second-Hand Tobacco Smoke in Never Smokers Is a Significant Risk Factor for Coronary Artery Calcification." *JACC Cardiovascular Imaging* (March 13, 2013) (e-pub).

16. "EPA Urges Home Radon Testing/Protect Your Family from Lung Cancer Caused by Exposure to Radon in Your Home." Environmental Protection Association (January 15, 2015), http://yosemite.epa.gov/opa/admpress.nsf/0/7D2B0496C1FDEA8785257DCE005C95E7

17. "Blood Lead Levels in Children Aged 1–5 Years—United States, 1999–2010." *Morbidity and Mortality Weekly Report* vol. 62, no. 13 (April 5, 2013): pp. 245–248.

18. Khanna, M. M. "Boys, not girls, are negatively affected on cognitive tasks by lead exposure: a pilot study." *J Environ Health* vol. 77, no. 6 (January-February 2015): pp. 72–77.

19. Stein, Y. et al. "Electromagnetic Radiation and Health: Human Indicators." In *Environmental Indicators* Springer edited by Robert H. Arman and Osmo Haminen (2015): pp. 1025–1046.

20. Naeem, Z. "Health risks associated with mobile phone use." *International Journal of Health Sciences* (2015), ijhs.org.sa.

21. Moshammer, H. et al. "Early prognosis of noise-induced hearing loss. *Occupational & Environmental Medicine* (2015). oem.bmj.com.

22. "Should You Be Screened for a Hearing Problem?" *Harvard Women's Health Watch* vol. 20, no. 5 (January 2013): p. 3. www.health.harvard.edu.

Chapter 20

1. http://www.helpage.org/global-agewatch/

2. http://www.census.gov

3. http://www.aoa.gov/aoaroot/aging_statistics/index.aspx

4. GBD 2013 Mortality and Causes of Death Collaborators. "Global, regional, and national age-sex specific all-cause and cause-specific mortality for 240 causes of death, 1990–2013: a systematic analysis for the Global Burden of Disease Study 2013." *The Lancet* vol. 14 (December 17, 2014): pp. 61682. pii: S0140–6736.

5. "U.S. Seniors' Health Poorest, Global Survey Shows," HealthDay, MedlinePlus.gov (November 19, 2014).

6. http://www.census.gov

7. *National Research Council and Institute of Medicine, U.S. Health in International Perspective. Shorter Lives, Poorer Health.* Panel on Understanding Cross-National Health Differences among High-Income Countries, Steven H. Woolf and Laudan Aron (eds.). Committee on Population, Division of Behavioral and Social Sciences and Education, and Board on Population Health and Public Health Practice, Institute of Medicine. Washington, DC: The National Academies Press (2013).

8. Jha, P., et al. "21ˢᵗ- Century Hazards of Smoking and Benefits of Cessation in the United States." *New England Journal of Medicine,* vol. 368, no. 4, (January 24, 2013) pp. 341–350.

9. Rippon, I. and Steptoe, A. "Feeling Old vs Being Old: Associations Between Self-perceived Age and Mortality." *JAMA Intern Med.* vol. 175, no. 2 (February 1, 2015): pp. 307–309.

10. Steptoe, A., et al. "Enjoyment of Life and Declining Physical Function at Older Ages: A Longitudinal Cohort Study." *Canadian Medical Association Journal* (January 20, 2014).

11. Holtermann, A., et al. "Does the Benefit on Survival from Leisure Time Physical Activity Depend on Physical Activity at Work? A Prospective Cohort Study." *PLoS One.* vol. 8, no. 1 (2013): p. e54548.

12. Flegal, K. M., et al. "Association of All-Cause Mortality with Overweight and Obesity Using Standard Body Mass Index Categories: A Systematic Review and Meta-analysis." *JAMA.* vol. 309, no. 1 (January 2, 2013) pp. 71–82.

13. Crous-Bou, M. et al. "Mediterranean diet and telomere length in Nurses' Health Study: population based cohort study." *BMJ.* vol. 349 (December 2, 2014): p. g6674.

14. Gold, B. T., et al. "Lifelong Bilingualism Maintains Neural Efficiency for Cognitive Control in Aging." *Journal of Neuroscience* vol. 33, no. 2 (January 9, 2013): pp. 387–396.

15. Scullin, M. K. and Bliwise, D. L. "Sleep, Cognition, and Normal Aging: Integrating a Half-Century of Multidisciplinary Research." *Perspect Psychol Sci.* vol. 10, no. 1 (January 2015): pp. 97–137

16. Smart, E. L. et al. "Occupational complexity and lifetime cognitive abilities. Neurology." vol. 9, no. 83(24) (December 2014): pp. 2285–2291.

17. "Practice Bulletin No 141: Management of Menopausal Symptoms." *Obstetrics & Gynecology,* vol. 123, no. 1 (January 2014): pp. 202–216.

18. Roussou, J. F., et al. "Lessons Learned from the Women's Health Initiative Trials of Menopausal Hormone Therapy." *Obstetrics and Gynecology* vol. 121, no. 1 (January 2013): pp. 172–176.

19. Collaborative Group of Epidemiological Studies of Ovarian Cancer. "Menopause Hormone Use and Ovarian Cancer Risk" *The Lancet*, published online February 15, 2015.

20. "Practice Bulletin No. 141: Management of Menopausal Symptoms."

21. Dumanski, J. P. et al. "Mutagenesis. Smoking is associated with mosaic loss of chromosome Y." *Science* vol. 347, no. 6217 (January 2, 2015): pp. 81–83. doi: 10.1126/science.1262092. Epub December 4, 2014.

22. Layton, J. B., et al. "Testosterone Lab Testing and Initiation in the United Kingdom and the United States, 2000–2011." *Journal of Clinical Endocrinology & Metabolism* (January 1, 2014).

23. Finkle, W. D., et al. "Increased Risk of Non-fatal Myocardial Infarction Following Testosterone Therapy Prescription in Men." *PLoS One* vol 9, no. 1 (January 29, 2014).

24. Preidt, Robert. "40 Percent of Seniors Report Having a Disability" MedlinePlus, *Healthday.* http://www.nlm.nih.gov/medlineplus/news/fullstory_149749.html.

25. American Psychiatric Association. *Diagnostic and Statistical Manual of Mental Disorders (DSM-5).* Washington, DC: American Psychiatric Association (2013).

26. van der Zwaluw, N. L. et al. "Results of 2-year vitamin B treatment on cognitive performance: secondary data from an RCT." *Neurology* vol. 83, no. 23 (December 2, 2014): pp. 2158–66.

27. Zissimopoulos, J. et al. "The Value of Delaying Alzheimer's Disease Onset Forum for Health Economics and Policy." ISSN (Online) 1558-9544, November 2014.

28. Chapman, S. B., et al. "Shorter Term Aerobic Exercise Improves Brain, Cognition, and Cardiovascular Fitness in Aging." *Frontiers of Aging Neuroscience* vol. 5 (November 2013): p. 75.

29. Stefansson, H., et al. "Variant of TREM2 Associated with the Risk of Alzheimer's Disease." *New England Journal of Medicine.* vol. 368, no. 2 (January 10, 2013): pp. 107–116.

30. Zissimopoulos, J. et al. The Value of Delaying Alzheimer's Disease Onset Forum.

31. Rao, J. K. "Completion of Advance Directives Among U.S. Consumers." *American Journal of Preventive Medicine*, vol. 46, no. 1 (January 2014): pp. 65–70.

32. Farabaugh, A., et al. "Depression and Suicidal Ideation in College Students." *Psychopathology* vol. 45, no. 4 (2012): pp. 228–234.

33. Kübler-Ross, Elisabeth. *Death: The Final Stage of Growth.* Englewood Cliffs, NJ: Prentice-Hall (1975).

34. Singer, A. E. et al. "Symptom trends in the last year of life from 1998 to 2010: a cohort study." *Ann Intern Med.* vol. 162, no. 3 (February 3, 2015): pp. 175–83.

35. Pirie, K., et al. "The 21ˢᵗ Century Hazards of Smoking and Benefits of Stopping: A Prospective Study of One Million Women in the UK." *The Lancet* vol. 381. no. 9861 (January 12, 2013): pp. 133–141.

Index

anger
   death and, 612
   epidemic, 85–86
   heart disease and, 463–464
   rape, 563
angina, 466
angina pectoris, 466
anorexia nervosa, 197–198
Antabuse, 409
antagonistic, 354
"anterograde amnesia," 374
antibiotics
   defined, 492
   excessive prescribing of, 502
   oral contraceptives and, 300
antibodies, 493
antidepressants, 57–58
antigens, 495
antioxidants, 150–151
antiviral drugs, 492
anus, 139
anxiety disorders
   characterization of, 58–59
   small penis, 254
   social phobia, 110
   social physique, 193
aorta, 461
aphrodisiacs, 272–273
appetite receptors, 187
arteriosclerosis, 465–466
artificial insemination, 315
artificial sweeteners, 190
asbestos, 584
ascorbic acid, 149
aspirin
   cardiovascular benefits of, 464–465
   colorectal cancer prevention, 481
   risks from, 356
   stroke prevention, 471
assertiveness, 30–31
assisted suicide, 614–615
asthma, 482
atherosclerosis, 465–466
athletic shoes, 233–234
Atkins, 188
atrium, 460
attention-deficit/hyperactivity
      disorder (ADHD)
   characterization of, 61
   drugs for, 362
   treatment of, 61–62
attitudes, 96
attraction, 118
autism spectrum disorder, 62
autoimmune disorders, 499
autonomy, 30
autopsies, 615–616
autoscopy, 614
aversion therapy, 433
axon terminal, 49

axons, 48–49
Ayurveda, 534–535

B

B cells, 495–496
babesiosis, 509
bacteria. *See individual species*
bacterial vaginosis, 336, 511
baking soda, 228
ballistic stretching, 230
banding surgery, 192
barbiturates, 374–375
bargaining, 612
barrier contraceptives
   cervical cap, 297–298
   condoms, 290, 292–294, 325–327
   diaphragm, 296–297
   effectiveness of, 292
   nonprescription, 290
   spermicides/films, 295–296
   sponges, 294–295
basal cells, 475
basal metabolic rate (BMR), 139
bath salts, 366–367
behavior
   alcohol's effects on, 403–404
   gender differences in, 8
   healthy, 6
   risky, 12
   sexual, 257–260
behavioral change
   HBM model of, 14–15
   predisposing factors, 14
   processes of, 17
   self-affirmation theory of, 15
   self-determination theory of, 15
   suggestions for, 19
   transtheoretical model of, 15–18
   understanding, 13
behavioral therapy, 70
benign pro static hypertrophy, 604
benzodiazepines, 374–375
beta-carotene, 150
bias crimes, 559
bidis, 431
Biggest Loser Club, 189
bile duct, 139
binge drinking, 391–392
binge eating, 92, 196
bioelectrical impedance analysis
      (BIA), 182
biofeedback, 94
biological factors, 8
biotin, 149
bipolar disorder, 58
birth control. *See* contraception
birth control pills. *See* oral
      contraceptives
birth outcomes, 4
bisexuality, 261

black cohosh, 604
blastocyst, 282–283
blended families, 129
blood
   clots, 469
   red cell count, 468
   tests, 528
   thinners, 470–471
blood alcohol concentration (BAC)
   defined, 398
   factors affecting, 400
   formula of, 398–399
blood circulation, 461
blood glucose
   function of, 449
   high, 446
   levels, tests for, 452
blood pressure. *See also*
      hypertension
   definition of, 454
   healthy, 456
   lowering, 456–457
   regulation of, 454
BMPEA, 536
"boarding-school amenorrhea," 253
Bod Pod, 182
body art, 533
body composition, 206
body fat, 182, 446
body image, 193–194
body language, 108–109
body mass index (BMI)
   cancer risk, 473
   defined, 178
   ranges of, 180–181
bodywork, 536
bone density, 211–212, 529
Borrelia burgdorferi, 509
botulinum. *See Clostridium
      botulinum*
brain
   adolescent's, 50
   aging, 601–602
   alcohol's effects on, 403–404, 408
   anatomical parts of, 48–49
   cannabinoid effects, 363
   chemistry, 66
   methamphetamine and, 371
   sex differences in, 50
   stroke effects on, 470
   synapses, 49
brain death, 611
brain-gut axis, 92
breast augmentation, 532
breast cancer
   incidents, 476
   risks factors, 477
   screening, 478
   treatments, 478–479

avian, 510
prevention of, 503
transmission of, 502
viruses, 492
informed consent, 530
inhalants, 377–378
injuries
exercise, 239
prevention, 228
repetitive motion, 553
U.S. incidences of, 4
unintentional, 548–549
inline skating, 222
inpatient care, 539
insomnia, 39
insulin resistance, 450
integrative medicine, 534
intellectual health
defined, 3
fitness and, 207
sexuality and, 246
stress and, 79
intercourse, 266, 283–284
intergroup stress, 83
internals, 18
Internet. *See also* social networks
diet programs on, 189
drugs sold on, 358–359, 366
health information on, 520–521
risks of, 113–115
interpersonal therapy (IPT), 70
interval training, 220–221
interventions, 378
intimacy
decisions about, 255–256
defined, 117, 246
prevalence of, 117
intoxication, 360
intraepithelial neoplasia, 330
intramuscular, 352
intrauterine devices (IUDs), 303
intravenous, 352
iodine, 154
ionizing radiation, 587
IPT. *See* interpersonal therapy
(IPT)
iron, 153
ischemic stroke, 469
isokinetic contraction, 224
isometric contraction, 224
isotonic contraction, 224

J
Jeanne Clery Disclosure of Campus
Security Policy and Campus
Crime Statistics Act, 558
Jenny Craig, 188
job stress, 86–87
jogging, 220–221
journaling, 94
"juggler family," 129

K
Karvonen formula, 218
ketamine, 376–377
ketones, 449
khat, 365–366
kick-boxing, 221
kreteks, 431

L
labia majora, 249
labia minora, 249
labor (childbirth), 314–315
laparoscopy, 307
LARCs. *See* long-acting reversible
contraceptives (LARCs)
large intestine, 139
LASIK (laser-assisted in situ
keratomileusis), 531–532
laxatives, 357
LCSWs. *See* licensed clinical social
workers (LCSWs)
lead, 584
leptin, 187
leukemia, 475
lice, 335
licensed clinical social workers
(LCSWs), 69
licensed practical nurses, 538
life change events, 80
life expectancy
exercise and, 211
healthy, 4
projecting, 598–599
"lifestyle" diets, 138
liking, 118
lipoproteins
defined, 447
profiles, 458–459
stroke and, 469
liposuction, 532
listening, 107
Listeria spp., 168
listeriosis, 169
liver
alcohol's effects on, 403
diseases, 408
function, 139
living wills, 608
locus of control, 18, 85
loneliness, 109–110
long-acting reversible contraceptives
(LARCs), 302–304
Lose it!, 189
loudness, 588
love. *See* romantic love
love triangle, 118
low-carbohydrate diets, 187–188
low-density lipoproteins,
184, 458
low-fat diets, 187–188
lower back pain, 232–233, 529

LSD (lysergic acid diethylamide), 376,
464
luteinizing hormone (LH), 247, 252
Lybrel, 301
Lyme disease, 509
lymph nodes, 495–496
lymphoma, 475

M
macronutrients, 139
macrophages, 495
magnesium, 153
mainstream smoke, 435
maintenance stage, 17
major depressive disorder, 57
major diseases, 443–488. *See also*
specific conditions
asthma, 482
cancer, 471–481
cardiometabolic-associated, 444–448
cardiovascular, 460–465
diabetes, 449–454
epilepsy, 481–482
hypertension, 454–458
metabolic syndrome, 448–449
overview of, 443–444
suicide and, 66
ulcers, 482–483
malaria, 493
male sexual anatomy, 253–254
mammography, 478, 529
manganese, 154
marijuana
characterization of, 363
dependence/withdrawal, 365
heart disease and, 464
legalized, 365
stroke and, 469
synthetic, 366
marital rape, 563
marriage
benefits of, 125
conflict in, 127
demographics, 124
equality, 125–126
issues in, 126
preparation for, 124–125
saving, 127–128
weight gain from, 184
marriage and family therapist, 69
masochism, 274
mass murder, 556
massage therapy, 536
mastectomy, 478
masturbation, 265
matrix model, 374
mature love, 119
Mayo Clinic, 521
ME/CFS. *See* Myalgic
encephalomyelitis/chronic fatigue
syndrome (ME/CFS)

sports drinks, 236
squamous cells, 475
squeeze ejaculation, 271–272
stability balls, 233
stair climbing, 222
stalking, 561
Staphylococcus aureus,
    508–509
starches, 141
static flexibility, 228
static stretching, 229
sterilization, 306–307
steroids. *See* anabolic steroids
stimulants
    amphetamines, 369–370
    characterization of, 369
    cocaine, 372–374
    methamphetamine, 370–372
    prescription, 362
stimulus control therapy, 39
STIs. *See* sexually transmitted
    infections
stomach, 139
stop-smoking groups, 433
stop-start ejaculation, 271
stranger rape, 565
strength. *See* muscular fitness
Streptococcus sanguis, 464
stress, 77–104
    accidents-related to, 549
    age factors, 83
    alcoholism and, 408
    APA report on, 80–81
    characterization of, 78
    college student's, 81–85
    combat-related, 65
    counseling, 466
    depression and, 55
    economic, 85–86
    effects of, 79
    exercise for, 212–213
    gender differences in, 82
    health effects of, 87
    heart disease and, 463
    immunity and, 497–498
    inoculation to, 96
    job, 86–87
    management of, 93–97, 100
    physical effects of, 89, 91–92
    posttraumatic, 88–89
    prevention of, 84, 97–99
    psychological responses to, 93
    symptoms of, 92–93
    test, 85
    theories of, 91
stress response, 90
stressors
    anger as, 85–86
    defined, 78
    positive, 78–79
    traumatic life events, 87–88

types of, 80
uncontrollable, 497
stretching
    athletic performance and, 230–231
    for lower back pain, 232–233
    pre-exercise, 231
    types of, 229–230
    warming up and, 230
strokes
    cerebral effects of, 470
    characterization of, 468
    cigarette smoking and, 427–428
    excessive weight and, 184
    risk factors, 468–469
    treatment for, 470–471
    types of, 469–470
subcutaneous, 352
substance abuse. *See also* addictions;
    alcoholism
    on campus, 349–351
    decline in, 345–346
    mortality and, 4
    prevention of, 361
    suicide and, 65
    symptoms of, 359
    treatments for, 378–379
substance use disorders
    causes of, 360–361
    dependence, 359–360
    dual diagnoses, 360
    intoxication, 360
    polyabuse, 360
    withdrawal, 360
suction curettage, 308–309
sudden infant death syndrome (SIDS),
    420
sugar. *See* simple carbohydrates
suicidal behavior disorder, 65
suicide
    assisted, 614–615
    causes of, 64–66
    incidence of, 63–64
    prevention, 66
    rational, 614
    risks factors for, 65
superficial frostbite, 238
supplements. *See* dietary supplements
surgery
    cosmetic, 532–533
    obesity, 191–192, 454
    vision, 531–532
sustainability, 578–579
swimming, 221
swine flu, 503
synapses, 49
Syndrome X. *See* metabolic syndrome
synergistic, 354
syphilis, 334–335
systemic disease, 497
systole, 460
systolic blood pressure, 447

T cells, 495–496
t'ai chi, 232
tar (tobacco), 326
teaching hospitals, 539
teenagers
    brains of, 50
    lonely, 110
    pregnancy among, 4
    shyness among, 110
    smoking by, 421
tend and befriend, 90
tennis, 222
terminal illness, 613
termination change, 17
tertiary care, 538
test stress, 85
testes, 253
testicular cancer, 480
testosterone, 247, 604
texting, 550
therapy
    practitioners of, 68–69
    selection of, 69
    types of, 68–69
thiamin, 148
thirdhand smoke, 581
thrill seeking, 549
time management, 97–98
tissue-type plasminogen activator, 471
tobacco, 419–441. *See also* cigarette
    smoking
    byproducts of, 426
    college control policies, 424
    emerging products, 429–431
    immediate effects of, 425–426
    noncigarette, 431
    overview of, 419–420
    quitting, 432–435
    risks from, 12
    smokeless, 432
tobacco use disorder, 422, 446
toxic shock syndrome, 253
toxicity, 352
Toxoplasma spp., 168
training. *See* physical conditioning
trans fat, 146
trans-fatty acids, 146
transgender, 263
transient ischemic attacks (TIAs),
    469–470
transtheoretical model, 16–17
transvestism, 273
traumatic life events, 87–88, 391
treadmills, 220
trichomoniasis, 335–336, 511
triglycerides, 447, 458
tubal ligation, 306
tubal occlusion, 306
tuberculosis (TB), 508
12 step program, 379, 410

two-carrier couples, 126
Tylenol, 356–357
Tylenol PM, 357
type A personalities, 464
type C personalities, 464
type D personalities, 464

U

ulcers, 482–483
ultraviolet light, 475
university social climate stress, 83
unsaturated fats, 146
upper respiratory infections, 500,
    502–503
urethra, 249, 254
urethritis, 511
urinalysis, 528
urinary tract infections, 511
uterus, 249

V

vaccinations
    adult, 499–500
    HPV, 329–330
    influenza, 503–503
    meningitis, 504
vagina, 249
vaginal contraceptive films (VCF),
    295–296
vaginal infections, 510–511
vaginal spermicides, 295–296
vaginismus, 272
Valacyclovir, 331
values, 32–33
varenicline, 434
vas deferens, 254
vasectomy, 306
vectors, 492
vegetables
    benefits of, 155
    color-coding, 157
    consumption of, 156
vegetarian diets, 159–160
ventricles, 460
Vicodin, 362
victims
    sexual, 390–391
    violence, 566–567

violence
    campus, 557–558
    forms of, 561
    gun, 555–557
    hate-based, 559
    hazing as, 558
    helping victims of, 566–567
    homicides, 4
    incidence of, 554–555
    intimate partner, 119–120, 561–562
    sexual, 560–566
    warning signs of, 555
virtual support, 67–68
viruses, 492
vision surgery, 531–532
visualization, 94
vital signs, 524
vitamins
    A, 149
    B complex, 148, 157
    C, 149
    D, 147, 150–152
    deficiencies, 408
    E, 150
    fat-soluble, 149–150
    function of, 147
    K, 150
    water-soluble, 148–150
volunteerism, 111
voyeurism, 273

W

waist circumference, 181–182
waist-to-hip ratio (WHR), 182
walking, 220
warfarin, 470–471
warm-up, 219, 230
water
    benefits of, 163
    bottled, 580
    function of, 141
    physical activity and, 236
    pollution, 579–585
    requirements for, 140
    tap, 162
water pipes, 429–431
waterborne diseases, 494
WebMD, 521

weight, 177–203
    alcohol's effects on, 403
    body image and, 193–194
    gains, in college, 178–180
    healthy, 180–182
    management of, 186–188, 459
    measures of, 180–182
    sleep and, 37
    status, 5
weight loss
    CAM treatments for, 189–190
    cigarette smoking for, 422
    common traps, 190
    diets, 187–188
    exercise for, 189, 212
    maintaining, 190–191
    programs, 188–191
Weight Watchers, 188
well-being scale, 42–43
Wellbutrin, 434
wellness, 2
Wernicke-Korsakoff syndrome, 408
West Nile virus, 494, 509–510
withdrawal
    alcohol, 409
    benzodiazepines/barbiturates, 374
    cocaine, 373
    defined, 360
    methamphetamine, 371–372
    opioid, 376
within-group stress, 83
Women's Health Initiative, 32
workplace safety, 552–554

X

X chromosomes, 247
x-rays, 528, 587–588

Y

Y chromosomes, 247
Yerkes-Dodson law, 91
yoga, 95–96, 231

Z

zinc, 153
Zumba, 222
Zyban, 434
zygote, 282–283